SHIELDS

Textbook of Glaucoma

SIXTH EDITION

SENIOR AUTHOR

R. RAND ALLINGHAM, MD
Richard and Kit Barkhouser Professor of Ophthalmology
Duke University School of Medicine
Chief, Glaucoma Service
Duke Eye Center
Durham, North Carolina, USA

ASSOCIATE AUTHORS

KARIM F. DAMJI, MD, MBA
Professor of Ophthalmology
University of Alberta—Faculty of Medicine & Dentistry
Director, Ophthalmology Fellowship Programs
Royal Alexandra Hospital
Edmonton, Alberta, Canada

SHARON F. FREEDMAN, MD
Professor of Ophthalmology and Pediatrics
Duke University School of Medicine
Chief, Pediatric Ophthalmology and Strabismus Service
Duke Eye Center
Durham, North Carolina, USA

SAYOKO E. MOROI, MD, PHD
Associate Professor of Ophthalmology and Visual Sciences
University of Michigan Medical School
Director, Glaucoma Fellowship Program
The University of Michigan W. K. Kellogg Eye Center
Ann Arbor, Michigan, USA

DOUGLAS J. RHEE, MD
Assistant Professor of Ophthalmology
Harvard Medical School
Associate Chief, Practice Development
Massachusetts Eye and Ear Infirmary
Boston, Massachusetts, USA

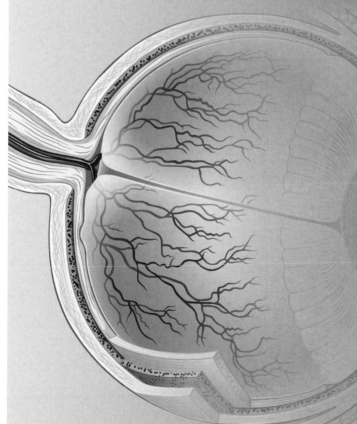

Wolters Kluwer | Lippincott Williams & Wilkins
Health

Philadelphia · Baltimore · New York · London
Buenos Aires · Hong Kong · Sydney · Tokyo

Senior Executive Editor: Jonathan W. Pine, Jr.
Senior Product Manager: Emilie Moyer
Vendor Manager: Bridgett Dougherty
Senior Manufacturing Manager: Benjamin Rivera
Senior Marketing Manager: Lisa Lawrence
Senior Designer: Stephen Druding
Production Service: MPS Limited, a Macmillan Company

Two Commerce Square
2001 Market Street
Philadelphia, PA 19103 USA
LWW.com

Printed in China

Library of Congress Cataloging-in-Publication Data

Shields textbook of glaucoma. — 6th ed. / R. Rand Allingham ... [et al.].
   p. ; cm.
   Other title: Textbook of glaucoma
  Includes bibliographical references and index.
  Summary: "Thoroughly updated, and now in full color, Shields Textbook of Glaucoma, Sixth Edition, is a clinically focused and practical textbook for general ophthalmologists treating patients with glaucoma. This classic text offers a rational approach to the medical and surgical management of glaucoma and presents a total care plan for the patient. This edition has new or reconfigured chapters—including those on principles of medical therapy and management; cholinergic stimulators and hyperosmotic agents; neuroprotection and other investigational drugs; and molecular genetics and pharmacogenomics of the glaucomas. The book examines new technologies for intraocular pressure assessment and current diagnostic technologies, such as optical coherence tomography, spectral-domain OCT, Heidelberg retina tomograph, and GDx. Noted experts detail advances in surgical treatment of glaucoma, including new glaucoma implants and angle surgery. Coverage also includes advances in genetics of glaucomatous diseases. A companion website includes the fully searchable text and an image bank"—Provided by pub-lisher.
  ISBN 978-0-7817-9585-2 (alk. paper)
  1. Glaucoma. I. Allingham, R. Rand. II. Shields, M. Bruce. Textbook of glaucoma. III. Title: Textbook of glaucoma.
  [DNLM: 1. Glaucoma. WW 290]
  RE871.S447 2011
  617.7'41—dc22

2010031608

To purchase additional copies of this book, call our customer service department at (800) 638-3030 or fax orders to (301) 223-2320. International customers should call (301) 223-2300.

Visit Lippincott Williams & Wilkins on the Internet: at LWW.com. Lippincott Williams & Wilkins customer service representatives are available from 8:30 am to 6 pm, EST.

10 9 8 7 6 5 4 3 2 1

Contents

Most of us, as we approach the "golden years" of life, can look back with joy and pride on how we watched our children grow from infancy through adolescence to adulthood, with accomplishments well beyond the ability of their parents. My feelings are much the same with this book. During its infancy in the early 1980s, it was small and naïve, and it grew slowly over the next 20 years, due in large measure to kind encouragement from generous readers. But the day came, as we crossed into the new century, when I could no longer fully provide for the book—the remarkable advances in glaucoma on so many fronts were exceeding my ability to keep up—and I was fortunate to have an extended family step in and author the fifth, and now this sixth, edition.

When I first approached each of them with the request to assume authorship of the book, to the person they did not hesitate to agree (at least they showed no outward hesitation), for which I will always be profoundly grateful. And it truly has been a family affair. My Duke partner and longtime friend, Dr. R. Rand Allingham, graciously agreed to serve as managing author, despite his heavy load as Chief of the Duke Glaucoma Service, and skillfully guided the preparation of the latest two editions. Three of the authors, in whom I take great pride, are former Duke glaucoma fellows who have gone on to become leaders in our profession at major universities: Drs. Karim F. Damji, University of Alberta; Sharon F. Freedman, Duke University; and Sayoko E. Moroi, University of Michigan. The final author of the fifth edition was my Yale partner, Dr. George Shafranov, who has since gone into private practice and has been replaced in the sixth edition by Dr. Douglas J. Rhee, also a rising star at the Massachusetts Eye and Ear Infirmary in the fine tradition of Drs. Paul A. Chandler and W. Morton Grant.

Each of these talented friends has added immensely to the editions in their areas of expertise, and I am grateful to them not only for taking the time from their busy practices to perpetuate this textbook but also for truly raising it to a new level. Sales of the fifth edition have approached 9000, which is quite remarkable (I felt good if we broke 2000 with the earlier editions). This success is undoubtedly due to the contributions of the team of authors. They not only updated all the chapters with the latest advances but also added new chapters on molecular genetics and clinical epidemiology and expanded information on evolving technologies, including ultrasound and image analysis. They updated information on the clinical forms of glaucoma, most notably exfoliation syndrome, and greatly enhanced the chapters on filtering surgery, glaucoma drainage-device surgery, and glaucoma surgery for children.

While the fifth edition was a vast improvement over the previous ones, the sixth edition offers even more. Two special features are the addition of color illustrations throughout the book and the accompanying Internet version (the latter is an example of how times are changing, since the Internet was not even heard of when the book began).

A goal of this book from the beginning has been to base the content on a moderately extensive bibliography of both the classic and recent literature and to provide balanced viewpoints where controversy exists. The authors have adhered admirably to this goal, and I hope it will continue to be the foundation of any future editions. Another strength of the book is its limited number of authors. Multiple-author textbooks, which are in the majority today, have the advantage of providing viewpoints by many individuals in their area of expertise, but a book that is written, rather than edited, by a small number of authors provides the advantages of more cohesiveness and consistent style throughout the book. This means more work for each author, several of whom were responsible for a dozen chapters or more, but I hope that this feature can also be perpetuated in future editions.

And so my hat is off to Rand, Karim, Sharon, Sy, and Doug for this latest accomplishment. I also want to again thank Mr. Jonathan Pine and all those at Lippincott Williams & Wilkins for their continued support over these past 30 years. Now I will sit back, like the proud parent, and watch with profound gratitude and admiration as these good friends continue to advance our understanding of glaucoma for the ultimate goal of preserving the precious gift of sight in our patients.

M. Bruce Shields

Preface

Nearly 30 years have passed since *A Study Guide for Glaucoma* was published by M. Bruce Shields in 1982. The first edition of the series that we now know as *Shields Textbook of Glaucoma*, has been embraced by generations of practitioners at all levels of training. No small measure of this book's popularity is the fact that it has become the leading subspecialty textbook on the subject of glaucoma. This should come as no surprise since the core qualities of simple organization and ease to read were adroitly established by Bruce Shields himself.

Over the past few decades, we have witnessed a logarithmic expansion of information in all areas of science and medicine. This certainly has been the case for the subspecialty of glaucoma, where our complete armamentarium consisted of three drugs after which surgery was the next step. Ironically, the mainstay of our treatment 30 years ago—pilocarpine, epinephrine, and systemic carbonic anhydrase inhibitors—is seldom, if ever, used today. Now, joining timolol, prostaglandin analogs, α_2-agonists, and topical carbonic anhydrase inhibitors is a multitude of laser surgical treatments, with many more therapeutic interventions in development. Similarly, technology for diagnosing and following glaucoma has undergone major changes. Optical coherence tomography is an increasingly used technology that will likely replace fundus photography as a mainstay to diagnose and monitor glaucoma. Keeping up with the broad advance in technology and treatment strategy is challenging but is essential if we are to utilize this knowledge effectively for patient care.

It has been a great joy seeing how *Shields Textbook of Glaucoma* is also evolving. It is immediately apparent that the sixth edition, like the field of glaucoma itself, continues to evolve. With the incorporation of full color, there is a sharper sense of what one sees clinically. Additionally, *Shields* has taken its place on the Internet, making it accessible almost anywhere or anytime. With increasing types of data, the ability to analyze and utilize multiple types of information will only increase. The need to have rapid and accurate information immediately at hand is becoming essential to the practice of medicine as the demands for higher efficiency and efficacy continue.

As you open the sixth edition of *Shields Textbook of Glaucoma*, we hope you, the reader, will appreciate the efforts of a dedicated team that values the tradition that was started so long ago.

R. Rand Allingham

ACKNOWLEDGMENTS

It has been a great pleasure and an honor to serve as the senior author of the sixth edition of *Shields Textbook of Glaucoma*. What would seem a daunting task has been an exciting and enjoyable journey. This landmark work, initiated almost 3 decades ago by Bruce Shields, has become the leading textbook on glaucoma worldwide. What Bruce did himself now takes a dedicated and talented team. I have had the honor of sharing this journey with four seasoned and gifted authors, Karim, Doug, Sy, and Sharon. Remarkably, this group has managed to keep the passion and spirit of this great work. This is no small undertaking when one considers the tidal wave of new information and technology that has occurred over the intervening years.

To assist us in this process has been the addition of a talented new member on our team, Cris Coren, our manager, copyeditor, and amazing "fix it" person! Cris was selected and elected to this position by unanimous decree of the authors and editor. She has seamlessly edited text, managed references and figures, improved flow, and organized the authorship and editing process. Being a stickler for detail, Cris refined the language and structure of Shields, not unlike a conductor for a symphony. In brief, Cris has made this edition of Shields better while making the journey a true pleasure.

Of course, none of this would be possible without the many dedicated and talented persons at Lippincott Williams & Wilkins who have shepherded this process from the beginning. Not only is this the first complete four-color edition, it is also the first to have an online version. This enhances the value to our readership and allows us to pursue new content in an increasingly wireless society. In particular, I would like to thank Eric Johnson at Red Act Group for his steady encouragement and wise counsel; Emilie Moyer, who has worked her magic on the appearance and "feel" of this edition; Jonathan Pine, a seasoned veteran at LWW whose oversight and guiding hand have been crucial to our success over the years; and Purnima Narayanan and the talented compositor and copyeditor teams at MPS Limited, a Macmillan Company, for their exceptional attention to detail and professionalism. Thanks as well to Julie Cancio Harper, our "permissions guru," for help with copyright clearance; and Beth Jenkinson and Ryan McCammon, for valuable editorial assistance.

Of course, all success derives from family and friends. Bruce Shields remains the person I come to for advice, counsel, and a heart-to-heart. Thank you, dear friend, for these many years together and those to come! My undying gratitude goes to Robin Goodwin, who has, most would say miraculously, kept order in my professional life at Duke for over 17 years. Erin, my daughter and soon-to-be English professor, who has been my "in-house" resource for all things literate! Michael, my son and evolving ophthalmologist and scientist, I can only imagine how the world of Ophthalmology will change in your lifetime. Of course, Anna, my wife, whose patience, understanding, and support have been central to this and so many other undertakings.

Finally, I wish to thank all of you who read and benefit from the knowledge contained in these pages. Your kind and constructive comments are critically important to us as we strive to provide lucid and useful information that will help those who suffer from glaucoma.

RAND ALLINGHAM

I am grateful to Bruce and Rand for having provided the opportunity to participate in this undertaking, which I regard as a privilege and an honor. I consider them exemplars par excellence. I have also enjoyed collaborating with my coauthors and have learned many new things from them. Over the years, residents and fellows, particularly from the Universities of Ottawa and Alberta, have offered many helpful suggestions. I am thankful for their feedback and hope that users of this book continue to provide input. My wife, Salima, daughters, Safeera, Nabeeha, and my parents, Fateh and Gulshan Damji, have provided incredible inspiration. I am particularly indebted to Salima, whose extraordinary strength, encouragement, and understanding have made it a joy to dedicate time and effort to this endeavor.

KARIM DAMJI

I express my gratitude to my husband, Neil, and to our wonderful children, Rebecca and Benjamin, for unwavering encouragement and support. I am grateful to Rand and Bruce for the privilege of participating in this wonderful creation; to my coauthors for continuing to teach me so much about glaucoma; to Cris Coren for making the process seamless and simple; and to Bruce Shields, my mentor, inspiration, and friend.

SHARON FREEDMAN

To my husband, Mike Fetters, and my four sons, Kori, Tomo, Kazu, and Taka, for understanding and supporting my contributions to this book. I am grateful to Gale Oren and her staff for medical information and literature, Richard Hackel and the photography staff for their support of this project, my coauthor colleagues and Cris Coren for their patience and support of this project, and my mentor and friend Bruce Shields.

SAYOKO ("SY") MOROI

I would like to thank my lovely wife, Tina, for your continual support, patience, and encouragement. To our daughters, Ashley and Alyssa, whose smiles and laughter bless our lives. To my father and mother, Dennis and Serena Rhee, for your support and guidance. To Susan Rhee, for your understanding, and to all my families—Rhee, Chang, Kim, and Chomakos. Finally, to my friends and coauthors, for the honor of working with you, and to Bruce Shields, our inspiration.

DOUGLAS RHEE

Introduction: An Overview of Glaucoma

HISTORICAL BACKGROUND

Although our modern understanding of glaucoma dates back only to the mid-19th century, this group of disorders was apparently recognized by the Greeks as early as 400 BC. In Hippocratic writings, it appears as "glaucosis," in reference to the bluish-green hue of the affected eye (1). This term, however, was also applied to a larger group of blinding conditions that included cataracts. Although an association with elevated intraocular pressure (IOP) is found in 10th-century Arabian writings, it was not until the 19th century that glaucoma was clearly recognized as a distinct group of ocular disorders.

SIGNIFICANCE OF GLAUCOMA

Glaucoma is a leading cause of irreversible blindness throughout the world. World Health Organization statistics, published in 1995, indicate that glaucoma accounts for blindness in 5.1 million persons, or 13.5% of global blindness (behind only cataracts and trachoma at 15.8 million persons, or 41.8% of global blindness, and 5.9 million, or 15.5%, respectively) (2). Worldwide, it has become the second most common cause of bilateral blindness. Open-angle glaucoma and angle-closure glaucoma were estimated to affect approximately 66.8 million persons by the year 2000, with 6.7 million experiencing bilateral blindness (3).

In the United States, glaucoma is the second leading cause of blindness and the most frequent cause of blindness among African Americans. The U.S. Department of Commerce's Bureau of the Census 1990 population data (provided by the National Society to Prevent Blindness in 1993) estimated the total number of glaucoma cases among persons 40 years of age or older to be 0.5 million (5.6%) among African Americans and 1.5 million (1.7%) among whites and others (including Hispanics, Asians, and Native Americans). Glaucoma is also the second most common reason for ambulatory visits to ophthalmologists in the United States by Medicare beneficiaries and is the leading cause of such visits among African Americans. An analysis of a random 5% subsample of 1991 Medicare beneficiaries (National Claims History File—Part B) revealed approximately 223 office visits for glaucoma per 1000 patients among African Americans and 154 such visits for whites (compared with 136 and 194 office visits, respectively, for cataracts) (4). Although glaucoma more commonly affects older adults, it occurs in all segments of society, with significant health and economic consequences (5), making it a major public health problem.

A DEFINITION OF GLAUCOMA

A Group of Diseases

The most fundamental fact concerning glaucoma is that it is not a single disease process. Rather, it is a large group of disorders characterized by widely diverse clinical and histopathologic manifestations. This point is not commonly appreciated by the general public, or even by a portion of the medical community, which frequently leads to confusion. For example, a patient may have difficulty understanding why she has no symptoms with her glaucoma, when a friend experienced sudden pain and redness with a disease of the same name. Another individual may avoid the use of cold medications because the package inserts cautions against its use in patients with glaucoma, but this caution is only warranted for certain types of glaucoma.

Terminology

The term glaucoma should be used only in reference to the entire group of disorders, just as the term cancer is used to refer to another discipline of medicine that encompasses many diverse clinical entities with certain common denominators. When referring to a diagnosis, one of the more precise terms, such as chronic open-angle glaucoma, should be used to indicate the specific type of glaucoma that the individual is believed to have.

Common Denominator

The common denominator of the glaucomas is a characteristic optic neuropathy, which derives from various risk factors that include but are not limited to increased IOP (6). Although elevated IOP is clearly the most frequent causative risk factor for glaucomatous optic atrophy, it is not the only factor; therefore, to define glaucoma on the basis of ocular tension is unwise and in many instances misleading. Nevertheless, aqueous humor dynamics, which are integrally related to ocular pressure, are critical to our understanding of glaucoma, not only because they are the most common and best understood of the causative risk factors for glaucoma but also because they are presently the only factors that can be controlled to prevent progressive optic neuropathy.

At present, current classifications of glaucoma are based on the multitude of initiating events that ultimately leads to elevated IOP or the alterations in aqueous humor dynamics that are directly responsible for the pressure increase. As continuous research expands modern knowledge of the various factors leading to glaucomatous optic neuropathy, both classifications of glaucoma and approaches to management will no doubt change. The unraveling of the genetic underpinnings of glaucoma continues at an accelerating rate. Most forms of this group of diseases are extremely complex. In the end, however, this knowledge will greatly alter how we classify and treat the various forms of glaucoma. For now, the most important point to recognize is that glaucomatous optic neuropathy causes progressive loss of the visual field, which can lead to total, irreversible blindness if the condition is not diagnosed and treated properly. In Section I, three crucial parameters—IOP, the optic nerve, and the visual field—are considered as they relate to our current understanding of glaucoma.

Prevention of Blindness from Glaucoma

Once the blindness of glaucoma has occurred, there is no known treatment that will restore the lost vision. In nearly all cases, however, blindness due to glaucoma is preventable. This prevention requires early detection and proper treatment. Detection depends on the ability to recognize the early clinical manifestations of the various glaucomas. Section II discusses the many forms of glaucoma and the clinical and histopathologic features by which they are characterized. Appropriate treatment requires an understanding of the pathogenic mechanisms involved, as well as a detailed knowledge of the drugs and operations that are used to control the IOP. Section III considers the medical and surgical modalities that are used in the treatment of glaucoma.

REFERENCES

1. Fronimopoulos J, Lascaratos J. The terms glaucoma and cataract in the ancient Greek and Byzantine writers. *Doc Ophthal.* 1991;77(4):369–375.
2. Thylefors B, Négrel AD, Pararajasegaram R, et al. Global data on blindness [review]. *Bull World Health Org.* 1995;73(1):115–121.
3. Quigley HA. Number of people with glaucoma worldwide [review]. *Br J Ophthal.* 1996;80(5):389–393.
4. Javitt JC. Ambulatory visits for eye care by Medicare beneficiaries. *Arch Ophthal.* 1994;112(8):1025.
5. Leske MC. The epidemiology of open-angle glaucoma: a review. *Am J Epidemiol.* 1983;118(2):166–191.
6. Van Buskirk EM, Cioffi GA. Glaucomatous optic neuropathy [review]. *Am J Ophthal.* 1992;113(4):447–452.

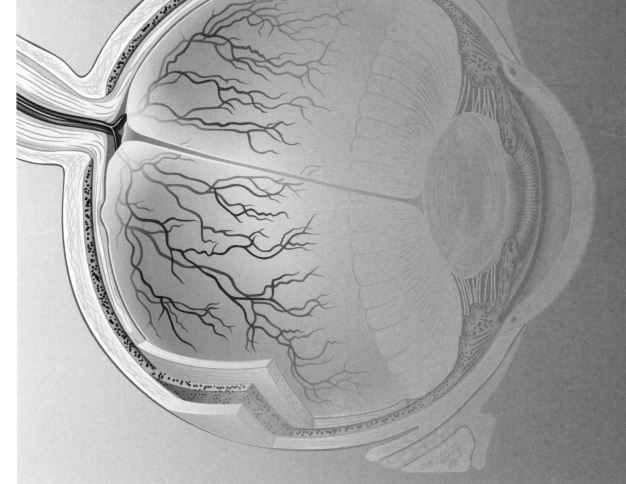

The Basic Aspects of Glaucoma

Cellular and Molecular Biology of Aqueous Humor Dynamics

The study of glaucoma deals with factors involved in the pathophysiology of progressive optic neuropathy characterized by "cupping" of the optic disc. These factors include the following disciplines: (a) clinical epidemiology, (b) clinical research and outcome studies, (c) pharmacology of glaucoma therapeutics, (d) genetics, (e) embryology and development of ocular structures, and (f) basic science investigations of the anterior and posterior segments of the ocular structures relevant to glaucoma. Because the role of lowering intraocular pressure (IOP) as a treatment of glaucoma has been substantiated by several prospective, randomized clinical trials (see Chapter 27), a logical place to begin this study is with an overview of the basic anatomy of the structural determinants responsible for aqueous

humor dynamics. The basic anatomy of the optic nerve, retina, and choroid is presented in Chapter 4.

OVERVIEW OF THE ANATOMY

Aqueous humor has multiple physiologic functions throughout the various ocular structures. The two main structures related to aqueous humor dynamics are the ciliary body, the site of aqueous humor production, and the limbal region, which includes the trabecular meshwork, the principal site of aqueous humor outflow. **Figure 1.1** shows the close relationship between these two structures and the surrounding anatomy.

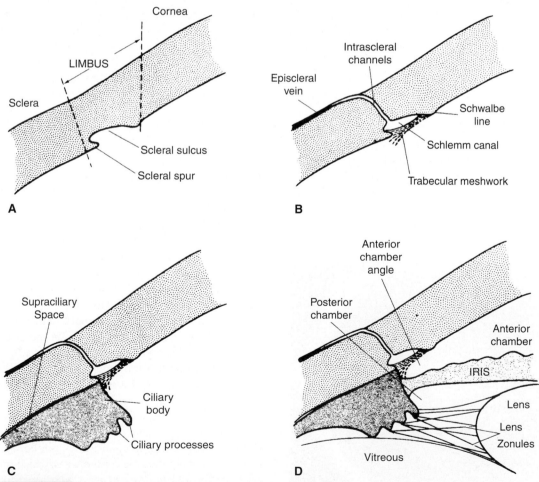

Figure 1.1 Stepwise construction of a schematic model, depicting the relationship of structures involved in aqueous humor dynamics. **A:** Limbus. **B:** Main route of aqueous humor outflow ("conventional" or trabecular outflow). **C:** Ciliary body (site of aqueous humor production and other outflow route of "unconventional" or uveoscleral outflow). **D:** Iris and lens.

The limbus is the transition zone between the cornea and the sclera. On the inner surface of the limbus is an indentation; the scleral sulcus, which has a sharp posterior margin; the scleral spur; and a sloping anterior wall that extends to the peripheral cornea.

A sieve-like structure, the trabecular meshwork, bridges the scleral sulcus and converts it into a tube, called the Schlemm canal. Where the meshwork inserts into the peripheral cornea, a ridge is created, known as the Schwalbe line. The Schlemm canal is connected by intrascleral channels to the episcleral veins. The trabecular meshwork, Schlemm canal, and the intrascleral channels make up the main route of aqueous humor outflow.

The ciliary body attaches to the scleral spur and creates a potential space, the supraciliary space, between itself and the sclera. On cross section, the ciliary body has the shape of a right triangle, and the ciliary processes (the actual site of aqueous humor production) occupy the innermost and anterior-most portion of this structure in the region called the pars plicata (or corona ciliaris). The pars plicata region is also composed of smooth muscle, which serves the important functions of accommodation and uveoscleral outflow. The ciliary processes consist of 70 to 80 radial ridges (major ciliary processes), between which are interdigitated an equal number of smaller ridges (minor or intermediate ciliary processes) (1) (**Fig. 1.2**). The posterior portion of the ciliary body, called the pars plana (or orbicularis ciliaris), has a flatter inner surface and joins the choroid at the ora serrata.

The anterior–posterior length of the ciliary body in the adult eye ranges from 4.6 to 5.2 mm nasally to 5.6 to 6.3 mm temporally, according to various reports, with the pars plana accounting for approximately 75% of the total length. The most rapid phase of growth of the proportions of the pars plana occurs between 26 and 35 weeks' gestation (2). At birth, these measurements are 2.6 to 3.5 mm nasally and 2.8 to 4.3 mm temporally, and they reach three fourths of the adult dimensions by 24 months, with a constant ratio between pars plicata and pars plana (3).

The iris inserts into the anterior side of the ciliary body, leaving a variable width of the latter structure visible between the root of the iris and the scleral spur, referred to as the ciliary body band. The lens is suspended from the ciliary body by zonules and separates the vitreous posteriorly from the aqueous humor anteriorly. The iris separates the aqueous humor compartment into a posterior and an anterior chamber, and the angle formed by the iris and the cornea is called the anterior chamber angle. Further details regarding the gonioscopic appearance of the anterior chamber angle are considered in Chapter 3.

With this basic outline of the anatomic structures that regulate aqueous humor dynamics, it is important to review the development of these structures and other structures of the eye. Current clinical training teaches clinicians to subclassify various ocular disease phenotypes among patients who have "outside" ocular abnormalities (or ocular phenotypes) that often have a strong genetic component, which is discussed in Chapter 8. (Another useful resource for information on human diseases with a genetic component is "Online Mendelian Inheritance in Man," or OMIM. It can be accessed at www.ncbi.nlm.nih.gov.) As more disease genes are identified, the clinical phenotypic presentations, which are an "outside in" approach to understand disease, will merge with an "inside out" approach, whereby identified gene mutations and risk alleles are related to the ocular and systemic phenotypes. Our knowledge of the human genome, which has approximately 30,000 genes (4), and proteinomics (5), which is the study of proteins, will provide a blueprint for understanding individual variations in eye anatomy and ocular disease presentations (6).

EMBRYOLOGY OF THE EYE

The eye shows incredible diversity among the various phyla from simple eye spots, through compound eyes, to complex structures with a single lens and photoreceptor arrays (7). The developmental biology of the vertebrate eye from surface ectoderm, neural crest, and mesodermal mesenchyme has been extensively investigated (8). An overall schematic of eye development is summarized in **Figure 1.3**. The tissue origin of the various ocular structures is summarized in **Table 1.1**.

Ocular development from these three tissue sources involves complex, specific cell growth, and differentiation processes, which are not fully understood. These complex processes involve carefully timed expression of various growth factors and their receptors, other signaling molecules and their pathways, transcription factors, and structural components (9). In general, the genes that regulate development can be categorized into different functional classes as follows: (a) structural genes, such as cytoskeletal components, which may be considered as "housekeeping" genes that carry out ubiquitous biochemical and structural functions; (b) regulatory genes, such as transcription factors (i.e., molecular switches that control mRNA production by other genes) and cell signaling molecules, which mainly determine specialized expression of

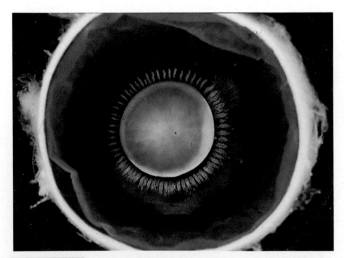

Figure 1.2 Gross anatomic view of the inside view of the anterior segment showing the radial ridges of the ciliary processes at the pars plicata portion of the ciliary body.

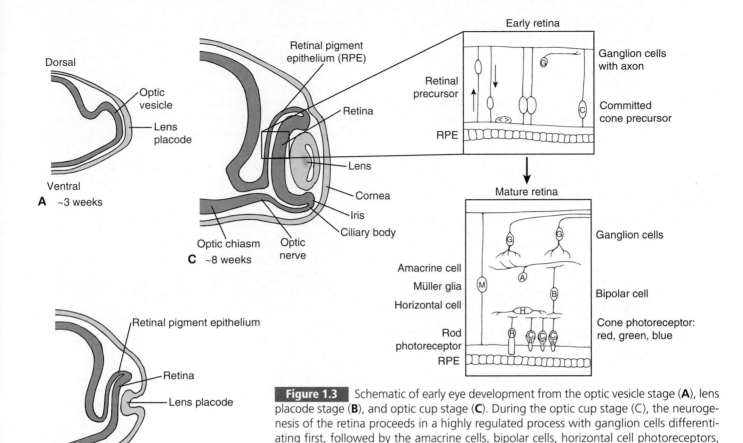

Figure 1.3 Schematic of early eye development from the optic vesicle stage (**A**), lens placode stage (**B**), and optic cup stage (**C**). During the optic cup stage (C), the neurogenesis of the retina proceeds in a highly regulated process with ganglion cells differentiating first, followed by the amacrine cells, bipolar cells, horizontal cell photoreceptors, and Müller (glial) cells. (Modified from Traboulsi EI, ed. *Genetic Diseases of the Eye*; 1998:12, 15. By permission of Oxford University Press.)

Table 1.1	Derivatives of Embryonic Tissues		
Neuroectoderm	**Cranial Neural Crest Cells**	**Surface Ectoderm**	**Mesoderm**
Neurosensory retina	Corneal stroma and endothelium	Epithelium, glands, cilia of skin of lids, and caruncle	Fibers of extraocular ; muscles endothelial lining of all orbital and ocular blood vessels; temporal portion of sclera; vitreous
Retinal pigment epithelium	Sclera (see also mesoderm)	Conjunctival epithelium	
Pigmented ciliary epithelium	Trabecular meshwork	Lens	
Nonpigmented ciliary epithelium	Sheaths and tendons of extraocular muscles	Lacrimal gland and drainage system	
Pigmented iris epithelium	Connective tissues of iris	Vitreous	
Sphincter and dilator muscles of iris	Ciliary muscles		
Optic nerve, axons, and glia	Choroidal stroma		
Vitreous	Melanocytes (uveal and epithelial)		
	Meningeal sheaths of the optic nerve		
	Schwann cells of ciliary nerves		
	Ciliary ganglion		
	Most orbital bones, cartilage, and connective tissue of the orbit		
	Muscular layer and connective tissue sheaths of all ocular and orbital vessels		

genes; and (c) cell-specific genes encoding for specialized proteins of a particular cell type within an organ, such as the unique proteins expressed in the photoreceptors. Abnormalities in expression of the individual genes or interaction among multiple genes caused by gene mutations or altered expression can lead to congenital defects and human disease (**Table 1.2**).

The following regulatory genes have been grouped into large families of transcription factors: homeobox genes, zinc finger genes, and helix-loop-helix genes. Homeobox genes encode for a 60-amino acid DNA-binding element and specifically determine the target gene for a transcription factor. These genes are frequently involved in determining the regional identity of the embryo or individual fate and differentiation of cells (10). Examples of homeobox genes include the *PAX* family and *POU* domain family. The zinc finger family of genes is thought to be the most abundant of the transcription factors. These genes

Table 1.2	Selected Genes Involved in Vertebrate Eye Development			
Gene (Gene Family)	**Function**	**Tissue Expression**	**Animal Model**	**Human Disease**
BMP4 (TGF-β)	Regulatory	Optic primordium	Mouse anterior segment dysgenesis, IOP, abnormal teeth	Not reported
BMP7 (TGF-β)	Regulatory	Optic primordium, cornea, kidney, skeleton	Mouse knockout—microphthalmia Mouse polydactyly	Not reported
Brn3B (POU Domain)	Regulatory	Retinal ganglion cells	Mouse knockout—optic nerve Mouse hypoplasia	Not reported
Chx10 (Homeobox)	Transcription factor	Retina, brain	Mouse ocular retardation	Microphthalmia, cataracts, abnormal iris sclerocornea
CRB1	Structural	Retina	*Drosophila* photoreceptor abnormalities	Leber congenital amaurosis, retinitis pigmentosa
CYP1B1	Regulatory		Mouse anterior segment dysgenesis	Congenital glaucoma
γ-crystallin (βγ-crystallins)	Structural	Lens	Mouse eye lens obsolescence (Elo), cataract	Coppock cataract, congenital lamellar, punctate, and nuclear
FoxC1 *(FKHL7/FREAC3)* (Bicoid homeobox)	Regulatory	Anterior segment of the eye	Mouse hydrocephalus, skeletal and eye abnormalities	Axenfeld–Rieger syndrome, anterior segment dysgenesis
LMX1B (Homeodomain)	Regulatory	Anterior segment of the eye	Mouse microphthalmia	Nail–patella syndrome with COAG
Math3 (Basic HLH)	Regulatory			
Mi (Basic HLH)	Regulatory	Retinal pigment epithelium, pigment cells	Mouse microphthalmia	Waardenburg syndrome, type II Tietz Albinism–deafness syndrome
Myoc	Structural	Trabecular meshwork, ciliary body, iris muscle[a]	Fluid discharge in the *Drosophilas*	Juvenile glaucoma
NR2E3	Regulatory	Retina	Mouse retinal degeneration	Enhanced S cone syndrome, Goldmann–Favre syndrome
ocrl-1 (Inositol phosphatase)	Regulatory	Lens, brain, kidney function	Mouse knockout without Lowe syndrome phenotype	Lowe syndrome
Optx2 (Bicoid)		Retina	Mouse pituitary, retinal, and optic nerve hypoplasia	Anophthalmia
Otx1/2 (Homeobox)	Regulatory	Iris and ciliary epithelium, ocular surface	Mouse knockout—brain seizures; mouse lacrimal gland missing	Not reported

Table 1.2 (Continued)				
Gene (Gene Family)	**Function**	**Tissue Expression**	**Animal Model**	**Human Disease**
Otx2 (Homeobox)	Regulatory	Retinal pigment epithelium, optic nerve	Mouse knockout—lethal	Not reported
Pax2 (Homeobox)	Regulatory	Early optic nerve, kidney defects	Mouse knockout—eye, kidney	Renal-coloboma syndrome
Pax6 (Homeobox)	Regulatory	Lens, retina, nose, brain	Mouse small eye, *Drosophila* "eyeless"	Aniridia, anophthalmia, Peters anomaly, brain, nose defects, optic nerve hypoplasia, coloboma, microphthalmia
PITX2 (Bicoid homeobox)	Regulatory	Brain, pituitary, ocular mesenchyme, cardiac mesenchyme, neural crest	Chicken, frog, mouse situs inversus	Axenfeld–Rieger syndrome
POU (Brn3, RPF-1)	Regulatory	Retinal ganglion cells	Mouse knockout—ganglion cell hypoplasia	Not reported
Thyroid receptor (TR)	Regulatory	Oligodendrocytes	Mouse ganglion cell degeneration	Not reported
Xath5 (Basic HLH)	Regulatory			

[a]Skeletal muscle, heart, stomach, thyroid, trachea, bone marrow, thymus, prostate, small intestine, colon, lung, pancreas, testis, ovary, spinal cord, lymph node, and adrenal gland.
TGF-β, transforming growth factor beta; IOP, intraocular pressure; COAG, chronic open-angle glaucoma; HLH, helix-loop-helix.

share a common motif of a zinc atom binding to a group of histidine and cysteine amino acids and holding together a small loop of amino acids. Examples of this gene family include the retinoic acid receptors (RAR) and retinoid X receptor (RAX), which direct the binding of retinoic acid. Mutations in these receptors have been associated with abnormal eye development (11). The helix-loop-helix family of genes is characterized by two helical DNA-binding domains held together by a special domain or region called as "leucine zipper" (12).

The role for these various structural, regulatory, and cell-specific genes in ocular development has been most extensively examined thus far in the retina, which is highly complex and only partially understood (12). Although not as extensively studied as retinal development, the anterior ocular segment, including the ciliary body and lens (13), also has important and complex roles in the development of the normal eye. The tissue origins of the ciliary epithelium, ciliary smooth muscle, and lens are listed in Table 1.1. The lens induces differentiation of ciliary epithelium at the edge of the optic cup (Fig. 1.3), and the iris develops later from the edge of the optic cup. The ciliary muscle and stroma differentiate after the ciliary epithelium is formed. It is not clear when during gestation the ciliary epithelium becomes active to secrete aqueous humor, but it is assumed to start very early after formation (14). As the IOP increases, the eye grows. It is also believed that the increase in IOP provides the force to generate ciliary folds in the ciliary body and to change the shape of the cornea (15).

Abnormalities in the development of the anterior chamber angle, or anterior segment dysgenesis, are exemplified in Axenfeld–Rieger syndrome (see Chapter 14). Thus far, genes that have been shown most frequently to cause anterior segment dysgenesis encode transcription factors that are important in early development. These transcription factors include *PITX2*, *PITX3*, *PAX6*, *FOXC1*, *FOXC2*, and *FOXC3* (16). In transgenic mice, the cell signaling molecule, bone morphogenetic proteins, and related signaling molecules play an important role in normal development of the anterior segment (17).

An approach to study embryology of ocular structures is using data obtained through bioinformatics—a discipline that integrates the study of genes, pathways, and function. Gene expression data, also known as transcript or mRNA expression, may be gleaned in discrete ocular tissues and at various time points in development (18). Such a "global" overview of gene expression in these discrete ocular tissues enables us to hypothesize and to design studies to answer some fundamental cell biology questions about these ocular structures. By comparing and contrasting the gene expression profiles of these discrete ocular tissues at various stages of development and the impact of environmental exposures, we will understand the function of these eye structures at the cellular and molecular level (see further discussion in Chapter 8).

BIOLOGY OF AQUEOUS HUMOR INFLOW

The regulation of IOP is a complex physiologic trait that depends on (a) production of aqueous humor, (b) resistance to aqueous humor outflow, and (c) episcleral venous pressure.

To reduce this highly complex and only partially understood situation to its simplest form, IOP is a function of the rate at which aqueous humor enters the eye (inflow) and the rate at which it leaves the eye (outflow). When inflow equals outflow, a steady state exists, and the pressure remains constant. The remainder of this chapter deals with these inflow and outflow parameters and their complex interrelationships with the IOP.

Cellular Organization of the Ciliary Body and the Ciliary Processes

The ciliary body is one of three portions of the uveal tract, or vascular layer of the eye; the other two structures in this system are the iris and choroid. The ciliary body is composed of (a) muscle, (b) vessels, (c) epithelia lining the ciliary processes, and (d) nerve terminals from the autonomic nervous system (**Fig. 1.4**).

Ciliary Body Muscle

The ciliary muscle consists of two main portions: the longitudinal and the circular fibers (Fig. 1.4). The longitudinal fibers attach the ciliary body to the limbus at the scleral spur. This portion of muscle then runs posteriorly to insert into the suprachoroidal lamina (fibers connecting choroid and sclera) as far back as the equator or beyond. The circular fibers occupy the anterior and inner portions of the ciliary body and run parallel to the limbus. One-third portion of the ciliary muscle has been described as radial fibers, which connect the longitudinal and circular fibers. The physiologic function and pharmacologic action of parasympathomimetic agents as they relate to the ciliary muscle are discussed in Chapter 32.

Ciliary Body Vessels

On the basis of studies in primate and human eyes, the vessels of the ciliary body appear to have a complex arrangement with collateral circulation on at least three levels (19,20): (a) The anterior ciliary arteries on the surface of the sclera send out

lateral branches that supply the episcleral plexus and anastomose with branches from adjacent anterior ciliary arteries to form an episcleral circle. (b) The anterior ciliary arteries then perforate the limbal sclera. In the ciliary muscle, branches of these arteries anastomose with each other as well as with branches from the long posterior ciliary arteries to form the intramuscular circle. Divisions of the anterior ciliary arteries also provide capillaries to the ciliary muscle and iris and send recurrent ciliary arteries to the anterior choriocapillaris. (c) The major arterial circle lies near the iris root anterior to the intramuscular circle and is actually the least consistent of the three collateral systems. Although the primate studies reveal a contribution from perforating anterior ciliary arteries, microvascular casting studies of human eyes, as well as several nonprimate animals, indicate that this "circle" is formed primarily, if not exclusively, by paralimbal branches of the long posterior ciliary arteries, which begin dividing in the anterior choroid. In any case, the major arterial circle is the immediate vascular supply of the iris and ciliary processes.

Each ciliary process in primates is supplied by two branches from the major arterial circle: the anterior and posterior ciliary process arterioles (20) (**Fig. 1.5**). Anterior ciliary process arterioles supply the anterior and marginal (innermost) aspects of the major ciliary processes. These arterioles have luminal constrictions before producing irregularly dilated capillaries within the processes, suggesting precapillary arteriolar sphincters. This may represent the anatomic site of adrenergic neural influence on aqueous humor production by regulation of blood flow through the ciliary processes. The posterior ciliary process arterioles supply the central, basal, and posterior aspects of the major ciliary processes, as well as all portions of the minor processes. These arterioles are of larger caliber than the anterior arterioles and lack the constrictions seen in the latter vessels. Both populations of arterioles have interprocess anastomoses.

Vascular casting studies of capillary networks in the ciliary processes of human eyes suggest three different vascular territories with discrete arterioles and venules (19). The first is located at the anterior end of the major ciliary processes and is drained posteriorly by venules without significant connections to other venules in the ciliary processes. The second is in the center of the major processes, whereas the third capillary network occupies the minor processes and posterior third of the major processes. Both of the latter territories are drained by marginal venules, which are situated at the inner edge of the major processes. It is thought that these three vascular territories may reflect a functional differentiation in the process of aqueous humor production. Venous drainage is into choroidal veins, either from the posterior aspects of the major and minor processes or by direct communication from the interprocess connections (**Fig. 1.6**).

Ciliary Processes

The functional unit responsible for aqueous humor secretion is the ciliary process, which is composed of (a) capillaries, (b) stroma, and (c) epithelia (Figs. 1.4 and 1.6). The ciliary process capillaries occupy the center of each process. The thin endothelium has false "porous" areas of fused plasma

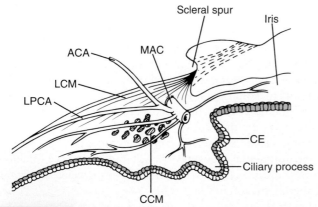

Figure 1.4   Schematic of the three major components of the ciliary body: (1) the ciliary muscle, composed of longitudinal (*LCM*), radial, and circular (*CCM*) fibers; (2) the vascular system, formed by branches of the anterior ciliary arteries (*ACA*) and long posterior ciliary arteries (*LPCA*), which form the major arterial circle (*MAC*); and (3) the ciliary epithelium (*CE*), composed of an outer pigmented and an inner nonpigmented layer.

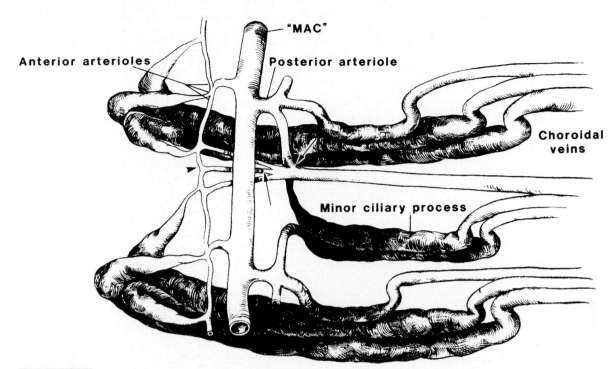

Figure 1.5 Schematic of vascular interconnections of two contiguous major ciliary processes. Lateral anterior arteriolar branches join to form interprocess capillary networks (*arrowhead*), which provide communication between major processes. Laterally directed posterior arterioles form posterior interprocess networks through which the minor ciliary processes receive blood. In addition, both anterior and posterior interprocess networks drain directly into the choroidal veins (*arrows*). *MAC*, major arterial circle. (From Morrison JC, Van Buskirk EM. Ciliary process microvasculature of the primate eye. *Am J Ophthalmol*. 1984;97:372–383, with permission.)

membranes with absent cytoplasm, which may be the site of increased permeability. A basement membrane surrounds the endothelium, and mural cells, or pericytes, are located within the basement membrane (21).

A very thin stroma surrounds the capillary networks and separates them from the epithelial layers. The stroma is composed of ground substance, consisting of mucopolysaccharides, proteins, and plasma solutes (except those of large molecular size); very few collagen connective tissue fibrils, especially

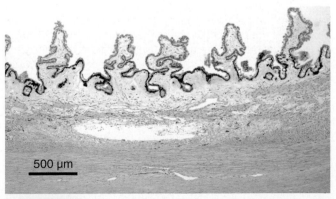

Figure 1.6 Light microscopic view of ciliary processes, sectioned perpendicular to radial ridges, showing major ciliary processes and minor ciliary processes from a human eye stained with toluidine blue.

collagen type III (22); and migrating cells of connective tissue and blood origin (21). Tubular microfibrils with and without elastin have been demonstrated in bovine ciliary body, especially in the stroma of the pars plana, in relation to zonules (23).

Two layers of ciliary epithelium surround the stroma, with the apical surfaces of the two cell layers in apposition to each other (**Fig. 1.7**). The pigmented epithelium has numerous melanin granules in the cytoplasm and an atypical basement membrane on the stromal side.

In the nonpigmented epithelium, the basement membrane is composed of glycoproteins that are immunoreactive for laminin and collagen types I, III, and IV (24). This membrane, which faces the aqueous humor, is also called the internal limiting membrane and fuses with the zonules. The nonpigmented epithelium stains less intensely than the pigmented layer for cytokeratin 18 but more so for vimentin, with the predominant distribution in the crests of the pars plicata and the posterior pars plana (25). It also stains with antibodies against S-100 protein (22). Another molecule with restricted expression in the nonpigmented cells are the water channels aquaporin-1, which is also expressed in trabecular meshwork endothelium, and aquaporin-4 (26). In transgenic knockout mice, which do not express these water channels, IOP is significantly reduced compared within the wild-type mice, whose water channels are normally expressed. The mechanism of IOP lowering is through reduction in decreasing aqueous humor production, but not in outflow. Although these genetically modified mice have a

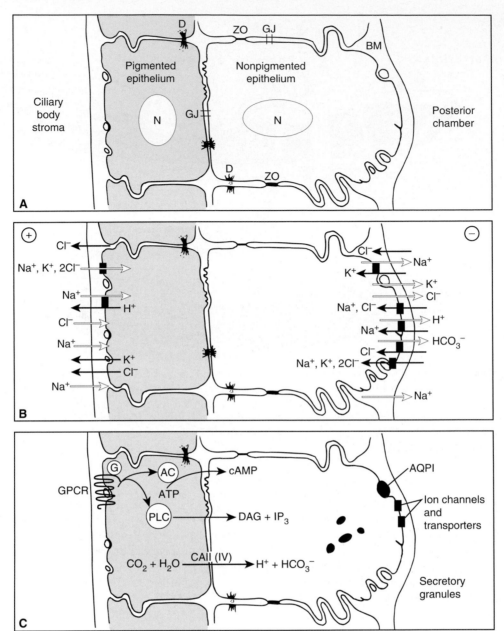

Figure 1.7   Schematic of the ciliary epithelium summarizing the histology and junctional complexes (**A**), physiology of ionic transport mechanisms (**B**), transmembrane signaling and enzymatic pathways and other paracrine functions (**C**). **A:** The ciliary epithelium is composed of two layers containing nuclei (*N*) with an outer pigmented layer (facing the stroma of the ciliary process) and inner nonpigmented layer (facing and lining the posterior chamber). Apical surfaces are in apposition to each other. Basement membrane (*BM*) lines the bilayer and constitutes the internal limiting membrane on the inner surface. The nonpigmented epithelium is characterized by mitochondria, zonula occludens (*ZO*), and lateral and surface interdigitations. The pigmented epithelium contains numerous melanin granules. Additional intercellular junctions include desmosomes (*D*) and gap junctions (*G*). **B:** Overall, there is a net secretion (*open arrows*) of the cations (Na^+, K^+, and H^+) and anions (Cl^- and HCO_3^-), but there is also some absorption (*solid arrows*) of these ions. The net effect is a negative charge ($\ominus$) toward the posterior chamber relative to the ciliary body stroma ($\oplus$). The transfer of these ions proceeds primarily through a transcellular route, or transport across the bilayer through some ion channels and transporters (*black rectangles*) Transfer also occurs to a lesser extent through the paracellular route, or between the cells. **C:** Aqueous humor secretion is highly regulated by multiple transmembrane receptor-mediated pathways (*GPCR*, G-protein coupled receptor; *G*, G-protein; *AC*, adenylate cyclase; *ATP*, adenosine triphosphate; *cAMP*, cyclic adenosine monophosphate; *PLC*, phospholipase C; *PI*, phosphatidyl inositol; *DAG*, diacyl glycerol; *IP_3*, inositol trisphosphate), enzymatic-mediated pathways (*CA*, carbonic anhydrase type II [and possibly type IV]), and specialized transporters, such as the aquaporin type I channel (*AQP1*), which has restricted expression in the nonpigmented ciliary epithelium. The precise localization to pigmented versus nonpigmented and orientation on apical versus basolateral surfaces are unknown for these pathways; thus, they are represented in a bilayer couplet. Other potential paracrine functions of the ciliary epithelium include secretion of small peptides (*granules*).

phenotype of lower IOP, patients with aquaporin-1 mutations have normal IOP (27).

A variety of intercellular junctions connect adjacent cells within each epithelial layer, as well as the apical surfaces of the two layers (28). Such junctions include gap junctions, which are expressed by the pigmented cells, the nonpigmented cells and the pigmented–nonpigmented cells, and tight junctions or zonula occludens, which are expressed between the nonpigmented cells. It is primarily the zonula occludens in the nonpigmented ciliary epithelium that creates an effective barrier to intermediate and high-molecular-weight substances, such as proteins.

Electrophysiologic studies of rabbit ciliary epithelium suggest that all of the cells in the epithelium function as a syncytium (29). Tight junctions create a permeability barrier between the nonpigmented epithelial cells, which forms part of the blood–aqueous barrier. These tight junctions are said to be the "leaky" type, in contrast to the "nonleaky" type in the blood–retinal barrier, and may be the main diffusional pathways for water and ion flow. Microvilli separate the two layers of epithelial cells. In addition, "ciliary channels" have been described as spaces between the two epithelial layers. These channels may be related to the formation of aqueous humor in that they develop between the fourth and sixth months of gestation, corresponding to the start of aqueous humor production.

The Autonomic Innervation of the Ciliary Body

Both sympathetic and parasympathetic nerve endings innervate the ciliary body (30). The sympathetic fibers synapse in the superior cervical ganglion, and the postsynaptic fibers are distributed to the ciliary body vessels. Because the ciliary epithelium is not innervated, it is thought that the catecholamine neurotransmitters released from the sympathetic nerve endings "diffuse" to the adrenergic receptors on the ciliary epithelium. Stimulation of these receptors increases aqueous humor secretion by the ciliary epithelium (discussed further in the section on Molecular Mechanisms and Regulation of Aqueous Humor Production).

The parasympathetic fibers originate from the Edinger-Westphal nucleus to innervate the ciliary muscles. Stimulation of these nerve fibers releases acetylcholine, which then stimulates the cholinergic receptors on the ciliary muscle. These activated receptors cause the ciliary muscle to contract, causing accommodation by changing the shape of the crystalline lens. In addition, ciliary muscle contraction reduces resistance to conventional aqueous humor outflow, or trabecular outflow, and may also affect unconventional aqueous humor outflow, or uveoscleral outflow. The effect of the cholinergic pathway on the trabecular outflow pathway is used pharmacologically in the treatment of glaucoma and is discussed in Chapter 32.

Molecular Mechanisms and Regulation of Aqueous Humor Production

Aqueous humor is a dynamic intraocular fluid that is vital to the health of the eye. The precise localization of aqueous humor production appears to be in the anterior portion of the pars plicata along the tips or crests of the ciliary processes (Fig. 1.2). This region has increased basal and lateral interdigitations, mitochondria, and rough endoplasmic reticulum in the nonpigmented ciliary epithelium; more numerous fenestrations in the capillary endothelium; a thinner layer of ciliary stroma; and an increase in cell organelles and gap junctions between pigmented and nonpigmented epithelia (30).

Aqueous humor is derived from plasma within the capillary network of the ciliary processes. The circulating aqueous humor enters the posterior chamber and flows around the lens and through the pupil into the anterior chamber. Within the anterior chamber, a temperature gradient (cooler toward the cornea) creates a convection flow pattern, which may occasionally be visualized clinically when a patient has inflammation with circulating inflammatory cells. Initially, to reach the posterior chamber, the various constituents of aqueous humor must traverse the three tissue components of the ciliary processes, that is, the capillary wall, stroma, and epithelial bilayer. The principal barrier to transport across these tissues is the cell membrane and related junctional complexes of the nonpigmented epithelial layer, and substances appear to pass through this structure by the following processes: (a) diffusion (lipid-soluble substances are transported through the lipid portions of the membrane proportional to a concentration gradient across the membrane), (b) ultrafiltration (water and water-soluble substances, limited by size and charge, flow through theoretical "micropores" in the protein of the cell membrane in response to an osmotic gradient or hydrostatic pressure), or (c) secretion (substances of larger size or greater charge are actively transported across the cell membrane). The latter process is mediated by transporters, which are proteins in the membrane, and requires the expenditure of energy generated by adenosine triphosphate (ATP) hydrolysis (29).

Basic Physiologic Processes

The following simplified three-part scheme describes the basic physiologic processes involved in aqueous humor production.

Accumulation of Plasma Reservoir

First, tracer studies suggest that most plasma substances pass easily from the capillaries of the ciliary processes, across the stroma, and between the pigmented epithelial cells before accumulating behind the tight junctions of the nonpigmented epithelium (30). This movement takes place primarily by diffusion and ultrafiltration. Drugs that alter perfusion of the ciliary blood vessels may exert their influence on IOP at this level (20).

Transport across Blood–Aqueous Barrier

Second, as mentioned previously, active secretion is a major contributor to aqueous humor formation (29). This active transport takes place through selective transcellular movement of certain cations, anions, and other substances across the blood–aqueous barrier formed by the tight junctions between the nonpigmented epithelium (Fig. 1.7). The process of aqueous humor secretion is mediated by transferring NaCl from the ciliary body stroma to the posterior chamber with water passively following. This secretion occurs in three steps by uptake of NaCl from stroma to pigment epithelial cells by electroneutral transporters, by passage of NaCl from pigmented to nonpigmented cells through gap junctions, and finally by release of Na^+ and Cl^- through Na^+,K^+-activated ATPase and Cl^- channels, respectively.

At the first step of NaCl secretion, rabbit in vitro studies demonstrated that paired activity of Na^+/H^+ and Cl^-/HCO_3^- antiports may be the dominant mechanism in the pigmented epithelium. At the opposite nonpigmented epithelial surface, release of Na^+ through Na^+,K^+-activated ATPase with the accompanying release of Cl^- through ion channels is enhanced by agonists of A3 adenosine receptors (A3ARs). These mechanisms were confirmed in vivo in a mouse model that showed that inhibitors of Na^+/H^+ antiports lower IOP and that A3AR agonists and antagonists raise and lower IOP, respectively.

Carbonic anhydrase mediates the transport of bicarbonate across the ciliary epithelium through a rapid interconversion between HCO_3^- and CO_2 (see details in Chapter 31). Bicarbonate formation influences fluid transport through its effect on Na^+, possibly by regulating the pH for optimum active transport of Na^+ (31).

Other transported substances (see "Function and Composition of Aqueous Humor") include ascorbic acid, which is secreted against a large concentration gradient by the sodium-dependent vitamin C transporter 2, or SVCT2 (32), and certain amino acids, which are secreted by at least three carriers (33).

Osmotic Flow

Third, the osmotic gradient across the ciliary epithelium, which results from the active transport of the above substances, favors the movement of other plasma constituents by ultrafiltration and diffusion. The mechanisms by which water moves from the ciliary body stroma, across the ciliary epithelium, and into the posterior chamber are complex and only partially understood. There is evidence that Na^+ is the driving cationic force (29). Supporting this concept is the restricted expression of the water channels, aquaporin-1 and aquaporin-4, in the nonpigmented ciliary epithelium (26). A specific water channel antagonist has not yet been identified. The functional significance of these channels has not been extensively studied and the rare individuals with mutations of the gene encoding these water channels have a normal IOP (55).

Rate of Aqueous Humor Production

The turnover of aqueous humor within the anterior chamber is estimated to be approximately 1.0% to 1.5% of the anterior chamber volume per minute (34). The rate at which aqueous humor is formed (inflow) is measured in microliters per minute (as discussed in Chapter 2). By using the technique of scanning ocular fluorophotometry in more than 519 healthy persons, the mean (±standard deviation [SD]) rate of aqueous humor flow between 8 AM and noon was 3.0 ± 0.8 μL/min (35). The normal range (i.e., 95% of the sample) was 1.5 to 4.5 μL/min and showed a Gaussian distribution of flow rates. In 490 persons, the afternoon flow rate decreased to 2.7 ± 0.6 μL/min, while the mean rate in 180 persons between midnight and 6 AM was 1.3 ± 0.4 μL/min, with a range of 0.4 to 2.1 μL/min. A later study showed that individuals show concordance in aqueous humor flow, whereby those individuals who show a high aqueous flow in the morning also show a lower but relative higher flow at night (36). These changes in aqueous humor flow throughout the day reflect a biological pattern, also known as circadian rhythm, but the changes in this flow cannot account alone for the circadian patter in IOP (see modified Goldmann equation in Chapter 3) (37).

Circadian Rhythm of Aqueous Humor Flow

As noted above, there is a circadian rhythm of aqueous humor flow in humans, with rates during sleep being approximately one half of those in the morning. The mechanisms that control this biological rhythm are only partly understood and cannot be overcome entirely by light, ambulation, or activity level. The hormonal basis for the diurnal fluctuation in the rate of aqueous humor flow, or circadian rhythm, in humans is not completely understood (35). The strongest evidence suggests that physiologic changes in the level of circulating epinephrine available to the ciliary epithelia are the major driving force. Topical epinephrine has been shown to stimulate flow by 19% during the day and by 47% during the evening. Norepinephrine has also been shown to stimulate flow, but not as effectively as epinephrine. In patients who have had surgical adrenalectomy, a normal circadian rhythm of aqueous humor flow persists. In patients with Horner syndrome, where there is reduced or absent sympathetic innervation on one side, the circadian flow pattern is maintained. Systemically administered melatonin, hormones related to pregnancy, and antidiuretic hormone also do not appear to influence the normal circadian rhythm of flow. The effect of corticosteroids is more complex, in that exogenous corticosteroid appears to augment the effect of epinephrine-mediated stimulation of flow.

Other Factors Influencing Aqueous Humor Flow

Aqueous humor flow is also reduced in patients with diabetes mellitus, regardless of type (38). In myotonic dystrophy, the relative hypotony has been attributed to both reduction inflow rate and enhanced uveoscleral outflow route through the atrophic ciliary muscle (39). This causes a decrease in inflow (96), possibly related to a disruption in ciliary epithelium (97). Aqueous humor production can be reduced with inflammation (iridocyclitis) and by cyclodialysis (40).

In comparing different types of glaucoma, there are similar aqueous humor flow rates in patients with normal-tension glaucoma and healthy persons (41). Patients with ocular hypertension showed flow patterns similar to those of healthy persons during the morning hours, but the IOP and resistance to outflow values were higher in the patients with ocular hypertension (42). In patients with pigment dispersion syndrome, aqueous humor flow rate was slightly higher than in control participants because of the larger volume of the anterior chamber in the patients than in the controls (43). In patients with chronic open-angle glaucoma (COAG), aqueous humor flow during sleep was higher than in controls (44).

With aging, there is a decline in aqueous humor production—2.4% to 3.2% per decade after 10 years of age (45). There appears to be a trend of lower flow in women than in men, but this may be related to small differences in the size of the ocular structures (35). An elevation of IOP was once thought to be associated with a decline in aqueous humor production, which was referred to as "pseudofacility," but it is now understood that aqueous humor flow is pressure insensitive (35). The osmotic stress of drinking 1000 mL of water is associated with a significant increase in aqueous humor flow after 90 minutes (46). Caffeine does not have any clinically significant effect on aqueous humor flow in the normal human eye (47).

The pharmacologic agents that reduce aqueous humor flow in the treatment of glaucoma are discussed in Section III. These agents include the β-adrenergic receptor antagonists or β-blockers (see Chapter 29), the nonspecific adrenergic and selective α_2-adrenergic receptor agonists (Chapter 30), and the carbonic anhydrase inhibitors (Chapter 31).

Function and Composition of Aqueous Humor

Function

The circulating aqueous humor has at least the following functions: (a) maintaining proper IOP, which is important in early ocular development as well as in maintaining globe integrity throughout life; (b) providing substrates and removing metabolites from the cornea, lens, and trabecular meshwork; (c) delivering high concentrations of ascorbate; (d) participating in local paracrine signaling and immune responses; and (e) providing a colorless and transparent medium as a part of the eye's optical system.

Composition

The following statements, summarized in **Table 1.3**, describe the general characteristics of aqueous humor, expressed relative to plasma. Aqueous humor of both the anterior and the posterior chambers is slightly hypertonic compared with plasma. It is acidic, with a pH of 7.2 in the anterior chamber (48). The two most striking characteristics of aqueous humor are (a) a marked excess of ascorbate (15 times greater than that of arterial plasma) and (b) a marked deficit of protein (0.02% in aqueous humor compared with 7% in plasma) (32,49–51).

To illustrate the constant metabolic interchanges that occur with various ocular tissues, the cornea takes glucose and oxygen from the aqueous humor and releases lactic acid and a small amount of CO_2 into the aqueous humor (52). The lens takes up glucose, K^+, and amino acids from the aqueous humor and generates lactate and pyruvate; however, close similarities in aqueous humor composition between the phakic and aphakic eye of the same individual suggest that lens metabolism has practically no influence on the composition of aqueous humor (53). The exchange between the vitreous and retina with aqueous humor has been shown for amino acids and glucose passing into the vitreous from the aqueous humor (33).

The relative concentrations of free amino acids in human aqueous humor vary, with ratios of aqueous humor to plasma

Table 1.3	General Character of Human Aqueous Humor (Expressed Relative to Plasma)
Slightly hypertonic	
Acidic	
Marked excess of ascorbate	
Marked deficit of protein	

Slight excess of
    Chloride
    Lactic acid[a]	

Slight deficit of
    Sodium (rabbit study)
    Bicarbonate[a]
    Carbon dioxide
    Glucose	

Other reported constituents/features
    Amino acids (variable concentrations)
    Sodium hyaluronate
    Norepinephrine	

Coagulation properties	
Tissue plasminogen activator	
Latent collagenase activity	

[a]Varies with measurement technique.

concentrations ranging from 0.08 to 3.14, supporting the concept of active transport of amino acids (54). The concentrations of most other ions and non-electrolytes are very close to those in the plasma, and conflicting statements in the literature primarily represent differences with regard to species and measurement techniques. In general, human aqueous humor has a slight excess of chloride and a deficiency of bicarbonate and CO_2 (48,55). Lactic acid is reported to be in relative excess in human aqueous humor, although this determination varies widely with the technique of measurement. Sodium in rabbits and glucose in human eyes show a relative deficiency in the aqueous humor (54).

Other molecules that have been identified in human aqueous humor may be considered potential paracrine signaling molecules (56), meaning that these molecules are circulated and distributed to local tissues. Sodium hyaluronate, a glycosaminoglycan, was reported to have a mean value of 1.14 ± 0.46 mg/g in human aqueous humor obtained before cataract extraction, with no substantial difference in patients with diabetes or glaucoma (57). Signaling molecules, such as the catecholamine, norepinephrine, and nitric oxide, have been identified in human aqueous humor (58,59). Various components of the coagulation and anticoagulation pathways may be present in human aqueous humor (60), with an overall trend toward fibrinolytic activity. Various components involved in the maintenance of extracellular matrix have been detected in aqueous humor, which may influence the trabecular meshwork activity and subsequently the IOP (61). Several growth factors, which are polypeptides involved in the homeostatic balance of cells in a tissue, have been detected in human aqueous humor, and receptors for many of these factors have been identified on appropriate target tissues, such as trabecular meshwork and cornea (56). Of interest, myocilin has been detected in normal aqueous humor, but it is absent in the aqueous humor of patients with myocilin-associated glaucoma (62).

BIOLOGY OF AQUEOUS HUMOR OUTFLOW

As noted earlier, most of the aqueous humor leaves the eye at the anterior chamber angle through the system consisting of trabecular meshwork, the Schlemm canal, intrascleral channels, and episcleral and conjunctival veins. This pathway is referred to as the conventional or trabecular outflow. In the unconventional or uveoscleral outflow, aqueous humor exits by passing through the root of the iris, between the ciliary muscle bundles, then through the suprachoroidal–scleral tissues.

The relative contribution of these outflow pathways depends on the species studied. Furthermore, there is an age-dependent change in aqueous humor outflow in both the trabecular and the uveoscleral pathways. In general, the trabecular outflow in human eyes accounts for approximately 70% to 95% of the aqueous humor egress from the eye, with the lower values corresponding to younger eyes and the higher values corresponding to older eyes (63). The other 5% to 30% of the aqueous humor leaves primarily by the uveoscleral outflow pathway, with a decline in the contribution of this pathway with age (64). Whereas both total outflow facility and trabecular outflow facility also decline with age, the relative contributions of trabecular and uveoscleral outflow show an age-related shift, with a relative increase in the contribution in the trabecular pathway. Because uveoscleral outflow is relatively independent of IOP in the physiologic range, decreased uveoscleral outflow and increased trabecular outflow resistance with age simply mean that IOP must increase sufficiently to drive a higher proportion of total flow (which remains rather constant with age) across the increased trabecular resistance.

Cellular Organization of the Trabecular Outflow Pathway

Scleral Spur

The posterior wall of the scleral sulcus is formed by a group of fibers, the scleral roll, which run parallel to the limbus and project inward to form the scleral spur (Fig. 1.1), which is composed of 75% to 80% collagen and 5% elastic tissue (65). Myofibroblast-like scleral spur cells, in close association with varicose axons characteristic of mechanoreceptor nerve endings, suggest there is a mechanism for measuring stress or strain in the scleral spur, as might occur with ciliary muscle contraction or changes in IOP (66).

Schwalbe Line

Just anterior to the apical portion of the trabecular meshwork is a smooth area, which varies in width from 50 to 150 μm and has been called zone S (67). The anterior border of this zone consists of the transition from trabecular to corneal endothelium and the thinning and termination of the Descemet membrane. The posterior border is demarcated by a discontinuous elevation, called the Schwalbe line, which appears to be formed by the oblique insertion of uveal trabeculae into limbal stroma. Clusters of secretory cells, called Schwalbe line cells, have been observed just beneath this ridge in monkey eyes and are believed to produce a phospholipid material that facilitates aqueous humor flow through the canalicular system (68).

Trabecular Meshwork

As previously discussed, the scleral sulcus is converted into a circular channel, called the Schlemm canal, by the trabecular meshwork. This tissue consists of a connective tissue core surrounded by endothelium and may be divided into three portions: (a) uveal meshwork; (b) corneoscleral meshwork; and (c) juxtacanalicular tissue, which is sometimes referred to as the cribriform layer (**Fig. 1.8**) (63).

Uveal Meshwork

This innermost portion is adjacent to the aqueous humor in the anterior chamber and is arranged in bands or ropelike trabeculae that extend from the iris root and ciliary body to the peripheral cornea. The arrangement of the trabecular bands creates irregular openings that vary in size from 25 to 75 μm across.

Corneoscleral Meshwork

This portion extends from the scleral spur to the anterior wall of the scleral sulcus and consists of sheets of trabeculae that are perforated by elliptical openings. These holes become progressively smaller as the trabecular sheets approach the Schlemm canal, with a diameter range of 5 to 50 μm. The anterior tendons of the longitudinal ciliary muscle fibers insert on the scleral spur and posterior portion of the corneoscleral meshwork. This anatomic arrangement suggests an important mechanical role for the cholinergic innervation of ciliary muscle on trabecular meshwork function.

Both the uveal and corneoscleral trabecular bands or sheets are composed of four concentric layers. First, an inner connective tissue core is composed of typical collagen fibers with the usual 640 Å periodicity. Indirect immunofluorescent studies of human trabecular meshwork indicate that the central core contains collagen types I and III and elastin (69). Second, "elastic" fibers are composed of otherwise typical collagen, arranged in a spiraling pattern with an apparent periodicity of 1000 Å. These spiral fibrils may wind loosely or tightly and may provide flexibility to the trabeculae. Third, "glass membrane" is a name given to the layer between the spiraling collagen and the basement membrane of the endothelium. It is a broad zone composed of delicate filaments embedded in a ground substance (70). Fourth, an outer endothelial layer provides a continuous covering over the trabeculae.

The trabecular endothelial cells are larger, are more irregular, and have less prominent borders than corneal endothelial cells. They are joined by gap junctions and desmosomes, which provide stability, but allow aqueous humor to freely traverse

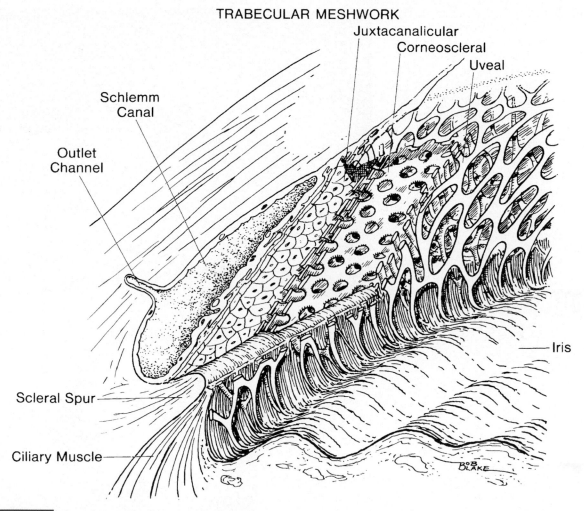

TRABECULAR MESHWORK

Figure 1.8 Three layers of trabecular meshwork (shown in cutaway views): uveal, corneoscleral, and juxtacanalicular.

the patent endothelial clefts (71). Two types of microfilaments have been found in the cytoplasm of human trabecular endothelium. Sixty Å filaments are located primarily in the cell periphery, around the nucleus, and in cytoplasmic processes. These appear to be actin filaments (72), which are involved in cell contraction and motility, phagocytosis, pinocytosis, and cell adhesion. Intermediate filaments of 100 Å are more numerous in the cells and are composed of vimentin and desmin, according to immunocytochemical studies of cultured human trabecular cells (73). These molecular markers in the trabecular endothelial cells suggest a myocyte or muscle cell-like phenotype, which further implies important contractile and motility functions.

Juxtacanalicular Tissue

This portion of the trabecular meshwork differs histologically from the other parts of the meshwork and has been given various names, including juxtacanalicular connective tissue, pore tissue, cribriform layer, and endothelial meshwork, depending on how one defines the anatomic limits of the tissue. In the broadest sense, this structure has three layers, discussed here beginning with the innermost portion. The inner trabecular

endothelial layer is continuous with the endothelium of the corneoscleral meshwork and might be considered as a part of this layer. The central connective tissue layer has variable thickness and is unfenestrated with several layers of parallel, spindle-shaped cells loosely arranged in a connective tissue ground substance (168,177). This tissue contains collagen type III but no collagen type I or elastin (69). Connective tissue cells in human and rabbit trabecular meshwork contain coated pits and coated vesicles in the plasma membrane, which are involved in receptor-mediated endocytosis (74).

The outermost portion of the trabecular meshwork—that is, the last tissue that aqueous humor must traverse before entering the canal—is the inner wall endothelium of the Schlemm canal. This endothelial layer has significant morphologic characteristics, which distinguish it from the rest of the endothelium in both the trabecular meshwork and in the Schlemm canal. The surface is bumpy due to protruding nuclei, cyst-like vacuoles, and fingerlike projections bulging into the canal (75,76). The fingerlike projections have been described as endothelial tubules with patent lumens, although there is lack of agreement as to whether they communicate between the anterior chamber and Schlemm canal (77). Actin filaments, as

Figure 1.9   A: Light microscopic view of the Schlemm canal (*SC*) and adjacent trabecular meshwork (*TM*) of normotensive Rhesus monkey eye. Trabecular wall of the Schlemm canal (*TW*) with prominent vacuolated cells (*arrows*); corneoscleral wall of the Schlemm canal (*CW*); collector channel (*CC*). (Toluidine blue stain, ×1030.) (From Tripathi RC. Ultrastructure of the trabecular wall of the Schlemm canal in relation to aqueous humor outflow. *Exp Eye Res.* 1968;7:335, with permission.) **B:** Electron microscopic view of trabecular wall of SC of normotensive human eye, showing vacuolated endothelial cells (*V*) containing flocculent material (*FL*). *OZ*, occluding zonules; *BM*, basement membrane; *OS*, open spaces in endothelial meshwork (×15,000). (From Tripathi RC. Ultrastructure of the trabecular wall of Schlemm's canal: a study of normotensive and chronic simple glaucomatous eyes. *Trans Ophthalmol Soc U K.* 1970;89:449–465, with permission.)

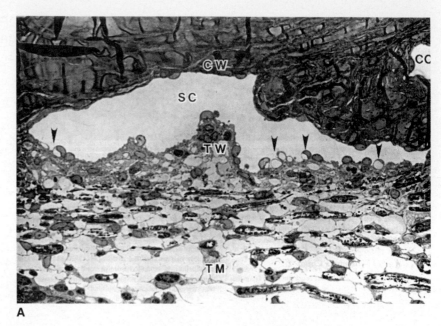

A

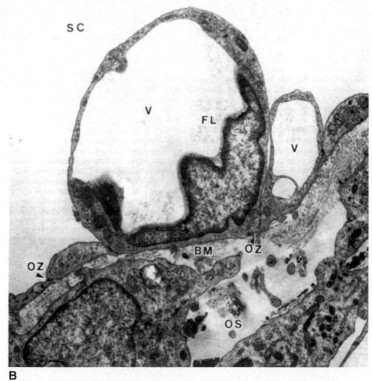

B

previously described in the uveal and corneoscleral trabecular endothelium, are also present in the inner wall endothelium of Schlemm canal (72).

The intercellular spaces are 150 to 200 Å wide and the adjacent cells are connected by various intercellular junctions. It is not clear as to how tightly these junctions maintain the intercellular connections, although they will open to permit the passage of red blood cells (78). Zonula occludens have been demonstrated in primate studies, which are traversed by meandering channels of extracellular space or slit pores, although it is estimated that this accounts for only a small fraction of the aqueous humor that leaves the eye by the conventional route (71).

Openings in the inner wall endothelium of the Schlemm canal have been described, and in general, the openings consist of minute pores and giant vacuoles that vary in size ranging from 0.5 to 2.0 μm (79) (**Fig. 1.9**). Evidence in support of their role in the transcellular outflow is based on injection of tracer elements into the anterior chamber with demonstration of the tracers in the vacuoles and pores (80). The observation that the concentration of tracer material in the giant vacuoles is not always the same as in the juxtacanalicular connective tissue suggests a dynamic system in which the vacuoles intermittently open and close to transport aqueous humor from the juxtacanalicular tissue to the Schlemm canal.

This transcellular transport has active and passive mechanisms. Indirect evidence for active transport includes the demonstration of enzymes and microscopic structures compatible with an active transport system in or near the endothelial layer (81,82). However, the bulk of evidence supports the theory of passive (pressure-dependent) transport, because the number and size of the vacuoles increase with progressive elevation of the IOP (83). It has been proposed that potential transcellular spaces exist in the inner wall endothelium of the Schlemm canal, which open as a system of vacuoles and pores, primarily in response to pressure, to transport aqueous humor from the juxtacanalicular connective tissue to the Schlemm canal. If intracellular transport through the inner wall endothelium of the Schlemm canal exists, it has been calculated, on the basis of the estimated size and total number of pores and giant vacuoles, that resistance to outflow through this system accounts for only a small fraction of the total resistance to aqueous humor outflow (84). It is also possible that only a portion of the juxtacanalicular tissue actually filters. It has been suggested that aqueous humor flows preferentially through those regions of the juxtacanalicular connective tissue nearest the inner wall pores creating a "funneling effect," which increases apparent flow resistance in the connective tissue by approximately 30-fold (85).

An alternative theory to that of transcellular transport is paracellular routes between the inner wall endothelial cells. Perfusion of monkey eyes with cationized ferritin revealed separation of adjacent cell membranes between tight junctions forming openings and tunnellike channels, which stained with the tracer indicating intercellular passage (86). These paracellular pathways were larger at higher perfusion pressure, and

apparent giant vacuoles were often dilatations of the paracellular spaces.

Of historical interest, the Sondermann canals, although originally described as endothelial-lined channels communicating between the Schlemm canal and intertrabecular spaces, have subsequently been interpreted as tortuous communications wandering irregularly and obliquely through the meshwork (87).

Schlemm Canal

This 360-degree, endothelial-lined channel averages 190 to 370 mm in diameter with occasionally branching into a plexus-like system (**Fig. 1.10**) (88). The endothelium of the outer wall is a single cell layer that is continuous with the inner wall endothelium but has a smoother surface with larger, less numerous cells and no pores (89). The outer wall also differs in having numerous, large outlet channels, which are described below. Smooth-muscle myosin-containing cells have been localized in the human aqueous humor outflow pathway adjacent to the collector channels, slightly distal to the outer wall of the Schlemm canal (90). Torus or liplike thickenings have been observed around the openings of the outlet channels, and septa have been noted to extend from these openings to the inner wall of the Schlemm canal, which presumably help keep the canal open (88). The endothelium is separated from the collagenous bundles of the limbus by a basement membrane and fibroblasts (89).

Episcleral and Conjunctival Veins

The Schlemm canal is connected to episcleral and conjunctival veins by a complex system of intrascleral channels (Fig. 1.10). The aqueous veins of Ascher (91), which are now more commonly referred to as collector channels (92), have been

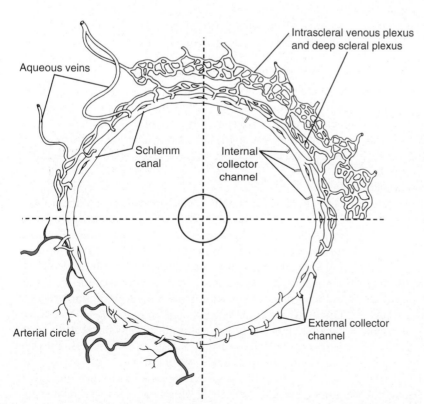

Figure 1.10 Schematic of aqueous humor outflow distal or beyond the "conventional" or trabecular pathway and into the canal of Schlemm. The canal divides into two or more portions intermittently. The drawing is divided into four portions by the dotted lines. The internal collector channels of Sondermann are labeled in the upper right sector as they extend into the trabecular meshwork. The external collector channels are seen in the upper and lower right sectors, arising from the canal and uniting with the deep intrascleral plexus of extending directly to the episcleral veins. The deep and intrascleral venous plexuses are external to the canal. In the upper left sector, an aqueous vein arises from the deep scleral plexus and another arises from the Schlemm canal and runs directly to the episcleral venous plexus. External collector veins are seen to arise from the canal and join the deep scleral plexus. In the lower left sector, the arteries of the deep sclera are seen to be in close relation to the canal of Schlemm. (Modified from Hogan MA, Alvarado J, Weddell J. *Histology of the Human Eye.* Philadelphia: WB Saunders; 1971, with permission.)

Labels in figure: Intrascleral venous plexus and deep scleral plexus; Aqueous veins; Schlemm canal; Internal collector channel; Arterial circle; External collector channel defined as originating at the outer wall of the Schlemm canal and terminating in episcleral and conjunctival veins in a lamination of aqueous humor and blood, referred to as the laminated vein of Goldmann. Two systems of intrascleral channels have been identified: (a) a direct system of large caliber vessels, which run a short intrascleral course and drain directly into the episcleral venous system, and (b) an indirect system of more numerous, finer channels, which form an intrascleral plexus before eventually draining into the episcleral venous system (88). The intrascleral aqueous channels do not connect with vessels of the uveal system, except for occasional fine communications with the ciliary muscle (93).

The aqueous vessels join the episcleral and conjunctival venous systems by several routes (91). Most aqueous vessels are directed posteriorly and drain into episcleral veins, whereas a few cross the subconjunctival tissue and drain into conjunctival veins. Some aqueous vessels proceed anteriorly to the limbus, with most running a short course parallel to the limbus before turning posteriorly to conjunctival veins. Casting studies in rabbit and dog eyes revealed a wide venous plexus in the limbic region of the episcleral vasculature anastomosing with a small arteriolar segment, the latter of which contains smooth-muscle cells that may have a role in regulating aqueous humor drainage by the episcleral venous plexus and subsequently influencing the IOP (94). In the rhesus monkey, the conjunctival vessels receiving aqueous humor drainage have a diameter consistent with that of capillaries, whereas most of the vessels in the episcleral plexus are the size of venules (95). Both types of vessels have simple walls composed of endothelium and a discontinuous layer of pericytes, through which tracer element (e.g., horseradish peroxidase) and presumably aqueous humor freely diffuse into subconjunctival and episcleral loose connective tissue. The episcleral veins drain into the cavernous sinus via the anterior ciliary and superior ophthalmic veins, whereas the conjunctival veins drain into superior ophthalmic or facial veins via the palpebral and angular veins (96).

Cellular Organization of the Uveoscleral Pathway

The unconventional outflow for aqueous humor outflow has not been studied as extensively as the trabecular outflow pathway. Historically, two unconventional pathways have been discriminated: (a) through the anterior uvea at the iris root, which is referred to the uveoscleral pathway, and (b) through transfer of fluid into the iris vessels and vortex veins, which has been described as uveovortex outflow.

Uveoscleral Outflow

Tracer studies have shown that aqueous humor passes through the root of the iris and interstitial spaces of the ciliary muscle to reach the suprachoroidal space (97). From there it passes to episcleral tissue via scleral pores surrounding ciliary blood vessels and nerves, vessels of optic nerve membranes, or directly through the collagen substance of the sclera. Studies with cynomolgus monkeys revealed a lower hydrostatic pressure in the suprachoroidal space than in the anterior chamber, and it was suggested that this

pressure differential is the driving force for uveoscleral outflow (98). The extracellular matrix of normal human ciliary muscle contains collagen types I, III, and IV; fibronectin; and laminin in association with muscle fibers and blood vessels, and it has been suggested that the biosynthesis and turnover of these glycoproteins may play an important role in resistance to flow within the unconventional pathways and in mediating the action of certain pharmacologic agents (99). This is discussed further in the following section on molecular mechanisms of outflow resistance and in Chapter 28 on prostaglandins.

Uveovortex Outflow

Tracer studies in primates have also demonstrated unidirectional flow into the lumen of iris vessel by vesicular transport, which is not energy dependent (100). The tracer can penetrate vessels of the iris, ciliary muscle, and anterior choroid to eventually reach the vortex veins; however, the role of net fluid movement into the iris vasculature is probably clinically insignificant (101). Some evidence suggests that there is a process of net osmotic resorption of some aqueous humor into the uveal venous circulation, driven by the high protein content in the blood in these vessels (102). The relative contribution for this fluid outflow pathway is not understood for the healthy eye, but it may be clinically relevant in an eye with nanophthalmos (103,104).

Molecular Mechanisms of Aqueous Humor Outflow Resistance

The biomechanical parameters and fluid hydrodynamics of the aqueous humor outflow pathways are complex. The technical challenges to study this important scientific discipline include the unique anatomy of these ocular tissues, the minute amounts of tissue available for study, and the difficulties in studying these tissues in vivo.

Resistance in the Trabecular Meshwork

Although the precise mechanism of resistance to conventional outflow is unknown, the following observations provide evidence that most resistance to conventional outflow, or trabecular outflow, is thought to be a combination of the inner wall endothelial layer and the adjacent juxtacanalicular tissues (63).

Perfusion Studies

Grant demonstrated that a 360-degree incision of the trabecular meshwork (trabeculotomy) eliminates approximately 75% of the normal outflow resistance (105). However, when such an eye is perfused at 7 mm Hg, the trabeculotomy eliminates only half the measured aqueous flow resistance (106). The remainder of the resistance to conventional aqueous humor outflow appears to be within the intrascleral outflow channels. One study in monkeys has suggested that 60% to 65% of outflow resistance is in the trabecular meshwork, 25% is in the inner one third to one half of the sclera, and 15% is in the outer one half to one third of the sclera (107).

Elevating IOP causes an increased resistance to aqueous humor outflow (108,109), which appears to be related to a collapse of the Schlemm canal due to distention of the trabecular meshwork, an increase in endothelial vacuoles with ballooning of the inner wall endothelial cells into the canal (83).

As might be expected from these observations, resistance to outflow is decreased by expanding the Schlemm canal. The trabecular meshwork has been described as a three-dimensional set of diagonally crossing collagen fibers, which respond to backward, inward displacement with a widening of the Schlemm canal (110). With either posterior depression of the lens or tension on the choroid (111,112), the tension on the trabecular meshwork caused an increased outflow facility, which appeared to be due to widening of the Schlemm canal and an increase in canal inner wall porosity. Further evidence for the effect of expanding the Schlemm canal may be supported by the IOP-lowering effect of viscocanalostomy (113). In contrast, after successful filtration surgery, there is a decrease in the size of the Schlemm canal, most likely due to underperfusion of the meshwork (114).

The pattern of aqueous humor circulation within the Schlemm canal is not fully understood. Perfusion studies in enucleated human adult eyes suggest that aqueous humor cannot flow more than 10 degrees within the canal (211), although there is less resistance to circumferential flow in infant eyes (212). However, studies of segmental blood reflux into the Schlemm canal imply that the canal is normally entirely open and that there is circumferential flow (213).

Other perfusion studies using tracer elements showed relatively free flow through the trabecular spaces and juxtacanalicular connective tissue until reaching the inner surface of the inner wall endothelium of the Schlemm canal. However, microspheres of smaller size than those used to determine flow dimensions in a perfused eye are captured by "sticky wall" interactions (115). This artifact may limit the information gained from perfusion studies concerning the dimensions of the flow-limiting passages in the conventional outflow system.

Morphology Changes

The normal human trabecular meshwork undergoes several changes with *age*. The general configuration changes from a long, wedge shape (Fig. 1.8) to a shorter, more rhomboidal form (116). The scleral spur becomes more prominent, the uveal meshwork becomes more compact, and localized closures in the Schlemm canal are present. The trabecular beams progressively thicken, and the endothelial cellularity declines at the rate of approximately 0.58% of cells per year, occasionally leading to trabecular denuding (117,118). A decrease in the number of giant vacuoles and of the cell count in the Schlemm canal is explained by an age-related reduction in the size of the Schlemm canal (119). In addition to these changes, the intertrabecular spaces narrow, and extracellular material increases, especially electron-dense plaques near the juxtacanalicular tissue that is associated with the ciliary muscle tendons inserting on the scleral spur (116,118) with age.

In COAG, there is a marked loss of trabecular meshwork cells leading to fusion and thickening of trabecular lamellae and a significant increase in electron-dense plaques compared with age-matched controls owing to components of the extracellular matrix that adhere to the sheaths of the elastic fibers and their connections to the inner wall endothelium (118). In steroid-induced glaucoma (also discussed further in the "Glucocorticoid Mechanisms" section), an increase in fine fibrillar material stains for collagen type IV in the subendothelial region of the Schlemm canal. In pigmentary glaucoma, cell loss is more prominent than in eyes with COAG presumably due to overload with pigment granules that were visible in remaining trabecular meshwork cells. The denuded trabecular meshwork areas were collapsed, and there were areas of disorganized cribriform regions and collapse of the Schlemm canal. These occluded areas had no pigment granules.

Extracellular Matrix

The extracellular matrix within basement membranes and stroma of the trabecular meshwork plays an important mechanism for regulating IOP. The extracellular matrix is composed of fibrillar and nonfibrillar collagens, elastin-containing microfibrils, matricellular and structural organizing proteins, glycosaminoglycans, and proteoglycans (120). The extracellular matrix of the outflow pathway is dynamic, undergoing constant turnover and remodeling in response to mechanically induced IOP stretching through cell adhesion proteins, cell surface receptors, associated binding proteins, certain cytokines, growth factors, and drugs (121).

The glycosaminoglycans have been extensively studied as a component of the extracellular matrix in the trabecular meshwork. Recently in an organ culture perfusion study, outflow facility was increased at least threefold in porcine eyes and 1.5-fold in human eyes by disrupting glycosaminoglycan biosynthesis with chlorate, an inhibitor of sulfation, and with β-xyloside, which provides a competitive nucleation point for addition of disaccharide units (122). In the control eyes, immunostaining for chondroitin and heparan sulfates was intensely staining the juxtacanalicular tissue region. In treated eyes, staining was severely reduced and showed prominent plaques.

Overall in the trabecular meshwork and endothelium of the Schlemm canal, fibrinolysis is favored as a protective mechanism against obstruction from fibrin and platelets (123). In addition to facilitating the resolution of fibrin clots, tissue plasminogen activator may also influence resistance to aqueous humor outflow under normal circumstances by altering the glycoprotein content of the extracellular matrix (84).

Glucocorticoid Mechanisms

The effects of glucocorticoids in the trabecular outflow pathway are complex, with both physiologic and pharmacologic implications. Glucocorticoids inhibit the synthesis of endogenous prostaglandins (124), which is clinically relevant because certain prostaglandins increase IOP in high doses but reduce ocular tension in moderate to low concentrations (see Chapter 28). Glucocorticoid receptors have been demonstrated in trabeculectomy specimens from human glaucomatous eyes, nonglaucomatous autopsy eyes, and cultured human trabecular cells (125,126). Glucocorticoids may influence the outflow facility by a direct effect on the extracellular matrix metabolism and the cytoskeleton (127,128).

The role of myocilin, previously called *TIGR*, expression in the trabecular outflow pathways is not fully understood, but it is clinically important given its role in juvenile glaucoma (see Chapter 8) (129). Some studies have shown that myocilin expression is increased in trabecular meshwork in response to dexamethasone (130), but it is curious that patients who have steroid-induced glaucoma do not have myocilin mutations (131).

Cellular and Cytoskeletal Mechanisms

The trabecular endothelial cells have been shown to phagocytize and degrade foreign material (132); to phagocytize pigment granules observed in eyes with pigmentary glaucoma (118); and to engulf debris, detach from the trabecular core, and leave in the Schlemm canal (78). A general mechanism that contributes to decreased function of trabecular meshwork cells is progressive accumulation of damaged proteins with age due to oxidative stress and to a decline in the cellular proteolytic machinery that eliminates misfolded and damaged proteins (133).

Altering trabecular meshwork resistance through the cytoskeleton has been shown in different experimental models. In a perfusion model with substances that are known to disrupt the microfilaments, such as cytochalasins, EDTA, or H-7, monkey eyes showed significantly reduced resistance to aqueous humor outflow, and histology showed alterations in the trabecular meshwork or inner wall of the Schlemm canal (134). In a perfusion model with sulfhydryl reagents, including iodoacetamide, *N*-ethylmaleimide, and ethacrynic acid, facility of outflow increased owing to an alteration of cell membrane sulfhydryl groups at multiple sites in the endothelial lining of the Schlemm canal and is not due to a metabolic inhibition (135–138).

Another mechanism by which sulfhydryl groups might modulate aqueous humor outflow involves hydrogen peroxide, a normal constituent of aqueous humor, which may reduce outflow through oxidative damage of the trabecular meshwork. Calf trabecular meshwork contains the sulfhydryl compound, glutathione, as well as the enzyme glutathione peroxidase, which catalyzes the reaction between glutathione and hydrogen peroxide, thereby detoxifying the latter and presumably protecting the meshwork from its harmful effects (139). In the pig eye, oxidative damage increases outflow facility at normal pressure but decreases it with elevated IOP, suggesting that elevated pressure may increase susceptibility of the outflow pathway to this form of stress (140).

Resistance to Unconventional Outflow

Our understanding of the unconventional outflow system is based more on physiology than on anatomy, and further study is needed to correlate function and anatomy in this system. In general terms, the uveoscleral pathway is characterized as "pressure independent," is reduced by cholinergic agonists (Chapter 32), decreases with aging, and is enhanced by prostaglandin drugs (Chapter 28) (97). In both humans and monkeys, there is a decline in uveoscleral outflow with aging (64,141). A potential explanation for the observed decline in uveoscleral outflow with aging is thickening of elastic fibers in the ciliary muscles (141).

Episcleral Venous Pressure

As discussed earlier in this chapter, another factor that contributes to the IOP is episcleral venous pressure. The precise interrelationship between episcleral venous pressure and aqueous humor dynamics is complex and is only partially understood. It has been commonly thought that for each mm Hg increase in episcleral venous pressure the IOP increases one mm Hg, although it may be that the magnitude of IOP increase is greater than the increase in venous pressure (142). The normal episcleral venous pressure is reported to be within the range of 8 to 11 mm Hg (143); however, these values are influenced considerably by the particular technique of measurement (as discussed in Chapter 3).

KEY POINTS

- Our understanding of the embryology of these ocular structures has advanced considerably from studies in human genetics, cellular and molecular biology, and transgenic animals.
- The basic chemistry of the aqueous humor is known. The multiple functions of this dynamic fluid include maintaining IOP, providing substrates and removing metabolites from the ocular structures, delivering high concentrations of ascorbate, participating in local paracrine signaling and immune responses, and providing a colorless and transparent medium as a part of the eye's optical system.
- We have considerable knowledge about the morphology of the ciliary body; however, we do not yet fully understand the molecular mechanisms that regulate circadian rhythm, hormonal effects, and aging impact on aqueous humor production.
- We have considerable knowledge about the morphology of the trabecular and uveoscleral outflow pathways in health and aging; however, we do not yet fully understand the molecular mechanisms that regulate outflow through these pathways. In general, it is thought that most resistance to outflow is due to a combination of the inner wall endothelial layer and adjacent juxtacanalicular tissues.

REFERENCES

1. Hogan M, Alvarado JA, Weddell JE. *Histology of the Human Eye.* Philadelphia: WB Saunders; 1971.
2. Hairston RJ, Maguire AM, Vitale S, et al. Morphometric analysis of pars plana development in humans. *Retina.* 1997;17(2):135–138.
3. Aiello AL, Tran VT, Rao NA. Postnatal development of the ciliary body and pars plana. A morphometric study in childhood. *Arch Ophthalmol.* 1992;110(6):802–805.
4. International Human Genome Sequencing Consortium. Finishing the euchromatic sequence of the human genome. *Nature.* 2004;431(7011): 931–945.
5. Lam TC, Chun RK, Li KK, et al. Application of proteomic technology in eye research: a mini review. *Clin Exp Optom.* 2008;91(1):23–33.
6. Wistow G. The NEIBank project for ocular genomics: data-mining gene expression in human and rodent eye tissues. *Prog Retin Eye Res.* 2006; 25(1):43–77.
7. Vopalensky P, Kozmik Z. Eye evolution: common use and independent recruitment of genetic components. *Philos Trans R Soc Lond B Biol Sci.* 2009;364(1531):2819–2832.

8. Barishak YR. *Embryology of the Eye and Its Adnexa.* 2nd ed. Basel, Switzerland: Karger; 2001.

9. Barishak RY, Ofri R. Embryogenetics: gene control of the embryogenesis of the eye. *Vet Ophthalmol.* 2007;10(3):133–136.

10. Beebe DC. Homeobox genes and vertebrate eye development. *Invest Ophthalmol Vis Sci.* 1994;35(7):2897–2900.

11. Kastner P, Grondona JM, Mark M, et al. Genetic analysis of RXR alpha developmental function: convergence of RXR and RAR signaling pathways in heart and eye morphogenesis. *Cell.* 1994;78(6):987–1003.

12. Livesey FJ, Cepko CL. Vertebrate neural cell-fate determination: lessons from the retina. *Nat Rev Neurosci.* 2001;2(2):109–118.

13. Zhao S, Chen Q, Hung FC, et al. BMP signaling is required for development of the ciliary body. *Development.* 2002;129(19):4435–4442.

14. Reichman EF, Beebe DC. Changes in cellular dynamics during the development of the ciliary epithelium. *Dev Dyn.* 1992;193(2):125–135.

15. Sellheyer K, Spitznas M. Surface morphology of the human ciliary body during prenatal development. A scanning electron microscopic study. *Graefes Arch Clin Exp Ophthalmol.* 1988;226(1):78–83.

16. Sowden JC. Molecular and developmental mechanisms of anterior segment dysgenesis. *Eye (Lond).* 2007;21(10):1310–1318.

17. Wordinger RJ, Clark AF. Bone morphogenetic proteins and their receptors in the eye. *Exp Biol Med (Maywood).* 2007;232(8):979–992.

18. Choy KW, Wang CC, Ogura A, et al. Genomic annotation of 15,809 ESTs identified from pooled early gestation human eyes. *Physiol Genomics.* 2006;25(1):9–15.

19. Funk R, Rohen JW. Scanning electron microscopic study on the vasculature of the human anterior eye segment, especially with respect to the ciliary processes. *Exp Eye Res.* 1990;51(6):651–661.

20. Morrison JC, DeFrank MP, Van Buskirk EM. Comparative microvascular anatomy of mammalian ciliary processes. *Invest Ophthalmol Vis Sci.* 1987;28(8):1325–1340.

21. Smelser GK. Electron microscopy of a typical epithelial cell and of the normal human ciliary process. *Trans Am Acad Ophthalmol Otolaryngol.* 1966;70(5):738–754.

22. Kitada S, Shapourifar-Tehrani S, Smyth RJ, et al. Characterization of human and rabbit pigmented and nonpigmented ciliary body epithelium. *Curr Eye Res.* 1991;10(5):409–415.

23. Bourge JL, Robert AM, Robert L, et al. Zonular fibers, multimolecular composition as related to function (elasticity) and pathology. *Pathol Biol (Paris).* 2007;55(7):347–359.

24. Marshall GE, Konstas AG, Abraham S, et al. Extracellular matrix in aged human ciliary body: an immunoelectron microscope study. *Invest Ophthalmol Vis Sci.* 1992;33(8):2546–2560.

25. Eichhorn M, Flugel C, Lutjen-Drecoll E. Regional differences in the distribution of cytoskeletal filaments in the human and bovine ciliary epithelium. *Graefes Arch Clin Exp Ophthalmol.* 1992;230(4):385–390.

26. Zhang D, Vetrivel L, Verkman AS. Aquaporin deletion in mice reduces intraocular pressure and aqueous fluid production. *J Gen Physiol.* 2002;119(6):561–569.

27. Preston GM, Smith BL, Zeidel ML, et al. Mutations in aquaporin-1 in phenotypically normal humans without functional CHIP water channels. *Science.* 1994;265(5178):1585–1587.

28. Raviola G, Raviola E. Intercellular junctions in the ciliary epithelium. *Invest Ophthalmol Vis Sci.* 1978;17(10):958–981.

29. Civan MM, Macknight AD. The ins and outs of aqueous humour secretion. *Exp Eye Res.* 2004;78(3):625–631.

30. Tamm ER, Lutjen-Drecoll E. Ciliary body. *Microsc Res Tech.* 1996;33(5):390–439.

31. Maren T. The rates of movement of Na^+, Cl^-, and HCO_3^- from plasma to posterior chamber: effect of acetazolamide and relation to the treatment of glaucoma. *Invest Ophthalmol.* 1976;15:356–364.

32. Tsukaguchi H, Tokui T, Mackenzie B, et al. A family of mammalian Na^+-dependent L-ascorbic acid transporters. *Nature.* 1999;399(6731):70–75.

33. Reddy VN. Dynamics of transport systems in the eye. Friedenwald Lecture. *Invest Ophthalmol Vis Sci.* 1979;18(10):1000–1018.

34. McLaren JW. Measurement of aqueous humor flow. *Exp Eye Res.* 2009;88(4):641–647.

35. Brubaker RF. Clinical measurements of aqueous dynamics: implications for addressing glaucoma. In: Civan MM, ed. *The Eye's Aqueous Humor, From Secretion to Glaucoma.* New York, NY: Academic Press; 1998:234–284.

36. Radenbaugh PA, Goyal A, McLaren NC, et al. Concordance of aqueous humor flow in the morning and at night in normal humans. *Invest Ophthalmol Vis Sci.* 2006;47(11):4860–4864.

37. Sit AJ, Nau CB, McLaren JW, et al. Circadian variation of aqueous dynamics in young healthy adults. *Invest Ophthalmol Vis Sci.* 2008;49(4):1473–1479.

38. Hayashi M, Yablonski ME, Boxrud C, et al. Decreased formation of aqueous humour in insulin-dependent diabetic patients. *Br J Ophthalmol.* 1989;73(8):621–623.

39. Walker SD, Brubaker RF, Nagataki S. Hypotony and aqueous humor dynamics in myotonic dystrophy. *Invest Ophthalmol Vis Sci.* 1982;22(6):744–751.

40. Pederson JE. Ocular hypotony. *Trans Ophthalmol Soc U K.* 1986;105 (pt 2):220–226.

41. Larsson LI, Rettig ES, Sheridan PT, et al. Aqueous humor dynamics in low-tension glaucoma. *Am J Ophthalmol.* 1993;116(5):590–593.

42. Ziai N, Dolan JW, Kacere RD, et al. The effects on aqueous dynamics of PhXA41, a new prostaglandin F2 alpha analogue, after topical application in normal and ocular hypertensive human eyes. *Arch Ophthalmol.* 1993;111(10):1351–1358.

43. Brown JD, Brubaker RF. A study of the relation between intraocular pressure and aqueous flow in the pigment dispersion syndrome. *Ophthalmology.* 1989;96(10):1468–1470.

44. Larsson LI, Rettig ES, Brubaker RF. Aqueous flow in open-angle glaucoma. *Arch Ophthalmol.* 1995;113(3):283–286.

45. Brubaker RF, Nagataki S, Townsend DJ, et al. The effect of age on aqueous humor formation in man. *Ophthalmology.* 1981;88(3):283–288.

46. Diestelhorst M, Krieglstein GK. The effect of the water-drinking test on aqueous humor dynamics in healthy volunteers. *Graefes Arch Clin Exp Ophthalmol.* 1994;232(3):145–147.

47. Adams BA, Brubaker RF. Caffeine has no clinically significant effect on aqueous humor flow in the normal human eye. *Ophthalmology.* 1990;97(8):1030–1031.

48. Becker B. Chemical composition of human aqueous humor: effects of acetazolamide. *AMA Arch Opthalmol.* 1957;57(6):793–800.

49. Reiss GR, Werness PG, Zollman PE, et al. Ascorbic acid levels in the aqueous humor of nocturnal and diurnal mammals. *Arch Ophthalmol.* 1986;104(5):753–755.

50. Barsotti MF, Bartels SP, Freddo TF, et al. The source of protein in the aqueous humor of the normal monkey eye. *Invest Ophthalmol Vis Sci.* 1992;33(3):581–595.

51. Haddad A, Laicine EM, de Almeida JC. Origin and renewal of the intrinsic glycoproteins of the aqueous humor. *Graefes Arch Clin Exp Ophthalmol.* 1991;229(4):371–379.

52. Gabelt BT, Kaufman PL. Aqueous humor hydrodynamics. In: Kaufman P, Alm A, eds. *Adler's Physiology of the Eye.* 10th ed. St. Louis: Mosby; 2003:237–289.

53. De Berardinis E, Tieri O, Iuglio N, et al. The composition of the aqueous humour of man in aphakia. *Acta Ophthalmol.* 1966;44:64–68.

54. De Berardinis E, Tieri O, Polzella A, et al. The chemical composition of the human aqueous humour in normal and pathological conditions. *Exp Eye Res.* 1965;4:179–186.

55. Davson H, Luck CP. A comparative study of the total carbon dioxide in the ocular fluids, cerebrospinal fluid, and plasma of some mammalian species. *J Physiol.* 1956;132(2):454–464.

56. Coca-Prados M, Escribano J. New perspectives in aqueous humor secretion and in glaucoma: the ciliary body as a multifunctional neuroendocrine gland. *Prog Retin Eye Res.* 2007;26(3):239–262.

57. Laurent UB. Hyaluronate in human aqueous humor. *Arch Ophthalmol.* 1983;101(1):129–130.

58. Trope GE, Rumley AG. Catecholamines in human aqueous humor. *Invest Ophthalmol Vis Sci.* 1985;26(3):399–401.

59. Carreiro S, Anderson S, Gukasyan HJ, et al. Correlation of in vitro and in vivo kinetics of nitric oxide donors in ocular tissues. *J Ocul Pharmacol Ther.* 2009;25(2):105–112.

60. Khodadoust AA, Stark WJ, Bell WR. Coagulation properties of intraocular humors and cerebrospinal fluid. *Invest Ophthalmol Vis Sci.* 1983;24(12):1616–1619.

61. Schlotzer-Schrehardt U, Lommatzsch J, Kuchle M, et al. Matrix metalloproteinases and their inhibitors in aqueous humor of patients with exfoliation syndrome/glaucoma and primary open-angle glaucoma. *Invest Ophthalmol Vis Sci.* 2003;44(3):1117–1125.

62. Gould DB, Reedy M, Wilson LA, et al. Mutant myocilin nonsecretion in vivo is not sufficient to cause glaucoma. *Mol Cell Biol.* 2006;26(22):8427–8436.

63. Tamm ER. The trabecular meshwork outflow pathways: structural and functional aspects. *Exp Eye Res.* 2009;88(4):648–655.

64. Toris CB, Yablonski ME, Wang YL, et al. Aqueous humor dynamics in the aging human eye. *Am J Ophthalmol.* 1999;127(4):407–412.

65. Moses RA, Grodzki WJ Jr, Starcher BC, et al. Elastin content of the scleral spur, trabecular mesh, and sclera. *Invest Ophthalmol Vis Sci.* 1978;17(8):817–818.

66. Tamm ER, Flugel C, Stefani FH, et al. Nerve endings with structural characteristics of mechanoreceptors in the human scleral spur. *Invest Ophthalmol Vis Sci.* 1994;35(3):1157–1166.

67. Spencer WH, Alvarado J, Hayes TL. Scanning electron microscopy of human ocular tissues: trabecular meshwork. *Invest Ophthalmol.* 1968;7(6):651–662.

68. Raviola G. Schwalbe line's cells: a new cell type in the trabecular meshwork of Macaca mulatta. *Invest Ophthalmol Vis Sci.* 1982;22(1):45–56.

69. Murphy CG, Yun AJ, Newsome DA, et al. Localization of extracellular proteins of the human trabecular meshwork by indirect immunofluorescence. *Am J Ophthalmol.* 1987;104(1):33–43.

70. Gong HY, Trinkaus-Randall V, Freddo TF. Ultrastructural immunocytochemical localization of elastin in normal human trabecular meshwork. *Curr Eye Res.* 1989;8(10):1071–1082.

71. Raviola G, Raviola E. Paracellular route of aqueous outflow in the trabecular meshwork and canal of Schlemm. A freeze-fracture study of the endothelial junctions in the sclerocorneal angel of the macaque monkey eye. *Invest Ophthalmol Vis Sci.* 1981;21(1 pt 1):52–72.

72. Gipson IK, Anderson RA. Actin filaments in cells of human trabecular meshwork and Schlemm's canal. *Invest Ophthalmol Vis Sci.* 1979; 18(6):547–561.

73. Iwamoto Y, Tamura M. Immunocytochemical study of intermediate filaments in cultured human trabecular cells. *Invest Ophthalmol Vis Sci.* 1988;29(2):244–250.

74. Diaz G, Orzalesi N, Fossarello M, et al. Coated pits and coated vesicles in the endothelial cells of trabecular meshwork. *Exp Eye Res.* 1982;35(2): 99–106.

75. Anderson DR. Scanning electron microscopy of primate trabecular meshwork. *Am J Ophthalmol.* 1971;71(1 pt 1):90–101.

76. Johnstone MA. Pressure-dependent changes in configuration of the endothelial tubules of Schlemm's canal. *Am J Ophthalmol.* 1974;78(4): 630–638.

77. Svedbergh B. Protrusions of the inner wall of Schlemm's canal. *Am J Ophthalmol.* 1976;82(6):875–882.

78. Grierson I, Lee WR. Erythrocyte phagocytosis in the human trabecular meshwork. *Br J Ophthalmol.* 1973;57(6):400–415.

79. Ethier CR. The inner wall of Schlemm's canal. *Exp Eye Res.* 2002; 74(2):161–172.

80. Tripathi RC. Mechanism of the aqueous outflow across the trabecular wall of Schlemm's canal. *Exp Eye Res.* 1971;11(1):116–121.

81. Tarkkanen A, Niemi M. Enzyme histochemistry of the angle of the anterior chamber of the human eye. *Acta Ophthalmol.* 1987;45:93.

82. Vegge T. Ultrastructure of normal human trabecular endothelium. *Acta Ophthalmol.* 1963;41:193–199.

83. Grierson I, Lee WR. Pressure-induced changes in the ultrastructure of the endothelium lining Schlemm's canal. *Am J Ophthalmol.* 1975;80(5): 863–884.

84. Ethier CR, Kamm RD, Palaszewski BA, et al. Calculations of flow resistance in the juxtacanalicular meshwork. *Invest Ophthalmol Vis Sci.* 1986;27(12):1741–1750.

85. Johnstone MA. The aqueous outflow system as a mechanical pump: evidence from examination of tissue and aqueous movement in human and non-human primates. *J Glaucoma.* 2004;13(5):421–438.

86. Epstein DL, Rohen JW. Morphology of the trabecular meshwork and inner-wall endothelium after cationized ferritin perfusion in the monkey eye. *Invest Ophthalmol Vis Sci.* 1991;32(1):160–171.

87. Ashton N, Brini A, Smith R. Anatomical studies of the trabecular meshwork of the normal human eye. *Br J Ophthalmol.* 1956;40(5):257–282.

88. Rohen JW, Rentsch FJ. [Morphology of Schlemm's canal and related vessels in the human eye]. *Albrecht Von Graefes Arch Klin Exp Ophthalmol.* 1968;176(4):309–329.

89. Fine BS. Structure of the trabecular meshwork and the canal of Schlemm. *Trans Am Acad Ophthalmol Otolaryngol.* 1966;70(5):777–790.

90. de Kater AW, Spurr-Michaud SJ, Gipson IK. Localization of smooth muscle myosin-containing cells in the aqueous outflow pathway. *Invest Ophthalmol Vis Sci.* 1990;31(2):347–353.

91. Ascher K. *The Aqueous Veins. Biomicroscopic Study of the Aqueous Humor Elimination.* Springfield, IL: Charles C Thomas; 1961.

92. Hoffmann F, Dumitrescu L. Schlemm's canal under the scanning electron microscope. *Ophthalmic Res.* 1971;2:37.

93. Jocson VL, Grant WM. Interconnections of blood vessels and aqueous vessels in human eyes. *Arch Ophthalmol.* 1965;73:707–720.

94. Rohen JW, Funk RHW. Functional morphology of the episcleral vasculature in rabbits and dogs: presence of arteriovenous anastomoses. *J Glaucoma.* 1994;3:51–57.

95. Raviola G. Conjunctival and episcleral blood vessels are permeable to blood-borne horseradish peroxidase. *Invest Ophthalmol Vis Sci.* 1983; 24(6):725–736.

96. Hayreh SS. Orbital vascular anatomy. *Eye (Lond).* 2006;20(10):1130–1144.

97. Alm A, Nilsson SF. Uveoscleral outflow—a review. *Exp Eye Res.* 2009;88(4):760–768.

98. Emi K, Pederson JE, Toris CB. Hydrostatic pressure of the suprachoroidal space. *Invest Ophthalmol Vis Sci.* 1989;30(2):233–238.

99. Weinreb RN, Toris CB, Gabelt BT, et al. Effects of prostaglandins on the aqueous humor outflow pathways. *Surv Ophthalmol.* 2002; 47(suppl 1):S53–S64.

100. Raviola G, Butler JM. Unidirectional transport mechanism of horseradish peroxidase in the vessels of the iris. *Invest Ophthalmol Vis Sci.* 1984;25(7):827–836.

101. Bill A. Blood circulation and fluid dynamics in the eye. *Physiol Rev.* 1975;55(3):383–417.

102. Pederson JE, Toris CB. Uveoscleral outflow: diffusion or flow? *Invest Ophthalmol Vis Sci.* 1987;28(6):1022–1024.

103. Brockhurst RJ. Vortex vein decompression for nanophthalmic uveal effusion. *Arch Ophthalmol.* 1980;98(11):1987–1990.

104. Uyama M, Takahashi K, Kozaki J, et al. Uveal effusion syndrome: clinical features, surgical treatment, histologic examination of the sclera, and pathophysiology. *Ophthalmology.* 2000;107(3):441–449.

105. Grant WM. Experimental aqueous perfusion in enucleated human eyes. *Arch Ophthalmol.* 1963;69:783–801.

106. Rosenquist R, Epstein D, Melamed S, et al. Outflow resistance of enucleated human eyes at two different perfusion pressures and different extents of trabeculotomy. *Curr Eye Res.* 1989;8(12):1233–1240.

107. Peterson WS, Jocson VL, Sears ML. Resistance to aqueous outflow in the rhesus monkey eye. *Am J Ophthalmol.* 1971;72(2):445–451.

108. Johnstone MA, Grant WG. Pressure-dependent changes in structures of the aqueous outflow system of human and monkey eyes. *Am J Ophthalmol.* 1973;75(3):365–383.

109. Brubaker RF. The effect of intraocular pressure on conventional outflow resistance in the enucleated human eye. *Invest Ophthalmol.* 1975; 14(4):286–292.

110. Moses RA, Arnzen RJ. The trabecular mesh: a mathematical analysis. *Invest Ophthalmol Vis Sci.* 1980;19(12):1490–1497.

111. Rosenquist RC Jr, Melamed S, Epstein DL. Anterior and posterior axial lens displacement and human aqueous outflow facility. *Invest Ophthalmol Vis Sci.* 1988;29(7):1159–1164.

112. Moses RA, Grodzki WJ Jr. Choroid tension and facility of aqueous outflow. *Invest Ophthalmol Vis Sci.* 1977;16(11):1062–1064.

113. Johnson DH, Johnson M. How does nonpenetrating glaucoma surgery work? Aqueous outflow resistance and glaucoma surgery. *J Glaucoma.* 2001;10(1):55–67.

114. Johnson DH, Matsumoto Y. Schlemm's canal becomes smaller after successful filtration surgery. *Arch Ophthalmol.* 2000;118(9):1251–1256.

115. Johnson M, Johnson DH, Kamm RD, et al. The filtration characteristics of the aqueous outflow system. *Exp Eye Res.* 1990;50(4):407–418.

116. McMenamin PG, Lee WR, Aitken DA. Age-related changes in the human outflow apparatus. *Ophthalmology.* 1986;93(2):194–209.

117. Alvarado J, Murphy C, Polansky J, et al. Age-related changes in trabecular meshwork cellularity. *Invest Ophthalmol Vis Sci.* 1981;21(5): 714–727.

118. Tektas OY, Lutjen-Drecoll E. Structural changes of the trabecular meshwork in different kinds of glaucoma. *Exp Eye Res.* 2009;88(4):769–775.

119. Ainsworth JR, Lee WR. Effects of age and rapid high-pressure fixation on the morphology of Schlemm's canal. *Invest Ophthalmol Vis Sci.* 1990;31(4):745–750.

120. Acott TS, Kelley MJ. Extracellular matrix in the trabecular meshwork. *Exp Eye Res.* 2008;86(4):543–561.

121. Luna C, Li G, Liton PB, et al. Alterations in gene expression induced by cyclic mechanical stress in trabecular meshwork cells. *Mol Vis.* 2009;15: 534–544.

122. Keller KE, Bradley JM, Kelley MJ, et al. Effects of modifiers of glycosaminoglycan biosynthesis on outflow facility in perfusion culture. *Invest Ophthalmol Vis Sci.* 2008;49(6):2495–2505.

123. Shuman MA, Polansky JR, Merkel C, et al. Tissue plasminogen activator in cultured human trabecular meshwork cells. Predominance of enzyme over plasminogen activator inhibitor. *Invest Ophthalmol Vis Sci.* 1988;29(3):401–405.

124. Weinreb RN, Polansky JR, Alvarado JA, et al. Arachidonic acid metabolism in human trabecular meshwork cells. *Invest Ophthalmol Vis Sci.* 1988;29(11):1708–1712.

125. Hernandez MR, Wenk EJ, Weinstein BI, et al. Glucocorticoid target cells in human outflow pathway: autopsy and surgical specimens. *Invest Ophthalmol Vis Sci.* 1983;24(12):1612–1616.

126. Weinreb RN, Bloom E, Baxter JD, et al. Detection of glucocorticoid receptors in cultured human trabecular cells. *Invest Ophthalmol Vis Sci.* 1981;21(3):403–407.

127. Hernandez MR, Weinstein BI, Wenk EJ, et al. The effect of dexamethasone on the in vitro incorporation of precursors of extracellular matrix components in the outflow pathway region of the rabbit eye. *Invest Ophthalmol Vis Sci.* 1983;24(6):704–709.

128. Clark AF, Wilson K, McCartney MD, et al. Glucocorticoid-induced formation of cross-linked actin networks in cultured human trabecular meshwork cells. *Invest Ophthalmol Vis Sci.* 1994;35(1):281–294.

129. Resch ZT, Fautsch MP. Glaucoma-associated myocilin: a better understanding but much more to learn. *Exp Eye Res.* 2009;88(4):704–712.

130. Lo WR, Rowlette LL, Caballero M, et al. Tissue differential microarray analysis of dexamethasone induction reveals potential mechanisms of steroid glaucoma. *Invest Ophthalmol Vis Sci.* 2003;44(2):473–485.

131. Fingert JH, Stone EM, Sheffield VC, et al. Myocilin glaucoma. *Surv Ophthalmol.* 2002;47(6):547–561.

132. Johnson DH, Richardson TM, Epstein DL. Trabecular meshwork recovery after phagocytic challenge. *Curr Eye Res.* 1989;8(11):1121–1130.

133. Liton PB, Gonzalez P, Epstein DL. The role of proteolytic cellular systems in trabecular meshwork homeostasis. *Exp Eye Res.* 2009;88(4):724–728.

134. Kaufman PL. Enhancing trabecular outflow by disrupting the actin cytoskeleton, increasing uveoscleral outflow with prostaglandins, and understanding the pathophysiology of presbyopia interrogating Mother Nature: asking why, asking how, recognizing the signs, following the trail. *Exp Eye Res.* 2008;86(1):3–17.

135. Epstein DL, Hashimoto JM, Anderson PJ, et al. Effect of iodoacetamide perfusion on outflow facility and metabolism of the trabecular meshwork. *Invest Ophthalmol Vis Sci.* 1981;20(5):625–631.

136. Epstein DL, Patterson MM, Rivers SC, et al. N-ethylmaleimide increases the facility of aqueous outflow of excised monkey and calf eyes. *Invest Ophthalmol Vis Sci.* 1982;22(6):752–756.

137. Epstein DL, Freddo TF, Bassett-Chu S, et al. Influence of ethacrynic acid on outflow facility in the monkey and calf eye. *Invest Ophthalmol Vis Sci.* 1987;28(12):2067–2075.

138. Lindenmayer JM, Kahn MG, Hertzmark E, et al. Morphology and function of the aqueous outflow system in monkey eyes perfused with sulfhydryl reagents. *Invest Ophthalmol Vis Sci.* 1983;24(6):710–717.

139. Nguyen KP, Chung ML, Anderson PJ, et al. Hydrogen peroxide removal by the calf aqueous outflow pathway. *Invest Ophthalmol Vis Sci.* 1988;29(6):976–981.

140. Yan DB, Trope GE, Ethier CR, et al. Effects of hydrogen peroxide-induced oxidative damage on outflow facility and washout in pig eyes. *Invest Ophthalmol Vis Sci.* 1991;32(9):2515–2520.

141. Gabelt BT, Kaufman PL. Changes in aqueous humor dynamics with age and glaucoma. *Prog Retin Eye Res.* 2005;24(5):612–637.

142. Brubaker RF. Determination of episcleral venous pressure in the eye. A comparison of three methods. *Arch Ophthalmol.* 1967;77(1):110–114.

143. Zeimer RC, Gieser DK, Wilensky JT, et al. A practical venomanometer. Measurement of episcleral venous pressure and assessment of the normal range. *Arch Ophthalmol.* 1983;101(9):1447–1449.

Intraocular Pressure and Tonometry

INTRAOCULAR PRESSURE

What Is Normal?

In individuals who are susceptible to glaucoma, "normal" intraocular pressure (IOP) may be defined as that pressure which does not lead to glaucomatous damage of the optic nerve head. Unfortunately, such a definition cannot be expressed in precise numerical terms because individuals show different susceptibility to optic nerve damage at given pressure levels that also depends on the underlying form of glaucoma (1,2). The best we can do is to describe the distribution of IOP in general populations to establish levels of risk for glaucoma within different pressure ranges. This chapter considers the distribution of IOP in the general population; the factors, other than glaucoma, that may influence IOP; and the clinical techniques for measuring IOP. (In Section II, the significance of various pressure levels in populations of patients with specific types of glaucoma is considered.)

Distribution in General Populations

One of the earliest studies on IOP distribution in the general population was based on Schiötz tonometry and showed an IOP distribution resembling a Gaussian curve with a skew toward the higher pressures. In 1958, Leydhecker and associates measured the IOP using Schiötz tonometry in 10,000 individuals with no known eye disease (3). The mean IOP (± standard deviation [SD]) was 15.5 ± 2.57 mm Hg, and two SDs above the mean was 20.5 mm Hg, which the authors interpreted as the upper limit of normal because approximately 95% of the area under a Gaussian curve lies between the mean ± 2 SD.

Subsequent population-based and epidemiologic studies have generally agreed with the findings of Leydhecker and colleagues, and are summarized in **Table 2.1**. Initially these results were used to interpret two subpopulations with a larger "normal" group and a smaller group of "glaucoma" patients who had higher IOPs (**Fig. 2.1**). However, we now know that IOP is a causative risk factor for glaucoma on the basis of evidence

Table 2.1 Reported IOP Distributions in General Populations			
Study[a]	**Individuals, n**	**Ages, y**	**Mean IOP ± SD, mm Hg**
MEASURED WITH SCHIÖTZ TONOMETERS			
Leydhecker et al., 1958 (3)	10,000	10–69	15.8 ± 2.57
Johnson, 1966 (14)	7577	>41	15.4 ± 2.65
Segal and Skwierczyńska, 1967 (15)	15,695	>30	15.3–15.9 (range, women) 15.0–15.2 (range, men)
MEASURED WITH APPLANATION TONOMETERS			
Armaly, 1965 (16)	2316	20–79	15.91 ± 3.14[b]
Perkins, 1965 (17)	2000	>40	15.2 ± 2.5 (OD); 14.9 ± 2.5 (OS)
Loewen et al., 1976 (18)	4661	9–89	17.18 ± 3.78
Ruprecht et al., 1978 (19)	8899	5–94	16.25 ± 3.45
Shiose and Kawase, 1986 (20)	75,545 (men); 18,158 (women)	<70; <70	14.60 ± 2.52; 15.04 ± 2.33
David et al., 1987 (21)	2504	≥40	14.93 ± 4.04
Klein et al., 1992 (22)	4856	43–86	15.4 ± 3.35

[a]Numbers in parentheses are reference numbers.
[b]Computed from data reported according to sex and age-groups. IOP, intraocular pressure; SD, standard deviation.

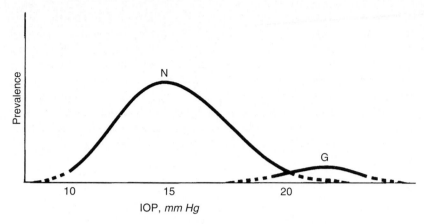

Figure 2.1 Theoretical distribution of IOPs in nonglaucoma (*N*) and glaucoma (*G*) populations, showing overlap between the two groups. *Dotted lines* represent uncertainty of extreme values in both populations.

from clinical trials (4–8). We also know that patients with glaucoma show different susceptibilities for disease progression at given pressure levels and based on the type of glaucoma (2). Thus, the previous simple notion that a patient's risk for glaucoma could be determined primarily on the basis of their IOP (Fig. 2.1) is now replaced with our understanding that IOP is a quantitative trait that is influenced by many factors (9). Although it is readily measured, IOP is a complex trait determined by aqueous humor flow, uveoscleral outflow, trabecular outflow, and episcleral venous pressure (10–15) (see details in Chapter 3).

Factors Affecting IOP

There have been many observations on factors that influence IOP (16–23). We should assimilate these important clinical observations from older studies with the evidence from the clinical trials, epidemiologic studies, and genetics. In addition, we should anticipate results from future studies designed to investigate the complex interactions between genetics and environment. Thus, it may be helpful to consider how these factors influence IOP on the basis of the categories of genetics, environment, and physiology.

Genetics

Early family studies provided evidence that IOP can be studied as a quantitative trait (24,25). In twin studies, IOP was observed to be more highly correlated between monozygotic than dizygotic twins (26,27). In addition, the mean IOP showed significantly higher concordance in twin-twin pairs, compared with twin-spouse pairs (27). Recently, studies have shown that heredity contributes to IOP (28–35).

Traditional genetic studies using linkage and genome-wide methods (see Chapter 8) led to the discovery of several loci, or chromosomal locations, for IOP. In the Blue Mountains Eye Study, commingling analysis of IOP supported that "a major gene" contributed to the variance of IOP (36). A family study showed significant linkage for IOP to chromosome 10q22 (37). An affected sibling pair study showed linkage to chromosomes 5q22 and 14q22 (38). In the Beaver Dam Eye Study, seven loci, on chromosomes 2, 5, 6, 7, 12, 15, and 19, were reported as

being linked to IOP (39). To date, however, no "IOP genes" have been reported in these chromosomal regions. The next steps will involve validating and excluding loci, identifying genes in these loci, cross-referencing to databases, and placing these genes in context with aqueous humor dynamics. It is expected that a combination of genes will be identified as having major and minor influences on IOP variation and variation in IOP response to glaucoma medications.

Environment

Thus far, the environmental factors observed to affect IOP may be categorized into physical, smoking, drug, and dietary exposures. Exposure to cold air reduces IOP, apparently because episcleral venous pressure is decreased (40). Reduced gravity causes a sudden, marked increase in IOP, apparently because of cephalad shifts in intravascular and extravascular body fluids (41).

Tobacco smoking causes a transient rise in the IOP immediately after smoking, possibly through a mechanism of vasoconstriction and elevated episcleral venous pressure (42). However, the direct risk of tobacco on chronic open-angle glaucoma (COAG) is not evident from epidemiologic and case–control studies (43,44).

The impact of various drugs, excluding antiglaucoma drugs (discussed in Section III), are considered in the general categories of general anesthesia, illicit drugs, and systemic medications. General anesthesia is usually associated with a reduction in the IOP (45), although some agents used for sedation, such as ketamine, do not lower IOP (46). The two situations in which the physician must be particularly concerned about anesthesia-induced alterations in IOP are (a) in the evaluation of infants and children and (b) in patients who have ocular trauma with a ruptured globe.

In infants and children examined under anesthesia for suspicion of congenital glaucoma, the main concern is to avoid the artificial reduction of IOP (as discussed earlier), which could mask a pathologic pressure elevation. In one study, the mean (± SD) IOP for children measured under halothane anesthesia was 7.8 ± 0.4 mm Hg at age 1 year, with a gradual increase of about 1 mm Hg per year of age to 11.7 ± 0.6 mm Hg at age 5 years (47).

When operating on an open eye, such as after penetrating injury or during intraocular surgery, the primary concern is to avoid sudden elevations of IOP that might lead to extrusion of ocular contents. Depolarizing muscle relaxants, such as succinylcholine and suxamethonium, cause a transient increase in IOP, possibly because of a combination of extraocular muscle contraction and intraocular vasodilation (45). In comparing intubation methods, the laryngeal mask airway causes less of an IOP risk, compared with tracheal intubation, and has the added advantage of less postintubation coughing and other symptoms (48,49).

Among the illicit drugs, heroin and marijuana lower the IOP (the latter is discussed further in Section III), whereas LSD (lysergic acid diethylamide) elevates the IOP (50,51).

Among the many systemic medications that may potentially affect IOP, the most relevant for clinical consideration include corticosteroids, anticholinergic agents, and unusual reaction to sulfonamides. Given the use of corticosteroids systemically for immunosuppression and dramatic increased intraocular use to treat retinal diseases, the potential risk of IOP elevation and steroid-induced glaucoma should be monitored in a patient receiving such treatment (see Chapter 23).

In general, the labels on systemic anticholinergics, antihistamines, decongestants, and psychiatric medications having some anticholinergic effects state warnings such as "contraindicated in patients with glaucoma." These warnings are meant to alert the patient and prescribing physician that use of these medications can precipitate pupillary block glaucoma or acute angle-closure glaucoma in patients with anatomically narrow angles (see Chapter 12) (52). Cases of acute angle-closure glaucoma have been reported with the use of scopolamine dermal patches for motion sickness, and the use of aerosolized atropine and ipratropium for chronic obstructive pulmonary disease (53–55). However, in patients with COAG, scopolamine was shown not to affect IOP (56). It would be expected that these other agents would not elevate IOP in patients with COAG.

The potential effects of dietary exposures on IOP have not been studied extensively (57). Acute doses of alcohol lower IOP, but the mechanism is not associated with a change in facility of aqueous outflow (58). The mechanism may be a combination of suppressed circulating antidiuretic hormone, leading to a reduction of net water movement into the eye, and direct inhibition of aqueous secretion (59). However, the clinical relevance of this acute effect is unknown since recent epidemiologic studies have not shown that alcohol consumption affects IOP or the risk for glaucoma (60–62).

Caffeine consumption may cause a slight, transient rise in IOP, although the levels associated with customary coffee drinking do not appear to cause a significant, sustained pressure elevation (63). There does not appear to be an overall population-based associated risk for glaucoma with caffeine consumption (64).

Recent epidemiologic studies have used validated nutritional surveys to analyze the association between certain dietary exposures and risk of COAG. In the Nurses' Health Study (with 76,200 respondents) and the Health Professionals Follow-up Study (40,284 participants), no strong association was found between antioxidant consumption and the risk of COAG (65). According to a women's health study of 1155 participants, a higher intake of certain fruits and vegetables may be associated with as much as a 69%-decreased risk of glaucoma (66). In a study comparing diets with sufficient and deficient intakes of omega-3 fatty acids since conception, those rats fed a sufficient omega-3 diet had decreased IOP with increasing age because of increased outflow facility, likely resulting from an increase in docosanoids (67).

Physiology

Sex

Overall, sex appears to have no major effect on IOP in the 20- to 40-year age-group. In older age-groups, the apparent rise in mean IOP with increasing age is greater among women than men, and coincides with the onset of menopause, whereas the increase in the standard deviation of the IOP distribution is equal between men and women in white populations (16,22). In a population-based Japanese study, IOP did not differ between women and men (68). In the Barbados Eye Study, which had a mixed population of participants, IOP was higher among women than men (69).

Age

IOP generally increases with age. Studies indicate that children have significantly lower pressures than adults do, although tonometric measurements may be influenced by the level of cooperation of the child if he or she is awake, the type of tonometer used to measure the IOP, and the general anesthetic when the child is asleep or sedated (47,70) (discussed earlier, under "Environment").

The reported mean ($\pm$ SD) IOP, by using only topical anesthesia for the tonometry, is 11.4 + 2.4 mm Hg in newborns and 8.4 + 0.6 mm Hg in infants younger than 4 months of age (47,71). In a study of 460 children between birth and 16 years of age using a noncontact tonometer, the mean IOP increased from 9.59 + 2.3 mm Hg at birth to 13.73 + 2.05 mm Hg at 3 to 4 years, with more stable measurements obtained thereafter (72). In another study, of 405 children between birth and 12 years, using the Perkins applanation tonometer, the mean IOP was 12.02 + 3.74 mm Hg (73). In this pediatric cohort, IOP showed a trend of increasing IOP with age (correlation coefficient [r] = 0.49) that approached adult IOP levels by 12 years of age; also observed were increased IOP with hyperopia (r = 0.69) and corneal thickness measured by pachymetry (r = 0.39). IOP was inversely proportional to axial length (r = –0.1).

Results of studies in premature infants have been conflicting, with mean IOPs of 18 mm Hg in one study and 10.13 to 10.17 mm Hg in another (74,75). The tonometer may also influence the results, with mean IOP measurements in 50 supine children younger than 5 years of 5.89 mm Hg with a handheld applanation tonometer and 14.76 mm Hg with a pneumotonometer (76). In a study of 77 children (132 eyes; mean age, 1 year, 7 months; range, 1 month to 60 months), mainly with retinopathy of prematurity (107 eyes), IOP was measured by using the Perkins, Schiötz, and Tono-Pen tonometers (70).

There was no significant difference between the mean IOPs obtained with the Tono-Pen and the Perkins, but the Schiötz measurements were significantly higher than those obtained with the Perkins and Tono-Pen tonometers.

In adults, the IOP distribution is Gaussian between 20 and 40 years of age (16), but tends to increase with advancing age (22). A study of 69,643 Japanese participants suggested that study design may influence the findings, in that a cross-sectional analysis showed a significant decrease in IOP with age, whereas a longitudinal analysis showed a significant increase (77). In a Malay Singapore cohort, IOP increased with age to the sixth decade, but with further increase in age there was a decrease in IOP, resulting in an inverted-U distribution pattern (78). Regression analysis showed that age, central cornea thickness (CCT), and systolic blood pressure were significant determinants of IOP in persons aged 40 to 80 years; CCT was a more important determinant in younger persons. In the white cohort of the Beaver Dam Eye Study, a population-based study of age-related eye diseases in persons aged 43 to 86 years, significant physiologic covariates on IOP with aging included systolic and diastolic blood pressures, body mass index, hematocrit, serum glucose, glycohemoglobin, cholesterol level, pulse, nuclear sclerosis, season, and time of day of the measurement (22).

In terms of aging effects on aqueous humor dynamics, studies have shown that there is reduced facility of aqueous outflow and uveoscleral outflow, and a decrease in aqueous production (79–81). Episcleral venous pressure does not appear to change significantly with advancing age (80,82).

Ethnicity

Clinical trials and population-based studies have shown that there is an increased risk for COAG among blacks, and for angle-closure glaucoma in certain Asian populations (83–85). However, with the current understanding of IOP as a causative risk factor for glaucoma and that a thin central cornea confers an increased risk for COAG, recent studies using regression analysis of multiple covariates found that black race is not an independent risk factor, although black individuals tend to have thinner corneas, greater cup-to-disc ratios, and higher IOP, which increase their risk (86). As we learn more about the biological and genomic correlates of the clinical risk factors for glaucoma, we will understand the basis of the earlier clinical observations of ethnoracial-based risk for glaucoma.

Refractive Error

In the infant eye, elevated IOP causes axial myopia as evident by buphthalmos (discussed further in Chapter 13). In older children, a positive correlation between IOP and both axial length of the globe and increasing degrees of myopia has been reported (21,87–89). Increasing IOP was also related to myopia in a study of 321 children (mean age, 9.8 years) (90). However, more recent studies have found no correlation between higher IOP and myopia in children (91,92).

In adults, it is still not known whether myopia is a risk factor for COAG. Some epidemiologic studies show no association (93), whereas other studies report a positive association between myopia and COAG (94–96). In the studies reporting an association between myopia and COAG, it is hard to know whether the higher pressures in this group reflect early glaucoma cases or a truly higher IOP distribution throughout the myopic population.

Diurnal and Postural Variation

Like many biological parameters, the IOP is subject to cyclic fluctuations throughout the day (97–99). In a study of 1062 persons middle-aged and older, the IOP was highest during the daytime (100). A study of 690 diurnal curves found that IOP peaked in the early morning for 40% of patients, and before noon in 65% (101). In a study of persons in China with (N = 59) and without (N = 67) ocular hypertension, IOP was highest in the morning (102).

More recent studies have taken into account postural variation in IOP and showed consistent elevation of IOP at nighttime (97,103), which is physiologically relevant because sleep occurs in the supine position. Whole-body, head-down tilt leads to a further increase in IOP, which correlates with the degree of inversion, is greater in glaucomatous eyes, and appears to be related to elevated episcleral venous pressure (104–106). Thus, obtaining clinical history on type of exercise—in particular, yoga and inversion—may be relevant for the patient with glaucoma. However, it is still unknown whether IOP changes induced by position contribute to optic nerve damage.

The obvious primary clinical value of measuring diurnal IOP variation is to avoid missing a pressure elevation with single readings; however, diurnal measurement is impractical in a busy clinical practice, and the logistics of obtaining the diurnal measurements is a practical concern. In any case, many physicians use a modified diurnal curve, by measuring the IOP in the office approximately every 2 hours from early morning to late afternoon or early evening. It has been suggested that measuring IOP in supine position during office hours estimates peak nocturnal IOP better than sitting measurements do (107).

In addition to trying to detect maximum IOP data as a risk for glaucoma, detecting large IOP fluctuations is also important. In a study of 64 patients with COAG and documented IOP less than 25 mm Hg over a mean follow-up of 5 years, patients were trained to perform 5 days of home self-tonometry (described later in this chapter) (108). Although mean home IOP and baseline office IOP were similar (16.4 ± 3.6 mm Hg and 17.6 ± 3.2 mm Hg, respectively), the diurnal IOP range and the IOP range over multiple days were significant risk factors for progression. The risk for visual field progression within 8 years among patients with a diurnal IOP range of 5.4 mm Hg was nearly six times as high as that among patients with IOP fluctuation of 3.1 mm Hg. Baseline office IOP had no predictive value.

The physiologic mechanisms that regulate diurnal IOP variation are complex. The IOP is regulated in part by adrenocortical steroids and catecholamines (109–111). The circadian rhythm of aqueous flow also does not appear to be influenced by plasma melatonin levels (112). In terms of circadian rhythm and the four parameters of aqueous humor dynamics, the reproducible circadian rhythm of higher aqueous humor flow in the morning compared with night does not solely explain the diurnal IOP variation (98,113,114).

Exertional Influences

Straining, as associated with the Valsalva maneuver, electroshock therapy, or playing a high-resistance musical instrument, has been reported to elevate the IOP (115–117). The mechanisms include elevated episcleral venous pressure, especially with the Valsalva maneuver; uveal engorgement; and possibly, increased orbicularis tone. Of particular clinical relevance is that overweight patients may have artificial IOP elevations when measured with Goldmann applanation tonometry, because they strain to reach the instrument; this can be overcome by measuring the pressure with the patient in a relaxed position, by using a Perkins tonometer (118).

Exercise has been shown to lower IOP in persons with and without glaucoma (119). The effect of aerobic exercise on IOP lowering is observed in patients receiving topical glaucoma medication (120). There is clinical relevance for taking an exercise history. For instance, in young patients with advanced congenital or juvenile glaucoma, exercise-induced decrease in central visual acuity and reduced foveal sensitivity on perimetry may occur transiently during exercise (121). Another example is that some patients with pigmentary dispersion syndrome or pigmentary glaucoma develop exercise-induced anterior chamber pigment dispersion with IOP elevation, which can be minimized with the use of low-dose pilocarpine before exercise (122); pilocarpine causes miosis, minimizing the contact between the midperipheral iris and zonules (see Chapter 31).

Several theories on mechanisms for exercise-induced IOP reduction have been investigated and include metabolic acidosis, and hypocapnia and blood lactate levels; exercise-induced IOP changes do not appear to be related to hydration status and other serology parameters, such as plasma osmolality (123–125). Clearly, the mechanisms involved in exercise-induced IOP reduction are complex and may differ between sedentary and conditioned patients, and between young and older patients. Regardless, future research should incorporate health behaviors that include nutritional intake, body mass index and obesity, exercise, smoking, and sleep apnea (126).

Eyelid and Eye Movement

Blinking has been shown to raise the IOP by 10 mm Hg, and hard eyelid squeezing may raise it to as high as 90 mm Hg (127). Voluntary eyelid fissure widening causes an increase in IOP of about 2 mm Hg, which may relate to an increased orbital volume from retraction of the upper eyelid into the orbit (128). Contraction of extraocular muscles also influences the IOP. There is an increase in IOP on up-gaze in healthy individuals, which is augmented by Graves infiltrative ophthalmopathy (129). During strabismus surgery, especially for eyes with thyroid ophthalmopathy, the IOP has been recorded to increase to as high as 84 mm Hg (130).

Intraocular Conditions

Some intraocular conditions may lead to a reduction in IOP. In the clinical setting of anterior uveitis without angle abnormalities, IOP may be reduced slightly. It has traditionally been thought that this is because of a decrease in aqueous humor formation (131), although anterior segment inflammation has also been shown to increase uveoscleral outflow in monkeys by reducing the density of collagen type I in the extracellular matrix of the ciliary body (132). Rhegmatogenous retinal detachment may also be associated with a reduced IOP, apparently because of reduced aqueous flow, as well as a shunting of aqueous from the posterior chamber, through the vitreous and retinal hole, into the subretinal space, and across the retinal pigment epithelium (131).

Systemic Conditions

On the basis of public health relevance, the two most common systemic diseases studied for potential contributory risk for glaucoma are hypertension and diabetes mellitus. The more recent epidemiology studies find a positive correlation between systemic hypertension and IOP in Latinos, Japanese, aging men, persons of mixed African descent, the Blue Mountains Eye Study cohort, and whites in the Beaver Dam Eye Study (88,99,133–136). In contrast, hypertension was not associated with glaucoma risk in Asian Indians (137). Retinal microvascular abnormalities seen with hypertension were not associated with risk for glaucoma among white participants in the Beaver Dam Eye Study (138). The mechanisms responsible for hypertension and risk for elevated IOP and glaucoma may involve a combination of ocular pulse pressure and ocular perfusion pressure (8,139,140).

The potential influence of diabetes on IOP and glaucoma risk is unclear on the basis of epidemiology, clinical trials, and large clinical studies. In a population-based study in 3280 Malay adults aged 40 to 80 years, diabetes and metabolic abnormalities were associated with a small increase in IOP but were not significant risk factors for glaucomatous optic neuropathy (141). In the Latino cohort of the Los Angeles Latino Eye Study, presence of type 2 diabetes and a longer duration of diabetes were independently associated with an increased risk for COAG (142). In a black cohort of African ancestry, diabetes was associated with increased IOP (134). In the Rotterdam Study and among an Asian Indian population, diabetes was not a risk factor for COAG (137,143).

An earlier study in dogs reported that retrolaminar pressure (i.e., pressure surrounding the optic nerve subarachnoid space) was lower, but dependent on cerebrospinal fluid (CSF) pressure (144). The investigators stated that the translaminar pressure gradient across the lamina cribrosa varied independently of IOP, and they hypothesized that this may be important in the pathophysiology of glaucoma. Subsequent clinical studies support this hypothesis. In a case–control study involving patients who had a lumbar puncture, the opening CSF pressure in 28 patients with COAG was 9.2 ± 2.9 mm Hg, which was significantly lower than that of the 49 controls, in whom the pressure was 13.0 ± 4.2 mm Hg (145). Another case–control study showed a glaucoma prevalence of 18.1% in patients with normal-pressure hydrocephalus and 5.6% in controls with hydrocephalus (146). In a prospective study, CSF pressure was lower in patients with COAG than in persons without COAG, and was lower among patients with normal-tension glaucoma than among those with high-pressure glaucoma (147).

Obesity and body mass index have also been associated with increased IOP (20,22,68,148). However, the relationship between obesity and increased body mass index and risk of glaucoma is not understood (149). In Graves disease, increased rate of ocular hypertension has been reported in several studies (150–153), and one study reported that such patients have normal corneal thickness (154). Although it is logical to hypothesize that thyroid hormone has some influence on IOP, the mechanism of this hormone on aqueous humor dynamics has not been elucidated (155,156).

Some case series and case–control studies have shown an increased rate of COAG in patients with sleep apnea (157,158). In myotonic dystrophy, the IOP is markedly low, which not only may be partially due to reduced aqueous production but also may be due to increased outflow, possibly by the uveoscleral route from atrophy of the ciliary muscles (159,160). Hyperthermia has been shown to cause an increased IOP (161). Patients with human immunodeficiency virus (HIV) have a relatively low mean IOP, which correlates with low CD4$^+$ T-lymphocyte counts and the presence and extent of cytomegalovirus retinitis (162).

TONOMETERS AND TONOMETRY

Classification of Tonometers

All clinical tonometers measure the IOP by relating a deformation of the globe to the force responsible for the deformation (163). The two basic types of tonometers differ according to the shape of the deformation: indentation and applanation (flattening).

Indentation Tonometers

The shape of the deformation with this type of tonometer is a truncated cone (**Fig. 2.2A**). The precise shape, however, is variable and unpredictable. In addition, these instruments displace a relatively large intraocular volume. As a result of these characteristics, conversion tables based on empirical data from in vitro and in vivo studies must be used to estimate the IOP. The prototype of this group, the Schiötz tonometer, was introduced in 1905.

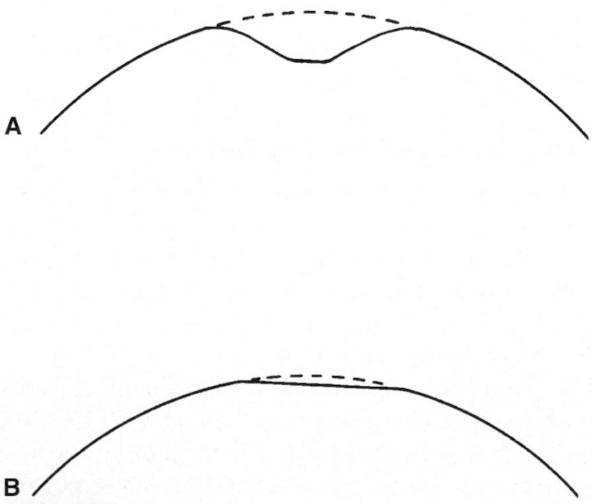

Applanation Tonometers

The shape of the deformation with these tonometers is a simple flattening (**Fig. 2.2B**), and because the shape is constant, its relationship to the IOP can, in most cases, be derived from mathematical calculations. The applanation tonometers are further differentiated on the basis of the variable that is measured.

Variable Force

This type of tonometer measures the force that is required to applanate (flatten) a standard area of the corneal surface. The prototype is the Goldmann applanation tonometer, which was introduced in 1954.

Variable Area

Other applanation tonometers measure the area of the cornea that is flattened by a known force (weight) (**Table 2.2**). The prototype in this group is the Maklakoff tonometer, which was introduced in 1885. The division between indentation and applanation tonometers, however, does not correlate entirely with the magnitude of intraocular volume displacement. Goldmann-type tonometers have relatively minimal displacement, whereas that with Maklakoff-type tonometers is sufficiently large to require the use of conversion tables.

Noncontact Tonometer

A third type of tonometer uses a puff of air to deform the cornea and measures the time or force of the air puff that is required to create a standard amount of corneal deformation. The prototype was introduced by Grolman in 1972.

Figure 2.2 Corneal deformation created by (**A**) indentation tonometers (a truncated cone) and (**B**) applanation tonometers (simple flattening).

Table 2.2	Applanation Tonometers with Variable Area
Tonometer	**Description/Use**
Maklakoff–Kalfa	Prototype
Applanometer	Ceramic endplates
Tonomat	Disposable endplates
Halberg tonometer	Transparent endplate for direct reading: multiple weights
Barraquer tonometer	Plastic tonometer for use in operating room
Ocular tension indicator	Uses Goldmann biprism and standard weight, for screening (measures above or below 21 mm Hg)
Glaucotest	Screening tonometer with multiple endplates for selecting different "cutoff" pressures

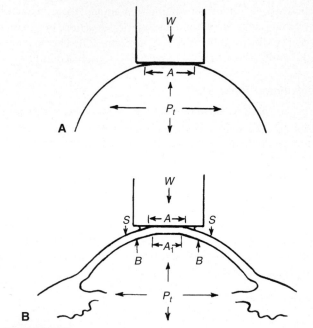

Figure 2.3   A: The Imbert–Fick law ($W = P_t \times A$). **B:** Modification of Imbert–Fick law for the cornea ($W + S = P_t \times A_1 + B$).

Next, we describe these various tonometers and their techniques, and compare their relative values and limitations.

Goldmann Applanation Tonometry

Basic Concept

Goldmann based his concept of tonometry on a modification of the Maklakoff–Fick law, also referred to as the Imbert–Fick law (164). This law states that an external force (W) against a sphere equals the pressure in the sphere (P_t) multiplied by the area flattened (applanated) by the external force (A) (**Fig. 2.3A**):

$$W = P_t \times A$$

The validity of the law requires that the sphere be (a) perfectly spherical, (b) dry, (c) perfectly flexible, and (d) infinitely thin. The cornea fails to satisfy any of these requirements, in that it is aspherical and wet, and neither perfectly flexible nor infinitely thin. The moisture creates a surface tension (S), and the lack of flexibility requires a force to bend the cornea (B), which is independent of the internal pressure. In addition, because the cornea has a central thickness of approximately 550 μm, the outer area of flattening (A) is not the same as the inner area (A_1). It was, therefore, necessary to modify the Imbert–Fick law in the following manner to account for these characteristics of the cornea (**Fig. 2.3B**):

$$W + S = P_t A_1 + B$$

When A_1 equals 7.35 mm², S balances B and W equals P_t. This internal area of applanation is obtained when the diameter of the external area of corneal applanation is 3.06 mm, which is used in the standard instrument. The volume of displacement produced by applanating an area with a diameter of 3.06 mm is approximately 0.50 mm³, so that P_t is very close to

P_0, and ocular rigidity does not significantly influence the measurement.

Description of Tonometer

The instrument is mounted on a standard slitlamp in such a way that the examiner's view is directed through the center of a plastic biprism, which is used to applanate the cornea. Two beam-splitting prisms within the applanating unit optically convert the circular area of corneal contact into semicircles. The prisms are adjusted so that the inner margins of the semicircles overlap when 3.06 mm of cornea is applanated. The biprism is attached by a rod to a housing, which contains a coil spring and series of levers that are used to adjust the force of the biprism against the cornea (**Fig. 2.4**).

Technique

The cornea is anesthetized with a topical preparation, and the tear film is stained with sodium fluorescein. With the cornea and biprism illuminated by a cobalt blue light from the slitlamp, the biprism is brought into gentle contact with the apex of the cornea (**Fig. 2.5**). The fluorescence of the stained tears facilitates visualization of the tear meniscus at the margin of contact between cornea and biprism. The fluorescent semicircles are viewed through the biprism, and the force against the cornea is adjusted until the inner edges overlap (**Fig. 2.6**). The influence of the ocular pulsations is seen when the instrument is properly positioned, and the excursions must be averaged to give the desired endpoint. The IOP is then read directly from a scale on the tonometer housing.

The staining of the tear film may be accomplished by instilling a drop of topical anesthetic and touching a fluorescein-impregnated paper strip to the tears in the lower cul-de-sac or using a commercial fluorescein solution combined with a topical anesthetic. With the commercial preparations, there is potential concern with bacterial contamination (165). When contaminated with *Pseudomonas* or *Staphylococcus*, a fluorescein preparation with the anesthetic, benoxinate, and the preservative, chlorobutanol (Fluress), regained sterility in the solution in 1 minute and on the dropper tip in 5 minutes, whereas sterility in preparations with proparacaine and thimerosal took at least 1 hour (166).

Sources of Error with Goldmann Tonometry

Tonometry has potential sources of error (167). The appropriate amount of fluorescein is important because the width of the semicircle meniscus influences the reading. Wider menisci cause falsely higher pressure estimates. Improper vertical alignment (one semicircle larger than the other) will also lead to a falsely high IOP estimate (Fig. 2.6).

The mathematical calculation for Goldmann applanation tonometry is based on a presumed average CCT of 520 μm. Deviations from the average CCT are a source of error with cornea edema underestimating the true IOP, whereas variations of CCT in normal corneas can lead to falsely higher pressure readings with thicker corneas and falsely lower ones with thinner corneas (168). After refractive surgery, the IOP is lower due

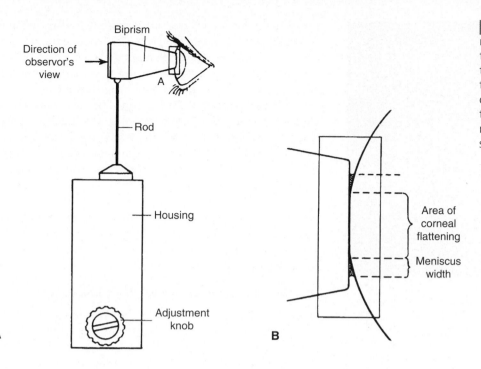

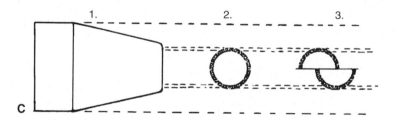

Figure 2.4 Goldmann-type applanation tonometry. **A:** Basic features of tonometer, shown in contact with patient's cornea. **B:** Enlargement shows tear film meniscus created by contact of biprism and cornea. **C:** View through biprism (*1*) reveals circular meniscus (*2*), which is converted into semicircles (*3*) by prisms.

to a thinner cornea as a result of laser-assisted in situ keratomileusis (LASIK) (169).

These latter observations have been evaluated to address the variance of CCTs in general populations and subgroups, including various glaucoma groups and the effect of refractive surgery

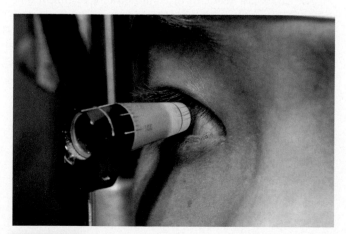

Figure 2.5 Technique of applanation tonometry with Goldmann tonometer.

influence the IOP measurements (170). From 300 datasets involving healthy eyes, the group-averaged CCT was 534 μm. From 230 datasets in which interindividual variance was reported, the group-averaged CCT (± SD) was 536 + 31 μm. There are ethnoracial differences, with thinner mean CCTs of 530 to 531 μm in one African–American population and 495 to 514 μm in a Mongolian population (171,172). A study in Japan revealed a mean of 552 μm among healthy persons (173). Individuals in the Ocular Hypertension Treatment Study (OHTS) had a mean CCT of 573.0 ± 39.0 μm, and 24% of the OHTS cohort had a CCT greater than 600 μm (174). Patients with normal-tension glaucoma have thinner mean CCTs of 514 to 521 μm (175).

This variance of CCT and its effect on the accuracy of IOP measurements raised questions as to what correction factor for the adjusted IOP measurement should be used when the CCT deviates from the assumed average, 520 μm. Ehlers and colleagues have published a table in which the average error is 0.7 mm Hg per 10 μ of deviation from the mean of 520 μ (168). Another study, however, revealed a smaller error, of 0.19 mm Hg per 10 μ (176), which is consistent with findings of a direct cannulation study (177). IOP measurements with the Tono-Pen are also affected by CCT, with reported errors of 0.29 mm Hg per

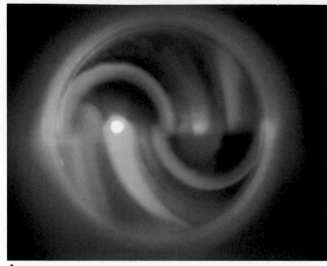

A

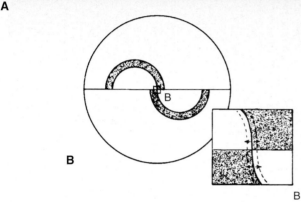

B

B

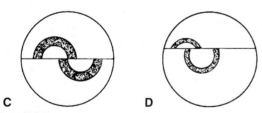

C   **D**

Figure 2.6   Semicircles of Goldmann-type applanation tonometry. **A:** Slitlamp view of Goldmann mires. **B:** Proper width and position. Enlargement (*B,* at right) depicts excursions of semicircles caused by ocular pulsations. **C:** Semicircles are too wide. **D:** Improper vertical and horizontal alignment.

10 μ in men and 0.12 mm Hg per 10 μ in women (178). However, there is a lack of general agreement on the correction factor that should be used for adjusting the IOP measured by Goldmann tonometry, when the CCT deviates from the norm (179).

Deviations of corneal curvature also influence IOP measurements, with an increase of approximately 1 mm Hg for every 3 diopters (D) of increase in corneal power (180). Marked corneal astigmatism produces an elliptical area of corneal contact. When the biprism is in the usual orientation, with the mires displaced horizontally, the IOP is underestimated for with-the-rule and overestimated for against-the-rule astigmatism, with approximately 1 mm Hg of error for every 4 D of astigmatism

(181). To minimize this error, the biprism may be rotated until the dividing line between the prisms is 45 degrees to the major axis of the ellipse, or an average may be taken of horizontal and vertical readings. An irregular cornea distorts the semicircles and interferes with the accuracy of the IOP estimates.

Prolonged contact of the biprism with the cornea leads to corneal injury, as manifested by staining, which makes multiple readings unsatisfactory. In addition, prolonged contact causes a decrease in IOP over a period of minutes, which is less pronounced in eyes with carotid occlusive disease, suggesting that it may be related to intraocular blood (182).

The Goldmann tonometer must be calibrated at least monthly. Instructions for quick, simple calibration come with the instrument. If the tonometer does not meet calibration specifications, it must be returned to the manufacturer or distributor for recalibration or repair.

Disinfection of Goldmann (and Other) Tonometers

With all tonometers that contact the eye, there is the risk of transmitting infection, such as the adenovirus of epidemic keratoconjunctivitis and herpes simplex virus type 1. In addition, there is the potential for transmitting more serious diseases, such as hepatitis and acquired immunodeficiency syndrome (AIDS) (183,184), although there is no evidence to suggest transmission of HIV by contact with tears.

Various techniques have been described for disinfecting tonometer tips (185,186). Adenovirus type 8 was removed or inactivated by soaking the applanation tip for 5 to 15 minutes in diluted sodium hypochlorite (1:10 household bleach), 3% hydrogen peroxide, or 70% isopropyl alcohol, or by wiping with alcohol, hydrogen peroxide, iodophor (povidone-iodine), or 1:1000 Merthiolate (187). Herpes simplex virus type 1 was eliminated by swabbing the applanation head with 70% isopropyl alcohol (188). Ten minutes of continuous rinsing in running tap water was reported to remove all detectable hepatitis B virus (HBV) surface antigen from contaminated tonometers (183), although another study showed that soap-and-water wash was the only disinfection method that removed all HBV DNA (189). Wiping with 3% hydrogen peroxide or 70% isopropyl alcohol swabs completely disinfected tonometer tips contaminated with HIV-1 (190).

The American Academy of Ophthalmology *Clinical statement on infection prevention in eye care services and operating areas and operating rooms* (http://one.aao.org/CE/PracticeGuidelines/ClinicalStatements_Content.aspx?cid=bfa87dce-adc9-4450-94a2-e49493154238) references the guidelines of the U.S. Centers for Disease Control and Prevention (186). With any technique, it is important to carefully remove the disinfectant from the contact surface before the next use, because alcohol and hydrogen peroxide each cause transient corneal defects.

Other Applanation Tonometers with Variable Force

The Maklakoff applanation tonometer was once popular in Russia and consisted of a dumbbell-shaped metal cylinder; it had a 10-mm diameter flat endplate of polished glass on either

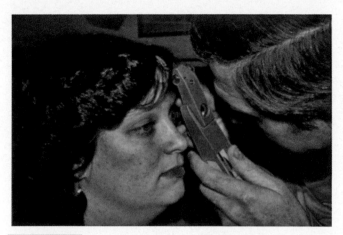

Figure 2.7 Applanation tonometry using the Perkins tonometer.

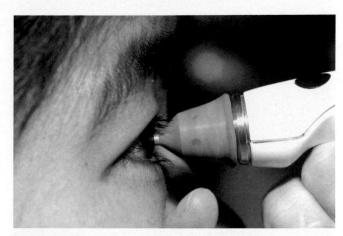

Figure 2.8 Technique of measuring IOP with handheld Tono-Pen.

end. A set of four such instruments were available, weighing 5, 7.5, 10, and 15 g. A dye suspension of Argyrol, glycerin, and water was applied to either endplate and, with the patient in a supine position and the cornea anesthetized, the instrument rested vertically on the cornea for 1 second. The resultant circular white imprint on the endplate corresponded to the area of cornea that was flattened. The diameter of the white area is measured with a transparent plastic measuring scale to 0.1 mm, and the IOP is read from a conversion table in the column corresponding to the weight used (191).

Although not commonly used now, the Perkins applanation tonometer uses the same biprism as the Goldmann applanation tonometer (192). The light source is powered by a battery and the force is varied manually. A counter balance makes it possible to use the instrument in either the vertical or horizontal position (**Fig. 2.7**). The Draeger applanation tonometer is similar to the Perkins tonometer, but uses a different biprism and has an electric motor that varies the force (193).

The original Mackay–Marg tonometer, which is no longer available, had a plate diameter of 1.5 mm surrounded by a rubber sleeve. The force required to keep the plate flush with the sleeve was electronically monitored and recorded on a paper strip (194). The most commonly used Mackay–Marg-type tonometer today is the Tono-Pen, a handheld instrument with a strain gauge that creates an electrical signal as the footplate flattens the cornea (195) (**Fig. 2.8**). A built-in single-chip microprocessor senses the proper force curves and averages 4 to 10 readings to give a final digital readout. It also provides the percentage of variability between the lowest and highest acceptable readings from 5% to 20%.

The pneumotonometer is similar to the Mackay–Marg in that a central sensing device measures the IOP, while the force required to bend the cornea is transferred to a surrounding structure. The sensor in this case, however, is air pressure, rather than an electronically controlled plunger (196). At one end of a pencil-like holder is a sensing nozzle, which has a 0.25-inch outer diameter and a 2.0-mm central chamber. The nozzle is covered with a Silastic diaphragm, and pressurized air in the central chamber exhausts at the face of the nozzle between the

orifice of the central chamber and the diaphragm. As the sensing nozzle touches the cornea and when the area of contact equals that of the central chamber, an initial inflection is recorded, which represents the IOP and the force required to bend the cornea (**Fig. 2.9**). With further enlargement of the corneal contact, the bending force is transferred to the face of the nozzle, which is interpreted as the actual IOP.

A newer applanation tonometer with a disposable cover, called the PASCAL tonometer, is available (**Fig. 2.10**). It repeatedly samples IOP 100 times per second in addition to ocular pulse amplitude and the systemic pulse rate (197). This portable slitlamp mounted device provides a digital output of the IOP and a graphic output of the ocular pressure pulse.

The noncontact tonometer was introduced by Grolman (198) and has the advantage over other tonometers of not touching the eye, other than with a puff of air. This instrument should not be confused with the pneumatic tonometers discussed earlier that require eye contact. After proper alignment of the patient, a puff of room air creates a constant force that momentarily deforms the central cornea, which is detected by an optoelectronic system of a transmitter, which directs a

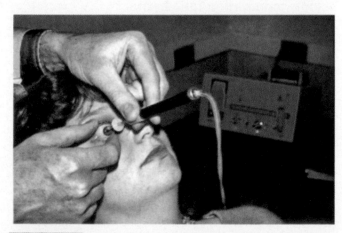

Figure 2.9 IOP measurement using a pneumotonometer.

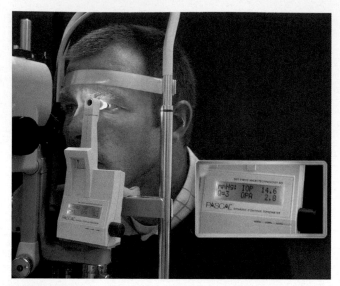

Figure 2.10 Measurement of IOP using the Pascal Dynamic Contour Tonometer.

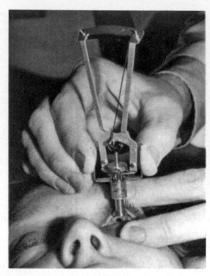

Figure 2.11 Technique of IOP measurement using Schiötz indentation tonometer.

collimated beam of light at the corneal vertex, and a receiver and detector, which accepts only parallel, coaxial rays reflected from the cornea. At the moment that the central cornea is flattened, the greatest number of reflected light rays are received, which is recorded as the peak intensity of light detected. The time from an internal reference point to the moment of maximum light detection is converted to IOP. With the newer instrument, additional data is provided on cornea hysteresis, which may be an indication of elasticity (199). The time interval for an average noncontact tonometer measurement is 1 to 3 milliseconds (1/500th of the cardiac cycle) and is random with respect to the phase of the cardiac cycle so that the ocular pulse becomes a significant variable—that is, unlike with some tonometers, it cannot be averaged. The probability that an instantaneous pressure measurement will lie within a given range of mean IOP increases as the number of tonometric measurements, averaged together, increases (200). For this reason, it is recommended that a minimum of three readings within 3 mm Hg be taken and averaged as the IOP.

Schiötz Indentation Tonometry

The prototype indentation tonometer is the Schiötz tonometer, which consists of a footplate that rests on the cornea and a weighted plunger that moves freely (except for the effect of friction) within a shaft in the footplate with the degree to which it indents the cornea is indicated by the movement of a needle on a scale. A 5.5-g weight is permanently fixed to the plunger, which can be increased to 7.5, 10, or 15 g by adding additional weights (**Fig. 2.11**). When the plunger indents the cornea, the baseline or resting pressure (P_0) is artificially raised to a new value (P_t). The change in pressure from P_0 to P_t is an expression of the resistance an eye offers to the displacement of a volume of fluid (V_c). Because the tonometer actually measures P_t, it is necessary to estimate P_0 for each scale reading and weight. Schiötz estimated P_0 by experiments in which a manometer

was attached to enucleated eyes by a cannula inserted through the optic nerve.

In the early days of indentation tonometry, the IOP values that were considered to be normal were considerably higher than today's accepted range, and it was not until Friedenwald's work that indentation tonometry acquired a mathematical basis (201). The formula has a single numerical constant, the coefficient of ocular rigidity (K), which is roughly an expression of the distensibility of the eye. He developed a nomogram for estimating K on the basis of two tonometric readings with different weights, and subsequent studies using applanation tonometry with different sized applanating areas have supported the accuracy of his formulations (202). On the basis of this formula and additional experiments, Friedenwald developed a set of conversion tables, referred to as the 1948 and 1955 tables for IOP. Subsequent studies indicated that the 1948 tables agree more closely with measurements by Goldmann applanation tonometry (203,204).

The basic technique involves positioning the patient in a supine position with a fixation target just overhead. The examiner separates the eyelids and gently rests the tonometer footplate on the anesthetized cornea in a position that allows free vertical movement of the plunger. When the tonometer is properly positioned, the examiner observes a fine movement of the indicator needle on the scale in response to the ocular pulsations. The scale reading should be taken as the average between the extremes of these excursions. It is customary to start with the fixed 5.5-g weight. However, if the scale reading is 4 or less, additional weight should be added to the plunger. A conversion table is then used to derive the IOP in mm Hg from the scale reading and plunger weight. Grant combined the concept of Schiötz tonometry with continuous electronic monitoring of the pressure for use in tonography (discussed in Chapter 3).

It is important to be aware of the potential sources of error with indentation tonometry. The accuracy depends on the assumption that all eyes respond the same way to the external force of indentation, which is not the case. Because conversion tables were based on an "average" coefficient of ocular rigidity (K), eyes that deviate significantly from this K value give false IOP measurements. The technique for determining K is based on the concept of differential tonometry, using two indentation tonometric readings with different weights, and the Friedenwald nomogram, as previously discussed. Another variable that affects accuracy is expulsion of intraocular blood during indentation tonometry (205). In addition, a relatively steep or thick cornea causes an increased displacement of fluid during indentation tonometry, which leads to a falsely high IOP reading (206).

Miscellaneous Tonometers

Rebound Tonometer

A new handheld tonometer, the Icare tonometer (Icare Finland, Helsinki) is able to measure IOP without the use of topical anesthetic (**Fig. 2.12**). IOP is determined by measuring the force produced by a small plastic probe as it rebounds from the cornea. This device has been assessed for use in children and adults. The rebound tonometer has been shown to have similar accuracy to the Tono-Pen, and it is comparable with Goldmann tonometry for IOPs over a reasonable range in adults. Icare was reported to be comfortable and highly reproducible for tonometry in healthy school-aged children (207). The Icare tonometer has already proven valuable as a screening tool in children (see Chapter 13). The ability to evaluate IOP without the use of topical anesthesia potentially provides the opportunity to monitor IOP at home.

IOP Monitoring Devices

In the diagnosis and management of glaucoma, there is need for an IOP telemetry device without artificially altering the pressure (208,209). Several prototypes—based on a contact lens, an implantable device, or a scleral band device (210,211)—have been developed. Such a lens will help us monitor and manage individuals who are susceptible to wide

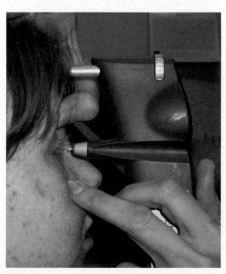

Figure 2.12 Measurement of IOP using the handheld Icare rebound tonometer.

IOP fluctuations, who have poor adherence to medical therapy, who perhaps are "poor responders" to medical therapy, and who have wide IOP fluctuations in the postoperative period (212).

Comparison of Tonometers

The most precise method for evaluating the accuracy of a tonometer is to compare it with manometric measurements of the cannulated anterior chamber. Although this technique is frequently used with animal and autopsy eyes, its use in large-scale human studies has been limited. The alternative is to compare the tonometer in question against the instrument that previous studies have shown to be the most accurate. In eyes with regular corneas, the Goldmann applanation tonometer is generally accepted as the standard against which other tonometers must be compared. Even with this instrument, however, inherent variability must be taken into account. When two readings were taken on the same eye with Goldmann tonometers in a short time frame, at least 30% of the paired readings differed by 2 and 3 mm Hg or more (213). In another study, intraobserver variation was 1.5 ± 1.96 mm Hg and interobserver variation was 1.79 ± 2.41 mm Hg, which could be reduced by 9% and 11%, respectively, by using the median value of three consecutive measurements (214).

Clinically, the most widely used methods for measuring IOP are by Goldmann applanation tonometry and with use of the Tono-Pen; the noncontact tonometer, Perkins tonometer, pneumotonometry, and the Schiötz tonometer are not used as much. In general, the Schiötz tonometer reads lower than the Goldmann, even when the postural influence on IOP is eliminated by performing both measurements in the supine position (215). The Perkins applanation tonometer compared favorably against the Goldmann tonometer (216). In a comparison of readings obtained by the Perkins tonometer, the Tono-Pen, and the Schiötz tonometer, the greatest agreement was between the Perkins and Tono-Pen tonometers in children under anesthesia (217).

The Tono-Pen has been compared favorably with manometric readings in human autopsy eyes (218,219). In clinical comparisons with Goldmann applanation readings, some studies found a good correlation, especially within the normal IOP range, although most studies agree that the Tono-Pen underestimates Goldmann IOP in the higher range and overestimates in the lower range (195,220).

In multiple comparative studies, readings taken with the pneumotonometer correlated closely with those obtained by using Goldmann tonometers, although the pneumotonometer readings tended to be higher (221,222). In comparing IOPs in eyes before and after LASIK for myopia, pneumotonometry showed less IOP lowering compared with Goldmann applanation tonometry after LASIK-induced cornea thinning, which was interpreted to mean that post-LASIK IOP measurements obtained by pneumotonometry were more reliable than those taken by Goldmann applanation (223). In cat eyes, pneumotonometry was more accurate than the Tono-Pen, compared to the set IOPs established by manometry (224).

Tonometry for Special Clinical Circumstances

Tonometry on Irregular Corneas

The accuracy of Goldmann and Tono-Pen tonometers and the noncontact tonometers is limited in eyes with irregular corneas. The pneumatic tonometer has been shown to be useful in eyes with diseased or irregular corneas (225). In eyes after penetrating keratoplasty, the Tono-Pen significantly overestimated Goldmann readings (226).

Tonometry over Soft Contact Lenses

It has been claimed that pneumotonometry and the Tono-Pen can measure with reasonable accuracy the IOP through bandage contact lenses (227,228). In cadaver eyes with four different brands of therapeutic contact lenses, readings from the pneumotonometer correlated well with manometrically determined IOP, whereas the Tono-Pen consistently underestimated the pressure (229).

Tonometry with Gas-Filled Eyes

Intraocular gas significantly affects scleral rigidity, rendering indentation tonometry particularly unsatisfactory. A pneumatic tonometer underestimated Goldmann IOP measurements in eyes with intravitreal gas, whereas measurement with the Tono-Pen compared favorably with Goldmann readings in eyes after pars plana vitrectomy and gas-fluid exchange (230). In a study of 50 eyes with irregular corneas after vitrectomy and air–gas-fluid exchange, readings with the Tono-Pen and pneumotonometer were highly correlated, although there was a mean difference of 1.4 mm Hg, with the Tono-Pen usually reading lower (220). A manometric study with human autopsy eyes indicated that both instruments significantly underestimated the IOP at pressures greater than 30 mm Hg (231).

Tonometry with Flat Anterior Chamber

In human autopsy eyes with flat anterior chambers, IOP readings from the Goldmann applanation tonometer, pneumotonometer, and Tono-Pen did not correlate well with manometrically determined pressures (232).

Tonometry in Eyes with Keratoprostheses

In patients at high risk for corneal transplant rejection, implantation of a keratoprosthesis is now a viable option for vision rehabilitation (233). However, given that most keratoprostheses have a rigid, clear surface, it is impossible to measure IOP by using applanation or indentation instruments. In such eyes, tactile assessment appears to be the most widely used method to estimate IOP (234).

KEY POINTS

- The mean IOP value in the general population is approximately 15 mm Hg, and two SDs to either side of the mean gives a "normal" range of roughly 10 to 20 mm Hg.

- IOP is a quantitative trait with a Gaussian distribution. IOP is an important consideration for diagnosis of glaucoma, for setting a target pressure (discussed further in Chapter 27), and for evaluating treatment outcomes.
- IOP is influenced by genetics, environment, and physiology.
- IOP is measured by essentially two different types of instruments that use either applanation methods, such as Goldmann tonometer, or indentation, like the Schiötz tonometer.

REFERENCES

1. Nemesure B, Honkanen R, Hennis A. Incident open-angle glaucoma and intraocular pressure. *Ophthalmology.* 2007;114(10):1810–1815.
2. Heijl A, Bengtsson B, Hyman L, et al. Early Manifest Glaucoma Trial Group. Natural history of open-angle glaucoma. *Ophthalmology.* 2009; 116(12):2271–2276.
3. Leydhecker W, Akiyama K, Neumann HG. Intraocular pressure in normal human eyes [in German]. *Klin Monbl Augenheilkd Augenarztl Fortbild.* 1958;133(5):662–670.
4. Gillespie BW, Musch DC, Guire KE, et al. The collaborative initial glaucoma treatment study: baseline visual field and test-retest variability. *Invest Ophthalmol Vis Sci.* 2003;44(6):2613–2620.
5. Nouri-Mahdavi K, Hoffman D, Coleman AL, et al. Predictive factors for glaucomatous visual field progression in the Advanced Glaucoma Intervention Study. *Ophthalmology.* 2004;111(9):1627–1635.
6. Gordon MO, Beiser JA, Brandt JD, et al. The Ocular Hypertension Treatment Study: baseline factors that predict the onset of primary open-angle glaucoma. *Arch Ophthalmol.* 2002;120(6):714–720.
7. Drance SM. The Collaborative Normal-Tension Glaucoma Study and some of its lessons. *Can J Ophthalmol.* 1999;34(1):1–6.
8. Leske MC, Heijl A, Hyman L, et al. Predictors of long-term progression in the early manifest glaucoma trial. *Ophthalmology.* 2007;114(11):1965–1972.
9. Iyengar SK. The quest for genes causing complex traits in ocular medicine: successes, interpretations, and challenges. *Arch Ophthalmol.* 2007; 125(1):11–18.
10. Brubaker RF. Clinical measurements of aqueous dynamics: implications for addressing glaucoma. In: Civan MM, ed. *The Eye's Aqueous Humor, From Secretion to Glaucoma.* New York,NY: Academic Press; 1998:234–284.
11. Toris CB, Koepsell SA, Yablonski ME, et al. Aqueous humor dynamics in ocular hypertensive patients. *J Glaucoma.* 2002;11(3):253–258.
12. Grant W. Tonographic method for measuring the facility and rate of aqueous flow in human eyes. *Arch Ophthalmol.* 1950;44:204–214.
13. Selbach JM, Posielek K, Steuhl KP, et al. Episcleral venous pressure in untreated primary open-angle and normal-tension glaucoma. *Ophthalmologica.* 2005;219(6):357–361.
14. Johnson LV. Tonographic survey. *Am J Ophthalmol.* 1966;61(4):680–689.
15. Segal P, Skwierczyńska J. Mass screening of adults for glaucoma. *Ophthalmologica.* 1967;153(5):336–348.
16. Armaly MF. On the distribution of applanation pressure. I. Statistical features and the effect of age, sex, and family history of glaucoma. *Arch Ophthalmol.* 1965;73:11–18.
17. Perkins ES. Glaucoma screening from a public health clinic. *Br Med J.* 1965;1(5432):417–419.
18. Loewen U, Handrup B, Redeker A. Results of a glaucoma mass screening program [in German]. *Klin Monbl Augenheilkd.* 1976;169(6):754–766.
19. Ruprecht KW, Wulle KG, Christl HL. Applanation tonometry within medical diagnostic "check-up" programs [in German]. *Klin Monbl Augenheilkd.* 1978;172(3):332–341.
20. Shiose Y, Kawase Y. A new approach to stratified normal intraocular pressure in a general population. *Am J Ophthalmol.* 1986;101(6):714–721.
21. David R, Zangwill L, Stone D, et al. Epidemiology of intraocular pressure in a population screened for glaucoma. *Br J Ophthalmol.* 1987;71(10): 766–771.
22. Klein BE, Klein R, Linton KL. Intraocular pressure in an American community. The Beaver Dam Eye Study. *Invest Ophthalmol Vis Sci.* 1992; 33(7):2224–2228.
23. Sultan MB, Mansberger SL, Lee PP. Understanding the importance of IOP variables in glaucoma: a systematic review. *Surv Ophthalmol.* 2009;54(6):643–662.
24. Armaly MF. The genetic determination of ocular pressure in the normal eye. *Arch Ophthalmol.* 1967;78(2):187–192.

25. Levene RZ, Workman PL, Broder SW, et al. Heritability of ocular pressure in normal and suspect ranges. *Arch Ophthalmol.* 1970;84(6):730–734.

26. Kalenak JW, Paydar F. Correlation of intraocular pressures in pairs of monozygotic and dizygotic twins. *Ophthalmology.* 1995;102(10):1559–1564.

27. Gottfredsdottir MS, Sverrisson T, Musch DC, et al. Chronic open-angle glaucoma and associated ophthalmic findings in monozygotic twins and their spouses in Iceland. *J Glaucoma.* 1999;8(2):134–139.

28. Zheng Y, Xiang F, Huang W, et al. Distribution and heritability of intraocular pressure in Chinese children: the Guangzhou twin eye study. *Invest Ophthalmol Vis Sci.* 2009;50(5):2040–2043.

29. Lee MK, Woo SJ, Kim JI, et al. Replication of glaucoma candidate gene on 5q22.1 for intraocular pressure in Mongolian populations: The GENDISCAN Project. *Invest Ophthalmol Vis Sci.* 2009; 51(3):1335–1340.

30. Carbonaro F, Andrew T, Mackey DA, et al. Repeated measures of intraocular pressure result in higher heritability and greater power in genetic linkage studies. *Invest Ophthalmol Vis Sci.* 2009;50(11):5115–5119.

31. Carbonaro F, Andrew T, Mackey DA, et al. Heritability of intraocular pressure: a classical twin study. *Br J Ophthalmol.* 2008;92(8):1125–1128.

32. van Koolwijk LM, Despriet DD, van Duijn CM, et al. Genetic contributions to glaucoma: heritability of intraocular pressure, retinal nerve fiber layer thickness, and optic disc morphology. *Invest Ophthalmol Vis Sci.* 2007;48(8):3669–3676.

33. Parssinen O, Era P, Tolvanen A, et al. Heritability of intraocular pressure in older female twins. *Ophthalmology.* 2007;114(12):2227–2231.

34. Klein BE, Klein R, Lee KE. Heritability of risk factors for primary open-angle glaucoma: the Beaver Dam Eye Study. *Invest Ophthalmol Vis Sci.* 2004;45(1):59–62.

35. Chang TC, Congdon NG, Wojciechowski R, et al. Determinants and heritability of intraocular pressure and cup-to-disc ratio in a defined older population. *Ophthalmology.* 2005;112(7):1186–1191.

36. Viswanathan AC, Hitchings RA, Indar A, et al. Commingling analysis of intraocular pressure and glaucoma in an older Australian population. *Ann Hum Genet.* 2004;68(pt 5):489–497.

37. Charlesworth JC, Dyer TD, Stankovich JM, et al. Linkage to 10q22 for maximum intraocular pressure and 1p32 for maximum cup-to-disc ratio in an extended primary open-angle glaucoma pedigree. *Invest Ophthalmol Vis Sci.* 2005;46(10):3723–3729.

38. Rotimi CN, Chen G, Adeyemo AA, et al. Genomewide scan and fine mapping of quantitative trait loci for intraocular pressure on 5q and 14q in West Africans. *Invest Ophthalmol Vis Sci.* 2006;47(8):3262–3267.

39. Duggal P, Klein AP, Lee KE, et al. Identification of novel genetic loci for intraocular pressure: a genomewide scan of the Beaver Dam Eye Study. *Arch Ophthalmol.* 2007;125(1):74–79.

40. Ortiz GJ, Cook DJ, Yablonski ME, et al. Effect of cold air on aqueous humor dynamics in humans. *Invest Ophthalmol Vis Sci.* 1988;29(1):138–140.

41. Mader TH, Gibson CR, Caputo M, et al. Intraocular pressure and retinal vascular changes during transient exposure to microgravity. *Am J Ophthalmol.* 1993;115(3):347–350.

42. Mehra KS, Roy PN, Khare BB. Tobacco smoking and glaucoma. *Ann Ophthalmol.* 1976;8(4):462–464.

43. Edwards R, Thornton J, Ajit R. Cigarette smoking and primary open angle glaucoma: a systematic review. *J Glaucoma.* 2008;17(7):558–566.

44. Charliat G, Jolly D, Blanchard F. Genetic risk factor in primary open-angle glaucoma: a case-control study. *Ophthalmic Epidemiol.* 1994;1(3):131–138.

45. Murphy DF. Anesthesia and intraocular pressure. *Anesth Analg.* 1985;64(5):520–530.

46. Blumberg D, Congdon N, Jampel H, et al. The effects of sevoflurane and ketamine on intraocular pressure in children during examination under anesthesia. *Am J Ophthalmol.* 2007;143(3):494–499.

47. Goethals M, Missotten L. Intraocular pressure in children up to five years of age. *J Pediatr Ophthalmol Strabismus.* 1983;20(2):49–51.

48. Lamb K, James MF, Janicki PK. The laryngeal mask airway for intraocular surgery: effects on intraocular pressure and stress responses. *Br J Anaesth.* 1992;69(2):143–147.

49. Akhtar TM, McMurray P, Kerr WJ. A comparison of laryngeal mask airway with tracheal tube for intra-ocular ophthalmic surgery. *Anaesthesia.* 1992;47(8):668–671.

50. Green K. Marihuana and the eye. *Invest Ophthalmol.* 1975;14(4):261–263.

51. Green K. Ocular effects of diacetyl morphine and lysergic acid diethylamide in rabbit. *Invest Ophthalmol.* 1975;14(4):325–329.

52. Lachkar Y, Bouassida W. Drug-induced acute angle closure glaucoma [review]. *Curr Opin Ophthalmol.* 2007;18(2):129–133.

53. Hamill MB, Suelflow JA, Smith JA. Transdermal scopolamine delivery system (TRANSDERM-V) and acute angle-closure glaucoma. *Ann Ophthalmol.* 1983;15(11):1011–1012.

54. Berdy GJ, Berdy SS, Odin LS, et al. Angle closure glaucoma precipitated by aerosolized atropine. *Arch Intern Med.* 1991;151(8):1658–1660.

55. Oksuz H, Tamer C, Akoglu S, et al. Acute angle-closure glaucoma precipitated by local tiotropium absorption. *Pulm Pharmacol Ther.* 2007; 20(6):627–628.

56. Maus TL, Larsson LI, Brubaker RF. Ocular effects of scopolamine dermal patch in open-angle glaucoma. *J Glaucoma.* 1994;3(3):190.

57. Pasquale LR, Kang JH. Lifestyle, nutrition, and glaucoma. *J Glaucoma.* 2009;18(6):423–428.

58. Pexczon JD, Grant WM. Glaucoma, alcohol, and intraocular pressure. *Arch Ophthalmol.* 1965;73:495–501.

59. Houle RE, Grant WM. Alcohol, vasopressin, and intraocular pressure. *Invest Ophthalmol.* 1967;6(2):145–154.

60. Doshi V, Ying-Lai M, Azen SP, et al. Sociodemographic, family history, and lifestyle risk factors for open-angle glaucoma and ocular hypertension. The Los Angeles Latino Eye Study. *Ophthalmology.* 2008;115(4):639–647.

61. Wang S, Wang JJ, Wong TY. Alcohol and eye diseases. *Surv Ophthalmol.* 2008;53(5):512–525.

62. Kang JH, Willett WC, Rosner BA, et al. Prospective study of alcohol consumption and the risk of primary open-angle glaucoma. *Ophthalmic Epidemiol.* 2007;14(3):141–147.

63. Peczon JD, Grant WM. Sedatives, stimulants, and intraocular pressure in glaucoma. *Arch Ophthalmol.* 1964;72:178–188.

64. Kang JH, Willett WC, Rosner BA, et al. Caffeine consumption and the risk of primary open-angle glaucoma: a prospective cohort study. *Invest Ophthalmol Vis Sci.* 2008;49(5):1924–1931.

65. Kang JH, Pasquale LR, Willett W, et al. Antioxidant intake and primary open-angle glaucoma: a prospective study. *Am J Epidemiol.* 2003;158(4):337–346.

66. Coleman AL, Stone KL, Kodjebacheva G, et al. Glaucoma risk and the consumption of fruits and vegetables among older women in the study of osteoporotic fractures. *Am J Ophthalmol.* 2008;145(6):1081–1089.

67. Nguyen CT, Bui BV, Sinclair AJ, et al. Dietary omega 3 fatty acids decrease intraocular pressure with age by increasing aqueous outflow. *Invest Ophthalmol Vis Sci.* 2007;48(2):756–762.

68. Fukuoka S, Aihara M, Iwase A, et al. Intraocular pressure in an ophthalmologically normal Japanese population. *Acta Ophthalmol.* 2008;86(4):434–439.

69. Leske MC, Connell AM, Wu SY, et al. Distribution of intraocular pressure. The Barbados Eye Study. *Arch Ophthalmol.* 1997;115(8):1051–1057.

70. Bordon AF, Katsumi O, Hirose T. Tonometry in pediatric patients: a comparative study among Tono-Pen, Perkins, and Schiötz tonometers. *J Pediatr Ophthalmol Strabismus.* 1995;32(6):373–377.

71. Radtke ND, Cohan BE. Intraocular pressure measurement in the newborn. *Am J Ophthalmol.* 1974;78(3):501–504.

72. Pensiero S, Da Pozzo S, Perissutti P, et al. Normal intraocular pressure in children. *J Pediatr Ophthalmol Strabismus.* 1992;29(2):79–84.

73. Sihota R, Tuli D, Dada T, et al. Distribution and determinants of intraocular pressure in a normal pediatric population. *J Pediatr Ophthalmol Strabismus.* 2006;43(1):14–18.

74. Musarella MA, Morin JD. Anterior segment and intraocular pressure measurements of the unanesthetized premature infant. *Metab Pediatr Syst Ophthalmol.* 1985;8(2 pt 3):53–60.

75. Spierer A, Huna R, Hirsh A, et al. Normal intraocular pressure in premature infants. *Am J Ophthalmol.* 1994;117(6):801–803.

76. Jaafar MS, Kazi GA. Normal intraocular pressure in children: a comparative study of the Perkins applanation tonometer and the pneumatonometer. *J Pediatr Ophthalmol Strabismus.* 1993;30(5):284–287.

77. Shiose Y. The aging effect on intraocular pressure in an apparently normal population. *Arch Ophthalmol.* 1984;102(6):883–887.

78. Wong TT, Wong TY, Foster PJ, et al. The relationship of intraocular pressure with age, systolic blood pressure, and central corneal thickness in an Asian population. *Invest Ophthalmol Vis Sci.* 2009;50(9):4097–4102.

79. Becker B. The decline in aqueous secretion and outflow facility with age. *Am J Ophthalmol.* 1958;46(5 pt 1):731–736.

80. Toris CB, Yablonski ME, Wang YL, et al. Aqueous humor dynamics in the aging human eye. *Am J Ophthalmol.* 1999;127(4):407–412.

81. Brubaker RF, Nagataki S, Townsend DJ, et al. The effect of age on aqueous humor formation in man. *Ophthalmology.* 1981;88(3):283–288.

82. Sultan M, Blondeau P. Episcleral venous pressure in younger and older subjects in the sitting and supine positions. *J Glaucoma.* 2003;12(4):370–373.

83. Racette L, Wilson MR, Zangwill LM, et al. Primary open-angle glaucoma in blacks: a review. *Surv Ophthalmol.* 2003;48(3):295–313.

84. Yip JL, Foster PJ, Gilbert CE, et al. Incidence of occludable angles in a high-risk Mongolian population. *Br J Ophthalmol.* 2008;92(1):30–33.

85. Lavanya R, Wong TY, Friedman DS, et al. Determinants of angle closure in older Singaporeans. *Arch Ophthalmol.* 2008;126(5):686–691.

86. Friedman DS, Wilson MR, Liebmann JM, et al. An evidence-based assessment of risk factors for the progression of ocular hypertension and glaucoma. *Am J Ophthalmol.* 2004;138(3 suppl):S19–S31.

87. Tomlinson A, Phillips CI. Applanation tension and axial length of the eyeball. *Br J Ophthalmol.* 1970;54(8):548–553.

88. Kawase K, Tomidokoro A, Araie M, et al. Ocular and systemic factors related to intraocular pressure in Japanese adults: the Tajimi study. *Br J Ophthalmol.* 2008;92(9):1175–1179.

89. David R, Zangwill LM, Tessler Z, et al. The correlation between intraocular pressure and refractive status. *Arch Ophthalmol.* 1985;103(12):1812–1815.

90. Quinn GE, Berlin JA, Young TL, et al. Association of intraocular pressure and myopia in children. *Ophthalmology.* 1995;102(2):180–185.

91. Manny RE, Deng L, Crossnoe C, et al. IOP, myopic progression and axial length in a COMET subgroup. *Optom Vis Sci.* 2008;85(2):97–105.

92. Lee AJ, Saw SM, Gazzard G, et al. Intraocular pressure associations with refractive error and axial length in children. *Br J Ophthalmol.* 2004;88(1):5–7.

93. Vijaya L, George R, Baskaran M, et al. Prevalence of primary open-angle glaucoma in an urban south Indian population and comparison with a rural population. The Chennai Glaucoma Study. *Ophthalmology.* 2008;115(4):648–654.

94. Xu L, Wang Y, Wang S, et al. High myopia and glaucoma susceptibility the Beijing Eye Study. *Ophthalmology.* 2007;114(2):216–220.

95. Suzuki Y, Iwase A, Araie M, et al. Risk factors for open-angle glaucoma in a Japanese population: the Tajimi Study. *Ophthalmology.* 2006;113(9):1613–1617.

96. Wong TY, Klein BE, Klein R, et al. Refractive errors, intraocular pressure, and glaucoma in a white population. *Ophthalmology.* 2003;110(1):211–217.

97. Bagga H, Liu JH, Weinreb RN. Intraocular pressure measurements throughout the 24 h. *Curr Opin Ophthalmol.* 2009;20(2):79–83.

98. Sit AJ, Nau CB, McLaren JW, et al. Circadian variation of aqueous dynamics in young healthy adults. *Invest Ophthalmol Vis Sci.* 2008;49(4):1473–1479.

99. Perlman JI, Delany CM, Sothern RB, et al. Relationships between 24h observations in intraocular pressure vs blood pressure, heart rate, nitric oxide and age in the medical chronobiology aging project. *Clin Ter.* 2007;158(1):31–47.

100. Giuffre G, Giammanco R, Dardanoni G, et al. Prevalence of glaucoma and distribution of intraocular pressure in a population. The Casteldaccia Eye Study. *Acta Ophthalmol Scand.* 1995;73(3):222–225.

101. David R, Zangwill L, Briscoe D, et al. Diurnal intraocular pressure variations: an analysis of 690 diurnal curves. *Br J Ophthalmol.* 1992;76(5):280–283.

102. Xi XR, Qureshi IA, Wu XD, et al. Diurnal variation of intraocular pressure in normal and ocular hypertensive subjects of China. *J Pak Med Assoc.* 1996;46(8):171–174.

103. Sit AJ, Liu JH. Pathophysiology of glaucoma and continuous measurements of intraocular pressure. *Mol Cell Biomech.* 2009;6(1):57–69.

104. Linder BJ, Trick GL, Wolf ML. Altering body position affects intraocular pressure and visual function. *Invest Ophthalmol Vis Sci.* 1988;29(10):1492–1497.

105. Weinreb RN, Cook J, Friberg TR. Effect of inverted body position on intraocular pressure. *Am J Ophthalmol.* 1984;98(6):784–787.

106. Friberg TR, Sanborn G, Weinreb RN. Intraocular and episcleral venous pressure increase during inverted posture. *Am J Ophthalmol.* 1987;103(4):523–526.

107. Mosaed S, Liu JH, Weinreb RN. Correlation between office and peak nocturnal intraocular pressures in healthy subjects and glaucoma patients. *Am J Ophthalmol.* 2005;139(2):320–324.

108. Asrani S, Zeimer R, Wilensky J, et al. Large diurnal fluctuations in intraocular pressure are an independent risk factor in patients with glaucoma. *J Glaucoma.* 2000;9(2):134–142.

109. Weitzman ED, Henkind P, Leitman M, et al. Correlative 24-hour relationships between intraocular pressure and plasma cortisol in normal subjects and patients with glaucoma. *Br J Ophthalmol.* 1975;59(10):566–572.

110. Maus TL, McLaren JW, Shepard JW Jr, et al. The effects of sleep on circulating catecholamines and aqueous flow in human subjects. *Exp Eye Res.* 1996;62(4):351–358.

111. Liu JH, Dacus AC. Endogenous hormonal changes and circadian elevation of intraocular pressure. *Invest Ophthalmol Vis Sci.* 1991;32(3):496–500.

112. Viggiano SR, Koskela TK, Klee GG, et al. The effect of melatonin on aqueous humor flow in humans during the day. *Ophthalmology.* 1994;101(2):326–331.

113. Brubaker RF. Flow of aqueous humor in humans [The Friedenwald Lecture]. *Invest Ophthalmol Vis Sci.* 1991;32(13):3145–3166.

114. Radenbaugh PA, Goyal A, McLaren NC, et al. Concordance of aqueous humor flow in the morning and at night in normal humans. *Invest Ophthalmol Vis Sci.* 2006;47(11):4860–4864.

115. Rafuse PE, Mills DW, Hooper PL, et al. Effects of Valsalva's manoeuvre on intraocular pressure. *Can J Ophthalmol.* 1994;29(2):73–76.

116. Epstein HM, Fagman W, Bruce DL, et al. Intraocular pressure changes during anesthesia for electroshock therapy. *Anesth Analg.* 1975;54(4):479–481.

117. Schuman JS, Massicotte EC, Connolly S, et al. Increased intraocular pressure and visual field defects in high resistance wind instrument players. *Ophthalmology.* 2000;107(1):127–133.

118. Dos Santos MG, Makk S, Berghold A, et al. Intraocular pressure difference in Goldmann applanation tonometry versus Perkins hand-held applanation tonometry in overweight patients. *Ophthalmology.* 1998;105(12):2260–2263.

119. Risner D, Ehrlich R, Kheradiya NS, et al. Effects of exercise on intraocular pressure and ocular blood flow: a review. *J Glaucoma.* 2009;18(6):429–436.

120. Natsis K, Asouhidou I, Nousios G, et al. Aerobic exercise and intraocular pressure in normotensive and glaucoma patients. *BMC Ophthalmol.* 2009;9:6.

121. Shah P, Whittaker KW, Wells AP, et al. Exercise-induced visual loss associated with advanced glaucoma in young adults. *Eye (Lond).* 2001;15(pt 5):616–620.

122. Haynes WL, Johnson AT, Alward WL. Effects of jogging exercise on patients with the pigmentary dispersion syndrome and pigmentary glaucoma. *Ophthalmology.* 1992;99(7):1096–1103.

123. Kypke W, Hermannspann U. Glaucoma physical activity and sport [in German]. *Klin Monbl Augenheilkd.* 1974;164(3):321–327.

124. Harris A, Malinovsky V, Martin B. Correlates of acute exercise-induced ocular hypotension. *Invest Ophthalmol Vis Sci.* 1994;35(11):3852–3857.

125. Martin B, Harris A, Hammel T, et al. Mechanism of exercise-induced ocular hypotension. *Invest Ophthalmol Vis Sci.* 1999;40(5):1011–1015.

126. Coleman AL, Kodjebacheva G. Risk factors for glaucoma needing more attention. *Open Ophthalmol J.* 2009;3:38–42.

127. Coleman DJ, Trokel S. Direct-recorded intraocular pressure variations in a human subject. *Arch Ophthalmol.* 1969;82(5):637–640.

128. Moses RA, Carniglia PE, Grodzki WJ Jr., et al. Proptosis and increase of intraocular pressure in voluntary lid fissure widening. *Invest Ophthalmol Vis Sci.* 1984;25(8):989–992.

129. Spierer A, Eisenstein Z. The role of increased intraocular pressure on upgaze in the assessment of Graves ophthalmopathy. *Ophthalmology.* 1991;98(10):1491–1494.

130. Raizman MB, Beck RW. Sustained increases in intraocular pressure during strabismus surgery. *Am J Ophthalmol.* 1986;101(3):308–309.

131. Pederson JE. Ocular hypotony. *Trans Ophthalmol Soc U K.* 1986;105(pt 2):220–226.

132. Sagara T, Gaton DD, Lindsey JD, et al. Reduction of collagen type I in the ciliary muscle of inflamed monkey eyes. *Invest Ophthalmol Vis Sci.* 1999;40(11):2568–2576.

133. Memarzadeh F, Ying-Lai M, Azen SP, et al. Associations with intraocular pressure in Latinos: the Los Angeles Latino Eye Study. *Am J Ophthalmol.* 2008;146(1):69–76.

134. Wu SY, Nemesure B, Hennis A, et al. Nine-year changes in intraocular pressure: the Barbados Eye Studies. *Arch Ophthalmol.* 2006;124(11):1631–1636.

135. Mitchell P, Lee AJ, Rochtchina E, et al. Open-angle glaucoma and systemic hypertension: the blue mountains eye study. *J Glaucoma.* 2004;13(4):319–326.

136. Klein BE, Klein R, Knudtson MD. Intraocular pressure and systemic blood pressure: longitudinal perspective: the Beaver Dam Eye Study. *Br J Ophthalmol.* 2005;89(3):284–287.

137. Vijaya L, George R, Paul PG, et al. Prevalence of open-angle glaucoma in a rural south Indian population. *Invest Ophthalmol Vis Sci.* 2005;46(12):4461–4467.

138. Klein R, Klein BE, Tomany SC, et al. The relation of retinal microvascular characteristics to age-related eye disease: the Beaver Dam eye study. *Am J Ophthalmol.* 2004;137(3):435–444.

139. Sung KR, Lee S, Park SB, et al. Twenty-four hour ocular perfusion pressure fluctuation and risk of normal-tension glaucoma progression. *Invest Ophthalmol Vis Sci.* 2009;50(11):5266–5274.

140. Hulsman CA, Vingerling JR, Hofman A, et al. Blood pressure, arterial stiffness, and open-angle glaucoma: the Rotterdam study. *Arch Ophthalmol.* 2007;125(6):805–812.

141. Tan GS, Wong TY, Fong CW, et al. Diabetes, metabolic abnormalities, and glaucoma. *Arch Ophthalmol.* 2009;127(10):1354–1361.

142. Chopra V, Varma R, Francis BA, et al. Type 2 diabetes mellitus and the risk of open-angle glaucoma the Los Angeles Latino Eye Study. *Ophthalmology.* 2008;115(2):227–232 e1.

143. de Voogd S, Ikram MK, Wolfs RC, et al. Is diabetes mellitus a risk factor for open-angle glaucoma? The Rotterdam Study. *Ophthalmology.* 2006; 113(10):1827–1831.

144. Morgan WH, Yu DY, Cooper RL, et al. The influence of cerebrospinal fluid pressure on the lamina cribrosa tissue pressure gradient. *Invest Ophthalmol Vis Sci.* 1995;36(6):1163–1172.

145. Berdahl JP, Allingham RR, Johnson DH. Cerebrospinal fluid pressure is decreased in primary open-angle glaucoma. *Ophthalmology.* 2008;115(5): 763–768.

146. Chang TC, Singh K. Glaucomatous disease in patients with normal pressure hydrocephalus. *J Glaucoma.* 2009;18(3):243–246.

147. Ren R, Jonas JB, Tian G, et al. Cerebrospinal fluid pressure in glaucoma: a prospective study. *Ophthalmology.* 2009; 117(2):259–266.

148. Akinci A, Cetinkaya E, Aycan Z, et al. Relationship between intraocular pressure and obesity in children. *J Glaucoma.* 2007;16(7):627–630.

149. Cheung N, Wong TY. Obesity and eye diseases. *Surv Ophthalmol.* 2007; 52(2):180–195.

150. Behrouzi Z, Rabei HM, Azizi F, et al. Prevalence of open-angle glaucoma, glaucoma suspect, and ocular hypertension in thyroid-related immune orbitopathy. *J Glaucoma.* 2007;16(4):358–362.

151. Boulos PR, Hardy I. Thyroid-associated orbitopathy: a clinicopathologic and therapeutic review. *Curr Opin Ophthalmol.* 2004;15(5):389–400.

152. He J, Wu Z, Yan J, et al. Clinical analysis of 106 cases with elevated intraocular pressure in thyroid-associated ophthalmopathy. *Yan Ke Xue Bao.* 2004;20(1):10–14.

153. Skalicky SE, Borovik AM, Masselos K, et al. Prevalence of open-angle glaucoma, glaucoma suspect, and ocular hypertension in thyroid related immune orbitopathy. *J Glaucoma.* 2008;17(3):249; author reply 249–250.

154. Konuk O, Aktas Z, Aksoy S, et al. Hyperthyroidism and severity of orbital disease do not change the central corneal thickness in Graves' ophthalmopathy. *Eur J Ophthalmol.* 2008;18(1):125–127.

155. Cross JM, Girkin CA, Owsley C, et al. The association between thyroid problems and glaucoma. *Br J Ophthalmol.* 2008;92(11):1503–1505.

156. Goldberg I. Thyroid eye disease and glaucoma. *J Glaucoma.* 2003;12(6): 494–496.

157. Bendel RE, Kaplan J, Heckman M, et al. Prevalence of glaucoma in patients with obstructive sleep apnoea—a cross-sectional case-series. *Eye (Lond).* 2008;22(9):1105–1109.

158. Mojon DS, Hess CW, Goldblum D, et al. High prevalence of glaucoma in patients with sleep apnea syndrome. *Ophthalmology.* 1999;106(5): 1009–1012.

159. Walker SD, Brubaker RF, Nagataki S. Hypotony and aqueous humor dynamics in myotonic dystrophy. *Invest Ophthalmol Vis Sci.* 1982;22(6): 744–751.

160. Khan AR, Brubaker RF. Aqueous humor flow and flare in patients with myotonic dystrophy. *Invest Ophthalmol Vis Sci.* 1993;34(11):3131–3139.

161. Shapiro A, Shoenfeld Y, Konikoff F, et al. The relationship between body temperature and intraocular pressure. *Ann Ophthalmol.* 1981;13(2): 159–161.

162. Arevalo JF, Munguia D, Faber D, et al. Correlation between intraocular pressure and CD4$^+$ T-lymphocyte counts in patients with human immunodeficiency virus with and without cytomegalovirus retinitis. *Am J Ophthalmol.* 1996;122(1):91–96.

163. Robert YC. What do we measure with various techniques when assessing IOP? *Surv Ophthalmol.* 2007;52(suppl 2):S105–S108.

164. Goldmann MH. Un nouveau tonometre a applanation. *Bull Soc Fr Ophthalmol.* 1954;67:474.

165. Palmberg R, Gutierrez YS, Miller D, et al. Potential bacterial contamination of eyedrops used for tonometry. *Am J Ophthalmol.* 1994;117(5): 578–582.

166. Duffner LR, Pflugfelder SC, Mandelbaum S, et al. Potential bacterial contamination in fluorescein-anesthetic solutions. *Am J Ophthalmol.* 1990; 110(2):199–202.

167. Whitacre MM, Stein R. Sources of error with use of Goldmann-type tonometers [Review]. *Surv Ophthalmol.* 1993;38(1):1–30.

168. Ehlers N, Bramsen T, Sperling S. Applanation tonometry and central corneal thickness. *Acta Ophthalmol (Copenh).* 1975;53(1):34–43.

169. Pepose JS, Feigenbaum SK, Qazi MA, et al. Changes in corneal biomechanics and intraocular pressure following LASIK using static, dynamic, and noncontact tonometry. *Am J Ophthalmol.* 2007;143(1):39–47.

170. Doughty MJ, Zaman ML. Human corneal thickness and its impact on intraocular pressure measures: a review and meta-analysis approach [Review]. *Surv Ophthalmol.* 2000;44(5):367–408.

171. La Rosa FA, Gross RL, Orengo-Nania S. Central corneal thickness of Caucasians and African Americans in glaucomatous and nonglaucomatous populations. *Arch Ophthalmol.* 2001;119(1):23–27.

172. Foster PJ, Baasanhu J, Alsbirk PH, et al. Central corneal thickness and intraocular pressure in a Mongolian population. *Ophthalmology.* 1998; 105(6):969–973.

173. Wu LL, Suzuki Y, Ideta R, et al. Central corneal thickness of normal tension glaucoma patients in Japan. *Jpn J Ophthalmol.* 2000;44(6): 643–647.

174. Brandt JD, Beiser JA, Kass MA, et al. Central corneal thickness in the Ocular Hypertension Treatment Study (OHTS). *Ophthalmology.* 2001; 108(10):1779–1788.

175. Copt RP, Thomas R, Mermoud A. Corneal thickness in ocular hypertension, primary open-angle glaucoma, and normal tension glaucoma [Comment]. *Arch Ophthalmol.* 1999;117(1):14–16.

176. Wolfs RC, Klaver CC, Vingerling JR, et al. Distribution of central corneal thickness and its association with intraocular pressure: the Rotterdam study. *Am J Ophthalmol.* 1997;123(6):767–772.

177. Whitacre MM, Stein RA, Hassanein K. The effect of corneal thickness on applanation tonometry. *Am J Ophthalmol.* 1993;115(5):592–596.

178. Dohadwala AA, Munger R, Damji KF. Positive correlation between tonopen intraocular pressure and central corneal thickness. *Ophthalmology.* 1998;105(10):1849–1854.

179. Brandt JD. Corneal thickness in glaucoma screening, diagnosis, and management. *Curr Opin Ophthalmol.* 2004;15(2):85–89.

180. Mark HH. Corneal curvature in applanation tonometry. *Am J Ophthalmol.* 1973;76(2):223–224.

181. Holladay JT, Allison ME, Prager TC. Goldmann applanation tonometry in patients with regular corneal astigmatism. *Am J Ophthalmol.* 1983; 96(1):90–93.

182. Bynke H, Wilke K. Repeated applanation tonometry in carotid occlusive disease. *Acta Ophthalmol (Copenh).* 1974;52(1):125–133.

183. Moniz E, Feldman F, Newkirk M, et al. Removal of hepatitis B surface antigen from a contaminated applanation tonometer. *Am J Ophthalmol.* 1981;91(4):522–525.

184. Ablashi DV, Sturzenegger S, Hunter EA, et al. Presence of HTLV-III in tears and cells from the eyes of AIDS patients. *J Exp Pathol.* 1987;3(4):693–703.

185. Nagington J, Sutehall GM, Whipp P. Tonometer disinfection and viruses. *Br J Ophthalmol.* 1983;67(10):674–676.

186. Rutala WA, Weber DJ. Healthcare Infection Control Practices Advisory Committee (HICPAC). *Guideline for Disinfection and Sterilization in Healthcare Facilities, 2008.* U.S. Centers for Disease Control and Prevention. Available at: www.cdc.gov/ncidod/dhqp/pdf/guidelines/Disinfection_Nov_2008.pdf. Accessed December 22, 2009.

187. Threlkeld AB, Froggatt JW III, Schein OD, et al. Efficacy of a disinfectant wipe method for the removal of adenovirus 8 from tonometer tips. *Ophthalmology.* 1993;100(12):1841–1845.

188. Ventura LM, Dix RD. Viability of herpes simplex virus type 1 on the applanation tonometer. *Am J Ophthalmol.* 1987;103(1):48–52.

189. Su CS, Bowden S, Fong LP, et al. Current tonometer disinfection may be inadequate for hepatitis B virus. *Arch Ophthalmol.* 1994;112(11): 1406–1407.

190. Pepose JS, Linette G, Lee SF, et al. Disinfection of Goldmann tonometers against human immunodeficiency virus type 1. *Arch Ophthalmol.* 1989; 107(7):983–985.

191. Posner A. An evaluation of the Maklakov applanation tonometer. *Eye Ear Nose Throat Mon.* 1962;41:377–378.

192. Perkins ES. Hand-held applanation tonometer. *Br J Ophthalmol.* 1965; 49(11):591–593.

193. Draeger J. Principle and clinical application of a portable applanation tonometer. *Invest Ophthalmol.* 1967;6(2):132–134.

194. Mackay RS, Marg E, Oechsli R. Automatic tonometer with exact theory: various biological applications. *Science.* 1960;131:1668–1669.

195. Kao SF, Lichter PR, Bergstrom TJ, et al. Clinical comparison of the Oculab Tono-Pen to the Goldmann applanation tonometer. *Ophthalmology.* 1987;94(12):1541–1544.

196. Durham DG, Bigliano RP, Masino JA. Pneumatic applanation tonometer. *Trans Am Acad Ophthalmol Otolaryngol.* 1965;69(6):1029–1047.

197. Kaufmann C, Bachmann LM, et al. Comparison of dynamic contour tonometry with goldmann applanation tonometry. *Invest Ophthalmol Vis Sci.* 2004;45(9):3118–3121.

198. Forbes M, Pico G Jr, Grolman B. A noncontact applanation tonometer. Description and clinical evaluation. *Arch Ophthalmol.* 1974;91(2): 134–140.

199. Touboul D, Roberts C, Kerautret J, et al. Correlations between corneal hysteresis, intraocular pressure, and corneal central pachymetry. *J Cataract Refract Surg.* 2008;34(4):616–622.

200. Moses RA, Arnzen RJ. Instantaneous tonometry. *Arch Ophthalmol.* 1983;101(2):249–252.

201. Friedenwald JS, Moses R. Modern refinements in tonometry. *Doc Ophthalmol.* 1950;4:335–362.

202. Moses RA, Tarkkanen A. Tonometry; the pressure-volume relationship in the intact human eye at low pressures. *Am J Ophthalmol.* 1959;47(1 pt 2): 557–563.

203. Anderson DR, Grant WM. Re-evaluation of the Schiötz tonometer calibration. *Invest Ophthalmol.* 1970;9(6):430–446.

204. Bayard WL. Comparison of Goldmann applanation and Schiötz tonometry using 1948 and 1955 conversion scales. *Am J Ophthalmol.* 1970; 69(6):1007–1009.

205. Hetland-Eriksen J. On tonometry. 2. Pressure recordings by Schiötz tonometry on enucleated human eyes. *Acta Ophthalmol (Copenh).* 1966; 44(1):12–19.

206. Friedenwald JS. Some problems in the calibration of tonometers. *Am J Ophthalmol.* 1948;31:935.

207. Sahin A, Basmak H, Niyaz L, et al. Reproducibility and tolerability of the ICare rebound tonometer in school children. *J Glaucoma.* 2007;16(2): 185–188.

208. Kakaday T, Hewitt AW, Voelcker NH, et al. Advances in telemetric continuous intraocular pressure assessment. *Br J Ophthalmol.* 2009;93(8): 992–996.

209. Sit AJ. Continuous monitoring of intraocular pressure: rationale and progress toward a clinical device. *J Glaucoma.* 2009;18(4):272–279.

210. Leonardi M, Pitchon EM, Bertsch A, et al. Wireless contact lens sensor for intraocular pressure monitoring: assessment on enucleated pig eyes. *Acta Ophthalmol.* 2009;87(4):433–437.

211. McLaren JW, Brubaker RF, FitzSimon JS. Continuous measurement of intraocular pressure in rabbits by telemetry. *Invest Ophthalmol Vis Sci.* 1996;37(6):966–975.

212. Wax MB, Camras CB, Fiscella RG, et al. Emerging perspectives in glaucoma: optimizing 24-hour control of intraocular pressure [Review]. *Am J Ophthalmol.* 2002;133(suppl)S1–S10.

213. Moses RA, Liu CH. Repeated applanation tonometry. *Am J Ophthalmol.* 1968;66(1):89–91.

214. Dielemans I, Vingerling JR, Hofman A, et al. Reliability of intraocular pressure measurement with the Goldmann applanation tonometer in epidemiological studies. *Graefes Arch Clin Exp Ophthalmol.* 1994;232(3):141–144.

215. Bengtsson B. Comparison of Schiötz and Goldmann tonometry in a population. *Acta Ophthalmol (Copenh).* 1972;50(4):445–457.

216. Krieglstein GK, Waller WK. Goldmann applanation versus hand-applanation and Schiötz indentation tonometry. *Albrecht Von Graefes Arch Klin Exp Ophthalmol.* 1975;194(1):11–16.

217. Gharaei H, Kargozar A, Raygan F, et al. Comparison of Perkins, Tono-Pen and Schiötz tonometers in paediatric patients under general anaesthesia. *East Mediterr Health J.* 2008;14(6):1365–1371.

218. Hessemer V, Rossler R, Jacobi KW. Comparison of intraocular pressure measurements with the Oculab Tono-Pen vs manometry in humans shortly after death. *Am J Ophthalmol.* 1988;105(6):678–682.

219. Boothe WA, Lee DA, Panek WC, et al. The Tono-Pen. A manometric and clinical study. *Arch Ophthalmol.* 1988;106(9):1214–1217.

220. Hines MW, Jost BF, Fogelman KL. Oculab Tono-Pen, Goldmann applanation tonometry, and pneumatic tonometry for intraocular pressure assessment in gas-filled eyes. *Am J Ophthalmol.* 1988;106(2):174–179.

221. Quigley HA, Langham ME. Comparative intraocular pressure measurements with the pneumatonograph and Goldmann tonometer. *Am J Ophthalmol.* 1975;80(2):266–273.

222. Jain MR, Marmion VJ. A clinical evaluation of the applanation pneumatonograph. *Br J Ophthalmol.* 1976;60(2):107–110.

223. Zadok D, Tran DB, Twa M, et al. Pneumotonometry versus Goldmann tonometry after laser in situ keratomileusis for myopia. *J Cataract Refract Surg.* 1999;25(10):1344–1348.

224. Stoiber J, Fernandez V, Lamar PD, et al. Ex vivo evaluation of Tono-Pen and pneumotonometry in cat eyes. *Ophthalmic Res.* 2006;38(1):13–18.

225. West CE, Capella JA, Kaufman HE. Measurement of intraocular pressure with a pneumatic applanation tonometer. *Am J Ophthalmol.* 1972;74(3): 505–509.

226. Geyer O, Mayron Y, Loewenstein A, et al. Tono-Pen tonometry in normal and in post-keratoplasty eyes. *Br J Ophthalmol.* 1992;76(9):538–540.

227. Rubenstein JB, Deutsch TA. Pneumotonometry through bandage contact lenses. *Arch Ophthalmol.* 1985;103(11):1660–1661.

228. Khan JA, LaGreca BA. Tono-Pen estimation of intraocular pressure through bandage contact lenses. *Am J Ophthalmol.* 1989;108(4): 422–425.

229. Mark LK, Asbell PA, Torres MA, et al. Accuracy of intraocular pressure measurements with two different tonometers through bandage contact lenses. *Cornea.* 1992;11(4):277–281.

230. Del Priore LV, Michels RG, Nunez MA, et al. Intraocular pressure measurement after pars plana vitrectomy. *Ophthalmology.* 1989;96(9): 1353–1356.

231. Lim JI, Blair NP, Higginbotham EJ, et al. Assessment of intraocular pressure in vitrectomized gas-containing eyes. A clinical and manometric comparison of the Tono-Pen to the pneumotonometer. *Arch Ophthalmol.* 1990;108(5):684–688.

232. Wright MM, Grajewski AL. Measurement of intraocular pressure with a flat anterior chamber. *Ophthalmology.* 1991;98(12):1854–1857.

233. Liu C, Hille K, Tan D, et al. Keratoprosthesis surgery. *Dev Ophthalmol.* 2008;41:171–186.

234. Chew HF, Ayres BD, Hammersmith KM, et al. Boston keratoprosthesis outcomes and complications. *Cornea.* 2009;28(9):989–996.

Gonioscopy and Other Techniques for Assessing the Anterior Segment

3

Assessment of the anatomy of the anterior chamber angle by gonioscopy is an essential part of the glaucoma evaluation. The drainage angle, as well as other structures in the anterior segment (namely, iris insertion and ciliary body anatomy), can also be assessed by using ultrasonographic and laser imaging techniques, and cycloscopy. In this chapter, we describe these techniques, and those involved in the assessment of aqueous humor dynamics. Although the methods in the latter category—specifically, tonography, fluorophotometry, and measurement of episcleral venous pressure—are not routinely used in clinical practice today, clinicians should be familiar with them because their results form our understanding of aqueous humor dynamics and the mechanism of action of glaucoma medications used to lower intraocular pressure (IOP).

GONIOSCOPY

This discussion of gonioscopy is limited to technique and normal anatomic findings, whereas abnormal findings on gonioscopic examination associated with the various forms of glaucoma are considered in Section II.

Historical Background

In 1907, Trantas visualized the angle in an eye with keratoglobus by indenting the limbus. He later coined the term gonioscopy. Salsmann introduced the goniolens in 1914, and Koeppe improved on it 5 years later by designing a steeper lens. Troncoso also contributed to gonioscopy by developing the gonioscope for magnification and illumination of the angle. In 1938, Goldmann introduced the gonioprism, and Barkan established the use of gonioscopy in the management of glaucoma. (More details on the history of gonioscopy are available in a review by Dellaporta (1).)

Principle of Gonioscopy

In healthy eyes, the angle cannot be visualized directly because of the optical principle known as the critical angle. The critical angle is related to the properties of light passing through media with different indices of refraction. When light passes from a medium with a greater index of refraction to one with a lesser index, the angle of refraction (r) is larger than the angle of incidence (i). When r equals 90 degrees, i is said to have attained the critical angle. When i exceeds the critical angle, the light is reflected back into the first medium. The critical angle for the cornea–air interface is approximately 46 degrees. Light rays coming from the anterior chamber angle exceed this critical angle and are therefore reflected back into the anterior chamber, preventing direct visualization of the angle (**Fig. 3.1A–D**).

The solution to this problem is to eliminate the cornea–air interface by using a goniolens or gonioprism. Because the index of refraction of a contact lens approaches that of the cornea, there is minimal refraction at the interface of these two media, which eliminates the optical effect of the front corneal surface. Therefore, light rays from the anterior chamber angle enter the contact lens and are then made to pass through the new contact lens–air interface by one of two basic designs. In direct gonioscopy, the anterior curve of the contact lens—the goniolens—is such that the critical angle is not reached, and the light rays are refracted at the contact lens–air interface. In indirect gonioscopy, the light rays are reflected by a mirror in the contact lens—the gonioprism—and leave the lens at nearly a right angle to the contact lens–air interface (**Fig. 3.1E,F**). (Commonly used goniolenses and gonioprisms are listed in **Table 3.1**, and some are shown in **Fig. 3.2**.)

Direct Gonioscopy

Instruments

The Koeppe lens is the prototype diagnostic goniolens and is available in different diameters and radii of posterior curvature. A gonioscope, or handheld biomicroscope, provides 15× to 20× magnification. The light source is usually a separate handheld unit, such as the Barkan focal illuminator, although it may be attached to the gonioscope.

Technique

Direct gonioscopy is performed with the patient in a supine position, preferably on a movable diagnostic table or chair. After applying a topical anesthetic, the goniolens is positioned on the cornea, with either balanced salt solution, a viscous preparation such as methylcellulose, or the patient's own tears between the goniolens and the patient's cornea. The examiner usually holds the gonioscope in one hand and a light source in the other (**Fig. 3.3**). Occasionally, an assistant may be needed to move the goniolens to the desired position. Alternatively, a gonioscope with mounted light source may be used, which allows the examiner to control the goniolens with the other hand. In either case, the examiner scans the anterior chamber angle by shifting his or her position until all 360 degrees have been studied. An excellent overview of direct gonioscopy, with guided video gonioscopy examinations, is available at http://www.gonioscopy.org/.

Figure 3.1 Principle of gonioscopy. **A:** Light ray is refracted when angle of incidence (*i*) at interface of two media with different indices of refraction (*n* and *n'*) is less than the critical angle. **B:** Angle of refraction (*r*) is 90 degrees when *i* equals the critical angle. **C:** Light is reflected when *i* exceeds the critical angle. **D:** Light from the anterior chamber angle exceeds the critical angle at the cornea–air interface and is reflected back into the eye. **E** and **F:** Contact lenses have an index of retraction (*n*) similar to that of the cornea, allowing light to enter the lens and then be refracted (goniolens) or reflected (gonioprism) beyond the contact lens–air interface.

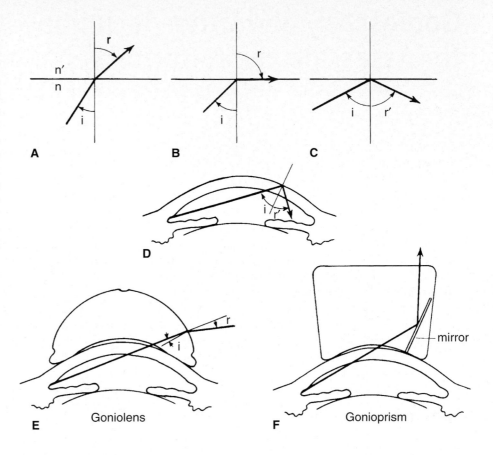

Table 3.1	Contact Lenses for Gonioscopy	
Lens	**Description/Use**	
Goniolenses (direct gonioscopy)		
Koeppe	Prototype diagnostic goniolens	
Richardson–Shaffer	Small Koeppe lens for use in infants	
Layden	For gonioscopic examination of premature infants	
Barkan	Prototype surgical goniolens	
Thorpe	Surgical and diagnostic lens for operating rooms	
Swan–Jacob	Surgical goniolens for use in children	
Gonioprisms (indirect gonioscopy)		
Goldmann single-mirror	Mirror inclined at 62 degrees for gonioscopy	
Goldmann three-mirror	One mirror for gonioscopy, two for retina; coated front surface available for laser use	
Zeiss four-mirror	All four mirrors inclined at 64 degrees for gonioscopy; requires holder (Unger); fluid bridge not required	
Posner four-mirror	Modified Zeiss four-mirror gonioprism with attached handle	
Sussman four-mirror	Handheld Zeiss-type gonioprism	
Thorpe four-mirror	Four gonioscopy mirrors, inclined at 62 degrees requires fluid bridge	
Ritch trabeculoplasty lens	Four gonioscopy mirrors, two inclined at 59 degrees and two at 62 degrees, with convex lens over two	
Latina trabeculoplasty lens	One mirror for trabeculoplasty	

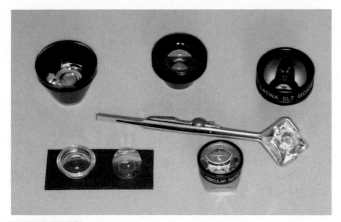

Figure 3.2 Representative indirect and direct goniolenses. Top row, from left to right: large Goldmann three-mirror indirect goniolens, small Goldmann three-mirror indirect goniolens, and Latina indirect goniolens. Middle row: Zeiss four-mirror indirect goniolens with Unger holder. Bottom row, from left: adult Koeppe direct goniolens, Leyden direct goniolens, and four-mirror Sussman indirect goniolens.

Indirect Gonioscopy

Instruments

The gonioprism and a slitlamp are the only instruments needed for indirect gonioscopy. Several types of goniolenses are available with a single mirror or multiple mirrors. The Goldmann single-mirror lens is tilted 62 degrees from the plano front surface, which allows examination of the anterior chamber angle. The Goldmann three-mirror lens contains two mirrors for examination of the fundus, and one for examination of the angle. Because of their 7.38-mm posterior radius of curvature, both Goldmann lenses require the use of a viscous material to fill the space between the cornea and the lens. In contrast, a modified Goldmann-type lens, with its 8.4-mm radius of curvature, requires no viscous

bridge (2). Goldmann-type lenses have also been modified with antireflection coating, allowing them to be used for laser trabeculoplasty.

In the Zeiss four-mirror lens, all the mirrors are tilted at 64 degrees for evaluation of the angle, eliminating the need to rotate the lens. The original four-mirror lens is mounted on a holding fork (an Unger holder), whereas newer models have a permanently attached holding rod (a Posner lens) or are held directly, such as the Sussman-style lenses (3). The posterior curvature of these four-mirror lenses is similar to that of the cornea, conveniently allowing the patient's own tears to be used as the fluid bridge. With the Goldmann- and Zeiss-type instruments, the anterior chamber angle is viewed "indirectly" through a mirror 180 degrees from the quadrant being viewed (**Fig. 3.4**). Some newer gonioprisms enable direct viewing of the angle (4,5).

Several types of lenses, including the Ritch trabeculoplasty lens and the Latina lens, are used in laser therapy (discussed in Section III).

Technique

The cornea is anesthetized and, with the patient positioned at the slitlamp, the gonioprism is placed against the cornea with or without a fluid bridge, depending on the posterior radius of

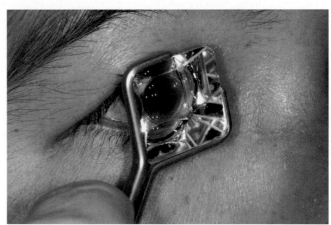

A

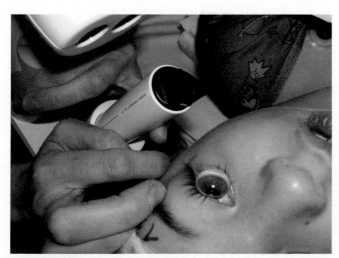

Figure 3.3 Technique of direct gonioscopy, by using a Koeppe goniolens and portable slitlamp, during an examination under anesthesia of a child's eye.

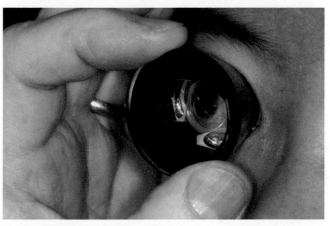

B

Figure 3.4 Technique of indirect gonioscopy with a Zeiss four-mirror lens (**A**) and a Goldmann three-mirror lens (**B**).

curvature of the instrument. The lens is then rotated to allow visualization of all 360 degrees of the angle, or the quadrants are studied with the four mirrors. Visualization into a narrow angle can be enhanced by manipulating the gonioprism—for example, asking the patient to look in the direction of the mirror being used. A web-based gonioscopy module with video, available at www.gonioscopy.org, is recommended for learning this technique (4).

Comparison of Direct and Indirect Gonioscopy

There is no unanimity of opinion on which basic method of gonioscopy is best. With direct gonioscopy, the height of the observer may be changed to look deeper into a narrow angle, whereas the gonioprism is limited in this regard by the height of the mirror. In addition, the goniolens may cause less distortion of the anterior chamber. Both features make it desirable when assessing the true depth of the anterior chamber angle (5). A major advantage of direct gonioscopy, especially with the infant Koeppe lenses, is its use in sedated or anesthetized patients, as in the examination of children. These lenses are also useful in examining the fundus through a small pupil with a direct ophthalmoscope.

In indirect gonioscopy, the slitlamp may provide better optics and lighting, which could be an advantage when looking for subtle details in the angle. Furthermore, the method requires fewer additional instruments and occupies less space than direct gonioscopy does. Indirect gonioscopy is also performed faster than direct gonioscopy is; this is particularly true with the Zeiss four-mirror lenses and modified Goldmann-type lenses, because no viscous bridge is required. Gonioprisms with a posterior radius of curvature closer to that of the anterior corneal surface may also reduce corneal distortion. Gonioprisms with taller mirrors facilitate visualization of narrow angles. Finally,

because of its relatively small diameter of corneal contact, the Zeiss four-mirror lens can also be used in "compressive gonioscopy" (6) (explained in Chapter 12).

Cleaning of Diagnostic Contact Lenses

Any instrument that contacts the eye creates the potential hazard of transmitting bacterial and viral infection. This issue is considered in more detail in Chapter 2. (Although Chapter 2 discusses instrument cleaning in the context of tonometry use, the same basic principles apply with diagnostic contact lenses (7).)

Gonioscopic Appearance of the Normal Anterior Chamber Angle

Starting at the root of the iris and progressing anteriorly toward the cornea, the following structures can be identified by gonioscopy in an adult with a normal angle (**Figs. 3.5** and **3.6**).

Ciliary Body Band

The ciliary body band is the portion of ciliary body visible in the anterior chamber as a result of the iris insertion into the ciliary body. The width of the band depends on the level of iris insertion, and tends to be wider in myopic eyes and narrower in hyperopic eyes. The color of the band is usually gray or dark brown.

Scleral Spur

This is the posterior lip of the scleral sulcus, which is attached to the ciliary body posteriorly and the corneoscleral meshwork anteriorly. It is usually seen as a prominent white line between the ciliary body band and functional trabecular meshwork,

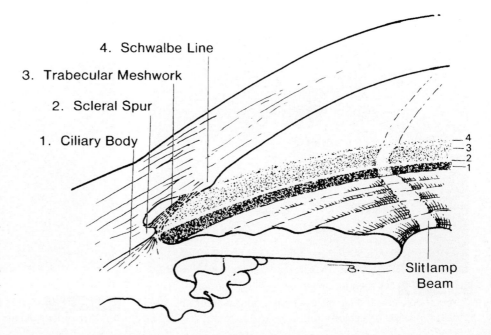

Figure 3.5 Normal adult anterior chamber angle showing gonioscopic appearance (*right*) and cross section of corresponding structures (*left*). 1. Ciliary body band; 2. scleral spur; 3. trabecular meshwork (degree of pigmentation varies); 4. Schwalbe line.

4. Schwalbe Line
3. Trabecular Meshwork
2. Scleral Spur
1. Ciliary Body
Slitlamp Beam

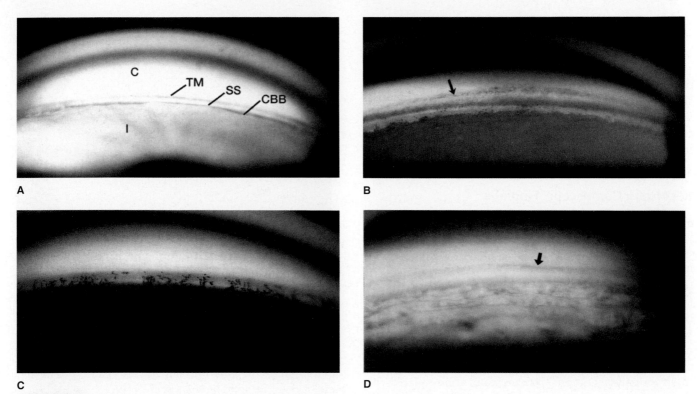

Figure 3.6 **A:** Going from the iris (*I*) to the cornea (*C*), the structures normally seen by gonioscopy in the open, adult anterio chamber angle are the ciliary body band (*CBB*), scleral spur (*SS*), and the functional portion of the trabecular meshwork (*TM*). **B:** In this eye, the ciliary body band is light gray; trabecular meshwork is heavily pigmented. The thinner, pigmented line above the meshwork (*arrow*) is the Schwalbe line, more easily seen in some eyes because of pigment buildup along the ridge, especially in the inferior quadrant. **C:** Whereas the ciliary body band may appear dark brown in some eyes (e.g., A, *above*), it may be a slate gray band in others, as seen in this image just above the iris root. Also note the numerous iris processes, which typically extend across the ciliary body band and scleral spur to the trabecular meshwork, which is medium brown in this image. **D:** Sometimes helpful in identifying the location of a lightly pigmented trabecular meshwork is blood reflux in the Schlemm canal (*arrow*).

unless it is obscured by dense uveal meshwork or excessive pigment dispersion. Variable numbers of fine, pigmented strands may frequently be seen crossing the scleral spur from the iris root to the functional meshwork. These are referred to as iris processes, and represent thickenings of the posterior uveal meshwork.

Functional Trabecular Meshwork

This is seen as a pigmented band just anterior to the scleral spur. Although the trabecular meshwork actually extends from the iris root to Schwalbe line, it may be considered in two portions: (a) the anterior part, between the Schwalbe line and the anterior edge of the Schlemm canal, which is involved to a lesser degree in aqueous outflow, and (b) the posterior (or functional) part, which is the remainder of the meshwork and is the primary site of aqueous outflow (especially that portion immediately adjacent to the Schlemm canal) (8).

The appearance of the functional meshwork varies considerably depending on the amount and distribution of pigment deposition. The trabecular meshwork has no pigment at birth, but with age, color develops, from faint tan to dark brown, depending on the degree of pigment dispersion in the anterior

chamber. The distribution of pigment may be homogeneous for 360 degrees in some eyes and irregular in others. In the functional portion of the meshwork, especially when lightly pigmented, blood reflux in the Schlemm canal may sometimes be seen as a red band.

Schwalbe Line

The Schwalbe line is the junction between the anterior chamber angle structures and the cornea. It is a fine ridge just anterior to the meshwork and is often identified by a small buildup of pigment, especially inferiorly. By using a thin slit beam at a slightly oblique angle, this line can be identified by the corneal wedge created by light wedge created at the junction between the inner light beam along the cornea endothelium and the outer light beam along the corneoscleral junction.

Normal Blood Vessels

Blood vessels are normally not seen in the angle, although loops from the major arterial circle may appear in front of the ciliary body band and less commonly over the scleral spur and trabecular meshwork. These vessels typically take a circumferential route in the angle.

In addition, an anterior ciliary artery may occasionally be seen as a more radially oriented vessel in the ciliary body band of lightly pigmented eyes. Circumferential and radial vessels may also occasionally be seen in the peripheral iris of lightly colored eyes. In a study of 100 patients with abnormal anterior chamber angle vascularization of unknown cause, 16 patients had normal angle vessels in both eyes and 10 patients had normal angle vessels in one eye (9). Radial vessels were more common in the peripheral iris, whereas the circumferential type was more common on the ciliary body band.

Recording Gonioscopic Findings

Various classification systems have been suggested for describing the width and appearance of the anterior chamber angle. However, descriptive words and drawings are probably the most useful technique for recording gonioscopic findings. The recorded data should include (a) configuration of the angle, (b) depth of the angle on the basis of the most posterior structure that can be seen, (c) degree of pigmentation, and (d) presence of abnormal structures. For example, a normal angle might be recorded as "wide open, with visualization to a wide ciliary body band for 360 degrees and moderate trabecular meshwork pigmentation." Drawings can also be placed on a chart with concentric circles to document more specific details.

CYCLOSCOPY

This technique allows direct visualization of ciliary processes under special circumstances, such as the presence of an iridectomy, wide iris retraction, aniridia, and some patients with aphakia. The main value of the technique is in conjunction with laser therapy to the ciliary processes (transpupillary cyclophotocoagulation, discussed in Section III).

HIGH-RESOLUTION ULTRASOUND BIOMICROSCOPY

Another useful clinical tool to examine the anterior ocular segment is ultrasound technology. Ultrasound echoes are produced from interfaces of fluids and tissues. The differences between fluid or tissue properties yield certain echo characteristics between the interfaces of various compartments or tissue densities. The echo is optimal when the acoustic wave is oriented perpendicular to the interface. Ultrasonographic techniques can provide information in the amplitude mode, or A-scan, or in the brightness mode, or B-scan.

In general, low-frequency ultrasonography allows deeper tissue penetration but lower resolution, compared with high-frequency ultrasonography, which provides higher resolution but shallower penetration. There is a wide range of frequencies currently in use in ophthalmology, from 10 MHz, to image the globe and orbit, through 20 MHz, which images from the cornea to the posterior lens, 35 to 50 MHz, which image from the cornea to the anterior lens, and 100 MHz, for imaging the

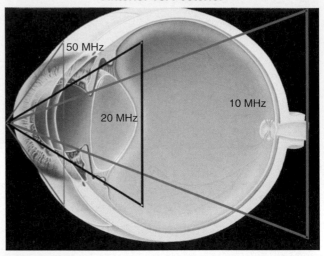

Anterior vs. Posterior

Figure 3.7 Schematic representation of penetration of acoustic sound waves by different ultrasound frequencies. (Modified with permission from Cynthia Kendall.)

cornea only (**Fig. 3.7**). Frequencies of 20 to 50 MHz, which are used to image the anterior segment, are referred to as high-resolution ultrasound biomicroscopy (10).

High-resolution ultrasound biomicroscopy allows for a noninvasive means of visualizing anterior ocular structures at high resolution. In the management of patients with glaucoma, high-resolution ultrasound biomicroscopy is helpful to define the anterior chamber angle anatomy, when it cannot be seen gonioscopically, as well as structure and relationships among the iris, ciliary body, crystalline lens, intraocular lens, and anterior vitreous. (The use of high-resolution ultrasound biomicroscopy in managing the various forms of glaucoma is considered in Section II.)

OPTICAL COHERENCE TOMOGRAPHY OF THE ANTERIOR SEGMENT

Introduced in 2006, anterior-segment optical coherence topography, or AS-OCT, provides a noncontact, noninvasive means to image the anterior chamber angle anatomy (11,12). The AS-OCT uses a 1310-nm wavelength, compared with the 820-nm wavelength for posterior-segment imaging. The AS-OCT has higher resolution, compared with high-resolution ultrasound biomicroscopy, for imaging structures in the iris and the angle anatomy. The AS-OCT is limited to imaging the cornea, anterior chamber, angle anatomy, and central portion of the lens through the pupil (**Fig. 3.8**). This instrument is unable to adequately image the anatomy of the ciliary body or tissue masses behind the iris.

AQUEOUS HUMOR DYNAMICS

There are several techniques used to measure and calculate the determinants of IOP, which include aqueous humor flow, facility of aqueous outflow, uveoscleral outflow, and episcleral

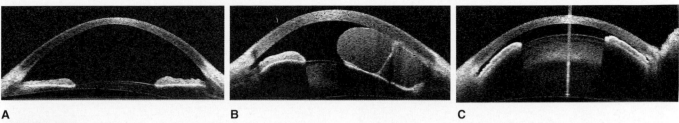

A   **B**   **C**

Figure 3.8   Montage of anterior-segment OCT images showing normal anterior segment (**A**), iris cyst (**B**), and subluxated lens with shallow anterior chamber and narrow angle (**C**).

venous pressure (13). These techniques include (a) fluorophotometry, a noninvasive and noncontact technique to measure the rate of fluorescein disappearance from the anterior segment and to calculate aqueous humor flow; (b) tonography, a noninvasive but contact technique to estimate the facility of aqueous outflow; and (c) the episcleral venometer, a noninvasive but contact technique to estimate episcleral venous pressure.

Mathematical Models for IOP

The mathematical relationship of the determinants of IOP is based on Poiseuille law that relates the velocity of flow (F) of fluid in a rigid tube to the following: the radius of the tube (r), the pressure drop per length of tube $[(P_1 - P_2)/1]$, and the coefficient of viscosity (η) of the fluid (http://hyperphysics.phy-astr.gsu.eu/hbase/ppois.html):

$$F = \pi r^4/8\eta \times (P_1 - P_2)/1\eta$$

In 1949, Goldmann applied Poiseuille law to aqueous outflow (14). Goldmann proposed that the rate of aqueous flow through the trabecular meshwork (F) is directly proportional to the IOP (P_0) minus the episcleral venous pressure (P_v) and inversely proportional to the resistance to outflow (R):

$$F = (P_0 - P_v)/R$$

Building on earlier observations by Pagenstecher (in 1878) and Schiotz (in 1905) that eye massage and repeated tonometry reduced IOP, Polak-van Gelder in 1911 described a technique of repeated tonometer applications for 1 to 2 minutes to differentiate healthy from glaucomatous eyes. Schoenberg modified this technique by using a continuous application of the tonometer while reading the pressure fall on the scale of the instrument. Later in 1950, Grant introduced tonography using electronic continuous IOP measurement and proposed an alternative factor to collectively express "outflow resistance" as the coefficient of outflow facility (C), which is reported in microliters per minute per millimeter of mercury in the following equation (15):

$F = C(P_0 - P_v)$ The C value is an expression of the degree to which a change in the IOP will cause a change in the rate of aqueous outflow, which is an indirect expression of the patency of the aqueous outflow system.

The Goldmann equation implied that aqueous flow in living ocular tissue could be expressed in the same linear terms as that of fluid in rigid tubes, which was subsequently proven inaccurate. Nevertheless, it has served for over 50 years as an adequate description of aqueous humor dynamics for clinical applications. Recent advances in glaucoma therapeutics, namely the prostaglandin agents (described in Chapter 28), have made it necessary to revise the equation and to reinterpret the meanings of its parameters to the following equation (13) presented in a form based on IOP, using the variables of aqueous flow (F_a), uveoscleral flow (F_u), trabecular outflow facility (C_t), and episcleral venous pressure (EVP):

$$IOP = [(F_a - F_u)/C_t] + EVP$$

Fluorophotometry

Fluorophotometry is the standard research technique by which the rate of aqueous humor flow is calculated under various circumstances, including the response to glaucoma drugs.

In brief, the fluorophotometry protocol involves instilling a given number of drops of saturated fluorescein topically, waiting for an appropriate period of time for steady state distribution of the fluorescein in the anterior segment structures of the cornea and anterior chamber, and then scanning the eye two or three times to obtain appropriate emission scans (16). Calculations are made on the basis of the change in fluorescein measured in the cornea and anterior chamber over time.

In a study of 519 subjects, there is a skewed normal distribution of aqueous humor flow measured between 8 AM and noon with an average of 2.97 μL/min (16). Among 180 normal subjects studied between midnight and 6 AM, there was decrease in aqueous humor flow to half of the morning flow value and with a narrower distribution of flow. A later study showed concordance of flow in normal subjects in the morning and night (17) meaning that individuals who had either low, medium, or high aqueous flow phenotypes in the morning showed the expected decrease in flow at night time, but also had a relatively low, medium, or high flow at night, respectively. This latter approach to characterize aqueous flow as a phenotype provides evidence that the factors that contribute to IOP can be studied as a quantitative trait (18). At present, there are no genetic markers for IOP variance, but genome-wide studies currently under way hold the promise of identifying such markers that may be important in identifying patients who have wide IOP fluctuation. In the future, such a molecular medicine approach (see Chapter 8) will help minimize glaucoma progression in patients with wide IOP fluctuation.

In general, aqueous humor flow decreases with age (16,19). Fluorophotometric studies suggest that aqueous production is relatively insensitive to long-term changes in IOP (20). It

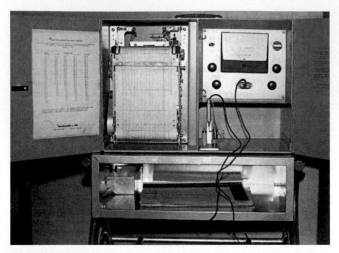

Figure 3.9 Tonography unit.

appears that the main mechanism involved in elevated IOP is alteration in outflow facility (21), which is related to increased resistance to outflow at the trabecular meshwork to a greater extent than the uveoscleral outflow, rather than a "hyper secreter," but the role of high aqueous flow phenotype in large IOP fluctuation is not known. Resistance to aqueous outflow increases with an increase in the IOP (the physiologic basis of which is discussed in Chapter 1). The tonographic result is that the *C* value of an eye decreases with increasing IOP (21), which is related to trabecular outflow, also described as conventional outflow, which is discussed in the next section on tonography.

At present, there is no method to measure uveoscleral outflow, also described as unconventional outflow. The influence of unconventional outflow on the tonographic results (discussed in the next section) is not fully understood. At present, the uveoscleral outflow is calculated on the basis of measurements derived from fluorophotometry and tonography (22,23).

Tonography

Tonography is a means of estimating the outflow facility by raising the IOP with an electronic indentation tonometer and observing the subsequent decay curve in the IOP over time, which is continuously recorded on a paper strip (**Figs. 3.9** and **3.10**). The elevated pressure causes an increased rate of aqueous outflow, leading to a change in the aqueous volume (*V*), which is inferred from Friedenwald tables (24).

In brief, the protocol involves measurements on a patient in a supine position. After measuring the IOP, a weighted tonometer raises the IOP from the baseline (P_0) to a new, higher level (P_t). Depending on the instrument, a 2- or 4-minute pressure tracing is recorded by gently applying the tonometer to the cornea and maintaining this position until a smooth tracing has been obtained. A good tracing will have fine oscillations and a gentle downward slope. If the slope is steeper or irregular during the first few seconds, which is not uncommon, the study is continued until a smooth tracing is obtained.

The slope of the tracing is estimated by placing a line through the middle of the oscillations. The change in IOP during this

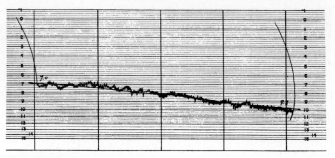

Figure 3.10 Tonographic tracing.

time is computed as an arithmetic average of pressure increments for successive half-minute intervals $[Ave.(P_t - P_0)]$. The scale readings are noted at the beginning and end of the tracing. P_0 and the change in scale readings over 4 minutes (*T*) are then used to obtain the *C* value from special tonographic tables derived from Grant's equation:

$$C = V/T[Ave.(P_t - P_0)]$$

The wave components of a tonographic tracing include (a) fine oscillations, which reflect the cardiac pulse; (b) large waves, which reflect the respiratory movement; and (c) still larger, irregular waves (Traube–Hering waves), which reflect periodic oscillations in the systemic blood pressure. Cardiac irregularities (e.g., extrasystole, bigeminy) can also cause irregularities in the tonographic tracing (25).

Aqueous production may decrease during the early phase of a rise in IOP, primarily because of an alteration in ultrafiltration (26). Any subsequent IOP drop in response to reduced production of aqueous creates an impression of increased outflow and is called pseudofacility. This may account for as much as 20% of the total *C* value. Tonography measures the total *C* value without distinguishing between true facility and pseudofacility.

In a study of 1379 eyes, Becker reported a mean *C* value of 0.28 μL/min/mm Hg in 909 healthy eyes (27). A low *C* value of less than 0.18 μL/min/mm Hg was found in 2.5% of healthy eyes, 65% of those with glaucoma (*N* = 250 eyes), and 20% of those with a family history of glaucoma (*N* = 220 eyes). An even lower *C* value, of less than 0.13 μL/min/mm Hg, was recorded for 0.15%, 3%, and 11%, respectively. The P_0/C ratio was 56 in the healthy populations. The proportion of participants with a high P_0/C ratio of greater than 100 was 2.5% among healthy eyes, 95% among those with glaucoma, and 31% in those with a family history of glaucoma. An even higher P_0/C ratio, of greater than 138, was found among 0.15% of healthy eyes, 50% of those with glaucoma and 14% of those with a family history of glaucoma.

In a study of 7577 eyes, the *C* value was found to decrease with age, with an average of 0.29 μL/min/mm Hg for those aged 41 to 45 years, compared with 0.25 μL/min/mm Hg in those aged 81 to 85 years (28). No differences by sex were found for any age-group.

The tonographic method has several sources of error. First, this technique was developed with several major assumptions.

The calculations assume that only the rate of aqueous outflow changes in response to a change in IOP. However, many other ocular parameters, such as ocular blood volume (29) and ocular rigidity, also respond to pressure change, and all of them can affect the tonographic result. Ocular rigidity is an expression of the "stretchability" of the eye and represents elasticity and viscoelastic properties of the eye (30–32). An average ocular rigidity coefficient of 0.013 mm Hg/μL was used for calculating the tonographic C value, which leads to a potential source of error because of significant interpatient variation in this parameter. For this reason, it is useful to check the pressure by applanation tonometry before performing the tonography and to compare this with the P_0 obtained with the indentation tonometer, to identify any major discrepancy in ocular rigidity. Another assumption was that the C value calculations from each minute did not differ significantly; however, this was shown to be invalid, with a trend toward highest values in the first minute and progressive reduction in the ensuing minutes (33). Last, the corneal curvature was assumed as an average of 7.8 mm, but variations in the cornea may significantly influence the pressure measurements.

Second, there were some instrumentation and operating issues that contributed as a source of error. The instrument was designed with a larger hole in the electronic tonometer footplate to prevent sticking. At low scale readings, the cornea may mold into the space between the plunger and hole, pushing the plunger up and leading to falsely high pressure readings (34). During the time of these studies, variations in line voltage could produce a drift in the IOP measurements, which was minimized with line voltage stabilizers and by avoiding magnetic fields.

Third, several patient factors influence tonography studies. The IOP has been shown to drop approximately 1 mm Hg in the fellow eye while tonography is being performed on the first eye. This consensual pressure drop was once thought to have a neural cause, but it was subsequently found to be secondary to the evaporation that results from keeping the eye open for fixation during the 4-minute test (35). In addition, eye movement affected IOP measurements, which was described as a "patient-relaxation effect" during the first 15 to 20 seconds after the tonometer is placed on the cornea. So, additional time was allowed for this before starting the 4-minute tracing.

Fourth, operator error, including improper cleaning leading to a sticky tonometer, calibration, or positioning of the instrument, and improper calculation of the tracing, can also lead to inaccurate results.

Measurement of Episcleral Venous Pressure

Various techniques have been developed for measuring the pressure in the episcleral veins. All of these work on the principle of correlating partial collapse of the vein with the force required to achieve the alteration in blood flow (36). A pressure-chamber technique uses a thin membrane stretched over the tip of a hollow applanating head, which is filled with air or saline. The pressure in the chamber is raised until the bulging membrane produces the desired visible change in the adjacent vessel. Most of these instruments are mounted on a slitlamp, although a portable pressure transducer has been developed to measure episcleral venous pressure with a patient in various body positions (37). When comparing a torsion balance instrument and a pressure chamber technique to direct cannulation of the episcleral vein, the pressure chamber method was found to be superior to the torsion technique (38).

The normal episcleral venous pressure is generally considered to be between 8 and 11 mm Hg. Two features that significantly influence the measured pressure are the selected endpoint and the choice of vessel. When a pressure chamber technique was compared to direct cannulation, a slight indentation, rather than an intermittent or sustained collapse of the vein lumen, gave the most accurate reading (39). It has been suggested that the best point of measurement is just distal to the junction of aqueous and episcleral veins, although this junction is often difficult to ascertain and it may be more practical to take all measurements 3 mm from the limbus (36).

Episcleral venous pressure rises an average of 1.25 mm Hg with the pressure elevation during tonography (40), which is usually corrected for in the formula by adding 1.25 to P_0. Episcleral venous pressure measurements throughout tonography indicate that the rise is greatest during the first half of tonography, with a return to a nearly pretonographic level by the end of the procedure and a mean change in episcleral venous pressure during this time of 0.44 mm Hg.

KEY POINTS

- Gonioscopy is an essential tool used to evaluate patients with glaucoma to assess the angle anatomy.
- High-resolution ultrasound biomicroscopy and anterior-segment OCT are imaging methods to evaluate the drainage angle. High-resolution ultrasound biomicroscopy can evaluate structures, such as the ciliary body and suspicious masses, behind the iris.
- Aqueous humor flow, trabecular outflow, uveoscleral outflow, and episcleral venous pressure are the four physiological components of IOP. Functional assessment of these dynamic components is possible using fluorophotometry, tonography, and venomanometry.

REFERENCES

1. Dellaporta A. Historical notes on gonioscopy. *Surv Ophthalmol.* 1975;20(2):137–149.
2. Kapetansky FM. A bubble-free goniolens. *Ophthalmic Surg.* 1988;19(6):414–416.
3. Sussman W. Ophthalmoscopic gonioscopy. *Am J Ophthalmol.* 1968;66(3):549.
4. Alward WLM. Available at: http://www.gonioscopy.org/. Iowa City; 2009.
5. Campbell DG. A comparison of diagnostic techniques in angle-closure glaucoma. *Am J Ophthalmol.* 1979;88(2):197–204.
6. Forbes M. Gonioscopy with corneal indentation. A method for distinguishing between appositional closure and synechial closure. *Arch Ophthalmol.* 1966;76(4):488–492.

7. Rutala WA, Weber DJ, Healthcare Infection Control Practices Advisory Committee (HICPAC). Guideline for disinfection and sterilization in healthcare facilities, 2008 U.S. Centers for Disease Control and Prevention. Available at: http://www.cdc.gov/ncidod/dhqp/pdf/guidelines/Disinfection_Nov_2008.pdf. Accessed December 22, 2009.

8. Inomata H, Tawara A. Anterior and posterior parts of human trabecular meshwork. *Jpn J Ophthalmol*. 1984;28(4):339–348.

9. Shihab ZM, Lee PF. The significance of normal angle vessels. *Ophthalmic Surg*. 1985;16(6):382–385.

10. Pavlin CJ, Foster FS. Ultrasound biomicroscopy. High-frequency ultrasound imaging of the eye at microscopic resolution. *Radiol Clin North Am*. 1998;36(6):1047–1058.

11. Radhakrishnan S, Huang D, Smith SD. Optical coherence tomography imaging of the anterior chamber angle. *Ophthalmol Clin North Am*. 2005;18(3):375–381.

12. Ahmed IK, Lee RH. Utilization of Visante OCT for glaucoma evaluations. In: Steinert RF, Huang D, eds. *Anterior Segment Optical Coherence Tomography*. Thorofare, NJ: SLACK Inc.; 2008:89–106.

13. Brubaker RF. Goldmann's equation and clinical measures of aqueous dynamics. *Exp Eye Res*. 2004;78(3):633–637.

14. Goldmann H. Augendruck and gluakom. Die Kammer-wasservenen und das Poiseuille'sche Gesetz. *Ophthalmologica*. 1949;118:496–519.

15. Grant W. Tonographic method for measuring the facility and rate of aqueous flow in human eyes. *Arch Ophthalmol*. 1950;44:204–214.

16. Brubaker RF. Clinical measurements of aqueous dynamics: implications for addressing glaucoma. In: Civan MM, ed. *The Eye's Aqueous Humor, From Secretion to Glaucoma*. New York, NY: Academic Press; 1998:234–284.

17. Radenbaugh PA, Goyal A, McLaren NC, et al. Concordance of aqueous humor flow in the morning and at night in normal humans. *Invest Ophthalmol Vis Sci*. 2006;47(11):4860–4864.

18. Iyengar SK. The quest for genes causing complex traits in ocular medicine: successes, interpretations, and challenges. *Arch Ophthalmol*. 2007;125(1):11–18.

19. Toris CB, Koepsell SA, Yablonski ME, et al. Aqueous humor dynamics in ocular hypertensive patients. *J Glaucoma*. 2002;11(3):253–258.

20. Carlson KH, McLaren JW, Topper JE, et al. Effect of body position on intraocular pressure and aqueous flow. *Invest Ophthalmol Vis Sci*. 1987; 28(8):1346–1352.

21. Moses RA. Constant pressure applanation tonography. 3. The relationship of tonometric pressure to rate of loss of ocular volume. *Arch Ophthalmol*. 1967;77(2):181–184.

22. Alm A, Nilsson SF. Uveoscleral outflow—a review. *Exp Eye Res*. 2009; 88(4):760–768.

23. Toris CB, Yablonski ME, Wang YL, et al. Aqueous humor dynamics in the aging human eye. *Am J Ophthalmol*. 1999;127(4):407–412.

24. Hetland-Eriksen J, Odberg T. Experimental tonography on enucleated human eyes. II. The loss of intraocular fluid caused by tonography. *Invest Ophthalmol*. 1975;14:944–947.

25. Haik GM, Francisco Perez L, Reitman HS, et al. Tonographic tracings in patients with cardiac rhythm disturbances. *Am J Ophthalmol*. 1970; 70(6):929–934.

26. Kupfer C. Clinical significance of pseudofacility. Sanford R. Gifford Memorial Lecture. *Am J Ophthalmol*. 1973;75(2):193–204.

27. Becker B. Tonography in the diagnosis of simple (open-angle) glaucoma. *Trans Am Ophthalmol Otololaryngol*. 1961;65:156–162.

28. Johnson LV. Tonographic survey. *Am J Ophthalmol*. 1966;61:680–689.

29. Fisher RF. Value of tonometry and tonography in the diagnosis of glaucoma. *Br J Ophthalmol*. 1972;56(3):200–204.

30. Johnson CS, Mian SI, Moroi S, et al. Role of corneal elasticity in damping of intraocular pressure. *Invest Ophthalmol Vis Sci*. 2007;48(6): 2540–2544.

31. Glass DH, Roberts CJ, Litsky AS, et al. A viscoelastic biomechanical model of the cornea describing the effect of viscosity and elasticity on hysteresis. *Invest Ophthalmol Vis Sci*. 2008;49(9):3919–3926.

32. Downs JC, Suh JK, Thomas KA, et al. Viscoelastic material properties of the peripapillary sclera in normal and early-glaucoma monkey eyes. *Invest Ophthalmol Vis Sci*. 2005;46(2):540–546.

33. Armaly MF. Continuity of the tonography curve. II. Analysis of 1-minute intervals of the clinical tonogram [in German]. *Klin Monbl Augenheilkd*. 1984;184(4):299–302.

34. Moses R. Tonometry-effect of tonometer footplate hole on scale reading; further studies. *AMA Arch Ophthalmol*. 1959;61(3):373–375.

35. Grant WM, English FP. An explanation for so-called consensual pressure drop during tonography. *Arch Ophthalmol*. 1963;69:314–316.

36. Zeimer RC, Gieser DK, Wilensky JT, et al. A practical venomanometer. Measurement of episcleral venous pressure and assessment of the normal range. *Arch Ophthalmol*. 1983;101(9):1447–1449.

37. Friberg TR. Portable transducer for measurement of episcleral venous pressure. *Am J Ophthalmol*. 1986;102(3):396–397.

38. Brubaker RF. Determination of episcleral venous pressure in the eye. A comparison of three methods. *Arch Ophthalmol*. 1967;77(1):110–114.

39. Gaasterland DE, Pederson JE. Episcleral venous pressure: a comparison of invasive and noninvasive measurements. *Invest Ophthalmol Vis Sci*. 1983;24(10):1417–1422.

40. Leith AB. Episcleral venous pressure in tonography. *Br J Ophthalmol*. 1963;47:271–278.

Optic Nerve, Retina, and Choroid

4

Glaucoma is characterized by progressive atrophy of the optic nerve head secondary to the loss of optic nerve fiber. Because it is this pathologic alteration that leads to the irreversible loss of vision, an understanding of glaucomatous optic atrophy is essential in the diagnosis and management of glaucoma.

ANATOMY AND HISTOLOGY

Terminology

In the context of a discussion on glaucoma, the optic nerve head is defined as the distal portion of the optic nerve that is directly susceptible to intraocular pressure (IOP) elevation. In this sense, the optic nerve head extends anteriorly from the retinal surface to the myelinated portion of the optic nerve that begins just behind the sclera, posterior to the lamina cribrosa. The term optic nerve head is generally preferred over optic disc because the latter suggests a flat structure without depth. However, the terms disc and papilla are frequently used when referring to the portion of the optic nerve head that is clinically visible by ophthalmoscopy (1). It is the optic nerve head and nerve fiber layer containing retinal ganglion cell (RGC) axons that are most clearly associated with glaucomatous vision loss (**Fig. 4.1**).

General Description

The optic nerve head comprises the nerve fibers that originate in the ganglion cell layer of the retina and converge upon the nerve head from all points in the fundus. At the surface of the nerve head, these RGC axons bend acutely to exit the globe through a fenestrated scleral canal, called the lamina cribrosa. In the nerve head, the axons are grouped into approximately 1000 fascicles, or bundles, and are supported by astrocytes. There is considerable variation in the size of the optic nerve head. In one study, the diameter varied from 1.18 to 1.75 mm (2). Other studies have revealed ranges of 0.85 to 2.43 mm in the shortest diameter and 1.21 to 2.86 mm in the longest (3), or a mean of 1.88 mm vertically and 1.77 mm horizontally (4). The disc area may range from 0.68 mm^2 to 4.42 mm^2 (3). In a large, population-based study, the average disc area was 2.42 mm^2 (5). In a different study, the average disc area was 2.56 mm^2 when measured by the Heidelberg retina tomograph (HRT) and 2.79 mm^2 by the analysis of disc photographs (6). When optic nerve head area and neuroretinal rim area were determined in 36 radial 10-degree segments on stereophotographs, cup area had stronger correlation with the disc area than the rim area, suggesting that correction for disc size may be more important for cup area than for rim area (7). Another study showed a positive correlation between the optic disc size and the thickness of the peripapillary retinal nerve fiber layer (RNFL) (8).

Studies using a confocal scanning laser tomograph showed that in healthy eyes the neuroretinal rim area and optic disc diameter have a higher correlation with the optic nerve head configuration than with age, sex, or refractive error (9). The diameter and the area may vary depending on the definition of the edge of the optic disc and methods of measurement (4,10,11). Therefore, some authors have suggested applying various formulas to correct magnification of images when comparing disc measurements on different instruments (12,13).

The diameter of the nerve expands to approximately 3 mm just behind the sclera, where the neurons acquire a myelin

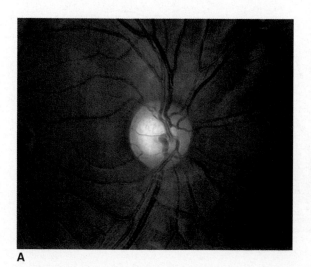

A

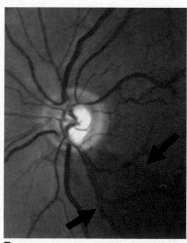

B

Figure 4.1 **A:** Optic nerve head with physiologic enlarged cupping demonstrating robust, symmetric, and healthy RNFL. **B:** Glaucomatous optic nerve showing an inferotemporal notch and corresponding loss of the RNFL that is appreciated by "baring" of the retinal vessels. The point of the (*arrows*) delimits the RNFL defect.

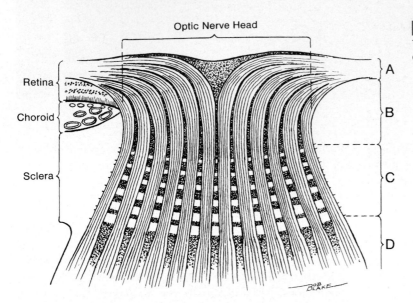

Optic Nerve Head

Retina

Choroid

Sclera

A
B
C
D

Figure 4.2   Divisions of the optic nerve head. **A:** Surface nerve fiber layer. **B:** Prelaminar region. **C:** Lamina cribrosa region. **D:** Retrolaminar region.

sheath. The optic nerve head is also the site of entry and exit of the retinal vessels. This vascular system supplies some branches to the optic nerve head, although the predominant blood supply for the nerve head comes from the ciliary circulation.

Divisions of the Optic Nerve Head

The nerve head may be arbitrarily divided into four portions from anterior to posterior (14) (**Fig. 4.2**).

Surface Nerve Fiber Layer

The innermost portion of the optic nerve head is composed predominantly of nerve fibers. In the rhesus monkey, this layer is 94% RGC axons and 5% astrocytes (15). The axonal bundles acquire progressively more interaxonal glial tissue in the intraocular portion of the nerve head as this structure is followed posteriorly (15).

Prelaminar Region

The prelaminar region is also called the anterior portion of the lamina cribrosa (16). The predominant structures at this level are nerve axons and astrocytes, with a significant increase in the quantity of astroglial tissue.

Lamina Cribrosa Region

This portion contains fenestrated sheets of scleral connective tissue and occasional elastic fibers. Astrocytes separate the sheets and line the fenestrae (16), and the fascicles of neurons leave the eye through these openings.

Retrolaminar Region

This area is characterized by a decrease in astrocytes and the acquisition of myelin that is supplied by oligodendrocytes. The axonal bundles are surrounded by connective tissue septa.

The posterior extent of the retrolaminar region is not clearly defined. An India ink study of monkey eyes showed nonfilling with the ink for 3 to 4 mm behind the lamina cribrosa when the IOP was elevated (17). However, a similar study using unlabeled microspheres showed an increased blood flow in the retrolaminar region close to the lamina even when the IOP was elevated high enough to stop retinal blood flow (18).

Vasculature

Arterial Supply

Posterior ciliary artery circulation is the main source of blood supply to the optic nerve head (19), except for the nerve fiber layer—which is supplied by the retinal circulation. The blood supply in the optic nerve head has a sectoral distribution (20). The four divisions of the optic nerve head correlate roughly with a four-part vascular supply (**Fig. 4.3**).

The surface nerve fiber layer is mainly supplied by arteriolar branches of the central retinal artery, which anastomose with vessels of the prelaminar region and are continuous with

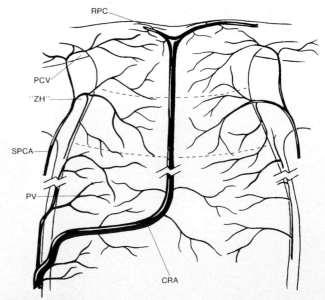

RPC

PCV

"ZH"

SPCA

PV

CRA

Figure 4.3   Vascular supply of the optic nerve head. *CRA*, central retinal artery; *RPC*, radial peripapillary capillaries; *PV*, pial vessels; *SPCA*, short posterior ciliary arteries; *PCV*, peripapillary choroidal vessels; *ZH*, "circle" of Zinn–Haller.

the peripapillary retinal and long radial peripapillary capillaries (14,19,21). The temporal region may also be supplied by one or more of the ciliary-derived vessels from the posterior ciliary artery circulation in the deeper prelaminar region, which may occasionally enlarge to form cilioretinal arteries (14). The cilioretinal artery, when present, usually supplies the corresponding sector of the surface layer (20). In elderly rhesus monkeys, central retinal artery occlusion for less than 100 minutes produced no apparent evidence of optic nerve damage. However, longer occlusion produced a variable degree of damage (22).

The prelaminar and laminar regions are supplied primarily by short posterior ciliary arteries, which form a perineural, circular arterial anastomosis at the scleral level, called the circle of Zinn–Haller (14,19,21,23). Branches from this circle penetrate the optic nerve to supply the prelaminar and laminar regions and the peripapillary choroid (19). The circle is not present in all eyes, in which case direct branches from the short posterior ciliary arteries supply the anterior optic nerve. The peripapillary choroid may also minimally contribute to anterior optic nerve (14,19,21,23).

The retrolaminar region is supplied by both the ciliary and retinal circulations, with the former coming from recurrent pial vessels. Medial and lateral perioptic nerve short posterior ciliary arteries anastomose to form an elliptical arterial circle around the optic nerve, which has also been referred to as the circle of Zinn–Haller (24,25). This perioptic nerve arteriolar anastomosis, which supplies the retrolaminar optic nerve, was found to be complete in 75% of 18 human eyes in one study (24). The central retinal artery provides centripetal branches from the pial system and frequently, but not always, gives off centrifugal vessels (20).

Continuity between small vessels from the retrolaminar region to the retinal surface has been observed (21), and the optic nerve head microvasculature is said to represent an integral part of the retina–optic nerve vascular system (23).

Capillaries

Although derived from both the retinal and ciliary circulations, the capillaries of the optic nerve head resemble more closely the features of retinal capillaries than of the choriocapillaris. These characteristics include (a) tight junctions, (b) abundant pericytes, and (c) nonfenestrated endothelium (23). They do not leak fluorescein and may represent a nerve–blood barrier, supporting the concept of the retina–nerve vasculature as a continuous system with the central nervous system (21,23). The capillaries decrease in number posterior to the lamina, especially along the margins of the larger vessels (26).

Venous Drainage

The venous drainage from the optic nerve head is almost entirely through the central retinal vein (19), although a small portion may occur through the choroidal system (27). Occasionally, these communications are enlarged as retinociliary veins, which drain from the retina to the choroidal circulation, or cilio-optic veins, which drain from the choroid to the central retinal vein (28).

Astroglial Support

Astrocytes provide a continuous layer between the nerve fibers and blood vessels in the optic nerve head (29). In the rhesus monkey, astrocytes occupy 5% of the nerve fiber layer, increase to 23% of the laminar region, and then decrease to 11% in the retrolaminar area (15). The astrocytes are joined by "gap junctions," which resemble tight junctions but have minute gaps between the outer membrane leaflets (30).

Thick- and thin-bodied astrocytes have been described. The thin-bodied astrocytes accompany the axons in the nerve fiber layer, and the thick-bodied astrocytes direct axons in the prelaminar region toward the laminar region (31).

The astroglial tissue also provides a covering for portions of the optic nerve head (**Fig. 4.4**). The internal limiting membrane of Elschnig separates the nerve head from the vitreous and is continuous with the internal limiting membrane of the retina (29,32–34). The central portion of the internal limiting membrane is referred to as the central meniscus of Kuhnt (33). Although the central meniscus of Kuhnt is traditionally described as a central thickening of the internal limiting membrane, ultrastructural studies of the monkey optic nerve head revealed a thinning of 20 nm centrally, which thickened to 70 nm peripherally (34). The Müller cells are a major constitutional element of the intermediary tissue of Kuhnt (35), which separates the nerve from the retina, whereas the border tissue of Jacoby separates the nerve from the choroid (16,33).

Astrocytes also play a major role in the remodeling of the extracellular matrix of the optic nerve head and synthesizing growth factors and other cellular mediators that may affect the axons of the RGCs and contribute to health or susceptibility to disease (36).

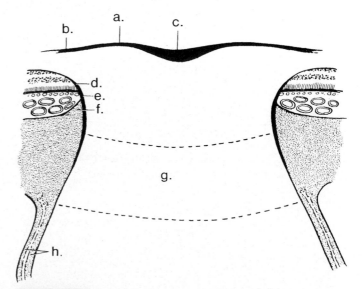

Figure 4.4 Supportive structures of the optic nerve head: internal limiting membrane of Elschnig (*a*); continuous with the internal limiting membrane of the retina (*b*); central meniscus of Kuhnt (*c*); intermediary tissue of Kuhnt (*d*); border tissue of Jacoby (*e*); border tissue of Elschnig (*f*); lamina cribrosa (*g*); meningeal sheaths (*h*).

Connective Tissue Support

Lamina Cribrosa

This structure is not simply a porous region of the sclera but also a specialized extracellular matrix that consists of fenestrated sheets of connective tissue and occasional elastic fibers lined by astrocytes (16,37). Astrocytes may respond to changes in IOP in glaucoma, leading to axonal loss and RGC degeneration at the level of lamina cribrosa (36). Extracellular matrix components in the lamina cribrosa differ from those in sclera or pial septa (38), which may be important in the pathogenesis of glaucomatous optic nerve damage. Hyaluronate was found surrounding the myelin sheaths in the retrolaminar nerve, playing an important role in the maintenance of the hydrodynamic properties of the extracellular matrix. Hyaluronate decreases with age and is further reduced in eyes with chronic open-angle glaucoma (COAG), possibly increasing susceptibility to elevated IOP (39). The lamina cribrosa has also been found to be significantly thinner in glaucomatous eyes than in nonglaucomatous eyes (40).

Analysis of the pores in the lamina cribrosa with a confocal scanning laser ophthalmoscope shows nearly round pores in the eyes with physiologic cupping, whereas eyes with COAG frequently have compressed pores (41). There are regional differences in the fenestration or pores through which the axons pass. The superior and inferior portions, compared with the nasal and temporal regions, have larger single pore areas and summed pore areas and thinner connective tissue and glial cell support (42–45) (**Fig. 4.5**). The ratio of single and summed pore areas

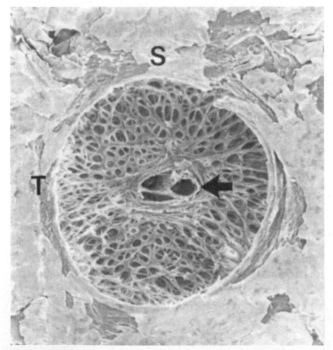

Figure 4.5 Gross anatomic photograph of lamina cribrosa showing central openings for central retinal vessels *(arrow)* and surrounding fenestrae of lamina for passage of axon bundles. Note larger size of fenestrae in superior and inferior quadrants. *S*, superior; *T*, temporal. (Courtesy of Harry A. Quigley, MD.)

between the laminar regions decreases with increasing lamina cribrosa area, but does not correlate with age or sex (45). A majority of RGC axons take a direct course through the lamina cribrosa (46), but about 10% of axons exit more peripherally, where the lamina cribrosa is more curvilinear, which may influence the regional susceptibility for glaucomatous optic nerve fiber loss (47). The size of the laminar openings for the retinal vessels does not correlate with the lamina cribrosa area (45).

As mentioned previously, the lamina cribrosa of the human optic nerve head contains a specialized extracellular matrix composed of collagen types I through VI, laminin, and fibronectin (48–50). Studies of young human donor eyes show that the cribriform plates are composed of a core of elastin fibers with a sparse, patchy distribution of collagen type III, coated with collagen type IV and laminin (48). Cell cultures of human lamina cribrosa reveal two cell types, which appear to synthesize this extracellular matrix (51). The expression of mRNA for collagen types I and IV in both fetal and adult human optic nerve heads suggests that these extracellular matrix proteins are synthesized in this tissue throughout life (52). Proteoglycans, which are macromolecular components of connective tissue believed to have a role in the organization of other extracellular matrix components and in the hydration and rigidity of tissue, have been identified in the cores of the laminar plates in association with collagen fibers (53,54). Cell adhesive proteins, including vitronectin and thrombospondin, have been found in human lamina cribrosa (38). Abnormalities of this extracellular matrix in the lamina cribrosa may influence optic nerve function and its susceptibility to glaucomatous damage caused by elevated IOP. Lamina cribrosa cells from glaucomatous eyes express more profibrotic genes than cells from normal lamina cribrosa do (55). These differences in extracellular matrix probably translate into difference in biomechanical properties (56,57).

Nerve Sheaths

A rim of connective tissue, the border tissue of Elschnig, occasionally extends between the choroid and optic nerve tissues, especially temporally (33) (Fig. 4.4). Posterior to the globe, the optic nerve is surrounded by meningeal sheaths (pia, arachnoid, and dura), which consist of connective tissue lined by meningothelial cells, or mesothelium (58). Lymphatic capillaries in the dura of the human optic nerve have been described (59). Vascularized connective tissue extends from the undersurface of the pia mater to form longitudinal septa, which partially separate the axonal bundles in the intraorbital portion of the optic nerve (33).

Axons

Retinal Nerve Fiber Layer

As the axons traverse the nerve fiber layer from the ganglion cell bodies to the optic nerve head, they are distributed in a characteristic pattern (**Fig. 4.6**). Fibers from the temporal periphery originate on either side of a horizontal dividing line, the median raphe, and arch above or below the fovea as the arcuate nerve fibers, while those from the central retina, the

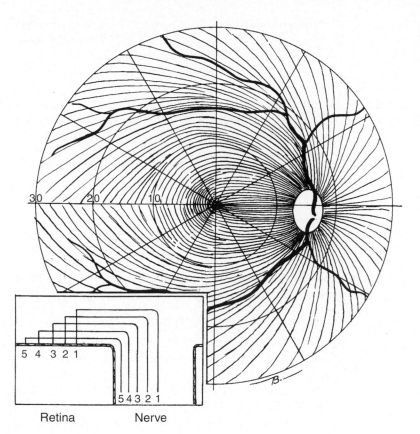

Figure 4.6 Distribution of retinal nerve fibers. Note arching above and below the fovea of fibers temporal to the optic nerve head. *Inset* depicts cross-sectional arrangement of axons, with fibers originating from peripheral retina running closer to choroid and periphery of optic nerve, while fibers originating nearer to the nerve head are situated closer to the vitreous and occupy a more central portion of the nerve.

papillomacular fibers, and the nasal fibers take a more direct path to the nerve head. The significance of this anatomy to the visual field defects of glaucoma is discussed in Chapter 5. The axons in monkeys and rabbits are grouped into fiber bundles by tissue tunnels composed of elongated processes of Müller cells (60–62). These bundles, especially on the temporal side, become larger as they approach the nerve head, primarily because of lateral fusion of bundles (63), and are normally visible by ophthalmoscopy as retinal striations (62). The axons in the bundles vary in size, with larger fibers coming from the more peripheral retina (63). One study also demonstrated that intra-RGC axons contain numerous bulb-shaped varicosities in humans of different ages (64).

Axons in Optic Nerve Head

The arcuate nerve fibers occupy the superior and inferior temporal portions of the optic nerve head, with axons from the peripheral retina taking a more peripheral position in the nerve head (Fig. 4.6) (65). The arcuate fibers are the most susceptible to early glaucomatous damage. The papillomacular fibers spread over approximately one third of the distal optic nerve, primarily inferior temporally, where the axonal density is higher (66,67). They intermingle with extramacular fibers, which may explain the retention of central vision in early glaucomatous optic atrophy.

The mean axonal population in the normal human optic nerve head, as measured by computed image analysis of sections throughout the nerve, ranges from approximately 700,000 fibers to 1.2 million fibers (67–70). The optic nerve

fiber count has been shown to increase significantly with the optic nerve head area in human and monkey eyes, although another study of human eyes showed no such correlation (69,71,72). A positive correlation has also been demonstrated between the retinal photoreceptor count and optic nerve area (73). The reported mean axonal fiber diameter ranges from 0.65 to 1.10 μm (67,68,74). Axons of all sizes are mixed throughout the nerve area, although higher mean diameters appear to be more common in the nasal segment (67).

EMBRYOLOGY OF THE RETINA AND OPTIC NERVE

The retina and optic nerve develop from the optic cup and the contiguous optic stalk (75–80).

The inner layer of the cup contains the pluripotent retinal progenitor cells, which differentiate in a specific chronologic sequence and defined histogenic order into the final seven retinal cell types (see Fig. 1.3 in Chapter 1). In general, the RGCs differentiate first (81,82), followed by the cone photoreceptors, amacrine cells, horizontal cells, and finally, the rod photoreceptors, bipolar cells, and Müller cells. Retinal neurogenesis starts in the central optic cup region and then fans out concentrically in a wavelike pattern into the periphery. There is a basic topographic organization of the optic cup with dorsoventral and nasotemporal patterning (83), which involves certain genetic cues, including that of the *Otx* genes (84).

The optic fissure of the optic stalk closes to convert it into a cylinder, into which the RGC axons grow. The lumen of the optic stalk is obliterated by axons by approximately the third fetal month. Apoptosis, or selective cell death, and cell cycle regulators are important in normal ocular development (85–87). The optic nerve axon count in humans peaks at approximately 3.7 million by fetal week 16 to 17 and then rapidly declines to near adult levels of around 1 million by term (88). Epithelial cells in the walls of the stalk differentiate into the neuroglia of the optic nerve. Mesenchymal tissue gives rise to the optic nerve septa in the third month and to the lamina cribrosa in the final month of gestation.

Key regulatory genes involved in the early development of the eye and the fate of retinal cells include *Pax6*, *Rx1*, *Six3/6*, *Lhx2*, and certain basic helix–loop–helix transcription factors. The expression of these genes and their effect on retinal neurogenesis and differentiation are considered "cell-intrinsic" mechanisms, whereas "extrinsic" mechanisms include thyroid hormones and their receptors, fibroblast growth factors and other "growth factors," hedgehog proteins, various neurotrophins, and nitric oxide (75,89–95).

The optic nerve cross-sectional area reaches 50% of the adult size by 20 weeks' gestation, 75% at birth, and 95% before 1 year of age (96). At birth, the optic nerve is nearly unmyelinated (97), and myelination, which proceeds from the brain to the eye during gestation, is largely completed in the retrolaminar region of the optic nerve by the first year of life (98). The connective tissue of the lamina cribrosa is also incompletely developed at birth, which may account for the increased susceptibility of the infant nerve head to glaucomatous cupping and its potential for reversible cupping (99). With increasing age, the cores of the cribriform plates enlarge, and the apparent density of collagen types I, III, and IV and elastin increases (100,101). Not only does elastin increase with age, but also elastic fibers become thicker, tubular, and surrounded by densely packed collagen fibers (101). Proteoglycan filaments in the human lamina cribrosa also decrease in length and diameter with age (102). Also with increasing age, there appears to be a progressive loss of axons with a decrease of the nerve fiber layer thickness (103,104) and a corresponding increase in the cross-sectional area occupied by the leptomeninges and fibrous septa (67–70). The loss of axons has been estimated to be between 4000 and 12,000 per year, with most studies nearer the lower figure (67,69,70,105). One study suggested a selective loss of large nerve fibers with age (68), although this has not been confirmed by others (67,74).

PATHOPHYSIOLOGY OF GLAUCOMATOUS OPTIC NERVE DAMAGE

Theories

The pathogenesis of glaucomatous optic atrophy has remained a matter of controversy since the mid-19th century, when two concepts were introduced in the same year. In 1858, Müller (106) proposed that the elevated IOP led to direct compression and death of the neurons (the mechanical theory), while von Jaeger (107) suggested that a vascular abnormality was the underlying cause of the optic atrophy (the vascular theory). In 1892, Schnabel (108) proposed another concept in the pathogenesis of glaucomatous optic atrophy, suggesting that atrophy of neural elements created empty spaces, which pulled the nerve head posteriorly (Schnabel cavernous atrophy).

Initially, the mechanical theory received the greatest support (109–111). This concept held sway through the first quarter of the 20th century until LaGrange and Beauvieux (112) popularized the vascular theory in 1925. In general, this belief held that glaucomatous optic atrophy was secondary to ischemia, whether the primary result of the elevated IOP or an unrelated vascular lesion (113–115). In 1968, however, the role of axoplasmic flow in glaucomatous optic atrophy was introduced (116), which revived support for the mechanical theory, but did not exclude the possible influence of ischemia.

Evidence

Continued investigation into the pathogenesis of glaucomatous optic atrophy has led to the following bodies of information.

Anatomic and Histopathologic Studies

Histopathologic observations of human eyes with glaucoma provide the most direct method of studying the alterations associated with glaucomatous optic atrophy, although they do not fully explain the mechanisms that caused the damage. One of the limiting factors has been that many of the specimens studied have come from eyes with advanced glaucomatous change, which led to possible misconceptions regarding the early pathogenic features. More recent studies, which have attempted to correlate clinical observations with histopathologic changes in optic nerve heads from eyes with varying stages of glaucoma, appear to clarify many of these points.

Glial Alterations

It was once suggested that loss of astroglial supportive tissue precedes neuronal loss (117), which was thought to explain the early and reversible cupping in infants (118). However, subsequent studies have shown that glial cells are not selectively lost in early glaucoma and are actually the only remaining cells after loss of axons in advanced cases (119,120).

Vascular Alterations

It was also once proposed that loss of small vessels in the optic nerve head accompanies atrophy of axons (121), and one histologic study suggested a selective loss of retinal radial peripapillary capillaries in eyes with chronic glaucoma (122). However, subsequent investigations revealed neither a correlation between atrophy of this vascular system and visual field loss nor a major selective loss of optic nerve head capillaries in human eyes with glaucoma (119,120,123,124). In animal models of optic atrophy, created by either sustained IOP elevation, sectioning of the optic nerve, or photocoagulation of the RNFL, the resulting disc pallor was not associated with a decrease in the ratio of capillaries to neural tissue, although the caliber of the vessels diminished (124–128). Instead, these studies showed a proliferation or reorganization of glial tissue, which obscures ophthalmoscopic visualization of the vessels (125,126,128).

Alterations of the Lamina Cribrosa

Backward bowing of the lamina cribrosa has long been recognized as a characteristic feature of late glaucomatous optic atrophy (129,130), and as an early change in the infant eye with glaucoma (99). Further study, however, has suggested that alterations in the lamina may actually be a primary event in the pathogenesis of glaucomatous optic atrophy. In enucleated human eyes, acute IOP elevation causes a backward bowing of the lamina (131,132), and similar changes are observed in primate glaucoma models (133,134) with compensatory remodeling and fibrosis (135).

Most of the posterior displacement occurred in the peripheral lamina cribrosa, corresponding to the region of early axonal loss (132). In a histopathologic evaluation of 25 glaucomatous human eyes, compression of successive lamina cribrosa sheets was the earliest detected abnormality, and backward bowing of the entire lamina occurred later and involved primarily the upper and lower poles (136).

In the early stages of adult glaucoma, the magnitude of backward bowing is not sufficient to explain the ophthalmoscopically observed cupping, but may be enough to produce a pressure gradient along the axoplasm of exiting optic nerve axons, compromise the circulation (137), and cause compression of the axons. It has been suggested that the structure of the lamina cribrosa may be an important determinant in the susceptibility of the optic nerve head to damage from elevated IOP (119,120). However, racial comparison of the relative connective tissue support and regional pore size of the lamina cribrosa did not explain the increased susceptibility of blacks to glaucomatous damage (138). The extracellular matrix

of the lamina cribrosa may play an important role in the progression of glaucomatous damage (139–141). In glaucomatous monkey eyes, increased collagen type IV and laminin lined the margins of the laminar beams (140,141), and collagen types I, III, and IV were found in the pores of the beams (140). Elastin, which is the major protein of elastic fibers and responsible for elastic recoil, appeared curled instead of straight and seemed disconnected from other elements of the connective tissue matrix in glaucomatous eyes of humans and monkeys (142). Elastin mRNA expression in human eyes with COAG suggests synthesis of abnormal elastic fibers (143). These changes may be secondary to long-standing elevation of IOP and may modify the course of glaucomatous optic atrophy.

Axonal Alterations

The actual cause of early optic nerve head cupping in glaucoma appears to be the loss of axonal tissue (119,120,144). Experimental models of primate eyes exposed to chronic IOP elevation suggest that the damage is associated with a posterior and lateral displacement of the lamina cribrosa, which compresses the axons and disrupts axoplasmic flow (145). The damage first involves axonal bundles throughout the nerve with somewhat greater involvement of the inferior and superior poles (136). With continued optic nerve damage, the susceptibility of the polar zones becomes more prominent (**Fig. 4.7**) (119,120,136,144). Histologic studies of both monkey and human optic nerves indicate that nerve fibers larger than the normal mean diameter atrophy more rapidly in glaucomatous eyes, although no fiber size is spared from damage (146,147). This preferential loss of large fibers appears to be due to a higher proportion of the fibers in

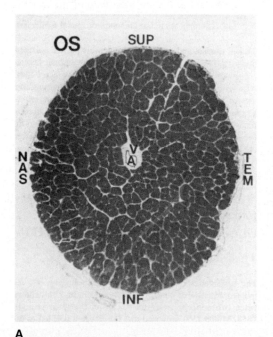
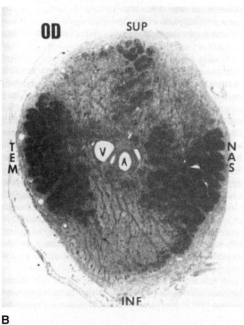

A   **B**

Figure 4.7   **A:** Light microscopic view of normal optic nerve head on cross section with darkly staining axon bundles and intervening glial supportive tissue surrounding openings for central retinal vessels. **B:** Light microscopic cross-sectional view of optic nerve head with glaucomatous atrophy showing loss of axon bundles predominantly in the inferior and superior quadrants (compare with normal nerve head in A). *INF*, inferior; *NAS*, nasal; *SUP*, superior; *TEM*, temporal. (Courtesy of Harry A. Quigley, MD.)

the inferior and superior poles, and an inherent susceptibility to injury by glaucoma (146,147).

In the retina of glaucomatous monkey eyes, there is also a selective loss of the larger ganglion cells in both the midperiphery and fovea, and it has been suggested that psychophysical testing should be aimed at these cells in the early stages of glaucoma (148,149). The same animal studies suggest that RGCs in glaucoma die by apoptosis, a genetically programmed process of cell death, characterized histologically by chromatin condensation and intracellular fragmentation (150). This apoptosis is possibly related to loss of trophic influences resulting from inhibited transmission of neurotrophic signals from axon terminals to neuronal cell bodies; histologic studies have also shown a significant decrease of corpora amylacea, which are homogeneous oval bodies believed to correlate with axonal degeneration, in RGCs and the optic nerve of human eyes with advancing stages of glaucoma (151,152). One study revealed a significant reduction in photoreceptor count in human eyes with angle-closure glaucoma associated with trauma (153), although this was not observed in human eyes with COAG or in monkey eyes with experimental glaucoma (154,155).

Secondary degeneration has been reported to occur after experimental injury of RGCs, causing loss of neighboring RGCs as an indirect effect of the injury and death of transected RGCs. Glutamate levels in the vitreous did not increase at 3 months after injury, suggesting the need for further investigations of the mechanisms of secondary degeneration (156).

Blood-Flow Studies

Blood flow in the optic nerve head of cats is relatively high compared with that in more posterior portions of the nerve, and autoregulation appears to compensate for alterations in mean arterial blood pressure (157). With elevation of IOP, blood flow in the optic nerve head, retina, and choroid of cat eyes is only slightly affected before the pressure is within 25 mm Hg of the mean arterial blood pressure, and flow in the lamina cribrosa is reduced only with extreme pressure elevations, again suggesting autoregulation in the optic nerve head (158). Another study, however, suggests that the electrical function of ganglion cell axons in cat eyes depends on the perfusion pressure and not on the absolute height of the IOP (159). Real-time analysis of optic nerve head oxidative metabolism in cats indicates that the metabolic response is dependent on IOP or mean arterial pressure and that lowering the IOP can reverse metabolic dysfunction (160).

Short-term IOP elevation in monkey eyes did not alter optic nerve head blood flow until it exceeded 75 mm Hg, and long-term glaucoma in monkeys had no apparent influence on mean blood flow in the nerve head (161); others have shown that the threshold of IOP that is needed to affect blood flow is partly determined by the animal's systemic blood pressure (162). A study of oxygen tension in the monkey optic nerve head suggested that autoregulation compensates for changes in perfusion pressure (163), and a noninvasive phosphorescence imaging technique in cats revealed well-maintained oxygen tension in the optic nerve head and retina despite increasing IOP, until blood flow to the eye was stopped (164).

Blood-flow measurements in the optic nerve head of human eyes, using laser Doppler, demonstrate autoregulatory compensation to reduced perfusion pressure secondary to elevated IOP (165). In glaucomatous eyes, however, Doppler studies show reduced flow velocity in the nerve head (166–169). Blood flow of the optic nerve head lamina, rim area, and retrobulbar flow is decreased with increasing glaucomatous damage (170,171). Eyes with glaucoma also appear to have more diurnal fluctuation of optic nerve blood flow (172).

A technique of continuously monitoring disc brightness during and after an abrupt artificial elevation of IOP also showed that the extent to which a glaucomatous eye can adjust to the pressure changes is significantly reduced from that of nonglaucomatous eyes (173). Diminished autoregulatory response to postural changes in the retinal vasculature of patients with glaucoma is also seen (174). Age may influence the vascular responses to IOP. One study showed that major retinal vessels at the disc border increased in caliber in response to IOP reduction in patients with COAG who were 55 years or younger, but not after that age (175). In children, intracranial pressure also affects optic nerve blood flow (176). It may be that ischemia of the optic nerve head in glaucoma involves faulty autoregulation, which may worsen with age and is also affected by systemic blood pressure and intracranial blood pressure (158,177,178). Molecules such as endothelin and nitric oxide are being investigated for their possible role in the normal and altered autoregulatory responses (179,180).

Fluorescein Angiography

Normal Fluorescein Pattern

The normal fluorescein pattern of the optic nerve head is usually described as having three phases (14):

In the first phase, an initial filling, or preretinal arterial, phase is thought to represent filling of the prelaminar and lamina cribrosa regions by the posterior ciliary arteries. Fluorescein in the retrobulbar vessels may also contribute to this phase (181).

The peak fluorescence, or retinal arteriovenous phase, is primarily due to filling of the dense capillary plexus on the nerve head surface from retinal arterioles. With increasing age, there is a decrease in the filling time of both the retinal and choroidal circulations (182).

A late phase consists of 10 to 15 minutes of delayed staining of the nerve head, probably because of fluorescein in the connective tissue of the lamina cribrosa. Tracer studies in monkeys suggest that the leakage may come from the adjacent choroid (183).

Effect of Artificially Elevated IOP

The effect of artificially elevated IOP on the fluorescein angiographic pattern has provided an understanding of the relative vulnerability of ocular vessels to elevated pressure in the normal and glaucomatous eyes. There is a general delay in the entire ocular circulation in response to an elevation of the IOP. The prelaminar portion of the nerve head appears to be the most vulnerable portion of the ocular vascular system to elevated pressure in monkeys (14,184).

Studies regarding the vulnerability of the peripapillary choroid to IOP elevation have provided conflicting results. Fluorescein angiography of monkey eyes has suggested a marked susceptibility of this vascular system to elevated pressure (14,184), and fluorescein studies of human eyes with glaucoma have shown similar delays in peripapillary choroidal filling (184–188). The delay appears to be sensitive to elevated IOP (185). It has been suggested that this vascular disturbance of the peripapillary choroid contributes to glaucomatous optic atrophy (187). However, fluorescein angiographic studies of normal human eyes have shown similar delayed or irregular choroidal filling at normal pressures (189,190), and the peripapillary choroidal capillaries of normal human eyes were relatively resistant to artificial pressure elevations (191). Furthermore, a fluorescein study of patients with low-tension glaucoma or COAG provided no evidence that hypoperfusion of the peripapillary choroid contributed to optic nerve hypoperfusion (192).

A selective nonfilling of the retinal radial peripapillary capillaries during India ink perfusion has been demonstrated in cats (193). As previously discussed, however, histopathologic observations differ regarding alterations of this vascular system in glaucomatous eyes (122,123). Most studies of monkey and normal human eyes have shown the choroidal circulation in general to be more vulnerable than that of the retina to elevated IOP (14,184,187,194), although one study found the two systems to fill at the same level of increased pressure (195). Regional differences in circulation of the optic nerve head, retina, and peripapillary choroid have been reported (196).

Studies of Glaucomatous Eyes

Fluorescein angiographic studies of glaucomatous and nonglaucomatous eyes have revealed two types of filling defects of the optic nerve head: (a) persisting hypoperfusion and (b) transient hypoperfusion (192,197).

Persisting hypoperfusion, or absolute filling defects, is more common in eyes with glaucoma, especially low-tension glaucoma, and are said to correlate with visual field loss (192,197,198). The characteristics of a filling defect include decreased blood flow, a smaller vascular bed, narrower vessels, and increased permeability of the vessels (199). The filling defect may be either focal or diffuse. The former is thought to reflect susceptible vasculature with or without elevated IOP, and is the typical defect in low-tension glaucoma (192). Focal defects occur primarily in the inferior and superior poles of the optic nerve head (197,198,200). In glaucomatous eyes, they are most often seen in the wall of the cup, whereas in nonglaucomatous eyes they occur more commonly in the floor of the cup (201). The diffuse defect is thought to represent prolonged pressure elevation (192).

The nature of the defect in COAG is thought to be specific, and fluorescein angiography of the optic nerve head may help to differentiate COAG from other conditions that have similar clinical changes in the optic disc (202). Computed image analysis has been used to objectively quantify fluorescein angiograms of the optic disc and has shown that increases in fluorescein-filling defect areas correlate with glaucomatous progression (203).

In patients with low-tension glaucoma, retinal arteriovenous passage times are prolonged in fluorescein angiography, possibly from the increased resistance in the central retinal and posterior ciliary arteries. Arteriovenous passage correlated with the size of the optic nerve head, visual field indices, and contrast sensitivity (204).

Axoplasmic Flow

Physiology of Axoplasmic Flow

Axoplasmic flow, or axonal transport, refers to the movement of material (axoplasm) along the axon of a nerve (the dendrite may also have transport) in a predictable, energy-dependent manner. This movement has been characterized as having fast and slow components, although numerous intermediate rates may also exist (205). The fast phase moves approximately 410 mm/day in various species and may supply material to synaptic vesicles, the axolemma, and agranular endoplasmic reticulum of the axon; the slow phase moves at 1 to 3 mm/day and is believed to subserve growth and maintenance of axons (205). The flow of axoplasm may be orthograde (from retina to lateral geniculate body) or retrograde (lateral geniculate body to retina) (206).

Experimental Models of Axoplasmic Flow

Animal models (usually in monkeys) have been developed for studying axoplasmic flow by injecting radioactive amino acids, such as tritiated leucine, into the vitreous. In other animal models, the results may have less generalizability to human glaucoma because of species differences of the lamina cribrosa region; some animals do not have a lamina. The amino acid is incorporated into the protein synthesis of RGCs and then moves down the ganglion cell axon into the optic nerve, allowing histologic study of the orthograde movement of radioactively labeled protein (207). In addition, retrograde flow can be studied by observing the accumulation of certain unlabeled neuronal components, such as mitochondria by electron microscopy (208), or by injecting tracer elements, such as horseradish peroxidase into the lateral geniculate body and studying its movement toward the retina (209). These models can be used to study factors that cause abnormal blockade of axoplasmic flow, which may relate to glaucomatous optic atrophy in the human eye.

Influence of IOP on Axoplasmic Flow

Elevated IOP in monkey eyes causes obstruction of axoplasmic flow at the lamina cribrosa and the edge of the posterior scleral foramen (206,210–215). Axonal transport in monkey eyes with chronic IOP elevation is also preferentially decreased in the magnocellular layers of the dorsal lateral geniculate nucleus, to which the large RGCs project (216). The obstruction in general involves both the fast and slow phases, and the orthograde and retrograde components (206,211,213,214). In monkey eyes, the obstruction to fast axonal transport preferentially involves the superior, temporal, and inferior portions of the optic nerve head (217). The height and duration of pressure elevation influence the onset, distribution, and degree of axoplasmic obstruction in the optic nerve head (214,218,219). The mechanism by which elevated IOP leads to obstruction of axoplasmic flow is uncertain, but there are two popular theories: mechanical and vascular.

The mechanical theory suggests that physical alterations in the optic nerve head lead to misalignment of the fenestrae in the lamina cribrosa and may result in axoplasmic flow obstruction (116,130,214). In support of this hypothesis is the observation that elevated IOP leads to blockage of axonal transport despite an intact nerve head capillary circulation and an elevated arterial pO_2 (206,220). Furthermore, obstruction of axoplasmic flow has also been reported in response to ocular hypotony (211,213,221), leading some investigators to suggest that a pressure differential across the optic nerve head, whether due to a relative increase or decrease in IOP, causes mechanical changes with compression of the axonal bundles (211,213, 221,222). In the laminar portion of pig ganglion cell axons, cytoskeletal changes are seen before disruption of axoplasmic flow; the disruption of axoplasmic flow was observed to be greater in the axons of the periphery of the optic nerve, favoring a mechanical issue as the primary pathologic process (223).

In conflict with the mechanical theory is the observation that elevated intracranial pressure in monkeys neither caused obstruction of rapid axoplasmic flow nor prevented it in response to elevated IOP, despite reduction in the pressure gradient across the lamina (224). This suggests that more than a simple mechanical or hydrostatic mechanism may be involved with obstruction of axoplasmic flow in response to elevated IOP (224). Also against the simple mechanical theory are the observations that axon damage is diffuse within bundles, rather than focal, as might be expected with a kinking effect (225), and the location of transport interruption does not correlate with the cross-sectional area of fiber bundles, the shape of the laminar pores, or the density of interbundle septa (226,227).

The vascular theory suggests that ischemia at least plays a role in the obstruction of axoplasmic flow in response to elevated IOP. Interruption of the short posterior ciliary arteries in monkeys has been reported to block both slow and fast axoplasmic flow, although it did not cause glaucomatous cupping (228–230). Central retinal artery occlusion has been associated with obstruction of rapid orthograde and retrograde axonal transport (231). Furthermore, accumulation of tracer at the lamina cribrosa was inversely proportional to the perfusion pressure in cat eyes (232), and IOP-induced blockage of axonal transport was increased in eyes with angiotensin-induced systemic hypertension (233). In monkey eyes with elevated IOP, leakage from microvasculature of the nerve head has been associated with blockade of axonal transport at the lamina cribrosa (234).

Arguing against a vascular mechanism for pressure-induced obstruction of axoplasmic flow is the observation that ligation of the right common carotid artery in monkeys, which reduced the estimated ophthalmic artery pressure by 10 to 20 mm Hg, does not significantly affect the extent to which IOP elevation interrupts axonal transport (235). When obstruction to retrograde axoplasmic flow was studied in rat eyes, a direct relationship with IOP was still found, although the influence of the blood circulation was removed and the lamina cribrosa is only a single laminar sheet (209). It may be, therefore, that factors other than, or in addition to, ischemia and kinking of axons by a multilayered lamina cribrosa are involved in the IOP-induced obstruction to axoplasmic flow.

One study has found that partial constriction of axoplasmic flow may be present at the lamina cribrosa in orthograde and retrograde directions, and that accumulations of mitochondria at that level were more common in unmyelinated axons than in adjacent, myelinated axons. The authors suggested that the constriction may be a factor in glaucoma wherein IOP is not elevated (236). Endothelin-1, which produces vasoconstriction, reduces fast axonal transport in rats (237).

The effects on axoplasmic flow in the laminar region that are seen in monkeys with experimental glaucoma are similar to those seen in one of the few species to develop spontaneous glaucoma, the American Cocker Spaniel (238).

Cerebrospinal Fluid Pressure and Glaucomatous Optic Neuropathy

Anatomically, the cerebrospinal fluid (CSF) extends anteriorly in the optic nerve sheath and the subarachnoid space to the posterior aspect of the lamina cribrosa. Although IOP has been known to play a role in glaucomatous optic neuropathy, only relatively recently has there been speculation about any effect the CSF pressure may have (239,240). Studies in dogs have shown that the biomechanical effect of altering CSF pressure on the lamina cribrosa is equal to or greater than an equivalent change in IOP (241). Studies of the optic nerve architecture in human eyes have shown that the lamina cribrosa is relatively thin and bowed posteriorly in human eyes with glaucoma (40,242) (**Fig. 4.8**). A recent retrospective study found that the CSF pressure in patients with COAG was significantly decreased (243). In a subsequent study, CSF pressure was also lower in patients with normal-tension glaucoma and higher in patients with ocular hypertension, compared with control participants (244). A prospective study confirmed that persons with COAG have significantly lower CSF pressures than controls do; in addition, CSF pressure was lower in patients with normal-tension glaucoma than in patients with COAG (245). In this study, IOP, CSF pressure, and blood pressure were positively correlated, suggesting a dynamic interplay among these factors. Although preliminary, these studies suggest that translaminar pressure—the difference between IOP and CSF pressure—plays an important role in the pathogenesis of glaucomatous optic neuropathy.

Electrophysiologic Studies

When the IOP is artificially elevated in healthy human eyes, a significant reduction in the amplitudes of electroretinographic components and visual-evoked potentials occurs only when the pressure approaches or exceeds the ophthalmic blood pressure (246,247). However, the perfusion-pressure amplitude curve of the visual-evoked potential in normal eyes showed a kink, suggestive of vascular autoregulation, which was not observed in patients with glaucoma (248), again pointing to a possible deficiency in autoregulation in glaucoma. As previously noted, the electrical function of RGCs in cat eyes was found to depend more on perfusion pressure than the absolute height of the IOP (159).

The pattern electroretinography is believed to originate in the RGCs and is expected to be reduced in glaucoma. Therefore, it might be used to detect ganglion cell loss, but it failed

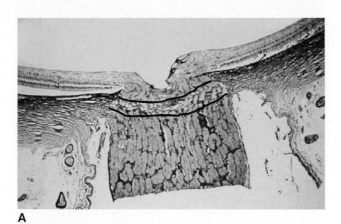
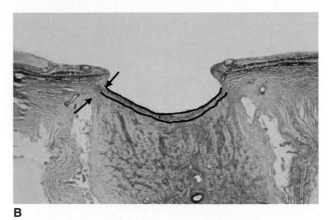

Figure 4.8 **A:** Histologic section (PAS) of the optic nerve in a nonglaucomatous eye. The lamina cribrosa is indicated. **B:** Histologic section of the optic nerve in a glaucomatous eye. Compared with A, the lamina cribrosa is thinner and bowed posteriorly. Note the reduction in distance between the subarachnoid space, containing cerebrospinal fluid, and the laminar tissues. (Reproduced from Jonas JB, Berenshtein E, Holbach L. Anatomic relationship between lamina cribrosa, intraocular space, and cerebrospinal fluid space. *Invest Ophthalmol Vis Sci.* 2003;44:5189–5195, with permission.)

to separate glaucoma patients from healthy individuals when used alone (249). However, a study of patients with ocular hypertension showed that pattern electroretinographic amplitude correlates with various optic disc morphometric parameters, particularly in sectors considered to be at risk for early glaucomatous damage (250). Although still early in its development, pattern electroretinography, as well as multifocal electroretinography, shows promise in the roles of diagnosis and functional assessment of ganglion cell loss (251–254).

Comparison with Nonglaucomatous Optic Atrophy

Studies of other ocular disorders provide some indirect insight into the possible mechanism of glaucomatous optic atrophy. For example, a histopathologic study of severe peripapillary choroidal atrophy revealed a normal optic nerve head, suggesting that the vascular supply of these two structures may be independent (255). Studies of nonglaucomatous optic atrophy have been used both to support and to refute an ischemic basis for glaucomatous optic atrophy. In patients with anterior ischemic optic neuropathy, cupping similar to that seen in glaucoma is frequently observed when the ischemia is due to giant cell arteritis, but it is less common in nonarteritic cases (256–258). These observations have led to the suggestion that glaucoma and anterior ischemic optic neuropathy have the same vasogenic basis of optic nerve damage, but differ according to the rate of change (256). It has also been suggested that acute ischemic optic neuropathy may be one of several mechanisms of optic nerve disease in chronic glaucoma (259). If this is true, the difference in visual field loss suggests that there is also a difference in the nature or distribution of the ischemia (258). In addition, the pattern of optic nerve fiber loss in nonarteritic anterior ischemia optic neuropathy involves primarily the superior half of the nerve and is unlike that found in glaucoma (260).

In contrast to the studies already described, a review of 170 eyes with nonglaucomatous optic atrophy of various etiologies revealed a small but significant increase in cupping (261).

However, the cups were morphologically different from those seen in glaucoma, which was suggested as evidence against a vascular etiology in glaucomatous cupping. Furthermore, a study of 18 patients with vasogenic shock and poor peripheral tissue perfusion revealed no evidence of glaucomatous optic nerve head or visual field change (262).

Cavernous atrophy of the optic nerve, as originally described by Schnabel (108), has been considered to be a form of glaucomatous optic atrophy caused by severe elevations of IOP. However, this also occurs in patients with normal pressures, in which case it may represent an aging change associated with generalized arteriosclerosis and a chronic vascular occlusive disease of the proximal optic nerve (263,264).

Conclusions Regarding Pathophysiology

The present evidence suggests that obstruction to axoplasmic flow may be involved in the pathogenesis of glaucomatous optic atrophy. However, it is still unclear whether mechanical or vascular factors are primarily responsible for this obstruction, or whether other alterations are also important in the ultimate loss of axons. All of these factors may be involved to some degree, or there may be more than one mechanism of optic atrophy in eyes with glaucoma (197,265). For example, the observed differences in glaucomatous visual field defects between patients with low-tension and high-tension glaucomas have led to the suggestion that ischemia may be the predominant factor in those glaucomas at the lower end of the IOP scale, whereas a more direct mechanical effect of the pressure may prevail in cases with higher IOP (266).

CLINICAL APPEARANCE OF OPTIC NERVE HEAD

While investigators continue to study the pathophysiology of glaucomatous optic atrophy, the practicing physician has a responsibility to become thoroughly familiar with the clinical morphology of this condition, because it provides the most reliable early evidence of damage in glaucoma.

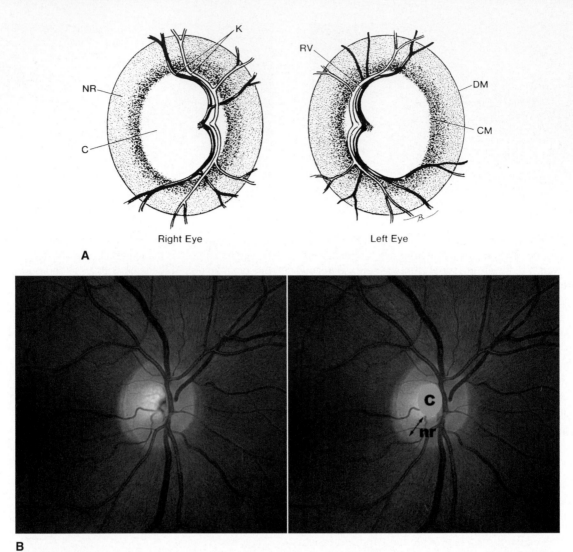

Right Eye   Left Eye

A

B

Figure 4.9 Normal optic nerve heads. **A:** Note that size of cups is symmetric between the two eyes and that neural rims are even for 360 degrees. *C*, cup; *CM*, cup margin; *DM*, disc margin; *K*, kinking of vessels at cup margin; *NR*, neural rim; *RV*, retinal vessels. **B:** Fundus photo of a normal right eye. *C*, approximation of the cup; *NR*, neural rim.

Morphology of the Normal Optic Nerve Head

To recognize pathologic alterations of the optic nerve head, one must first be familiar with the wide range of normal variations.

General Features

The ophthalmoscopic appearance of the optic nerve head is generally that of a vertical oval, although there is considerable variation in size and shape. Clinical studies have revealed a greater than sixfold difference in the area of normal nerve heads (267,268), which is consistent with histologic studies cited earlier (2–4). The central portion of the disc usually contains a depression, the cup, and an area of pallor, which represents a partial or complete absence of axons, with exposure of the lamina cribrosa. Although the size and location of cup and pallor are normally the same, this is not always the case, especially in disease states (121), and these two parameters should not be thought of as being synonymous. The tissue between the cup and disc margins is referred to as the neural rim. It represents the location of the bulk of the axons and normally has an orange-red color because of the associated capillaries. Retinal vessels ride up the nasal wall of the cup, often kinking at the cup margin before crossing the neural rim to the retina (**Fig. 4.9**).

Physiologic Neural Rim

By tradition, more is said about the cup than the neural rim of normal and glaucomatous optic nerve heads. However, it is actually alterations in the neural rim of an eye with glaucoma that lead to changes in the cup and to loss of visual field. The cup-to-disc ratio is only an indirect measure of the amount of neural tissue in the optic nerve head and may be misleading, because a larger diameter of the nerve head may be associated with a thinner neural rim width and larger cup size despite a stable number of axons (269,270). It is important, therefore, to pay close attention to the appearance of the neural rim.

The neural rim of the normal optic nerve head is typically broadest in the inferior quadrant, followed by the superior

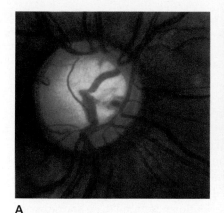

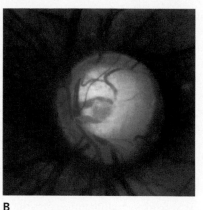

A   **B**

Figure 4.10 Gray crescents in the optic nerve head of a patient with large physiologic cups. The thin crescent is seen just inside the scleral lip in the temporal quadrant of the right eye (**A**) and the inferotemporal quadrant of the left (**B**).

and then the nasal rims, with the temporal rim being the thinnest (267). Several studies have attempted to correlate the area of the neural rim with that of the disc, and there is general agreement that the two are positively correlated—that is, larger discs have larger neural rim areas (267,271–273). However, the contour of the cup influences this correlation, in that the relative rim area is typically larger in discs with flat temporal sloping than in those with circular steep cups (273). The increase in neural rim area with increasing disc area appears to be due, at least in part, to a greater number of ganglion cell axons (4).

Several factors can interfere with the interpretation of the neural rim width. A gray crescent in the optic nerve head has been described, which typically is slate gray and located in the temporal or inferotemporal periphery of the neural rim (274). It is more common in blacks and apparently represents a variation of the normal anatomy. However, mistaking the gray crescent for a peripapillary pigmented crescent could result in the physiologic neural rim's being misinterpreted as pathologically thin in that area (**Fig. 4.10**).

Another source of error in interpreting the neural rim is the optic nerve head in myopia, in which the oblique insertion of the nerve may lead to distortion of the temporal neural rim from ophthalmoscopic view, suggesting pathologic thinning of this tissue (**Fig. 4.11**). Other features of highly myopic discs that may interfere with interpretation include a relatively large disc area; a shallower-than-usual cup, which may mask the deepening of the cup in glaucoma; and a temporal peripapillary crescent, which may be confused with peripapillary pigmentary changes that are seen more frequently around some glaucomatous discs (275).

The rim area appears to decline with age and with increasing IOP (276,277). It has also been observed that patients with diabetes mellitus may have an increase in the neural rim over time, which could be due to nerve swelling (278).

Physiologic Peripapillary Retina
Retinal Nerve Fiber Layer

Striations in the RNFL are normally seen ophthalmoscopically as light reflexes from bundles of nerve fibers (62,279) (Fig. 4.1).

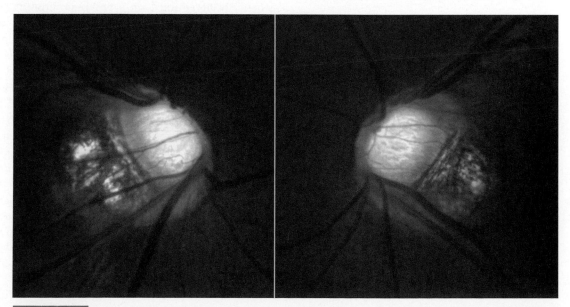

Figure 4.11 Oblique insertion of optic nerve heads in myopic eyes can obfuscate the interpretation of the neuroretinal rim and creates a wide temporal peripapillary crescent. In this case, the asymmetry and loss of the superonasal rim of the right eye corresponds to glaucomatous damage.

They are visible only after the bundles reach a critical thickness and are consequently seen best in the posterior pole and peripapillary regions, especially at the vertical poles of the disc and extending temporally from them (280). Under white light, the nerve fiber layer appears as a whitish haze over the retina and retinal vessels. In one large study, the RNFL was most visible in the inferior temporal arcade, followed by the superior temporal arcade, then the temporal macular area, and finally the nasal area (281). The nerve fiber layer has been noted to decrease with age (104,281). The visibility of the nerve fiber layer has been shown to correlate with the width of the neural rim and the caliber of the retinal artery (282). The relative height of the nerve fiber layer, especially when combined with visual field mean defect, has been shown to discriminate best between glaucomatous and nonglaucomatous eyes (283).

Peripapillary Pigmentary Variations

The normal optic nerve head may be surrounded by zones that vary in width, circumference, and pigmentation. A clinicopathologic study has revealed several clinical configurations with anatomic correlations (284,285). A scleral lip, which appears commonly as a thin, even, white rim that marks the disc margin, usually for the full 360 degrees, represents an anterior extension of sclera between the choroid and optic nerve head. A chorioscleral crescent, also called zone beta (**Fig. 4.12**), is a broader but more irregular and incomplete area of depigmentation, which represents a retraction of retinal pigment epithelium from the disc margin, often associated with a thinning or absence of choroid next to the disc, with exposure of the sclera. It is commonly seen with a tilted scleral canal, as in myopia. Large zone beta area–to–disc area ratio was found to be associated with an increased risk for glaucomatous damage in patients with ocular hypertension (286). A peripapillary crescent of increased pigmentation has been called zone alpha and may represent a malposition of the embryonic fold with a double layer or irregularity

of retinal pigment epithelium. It may be peripheral to zone beta or may be adjacent to the disc if the zone beta is absent.

Physiologic Cup
Size

The size of the optic nerve head cup, which is commonly described as the horizontal and vertical cup-to-disc ratio, varies considerably in the normal population, possibly because of normal variation in disc diameter (4). Reports of cup-to-disc ratio distribution in the general population differ according to the examination technique used. When the discs were studied by direct ophthalmoscopy, the distribution was found to be nongaussian, with most eyes having a cup-to-disc ratio of 0.0 to 0.3 and only 1% to 2% being 0.7 or greater (287). However, when stereoscopic views were used, a gaussian distribution was found with a mean cup-to-disc ratio of 0.4, and approximately 5% were 0.7 (288). In another study, the two techniques of optic nerve head evaluation were compared, and stereoscopic examination with a Hruby lens gave consistently larger cup-to-disc ratio estimates, with a mean of 0.38, compared with 0.25 by direct ophthalmoscopy (289). The investigators noted that the disparity between estimated cup-to-disc ratios for the same eye at different times seldom exceeds 0.2, so that the documentation of such a difference over time should be viewed with suspicion (289). Also of note, physiologic cups tend to be symmetric between the two eyes of the same individual (287–291), with a cup-to-disc ratio difference of greater than 0.2 between fellow eyes occurring in only 1% to 6% of the normal population but in 24% of patients with COAG (287,292). However, asymmetry alone was not found useful in identifying patients with COAG (292).

The size of the physiologic cup is frequently similar to that of the individual's parents and siblings (287,293,294). In other cases, the large cup may be the earliest sign of glaucoma in relatives (295). The size of the physiologic cup is thought to be genetically determined on a polygenic, multifactorial basis (287,296). The heritability has been estimated at two thirds, with the remaining variance attributed to environmental factors (294). Therefore, examining other family members is helpful in distinguishing between a large physiologic cup and glaucomatous cupping. The physiologic cup-to-disc ratio does not appear to correlate with a family history of COAG (287,297), although some studies have suggested a weak correlation with higher IOP, abnormal tonographic outflow facilities, or highly positive pressure responses to topical corticosteroid use (269,288,297–299). Other studies, looking primarily at disc area, showed significantly larger discs in patients with normal-tension glaucoma than in patients with COAG or control participants, and suggested that large discs have increased susceptibility to glaucomatous damage at normal pressures (300,301). However, another study found no apparent differences between COAG and normal-tension glaucoma in morphometric parameters measured by scanning laser ophthalmoscopy (302).

Most studies have shown no significant correlation between age and the size of the physiologic cup (5,267,293,303), whereas other investigations suggest that both the cup and pallor do enlarge slightly with increasing age (269,288,289,304,305). Any

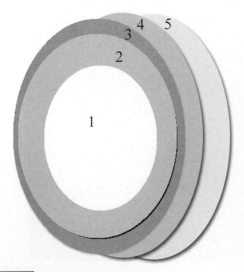

Figure 4.12 Zones of the optic nerve head and peripapillary pigmentation. 1. Cup. 2. Neuroretinal rim. 3. Scleral lip. 4. Zone beta. 5. Zone alpha.

enlargement of the cup with age is gradual and should not be confused with the more rapid progression of glaucomatous cupping.

Racial differences in optic nerve head parameters have been shown, with African-Americans having a larger disc and cup-to-disc ratio than whites (303,306–309). This racial difference has also been demonstrated in children (310). Cup area and depth were larger in African-Americans than in whites in one study; however, structural characteristics of the optic nerve head associated with glaucoma were independent of differences in disc area (309).

Most studies have found no correlation between cup size and sex (287,288,293,294), although one investigation revealed larger relative areas of pallor in white male patients than in white female patients (305), and others showed that men had slightly larger discs than women (5,303). Refractive errors do not appear to correlate with the diameter of the physiologic cup (267,269,287,293,303), although a study of highly myopic eyes (>8.00 diopters [D]) revealed a significant correlation between refraction and disc size (275).

In the differential diagnosis of glaucomatous optic atrophy, it is important to distinguish between a large physiologic cup and glaucomatous enlargement of the cup (**Fig. 4.13**). One distinguishing feature is symmetry of cup size between the right and left eyes in the physiologic state, taking into consideration the normal variations. Another helpful feature is the configuration of the cup and neural rim and the appearance of the peripapillary pigmentation and RNFL, which are the same in eyes with large or normal-size physiologic cups (311). The most important feature, however, is documented progressive cup enlargement, which is highly suggestive of glaucoma.

Shape

The shape of the physiologic cup is roughly correlated with the shape of the disc, which means that the margins of cup and disc tend to run more or less parallel (312). However, as previously noted, the inferior neural rim is the broadest of the four quadrants, followed by the superior, nasal, and temporal rims (267). Consequently, the cup has a horizontally oval shape in most normal eyes; thus, a vertical cup-to-disc ratio greater than the horizontal cup-to-disc ratio should be considered suspicious (267,289).

Morphology of Glaucomatous Optic Atrophy

The disc changes associated with glaucoma are typically progressive and asymmetric and present in various characteristic clinical patterns. It may be helpful to think of these in three categories: (a) disc patterns, (b) vascular signs, and (c) peripapillary changes.

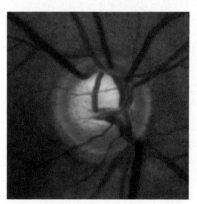
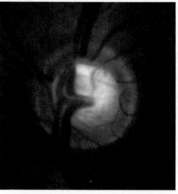

Figure 4.13 **A:** Large physiologic optic nerve head cups that are symmetrical and intact. **B:** Corresponding OCT image shows normal retinal NFL measurements.

A

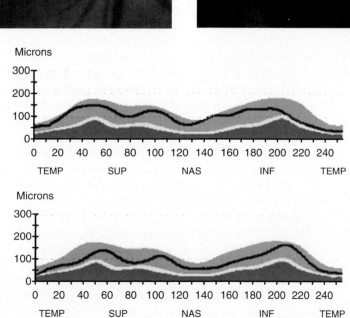

B

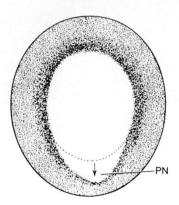

Figure 4.14 Inferior enlargement of cup (*arrow*) from original cup margin (*dotted line*) in glaucomatous optic atrophy, creating a polar notch (*PN*).

Disc Patterns of Glaucomatous Optic Atrophy

As bundles of axons are destroyed in an eye with glaucoma, the neural rim begins to thin in one of several patterns. One study, using confocal scanning laser ophthalmoscopy, found that half of patients with early glaucoma had smaller disc area with focal rim damage or no detectable damage, and the other half had larger discs with diffuse rim damage (313).

Focal Atrophy

Selective loss of neural rim tissue in glaucoma occurs primarily in the inferotemporal region of the optic nerve head and, to a somewhat lesser extent, in the superotemporal sector in the early stages of damage, which leads to enlargement of the cup in a vertical or oblique direction (314–324) (**Fig. 4.14**). In contrast to the normal optic nerve head, the inferior temporal rim in the glaucomatous eye is usually thinner than the superior temporal area, and the horizontal-to-vertical cup-to-disc ratio is reduced (321,322). The neural rim area is typically smaller in glaucomatous discs than in nonglaucomatous discs, and this is a better parameter than cup-to-disc ratio in distinguishing eyes with early glaucoma from healthy eyes (321,325,326). As previously noted, however, the wide range of neural rim areas in normal eyes even limits the usefulness of this parameter. As the glaucomatous process continues, the temporal neural rim is typically involved after the vertical poles, with the nasal quadrant being the last to be destroyed (322).

The focal atrophy of the neural rim often begins as a small, discrete defect, usually in the inferotemporal quadrant, which has been referred to as polar notching, focal notching, or pitlike changes (316–319). As the focal defect enlarges and deepens, it may develop a sharp nasal margin (316). When the local thinning of neural rim tissue reaches the disc margin (i.e., no visible neural rim remains in that area), a sharpened rim is said to be produced. If a retinal vessel crosses the sharpened rim, it will bend sharply at the edge of the disc, creating what has been termed bayoneting at the disc edge.

Concentric atrophy

In contrast to focal atrophy, glaucomatous damage may less commonly lead to enlargement of the cup in concentric circles, which are sometimes horizontal, but are more often directed infratemporally or superotemporally (317). Because the loss of neural rim tissue usually begins temporally and then progresses circumferentially toward these poles, this has been called temporal unfolding (316,317). In one study, this generalized expansion of the cup, with retention of its "round" appearance, was the most common form of early glaucomatous damage (327). Because distinguishing this type of glaucomatous cup from a physiologic cup is difficult, it is important to compare the cup in the fellow eye for symmetry and to study serial photographs for evidence of progressive change.

A thinning of the neural rim may be seen as a crescentic shadow adjacent to the disc margin as the intense beam of a direct ophthalmoscope passes across the neural rim (328). The histologic explanation for this phenomenon is uncertain, but it is thought to be associated with early glaucomatous damage and should not be confused with the previously discussed gray crescent in the optic nerve head (274,329).

Deepening of the Cup

In some cases, the predominant pattern of early glaucomatous optic atrophy is a deepening of the cup, which has been said to occur only when the lamina is not initially exposed (330). This may produce the picture of overpass cupping, in which vessels initially bridge the deepened cup and later collapse into it (316,317). Exposure of the underlying lamina cribrosa by the deepening cup is often recognized by the gray fenestra of the lamina, which has been referred to as the laminar dot sign (316). In most cases, the fenestrae of the lamina cribrosa have a dotlike appearance on ophthalmoscopy, although some are more striate and the latter configuration may have a higher association with glaucoma (331,332).

Pallor–Cup Discrepancy

In the early stages of glaucomatous optic atrophy, enlargement of the cup may progress ahead of that of the area of pallor. This biphasic pattern differs from other causes of optic atrophy in which the area of pallor is typically larger than the cup (121). A potential pitfall in interpreting optic nerve head cupping is to look only at the area of pallor and miss the larger area of cupping. The latter can usually be recognized by observing kinking of vessels at the cup margin or by examining the disc with stereoscopic techniques. Although the pallor–cup discrepancy is typical and strongly suggests glaucomatous cupping, it may also be seen in some normal optic nerve heads (333).

Pallor–cup discrepancy may occur with diffuse or focal enlargement of the cup. Saucerization refers to a pattern of early glaucomatous change in which diffuse, shallow cupping extends to the disc margins with retention of a central pale cup (**Figs. 4.15** and **4.16**) and may be an early sign of glaucoma (334,335). Focal saucerization refers to a more localized shallow, sloping cup, usually in the inferotemporal quadrant (317). The retention of normal neural rim color in the area of focal saucerization has been called the tinted hollow (316). As the glaucomatous damage progresses, the color is replaced by a grayish hue, termed the shadow sign, or by the laminar dot sign (**Figs. 4.17** and **4.18**).

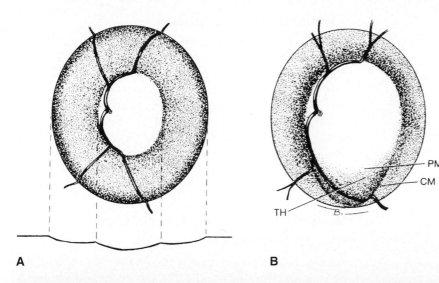

A

B

PM

CM

TH

B.

Figure 4.15 Glaucomatous optic atrophy. Pallor–cup discrepancy. **A:** Saucerization with corresponding cross-sectional view. **B:** Focal saucerization with tinted hollow *(TH)* between pallor margin *(PM)* and cup margin *(CM)*. Note kinking of vessels in both cases.

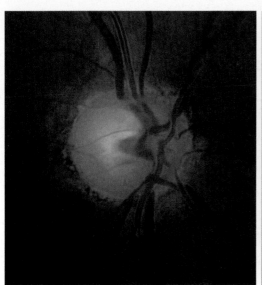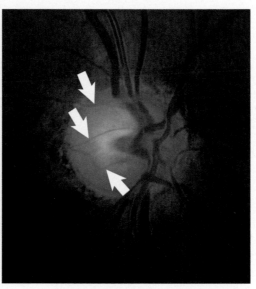

A

Figure 4.16 **A:** Saucerization of optic nerve head, evidenced by gradual sloping of vessels *(arrowheads)*. **B:** Topographic map using confocal scanning laser ophthalmoscopy (HRT-II) of the same optic nerve shows the loss of neuroretinal tissue. The vessel path gives the appearance of saucerization.

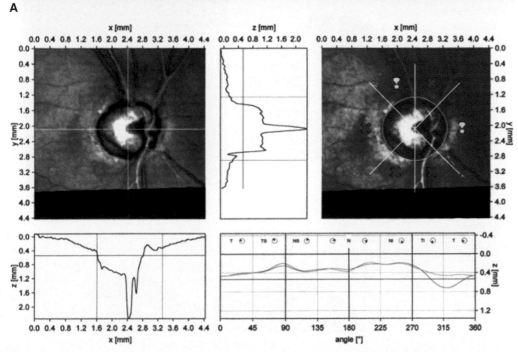

B

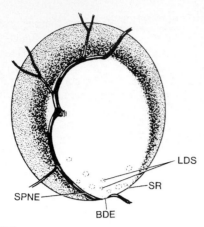

Figure 4.17 Inferotemporal loss of neural rim in glaucomatous optic atrophy, creating a sharpened rim *(SR)* at the disc margin, a sharpened polar nasal edge *(SPNE)* along the cup margin, bayoneting at the disc edge *(BDE)* where the vessels cross the sharpened rim, and laminar dot sign *(LDS)* due to exposure of fenestrae in lamina cribrosa.

Advanced Glaucomatous Cupping

If the progressive changes of glaucomatous optic atrophy are not arrested by appropriate measures to reduce the IOP, the typical course is eventual loss of all neural rim tissue. The ultimate result is total cupping, which is seen clinically as a white disc with loss of all neural rim tissue and bending of all vessels at the margin of the disc (**Fig. 4.19**). This has also been called bean-pot cupping, because the cross section of a histologic specimen reveals extreme posterior displacement of the lamina cribrosa and undermining of the disc margin (**Fig. 4.20**) (317,318).

Vascular Signs of Glaucomatous Optic Atrophy

Optic Disc Hemorrhages

Splinter hemorrhages, usually near the margin of the optic nerve head (**Figs. 4.21** and **4.22**), are a common feature of glaucomatous damage (336–339). They occur more commonly

Figure 4.18 **A:** Thinning of neural rim and "bayoneting" of a blood vessel at the site of a hemorrhage 2 years earlier. **B:** Corresponding visual field. Note the development of a superior paracentral scotoma. (From Jindal A, Fudemberg S. Primary open-angle glaucoma [Chapter 52]. In: Tasman W, Jaeger EA, eds. *Duane's Clinical Ophthalmology*. Vol 3. Philadelphia: Lippincott Williams & Wilkins; 2010.)

Figure 4.19 **A:** Advanced glaucomatous optic atrophy with nearly total cupping of the optic nerve head associated with the presence of shunt vessels inferotemporally and nasally. **B:** Confocal scanning laser ophthalmoscopic topography demonstrates only a small amount of nasal rim remaining.

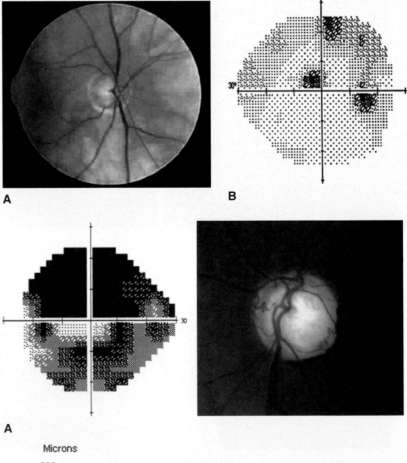

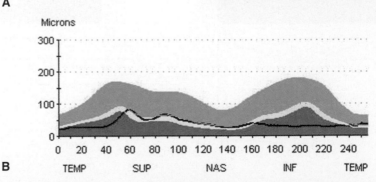

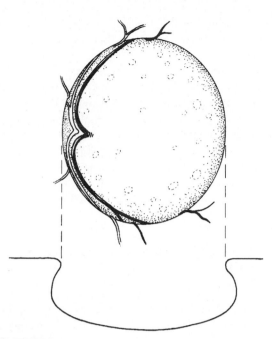

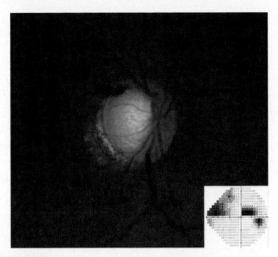

Figure 4.22 Splinter ("Drance") hemorrhage in glaucomatous optic nerve. *Inset* shows the corresponding automated achromatic visual field with nasal step and superior arcuate defect affecting the papillomacular bundle.

Figure 4.20 Advanced glaucomatous optic atrophy with total (bean-pot) cupping, shown best in cross-sectional view.

in patients with normal-tension glaucoma than in patients with COAG or suspected glaucoma, with cumulative incidences of 35.3%, 10.3%, and 10.4%, respectively (338). They tend to come and go, so that they may be seen on one visit and be gone the next, only to reappear at a later date in the same or a new location (340). One study has shown that 95.3% of disc hemorrhages were localized on or within 2 clock hours of an RNFL defect (341). Although they typically cross the disc margin, the papillary portion often disappears first during resorption, leaving the appearance of an extrapapillary hemorrhage (340). The most common location is the inferior quadrant, although they may be seen superiorly or at any other point around the disc margin. They are seen most often in the early to middle stages

of glaucomatous damage and decline in frequency with advanced damage, rarely appearing in quadrants with absent neural rim (339); however, a thin neuroretinal rim was found to be a risk factor for the development of optic disc hemorrhages (342). Although not pathognomonic of glaucoma, disc hemorrhages are a significant finding, because they may be the first sign of glaucomatous damage, often preceding RNFL defects, notches in the neural rim, and glaucomatous visual field defects (343–346). They are especially suggestive of glaucoma when associated with high IOP (347). However, as previously noted, disc hemorrhages commonly occur with minimal pressure elevation or in eyes with normal-tension glaucoma (338,348). If the glaucoma patient also has diabetes, disc hemorrhages are more common. Disc hemorrhages occur more commonly in diabetic versus nondiabetic patients with glaucoma (349,350). Although disc hemorrhages are not invariably associated with an increased rate of disc damage, they are often associated with progressive changes of the visual field and should be viewed as a sign that the glaucoma may be out of control (336,337, 347,350–354). It has also been noted that patients with high-tension glaucoma and disc hemorrhages have a significantly higher prevalence of neurosensorial dysacousia than those without hemorrhages do, which was thought to suggest a common vascular denominator in both conditions (355).

Tortuosity of Retinal Vessels

Tortuosity of retinal vessels on the disc may be seen with advanced glaucomatous optic atrophy, and in some cases with only moderate damage. It is believed to represent loops of collateral vessels in response to chronic central retinal vessel occlusion (356). Venovenous anastomoses associated with chronic branch retinal vessel occlusion, and the typical picture of acute central retinal vessel occlusion with massive flame hemorrhages, also occur with increased frequency in eyes with chronic glaucoma (356). Asymptomatic venous stasis changes on the disc, which are seen as enlargement of collateral vessels, have been estimated to occur in

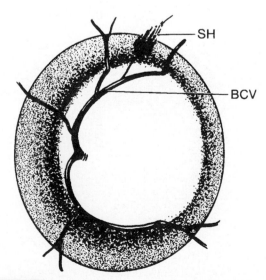

Figure 4.21 Vascular changes in glaucomatous optic atrophy. *SH*, splinter hemorrhage; *BCV*, baring of circumlinear vessel.

3% of patients with early to moderate glaucoma, and may be associated with progression of glaucomatous optic atrophy (357).

Cilioretinal Arteries

One study of 20 patients with bilateral symmetric COAG and unilateral cilioretinal arteries revealed a larger cup-to-disc ratio and more visual field damage in the eye with the cilioretinal artery (358). However, a similar study did not support this observation (359), whereas another suggested that glaucomatous eyes with one or more temporal cilioretinal arteries were more likely to retain central visual field than similar eyes with no cilioretinal artery (360).

Location of Retinal Vessels   The location of retinal vessels in relation to the cup may also have some diagnostic value. The significance of overpass cupping, in which vessels bridge a cup that is becoming deeper (316,317), is mentioned previously. Another vessel sign with some diagnostic value has been called baring of the circumlinear vessel (361,362). In many normal optic nerve heads, one or two vessels may curve to outline a portion of the physiologic cup. With glaucomatous enlargement of the cup, these circumlinear vessels may be "bared" from the margin of the cup (Fig. 4.21). This sign may occasionally be seen with nonglaucomatous disorders of the optic nerve and in some individuals with physiologic cups (362,363), although its presence in a glaucoma suspect group was associated with the development of visual field loss (364).

It was once taught that nasal displacement of the retinal vessels on the optic nerve head was a sign of glaucomatous cupping. However, because these vessels enter and leave the eye along the nasal margin of the cup, their location on the disc is a function of cup size, whether physiologic or glaucomatous, and does not provide a useful diagnostic parameter (298). On the other hand, the vertical eccentricity of the central retinal vessel trunk (where the vessels enter and leave through the disc) may be related to the course of glaucomatous optic atrophy (365). In one study, neural rim loss was more likely to occur in the vertical quadrant that was further from the trunk (366).

Retinal vessels beyond the disc margins may also undergo changes in glaucoma. One study showed proximal constriction (narrowing of retinal arteries near the disc) in 42% of patients with high-tension and normal-tension glaucoma, which correlated with the sectors of greatest cupping (367). General arterial narrowing (throughout the retinal course) was seen in 52% to 78%, corresponding to the overall severity of optic nerve damage. However, similar findings were also seen in patients with nonarteritic anterior ischemic optic neuropathy.

Peripapillary Changes Associated with Glaucomatous Optic Atrophy

Nerve Fiber Bundle Defects

The loss of axonal bundles, which leads to the neural rim changes of glaucomatous optic atrophy, also produces visible defects in the RNFL. These appear as dark stripes or wedge-shaped defects of varying width in the peripapillary area, paralleling the normal retinal striations, or as diffuse loss of the striations (368–371) (**Fig. 4.23**). They often follow disc hemorrhages and correlate highly with visual field changes, neural rim area, and fluorescein-filling defects (343,368–374). RNFL defects are also seen in many neurologic disorders, as well as in patients with ocular hypertension and healthy individuals. However, attention to the appearance of the defects in glaucoma has improved the sensitivity and specificity of this finding, and several studies have shown RNFL defects to be the most useful parameter in the early detection of glaucomatous damage (375–378). The diffuse loss is more common in patients with glaucoma than in patients with ocular hypertension (379), but it is also more common among persons with ocular hypertension than among those with normal IOPs (380). Localized defects

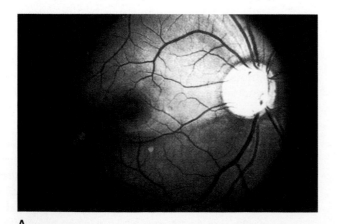
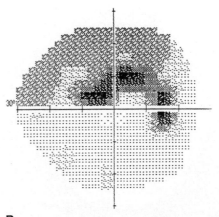

A   **B**

Figure 4.23   Nerve fiber layer defect in glaucoma. **A:** Inferior nerve fiber layer wedge defect. **B:** Corresponding superior visual field defect. (From Kwon YH, Caprioli J. Primary open-angle glaucoma [Chapter 52]. In: Tasman W, Jaeger EA, eds. *Duane's Clinical Ophthalmology.* Vol 3. Philadelphia: Lippincott Williams & Wilkins.)

are more directly associated with localized visual field loss than is the case with diffuse nerve loss (381). Either localized or diffuse loss may be the initial sign of glaucomatous damage (382).

Peripapillary Pigmentary Disturbance

Peripapillary pigmentary disturbance is frequently associated with glaucomatous optic atrophy, but is also seen with other conditions, such as myopia and aging changes. As previously noted, several variations of peripapillary pigmentary change may be seen in healthy eyes. The scleral lip, or peripapillary halo, is a narrow, homogenous light band at the edge of the disc. The incidence of prominent halos is higher in glaucoma, although the average degree of halos is statistically the same as in nonglaucomatous eyes (383). Peripapillary atrophy (both zone beta and zone alpha, as previously described) occurs more frequently and is larger in eyes with glaucomatous damage than in normal eyes, and it has been observed to progressively enlarge in eyes with glaucoma (384–387). It increases with decreasing neural rim area and correlates with the quadrants of the greatest rim loss (388). There is evidence that the absence of peripapillary atrophy may be associated with a decreased risk of glaucomatous damage among patients with ocular hypertension (389,390).

Reversal of Glaucomatous Cupping

It is generally taught that glaucomatous damage of the optic nerve head and visual field is an irreversible process. Although this may be true in many cases, especially when associated with actual loss of axons, there are situations in which glaucomatous damage may be at least partially reversible. Because of increased elasticity of their sclera, this is most commonly observed in children with early stages of glaucoma, particularly during the first year of life, when the IOP is successfully lowered surgically (391,392). However, improvement in the cup, neural rim, and even the nerve fiber layer height have been described in adults after a marked reduction in IOP by surgical or medical means (393–399). It is important to point out that "reversal of cupping" represents a mechanical effect of IOP reduction and not an increase in neuroretinal tissue.

DIFFERENTIAL DIAGNOSIS OF GLAUCOMATOUS OPTIC ATROPHY

Normal Variations

Normal variations in the physiologic cup, the neural rim, and the peripapillary retina, as discussed earlier in this chapter, may be confused with the changes of glaucoma. In addition, developmental anomalies and nonglaucomatous optic atrophies may be sources of diagnostic confusion.

Developmental Anomalies

Colobomas of the optic nerve head can simulate glaucomatous cupping. The defect may involve the entire disc, which is enlarged and excavated (400,401) (**Fig. 4.24**). In some cases, the diagnostic problem is compounded by associated field defects, which may resemble those of glaucoma, but are typically not progressive. A variation of optic nerve head colobomas, called the morning glory syndrome, is characterized by a large funnel-shaped staphylomatous coloboma of the nerve head and peripapillary region with white central tissue, elevated peripapillary pigment disturbance, and multiple radially oriented retinal vessels (402–404). Morning glory syndrome is typically seen only in one eye and is usually not inherited; however, bilateral cases, which may be hereditary, have been reported (405,406).

Another optic nerve head anomaly that may represent an atypical coloboma is the congenital pit (403,404). This is a localized, pale depression, usually near the temporal or inferotemporal margin of the disc, although it may be found in any area of the nerve head, and there may be two, or even three, pits in some eyes. These anomalies may have associated visual disturbance resulting from macular or extramacular serous detachment (407), in which the optic disc pit may act as a conduit for fluid flow from the schisis cavity into the subarachnoid space (408). The serous detachment may resolve spontaneously (409). Cases have also been reported in which congenital pits were noted to enlarge when observed for many years (410).

Tilted disc syndrome is a congenital anomaly in which the optic disc is tilted on its horizontal axis, with inferior chorioretinal hypoplasia (411). Although tilted disc syndrome is less

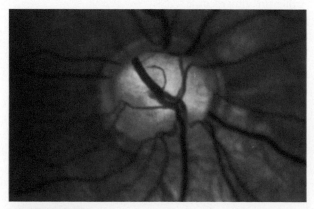
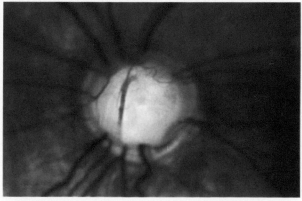

Figure 4.24 Colobomas of the optic nerve heads can simulate glaucomatous cupping. This patient would appear to have nearly total cupping and pallor, and yet the IOP was low normal and the visual fields were full with normal central vision.

likely than the colobomas to be confused with glaucoma, it can interfere with the recognition of glaucomatous damage, which is compounded by superotemporal visual field loss.

Nonglaucomatous Optic Nerve Atrophy

Ophthalmologists cannot always distinguish between glaucomatous and nonglaucomatous optic atrophy on the basis of the optic disc appearance alone (412). Parameters that are most useful in making this differentiation include pallor of the neural rim in nonglaucomatous eyes and obliteration of the rim in glaucoma (413). Nonglaucomatous conditions that may cause acquired cupping include anterior ischemic optic neuropathy (as previously discussed), especially when the ischemia is due to arteritis (256–258). A similar entity has been described in which infarction of the optic nerve head caused shallow cupping infratemporally, associated with arcuate field defects (414). This differed from glaucoma in that it was not progressive. Acquired cupping may also occur with compressive lesions of the optic nerve, such as an intracranial aneurysm, which was reported to cause cupping indistinguishable from that of early glaucoma (415). Nonglaucomatous optic neuropathies are also associated with loss of the RNFL, but with minimal cupping (416).

EVALUATION TECHNIQUES

Progressive cupping of the optic nerve head in a patient with glaucoma is the most reliable indicator that the IOP is not being adequately controlled. It is essential, therefore, to evaluate and record the appearance of the nerve head in a way that will accurately reveal subtle glaucomatous changes over the course of follow-up evaluations. In current practice, this involves careful evaluation in the office combined with photographic documentation. In addition, newer automated techniques may provide more precise methods of observation.

Office Evaluation and Recording of the Optic Nerve

In the clinical evaluation of the optic nerve head, the direct ophthalmoscope is occasionally useful, especially when evaluating the nerve fiber layer with a red-free filter. However, this technique does not permit detection of many of the glaucomatous changes in the nerve head and peripapillary area, and the most useful office approach is to carefully study these structures with stereoscopic methods. The most useful stereoscopic technique involves use of a slitlamp and an auxiliary fundus lens, such as the Goldmann contact lens, the handheld 78-D lens or 90-D lens (**Fig. 4.25**), or the Hruby lens slitlamp attachment. Each of these systems provides the advantages of magnification and stereopsis. However, because the lateral and axial magnifications are unequal, there is a certain amount of image distortion, with the Goldmann and handheld lenses producing a decrease in apparent depth and the Hruby lens producing a slight increase (417).

Several methods have been described for estimating the size of the disc and neural rim. These include use of (a) a direct

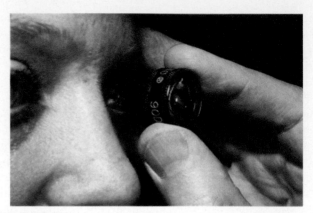

Figure 4.25 A 90-D lens used with slitlamp for stereoscopic indirect ophthalmoscopic evaluation of optic nerve head.

ophthalmoscope, using either the graticule incorporated in the instrument or the smallest round white light spot of the Welch Allyn direct ophthalmoscope, which projects a 1.5-mm diameter spot on the retina in most eyes (418,419); (b) an indirect ophthalmoscope with a spacing device on the condensing lens that allows measurement of the disc image with calipers (420,421); and (c) a Haag–Streit slitlamp with a 90-D lens or contact lens (422–424), in which the height of the slit beam is adjusted to coincide with the disc edges and is then read off the scale. When compared with more quantitative measurements, such as planimetry, these techniques provide reasonably accurate estimates, especially when appropriate correction factors are considered.

Subjective estimates of cup dimensions vary greatly, even among expert observers (425–428). These can be improved by paying attention to the many complex optic nerve head and peripapillary retinal parameters associated with glaucomatous damage and to the need for standardized methods for interobserver evaluation of the optic disc (427,429,430). Detailed drawings should include the area of cupping and pallor in all quadrants, the position and kinking of major vessels, splinter hemorrhages, and peripapillary changes. However, no degree of attention to detail is sufficient to detect subtle changes in all cases, and the office evaluation should be considered only as an adjunct to the indispensable use of photographic records or other imaging records.

Photographic Techniques
Two-Dimensional Photographs

Two-dimensional photographs, whether color or black-and-white, have the advantages of simplicity and lower cost, compared with stereophotographs and computed images. In addition, the relative dimensions of the pallor and cup can be measured directly on the photograph (431,432). Although one study found monocular and stereoscopic photographs to afford similar levels of accuracy (433), the former technique is frequently limited by the inability to precisely determine the cup margins. The projection of fine parallel lines onto the disc has been suggested as a way to improve recognition of the cup contours on two-dimensional photographs and stereophotographs (434,435). Techniques have also been developed to electronically scan black-and-white disc photos to obtain an objective measure of the amount of optic disc pallor (436,437). The main value of two-dimensional photos in the future may be to document the RNFL. Special techniques to enhance the subtle details of this parameter include monochromatic (red-free) filters and high-resolution film, crosspolarization photography, a wide-angle fundus camera, a spectral reflectance, and a charge-coupled device with digital filtering (438–446). The use of nerve fiber layer photography compared favorably with other glaucoma-screening methods in a general medical clinic setting (442).

Stereoscopic Photographs

A more reliable method for recording disc cupping and the other aspects of glaucomatous optic atrophy is the use of color stereophotographs. Stereophotographs can be obtained by taking two photos in sequence, either by manually repositioning the camera or by using a sliding carriage adapter (Allen separator), or by taking simultaneous photos with two cameras that utilize the indirect ophthalmoscopic principle (Donaldson stereoscopic fundus camera) or a twin-prism separator (447–450). These three techniques were compared for reproducibility, and the Donaldson camera was found to be superior (451). However, use of a simultaneous stereo camera, which provides the stereo pair on two halves of the same frame (Nidek 3Dx), had significantly better overall mean stereoscopic quality than the Donaldson camera (452). Transparencies from the Nidek camera can also be used to create lenticular images, which are single prints on a unique, photosensitized plastic base that produces a three-dimensional image without use of a stereoviewer (453). Although simultaneous stereophotography may be optimal for assessing the optic nerve head, no manufacturers currently make these cameras.

Ultrasonography

Ultrasound can be used to detect glaucomatous cupping of 0.7 cup-to-disc ratio or greater (454).

Computed Analysis of the Optic Nerve Head and RNFL

Historical Perspective

Even the most sophisticated fundus photographs are limited in their clinical value by the qualitative, subjective interpretation of the images (426). Efforts to refine the assessment of these subtle findings have included quantitative analyses of optic nerve head topography and pallor, and RNFL height or thickness. These techniques were initially performed manually (455), which was time consuming and impractical for routine clinical practice. With the advent of computers and newer imaging technologies, however, applying these concepts to the clinical management of glaucoma is now a possibility.

The concept of computed image analysis of the optic nerve head was pioneered by Dr. Bernard Schwartz, who developed prototypes for analysis of contour and pallor of the disc (456).

Early instruments used the basic principle of stereopsis, in which disparity between corresponding points of stereo pair images was used to generate contour lines and three-dimensional contour maps (stereophotogrammetry). Commercial instruments in this category were the Rodenstock optic nerve head analyzer (457–459), the Topcon Imagenet (460), and the Humphrey retinal analyzer (461). The Topcon Imagenet and Humphrey retinal analyzer measured disparity between existing structures in the stereo images, whereas the optic nerve head analyzer used projected light stripes on the disc to measure image disparity. Stereochronoscopy used the stereoscopic principle to detect subtle changes in photographs of a disc taken at different times (462–464). If any progression of the cupping has occurred, the disparity in the cup margins of the superimposed photographs would produce a stereoscopic effect. A modification of this concept, referred to as stereo chronometry, used a stereoplotter to measure the changes created by the two photographs (465). Other modifications for detecting differences in serial fundus photographs involve analysis of flicker while alternately viewing one photograph and then the other, and electronic subtraction, in which areas of disparity between the two images are enhanced (464,466,467).

Colorimetric measurements have also been studied to detect reduced or changing color intensity of the optic nerve head (468–471). A photographic technique has also been developed to permit quantitative evaluation of the relative brightness of the illuminated optic nerve head (472).

In another technology, rasterstereography, a series of horizontal dark-light line pairs are projected on the disc and peripapillary retina at a fixed angle and the computer scans a video image of the lines in a raster fashion. Raster refers to a scanning pattern that moves from side to side and from top to bottom (the same scanning pattern used in confocal laser scanning). Because the lines are deflected proportional to the height or depth of the disc and retinal surfaces, a computer algorithm can translate the deflections into depth numbers and create a topographic map.

An image analyzer that used the rasterstereography concept was the Glaucoma-Scope, which is no longer available (473,474). It projected a near infrared light in parallel stripes on the nerve head. The computer analyzed the data points to generate depth measures, which were displayed in microns relative to reference planes. In the initial set of measurements, the actual depth measures were provided, while follow-up studies showed only change of more than 50 μm from baseline.

Despite reasonable reproducibility and accuracy, these instruments never achieved widespread clinical use primarily because of technical complexity, the size and cost of the instrument, and the need for relatively wide pupillary dilatation and clear media. Nevertheless, the experience gained through the study of these instruments provided the basis for much of our understanding of computed image analysis of the optic nerve head and of the potential for clinical application of newer instruments and techniques in the management of glaucoma.

Over the past decade, several commercially available instruments have been described. These instruments use newer techniques, such as confocal laser scanning ophthalmoscopy and polarimetry, optical coherence tomography (OCT), and the retinal thickness analyzer. Imaging and computed data processing allow for precise three-dimensional in vivo measurements. However, computed results should always be evaluated in a clinical context (475).

Measure of Clinical Utility

For a structural test to be diagnostically useful, it should be able to (a) differentiate between healthy and glaucomatous eyes, (b) detect glaucomatous changes earlier than functional changes (i.e., preperimetric glaucoma—when psychophysical testing does not show an abnormality), and (c) detect progression of disease.

Optic Nerve Topography

Principles of Confocal Scanning Laser Tomography

Confocal scanning laser ophthalmoscopy is a technique for obtaining high-resolution images by using a focused laser beam to scan over the area of the fundus to be imaged. Only a small spot on the fundus is illuminated at any instant, and the light reflected determines the brightness of the corresponding pixel on a computer monitor. To improve contrast, a pinhole, or confocal aperture, is placed in front of the photodetector to eliminate scattered light (**Fig. 4.26**). The aperture is conjugate to the laser focus, and the resulting image is said to be confocal. The instantaneous volume of tissue from which reflected light is accepted by the confocal aperture is called a voxel, and the smaller the aperture, the smaller the voxel and the higher the resolution of the image. By scanning the fundus with the laser in a raster pattern, a two-dimensional image can be built up as an array of pixels. If a series of confocal scanning laser ophthalmoscopy images are obtained at successive planes of depth in the tissue, these can be used to construct a three-dimensional image, or confocal scanning laser tomography.

The prototype in this category of instruments was the laser tomographic scanner (476,477). Although the laser tomographic scanner is no longer commercially available, new-generation units were developed from the original laser tomographic scanner and are similar in basic design.

The HRT-II and HRT-III (**Fig. 4.27**) are completely automatic instruments designed to be used in routine clinical practice for study of optic nerve head morphology. They are based on the original HRT, which has had the most extensively re-

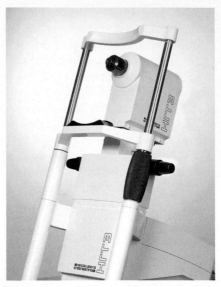

Figure 4.27   HRT-III. (Courtesy of Heidelberg Engineering.)

ported evaluation and was found to have reproducibility of stereometric parameters comparable with the original HRT (478). The HRT-II uses a 675-nm diode laser as a light source to measure the reflectivity of millions of points in multiple consecutive focal planes in 0.024 second per plane. The first section image is located above the reflection of the first retinal vessel, and the last is beyond the bottom of the optic nerve head cup, with 16 confocal images acquired per 1 mm of the scan depth, achieving high spatial resolution. The computer then converts the acquired data to a single topographic image with 384×384 data points (pixels) within a 15-degree area. The calculated image is then used to produce quantitative measurements of morphometric parameters of the disc that can be used to classify the nerve as normal or glaucomatous, or to compare topography images to quantify progression of glaucoma.

For the HRT to calculate these parameters, several preliminary steps are performed. First, a reference ring with an outer diameter of 94% and a width of 3% of the acquired image is placed on the image to define the retinal surface. The absolute height of that surface is then calculated, relative to the focal plane of the eye, and the mean height of that retinal reference ring is used to calculate the relative coordinate system, or reference plane. A correction for tilt is also made. Another surface, called the curved surface, is then defined after a contour line is drawn around the border of the optic disc. Topographic measurements are then calculated.

Because the magnitude of morphometric parameter values depends strongly on the chosen reference plane (479), defining the plane becomes a critical issue. Theoretical and practical problems have complicated the choice of the reference plane. Various modifications of the position of the reference plane have been offered to compensate for possible thinning of the retina during the course of glaucoma (480,481). The HRT software automatically defines a reference plane parallel to the peripapillary retinal surface and 50 μm posterior to the retinal surface at the papillomacular bundle (479,482). The rationale for this definition is that, during development of glaucoma, the

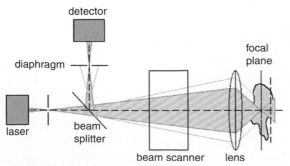

Figure 4.26   Principles of confocal scanning laser ophthalmoscopy.

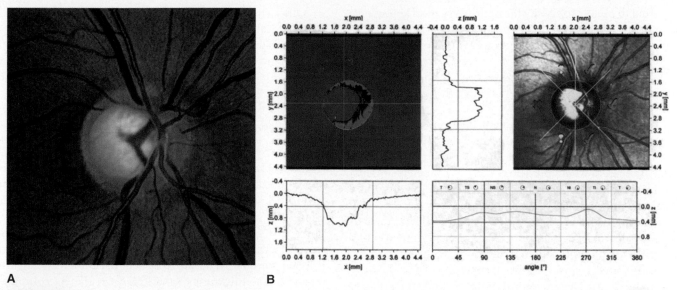

Figure 4.28 **A:** Color photograph of a right optic nerve. **B:** Corresponding image from an HRT-II. The reference planes are the *red lines*.

nerve fibers at the papillomacular bundle remain intact longest, and the nerve fiber layer thickness at that location is approximately 50 μm. All structures located below the reference plane are considered to be the cup, and all structures located above the reference plane and within the contour line are considered to be the rim (**Fig. 4.28**). The cup of the optic nerve head is displayed in red, and the rim is displayed in blue and green. The distance between the reference plane and the retinal surface is used to measure the mean RNFL thickness.

Evaluation of Accuracy and Reproducibility of Confocal Scanning Laser Tomography

Numerous reproducibility studies have been reported for the HRT (483–488), revealing acceptably low variability. Tests that are reproducible will have a higher chance of detecting progression over time. Highly reproducible topographic data can be obtained with a nondilated pupil (485), although the accuracy and reproducibility declined when the pupil was very small or very dilated (489). It has been suggested that reproducibility can be improved in general by using a series of three examinations (483).

An accuracy study performed with the laser tomographic scanner by using a plastic model eye revealed low-average relative errors for diameter and depth (477). However, vertical disc diameter measurements with the HRT were significantly smaller than those obtained with planimetric methods (490). The reproducibility of the stereometric parameters was evaluated in different clinical studies in normal and glaucomatous eyes, and measurements were found to be highly reproducible (491), with typical coefficients of variation for area, volume, and depth measurements of about 5% (486,487).

One lesson learned from the study of image analysis of the optic nerve head is that traditional parameters, such as cup-to-disc ratio and neural rim area, are inadequate for interpreting the subtle findings in the disc and peripapillary retina in healthy and diseased states. To address this problem, the HRT provides

a wide range of two-dimensional and three-dimensional information on the disc and peripapillary retina, which is displayed on a monitor and in hard copy. One of these parameters is referred to as cup shape measure, previously known as the third moment. This parameter relates to the frequency distribution of depth values relative to the curved surfaces inside the disc area and is a function of the overall shape of the optic nerve head. It was found to be the most useful indicator of the degree of glaucomatous optic nerve damage and early glaucomatous visual field loss (492,493). In one study, the cup shape measure was the only parameter associated with changes in visual field (494). Other useful morphometric parameters include rim area, variation of height of contour line, and RNFL thickness (495). Less useful parameters include disc area, cup area, cup and rim volume, and mean and maximum cup depth. Optic nerve head parameters obtained by the HRT may be affected by age, refraction, or disc area (494,496). Rim volume appears to be the only parameter unaffected by these factors (496).

The sensitivity and specificity of the various HRT topographic parameters vary significantly. In general, the sensitivities have been reported in the low-80s to -90s (%), with specificity ranging from the low-80s to the mid-90s (%) (497–503). Except in eyes with advanced glaucomatous damage, classifying an individual eye as normal or glaucomatous is difficult to do with absolute certainty on the basis of single HRT parameters.

For better discrimination between normal and abnormal optic discs, the HRT software performs statistical analyses to allow a comparison between the examined optic disc and a database of normal eyes. Multivariate analysis methods that use combinations of individual parameters to classify an individual eye into a "normal" or a "glaucoma" group have been proposed (493,495,504–507). These studies have shown that, when the cup shape measure, rim volume, and retinal surface height variation are analyzed together, they appear to be the most important parameters to differentiate between normal and glaucomatous optic nerve heads. HRT-II was also reported to be able to classify the optic nerve head appearance as "normal," "borderline," or "outside normal limits" on the basis of the ratio of rim area to disc area (Moorfields regression analysis) (508). However, in a prospective study, multivariate analysis and Moorfields regression analysis did not discriminate as well between patients with glaucoma and control participants (509).

Another method to detect glaucomatous change is the ranked-segment distribution curve analysis (510). To perform this analysis, the optic nerve head is divided into 36 sectors, each 10 degrees wide. The stereometric parameters are then calculated for each segment, sorted in descending order, and displayed as a graphic representation of the optic nerve head configuration. From a population of normal eyes, ranked-segment distribution curves for the 5th and 95th percentiles are calculated, and a patient's ranked-segment distribution curve is plotted against the normal curves.

In the Ocular Hypertension Treatment Study (OHTS) and the Early Manifest Glaucoma Trial (EMGT), conversion from ocular hypertension to glaucoma was by optic nerve criterion in 40% to 50% of cases (511,512). In an ancillary study of OHTS involving use of confocal scanning laser ophthalmoscopy, large cup–disc area, mean cup depth, mean height contour, and cup volume had a positive predictive value between 14% and 40% for the development of COAG from ocular hypertension (513).

Progression in glaucoma may be detected by calculating a change probability map (514), which uses three images acquired during the baseline and three images during the follow-up examination. The six images are aligned and normalized to each other. Each image cluster of 4 by 4 adjacent height measurements or pixels is then combined to create so-called superpixels, with 48 baseline height measurements and 48 follow-up height measurements. Then the variability of the baseline measurements is compared with the combined variability of the baseline and follow-up measurements at each superpixel. The resulting probability maps are displayed in color codes. White superpixels indicate no significant change; dark-brown superpixels indicate that the surface height has changed significantly, with an error probability of less than 5% (514).

As mentioned previously, HRT can distinguish discs with specific appearances that include focal ischemia, myopic glaucomatous changes, senile sclerotic changes, and generalized cup enlargement by comparing mean values for certain optic disc variables (515). However, the ability to detect glaucomatous damage varies considerably with the disc appearance. In studies of patients with ocular hypertension and patients with glaucoma, the HRT and visual field tests had fair to poor agreement in detecting glaucoma (516). Therefore, in the clinical setting, caution should be used when interpreting HRT results on the basis of multivariate discriminant analysis or ranked-segment distribution curves. Clinical optic disc evaluation remains the most important method of detecting or following up patients with glaucoma, although information obtained with the HRT may have adjunctive value, and further refinement of the instrument may increase its value.

Other confocal laser scanners, including the Rodenstock 101 confocal scanning laser ophthalmoscope, are no longer commercially available. OCT can also be used to generate a topographic map. At the time of publication, the absence of a normative database for comparison limits the clinical utility of OCT for optic nerve topography.

Retinal Nerve Fiber Layer Imaging
Confocal Scanning Laser Polarimetry

A confocal scanning laser polarimeter combines the concept of a confocal scanning laser and polarimetry to measure the RNFL thickness (517). Based on the assumption that the RNFL is birefringent, caused by the parallel microtubules in the nerve fibers (518,519), a polarized diode laser light (780 nm) is changed when it penetrates the tissue. This change in the state of polarization is referred to as retardation and is linearly related to the thickness of the RNFL (518). The computer provides thickness data for concentric circles around the disc margin. The initial versions of this instrument—the Nerve Fiber Analyzer (NFA)-I and NFA-II—have since been upgraded several times. The current version, known as GDxPRO (**Fig. 4.29**), allows comparison of an individual's data against a large normative database.

In one study, the location of the peak retardation values was found to be in agreement with the values of RNFL thickness published for humans, but the retardation values around the disc were different from the anatomic data. The authors concluded that discrepancies between the retardation and anatomic data should be recognized in the clinical interpretation of polarimetric data (520). Differences of the corneal polarization axis naturally exist in healthy and glaucomatous eyes; therefore, influence of corneal birefringence should be properly compensated (521,522). The variable corneal compensator individually corrects for polarization induced by the cornea and the lens (523–527), improving the ability of GDx to discriminate between glaucomatous and healthy eyes. In general, the reported sensitivity and specificity of scanning laser polarimetry to detect glaucoma are above 80% (503,528,529).

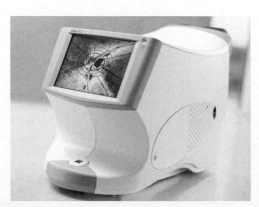

Figure 4.29 GDxPRO, a portable scanning laser polarimeter. (Courtesy of Carl Zeiss Meditec, Inc.)

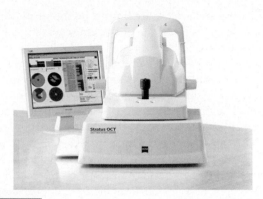

Figure 4.30 Stratus OCT. (Courtesy of Carl Zeiss Meditec, Inc.)

Optical Coherence Tomography

OCT was developed in the early 1990s and became available to ophthalmologists in 1996. A second-generation instrument was introduced in 2000, and a third-generation instrument, the Stratus OCT (**Fig. 4.30**), was introduced in 2002, achieving an increase in imaging speed and resolution. Later in the decade, several spectral-domain OCT machines (**Fig. 4.31**) became widely available. The first three generations of OCT are referred to as time-domain OCT.

The principle of OCT involves a low-coherence infrared (843-nm) diode light source, which is divided into reference and sample paths. Reflected sample light from the patient's eye creates an interference signal with the reference beam, which is detected in a fiber-optic interferometer. Cross-sectional images of the retina and disc are then constructed from a sequence of signals, similar to that of an ultrasound B-mode (530). Instead of sound waves, however, the OCT uses low-coherence light to quantify RNFL thickness, by measuring the difference in delay of backscattered light from the RNFL inside the imaged tissue. RNFL can be differentiated from other retinal layers with an algorithm that detects the anterior edge of retinal pigment epithelium and determines the photoreceptor layer position. Each resulting image consists of RNFL thickness measurements along a 360-degree circle around the optic disc (531). Multiple studies

have demonstrated that RNFL thickness can be accurately measured with the OCT (532–537), however it was suggested that earlier versions of the OCT may have underestimated RNFL thickness (538). One study compared RNFL thickness measurements using the first generations of OCT, NFA, and HRT and achieved the most reliable results with the NFA, followed by HRT (539). However, other studies showed that the third generation of OCT was similar to scanning laser polarimetry and HRT in differentiating glaucomatous eyes from healthy eyes (540,541). Unlike confocal scanning laser tomography, the OCT does not require a reference plane. Results of RNFL thickness measurements may vary with different instruments.

The final resolution of OCT is determined by transverse and axial resolution; transverse resolution is determined by the spacing of the A-scan and is ultimately limited by the optics of ocular tissue. Axial resolution varies by wavelength and bandwidth of the light source. Current models of time-domain and spectral-domain OCT use the same diode light sources. Some ultrahigh-resolution ophthalmic OCT scanners are based on a commercially available titanium–sapphire laser. This system enables in vivo cross-sectional retinal imaging with axial resolution of approximately 1 to 3 μm, compared with approximately 10 μm for the OCT3 (542,543). These OCT devices that use the titanium–sapphire laser sources are not commercially available because of prohibitive costs of the laser. Spectral-domain OCT does not rely on a beam splitter or moving reference mirror; instead, all of the reflected light returns to a spectrometer, and the wavelengths are converted by Fourier transformation to generate the images. This allows higher resolution than a time-domain OCT does, and faster acquisition time. Theoretically, the faster acquisition time should reduce the induced artifact from patients' eye movement, compared with OCT3.

OCT3 has a normative database and can differentiate glaucomatous and nonglaucomatous eyes with reported sensitivities and specificities generally ranging from the upper-60s to mid-80s (%) and the low-80s to -90s (%), respectively (497–500). Thin OCT measurements are associated with the conversion of suspected glaucoma to glaucoma (544). The utility of OCT3 for determining progression in

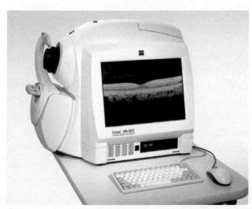

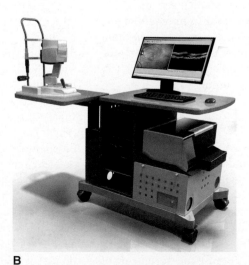

Figure 4.31 Two examples of spectral-domain OCT machines. **A:** Cirrus HD-OCT. (Courtesy of Carl Zeiss Meditec, Inc.) **B:** Spectralis OCT. (Courtesy of Heidelberg Engineering.)

A   **B**

advance of functional testing is less clear. At the time of publication, comparison of spectral-domain OCT to OCT3 with regard to diagnosing glaucoma and progression of glaucoma has not yet been established.

Retinal Thickness Analyzer

The retinal thickness analyzer is another computerized system for measuring the retina thickness. It projects a laser beam onto the retina, and a fundus camera observes reflections from internal limiting membrane and in the retina until the light reaches the retinal pigment epithelium. The profile of light intensity contains peak reflections from the internal limiting membrane and the retinal pigment epithelium, and the thickness of the retina is calculated from the distance between the two peaks. The retinal thickness analyzer may be useful in glaucoma management to monitor retinal thickness (545,546).

Clinical Value of Image Analyzers

In the few studies that have directly compared the different structural imaging technologies, OCT3 had better sensitivity and specificity, compared with the HRT-II and scanning laser polarimetry (528,529). Early in the course of the disease process, these structural imaging technologies are very helpful in differentiating glaucomatous damage before achromatic (i.e., white-on-white) visual field change. Perhaps the most useful application is a negative result on a structural test in a patient with suspected glaucoma; it can be reassuring that no disease is detectable when visual field and structural testing find no abnormality. No single test has absolute sensitivity and specificity. When used alone, HRT, GDx, and OCT summary data reports may help differentiate between healthy eyes and glaucomatous eyes with mild to moderate visual field loss, although none of the instruments provided enough sensitivity and specificity to be used as a screening tool for early glaucoma (547). A combination of the best parameters from the three imaging methods significantly improves this capability (541) (**Fig. 4.32**). Information obtained with HRT, GDx, and OCT allows combining qualitative data with graphic visual information and quantitative data, and, with improved sensitivity and specificity of these instruments, the summary data reports may better assist the physician in the management of patients with glaucoma (531).

At this time, none of these structural technologies alone can be relied on to ascertain glaucomatous progression without corroborating evidence. However, these technologies continue to evolve and improve rapidly. At the time of publication, HRT-III and spectral domain are at the beginning of their use.

Techniques for Blood-Flow Measurement

Early studies on ocular blood flow are discussed earlier; they relate to the pathophysiology of glaucomatous optic neuropathy. This section considers new techniques for measuring ocular blood flow, which may one day have clinical application. Although studies have shown deficient blood flow in at least 50% of patients with normal-tension glaucoma, direct evidence that vascular factors contribute to the development of glaucoma optic neuropathy is lacking, because measurements of the optic nerve blood flow are limited by the small caliber of blood vessels and the volume of the optic nerve tissue being studied (548–550).

In the past two decades, several methods have been developed to facilitate quantitative, comprehensive study of retinal, choroidal, and retrobulbar circulations. These techniques include vessel caliber assessment, pulsatile ocular blood-flow measurement, scanning laser fluorescein and indocyanine green (ICG) angiography of the peripapillary choroid and the retinal circulation, laser Doppler flowmetry, confocal scanning laser Doppler flowmetry, and color Doppler imaging (551). To fully assess optic nerve circulation, these techniques should be combined because no single technology can adequately describe the complex hemodynamics of the eye.

Angiography

New imaging technologies allow us to detect and follow very subtle changes of the structure and perfusion of the optic nerve head. These and other technologies may enhance the ability to diagnose and monitor glaucomatous disc damage (552).

Confocal scanning laser ophthalmoscopy can enhance angiographic examination of small vessels of the optic nerve head using fluorescein or ICG (553). The confocal scanning laser ophthalmoscopy allows acquisition of images of the retinal circulation and late leakage sites. Optical subtraction of the light contribution of the retinal circulation allows examination of the choroidal circulation and vice versa. At least three advantages of confocal scanning laser ophthalmoscopy over conventional instruments have been described as follows: (a) excellent visualization of the retinal circulation, (b) optical subtraction of retinal circulation, and (c) acquisition and processing of all data digitally with easy data exchange. This technology may potentially produce a three-dimensional map of the retinal and choroidal vasculature (554).

Heidelberg retina angiograph (HRA and HRA-II), which combines confocal scanning laser ophthalmoscopy technology with ICG and fluorescein angiography, is commercially available. With this instrument, several changes may be seen in peripapillary capillary vessels at the different glaucomatous stages. Persons with early glaucomatous damage have an increase of the cup area, secondary to a reduction of the neuroretinal rim area, and ICG angiography shows an increase in prepapillary plexus visualization, which may be caused by increased blood flow while autoregulation is still functioning. Some patients with advanced glaucoma show significant capillary dropout on ICG angiography (555).

The HRA can demonstrate the superficial and deep blood supply of the optic nerve, and simultaneous ICG and fluorescein angiography, and visualization of separate circulations in different planes. The technique allows overlaying ICG and fluorescein images or comparison of them side by side (556). One prospective study evaluated the correlation between the vascular supply of the optic nerve and visual fields. In eyes with a normal visual field, a diffuse microvascular filling pattern of the optic disc area was apparent with no filling defects, whereas angiography of glaucomatous eyes had good correlation with the visual field defect location (557).

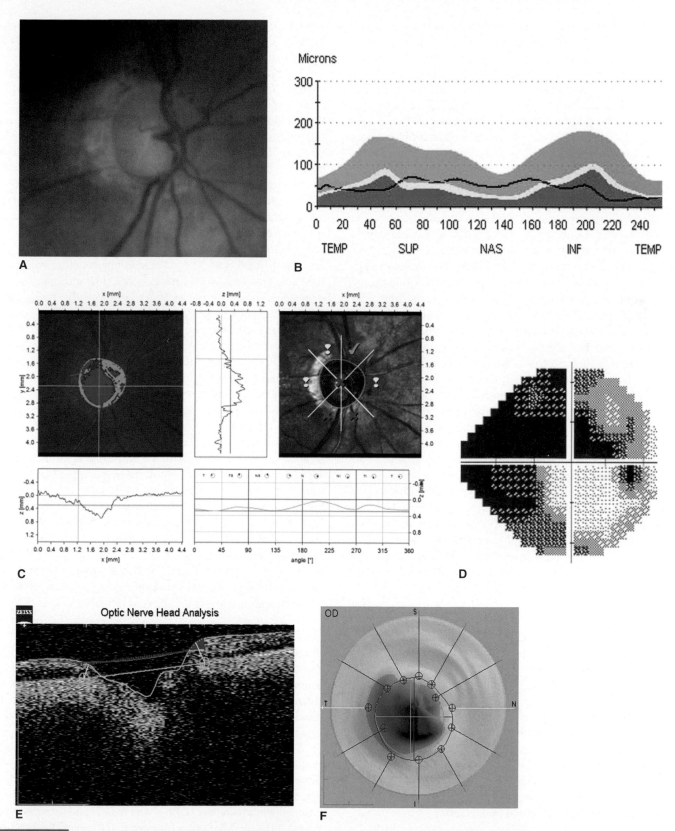

Figure 4.32 **A:** Color photograph of a glaucomatous optic nerve head showing advanced loss of the neuroretinal rim, especially inferotemporally. Peripapillary atrophy, arteriolar narrowing, and bayoneting of the retinal arterioles are also present. **B:** Corresponding OCT shows preservation of the nasal RNFL, but significant loss temporally. **C:** Topographic map by confocal scanning laser ophthalmoscopy of the same optic nerve. The *red x* denotes areas of neuroretinal rim thickness less than the normative database; the *yellow !* denotes areas of neuroretinal rim thickness in the border zone of normal in the same normative database. **D:** Corresponding automated achromatic visual field showing a near superior altitudinal defect and dense inferior arcuate and nasal step defect. **E:** Cross section of the optic nerve head by OCT. **F:** Topographic map by OCT of the same optic nerve.

When the optic disc and peripapillary region was evaluated by modified ICG confocal scanning laser ophthalmoscopy angiography, the hypofluorescent areas in the peripapillary region were more common in eyes with glaucoma; however, hypofluorescent halos that were extending around the optic disc margins did not correlate with any of the study factors. Hypofluorescence was demonstrated in 68% of glaucomatous eyes, compared with 20% of control eyes (558). These observations are similar to those of earlier fluorescein angiographic studies that were previously discussed.

Color Doppler Imaging

The normal vascular anatomy of the eye and orbit, and various conditions with vascular abnormalities, has been studied with the color Doppler imaging, which allows simultaneous imaging with real-time ultrasound and superimposed color-coded vascular flow, allowing visualization of vessels previously beyond the resolution of conventional imaging, such as those in the orbit (559). Combining B-scan ultrasonography and Doppler waveform analysis, color Doppler imaging has been reported to allow noninvasive examination of blood velocity and vascular resistance in the ophthalmic, short posterior ciliary, and central retinal arteries in patients with COAG or normal-tension glaucoma (167).

One investigative team, using color Doppler imaging to evaluate the blood flow in the ophthalmic, posterior ciliary, and central retinal arteries, found significantly reduced mean systolic peak flow velocity in the ophthalmic artery in patients with glaucoma, compared with controls. In patients with glaucoma who had uncontrolled IOP, there was a reduction of end-diastolic flow velocities and an increase of resistivity index in ciliary arteries and the central retinal artery (560). The color Doppler imaging showed a significant decrease in the mean end-diastolic velocity and an increase in the mean resistive index in all blood vessels in patients with glaucoma (561). There were no differences between the patients with COAG and those with normal-tension glaucoma (169).

Another study, testing the reproducibility of the central retinal artery velocity measurements by using color Doppler imaging, showed that large differences existed in measured central retinal artery velocity, depending on the location of the measurement, and that color-flow thresholding was valuable in locating the optimal location for pulsed Doppler spectral recording (562).

The high reproducibility of the color Doppler imaging technique for the peak-systolic and end-diastolic velocities and for the resistance index, taken in the central retinal artery, the ophthalmic artery, and the short posterior ciliary arteries, is suggestive to support the validity of using color Doppler imaging in a clinical setting to measure the hemodynamic parameters of small retrobulbar blood vessels (563).

Laser Doppler Flowmetry

Laser Doppler flowmetry was introduced in 1972 to provide a noninvasive method to measure the perfusion of ocular tissues at individual discrete locations (564). It has been used in experimental and clinical studies (565). This technology can measure blood cell velocity in a volume of tissue and derive an estimate of volumetric blood flow. Laser Doppler flowmetry has also been used to measure microcirculatory blood flow in neural tissue, muscles, skin, bone, and intestine (566,567).

The principle is to measure the Doppler shift, which is the change of frequency that light undergoes when reflected by moving objects, such as red blood cells. Because the velocity of the red blood cells is extremely low, compared with the speed of light, it is not possible to directly measure the resulting alteration in the frequency or color of the light. However, laser Doppler flowmetry provides an indirect method, in which the low-power coherent laser light that is scattered or reflected by moving red blood cells undergoes a Doppler frequency shift, while light reflected from surrounding tissue remains in its original frequency. The two coherent components of light, with only slightly different frequencies, interfere and result in a phenomenon called beat. This reflected light, together with laser light scattered from static tissue, is detected and processed to provide a blood-flow measurement. As a result, the Doppler shift of the light frequency is translated to an intensity oscillation, which can be measured. The laser Doppler flowmeter uses monochromatic light emitted from a low-power laser. Measurement of the erythrocyte movement is recorded continuously in the outer layer of the tissue under study, with no influence on physiologic blood flow. The output value is defined as the number of red blood cells times their velocity and is reported as microcirculatory perfusion units.

To obtain the measurement, a low-intensity laser beam is directed to a certain location of the retina and is scanned across a tissue surface in a raster fashion using a moving mirror. The intensity of the light reflected and scattered at that location is measured typically over several seconds. The amplitude of measured intensity is proportional to the number of moving particles, and the frequency of the intensity is proportional to the velocity of the particles. The results are interpreted as a frequency distribution of the number of moving red blood cells and their velocity, providing a simple and quantitative description of the blood flow at the selected retinal location.

Scanning Laser Doppler Flowmetry

Blood flow can be measured by combining laser Doppler flowmetry with confocal scanning laser (568–571). The method is noninvasive and results are rapidly obtained, but it requires clear optical media and good fixation and is highly sensitive to illumination changes and eye movement; in addition, it measures blood flow in a relatively small velocity range (572).

The Heidelberg retinal flowmeter, the model currently available, performs laser Doppler measurements in a two-dimensional array of points, resulting in two-dimensional perfusion maps. During an examination with the Heidelberg retinal flowmeter, a laser beam enters the eye and focuses on the retinal surface by the optical properties of the eye. The direction of the laser beam entering the eye is periodically changed in two directions by two oscillating mirrors, so that a two-dimensional region of the retina is scanned line by line. The scan field is 10 degrees wide and 2.5 degrees high, corresponding to a size of 2.88 mm × 0.72 mm. During the scan along one line, the reflected light intensity at 256 pixels is measured and digitized sequentially. Each of the 64 total lines is scanned 128 times, with the total acquisition time of about 2.5 seconds. After the scanning is complete, for each of the 256 × 64 locations, there are 128 measurements of the reflected light intensity versus time. When the analysis is performed at each measured location, the result is a matrix of 256 × 64, or 16,384 pixels (perfusion map), which provides perfusion measurements. For visualization, low perfusion values are displayed in dark colors and high perfusion in light colors, resulting in a color-coded two-dimensional perfusion map, with the parameters of (a) volume, (b) flow, and (c) velocity. The highest flow values occur in the larger vessels. Because of the dual blood-flow supply in the optic nerve and the limited penetration of the laser, the instrument primarily measures the microcirculation in the nerve fiber layer of the anterior optic nerve, which is largely supplied by the central retinal artery rather than the ciliary circulation (573). Blood flow in the laminar and retrolaminar regions makes only a small contribution to the measurements.

The Heidelberg retinal flowmeter has allowed demonstration in healthy volunteers that ocular blood flow increases while inhaling carbogen and decreases while inhaling oxygen or after increasing IOP to 50 mm Hg with a suction cup (574). Although IOP values were significantly reduced by the use of betaxolol and timolol, blood-flow values were significantly decreased only in the timolol group.

Laser Speckle Flowmetry

Laser speckle is seen when coherent laser light is scattered from a diffuse object. If instead of being stationary the illuminated object consists of individual moving red blood cells, the speckle pattern fluctuates randomly. The intensity of these fluctuations provides information about the velocity of the object producing the scatter. The structure of the pattern that changes according to blood-flow velocity is called "blurring," and a square blur rate is an index of blood velocity, calculated by a computer.

One prospective study compared blood-flow measurements in the optic nerve head by laser speckle flowmetry with confocal scanning laser Doppler flowmetry. There was only a weak correlation between the blood-flow indexes, as measured by laser speckle flowmetry and scanning laser Doppler flowmetry because of basic differences in the principles of measurement (575).

Another study has shown significant differences in optic nerve head blood flow in healthy volunteers between the right and left eyes and between the superior and inferior temporal neuroretinal rims using laser speckle flowmetry. These normal data may be useful in understanding the physiology of ocular hemodynamics (576).

Magnetic Resonance Imaging

Qualitative analysis of the perfusion of the human optic nerve with magnetic resonance imaging (MRI) may be used to study optic nerve blood-flow abnormalities (577). MRI can also be used to quantify changes in the optic nerve microcirculation. T2-weighted MRI in rats provided quantification of optic nerve blood flow and has shown that dopaminergic substances increase optic nerve blood flow (578).

The Possible Future of Imaging

Exciting areas of innovation are the structural imaging of RGC bodies and the imaging of individual ganglion cell stress and death (579–585). These areas are still in experimental development, but may be clinically relevant in the future.

KEY POINTS

- The optic nerve head comprises axons from the RGCs, as well as blood vessels and astroglial and collagen support. The normal optic nerve head has considerable variation in size and surface contour.
- The pathogenesis of glaucomatous optic atrophy appears to involve obstruction of axoplasmic flow, although whether this is a direct mechanical effect of elevated IOP or secondary to vascular changes is unclear.
- Glaucomatous optic atrophy is characterized clinically by a progressive, asymmetric loss of neural rim tissue, which is manifested by an enlargement in the area of cupping and pallor. This most often extends in a focal direction, producing early thinning of the inferior and superior portions of the neural rim. Enlargement of the cup often precedes that of the area of pallor, creating a pallor–cup discrepancy. Other important signs of glaucomatous optic atrophy are disc hemorrhages and peripapillary nerve fiber bundle defects.
- The differential diagnosis of glaucomatous optic atrophy includes normal variations, developmental anomalies, and nonglaucomatous causes of acquired cupping.
- Techniques for evaluating the optic nerve head include a careful office examination and photographic documentation, although newer techniques, such as computed image analysis and blood-flow measures, may provide more precise methods of observation in the clinical management of glaucoma.

REFERENCES

1. Jonas JB, Budde WM, Panda-Jonas S. Ophthalmoscopic evaluation of the optic nerve head. *Surv Ophthalmol.* 1999;43:293–320.
2. Kronfeld PC. Normal variations of the optic disc as observed by conventional ophthalmoscopy and their anatomic correlations. *Trans Am Acad Ophthalmol Otolaryngol.* 1976;81:214–216.
3. Jonas JB, Gusek GC, Guggenmoos-Holzmann I, et al. Size of the optic nerve scleral canal and comparison with intravital determination of optic disc dimensions. *Graefes Arch Clin Exp Ophthalmol.* 1988;226:213–215.
4. Quigley HA, Brown AE, Morrison JD, et al. The size and shape of the optic disc in normal human eyes. *Arch Ophthalmol.* 1990;108:51–57.
5. Ramrattan RS, Wolfs RC, Jonas JB, et al. Determinants of optic disc characteristics in a general population: The Rotterdam Study. *Ophthalmology.* 1999;106:1588–1596.
6. Jonas JB, Mardin CY, Grundler AE. Comparison of measurements of neuroretinal rim area between confocal laser scanning tomography and planimetry of photographs. *Br J Ophthalmol.* 1998;82:362–366.
7. Budde WM, Jonas JB, Martus P, et al. Influence of optic disc size on neuroretinal rim shape in healthy eyes. *J Glaucoma.* 2000;9:357–362.
8. Funaki S, Shirakashi M, Abe H. Relation between size of optic disc and thickness of retinal nerve fibre layer in normal subjects. *Br J Ophthalmol.* 1998;82:1242–1245.
9. Kashiwagi K, Tamura M, Abe K, et al. The influence of age, gender, refractive error, and optic disc size on the optic disc configuration in Japanese normal eyes. *Acta Ophthalmol Scand.* 2000;78:200–203.

10. Hellstrom A, Svensson E. Optic disc size and retinal vessel characteristics in healthy children. *Acta Ophthalmol Scand.* 1998;76:260–267.

11. Wolfs RC, Ramrattan RS, Hofman A, et al. Cup-to-disc ratio: ophthalmoscopy versus automated measurement in a general population—The Rotterdam Study. *Ophthalmology.* 1999;106:1597–1601.

12. Garway-Heath DF, Rudnicka AR, Lowe T, et al. Measurement of optic disc size: equivalence of methods to correct for ocular magnification. *Br J Ophthalmol.* 1998;82:643–649.

13. Meyer T, Howland HC. How large is the optic disc? Systematic errors in fundus cameras and topographers. *Ophthalmic Physiol Opt.* 2001; 21:139–150.

14. Hayreh SS. Anatomy and physiology of the optic nerve head. *Trans Am Acad Ophthalmol Otolaryngol.* 1974;78:OP240–OP254.

15. Minckler DS, McLean IW, Tso MO. Distribution of axonal and glial elements in the rhesus optic nerve head studied by electron microscopy. *Am J Ophthalmol.* 1976;82:179–187.

16. Anderson DR. Ultrastructure of human and monkey lamina cribrosa and optic nerve head. *Arch Ophthalmol.* 1969;82:800–814.

17. Hamasaki DI, Fujino T. Effect of intraocular pressure on ocular vessels: filling with India ink. *Arch Ophthalmol.* 1967;78:369–379.

18. Geijer C, Bill A. Effects of raised intraocular pressure on retinal, prelaminar, laminar, and retrolaminar optic nerve blood flow in monkeys. *Invest Ophthalmol Vis Sci.* 1979;18:1030–1042.

19. Onda E, Cioffi GA, Bacon DR, et al. Microvasculature of the human optic nerve. *Am J Ophthalmol.* 1995;120:92–102.

20. Hayreh SS. The blood supply of the optic nerve head and the evaluation of it—myth and reality. *Prog Retin Eye Res.* 2001;20:563–593.

21. Lieberman MF, Maumenee AE, Green WR. Histologic studies of the vasculature of the anterior optic nerve. *Am J Ophthalmol.* 1976;82:405–423.

22. Hayreh SS, Jonas JB. Optic disk and retinal nerve fiber layer damage after transient central retinal artery occlusion: an experimental study in rhesus monkeys. *Am J Ophthalmol.* 2000;129:786–795.

23. Anderson DR, Braverman S. Reevaluation of the optic disk vasculature. *Am J Ophthalmol.* 1976;82:165–174.

24. Olver JM, Spalton DJ, McCartney AC. Quantitative morphology of human retrolaminar optic nerve vasculature. *Invest Ophthalmol Vis Sci.* 1994;35:3858–3866.

25. Ko MK, Kim DS, Ahn YK. Morphological variations of the peripapillary circle of Zinn-Haller by flat section. *Br J Ophthalmol.* 1999;83:862–866.

26. Goder G. The capillaries of the optic nerve. *Am J Ophthalmol.* 1974;77:684–689.

27. Hayreh SS. Blood flow in the optic nerve head and factors that may influence it. *Prog Retin Eye Res.* 2001;20:595–624.

28. Zaret CR, Choromokos EA, Meisler DM. Cilio-optic vein associated with phakomatosis. *Ophthalmology.* 1980;87:330–336.

29. Anderson DR, Hoyt WF, Hogan MJ. The fine structure of the astroglia in the human optic nerve and optic nerve head. *Trans Am Ophthalmol Soc.* 1967;65:275–305.

30. Quigley HA. Gap junctions between optic nerve head astrocytes. *Invest Ophthalmol Vis Sci.* 1977;16:582–585.

31. Trivino A, Ramirez JM, Salazar JJ, et al. Immunohistochemical study of human optic nerve head astroglia. *Vision Res.* 1996;36:2015–2028.

32. Anderson DR. Ultrastructure of the optic nerve head. *Arch Ophthalmol.* 1970;83:63–73.

33. Anderson DR, Hoyt WF. Ultrastructure of intraorbital portion of human and monkey optic nerve. *Arch Ophthalmol.* 1969;82:506–530.

34. Heegaard S, Jensen OA, Prause JU. Structure of the vitread face of the monkey optic disc (*Macaca mulatta*): SEM on frozen resin-cracked optic nerve heads supplemented by TEM and immunohistochemistry. *Graefes Arch Clin Exp Ophthalmol.* 1988;226:377–383.

35. Hirata A, Kitaoka T, Ishigooka H, et al. Cytochemical studies of transitional area between retina and optic nerve. *Acta Ophthalmol (Copenh).* 1991;69:71–75.

36. Hernandez MR, Miao H, Lukas T. Astrocytes in glaucomatous optic neuropathy. *Prog Brain Res.* 2008;173:353–373.

37. Brooks DE, Komaromy AM, Kallberg ME. Comparative optic nerve physiology: implications for glaucoma, neuroprotection, and neuroregeneration. *Vet Ophthalmol.* 1999;2:13–25.

38. Fukuchi T, Ueda J, Abe H, et al. Cell adhesion glycoproteins in the human lamina cribrosa. *Jpn J Ophthalmol.* 2001;45:363–367.

39. Gong H, Ye W, Freddo TF, et al. Hyaluronic acid in the normal and glaucomatous optic nerve. *Exp Eye Res.* 1997;64:587–595.

40. Jonas JB, Berenshtein E, Holbach L. Anatomic relationship between lamina cribrosa, intraocular space, and cerebrospinal fluid space. *Invest Ophthalmol Vis Sci.* 2003;44:5189–5195.

41. Maeda H, Nakamura M, Yamamoto M. Morphometric features of laminar pores in lamina cribrosa observed by scanning laser ophthalmoscopy. *Jpn J Ophthalmol.* 1999;43:415–421.

42. Quigley HA, Addicks EM. Regional differences in the structure of the lamina cribrosa and their relation to glaucomatous optic nerve damage. *Arch Ophthalmol.* 1981;99:137–143.

43. Radius RL, Gonzales M. Anatomy of the lamina cribrosa in human eyes. *Arch Ophthalmol.* 1981;99:2159–2162.

44. Radius RL. Regional specificity in anatomy at the lamina cribrosa. *Arch Ophthalmol.* 1981;99:478–480.

45. Jonas JB, Mardin CY, Schlotzer-Schrehardt U, et al. Morphometry of the human lamina cribrosa surface. *Invest Ophthalmol Vis Sci.* 1991;32: 401–405.

46. Morgan JE, Jeffery G, Foss AJ. Axon deviation in the human lamina cribrosa. *Br J Ophthalmol.* 1998;82:680–683.

47. Dichtl A, Jonas JB, Naumann GO. Course of the optic nerve fibers through the lamina cribrosa in human eyes. *Graefes Arch Clin Exp Ophthalmol.* 1996;234:581–585.

48. Hernandez MR, Luo XX, Igoe F, et al. Extracellular matrix of the human lamina cribrosa. *Am J Ophthalmol.* 1987;104:567–576.

49. Rehnberg M, Ammitzboll T, Tengroth B. Collagen distribution in the lamina cribrosa and the trabecular meshwork of the human eye. *Br J Ophthalmol.* 1987;71:886–892.

50. Goldbaum MH, Jeng SY, Logemann R, et al. The extracellular matrix of the human optic nerve. *Arch Ophthalmol.* 1989;107:1225–1231.

51. Hernandez MR, Igoe F, Neufeld AH. Cell culture of the human lamina cribrosa. *Invest Ophthalmol Vis Sci.* 1988;29:78–89.

52. Hernandez MR, Wang N, Hanley NM, et al. Localization of collagen types I and IV mRNAs in human optic nerve head by in situ hybridization. *Invest Ophthalmol Vis Sci.* 1991;32:2169–2177.

53. Caparas VL, Cintron C, Hernandez-Neufeld MR. Immunohistochemistry of proteoglycans in human lamina cribrosa. *Am J Ophthalmol.* 1991;112:489–495.

54. Sawaguchi S, Yue BY, Fukuchi T, et al. Sulfated proteoglycans in the human lamina cribrosa. *Invest Ophthalmol Vis Sci.* 1992;33:2388–2398.

55. Kirwan RP, Wordinger RJ, Clark AF, et al. Differential expression patterns between normal and glaucomatous human lamina cribrosa cells. *Mol Vis.* 2009;15:76–88.

56. Thornton IL, Dupps WJ, Roy AS, et al. Biomechanical effects of intraocular pressure elevation on optic nerve/lamina cribrosa before and after peripapillary scleral collagen cross-linking. *Invest Ophthalmol Vis Sci.* 2009;50:1227–1233.

57. Sigal IA, Ethier CR. Biomechanics of the optic nerve head. *Exp Eye Res.* 2009;88:799–807.

58. Anderson DR. Ultrastructure of meningeal sheaths: normal human and monkey optic nerves. *Arch Ophthalmol.* 1969;82:659–674.

59. Killer HE, Laeng HR, Groscurth P. Lymphatic capillaries in the meninges of the human optic nerve. *J Neuroophthalmol.* 1999;19:222–228.

60. Radius RL, Anderson DR. The histology of retinal nerve fiber layer bundles and bundle defects. *Arch Ophthalmol.* 1979;97:948–950.

61. Radius RL, Anderson DR. The course of axons through the retina and optic nerve head. *Arch Ophthalmol.* 1979;97:1154–1158.

62. Radius RL, de Bruin J. Anatomy of the retinal nerve fiber layer. *Invest Ophthalmol Vis Sci.* 1981;21:745–749.

63. Ogden TE. Nerve fiber layer of the primate retina: morphometric analysis. *Invest Ophthalmol Vis Sci.* 1984;25:19–29.

64. Wang L, Dong J, Cull G, et al. Varicosities of intraretinal ganglion cell axons in human and nonhuman primates. *Invest Ophthalmol Vis Sci.* 2003;44:2–9.

65. Minckler DS. The organization of nerve fiber bundles in the primate optic nerve head. *Arch Ophthalmol.* 1980;98:1630–1636.

66. Hoyt WF, Luis O. Visual fiber anatomy in the infrageniculate pathway of the primate. *Arch Ophthalmol.* 1962;68:94–106.

67. Mikelberg FS, Drance SM, Schulzer M, et al. The normal human optic nerve: axon count and axon diameter distribution. *Ophthalmology.* 1989;96:1325–1328.

68. Repka MX, Quigley HA. The effect of age on normal human optic nerve fiber number and diameter. *Ophthalmology.* 1989;96:26–32.

69. Mikelberg FS, Yidegiligne HM, White VA, et al. Relation between optic nerve axon number and axon diameter to scleral canal area. *Ophthalmology.* 1991;98:60–63.

70. Jonas JB, Schmidt AM, Muller-Bergh JA, et al. Human optic nerve fiber count and optic disc size. *Invest Ophthalmol Vis Sci.* 1992;33:2012–2018.

71. Jonas JB, Schmidt AM, Muller-Bergh JA, et al. Optic nerve fiber count and diameter of the retrobulbar optic nerve in normal and glaucomatous eyes. *Graefes Arch Clin Exp Ophthalmol.* 1995;233:421–424.

72. Quigley HA, Coleman AL, Dorman-Pease ME. Larger optic nerve heads have more nerve fibers in normal monkey eyes. *Arch Ophthalmol.* 1991;109:1441–1443.

73. Panda-Jonas S, Jonas JB, Jakobczyk M, et al. Retinal photoreceptor count, retinal surface area, and optic disc size in normal human eyes. *Ophthalmology.* 1994;101:519–523.

74. Johnson BM, Miao M, Sadun AA. Age-related decline of human optic nerve axon populations. *Age.* 1987;10:5.

75. Marquardt T, Gruss P. Generating neuronal diversity in the retina: one for nearly all. *Trends Neurosci.* 2002;25(1):32–38.

76. Adler R. A model of retinal cell differentiation in the chick embryo [review]. *Prog Retin Eye Res.* 2000;19(5):529–557.

77. Livesey FJ, Cepko CL. Vertebrate neural cell-fate determination: lessons from the retina. *Nat Rev Neurosci.* 2001;2(2):109–118.

78. Sharma RK, Johnson DA. Molecular signals for development of neuronal circuitry in the retina. *Neurochem Res.* 2000;25(9–10):1257–1263.

79. Malicki J. Harnessing the power of forward genetics—analysis of neuronal diversity and patterning in the zebrafish retina. *Trends Neurosci.* 2000;23(11):531–541.

80. Perron M, Harris WA. Determination of vertebrate retinal progenitor cell fate by the Notch pathway and basic helix-loop-helix transcription factors [review]. *Cell Mol Life Sci.* 2000;57(2):215–223.

81. Xiang M, Zhou H, Nathans J. Molecular biology of retinal ganglion cells. *Proc Natl Acad Sci USA.* 1996;93(2):596–601.

82. Sernagor E, Eglen SJ, Wong RO. Development of retinal ganglion cell structure and function. *Prog Retin Eye Res.* 2001;20(2):139–174.

83. Pichaud F, Treisman J, Desplan C. Reinventing a common strategy for patterning the eye. *Cell.* 2001;105(1):9–12.

84. Martinez-Morales JR, Signore M, Acampora D, et al. Otx genes are required for tissue specification in the developing eye. *Development.* 2001;128(11):2019–2030.

85. Cellerino A, Bahr M, Isenmann S. Apoptosis in the developing visual system. *Cell Tissue Res.* 2000;301(1):53–69.

86. de la Rosa EJ, de Pablo F. Cell death in early neural development: beyond the neurotrophic theory. *Trends Neurosci.* 2000;23(10):454–458.

87. Dyer MA, Cepko CL. p27Kip1 and p57Kip2 regulate proliferation in distinct retinal progenitor cell populations. *J Neurosci.* 2001;21(12):4259–4271.

88. Provis JM, van Driel D, Billison FAB, et al. Human fetal optic nerve: overproduction and elimination of retinal axons during development. *J Comp Neurol.* 1985;238:92–100.

89. Mathers PH, Grinberg A, Mahon KA, et al. The Rx homeobox gene is essential for vertebrate eye development. *Nature.* 1997;387(6633):603–607.

90. Baas D, Legrand C, Samarut J, et al. Persistence of oligodendrocyte precursor cells and altered myelination in optic nerve associated to retina degeneration in mice devoid of all thyroid hormone receptors. *Proc Natl Acad Sci U S A.* 2002;99(5):2907–2911.

91. Forrest D, Reh TA, Rusch A. Neurodevelopmental control by thyroid hormone receptors. *Curr Opin Neurobiol.* 2002;12(1):49–56.

92. Russell C. The roles of hedgehogs and fibroblast growth factors in eye development and retinal cell rescue. *Vision Res.* 2003;43(8):899–912.

93. Tripathi BJ, Tripathi RC, Livingston AM, et al. The role of growth factors in the embryogenesis and differentiation of the eye. *Am J Anat.* 1991;192(4):442–471.

94. Bennett JL, Zeiler SR, Jones KR. Patterned expression of BDNF and NT-3 in the retina and anterior segment of the developing mammalian eye. *Invest Ophthalmol Vis Sci.* 1999;40(12):2996–3005.

95. Hardy P, Dumont I, Bhattacharya M, et al. Oxidants, nitric oxide, and prostanoids in the developing ocular vasculature: a basis for ischemic retinopathy. *Cardiovasc Res.* 2000;47(3):489–509.

96. Rimmer S, Keating C, Chou T, et al. Growth of the human optic disk and nerve during gestation, childhood, and early adulthood. *Am J Ophthalmol.* 1993;116:748–753.

97. Dolman CL, McCormick, Drance SM. Aging of the optic nerve. *Arch Ophthalmol.* 1980;98:2053–2058.

98. Magoon EH, Robb RM. Development of myelin in human optic nerve and tract: a light and electron microscopic study. *Arch Ophthalmol.* 1981;99:655–659.

99. Quigley HA. The pathogenesis of reversible cupping in congenital glaucoma. *Am J Ophthalmol.* 1977;84:358–370.

100. Hernandez MR, Luo XX, Andrzejewska W, et al. Age-related changes in the extracellular matrix of the human optic nerve head. *Am J Ophthalmol.* 1989;107:476–484.

101. Hernandez MR. Ultrastructural immunocytochemical analysis of elastin in the human lamina cribrosa: changes in elastic fibers in primary open-angle glaucoma. *Invest Ophthalmol Vis Sci.* 1992;33:2891–2903.

102. Sawaguchi S, Yue BY, Fukuchi T, et al. Age-related changes of sulfated proteoglycans in the human lamina cribrosa. *Curr Eye Res.* 1993;12:685–692.

103. Alamouti B, Funk J. Retinal thickness decreases with age: an OCT study. *Br J Ophthalmol.* 2003;87:899–901.

104. Toprak AB, Yilmaz OF. Relation of optic disc topography and age to thickness of retinal nerve fiber layer as measured using scanning laser polarimetry, in normal subjects. *Br J Ophthalmol.* 2000;84:473–478.

105. Kerrigan-Baumrind LA, Quigley HA, Pease ME, et al. Number of ganglion cells in glaucoma eyes compared with threshold visual field tests in the same persons. *Invest Ophthalmol Vis Sci.* 2000;41:741–748.

106. Müler H. Anatomische Beitrage zur Ophthalmologie: Ueber Nervean-Veranderungen an der Eintrittsstelle des Schnerven. *Arch Ophthalmol.* 1858;4:1.

107. von Jaeger E. Ueber Glaucom und seine Heilung durch Iridectomie. *Z Ges der Aerzte zu Wien.* 1858;14:465.

108. Schnabel J. Das glaucomatose Sehnervenleiden. *Archiv für Augenheilkunde.* 1892;XXIV:273.

109. Laker C. Ein experimenteller Beitrag zur Lehre von der glaukomatosen Excavation. *Klin Monatsbl Augenheilkd.* 1886;24:187.

110. Schreiber L. Ueber Degeneration der Netzhaut naut experimentellen und pathologisch-anatomischen Untersuchungen. *Graefes Arch Clin Exp Ophthalmol.* 1906;64:237.

111. Fuchs E. Ueber die Lamina cribrosa. *Graefes Arch Clin Exp Ophthalmol.* 1916;91:435.

112. LaGrange F, Beauvieux J. Anatomie de l'excavation glaucomateuse. *Arch Ophthalmol (Paris).* 1925;42:129.

113. Duke-Elder S. Fundamental concepts in glaucoma. *Arch Ophthalmol.* 1949;42:538–545.

114. Duke-Elder S. The problems of simple glaucoma. *Trans Ophthalmol Soc U K.* 1962;82:307.

115. Gafner F, Goldman H. Experimentelle Untersuchungen über den Zusammenhang von Augendrucksteigerung und Gesichtsfeldschadigung. *Ophthalmologica.* 1955;130:357.

116. Lampert PW, Vogel MH, Zimmerman LE. Pathology of the optic nerve in experimental acute glaucoma: electron microscopic studies. *Invest Ophthalmol.* 1968;7:199–213.

117. Shaffer RN. The role of the astroglial cells in glaucomatous disc cupping. *Doc Ophthalmol.* 1969;26:516–525.

118. Shaffer RN, Hetherington J Jr. The glaucomatous disc in infants: a suggested hypothesis for disc cupping. *Trans Am Acad Ophthalmol Otolaryngol.* 1969;73:923–935.

119. Quigley HA, Green WR. The histology of human glaucoma cupping and optic nerve damage: clinicopathologic correlation in 21 eyes. *Ophthalmology.* 1979;86:1803–1830.

120. Quigley HA, Addicks EM, Green WR, et al. Optic nerve damage in human glaucoma. II. The site of injury and susceptibility to damage. *Arch Ophthalmol.* 1981;99:635–649.

121. Schwartz B. Cupping and pallor of the optic disc. *Arch Ophthalmol.* 1973;89:272–277.

122. Kornzweig AL, Eliasoph I, Feldstein M. Selective atrophy of the radial peripapillary capillaries in chronic glaucoma. *Arch Ophthalmol.* 1968;80:696–702.

123. Daicker B. Selective atrophy of the radial peripapillary capillaries and visual field defects in glaucoma [in German]. *Albrecht Von Graefes Arch Klin Exp Ophthalmol.* 1975;195:27–32.

124. Quigley HA, Hohman RM, Addicks EM, et al. Blood vessels of the glaucomatous optic disc in experimental primate and human eyes. *Invest Ophthalmol Vis Sci.* 1984;25:918–931.

125. Quigley HA, Hohman RM, Addicks EM. Quantitative study of optic nerve head capillaries in experimental optic disk pallor. *Am J Ophthalmol.* 1982;93:689–699.

126. Quigley HA, Anderson DR. The histologic basis of optic disk pallor in experimental optic atrophy. *Am J Ophthalmol.* 1977;83:709–717.

127. Henkind P, Bellhorn R, Rabkin M, et al. Optic nerve transection in cats. II. Effect on vessels of optic nerve head and lamina cribrosa. *Invest Ophthalmol Vis Sci.* 1977;16:442–447.

128. Radius RL, Anderson DR. The mechanism of disc pallor in experimental optic atrophy: a fluorescein angiographic study. *Arch Ophthalmol.* 1979;97:532–535.

129. Hayreh SS. Pathogenesis of cupping of the optic disc. *Br J Ophthalmol.* 1974;58:863–876.

130. Emery JM, Landis D, Paton D, et al. The lamina cribrosa in normal and glaucomatous human eyes. *Trans Am Acad Ophthalmol Otolaryngol.* 1974;78:OP290–OP297.

131. Levy NS, Crapps EE. Displacement of optic nerve head in response to short-term intraocular pressure elevation in human eyes. *Arch Ophthalmol.* 1984;102:782–786.

132. Yan DB, Coloma FM, Metheetrairut A, et al. Deformation of the lamina cribrosa by elevated intraocular pressure. *Br J Ophthalmol.* 1994;78:643–648.

133. Radius RL, Pederson JE. Laser-induced primate glaucoma. II. Histopathology. *Arch Ophthalmol.* 1984;102:1693–1698.

134. Coleman AL, Quigley HA, Vitale S, et al. Displacement of the optic nerve head by acute changes in intraocular pressure in monkey eyes. *Ophthalmology.* 1991;98:35–40.

135. Roberts MD, Grau V, Grimm J, et al. Remodeling of the connective tissue microarchitecture of the lamina cribrosa in early experimental glaucoma. *Invest Ophthalmol Vis Sci.* 2009;50:681–690.

136. Quigley HA, Hohman RM, Addicks EM, et al. Morphologic changes in the lamina cribrosa correlated with neural loss in open-angle glaucoma. *Am J Ophthalmol.* 1983;95:673–691.

137. Anderson DR. Introductory comments on blood flow autoregulation in the optic nerve head and vascular risk factors in glaucoma. *Surv Ophthalmol.* 1999;43(suppl 1):S5–S9.

138. Dandona L, Quigley HA, Brown AE, et al. Quantitative regional structure of the normal human lamina cribrosa: a racial comparison. *Arch Ophthalmol.* 1990;108:393–398.

139. Hernandez MR, Andrzejewska WM, Neufeld AH. Changes in the extracellular matrix of the human optic nerve head in primary open-angle glaucoma. *Am J Ophthalmol.* 1990;109:180–188.

140. Morrison JC, Dorman-Pease ME, Dunkelberger GR, et al. Optic nerve head extracellular matrix in primary optic atrophy and experimental glaucoma. *Arch Ophthalmol.* 1990;108:1020–1024.

141. Fukuchi T, Sawaguchi S, Hara H, et al. Extracellular matrix changes of the optic nerve lamina cribrosa in monkey eyes with experimentally chronic glaucoma. *Graefes Arch Clin Exp Ophthalmol.* 1992;230:421–427.

142. Quigley HA, Brown A, Dorman-Pease ME. Alterations in elastin of the optic nerve head in human and experimental glaucoma. *Br J Ophthalmol.* 1991;75:552–557.

143. Hernandez MR, Yang J, Ye H. Activation of elastin mRNA expression in human optic nerve heads with primary open-angle glaucoma. *J Glaucoma.* 1994;3:214–215.

144. Vrabec F. Glaucomatous cupping of the human optic disk: a neuro-histologic study. *Albrecht von Graefes Arch Klin Exp Ophthalmol.* 1976;198:223–234.

145. Quigley HA, Addicks EM. Chronic experimental glaucoma in primates. II. Effect of extended intraocular pressure elevation on optic nerve head and axonal transport. *Invest Ophthalmol Vis Sci.* 1980;19:137–152.

146. Quigley HA, Sanchez RM, Dunkelberger GR, et al. Chronic glaucoma selectively damages large optic nerve fibers. *Invest Ophthalmol Vis Sci.* 1987;28:913–920.

147. Quigley HA, Dunkelberger GR, Green WR. Chronic human glaucoma causing selectively greater loss of large optic nerve fibers. *Ophthalmology.* 1988;95:357–363.

148. Glovinsky Y, Quigley HA, Dunkelberger GR. Retinal ganglion cell loss is size dependent in experimental glaucoma. *Invest Ophthalmol Vis Sci.* 1991;32:484–491.

149. Glovinsky Y, Quigley HA, Pease ME. Foveal ganglion cell loss is size dependent in experimental glaucoma. *Invest Ophthalmol Vis Sci.* 1993;34:395–400.

150. Quigley HA, Nickells RW, Kerrigan LA, et al. Retinal ganglion cell death in experimental glaucoma and after axotomy occurs by apoptosis. *Invest Ophthalmol Vis Sci.* 1995;36:774–786.

151. Kubota T, Holbach LM, Naumann GO. Corpora amylacea in glaucomatous and non-glaucomatous optic nerve and retina. *Graefes Arch Clin Exp Ophthalmol.* 1993;231:7–11.

152. Kubota T, Naumann GO. Reduction in number of corpora amylacea with advancing histological changes of glaucoma. *Graefes Arch Clin Exp Ophthalmol.* 1993;231:249–253.

153. Panda S, Jonas JB. Decreased photoreceptor count in human eyes with secondary angle-closure glaucoma. *Invest Ophthalmol Vis Sci.* 1992;33:2532–2536.

154. Kendell KR, Quigley HA, Kerrigan LA, et al. Primary open-angle glaucoma is not associated with photoreceptor loss. *Invest Ophthalmol Vis Sci.* 1995;36:200–205.

155. Wygnanski T, Desatnik H, Quigley HA, et al. Comparison of ganglion cell loss and cone loss in experimental glaucoma. *Am J Ophthalmol.* 1995;120:184–189.

156. Levkovitch-Verbin H, Quigley HA, Kerrigan-Baumrind LA, et al. Optic nerve transection in monkeys may result in secondary degeneration of retinal ganglion cells. *Invest Ophthalmol Vis Sci.* 2001;42:975–982.

157. Weinstein JM, Duckrow RB, Beard D, et al. Regional optic nerve blood flow and its autoregulation. *Invest Ophthalmol Vis Sci.* 1983;24:1559–1565.

158. Sossi N, Anderson DR. Effect of elevated intraocular pressure on blood flow: occurrence in cat optic nerve head studied with iodoantipyrine I 125. *Arch Ophthalmol.* 1983;101:98–101.

159. Grehn F, Prost M. Function of retinal nerve fibers depends on perfusion pressure: neurophysiologic investigations during acute intraocular pressure elevation. *Invest Ophthalmol Vis Sci.* 1983;24:347–353.

160. Novack RL, Stefansson E, Hatchell DL. Intraocular pressure effects on optic nerve-head oxidative metabolism measured in vivo. *Graefes Arch Clin Exp Ophthalmol.* 1990;228:128–133.

161. Quigley HA, Hohman RM, Sanchez R, et al. Optic nerve head blood flow in chronic experimental glaucoma. *Arch Ophthalmol.* 1985;103:956–962.

162. Liang Y, Downs JC, Fortune B, et al. Impact of systemic blood pressure on the relationship between intraocular pressure and blood flow in the optic nerve head of nonhuman primates. *Invest Ophthalmol Vis Sci.* 2009;50:2154–2160.

163. Ernest JT. Pathogenesis of glaucomatous optic nerve disease. *Trans Am Ophthalmol Soc.* 1975;73:366–388.

164. Shonat RD, Wilson DF, Riva CE, et al. Effect of acute increases in intraocular pressure on intravascular optic nerve head oxygen tension in cats. *Invest Ophthalmol Vis Sci.* 1992;33:3174–3180.

165. Riva CE, Hero M, Titze P, et al. Autoregulation of human optic nerve head blood flow in response to acute changes in ocular perfusion pressure. *Graefes Arch Clin Exp Ophthalmol.* 1997;235:618–626.

166. Rojanapongpun P, Drance SM, Morrison BJ. Ophthalmic artery flow velocity in glaucomatous and normal subjects. *Br J Ophthalmol.* 1993;77:25–29.

167. Sergott RC, Aburn NS, Trible JR, et al. Color Doppler imaging: methodology and preliminary results in glaucoma [review]. *Surv Ophthalmol.* 1994;38(suppl):S65–S70.

168. Hamard P, Hamard H, Dufaux J, et al. Optic nerve head blood flow using a laser Doppler velocimeter and haemorheology in primary open-angle glaucoma and normal pressure glaucoma. *Br J Ophthalmol.* 1994;78:449–453.

169. Rankin SJ, Walman BE, Buckley AR, et al. Color Doppler imaging and spectral analysis of the optic nerve vasculature in glaucoma. *Am J Ophthalmol.* 1995;119:685–693.

170. Harju M, Vesti E. Blood flow of the optic nerve head and peripapillary retina in exfoliation syndrome with unilateral glaucoma or ocular hypertension. *Graefes Arch Clin Exp Ophthalmol.* 2001;239:271–277.

171. Deokule S, Vizzeri G, Boehm AG, et al. Correlation among choroidal, peripapillary, and retrobulbar vascular parameters. *Am J Ophthalmol.* 2009;147:736–743.

172. Pemp B, Georgopoulos M, Vass C, et al. Diurnal fluctuation of ocular blood flow parameters in patients with primary open-angle glaucoma and healthy subjects. *Br J Ophthalmol.* 2009;93:486–491.

173. Robert Y, Steiner D, Hendrickson P. Papillary circulation dynamics in glaucoma. *Graefes Arch Clin Exp Ophthalmol.* 1989;227:436–439.

174. Feke GT, Pasquale LR. Retinal blood flow response to posture changes in glaucoma patients compared with healthy subjects. *Ophthalmology.* 2008;115:246–252.

175. Shin DH, Tsai CS, Parrow KA, et al. Intraocular pressure-dependent retinal vascular change in adult chronic open-angle glaucoma patients. *Ophthalmology.* 1991;98:1087–1092.

176. Miller MM, Chang T, Keating R, et al. Blood flow velocities are reduced in the optic nerve of children with elevated intracranial pressure. *J Child Neurol.* 2009;24:30–35.

177. Pillunat LE, Anderson DR, Knighton RW, et al. Auto regulation of human optic nerve head circulation in response to increased intraocular pressure. *Exp Eye Res.* 1997;64:737–744.

178. Ulrich WD, Ulrich C, Bohne BD. Deficient autoregulation and lengthening of the diffusion distance in the anterior optic nerve circulation in glaucoma: an electro-encephalo-dynamographic investigation. *Ophthalmic Res.* 1986;18:253–259.

179. Bhauhan BC. Endothelin and its potential role in glaucoma. *Can J Ophthalmol.* 2008;43:356–360.

180. Mozaffarieh M, Grieshaber MC, Flammer J. Oxygen and blood flow: players in the pathogenesis of glaucoma. *Mol Vis.* 2008;14:224–233.

181. Ernest JT, Archer D. Fluorescein angiography of the optic disk. *Am J Ophthalmol.* 1973;75:973–978.

182. Schwartz B, Kern J. Age, increased ocular and blood pressures, and retinal and disc fluorescein angiogram. *Arch Ophthalmol.* 1980;98:1980–1986.

183. Tso MO, Shih CY, McLean IW. Is there a blood-brain barrier at the optic nerve head? *Arch Ophthalmol.* 1975;93:815–825.

184. Hayreh SS. Optic disc changes in glaucoma. *Br J Ophthalmol.* 1972;56:175–185.

185. Rosen ES, Boyd TA. New method of assessing choroidal ischemia in open-angle glaucoma and ocular hypertension. *Am J Ophthalmol.* 1970;70:912–921.

186. Raitta C, Sarmela T. Fluorescein angiography of the optic disc and the peripapillary area in chronic glaucoma. *Acta Ophthalmol (Copenh).* 1970;48:303–308.

187. Blumenthal M, Gitter KA, Best M, et al. Fluorescein angiography during induced ocular hypertension in man. *Am J Ophthalmol*. 1970;69:39–43.

188. Hayreh SS. The pathogenesis of optic nerve lesions in glaucoma. *Trans Am Acad Ophthalmol Otolaryngol*. 1976;81:197–213.

189. Oosterhuis JA, Boen-Tan TN. Choroidal fluorescence in the normal human eye. *Ophthalmologica*. 1971;162:246–260.

190. Evans PY, Shimizu K, Limaye S, et al. Fluorescein cineangiography of the optic nerve head. *Trans Am Acad Ophthalmol Otolaryngol*. 1973;77:OP260–OP273.

191. Best M, Toyofuku H. Ocular hemodynamics during induced ocular hypertension in man. *Am J Ophthalmol*. 1972;74:932–939.

192. Hitchings RA, Spaeth GL. Fluorescein angiography in chronic simple and low-tension glaucoma. *Br J Ophthalmol*. 1977;61:126–132.

193. Alterman M, Henkind P. Radial peripapillary capillaries of the retina. II. Possible role in Bjerrum scotoma. *Br J Ophthalmol*. 1968;52:26–31.

194. Blumenthal M, Best M, Galin MA, et al. Ocular circulation: analysis of the effect of induced ocular hypertension on retinal and choroidal blood flow in man. *Am J Ophthalmol*. 1971;71:819–825.

195. Archer DB, Ernest JT, Krill AE. Retinal, choroidal, and papillary circulations under conditions of induced ocular hypertension. *Am J Ophthalmol*. 1972;73:834–845.

196. Schwartz B, Harris A, Takamoto T, et al. Regional differences in optic disc and retinal circulation. *Acta Ophthalmol Scand*. 2000;78:627–631.

197. Spaeth GL. Fluorescein angiography: its contributions towards understanding the mechanisms of visual loss in glaucoma. *Trans Am Ophthalmol Soc*. 1975;73:491–553.

198. Schwartz B, Rieser JC, Fishbein SL. Fluorescein angiographic defects of the optic disc in glaucoma. *Arch Ophthalmol*. 1977;95:1961–1974.

199. Sonty S, Schwartz B. Two-point fluorophotometry in the evaluation of glaucomatous optic disc. *Arch Ophthalmol*. 1980;98:1422–1426.

200. Fishbein SL, Schwartz B. Optic disc in glaucoma: topography and extent of fluorescein filling defects. *Arch Ophthalmol*. 1977;95:1975–1979.

201. Adam G, Schwartz B. Increased fluorescein filling defects in the wall of the optic disc cup in glaucoma. *Arch Ophthalmol*. 1980;98:1590–1592.

202. Talusan E, Schwartz B. Specificity of fluorescein angiographic defects of the optic disc in glaucoma. *Arch Ophthalmol*. 1977;95:2166–2175.

203. Tuulonen A, Nagin P, Schwartz B, et al. Increase of pallor and fluorescein-filling defects of the optic disc in the follow-up of ocular hypertensives measured by computerized image analysis. *Ophthalmology*. 1987;94:558–563.

204. Arend O, Remky A, Plange N, et al. Capillary density and retinal diameter measurements and their impact on altered retinal circulation in glaucoma: a digital fluorescein angiographic study. *Br J Ophthalmol*. 2002;86:429–433.

205. Minckler DS, Tso MO. A light microscopic, autoradiographic study of axoplasmic transport in the normal rhesus optic nerve head. *Am J Ophthalmol*. 1976;82:1–15.

206. Minckler DS, Bunt AH, Johanson GW. Orthograde and retrograde axoplasmic transport during acute ocular hypertension in the monkey. *Invest Ophthalmol Vis Sci*. 1977;16:426–441.

207. Taylor AC, Weiss P. Demonstration of axonal flow by the movement of tritium-labeled protein in mature optic nerve fibers. *Proc Natl Acad Sci U S A*. 1965;54:1521–527.

208. Weiss P, Pillai A. Convection and fate of mitochondria in nerve fibers: axonal flow as vehicle. *Proc Natl Acad Sci U S A*. 1965;54:48–56.

209. Johansson JO. Inhibition of retrograde axoplasmic transport in rat optic nerve by increased IOP in vitro. *Invest Ophthalmol Vis Sci*. 1983;24:1552–1558.

210. Anderson DR, Hendrickson A. Effect of intraocular pressure on rapid axoplasmic transport in monkey optic nerve. *Invest Ophthalmol*. 1974;13:771–783.

211. Minckler DS, Tso MO, Zimmerman LE. A light microscopic, autoradiographic study of axoplasmic transport in the optic nerve head during ocular hypotony, increased intraocular pressure, and papilledema. *Am J Ophthalmol*. 1976;82:741–757.

212. Quigley H, Anderson DR. The dynamics and location of axonal transport blockade by acute intraocular pressure elevation in primate optic nerve. *Invest Ophthalmol*. 1976;15:606–616.

213. Minckler DS, Bunt AH, Klock IB. Radioautographic and cytochemical ultrastructural studies of axoplasmic transport in the monkey optic nerve head. *Invest Ophthalmol Vis Sci*. 1978;17:33–50.

214. Quigley HA, Guy J, Anderson DR. Blockade of rapid axonal transport: effect of intraocular pressure elevation in primate optic nerve. *Arch Ophthalmol*. 1979;97:525–531.

215. Sakugawa M, Chihara E. Blockage at two points of axonal transport in glaucomatous eyes. *Graefes Arch Clin Exp Ophthalmol*. 1985;223:214–218.

216. Dandona L, Hendrickson A, Quigley HA. Selective effects of experimental glaucoma on axonal transport by retinal ganglion cells to the dorsal lateral geniculate nucleus. *Invest Ophthalmol Vis Sci*. 1991;32:1593–1599.

217. Radius RL. Distribution of pressure-induced fast axonal transport abnormalities in primate optic nerve: an autoradiographic study. *Arch Ophthalmol*. 1981;99:1253–1257.

218. Quigley HA, Anderson DR. Distribution of axonal transport blockade by acute intraocular pressure elevation in the primate optic nerve head. *Invest Ophthalmol Vis Sci*. 1977;16:640–644.

219. Gaasterland D, Tanishima T, Kuwabara T. Axoplasmic flow during chronic experimental glaucoma. 1. Light and electron microscopic studies of the monkey optic nerve head during development of glaucomatous cupping. *Invest Ophthalmol Vis Sci*. 1978;17:838–846.

220. Quigley HA, Flower RW, Addicks EM, et al. The mechanism of optic nerve damage in experimental acute intraocular pressure elevation. *Invest Ophthalmol Vis Sci*. 1980;19:505–517.

221. Minckler DS, Bunt AH. Axoplasmic transport in ocular hypotony and papilledema in the monkey. *Arch Ophthalmol*. 1977;95:1430–436.

222. Tso MO. Axoplasmic transport in papilledema and glaucoma. *Trans Am Acad Ophthalmol Otolaryngol*. 1977;83:771–777.

223. Balaratnasingam C, Morgan WH, Bass L, et al. Time-dependent effects of elevated intraocular pressure on optic nerve head axonal transport and cytoskeletal changes. *Invest Ophthalmol Vis Sci*. 2008;49:986–999.

224. Anderson DR, Hendrickson AE. Failure of increased intracranial pressure to affect rapid axonal transport at the optic nerve head. *Invest Ophthalmol Vis Sci*. 1977;16:423–426.

225. Radius RL, Anderson DR. Rapid axonal transport in primate optic nerve: distribution of pressure-induced interruption. *Arch Ophthalmol*. 1981;99:650–654.

226. Radius RL, Bade B. Axonal transport interruption and anatomy at the lamina cribrosa. *Arch Ophthalmol*. 1982;100:1661–1664.

227. Radius RL. Pressure-induced fast axonal transport abnormalities and the anatomy at the lamina cribrosa in primate eyes. *Invest Ophthalmol Vis Sci*. 1983;24:343–346.

228. Levy NS, Adams CK. Slow axonal protein transport and visual function following retinal and optic nerve ischemia. *Invest Ophthalmol*. 1975;14:91–97.

229. Levy NS. The effect of interruption of the short posterior ciliary arteries on slow axoplasmic transport and histology within the optic nerve of the rhesus monkey. *Invest Ophthalmol*. 1976;15:495–499.

230. Radius RL. Optic nerve fast axonal transport abnormalities in primates: occurrence after short posterior ciliary artery occlusion. *Arch Ophthalmol*. 1980;98:2018–2022.

231. Radius RL, Anderson DR. Morphology of axonal transport abnormalities in primate eyes. *Br J Ophthalmol*. 1981;65:767–777.

232. Radius RL, Bade B. Pressure-induced optic nerve axonal transport interruption in cat eyes. *Arch Ophthalmol*. 1981;99:2163–2165.

233. Sossi N, Anderson DR. Blockage of axonal transport in optic nerve induced by elevation of intraocular pressure: effect of arterial hypertension induced by angiotensin I. *Arch Ophthalmol*. 1983;101:94–97.

234. Radius RL, Anderson DR. Breakdown of the normal optic nerve head blood-brain barrier following acute elevation of intraocular pressure in experimental animals. *Invest Ophthalmol Vis Sci*. 1980;19:244–255.

235. Radius RL, Schwartz EL, Anderson DR. Failure of unilateral carotid artery ligation to affect pressure-induced interruption of rapid axonal transport in primate optic nerves. *Invest Ophthalmol Vis Sci*. 1980;19:153–157.

236. Hollander H, Makarov F, Stefani FH, et al. Evidence of constriction of optic nerve axons at the lamina cribrosa in the normotensive eye in humans and other mammals. *Ophthalmic Res*. 1995;27:296–309.

237. Wang X, Baldridge WH, Chauhan BC. Acute endothelin-1 application induces reversible fast axonal transport blockade in adult rat optic nerve. *Invest Ophthalmol Vis Sci*. 2008;49:961–967.

238. Iwabe S, Moreno-Mendoza NA, Trigo-Tavera F, et al. Retrograde axonal transport obstruction of brain-derived neurotrophic factor (BDNF) and its TrkB receptor in the retina and optic nerve of American Cocker Spaniel dogs with spontaneous glaucoma. *Vet Ophthalmol*. 2007;(suppl 1):12–19.

239. Volkov VV. Essential element of the glaucomatous process neglected in clinical practice [in Russian]. *Oftalmol Zh*. 1976;31:500–504.

240. Yang Y, Yu M, Zhu J, et al. Role of cerebrospinal fluid in glaucoma: pressure and beyond. *Med Hypotheses*. 2010;74(1):31–34.

241. Morgan WH, Yu DY, Alder VA, et al. The correlation between cerebrospinal fluid pressure and retrolaminar tissue pressure. *Invest Ophthalmol Vis Sci*. 1998;39:1419–1428.

242. Jonas JB, Berenshtein E, Holbach L. Lamina cribrosa thickness and spatial relationships between intraocular space and cerebrospinal fluid space in highly myopic eyes. *Invest Ophthalmol Vis Sci*. 2004;45:2660–2665.

243. Berdahl JP, Allingham RR, Johnson DH. Cerebrospinal fluid pressure is decreased in primary open-angle glaucoma. *Ophthalmology*. 2008;115:763–768.

244. Berdahl JP, Fautsch MP, Stinnett SS, et al. Intracranial pressure in primary open angle glaucoma, normal tension glaucoma, and ocular hy-

pertension: a case-control study. *Invest Ophthalmol Vis Sci.* 200;49:5412–5418.

245. Ren R, Jonas JB, Tian G, et al. Cerebrospinal fluid pressure in glaucoma: a prospective study. *Ophthalmology.* 2010;117(2):259–266.

246. Sipperley J, Anderson DR, Hamasaki D. Short-term effect of intraocular pressure elevation on the human electroretinogram. *Arch Ophthalmol.* 1973;90:358–360.

247. Bartl G. The electroretinogram and the visual evoked potential in normal and glaucomatous eyes [in German]. *Albrecht von Graefes Arch Klin Exp Ophthalmol.* 1978;207:243–269.

248. Pillunat LE, Stodtmeister R, Wilmanns I, et al. Autoregulation of ocular blood flow during changes in intraocular pressure: preliminary results. *Graefes Arch Clin Exp Ophthalmol.* 1985;223:219–223.

249. Breidenbach K, Neppert B, Dannheim F, et al. Pattern electroretinography in routine clinical diagnosis of open-angle glaucoma [in German]. *Ophthalmologe.* 1996;93:451–455.

250. Colotto A, Salgarello T, Falsini B, et al. Pattern electroretinogram and optic nerve topography in ocular hypertension. *Acta Ophthalmol Scand.* 1998;227:27–28.

251. Bowd C, Vizzeri G, Tafreshi A, et al. Diagnostic accuracy of pattern electroretinogram optimized for glaucoma. *Ophthalmology.* 2009;116:437–443.

252. Bach M, Hoffman MB. Update on the pattern electroretinogram in glaucoma [review]. *Optom Vis Sci.* 2008;85:386–395.

253. Fredette MJ, Anderson DR, Porciatti V, et al. Reproducibility of pattern electroretinogram in glaucoma patients with a range of severity of disease with the new glaucoma paradigm. *Ophthalmology.* 2008;115:957–963.

254. Asano E, Mochizuki K, Swanda A, et al. Decreased nasal-temporal asymmetry of the second-order kernel response of multifocal electroretinograms in eyes with normal-tension glaucoma. *Jpn J Ophthalmol.* 2007;51:379–389.

255. Weiter J, Fine BS. A histologic study of regional choroidal dystrophy. *Am J Ophthalmol.* 1977;83:741–750.

256. Hayreh SS. *Anterior Ischemic Optic Neuropathy.* New York, NY: Springer-Verlag; 1975.

257. Quigley H, Anderson DR. Cupping of the optic disc in ischemic optic neuropathy. *Trans Am Acad Ophthalmol Otolaryngol.* 1977;83:755–762.

258. Sebag J, Thomas JV, Epstein DL, et al. Optic disc cupping in arteritic anterior ischemic optic neuropathy resembles glaucomatous cupping. *Ophthalmology.* 1986;93:357–361.

259. Hitchings RA. The optic disc in glaucoma. III: diffuse optic disc pallor with raised intraocular pressure. *Br J Ophthalmol.* 1978;62:670–675.

260. Quigley HA, Miller NR, Green WR. The pattern of optic nerve fiber loss in anterior ischemic optic neuropathy. *Am J Ophthalmol.* 1985;100:769–776.

261. Radius RL, Maumenee AE. Optic atrophy and glaucomatous cupping. *Am J Ophthalmol.* 1978;85:145–153.

262. Jampol LM, Board RJ, Maumenee AE. Systemic hypotension and glaucomatous changes. *Am J Ophthalmol.* 1978;85:154–159.

263. Brownstein S, Font RL, Zimmerman LE, et al. Nonglaucomatous cavernous degeneration of the optic nerve: report of two cases. *Arch Ophthalmol.* 1980;98:354–358.

264. Giarelli L, Falconieri G, Cameron JD, et al. Schnabel cavernous degeneration: a vascular change of the aging eye. *Arch Pathol Lab Med.* 2003;127:1314–1319.

265. Spaeth GL. *The Pathogenesis of Nerve Damage in Glaucoma: Contributions of Fluorescein Angiography.* New York, NY: Grune & Stratton; 1977.

266. Caprioli J, Spaeth GL. Comparison of visual field defects in the low-tension glaucomas with those in the high-tension glaucomas. *Am J Ophthalmol.* 1984;97:730–737.

267. Jonas JB, Gusek GC, Naumann GO. Optic disc, cup and neuroretinal rim size, configuration and correlations in normal eyes. *Invest Ophthalmol Vis Sci.* 1988;29:1151–1158.

268. Jonas JB, Gusek GC, Guggenmoos-Holzmann I, et al. Variability of the real dimensions of normal human optic discs. *Graefes Arch Clin Exp Ophthalmol.* 1988;226:332–336.

269. Bengtsson B. The alteration and asymmetry of cup and disc diameters. *Acta Ophthalmol (Copenh).* 1980;58:726–732.

270. Balazsi AG, Drance SM, Schulzer M, et al. Neuroretinal rim area in suspected glaucoma and early chronic open-angle glaucoma: correlation with parameters of visual function. *Arch Ophthalmol.* 1984;102:1011–1014.

271. Caprioli J, Miller JM. Optic disc rim area is related to disc size in normal subjects. *Arch Ophthalmol.* 1987;105:1683–1685.

272. Britton RJ, Drance SM, Schulzer M, et al. The area of the neuroretinal rim of the optic nerve in normal eyes. *Am J Ophthalmol.* 1987;103:497–504.

273. Jonas JB, Gusek GC, Guggenmoos-Holzmann I, et al. Correlations of the neuroretinal rim area with ocular and general parameters in normal eyes. *Ophthalmic Res.* 1988;20:298–303.

274. Shields MB. Gray crescent in the optic nerve head. *Am J Ophthalmol.* 1980;89:238–244.

275. Jonas JB, Gusek GC, Naumann GO. Optic disk morphometry in high myopia. *Graefes Arch Clin Exp Ophthalmol.* 1988;226:587–590.

276. Tsai CS, Ritch R, Shin DH, et al. Age-related decline of disc rim area in visually normal subjects. *Ophthalmology.* 1992;99:29–35.

277. Varma R, Hilton SC, Tielsch JM, et al. Neural rim area declines with increased intraocular pressure in urban Americans. *Arch Ophthalmol.* 1995;113:1001–1005.

278. Klein BE, Moss SE, Klein R, et al. Neuroretinal rim area in diabetes mellitus. *Invest Ophthalmol Vis Sci.* 1990;31:805–809.

279. Radius RL. Thickness of the retinal nerve fiber layer in primate eyes. *Arch Ophthalmol.* 1980;98:1625–1629.

280. Quigley HA, Addicks EM. Quantitative studies of retinal nerve fiber layer defects. *Arch Ophthalmol.* 1982;100:807–814.

281. Jonas JB, Nguyen NX, Naumann GO. The retinal nerve fiber layer in normal eyes. *Ophthalmology.* 1980;96:627–632.

282. Jonas JB, Schiro D. Visibility of the normal retinal nerve fiber layer correlated with rim width and vessel caliber. *Graefes Arch Clin Exp Ophthalmol.* 1993;231:207–211.

283. Caprioli J. Discrimination between normal and glaucomatous eyes. *Invest Ophthalmol Vis Sci.* 1992;33:153–159.

284. Fantes FE, Anderson DR. Clinical histologic correlation of human peripapillary anatomy. *Ophthalmology.* 1989;96:20–25.

285. Jonas JB, Konigsreuther KA, Naumann GO. Optic disc histomorphometry in normal eyes and eyes with secondary angle-closure glaucoma. II. Parapapillary region. *Graefes Arch Clin Exp Ophthalmol.* 1992;230:134–139.

286. Tezel G, Kolker AE, Kass MA, et al. Parapapillary chorioretinal atrophy in patients with ocular hypertension. I. An evaluation as a predictive factor for the development of glaucomatous damage. *Arch Ophthalmol.* 1997;115:1503–1508.

287. Armaly MF. Genetic determination of cup/disc ratio of the optic nerve. *Arch Ophthalmol.* 1967;78:35–43.

288. Schwartz JT, Reuling FH, Garrison RJ. Acquired cupping of the optic nerve head in normotensive eyes. *Br J Ophthalmol.* 1975;59:216–222.

289. Carpel EF, Engstrom PF. The normal cup-disk ratio. *Am J Ophthalmol.* 1981;91:588–597.

290. Fishman RS. Optic disc asymmetry: a sign of ocular hypertension. *Arch Ophthalmol.* 1970;84:590–594.

291. Holm OC, Becker B, Asseff CF, et al. Volume of the optic disk cup. *Am J Ophthalmol.* 1972;73:876–881.

292. Ong LS, Mitchell P, Healey PR, et al. Asymmetry in optic disc parameters: the Blue Mountains Eye Study. *Invest Ophthalmol Vis Sci.* 1999;40:849–857.

293. Hollows FC, McGuiness R. The size of the optic cup. *Trans Ophthalmol Soc Aust.* 1966;25:33–38.

294. Bengtsson B. The inheritance and development of cup and disc diameters. *Acta Ophthalmol (Copenh).* 1980;58:733–739.

295. Wolfs RC, Klaver CC, Ramrattan RS, et al. Genetic risk of primary open-angle glaucoma: population-based familial aggregation study. *Arch Ophthalmol.* 1998;116:1640–1645.

296. Teikari JM, Airaksinen JP. Twin study on cup/disc ratio of the optic nerve head. *Br J Ophthalmol.* 1992;76:218–220.

297. Armaly MF, Sayegh RE. The cup-disc ratio: the findings of tonometry and tonography in the normal eye. *Arch Ophthalmol.* 1969;82:191–196.

298. Armaly MF. The optic cup in the normal eye. I. Cup width, depth, vessel displacement, ocular tension and outflow facility. *Am J Ophthalmol.* 1969;68:401–407.

299. Becker B. Cup-disk ratio and topical corticosteroid testing. *Am J Ophthalmol.* 1970;70:681–685.

300. Jonas JB. Size of glaucomatous optic discs. *Ger J Ophthalmol.* 1992;1:41–44.

301. Burk RO, Rohrschneider K, Noack H, et al. Are large optic nerve heads susceptible to glaucomatous damage at normal intraocular pressure? A three-dimensional study by laser scanning tomography. *Graefes Arch Clin Exp Ophthalmol.* 1992;230:552–560.

302. Iester M, Mikelberg FS. Optic nerve head morphologic characteristics in high-tension and normal-tension glaucoma. *Arch Ophthalmol.* 1999;117:1010–1013.

303. Varma R, Tielsch JM, Quigley HA, et al. Race-, age-, gender-, and refractive error-related differences in the normal optic disc. *Arch Ophthalmol.* 1994;112:1068–1076.

304. Schwartz B. Optic disc changes in ocular hypertension. *Surv Ophthalmol.* 1980;25:148–154.

305. Schwartz B, Reinstein NM, Lieberman DM. Pallor of the optic disc: quantitative photographic evaluation. *Arch Ophthalmol.* 1973;89:278–286.

306. Beck RW, Messner DK, Musch DC, et al. Is there a racial difference in physiologic cup size? *Ophthalmology.* 1985;92:873–876.

307. Chi T, Ritch R, Stickler D, et al. Racial differences in optic nerve head parameters. *Arch Ophthalmol.* 1989;107:836–839.

308. Tsai CS, Zangwill L, Gonzalez C, et al. Ethnic differences in optic nerve head topography. *J Glaucoma.* 1995;4:248–257.

309. Girkin CA, McGwin G Jr, McNeal SF, et al. Racial differences in the association between optic disc topography and early glaucoma. *Invest Ophthalmol Vis Sci.* 2003;44:3382–3387.

310. Mansour AM. Racial variation of optic disc size. *Ophthalmic Res.* 1991;23:67–72.

311. Jonas JB, Zach FM, Gusek GC, et al. Pseudoglaucomatous physiologic large cups. *Am J Ophthalmol.* 1989;107:137–144.

312. Tomlinson A, Phillips CI. Ovalness of the optic cup and disc in the normal eye. *Br J Ophthalmol.* 1974;58:543–547.

313. Emdadi A, Zangwill L, Sample PA, et al. Patterns of optic disk damage in patients with early focal visual field loss. *Am J Ophthalmol.* 1998;126:763–771.

314. Kirsch RE, Anderson DR. Clinical recognition of glaucomatous cupping. *Am J Ophthalmol.* 1973;75:442–454.

315. Weisman RL, Asseff CF, Phelps CD, et al. Vertical elongation of the optic cup in glaucoma. *Trans Am Acad Ophthalmol Otolaryngol.* 1973;77:OP157–OP161.

316. Read RM, Spaeth GL. The practical clinical appraisal of the optic disc in glaucoma: the natural history of cup progression and some specific disc-field correlations. *Trans Am Acad Ophthalmol Otolaryngol.* 1974;78:OP255–OP274.

317. Spaeth GL, Hitchings RA, Sivalingam E. The optic disc in glaucoma: pathogenetic correlation of five patterns of cupping in chronic open-angle glaucoma. *Trans Am Acad Ophthalmol Otolaryngol.* 1976;81:217–223.

318. Hitchings RA, Spaeth GL. The optic disc in glaucoma. I. Classification. *Br J Ophthalmol.* 1976;60:778–785.

319. Radius RL, Maumenee AE, Green WR. Pit-like changes of the optic nerve head in open-angle glaucoma. *Br J Ophthalmol.* 1978;62:389–393.

320. Betz P, Camps F, Collignon-Brach J, et al. Biometric study of the disc cup in open-angle glaucoma. *Graefes Arch Clin Exp Ophthalmol.* 1982;218:70–74.

321. Jonas JB, Gusek GC, Naumann GO. Optic disc morphometry in chronic primary open-angle glaucoma. I. Morphometric intrapapillary characteristics. *Graefes Arch Clin Exp Ophthalmol.* 1988;226:522–530.

322. Jonas JB, Fernandez MC, Sturmer J. Pattern of glaucomatous neuroretinal rim loss. *Ophthalmology.* 1993;100:63–68.

323. Shin DH, Lee MK, Briggs KS, et al. Intraocular pressure-related pattern of optic disc cupping in adult glaucoma patients. *Graefes Arch Clin Exp Ophthalmol.* 1992;230:542–546.

324. Garway-Heath DF, Ruben ST, Viswanathan A, et al. Vertical cup/disc ratio in relation to optic disc size: its value in the assessment of the glaucoma suspect. *Br J Ophthalmol.* 1998;82:1118–1124.

325. Airaksinen PJ, Drance SM, Schulzer M. Neuroretinal rim area in early glaucoma. *Am J Ophthalmol.* 1985;99:1–4.

326. Drance SM, Balazsi G. The neuro-retinal rim region in early glaucoma [in German]. *Klin Monatsbl Augenheilkd.* 1984;184:271–273.

327. Pederson JE, Anderson DR. The mode of progressive disc cupping in ocular hypertension and glaucoma. *Arch Ophthalmol.* 1980;98:490–495.

328. Cher I, Robinson LP. 'Thinning' of the neural rim of the optic nerve-head: an altered state, providing a new ophthalmoscopic sign associated with characteristics of glaucoma. *Trans Ophthalmol Soc UK.* 1973;93:213–242.

329. Cher I, Robinison LP. Thinning of the neural rim: a simple new sign of the optic disc related to glaucoma statistical considerations. *Aust J Ophthalmol.* 1974;2:27–34.

330. Portney GL. Photogrammetric analysis of the three-dimensional geometry of normal and glaucomatous optic cups. *Trans Am Acad Ophthalmol Otolaryngol.* 1976;81:239–246.

331. Susanna R Jr. The lamina cribrosa and visual field defects in open-angle glaucoma. *Can J Ophthalmol.* 1983;18:124–126.

332. Miller KM, Quigley HA. The clinical appearance of the lamina cribrosa as a function of the extent of glaucomatous optic nerve damage. *Ophthalmology.* 1988;95:135–138.

333. Shields MB. Problems in recognizing non-glaucomatous optic nerve head cupping. *Perspect Ophthalmol.* 1978;2:129.

334. Chandler PA, Grant WM. *Glaucoma.* Philadelphia: Lea & Febiger; 1977.

335. Phillips CI, Tsukahara S, Makino F, et al. Saucerisation (recession) of neuro-retinal rim is characteristic of glaucoma. *Jpn J Ophthalmol.* 1993;37:171–177.

336. Drance SM, Fairclough M, Butler DM, et al. The importance of disc hemorrhage in the prognosis of chronic open-angle glaucoma. *Arch Ophthalmol.* 1977;95:226–228.

337. Susanna R, Drance SM, Douglas GR. Disc hemorrhages in patients with elevated intraocular pressure: occurrence with and without field changes. *Arch Ophthalmol.* 1979;97:284–285.

338. Hendrickx KH, van den Enden A, Rasker MT, et al. Cumulative incidence of patients with disc hemorrhages in glaucoma and the effect of therapy. *Ophthalmology.* 1994;101:1165–1172.

339. Jonas JB, Xu L. Optic disk hemorrhages in glaucoma. *Am J Ophthalmol.* 1994;118:1–8.

340. Sonnsjo B. Glaucomatous disc haemorrhages photographed at short intervals. *Acta Ophthalmol (Copenh).* 1986;64:263–266.

341. Sugiyama K, Tomita G, Kitazawa Y, et al. The associations of optic disc hemorrhage with retinal nerve fiber layer defect and peripapillary atrophy in normal-tension glaucoma. *Ophthalmology.* 1997;104:1926–1933.

342. Jonas JB, Martus P, Budde WM, et al. Morphologic predictive factors for development of optic disc hemorrhages in glaucoma. *Invest Ophthalmol Vis Sci.* 2002;43:2956–2961.

343. Airaksinen PJ, Mustonen E, Alanko HI. Optic disc haemorrhages precede retinal nerve fibre layer defects in ocular hypertension. *Acta Ophthalmol (Copenh).* 1981;59:627–641.

344. Bengtsson B, Holmin C, Krakau CE. Disc haemorrhage and glaucoma. *Acta Ophthalmol (Copenh).* 1981;59:1–14.

345. Shihab ZM, Lee PF, Hay P. The significance of disc hemorrhage in open-angle glaucoma. *Ophthalmology.* 1982;89:211–213.

346. Bengtsson B. Optic disc haemorrhages preceding manifest glaucoma. *Acta Ophthalmol (Copenh).* 1990;68:450–454.

347. Diehl DL, Quigley HA, Miller NR, et al. Prevalence and significance of optic disc hemorrhage in a longitudinal study of glaucoma. *Arch Ophthalmol.* 1990;108:545–550.

348. Gloster J. Incidence of optic disc haemorrhages in chronic simple glaucoma and ocular hypertension. *Br J Ophthalmol.* 1981;65:452–456.

349. Poinoosawmy D, Gloster J, Nagasubramanian S, et al. Association between optic disc haemorrhages in glaucoma and abnormal glucose tolerance. *Br J Ophthalmol.* 1986;70:599–602.

350. Tuulonen A, Takamoto T, Wu DC, et al. Optic disk cupping and pallor measurements of patients with a disk hemorrhage. *Am J Ophthalmol.* 1987;103:505–511.

351. Heijl A. Frequent disc photography and computerized perimetry in eyes with optic disc haemorrhage: a pilot study. *Acta Ophthalmol (Copenh).* 1986;64:274–281.

352. Siegner SW, Netland PA. Optic disc hemorrhages and progression of glaucoma. *Ophthalmology.* 1996;103:1014–1024.

353. Drance S, Anderson DR, Schulzer M. Risk factors for progression of visual field abnormalities in normal-tension glaucoma. *Am J Ophthalmol.* 2001;131:699–708.

354. Ishida K, Yamamoto T, Sugiyama K, et al. Disk hemorrhage is a significantly negative prognostic factor in normal-tension glaucoma. *Am J Ophthalmol.* 2000;129:707–714.

355. Susanna R Jr, Basseto FL. Hemorrhage of the optic disc and neurosensorial dysacousia. *J Glaucoma.* 1992;1:248–253.

356. Hitchings RA, Spaeth GL. Chronic retinal vein occlusion in glaucoma. *Br J Ophthalmol.* 1976;60:694–699.

357. Tuulonen A. Asymptomatic miniocclusions of the optic disc veins in glaucoma. *Arch Ophthalmol.* 1989;107:1475–1480.

358. Shihab ZM, Beebe WE, Wentlandt T. Possible significance of cilioretinal arteries in open-angle glaucoma. *Ophthalmology.* 1985;92:880–883.

359. Lindenmuth KA, Skuta GL, Musch DC, et al. Significance of cilioretinal arteries in primary open-angle glaucoma. *Arch Ophthalmol.* 1988;106:1691–1693.

360. Lee SS, Schwartz B. Role of the temporal cilioretinal artery in retaining central visual field in open-angle glaucoma. *Ophthalmology.* 1992;99:696–699.

361. Herschler J, Osher RH. Baring of the circumlinear vessel: an early sign of optic nerve damage. *Arch Ophthalmol.* 1980;98:865–869.

362. Osher RH, Herschler J. The significance of baring of the circumlinear vessel: a prospective study. *Arch Ophthalmol.* 1981;99:817–818.

363. Sutton GE, Motolko MA, Phelps CD. Baring of a circumlinear vessel in glaucoma. *Arch Ophthalmol.* 1983;101:739–744.

364. Kasner O, Balazsi AG. Glaucomatous optic nerve atrophy: the circumlinear vessel revisited. *Can J Ophthalmol.* 1991;26:264–269.

365. Jonas JB, Budde WM, Nemeth J, et al. Central retinal vessel trunk exit and location of glaucomatous parapapillary atrophy in glaucoma. *Ophthalmology.* 2001;108:1059–1064.

366. Jonas JB, Fernandez MC. Shape of the neuroretinal rim and position of the central retinal vessels in glaucoma. *Br J Ophthalmol.* 1994;78:99–102.

367. Rader J, Feuer WJ, Anderson DR. Peripapillary vasoconstriction in the glaucomas and the anterior ischemic optic neuropathies. *Am J Ophthalmol.* 1994;117:72–80.

368. Sommer A, Miller NR, Pollack I, et al. The nerve fiber layer in the diagnosis of glaucoma. *Arch Ophthalmol.* 1977;95:2149–2156.

369. Sommer A, Pollack I, Maumenee AE. Optic disc parameters and onset of glaucomatous field loss. II. Static screening criteria. *Arch Ophthalmol.* 1979;97:1449–1454.

370. Quigley HA, Miller NR, George T. Clinical evaluation of nerve fiber layer atrophy as an indicator of glaucomatous optic nerve damage. *Arch Ophthalmol.* 1980;98:1564–1571.

371. Jonas JB, Schiro D. Localised wedge shaped defects of the retinal nerve fibre layer in glaucoma. *Br J Ophthalmol.* 1994;78:285–290.

372. Airaksinen PJ, Tuulonen A. Early glaucoma changes in patients with and without an optic disc haemorrhage. *Acta Ophthalmol (Copenh)* 1984;62:197–202.

373. Airaksinen PJ, Drance SM. Neuroretinal rim area and retinal nerve fiber layer in glaucoma. *Arch Ophthalmol.* 1985;103:203–204.

374. Nanba K, Schwartz B. Nerve fiber layer and optic disc fluorescein defects in glaucoma and ocular hypertension. *Ophthalmology.* 1988;95:1227–1233.

375. Quigley HA, Katz J, Derick RJ, et al. An evaluation of optic disc and nerve fiber layer examinations in monitoring progression of early glaucoma damage. *Ophthalmology.* 1992;99:19–28.

376. Jonas JB, Konigsreuther KA. Optic disk appearance in ocular hypertensive eyes. *Am J Ophthalmol.* 1994;117:732–740.

377. Sommer A, Katz J, Quigley HA, et al. Clinically detectable nerve fiber atrophy precedes the onset of glaucomatous field loss. *Arch Ophthalmol.* 1991;109:77–83.

378. Jonas JB, Fernandez MC, Naumann GO. Glaucomatous optic nerve atrophy in small discs with low cup-to-disc ratios. *Ophthalmology.* 1990;97:1211–1215.

379. Airaksinen PJ, Drance SM, Douglas GR, et al. Diffuse and localized nerve fiber loss in glaucoma. *Am J Ophthalmol.* 1984;98:566–571.

380. Sommer A, Quigley HA, Robin AL, et al. Evaluation of nerve fiber layer assessment. *Arch Ophthalmol.* 1984;102:1766–1771.

381. Airaksinen PJ, Drance SM, Douglas GR, et al. Visual field and retinal nerve fiber layer comparisons in glaucoma. *Arch Ophthalmol.* 1985;103:205–207.

382. Tuulonen A, Airaksinen PJ. Initial glaucomatous optic disk and retinal nerve fiber layer abnormalities and their progression. *Am J Ophthalmol.* 1991;111:485–490.

383. Wilensky JT, Kolker AE. Peripapillary changes in glaucoma. *Am J Ophthalmol.* 1976;81:341–345.

384. Jonas JB, Naumann GO. Parapapillary chorioretinal atrophy in normal and glaucoma eyes. II. Correlations. *Invest Ophthalmol Vis Sci.* 1989;30:919–926.

385. Buus DR, Anderson DR. Peripapillary crescents and halos in normal-tension glaucoma and ocular hypertension. *Ophthalmology.* 1989;96:16–19.

386. Jonas JB, Fernandez MC, Naumann GO. Parapapillary atrophy and retinal vessel diameter in nonglaucomatous optic nerve damage. *Invest Ophthalmol Vis Sci.* 1991;32:2942–2947.

387. Rockwood EJ, Anderson DR. Acquired peripapillary changes and progression in glaucoma. *Graefes Arch Clin Exp Ophthalmol.* 1988;226:510–515.

388. Jonas JB, Fernandez MC, Naumann GO. Glaucomatous parapapillary atrophy: occurrence and correlations. *Arch Ophthalmol.* 1992;110:214–222.

389. Kasner O, Feuer WJ, Anderson DR. Possibly reduced prevalence of peripapillary crescents in ocular hypertension. *Can J Ophthalmol.* 1989;24:211–215.

390. Stewart WC, Connor AB, Wang XH. Anatomic features of the optic disc and risk of progression in ocular hypertension. *Acta Ophthalmol Scand.* 1995;73:237–241.

391. Kessing SV, Gregersen E. The distended disc in early stages of congenital glaucoma. *Acta Ophthalmol (Copenh).* 1977;55:431–435.

392. Quigley HA. Childhood glaucoma: results with trabeculotomy and study of reversible cupping. *Ophthalmology.* 1982;89:219–226.

393. Pederson JE, Herschler J. Reversal of glaucomatous cupping in adults. *Arch Ophthalmol.* 1982;100:426–431.

394. Schwartz B, Takamoto T, Nagin P. Measurements of reversibility of optic disc cupping and pallor in ocular hypertension and glaucoma. *Ophthalmology.* 1985;92:1396–1407.

395. Greenidge KC, Spaeth GL, Traverso CE. Change in appearance of the optic disc associated with lowering of intraocular pressure. *Ophthalmology.* 1985;92:897–903.

396. Katz LJ, Spaeth GL, Cantor LB, et al. Reversible optic disk cupping and visual field improvement in adults with glaucoma. *Am J Ophthalmol.* 1989;107:485–492.

397. Funk J. Increase of neuroretinal rim area after surgical intraocular pressure reduction. *Ophthalmic Surg.* 1990;21:585–588.

398. Parrow KA, Shin DH, Tsai CS, et al. Intraocular pressure-dependent dynamic changes of optic disc cupping in adult glaucoma patients. *Ophthalmology.* 1992;99:36–40.

399. Yamada N, Tomita G, Yamamoto T, et al. Changes in the nerve fiber layer thickness following a reduction of intraocular pressure after trabeculectomy. *J Glaucoma.* 2000;9:371–375.

400. Jensen PE, Kalina RE. Congenital anomalies of the optic disk. *Am J Ophthalmol.* 1976;82:27–31.

401. Pagon RA. Ocular coloboma [review]. *Surv Ophthalmol.* 1981;25:223–236.

402. Kindler P. Morning glory syndrome: unusual congenital optic disk anomaly. *Am J Ophthalmol.* 1970;69:376–384.

403. Apple DJ, Rabb MF, Walsh PM. Congenital anomalies of the optic disc [review]. *Surv Ophthalmol.* 1982;27:3–41.

404. Brodsky MC. Congenital optic disk anomalies [review]. *Surv Ophthalmol.* 1994;39:89–112.

405. Deb N, Das R, Roy IS. Bilateral morning glory disc anomaly. *Indian J Ophthalmol.* 2003;51:182–183.

406. Nawratzki I, Schwartzenberg T, Zaubermann H, et al. Bilateral morning glory syndrome with midline brain lesion in an autistic child. *Metab Pediatr Syst Ophthalmol.* 1985;8:35–36.

407. Brown GC, Shields JA, Goldberg RE. Congenital pits of the optic nerve head. II. Clinical studies in humans. *Ophthalmology.* 1980;87:51–65.

408. Krivoy D, Gentile R, Liebmann JM, et al. Imaging congenital optic disc pits and associated maculopathy using optical coherence tomography. *Arch Ophthalmol.* 1996;114:165–170.

409. Yuen CH, Kaye SB. Spontaneous resolution of serous maculopathy associated with optic disc pit in a child: a case report. *J AAPOS.* 2002;6:330–331.

410. Theodossiadis G. Evolution of congenital pit of the optic disk with macular detachment in photocoagulated and nonphotocoagulated eyes. *Am J Ophthalmol.* 1977;84:620–631.

411. Brazitikos PD, Safran AB, Simona F, et al. Threshold perimetry in tilted disc syndrome. *Arch Ophthalmol.* 1990;108:1698–1700.

412. Trobe JD, Glaser JS, Cassady JC. Optic atrophy: differential diagnosis by fundus observation alone. *Arch Ophthalmol.* 1980;98:1040–1045.

413. Trobe JD, Glaser JS, Cassady J, et al. Nonglaucomatous excavation of the optic disc. *Arch Ophthalmol.* 1980;98:1046–1050.

414. Lichter PR, Henderson JW. Optic nerve infarction. *Am J Ophthalmol.* 1978;85:302–310.

415. Portney GL, Roth AM. Optic cupping caused by an intracranial aneurysm. *Am J Ophthalmol.* 1977;84:98–103.

416. Danesh-Meyer HV, Carroll SC, Ku JT, et al. Correlation of retinal nerve fiber layer measured by scanning laser polarimeter to visual field in ischemic optic neuropathy. *Arch Ophthalmol.* 2006;124:1720–1726.

417. Repka MX, Uozato H, Guyton DL. Depth distortion during slitlamp biomicroscopy of the fundus. *Ophthalmology.* 1986;93:47–51.

418. Romano JH. Graticule incorporated into an ophthalmoscope for the clinical evaluation of the cup/disc ratio. *Br J Ophthalmol.* 1983;67:214–215.

419. Gross PG, Drance SM. Comparison of a simple ophthalmoscopic and planimetric measurements of glaucomatous neuroretinal rim areas. *J Glaucoma.* 1995;4:314–316.

420. Montgomery DM. Measurement of optic disc and neuroretinal rim areas in normal and glaucomatous eyes: a new clinical method. *Ophthalmology.* 1991;98:50–59.

421. Montgomery DM. Clinical disc biometry in early glaucoma. *Ophthalmology.* 1993;100:52–56.

422. Ruben S. Estimation of optic disc size using indirect biomicroscopy. *Br J Ophthalmol.* 1994;78:363–364.

423. Spencer AF, Vernon SA. Repeatability and reproducibility of optic disc measurement with the Zeiss 4-mirror contact lens. *Ophthalmology.* 1996;103:163–167.

424. Jonas JB, Papastathopoulos K. Ophthalmoscopic measurement of the optic disc. *Ophthalmology.* 1995;102:1102–1106.

425. Shaffer RN, Ridgway WL, Brown R, et al. The use of diagrams to record changes in glaucomatous disks. *Am J Ophthalmol.* 1975;80:460–464.

426. Lichter PR. Variability of expert observers in evaluating the optic disc. *Trans Am Ophthalmol Soc.* 1976;74:532–572.

427. Varma R, Steinmann WC, Scott IU. Expert agreement in evaluating the optic disc for glaucoma. *Ophthalmology.* 1992;99:215–221.

428. Gaasterland DE, Blackwell B, Dally LG, et al. The Advanced Glaucoma Intervention Study (AGIS): 10. Variability among academic glaucoma subspecialists in assessing optic disc notching. *Trans Am Ophthalmol Soc.* 2001;99:177–184.

429. Tielsch JM, Katz J, Quigley HA, et al. Intraobserver and interobserver agreement in measurement of optic disc characteristics. *Ophthalmology.* 1988;95:350–356.

430. Coleman AL, Sommer A, Enger C, et al. Interobserver and intraobserver variability in the detection of glaucomatous progression of the optic disc. *J Glaucoma.* 1996;5:384–389.

431. Gloster J, Parry DG. Use of photographs for measuring cupping in the optic disc. *Br J Ophthalmol.* 1974;58:850–862.

432. Hitchings RA, Genio C, Anderton S, et al. An optic disc grid: its evaluation in reproducibility studies on the cup/disc ratio. *Br J Ophthalmol.* 1983;67:356–361.

433. Sharma NK, Hitchings RA. A comparison of monocular and 'stereoscopic' photographs of the optic disc in the identification of glaucomatous visual field defects. *Br J Ophthalmol.* 1983;67:677–680.

434. Cohan BE. Multiple-slit illumination of the optic disc. *Arch Ophthalmol.* 1978;96:497–500.

435. Kennedy SJ, Schwartz B, Takamoto T, et al. Interference fringe scale for absolute ocular fundus measurement. *Invest Ophthalmol Vis Sci.* 1983;24:169–174.

436. Schwartz B, Kern J. Scanning microdensitometry of optic disc pallor in glaucoma. *Arch Ophthalmol.* 1977;95:2159–2165.

437. Rosenthal AR, Falconer DG, Barrett P. Digital measurement of pallor-disc ratio. *Arch Ophthalmol.* 1980;98:2027–2031.

438. Frisen L. Photography of the retinal nerve fibre layer: an optimised procedure. *Br J Ophthalmol.* 1980;64:641–650.

439. Sommer A, D'Anna SA, Kues HA, et al. High-resolution photography of the retinal nerve fiber layer. *Am J Ophthalmol.* 1983;96:535–539.

440. Airaksinen PJ, Nieminen H. Retinal nerve fiber layer photography in glaucoma. *Ophthalmology.* 1985;92:877–879.

441. Peli E, Hedges TR III, McInnes T, et al. Nerve fiber layer photography: a comparative study. *Acta Ophthalmol (Copenh).* 1987;65:71–80.

442. Wang F, Quigley HA, Tielsch JM. Screening for glaucoma in a medical clinic with photographs of the nerve fiber layer. *Arch Ophthalmol.* 1994;112:796–800.

443. Sommer A, Kues HA, D'Anna SA, et al. Cross-polarization photography of the nerve fiber layer. *Arch Ophthalmol.* 1984;102:864–869.

444. Airaksinen PJ, Nieminen H, Mustonen E. Retinal nerve fibre layer photography with a wide angle fundus camera. *Acta Ophthalmol (Copenh).* 1982;60:362–368.

445. Knighton RW, Jacobson SG, Kemp CM. The spectral reflectance of the nerve fiber layer of the macaque retina. *Invest Ophthalmol Vis Sci.* 1989;30:2392–2402.

446. Richards DW, Janesick JR, Elliot ST, et al. Enhanced detection of normal retinal nerve-fiber striations using a charge-coupled device and digital filtering. *Graefes Arch Clin Exp Ophthalmol.* 1993;231:595–599.

447. Allen L. Ocular fundus photography: suggestions for achieving consistently good pictures and instructions for stereoscopic photography. *Am J Ophthalmol.* 1964;57:13–28.

448. Allen L. Stereoscopic fundus photography with the new instant positive print films. *Am J Ophthalmol.* 1964;57:539–543.

449. Donaldson DD. A new camera for stereoscopic fundus photography. *Trans Am Ophthalmol Soc.* 1964;62:429–458.

450. Saheb NE, Drance SM, Nelson A. The use of photogrammetry in evaluating the cup of the optic nerve head for a study in chronic simple glaucoma. *Can J Ophthalmol.* 1972;7:466–471.

451. Rosenthal AR, Kottler MS, Donaldson DD, et al. Comparative reproducibility of the digital photogrammetric procedure utilizing three methods of stereophotography. *Invest Ophthalmol Vis Sci.* 1977;16:54–60.

452. Greenfield DS, Zacharia P, Schuman JS. Comparison of Nidek 3Dx and Donaldson simultaneous stereoscopic disk photography. *Am J Ophthalmol.* 1993;116:741–747.

453. Minckler DS, Nichols T, Morales RB. Preliminary clinical experience with the Nidek 3Dx camera and lenticular stereo disc images. *J Glaucoma.* 1992;1:184.

454. Cohen JS, Stone RD, Hetherington J Jr, et al. Glaucomatous cupping of the optic disk by ultrasonography. *Am J Ophthalmol.* 1976;82:24–26.

455. Krohn MA, Keltner JL, Johnson CA. Comparison of photographic techniques and films used in stereophotogrammetry of the optic disk. *Am J Ophthalmol.* 1979;88:859–863.

456. Schwartz B. New techniques for the examination of the optic disc and their clinical application. *Trans Am Acad Ophthalmol Otolaryngol.* 1976;81:227–235.

457. Shields MB, Martone JF, Shelton AR, et al. Reproducibility of topographic measurements with the optic nerve head analyzer. *Am J Ophthalmol.* 1987;104:581–586.

458. Mikelberg FS, Airaksinen PJ, Douglas GR, et al. The correlation between optic disk topography measured by the video-ophthalmograph (Rodenstock analyzer) and clinical measurement. *Am J Ophthalmol.* 1985;100:417–419.

459. Miller E, Caprioli J. Regional and long-term variability of fundus measurements made with computer-image analysis. *Am J Ophthalmol.* 1991;112:171–176.

460. Varma R, Spaeth GL. The PAR IS 2000: a new system for retinal digital image analysis. *Ophthalmic Surg.* 1988;19:183–192.

461. Dandona L, Quigley HA, Jampel HD. Reliability of optic nerve head topographic measurements with computerized image analysis. *Am J Ophthalmol.* 1989;108:414–421.

462. Goldmann H, Lotmar W. Rapid detection of changes in the optic disc: stereo-chronoscopy. *Albrecht Von Graefes Arch Klin Exp Ophthalmol.* 1977;202:87–99.

463. Goldmann H, Lotmar W, Zulauf M. Quantitative studies in stereochronoscopy (Sc): application to the disc in glaucoma. II. Statistical evaluation. *Graefes Arch Clin Exp Ophthalmol.* 1984;222:82–85.

464. Berger JW, Patel TR, Shin DS, et al. Computerized stereochronoscopy and alternation flicker to detect optic nerve head contour change. *Ophthalmology.* 2000;107:1316–1320.

465. Takamoto T, Schwartz B. Stereochronometry: quantitative measurement of optic disc cup changes. *Invest Ophthalmol Vis Sci.* 1985;26:1445–1449.

466. Heijl A, Bengtsson B. Diagnosis of early glaucoma with flicker comparisons of serial disc photographs. *Invest Ophthalmol Vis Sci.* 1989;30:2376–2384.

467. Alanko H, Jaanio E, Airaksinen PJ, et al. Demonstration of glaucomatous optic disc changes by electronic subtraction. *Acta Ophthalmol (Copenh).* 1980;58:14–19.

468. Gloster J. The colour of the optic disc. *Doc Ophthalmol.* 1969;26:155–163.

469. Gloster J. Colorimetry of the optic disc. *Trans Ophthalmol Soc U K.* 1973;93:243–249.

470. Davies EW. Quantitative assessment of colour of the optic disc by a photographic method. *Exp Eye Res.* 1970;9:106–113.

471. Berkowitz JS, Balter S. Colorimetric measurement of the optic disk. *Am J Ophthalmol.* 1970;69:385–386.

472. Hendrickson P, Robert Y, Stockli HP. Principles of photometry of the papilla. *Arch Ophthalmol.* 1984;102:1704–1707.

473. Hoskins HD, Hetherington J, Glenday M, et al. Repeatability of the glaucoma-scope measurements of optic nerve head topography. *J Glaucoma.* 1994;3:17–27.

474. Pendergast SD, Shields MB. Reproducibility of optic nerve head topographic measurements with the glaucoma-scope. *J Glaucoma.* 1995;4:170–176.

475. Burk RO, Volcker HE. Current imaging of the optic disk and retinal nerve fiber layer [review]. *Curr Opin Ophthalmol.* 1996;7:99–108.

476. Weinreb RN, Dreher AW, Bille JF. Quantitative assessment of the optic nerve head with the laser tomographic scanner. *Int Ophthalmol.* 1989;13:25–29.

477. Dreher AW, Weinreb RN. Accuracy of topographic measurements in a model eye with the laser tomographic scanner. *Invest Ophthalmol Vis Sci.* 1991;32:2992–2996.

478. Uchida H, Tomita G, Kitazawa Y. Clinical evaluation of the Heidelberg Retina Tomograph II [in Japanese]. *Nippon Ganka Gakkai Zasshi.* 2000;104:826–829.

479. Burk RO, Vihanninjoki K, Bartke T, et al. Development of the standard reference plane for the Heidelberg retina tomograph. *Graefes Arch Clin Exp Ophthalmol.* 2000;238:375–384.

480. Miller JM, Caprioli J. An optimal reference plane to detect glaucomatous nerve fiber layer abnormalities with computerized image analysis. *Graefes Arch Clin Exp Ophthalmol.* 1992;230:124–128.

481. Park KH, Caprioli J. Development of a novel reference plane for the Heidelberg retina tomograph with optical coherence tomography measurements. *J Glaucoma.* 2002;11:385–391.

482. Vihanninjoki K, Burk RO, Teesalu P, et al. Optic disc biomorphometry with the Heidelberg Retina Tomograph at different reference levels. *Acta Ophthalmol Scand.* 2002;80:47–53.

483. Weinreb RN, Lusky M, Bartsch DU, et al. Effect of repetitive imaging on topographic measurements of the optic nerve head. *Arch Ophthalmol.* 1993;111:636–638.

484. Mikelberg FS, Wijsman K, Schulzer M. Reproducibility of topographic parameters obtained with the Heidelberg retina tomograph. *J Glaucoma.* 1993;2:101–112.

485. Lusky M, Bosem ME, Weinreb RN. Reproducibility of optic nerve head topography measurements in eyes with undilated pupils. *J Glaucoma.* 1993;2:104–109.

486. Rohrschneider K, Burk RO, Kruse FE, et al. Reproducibility of the optic nerve head topography with a new laser tomographic scanning device. *Ophthalmology.* 1994;101:1044–1049.

487. Janknecht P, Funk J. Optic nerve head analyser and Heidelberg retina tomograph: accuracy and reproducibility of topographic measurements in a model eye and in volunteers. *Br J Ophthalmol.* 1994;78:760–768.

488. Tomita G, Honbe K, Kitazawa Y. Reproducibility of measurements by laser scanning tomography in eyes before and after pilocarpine treatment. *Graefes Arch Clin Exp Ophthalmol.* 1994;232:406–408.

489. Janknecht P, Funk J. The Heidelberg Retina Tomograph: reproducibility and measuring errors in different pupillary widths using a model eye [in German]. *Klin Monatsbl Augenheilkd.* 1994;205:98–102.

490. Spencer AF, Sadiq SA, Pawson P, et al. Vertical optic disk diameter: discrepancy between planimetric and SLO measurements. *Invest Ophthalmol Vis Sci.* 1995;36:796–803.

491. Miglior S, Albe E, Guareschi M, et al. Intraobserver and interobserver reproducibility in the evaluation of optic disc stereometric parameters by Heidelberg Retina Tomograph. *Ophthalmology.* 2002;109:1072–1077.

492. Brigatti L, Caprioli J. Correlation of visual field with scanning confocal laser optic disc measurements in glaucoma. *Arch Ophthalmol.* 1995;113:1191–1194.

493. Mikelberg FS, Parfitt CM, Swindale NV, et al. Ability of the Heidelberg retina tomograph to detect early glaucomatous visual field loss. *J Glaucoma.* 1995;4:242–247.

494. Harju M, Vesti E. Scanning laser ophthalmoscopy of the optic nerve head in exfoliation glaucoma and ocular hypertension with exfoliation syndrome. *Br J Ophthalmol.* 2001;85:297–303.

495. Bathija R, Zangwill L, Berry CC, et al. Detection of early glaucomatous structural damage with confocal scanning laser tomography. *J Glaucoma.* 1998;7:121–127.

496. Nakamura H, Maeda T, Suzuki Y, et al. Scanning laser tomography to evaluate optic discs of normal eyes. *Jpn J Ophthalmol.* 1999;43:410–414.

497. Parikh RS, Parikh S, Sekhar GC, et al. Diagnostic capability of optical coherence tomography (Stratus OCT 3) in early glaucoma. *Ophthalmology.* 2007;114:2238–2243.

498. Mastrophasqua L, Brusini P, Carpineto P, et al. Humphrey matrix frequency doubling technology perimetry and optical coherence tomography measurement of the retinal nerve fiber layer thickness in both normal and ocular hypertensive subjects. *J Glaucoma.* 2006;15:328–335.

499. Manassakorn A, Nouri-Mahdavi K, Caprioli J. Comparison of retinal nerve fiber layer thickness and optic disk algorithms with optical coherence tomography to detect glaucoma. *Am J Ophthalmol.* 2006;141:105–115.

500. Nouri-Mahdavi K, Hoffman D, Tannenbaum DP, et al. Identifying early glaucoma with optical coherence tomography. *Am J Ophthalmol.* 2004;137:228–235.

501. Wollstein G, Garway-Heath DF, Fontana L, et al. Identifying early glaucomatous changes. Comparison between expert clinical assessment of optic disc photographs and confocal scanning ophthalmoscopy. *Ophthalmology.* 2000;107:2272–2277.

502. Reuss NJ, de Graaf M, Lemij HG. Accuracy of GDx VCC, HRT I, and clinical assessment of stereoscopic optic nerve head photographs for diagnosing glaucoma. *Br J Ophthalmol.* 2007;91:313–318.

503. Magacho L, Marcondes AM, Costa VP. Discrimination between normal and glaucomatous eyes with scanning laser polarimetry and optic disc topography. *Eur J Ophthalmol.* 2005;15:353–359.

504. Vihanninjoki K, Teesalu P, Burk RO, et al. Search for an optimal combination of structural and functional parameters for the diagnosis of glaucoma: multivariate analysis of confocal scanning laser tomograph, blue-on-yellow visual field and retinal nerve fiber layer data. *Graefes Arch Clin Exp Ophthalmol.* 2000;238:477–481.

505. Swindale NV, Stjepanovic G, Chin A, et al. Automated analysis of normal and glaucomatous optic nerve head topography images. *Invest Ophthalmol Vis Sci.* 2000;41:1730–742.

506. Iester M, Swindale NV, Mikelberg FS. Sector-based analysis of optic nerve head shape parameters and visual field indices in healthy and glaucomatous eyes. *J Glaucoma.* 1997;6:370–376.

507. Iester M, Mikelberg FS, Drance SM. The effect of optic disc size on diagnostic precision with the Heidelberg retina tomograph. *Ophthalmology.* 1997;104:545–548.

508. Wollstein G, Garway-Heath DF, Hitchings RA. Identification of early glaucoma cases with the scanning laser ophthalmoscope. *Ophthalmology.* 1998;105:1557–1563.

509. Ford BA, Artes PH, McCormick TA, et al. Comparison of data analysis tools for detection of glaucoma with the Heidelberg Retina Tomograph. *Ophthalmology.* 2003;110:1145–1150.

510. Asawaphureekorn S, Zangwill L, Weinreb RN. Ranked-segment distribution curve for interpretation of optic nerve topography. *J Glaucoma.* 1996;5:79–90.

511. Gordon MO, Beiser JA, Brandt JD, et al. The Ocular Hypertension Treatment Study: baseline factors that predict the onset of primary open-angle glaucoma. *Arch Ophthalmol.* 2002;120:714–720.

512. Miglior S, Zeyen T, Pfeiffer N, et al. Results of the European Glaucoma Prevention Study. *Ophthalmology.* 2005;112:366–375.

513. Zangwill LM, Weinreb RN, Beiser JA, et al. Baseline topographic optic disc measurements are associated with the development of primary open-angle glaucoma: the Confocal Scanning Laser Ophthalmoscopy Ancillary Study to the Ocular Hypertension Treatment Study. *Arch Ophthalmol.* 2005;123:1188–1197.

514. Chauhan BC, Blanchard JW, Hamilton DC, et al. Technique for detecting serial topographic changes in the optic disc and peripapillary retina using scanning laser tomography. *Invest Ophthalmol Vis Sci.* 2000;41:775–782.

515. Broadway DC, Drance SM, Parfitt CM, et al. The ability of scanning laser ophthalmoscopy to identify various glaucomatous optic disk appearances. *Am J Ophthalmol.* 1998;125:593–604.

516. Miglior S, Casula M, Guareschi M, et al. Clinical ability of Heidelberg retinal tomograph examination to detect glaucomatous visual field changes. *Ophthalmology.* 2001;108:1621–1627.

517. Weinreb RN, Shakiba S, Zangwill L. Scanning laser polarimetry to measure the nerve fiber layer of normal and glaucomatous eyes. *Am J Ophthalmol.* 1995;119:627–636.

518. Weinreb RN, Dreher AW, Coleman A, et al. Histopathologic validation of Fourier-ellipsometry measurements of retinal nerve fiber layer thickness. *Arch Ophthalmol.* 1990;108:557–560.

519. Knighton RW, Huang XR, Greenfield DS. Analytical model of scanning laser polarimetry for retinal nerve fiber layer assessment. *Invest Ophthalmol Vis Sci.* 2002;43:383–392.

520. Morgan JE, Waldock A. Scanning laser polarimetry of the normal human retinal nerve fiber layer: a quantitative analysis. *Am J Ophthalmol.* 2000;129:76–82.

521. Greenfield DS, Knighton RW, Huang XR. Effect of corneal polarization axis on assessment of retinal nerve fiber layer thickness by scanning laser polarimetry. *Am J Ophthalmol.* 2000;129:715–722.

522. Weinreb RN, Bowd C, Greenfield DS, et al. Measurement of the magnitude and axis of corneal polarization with scanning laser polarimetry. *Arch Ophthalmol.* 2002;120:901–906.

523. Greenfield DS, Knighton RW, Feuer WJ, et al. Correction for corneal polarization axis improves the discriminating power of scanning laser polarimetry. *Am J Ophthalmol.* 2002;134:27–33.

524. Weinreb RN, Bowd C, Zangwill LM. Scanning laser polarimetry in monkey eyes using variable corneal polarization compensation. *J Glaucoma.* 2002;11:378–384.

525. Weinreb RN, Bowd C, Zangwill LM. Glaucoma detection using scanning laser polarimetry with variable corneal polarization compensation. *Arch Ophthalmol.* 2003;121:218–224.

526. Bowd C, Zangwill LM, Weinreb RN. Association between scanning laser polarimetry measurements using variable corneal polarization compensation and visual field sensitivity in glaucomatous eyes. *Arch Ophthalmol.* 2003;121:961–966.

527. Garway-Heath DF, Greaney MJ, Caprioli J. Correction for the erroneous compensation of anterior segment birefringence with the scanning laser polarimeter for glaucoma diagnosis. *Invest Ophthalmol Vis Sci.* 2002;43:1465–1474.

528. Shah NN, Bowd C, Medeiros FA, et al. Combining structural and functional testing for detection of glaucoma. *Ophthalmology.* 2006;113:1593–1602.

529. Bowd C, Zangwill LM, Berry CC, et al. Detecting early glaucoma by assessment of retinal nerve fiber layer thickness and visual function. *Invest Ophthalmol Vis Sci.* 2001;42:1993–2003.

530. Hee MR, Izatt JA, Swanson EA, et al. Optical coherence tomography of the human retina. *Arch Ophthalmol.* 1995;113:325–332.

531. Sanchez-Galeana C, Bowd C, Blumenthal EZ, et al. Using optical imaging summary data to detect glaucoma. *Ophthalmology.* 2001;108:1812–1818.

532. Schuman JS, Hee MR, Puliafito CA, et al. Quantification of nerve fiber layer thickness in normal and glaucomatous eyes using optical coherence tomography. *Arch Ophthalmol.* 1995;113:586–596.

533. Schuman JS, Pedut-Kloizman T, Hertzmark E, et al. Reproducibility of nerve fiber layer thickness measurements using optical coherence tomography. *Ophthalmology.* 1996;103:1889–1898.

534. Kee C, Cho C. Evaluation of retinal nerve fiber layer thickness in the area of apparently normal hemifield in glaucomatous eyes with optical coherence tomography. *J Glaucoma.* 2003;12:250–254.

535. Aydin A, Wollstein G, Price LL, et al. Optical coherence tomography assessment of retinal nerve fiber layer thickness changes after glaucoma surgery. *Ophthalmology.* 2003;110:1506–1511.

536. Guedes V, Schuman JS, Hertzmark E, et al. Optical coherence tomography measurement of macular and nerve fiber layer thickness in normal and glaucomatous human eyes. *Ophthalmology.* 2003;110:177–189.

537. Baumann M, Gentile RC, Liebmann JM, et al. Reproducibility of retinal thickness measurements in normal eyes using optical coherence tomography. *Ophthalmic Surg Lasers.* 1998;29:280–285.

538. Jones AL, Sheen NJ, North RV, et al. The Humphrey optical coherence tomography scanner: quantitative analysis and reproducibility study of the normal human retinal nerve fibre layer. *Br J Ophthalmol.* 2001;85:673–677.

539. Klemm M, Rumberger E, Walter A, et al. Reproducibility of measuring retinal nerve fiber density: comparison of optical coherence tomography with the nerve fiber analyzer and the Heidelberg retinal tomography device [in German]. *Ophthalmologe.* 2002;99:345–351.

540. Zangwill LM, Bowd C, Berry CC, et al. Discriminating between normal and glaucomatous eyes using the Heidelberg Retina Tomograph, GDx Nerve Fiber Analyzer, and Optical Coherence Tomograph. *Arch Ophthalmol.* 2001;119:985–993.

541. Greaney MJ, Hoffman DC, Garway-Heath DF, et al. Comparison of optic nerve imaging methods to distinguish normal eyes from those with glaucoma. *Invest Ophthalmol Vis Sci.* 2002;43:140–145.

542. Drexler W, Sattmann H, Hermann B, et al. Enhanced visualization of macular pathology with the use of ultrahigh-resolution optical coherence tomography. *Arch Ophthalmol.* 2003;121:695–706.

543. Gloesmann M, Hermann B, Schubert C, et al. Histologic correlation of pig retina radial stratification with ultrahigh-resolution optical coherence tomography. *Invest Ophthalmol Vis Sci.* 2003;44:1696–1703.

544. Lalezary M, Medeiros FA, Weinreb RN, et al. Baseline optical coherence tomography predicts the development of glaucomatous change in glaucoma suspects. *Am J Ophthalmol.* 2006;142:576–582.

545. Zeimer R, Asrani S, Zou S, et al. Quantitative detection of glaucomatous damage at the posterior pole by retinal thickness mapping: a pilot study. *Ophthalmology.* 1998;105:224–231.

546. Asrani S, Challa P, Herndon L, et al. Correlation among retinal thickness, optic disc, and visual field in glaucoma patients and suspects: a pilot study. *J Glaucoma.* 2003;12:119–128.

547. Mistlberger A, Liebmann JM, Greenfield DS, et al. Assessment of optic disc anatomy and nerve fiber layer thickness in ocular hypertensive subjects with normal short-wavelength automated perimetry. *Ophthalmology.* 2002;109:1362–1366.

548. Geijssen HC, Greve EL. Vascular concepts in glaucoma [review]. *Curr Opin Ophthalmol.* 1995;6:71–77.

549. Cioffi GA, Wang L. Optic nerve blood flow in glaucoma [review]. *Semin Ophthalmol.* 1999;14:164–170.

550. Flammer J, Orgul S. Optic nerve blood-flow abnormalities in glaucoma [review]. *Prog Retin Eye Res.* 1998;17:267–289.

551. Harris A, Chung HS, Ciulla TA, et al. Progress in measurement of ocular blood flow and relevance to our understanding of glaucoma and age-related macular degeneration [review]. *Prog Retin Eye Res.* 1999;18:669–687.

552. Melamed S, Levkovitch-Verbin H. Laser scanning tomography and angiography of the optic nerve head for the diagnosis and follow-up of glaucoma [review]. *Curr Opin Ophthalmol.* 1997;8:7–12.

553. Weinreb RN, Bartsch DU, Freeman WR. Angiography of the glaucomatous optic nerve head. *J Glaucoma.* 1994;3(suppl 1):S55–S60.

554. Bartsch DU, Weinreb RN, Zinser G, et al. Confocal scanning infrared laser ophthalmoscopy for indocyanine green angiography. *Am J Ophthalmol.* 1995;120:642–651.

555. Marengo J, Ucha RA, Martinez-Cartier M, et al. Glaucomatous optic nerve head changes with scanning laser ophthalmoscopy. *Int Ophthalmol.* 2001;23:413–423.

556. Freeman WR, Bartsch DU, Mueller AJ, et al. Simultaneous indocyanine green and fluorescein angiography using a confocal scanning laser ophthalmoscope. *Arch Ophthalmol.* 1998;116:455–463.

557. Melamed S, Levkovitch-Verbin H, Krupsky S, et al. Confocal tomographic angiography of the optic nerve head in patients with glaucoma. *Am J Ophthalmol.* 1998;125:447–456.

558. O'Brart DP, de Souza LM, Bartsch DU, et al. Indocyanine green angiography of the peripapillary region in glaucomatous eyes by confocal scanning laser ophthalmoscopy. *Am J Ophthalmol.* 1997;123:657–666.

559. Baxter GM, Williamson TH, McKillop G, et al. Color Doppler ultrasound of orbital and optic nerve blood flow: effects of posture and timolol 0.5%. *Invest Ophthalmol Vis Sci.* 1992;33:604–610.

560. Galassi F, Nuzzaci G, Sodi A, et al. Color Doppler imaging in evaluation of optic nerve blood supply in normal and glaucomatous subjects. *Int Ophthalmol.* 1992;16:273–276.

561. Rankin SJ, Drance SM, Buckley AR, et al. Visual field correlations with color Doppler studies in open-angle glaucoma. *J Glaucoma.* 1996;5:15–21.

562. Dennis KJ, Dixon RD, Winsberg F, et al. Variability in measurement of central retinal artery velocity using color Doppler imaging. *J Ultrasound Med.* 1995;14:463–466.

563. Niwa Y, Yamamoto T, Kawakami H, et al. Reproducibility of color Doppler imaging for orbital arteries in Japanese patients with normal-tension glaucoma. *Jpn J Ophthalmol.* 1998;42:389–392.

564. Riva C, Ross B, Benedek GB. Laser Doppler measurements of blood flow in capillary tubes and retinal arteries. *Invest Ophthalmol.* 1972;11:936–944.

565. Riva CE, Harino S, Petrig BL, et al. Laser Doppler flowmetry in the optic nerve. *Exp Eye Res.* 1992;55:499–506.

566. Engelhart M, Petersen LJ, Kristensen JK. The local regulation of blood flow evaluated simultaneously by 133-xenon washout and laser Doppler flowmetry. *J Invest Dermatol.* 1988;91:451–453.

567. Phillips AR, Farrant GJ, Abu-Zidan FM, et al. A method using laser Doppler flowmetry to study intestinal and pancreatic perfusion during an acute intestinal ischaemic injury in rats with pancreatitis. *Eur Surg Res.* 2001;33:361–369.

568. Bohdanecka Z, Orgul S, Prunte C, et al. Influence of acquisition parameters on hemodynamic measurements with the Heidelberg retina flowmeter at the optic disc. *J Glaucoma.* 1998;7:151–157.

569. Lietz A, Hendrickson P, Flammer J, et al. Effect of carbogen, oxygen and intraocular pressure on Heidelberg retina flowmeter parameter 'flow' measured at the papilla. *Ophthalmologica.* 1998;212:149–152.

570. Chauhan BC, Smith FM. Confocal scanning laser Doppler flowmetry: experiments in a model flow system. *J Glaucoma.* 1997;6:237–245.

571. Kagemann L, Harris A, Chung HS, et al. Heidelberg retinal flowmetry: factors affecting blood flow measurement. *Br J Ophthalmol.* 1998;82:131–136.

572. Kagemann L, Harris A, Chung H, et al. Photodetector sensitivity level and Heidelberg retina flowmeter measurements in humans. *Invest Ophthalmol Vis Sci.* 2001;42:354–357.

573. Wang L, Cull G, Cioffi GA. Depth of penetration of scanning laser Doppler flowmetry in the primate optic nerve. *Arch Ophthalmol.* 2001;119:1810–1814.

574. Haefliger IO, Lietz A, Griesser SM, et al. Modulation of Heidelberg retinal flowmeter parameter flow at the papilla of healthy subjects: effect of carbogen, oxygen, high intraocular pressure, and beta-blockers. *Surv Ophthalmol.* 1999;43(suppl 1):S59–S65.

575. Yaoeda K, Shirakashi M, Funaki S, et al. Measurement of microcirculation in the optic nerve head by laser speckle flowgraphy and scanning laser Doppler flowmetry. *Am J Ophthalmol.* 2000;129:734–739.

576. Yaoeda K, Shirakashi M, Funaki S, et al. Measurement of microcirculation in optic nerve head by laser speckle flowgraphy in normal volunteers. *Am J Ophthalmol.* 2000;130:606–610.

577. Garcia GH, Donahue KM, Ulmer JL, et al. Qualitative perfusion imaging of the human optic nerve. *Ophthal Plast Reconstr Surg.* 2002;18:107–113.

578. Prunte C, Flammer J, Markstein R, et al. Quantification of optic nerve blood flow changes using magnetic resonance imaging. *Invest Ophthalmol Vis Sci.* 1995;36:247–251.

579. Leung CK, Lindsey JD, Chen L, et al. Longitudinal profile of retinal ganglion cell damage assessed with blue-light confocal scanning laser ophthalmoscopy after ischemic reperfusion injury. *Br J Ophthalmol.* 2009;93:964–968.

580. Leung CK, Weinreb RN. Experimental detection of retinal ganglion cell damage in vivo. *Exp Eye Res.* 2009;88:831–836.

581. Leung CK, Lindsey JD, Crowston JG, et al. Longitudinal profile of retinal ganglion cell damage after optic nerve crush with blue-light confocal scanning laser ophthalmoscopy. *Invest Ophthalmol Vis Sci.* 2008;49:4898–4902.

582. Leung CK, Lindsey JD, Crowston JG, et al. In vivo imaging of murine retinal ganglion cells. *J Neurosci Methods.* 2008;168:475–478.

583. Schmitz-Valckenberg S, Guo L, Maass A, et al. Real-time in vivo imaging of retinal cell apoptosis after laser exposure. *Invest Ophthalmol Vis Sci.* 2008;49:2773–2780.

584. Guo L, Salt TE, Maas A, et al. Assessment of neuroprotective effects of glutamate modulation on glaucoma-related retinal ganglion cell apoptosis in vivo. *Invest Ophthalmol Vis Sci.* 2006;47:626–633.

585. Cordeiro MF, Guo L, Luong V, et al. Real-time imaging of single nerve cell apoptosis in retinal neurodegeneration. *Proc Natl Acad Sci USA.*

5

Assessment of Visual Fields

Advances in the technology of visual field testing have changed our clinical perception of normal and abnormal fields of vision. For example, the two-dimensional presentation of concentric lines around the point of fixation has given way to three-dimensional displays in symbols and numerical values. However, the normal field of vision and the changes created by glaucoma are just the same as they were 100 years ago when Bjerrum discovered the arcuate scotoma using the back of his consulting room door as a background for his field testing. This chapter therefore first considers the normal field of vision and how it is altered by glaucomatous damage, and then reviews the instruments and techniques by which these parameters can be measured.

NORMAL VISUAL FIELD

A helpful way to begin the study of visual fields and the methods by which they are measured is to consider Traquair's classic analogy of "an island of vision surrounded by a sea of blindness" (**Fig. 5.1**). This three-dimensional concept can be reduced to quantitative values by plotting lines (isopters) at various levels around the island, or by measuring the height (sensitivity) at different points in the island of vision.

Boundaries

The shoreline of the island corresponds to the peripheral limits of the visual field, which normally measure, with maximum target stimulation, approximately 60 degrees above and nasal, 70 to 75 degrees below, and 100 to 110 degrees temporal to fixation (1). The typical configuration of the normal visual field, therefore, is a horizontal oval, often with a shallow inferonasal depression (Fig. 5.1). The shape is usually of greater diagnostic significance than the absolute size of the visual field is, because the latter is influenced by many physiologic and testing variables.

Contour

The peaks and valleys on the island correspond to areas of increased or decreased vision within the peripheral limits of the visual field. These contours can be mapped by recording the weakest light stimulus that can be seen at specific locations in the field of vision or by using test objects with reduced stimulus value to plot smaller isopters within the absolute boundaries. The area of maximum visual sensitivity in the normal field during photopic condition is at the point of fixation, corresponding to the foveola of the retina, and appears as a smoothly rising peak surrounded by a high plateau (2). The visual sensitivity

Figure 5.1 The normal visual field (right eye) is depicted as the Traquair "island of vision surrounded by a sea of blindness," with projections showing the peripheral limits (**A**) and the profile (**B**). Fixation (*f*) corresponds to the foveola of the retina, and the blind spot (*bs*) to the optic nerve head. The approximate dimensions of the absolute peripheral boundary of the visual field and the location of the blind spot are shown (**A**).

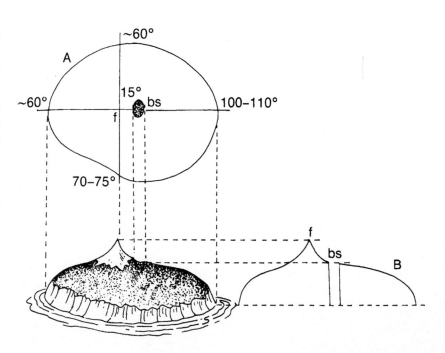

then tapers down more gradually until it again falls abruptly at the peripheral limits.

Blind Spot

Nerve fibers, collecting visual information from the retina, come together approximately 10 to 15 degrees nasally from the fovea. This region corresponds to the optic nerve head, and because there are no photoreceptors in this area, it creates a deep depression within the boundaries of the normal visual field, which is called the blind spot. Because the image formed on the retina is upside down and backward, the blind spot is located temporal to fixation. The blind spot has two portions: (a) an absolute scotoma and (b) a relative scotoma (3). The absolute scotoma corresponds to the actual optic nerve head and is seen as a vertical oval. Because the nerve head has no photoreceptors, this portion of the blind spot is independent of the test object stimulus value.

The relative scotoma surrounds the absolute portion and corresponds to peripapillary retina, which has reduced visual sensitivity, especially inferiorly and superiorly. In a study correlating the blind spot size to the area of the optic disc and peripapillary atrophy, the absolute scotoma included the peripapillary scleral ring and the peripapillary zone beta (see definitions in Chapter 4), whereas zone alpha was attributed to the relative scotoma (4).

VISUAL FIELD LOSS IN GLAUCOMA

Peripheral Loss

Defects along the peripheral boundaries of the visual field (i.e., peripheral nasal steps, vertical steps, and temporal sector defects) are most often found in association with scotomas in the more central arcuate area, although in some patients with early glaucomatous visual field loss, peripheral defects may be the only detectable abnormality (5–8). With automated static perimetry (discussed later), it has become common practice to measure only the central 24 to 30 degrees of the visual field, because of the increased time requirement with this technique. The question arises, therefore, as to how much information is being missed by ignoring the more peripheral portions of the field. In the presence of paracentral scotomas, peripheral measurements appear to add no significant information regarding the progression of visual field damage (9). In the initial diagnosis, however, a peripheral field defect, usually a nasal step, may be the only abnormality detected by automated perimetry in 3% to 11% of patients, depending on the testing method (10–13). To be clinically useful, the time required to obtain this information must not add excessively to the overall testing time; further study is needed to determine whether this can be achieved with newer programs for automated perimetry.

Localized Nerve Fiber Layer Defects

In glaucoma, structural damage to ganglion cells and their axons causes partial or complete functional loss in the area of damaged cells. The glaucomatous process typically causes initial damage to one or more axon bundles, creating a localized visual field defect. Focal defects, due to loss or impairment of retinal nerve fiber bundles, constitute the most definitive early evidence of visual field loss from glaucoma. The nature of the nerve fiber bundle defects relates to the retinal topography of these fibers, as discussed in Chapter 4.

Arcuate Defects

Bjerrum (pronounced *bee YER um*) described an arcuate visual defect, which he showed is strongly suggestive of glaucoma. This arcuate scotoma starts from the blind spot and arches above or below fixation, or both, to the horizontal median raphe, corresponding to the arcuate retinal nerve fibers (**Figs. 5.2A** and **5.3**). The nasal extreme of the arcuate area along the median raphe may come within 1 degree of fixation and extends nasally for 10 to 20 degrees (14). Early visual loss in glaucoma commonly occurs in this arcuate area, especially in the superior half, which correlates with the predilection of the inferior and superior temporal poles of the optic nerve head for early glaucomatous damage (14,15). As field defects develop within the arcuate area, they most often appear first as one or more localized defects, or paracentral scotomas (**Fig. 5.2B**). The typical pattern of progression of glaucomatous visual field defects is for a shallow paracentral depression to become denser and larger (16), eventually forming a central absolute defect, surrounded by a relative scotoma (17,18). The relative scotoma represents fluctuation that can be seen at the border of the physiologic blind spot and glaucomatous defects, but is significantly larger and more sloping in the latter (19). Occasionally, the early arcuate defect may connect with the blind spot and taper to a point in a slightly curved course, which has been referred to as a Seidel scotoma (**Fig. 5.2C**). As the isolated defects enlarge and coalesce, they form an arching scotoma that eventually fills the entire arcuate area from the blind spot to the median raphe, which is called an arcuate or Bjerrum scotoma (**Fig. 5.2D**). With further progression, a double arcuate (or ring) scotoma develops (**Fig. 5.2E**). The rate of visual field loss correlates with the size of the scotoma, in that, the larger the scotoma, the more rapidly it is likely to enlarge (20).

Although the arcuate defect is probably the most reliable early form of glaucomatous field loss, it is not pathognomonic, and the following additional causes must be considered, especially when the field and disc changes do not seem to correlate: chorioretinal lesions, optic nerve head lesions, anterior optic nerve lesions, and posterior lesions of the visual pathway (21–23) (**Table 5.1**). At times the arcuate defect involves the papillomacular nerve fiber bundle (**Fig. 5.4**).

Nasal Steps

The loss of retinal nerve fibers rarely proceeds at the same rate in the upper and lower portions of an eye. Consequently, a steplike defect is frequently created where the nerve fibers meet along the median raphe (**Fig. 5.5**). Because the superior field is involved somewhat more frequently than the inferior portion is in the early stages of glaucoma, the nasal step more often results from a greater defect above the horizontal midline, which is referred to as a superior nasal step. However, inferior nasal

Figure 5.2 Arcuate nerve fiber bundle defects. **A:** The arcuate (or Bjerrum) area is shown within the dotted lines. **B:** Superior paracentral scotoma, with central absolute defect surrounded by a relative scotoma. **C:** Seidel scotoma. **D:** Complete arcuate (Bjerrum) scotoma. **E:** Double arcuate (ring) scotoma with superior central nasal step. **F:** Vertical step (or hemianopic offset).

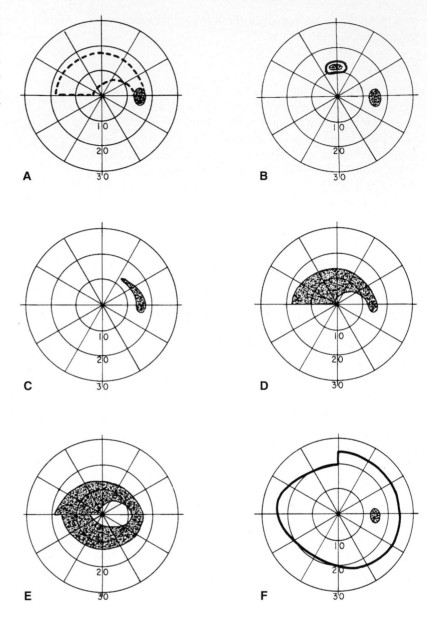

Figure 5.3 Grayscale of a SITA standard 24-2 achromatic visual field showing superior arcuate defect with corresponding inferior neuro-retinal thinning and retinal nerve fiber layer thinning.

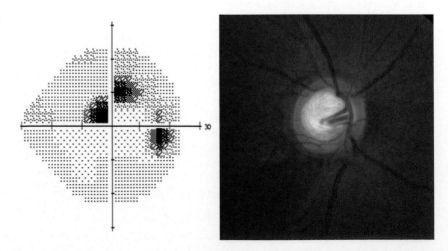

Table 5.1	Differential Diagnosis of Arcuate Scotomas

Chorioretinal lesions
  Juxtapapillary choroiditis and retinochoroiditis
  Myopia with peripapillary atrophy
  Retinal pigment epithelium and photoreceptor
    degeneration
  Retinal artery occlusions

Optic nerve head lesions
  Drusen
  Retinal artery plaques
  Chronic papilledema
  Papillitis
  Colobomas (including optic nerve pit)

Anterior optic nerve lesions
  Carotid and ophthalmic artery occlusion
  Ischemic infarct
  Cerebral arteritis
  Retrobulbar neuritis
  Electric shock
  Exophthalmos

Posterior lesions of the visual pathway
  Pituitary adenoma
  Opticochiasmatic arachnoiditis
  Meningiomas of the dorsum sella or optic foramen
  Progressive external ophthalmoplegia
  Pseudotumor cerebri

steps are not uncommon. Nasal steps are also distinguished by their central or peripheral location (5). A central nasal step is created at the side of an unequal double arcuate scotoma closest to fixation. Unequal contraction on the peripheral side of the defect, due to loss of corresponding bundles of peripheral arcuate nerve fibers, produces a defect that has been called the peripheral nasal step of Ronne. Nasal step often begins as an isolated scotoma in the nasal periphery (6). The shape of the peripheral nasal step with kinetic testing differs according to its distance from fixation and is not necessarily found in all isopters (18,24). Nasal step appears to be a common defect in acute and early chronic angle-closure glaucoma (25,26).

Vertical Step

A stepwise defect along the vertical midline, referred to as a vertical step (**Fig. 5.2F**) or hemianopic offset, is a less common feature of glaucomatous field loss than the nasal step is; it occurs in roughly 20% of cases (27,28). The mechanism of this field defect is not fully understood, although it may relate to segregation in the optic nerve head of axons from either side of the vertical midline (27). The defect more often appears on the nasal side of the vertical midline (**Fig. 5.6**). However, healthy eyes have also revealed greater sensitivity temporal to the hemianopic border, and it has been suggested that a small peripheral step at the vertical midline should arouse suspicion of glaucoma only if the defect is located temporally (29). It also has limited diagnostic value because most are associated with other glaucomatous field changes (28),

and the main significance of the observation is in distinguishing glaucomatous vertical midline defects from those caused by neurologic lesions.

Generalized and Central Depression of the Visual Field

The increased sensitivity with which newer instruments allow evaluation of vision is changing our understanding of the natural history of progressive visual field loss in glaucoma. Although defects related to loss of retinal nerve fiber bundles are the most familiar visual field changes induced by glaucoma, and central vision is typically one of the last regions to be totally lost, studies have shown mild central and diffuse reduction in the visual field even in the early stages of glaucoma (30–35). The mechanism for this is uncertain, although it appears to represent pressure-induced damage with diffuse nerve fiber loss, as evidenced by abnormal light-sense and flicker perimetry, which have been shown to accompany diffuse retinal nerve fiber layer (NFL) loss (33,34,36,37).

Central vision is typically preserved in the early course of glaucoma, but rarely it may be affected by a localized damage involving the fixation point. In these situations, other visual functions, such as visual acuity and color vision, may become abnormal. These central defects should be differentiated from macular disorders.

Although most studies agree that some patients with early glaucoma can have purely diffuse loss in the absence of other causes, other investigators have challenged this concept, suggesting that a generalized depression in glaucoma is rare and that these patients may have other causes for the diffuse loss of perimetric sensitivity, such as media opacity, miosis, or retinal dysfunction (30–32,34,38–42). In any case, the diagnostic value of this finding is currently limited by its nonspecific nature, but it should still be looked for and noted in the course of visual field testing and analysis. Although the measures of generalized reduction in visual function may one day be important in the early detection of glaucoma, they are too inconsistent and nonspecific at present to be of highly significant clinical value. In the future, they may acquire greater diagnostic significance as our knowledge of glaucomatous visual dysfunction expands. The following are some of the perimetric and other measures that can be used to evaluate generalized visual impairment in glaucoma.

Concentric Contraction

Generalized reduction in the visual field may become manifest as a decrease in sensitivity for specific retinal locations or as a concentric constriction of the visual field, both of which precede other detectable glaucomatous field defects in many patients (43,44). Isopter contraction, as an early field defect of glaucoma, is often more marked in the nasal field, which has been called "crowding of the peripheral nasal isopters" (45).

Enlargement of the Blind Spot

Enlargement of the blind spot, due to depression of peripapillary retinal sensitivity, is also considered to be an early glaucomatous field change. However, it may be seen with other optic nerve or

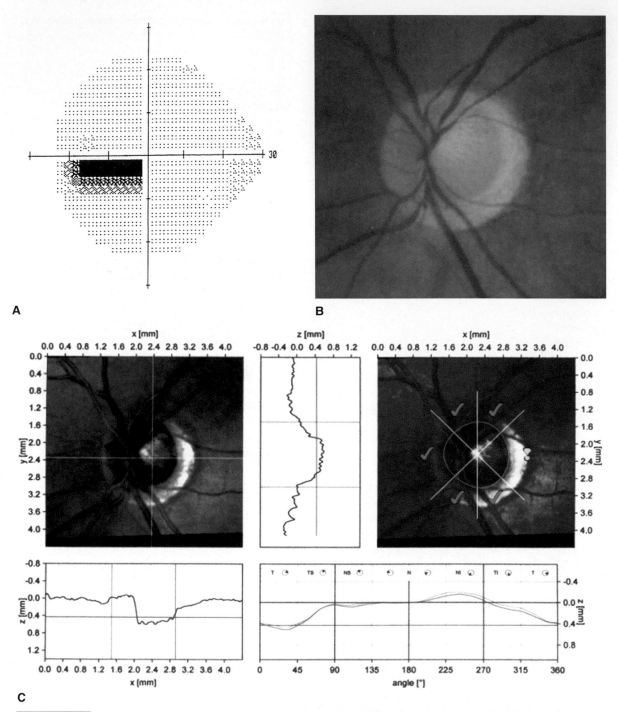

Figure 5.4   Grayscale of a SITA standard 24-2 achromatic visual field showing an arcuate defect involving the papillomacular nerve fiber bundle. The corresponding optic nerve with extensive temporal thinning and peripapillary atrophy. HRT-II Moorfields regression analysis calling attention to the temporal rim.

retinal disorders. One example has been called "acute idiopathic blind spot enlargement" and is related to multiple evanescent white-dot syndrome and possibly other retinal diseases (46–48). Enlargement of the blind spot can also be produced in healthy persons with threshold targets, so that it is not a pathognomonic sign of glaucoma (49). The relative portion of the blind spot depends on the stimulus value and varies with different testing methods. If the temporal margin of the relative blind spot comes close to the corresponding isopter (in kinetic perimetry), the two boundaries may artifactually become confluent, creating false

baring of the blind spot. In addition, because the reduced sensitivity of the peripapillary retina is greater in the upper and lower poles, test objects with small stimulus value may cause vertical elongation of the blind spot, which can break through the isopter, causing true baring of the blind spot (**Fig. 5.7**).

Angioscotomata

Angioscotomata are long, branching scotomas above and below the blind spot, which are presumed to result from shadows created by the large retinal vessels. Retinal vessels may

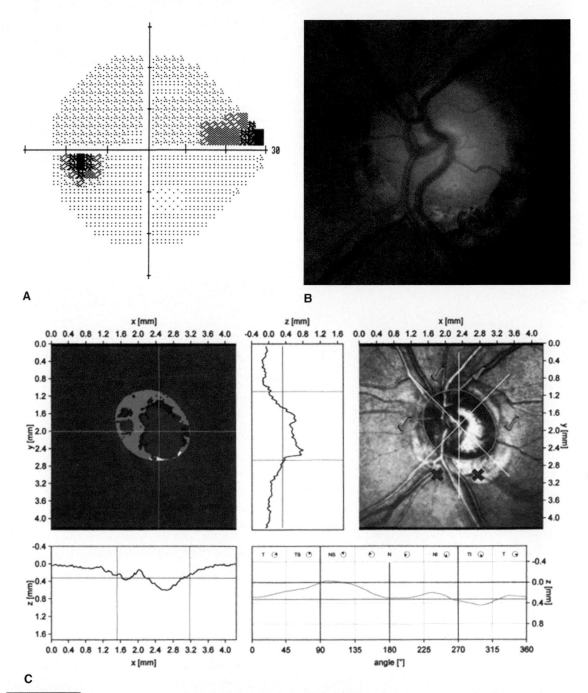

A

B

C

Figure 5.5 Grayscale of a SITA standard 24-2 achromatic visual field showing a nasal step. Optic nerve demonstrates significant inferior thinning, which is also called to attention by the HRT-II Moorfields regression analysis.

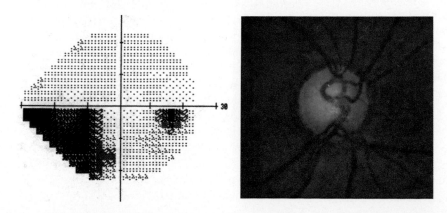

Figure 5.6 Grayscale of a SITA standard 24-2 achromatic visual field showing a vertical step.

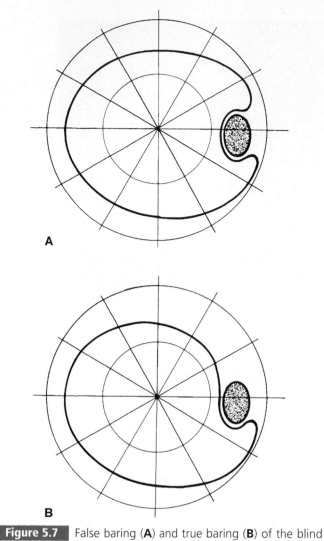

A

B

Figure 5.7 False baring (**A**) and true baring (**B**) of the blind spot.

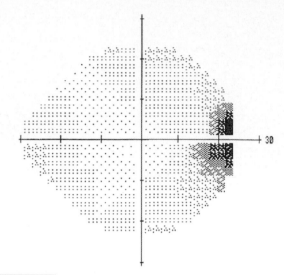

Figure 5.8 Grayscale of a SITA standard 24-2 achromatic visual field showing a temporal wedge defect.

have corresponding representation of angioscotomata in the visual cortex (50). Angioscotomata may represent an early glaucomatous field defect, although it is technically difficult to demonstrate and not highly diagnostic (51–54).

Temporal Sector Defect

Because the retinal nerve fibers nasal to the optic nerve head converge on the disc by a direct route, a lesion involving these fiber bundles produces a sector defect temporal to the blind spot (18,24) (**Fig. 5.8**). This defect usually appears later in the course of glaucomatous field loss (55), but can be the presenting visual field defect. With automated perimetry, glaucomatous defects temporal to the blind spot are not uncommon, but usually add significant information beyond findings of central field testing only in patients with late visual field loss (56).

Advanced Glaucomatous Field Defects

The natural history of progressive glaucomatous field loss involves the eventual development of a complete double arcuate scotoma, which coalesces nasally at the horizontal meridian (57)

and may extend to the peripheral limits in all areas except temporally. This results in a central island and a temporal island of vision in advanced glaucoma. With continued damage, these islands of vision progressively diminish in size until the tiny central island is totally extinguished, which may occur abruptly. Glaucoma surgery appears to accelerate the loss of the small central island in some patients, possibly because of the sudden change in intraocular pressure (IOP), although this complication does not occur frequently enough to constitute a contraindication to surgery in these patients (58). The temporal island of vision is more resistant and may persist long after central vision is lost. However, it, too, will eventually be destroyed if the glaucoma is not controlled, leaving the patient with no light perception.

Visual Field Changes in Normal-Tension Glaucoma

The nature of visual field defects may be influenced by the IOP, although reports on this are somewhat conflicting. In one study of patients with chronic open-angle glaucoma (COAG) who had early visual field loss, persons with diffuse depression had higher pressures than those with localized defects did (59) (**Fig. 5.9**). In addition, in some studies patients with COAG whose IOP has never exceeded approximately 21 mm Hg, commonly referred to as normal-tension (or low-tension) glaucoma, had scotomas with steeper slopes, greater depth, and closer proximity to fixation, compared with patients with COAG who had higher IOPs (60,61). In other studies, however, these two groups did not differ significantly when the same degree of optic nerve damage was present (62,63). Another study of normal-tension and high-tension glaucoma patients whose automated visual fields were matched to within a 0.3-dB mean deviation (explained later) revealed no significant difference in focal defects in the overall field or superior hemifield, but did show significantly more localized loss in the inferior hemifield among the normal-tension patients, supporting the hypothesis of a vascular mechanism in that group (64).

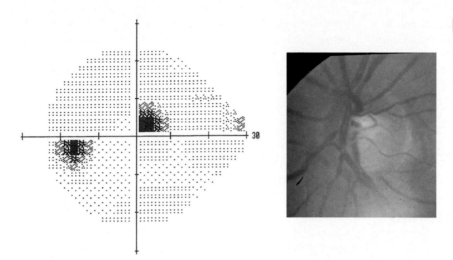

Figure 5.9 Grayscale of a SITA standard 24-2 achromatic visual field showing a paracentral defect from a patient with low-tension glaucoma. The optic nerve photograph demonstrates a corresponding notch inferiorly.

One study investigated the effect of trabeculectomy on the rate of visual field progression in patients with normal-tension glaucoma. The authors concluded that surgical lowering of IOP resulted in a decreased rate of visual field loss in the operated eye (65).

The Collaborative Normal-Tension Glaucoma Study investigators also concluded that IOP reduction decreases glaucoma progression in normal-tension glaucoma (66).

Visual Field Changes with Acute Pressure Elevation

The preceding discussions have dealt with field changes that are associated primarily with chronic forms of glaucoma. When the IOP elevation is sudden and marked, as in acute angle-closure glaucoma, various associated field changes have been reported, including general depression, early loss of central vision, arcuate scotomas, and enlargement of the blind spot (67). After the acute attack is brought under control, the fields return to normal in some patients, but other patients may have reduced color vision, generalized decreased sensitivity, or constriction of isopters, especially superiorly (68).

When the IOP is artificially elevated, by compression of the globe or administration of topical steroids, typical glaucomatous field defects or constriction of central isopters occur in some eyes (69–75). The changes are reversible when the IOP returns to normal and are dependent on the ocular perfusion pressure (73,74,76). This response to artificial pressure elevation is said to occur more commonly in patients with glaucoma (69,70,76)—especially normal-tension glaucoma (67)—although one study found no difference between patients with and without glaucoma (71).

Correlation between Optic Nerve Head and Visual Field Defects

In most patients with glaucoma, clinically recognizable disc changes precede detectable field loss, and the presence or absence of glaucomatous field defects can usually, but not always, be predicted from the appearance of the optic nerve head (77–82). Quigley and coworkers (83,84) attempted to correlate axon loss in the optic nerve head with visual field defects. Although limited by small sample size, their work suggested that not only does nerve fiber loss occur before reproducible field defects in some patients with elevated IOP, but the extent of axonal loss may be much greater than the corresponding visual field change. With standard perimetric techniques, 25% to 35% of the retinal ganglion cells may be lost in an eye with a normal field by the time reproducible early field defects are found (85), and 10% or fewer axons may remain by the stage of severe field loss (83). When correlating retinal ganglion cell atrophy with automated perimetry in patients with glaucoma, a 20% loss of cells, especially large ganglion cells in the central 30 degrees of the retina, correlated with a 5-dB sensitivity loss (discussed later), whereas a 40% loss corresponded with a 10-dB decrease, and some ganglion cells remained in areas with 0-dB sensitivity (84).

The nature of optic nerve head cupping can also be used to predict the type (in addition to the presence) of field loss. Extensive or focal absence of neural rim tissue, especially at the inferior or superior poles, is the most reliable indicator of visual field disturbance and is usually associated with a field defect in the corresponding arcuate area (79,86–89). In some eyes, field loss may occur before the pallor reaches the disc margin (86), and unusual cases have been reported with field damage despite round, symmetric cups (79). Quantitative measures of the retinal NFL also correlate with the visual field loss in patients with glaucoma (90).

The ability to predict impending glaucomatous visual field loss by the appearance of the optic nerve head is less accurate than correlating disc damage with established field loss. No single parameter or combination of parameters in glaucomatous optic atrophy is totally satisfactory for this purpose. The parameters that correlate best with visual field loss are magnification-corrected measurements of neuroretinal rim area and defects in the retinal NFL (91–99). Diffuse structural changes in the optic nerve head or retinal NFL are more often associated with diffuse depression of visual function, whereas localized changes correlate more with localized visual field changes (98). In some cases, the early field loss associated with retinal NFL defects can be detected with automatic perimetry when it has been missed with manual perimetry (100,101).

The correlation between optic nerve head and visual field defects in glaucoma is close enough to prompt a search for other underlying disease processes, such as neurologic disorders, if a correlation is not found. Nevertheless, the absence of a perfect correlation indicates that both disc and field examinations are essential in managing the glaucoma patient (102). In general, optic nerve head and retinal NFL changes have their greatest value in the early stages of glaucoma, whereas progressive visual field loss becomes the more useful guide to therapy in advanced cases (77,103).

BASIC PRINCIPLES OF VISUAL FIELD TESTING

Stimuli

The typical stimuli used in clinical perimetry are spots of light of various predefined combinations of diameter and intensity projected on the background. The visibility of the stimulus also depends on how far the eye is positioned from the screen and the brightness of the background. The other factors affecting perception of the stimulus include the length of time the stimulus is presented, the color of the stimulus and the background, whether kinetic or static techniques are used, and the condition of the eye and the patient.

The absolute light intensity is measured in units of luminance, called apostilbs, but the measured light sensitivity is expressed in logarithmic units referred to as decibels (dB), which provides a more linear relationship between visual perception and a change in light intensity. A decibel is 0.1 log-unit, so that a 10 dB represents a 10-fold decrease of the maximum stimulus of any specific perimeter, and a 20 dB represents a 100-fold stimulus attenuation. The maximum intensity of a perimeter has a value of 0 dB, meaning that the stimulus is not attenuated. Log-units and decibels are relative units, and resulting stimulus intensity is not the same for all instruments, but decibels represent the same percentage change of the intensity in all perimeters.

Stimulus Size

The standard target for kinetic and static perimetry is a white disc, the stimulus value of which can be adjusted by varying the target size or luminosity relative to that of the background. In healthy persons, the mean retinal sensitivity has been shown to increase with the increasing size of the test object (104). If the diameter of the smaller stimulus is increased, it may be as visible as the less intense larger stimulus, the phenomenon known as spatial summation. Usually, doubling the stimulus diameter has the same effect on the visibility of the stimulus as increasing its intensity by 5 dB (1).

Exposure Time

The exposure time will also affect the stimulus visibility. The stimulus presented over a longer period of time may become more visible, the phenomenon called temporal summation. However, after the temporal summation is complete, which happens typically after 0.1 second, the image is not seen any better. The Humphrey field analyzer uses a 0.2-second stimulus duration, which also helps prevent movement of the patient's gaze toward the stimulus. However, suprathreshold static targets should be presented for a longer time, usually 0.5 to 1 second, and test objects should be just above threshold for the area being tested.

Kinetic versus Static Perimetry

The threshold is theoretically the target that is just bright enough to be seen 50% of the time at that location (the differential light threshold). The stimulus that is below the threshold value cannot be seen. Kinetic perimetry defines threshold by moving the test object from a nonseeing (subthreshold) to a seeing (suprathreshold) area, and by recording the point at which it is first seen in relation to fixation (**Fig. 5.10A**). The procedure documents the boundaries of the visual field for the absolute limits and areas of relative differences in visual acuity within the field (**Fig. 5.11**). As previously noted, the boundaries, or contour lines, are called isopters. The size and shape of a particular isopter depend partly on the stimulus value of the corresponding test object.

Static perimetry involves the presentation of stationary test objects, by using suprathreshold or threshold presentations. Suprathreshold static presentation is an "on–off" technique in which a test object just above the anticipated threshold for the corresponding portion of the visual field is momentarily presented, and the points at which the patient fails to recognize the target are noted as visual field defects. It is a way of "spot checking" for areas of relative or absolute blindness, usually in the central visual field. The suprathreshold strategy is used mostly as a screening test.

Threshold static perimetry measures the relative intensity thresholds for the visual acuity of individual retinal points in the field of vision. The technique involves gradually increasing the target light from subthreshold intensity in small increments, and recording the level at which the patient first indicates recognition of the target (**Fig. 5.10B**), or decreasing

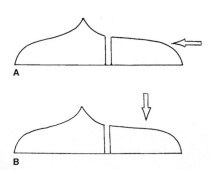

Figure 5.10 Standard techniques for measuring the visual field. In kinetic technique (**A**), test object moves from nonseeing to seeing area. Static technique (**B**) measures sensitivity of retina at a given point.

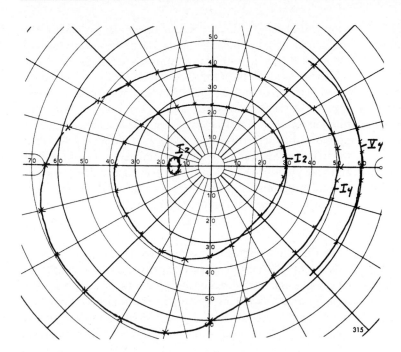

Figure 5.11 Example of manual kinetic perimetry showing two complete isopters (I_2 and I_4) and a third partial isopter (V_4) in nasal periphery with blind spot measured by I_2 target.

it from a suprathreshold level and recording the lowest stimulus value seen. The points are tested at predefined locations throughout the visual field, and the results are recorded as grayscale symbols and numerical sensitivity values in decibels (**Fig. 5.12**).

The kinetic stimuli are usually seen better than the static ones are, but when the stimulus is moved slowly, the results of kinetic and static perimetry are similar.

To minimize the patient's anticipation of when or where the next test object will appear, the presentation should be random, rather than following a predictable pattern, and the time between stimuli should be varied slightly. To avoid patient anxiety when testing in a nonseeing area, the examination should return periodically to a previously seen area.

For kinetic targets, a stimulus velocity of 4 degrees/sec appears to be optimal for all targets in the central and peripheral visual field, but a slower velocity of 2 degrees/sec may provide more reproducible results in some patients (105,106). The test object should always be moved from a nonseeing to a seeing area—that is, from the periphery toward fixation when outlining an isopter and from the center of the blind spot or a scotoma.

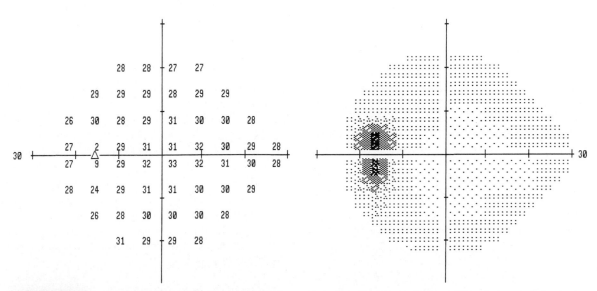

Figure 5.12 Examples of threshold static (standard automated) perimetry. Retinal sensitivity is measured at points throughout a portion of the visual field (central 24 to 30 degrees in this example). Results can be displayed in numerical values and symbols.

Threshold static perimetry has been shown to be more sensitive than kinetic perimetry is in detecting glaucomatous field loss (107,108). In one study of patients with COAG, a defect was found in one third of the cases with static perimetry that was missed by kinetic perimetry (109). In a long-term study of patients with ocular hypertension, 75% of those who developed glaucomatous damage had an abnormality detected by automated static perimetry (by using a hemifield test, explained later) 1 year before field loss was detected by manual perimetry, by using a combination of kinetic and static presentations (110).

When automated static perimetry was compared with Goldmann kinetic perimetry as a test for driving, a significant number of patients with severe field defects, detected by static perimetry, still met the standard for driving by the kinetic perimetry (111).

Because standard static threshold perimetry tests sensitivity near threshold, patients do not see approximately half the presented stimuli, and they may report that stimuli are too dim to see. Patients should be told that the limits of their seeing abilities are being tested and that barely seeing the stimuli is natural.

Background Illumination

Background illumination for manual perimetric techniques traditionally stimulates both rods and cones. The adapting field luminance currently used in static and kinetic perimetry is marginally photopic (e.g., 31.6 apostilbs), although the optimum luminance has yet to be established. One study suggested that the lower levels of background illumination may allow minor reductions in light transmission by the ocular media to produce significant changes in the recorded threshold sensitivity (112). In a comparison of scotopic and photopic fields, localized scotomas in patients with glaucoma were of equal depth, but diffuse scotopic defects significantly exceeded the photopic, supporting the concept that not all ganglion cell types are equally susceptible to glaucomatous damage (113). Scotopic defects were also found more often in patients with ocular hypertension or glaucoma than in healthy persons, and the defects were mainly in the superior hemifield (114).

With bowl perimeters, photometric adjustment should be made with the patient in place, because facial coloring affects luminosity. The most important principle regarding illumination is to keep the target and the background constant and reproducible from one examination to the next.

Physiologic Influences on Visual Fields

The following factors should be compensated for, if possible, or otherwise should be considered when interpreting the fields.

Pupil Size

Although decreased pupil size should have little effect on a patient's perception of a stimulus, because background and stimulus are affected equally, significant miosis may depress central and peripheral threshold sensitivities and exaggerate field defects (115), even after correction of induced myopia (116). One study

used neutral density filters to reduce the retinal illumination by the equivalent of halving the pupillary diameter, which reduced the mean threshold with two automated perimeters by 1.1 to 1.7 dB (117). In another study, use of pilocarpine worsened the visual field global indices, such as mean deviation and pattern standard deviation (explained later) (118). For this reason, the pupil size should be recorded with each field, and the influence of miosis should be considered when a field change is detected. Mydriasis has less influence on the visual field than miosis does, although pupillary dilatation with use of tropicamide, 1%, or no ocular medication in healthy persons reduced threshold sensitivity with automated perimetry in one study (119).

Age

Increasing age is also associated with reduced retinal threshold sensitivity (120). This effect starts as early as 20 years of age, progresses linearly throughout life, and involves the peripheral and superior areas more than the pericentric and inferior portions of the field (121,122). This age-related visual field sensitivity appears to be primarily due to neural loss rather than preretinal factors (123). Standard automated perimetry (SAP) protocols compensate for the effect of age by using age-bracketed databases.

Clarity of Ocular Media

Cataracts produce glare and change the intensity of the stimulus. Therefore, a cataract can cause or exaggerate central or peripheral field defects, which could be mistaken for the development or progression of glaucomatous field loss. Even minimal light scattering, as may be caused by an early cataract that has a relatively insignificant effect on visual acuity, may influence threshold measurements (124). As previously noted, this effect may be greater with lower levels of background illumination (112). Eyes with COAG and cataracts may have improvement of foveal sensitivity, visual field scores, and sometimes even a reversal of a partial or complete scotoma after cataract extraction (125–127). However, cataract surgery can also reveal mild and moderate field defects masked by cataracts (128,129). Nuclear cataracts depress central perimetric sensitivity more than peripheral sensitivity with both large and small targets, whereas nonnuclear cataracts influence central sensitivity more for small targets and peripheral sensitivity more for large targets (130). Attempts have been made to correlate visual field damage with lens opacity and visual acuity to aid clinicians in determining the significance of field change in patients with glaucoma and cataracts (131,132).

Reduced clarity of the ocular media from other causes, such as a corneal disturbance, a cloudy posterior lens capsule after cataract surgery, or vitreous opacities, may also affect the visual fields. Applanation tonometry before automated static threshold perimetry was found to have no detrimental effect on the visual field results (133).

Refractive Error and Retinal Blur

When the projected stimulus is not focused on the retina, the edge of the stimulus is blurred, contrast is decreased, and the stimulus may not be detected by the patient. The larger the stimulus, the less it is to be affected by the blur. Refractive errors primarily influence the central field (134). When a standard size III stimulus is used, refractive errors of 1 diopter (D) or less may not need to be corrected, because it usually will cause only slightly more than 1 dB of general reduction of sensitivity (135). Mild myopia requires no correction, unless the refractive error exceeds 3 D. Posterior staphylomas can create areas of relative myopia, called refraction scotomas, which may be confused with glaucomatous field defects, but can usually be eliminated with an appropriate refractive correction. Hyperopia has a greater influence on perimetric results, especially for the central field, and even small hyperopic refractive errors can significantly alter threshold sensitivity (134–136). Age tables are available to aid in determining the appropriate correction for presbyopia. A contact lens provides the best correction for the aphakic and highly myopic eyes (137), although spectacle correction can be used for the central 24 to 30 degrees with no correction for the peripheral field. Astigmatism should be corrected unless the cylinder is less than 1 D, in which case it can be included as the spherical equivalent.

Psychological Influences on Visual Fields

Patients' understanding of the test and their alertness, concentration, fixation, and cooperation all affect the results of visual field testing (138). A learning effect with automated perimetry may influence the results of a patient's first or second field test, suggesting that an initial field that does not agree with the clinical findings should be repeated (139–141). One study found that patients with refractive errors, especially those with myopia, had a larger learning effect than patients with emmetropia did (142). Another study found that moderate alcohol intake did not influence differential light sensitivity as tested by automated perimetry (143). With manual perimetry, the skill of the perimetrist influences the visual field test results (144).

Patient Fatigue

Full-threshold protocols take a long time to complete, and patients usually find visual field testing exhausting. Fatigue causes artificially decreased sensitivity in the areas of existent glaucomatous defect (145). Fatigue may also cause decreased performance in patients with glaucoma within central 10 degrees, and increased deterioration of the mean defect and localized loss in the periphery (146,147).

TECHNIQUES AND INSTRUMENTS FOR MEASURING THE FIELD OF VISION

Just as a cartographer maps the boundaries and topography of an island, so the perimetrist can measure both the peripheral limits of a visual field and the relative visual acuity of areas within those limits. This may be accomplished by using static or kinetic techniques with instruments that are computer assisted (automatic) or manually operated.

Automated Static Perimetry

Automated perimetry is accepted as the standard way of measuring the visual field. The standard protocol of static white-on-white stimuli is commonly known as SAP. A major limitation of tangent screens and arc perimeters (discussed later) was lack of standardization of the test objects and the background, and patient fixation. These needs were addressed in the era of standardization, which began in the middle of the 20th century with the contributions of Goldmann. The main problem that remained, however, was the subjectivity of the patient and the perimetrist. Although subjectivity of the patient has not been eliminated, the influence of the perimetrist was eliminated to variable degrees with the advent of automated perimetry in the 1970s. A wide variety of automated perimeters have been designed since then. Many of these are no longer commercially available, but current models represent modifications of the originals.

By reducing the influence of the perimetrist, automated perimetry improves the uniformity and reproducibility of visual fields. With these instruments, the perimetrist only ensures that the patient understands the testing procedure, is comfortably positioned at the perimeter, and adheres to the requirements of the test. In addition, the use of computers has provided new capabilities that are impossible with manual perimetry, including random presentation of targets, estimations of patient reliability, reduced variability, and statistical evaluation of data at many levels. With the recent introduction of efficient threshold strategies, automated perimetry is not only more accurate and informative but is also faster than manual perimetry.

Basic Components of Automated Perimeters

Automated perimeters have two main components: the perimetric unit and the control unit. The perimetric unit in most systems uses a bowl-type screen, similar to that of the Goldmann manual perimeter (discussed later).

The control unit provides interaction between the operator and the computer through a dialogue screen and a keyboard or light pen. The computer in the control unit provides and monitors instrumentation function according to the perimetrist's request, evaluates the patient's response, and processes data. The control unit also contains a printer, which provides a hard copy of the data in symbols and numeric values. Computers also store recorded information and can perform statistical analyses of the data in relation to the programmed normal database, or against previous fields for the same patient.

Static targets are used in most automated perimeters. Automated kinetic targets have also been evaluated and are provided on some automatic perimeters, although rarely used today, probably because of the high frequency of fixation errors and longer testing time (11–13,106,148,149). The targets may be projected onto the bowl, which is the current standard, or illuminated from light-emitting diodes (LEDs) or fiber optics in the perimetric bowl in earlier models. The former has the advantage of unlimited presentation locations on the screen, whereas the latter two have fixed positions in the bowl. In addition, the LEDs were recessed in dark cavities, which may allow perception by the most sensitive retinal areas of a stimulus that is of lower intensity than the background light (150,151). This "dark hole phenomenon" is associated with increased variability in retesting the threshold (150,151). Projected targets also have the advantage of allowing for change in size to alter the stimulus values. In practice, the size is usually kept constant, although larger targets may permit the measurement of visual function in areas that had been considered absolute scotomas with standard-sized stimuli (152). A larger target (size V stimulus) was found to be useful in patients with end-stage glaucoma (153). With all target systems, the patient usually presses a button to indicate when a target is seen, which is recorded by the computer.

The standard stimulus in most automated perimeters is a white light on a white background, which tests the patient's differential light sense.

Commercial Units

The first of the full-threshold perimeters to receive extensive study was called the Octopus. With each Octopus model, stimuli are projected onto a bowl, and fixation is monitored by the corneal light reflex method and a television view of the patient's eye. The models differ primarily according to computer capabilities. These automated perimeters were shown in early studies to compare favorably with manual perimetry and to frequently detect field loss missed with the Goldmann perimeter (154–156).

The Humphrey field analyzer and Humphrey field analyzer II also use projected stimuli on a bowl (**Fig. 5.13**). They monitor fixation by the Heijl–Krakau periodic blind spot check method and also by corneal light reflex in newer models. It is currently the most commonly used automated perimeter. It has also compared favorably with manual perimetry on the Goldmann perimeter, often detecting defects that the latter missed (157). In one study, however, patients preferred the Goldmann perimeter, whereas the technician favored the Humphrey (158). The Octopus and Humphrey units have been compared in several

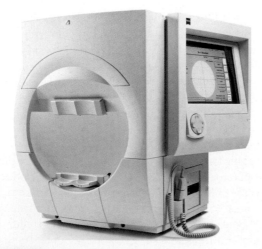

Figure 5.13 Humphrey Field Analyzer (HVAII). (Courtesy of Carl Zeiss Meditec, Inc.)

studies. In one study, both short- and long-term fluctuations (explained later) were greater with the Octopus (159). In another study, both automated perimeters identified slightly more defects by meridional threshold testing than the Tübingen manual perimeter did (160) (discussed later).

Test Patterns

A broad menu of test patterns is available with most instruments. The most commonly used are limited to the central 24 to 30 degrees, with a 6-degree separation between test locations. The 6-degree grid may miss the physiologic blind spot and small glaucomatous defects in a high percentage of cases, and it has been suggested that tighter grids should be used, especially in the central 10 to 28 degrees (161–163). Special programs are available to study smaller portions of the field with tighter grids. Programs are also available to study the peripheral field beyond 30 degrees in the nasal quadrant or for 360 degrees. The peripheral studies can be performed alone or in conjunction with a central field program and usually have wider target separation. Static testing of the peripheral nasal field has been shown to provide valuable additional information in detecting glaucomatous defects (164). Automated kinetic measurement of the peripheral field, especially nasally, was also found to provide useful information in many patients, in addition to the information obtained from central testing (11–13). One study of various factors that affect the reaction time during automated kinetic perimetry led to the suggestion that the test should be designed to adjust to individual patient responses, because other factors, such as eccentricity or luminance level, were found to have much smaller effect on reaction time within the central 30 degrees (106).

Testing Strategies

All fully automated perimeters take advantage of computer capabilities by using random presentation of the static targets to avoid patient anticipation of the next presentation sites. In addition, an adaptive technique is used, in which stimuli are presented according to the presumed normal retinal threshold contour (i.e., the relative differential light thresholds throughout the visual field), on the basis of age-corrected normal data or the patient's response to preliminary spot tests (**Fig. 5.14**). This approach, in comparison with the presentation of a constant stimulus value throughout a portion of the field, as with many manual techniques, improves the balance between sensitivity (the ability to detect defects) and specificity (the ability to detect normal areas). Fully automated perimeters provide suprathreshold and full-threshold measurements.

Suprathreshold Static Perimetry

Suprathreshold static perimeters present a stimulus brighter than the anticipated normal value for the corresponding retinal location. Some instruments simply indicate whether the target was seen, whereas others present a second, high-intensity target in nonseeing areas to distinguish between relative and absolute defects. In either case, however, these instruments are limited

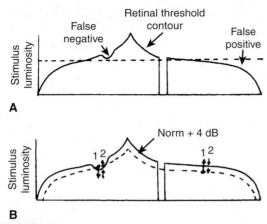

Figure 5.14 Adaptive strategy used in automated static perimetry. **A:** When a constant luminosity is presented throughout a portion of the visual field, true defects near fixation may be missed (false-negative), whereas more peripheral normal areas may be read as abnormal (false-positive). **B:** The adaptive strategy minimizes this by changing the stimulus value according to the retinal threshold contour. With full threshold programs, the retinal threshold is crossed by increasing or decreasing the stimulus value (1) and is then crossed a second time with smaller increments of change in luminosity (2).

to screening functions, in that they do not provide sufficient information about the depth or contour of a field defect to be used as a baseline study or for following up the patient during therapy. With the continued advances in automated perimetry, these suprathreshold strategies have been largely replaced by full-threshold strategies, although suprathreshold models may have value as screening devices. Improved algorithms have been suggested to improve performance of suprathreshold perimetry (165,166).

Full-Threshold Perimetry

Threshold static perimeters are capable of various testing strategies in addition to suprathreshold screening. The most commonly used programs measure the retinal threshold at 70 to 80 points within the central 24 to 30 degrees. A suprathreshold target is first presented, and the luminosity is then gradually increased or decreased until the patient's threshold is crossed—that is, the target comes into or goes out of view, respectively. The threshold is then crossed a second time with smaller increments of change in luminosity to refine the threshold determination. Many programs continuously adjust subsequent stimulus values according to prior measurements; for example, the level is increased when testing near a known scotoma on the basis of optimized algorithms. Special programs have been evaluated that automatically increase the density of test locations around defective areas, although the value of this approach has yet to be established (167,168). Other programs are designed to reduce testing time by adjusting the initial target values according to previous fields by the same patient or by thresholding only locations that are missed

with the suprathreshold target. The latter strategy, when compared with full-threshold programs, reduced the testing time by as much as two thirds but missed some defects that were detected with full thresholding (169,170).

Other Threshold-Testing Algorithms

FASTPAC. Another thresholding strategy to reduce testing time is the FASTPAC program of the Humphrey field analyzer, which estimates thresholding from a single threshold crossing in 3-dB increments, in contrast to the standard double threshold crossing with 4 and 2 dB. This strategy has been evaluated by several investigative teams, most of whom agree that it provides time reduction at some expense of accuracy and reliability (171–174).

Swedish Interactive Threshold Algorithm (SITA). In recent years, the relatively new threshold strategy known as SITA has become increasingly popular (175–182). This algorithm uses standard 24-2 or 30-2 patterns to assess the visual field on the basis of the probability analysis of the patterns of glaucomatous damage; it is more time efficient than standard threshold strategies. It significantly minimizes test time without significant reduction of data quality. Two versions of SITA are currently available: SITA Standard and SITA Fast. SITA Standard takes approximately half the time to complete, compared with the standard full-threshold program, and SITA Fast takes about half the time of the FASTPAC algorithm. SITA requires significant computer power during the test and is available only on newer Humphrey visual field analyzers.

SITA uses new concepts, such as visual field modeling, that utilizes frequency-of-seeing curves for patients with and without glaucoma. During the SITA test, a computer also produces an information index, which stops the test at the location being examined when threshold reaches a preselected level. The SITA method also makes more individual adjustments to patient response time. After the test is complete, the program makes additional, more precise recalculation of all thresholds measured and produces estimates of false-positive and false-negative response rates (1). One retrospective study found that defects assessed with SITA were often more pronounced, when compared with standard full-threshold perimetry, but there were essentially no significant differences in quality. Average time reduction by SITA Standard depended on the severity of glaucomatous stage. No significant time difference was found for advanced glaucoma, whereas normal fields using SITA were performed in half the time of full-threshold strategy. The reduction of test time reduces the fatigue factor and permits more frequent visual field examinations and thus a better detection of early glaucoma or progressing visual field damage (183).

Tendency-Oriented Perimetry (TOP). TOP is another fast strategy algorithm available on new Octopus perimeters (184,185). It also uses a computational approach to estimate threshold values by extrapolating information from surrounding test points. One study compared SITA Fast and TOP technologies, and found that the mean testing time for the TOP strategy was slightly more than 2.5 minutes, compared with approximately 4 minutes for SITA Fast (186). However, another report suggested that the TOP algorithm may not be able to spatially localize defects and accurately estimate sensitivity of visual field defects (187).

Patient Fixation

Patient fixation is monitored in various ways depending on the sophistication of the instrument. Some use a telescope, similar to the Goldmann manual perimeter, whereas others allow the operator to observe the patient's eye on a television screen. Automatic fixation monitoring is also incorporated into most units either by periodically retesting the patient's response in the previously determined blind spot (the Heijl–Krakau method) or by monitoring a light reflex from the patient's cornea. With the latter method, the computer can be programmed to stop the test whenever fixation is lost. Fixation is important, because eye movement has been shown to increase local short-term fluctuation and false-negative rates (188). However, maintaining fixation is difficult for many patients, and a new strategy of kinetic fixation, in which the fixation target is moved between stimuli, has been shown to improve threshold sensitivity (189). On the other hand, another study has found that kinetic fixation was associated with inaccurate fixation and underestimation of the absolute scotoma at the physiologic blind spot (148). New perimeters also use gaze tracking devices, which allow monitoring of the patient's gaze during the test.

Interpreting the Results and Analyzing Progression

Determining Test Reliability

Several strategies are used to document variability and reliability of test results. With most full-thresholding programs, a percentage of random locations are retested to determine the reproducibility at those points. As noted earlier, these variations are referred to as short-term fluctuation and are expressed as the square root of the variance. The patient's general reliability is assessed with a series of false-positives (patient responds when no target is presented) and false-negatives (patient does not respond to a stimulus of maximal intensity where a stimulus was previously reported to be seen), as well as the frequency of fixation losses and the number of stimuli required to complete the test. This current strategy of reliability indices has several problems. With the exception of the number of stimuli, all reliability parameters add to the testing time, which may actually reduce the patient's reliability. Furthermore, because each represents a limited sampling, the usefulness is questionable. Several evaluations of the Humphrey field analyzer, which uses the Heijl–Krakau blind-spot–checking method, revealed a high percentage of tests that were considered unreliable because the patient exceeded the established criteria for fixation losses (190–192). Suggestions for modifying reliability indices to reduce testing time have included estimating short-term

fluctuation from grids of single threshold determinations; using intermittent monitoring for patients who perform well during the first 1.5 minutes of testing; and substituting all indices with a new reliability parameter, which analyzes the inconsistency of responses to the standard thresholding algorithm (193–195).

As discussed earlier, there is a certain degree of short-term fluctuation in the retinal threshold sensitivity profile (or hill of vision) among healthy individuals, especially in the midperiphery and superior quadrant (196–198). In addition, each person with normal vision shows some variation from test to test, which is referred to as long-term fluctuation (198). However, both of these normal variations are more likely in glaucomatous visual fields and must be taken into account when attempting to interpret the significance of visual field data. Average total long-term fluctuation in patients with clinically stable glaucoma is similar to that in healthy persons (199). However, long-term fluctuation can be considerable in field areas with moderate loss of sensitivity (200). In addition, short-term fluctuation is increased around both physiologic and glaucomatous scotomas (19,201,202). Short- and long-term fluctuations are increased among older patients (203), and short-term fluctuation is often greatest in the patient's first automated field test, indicating the influence of experience (204). In one study, a change in mean sensitivity of approximately 5 to 7 dB between two successive fields was needed to have 95% confidence that the trend would be confirmed by the third field (205).

Printouts and Automated Analyses

In addition to providing indications of patient reliability, as noted above, the computer printout records the threshold for each retinal point tested along with various analyses of these measurements. The clinician can read computerized visual field printouts by looking primarily for NFL defects, such as paracentral and arcuate scotomas and nasal steps, in the grayscale, numerical values, or symbols representing a decibel range (**Fig. 5.15**). The Humphrey field analyzer also provides printouts in total deviation (Fig. 5.15A), which is the difference between the measured threshold for each retinal point tested and the age-corrected normal, and in pattern deviation (Fig. 5.15B), which is created from the total deviation by adjusting it an amount equal to an average of the 17 worst test points. This helps eliminate "background noise," such as the generalized depression of a cataract. Both total and pattern deviations are displayed in numeric and probability plots. Graphic methods have been devised to show the development of visual field defects by analyzing recorded visual fields and displaying changing areas as stripes (206), or triangles, or colored display of pointwise analysis, as in newer Progressor software (discussed later).

Global Indices

Static threshold data can be analyzed mathematically, allowing detection of more subtle visual field abnormalities. The statistical techniques used in this approach are referred to as visual field global indices (Fig. 5.15C). An average of all points

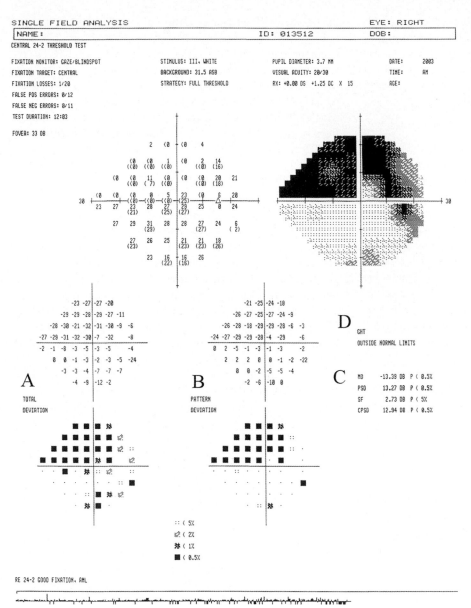

SINGLE FIELD ANALYSIS   EYE: RIGHT

NAME: ID: 013512   DOB:

CENTRAL 24-2 THRESHOLD TEST

FIXATION MONITOR: GAZE/BLINDSPOT   STIMULUS: III, WHITE   PUPIL DIAMETER: 3.7 MM   DATE: 2003
FIXATION TARGET: CENTRAL   BACKGROUND: 31.5 ASB   VISUAL ACUITY: 20/30   TIME: AM
FIXATION LOSSES: 1/20   STRATEGY: FULL THRESHOLD   RX: +0.00 DS +1.25 DC X 15 AGE:
FALSE POS ERRORS: 0/12
FALSE NEG ERRORS: 0/11
TEST DURATION: 12:03

FOVEA: 33 DB

Figure 5.15 Computer printout of visual field of a right eye, measured by automated static technique, showing superior arcuate scotoma and nasal step. **A:** Total deviation. **B:** Pattern deviation. **C:** Global indices. **D:** Glaucoma hemifield test.

in the total deviation is referred to as mean deviation. These indices primarily reflect diffuse changes. One way to detect localized defects is to calculate the number of threshold values that deviate significantly from the age-corrected normal, which is called pattern standard deviation. Corrected pattern standard deviation takes into account the short-term fluctuations.

Short-Term Fluctuations

The visibility of the stimulus in standard static perimetry is typically adjusted by changing its intensity. Although in the laboratory threshold sensitivity is considered to be the stimulus intensity at which the patient responds 50% of the time, it is impractical to measure threshold so precisely in the clinical situation. Standard static threshold perimetry estimates the threshold sensitivity with approximately 2 dB of precision by presenting the stimuli in increments to a certain location in the retina and recording the value of the weakest stimulus seen. In some protocols, this process is repeated in random locations. The difference between the patient's responses at the same location during the same session may be used to calculate the standard deviation of the threshold values, called the short-term fluctuation or intratest variability.

Long-Term Fluctuation

The difference in threshold values in the same location between separate sessions is called the long-term fluctuation. This typically represents physiologic rather than glaucomatous changes in visual function over time. Although long-term fluctuation is not quantified in routine clinical perimetry, it should be considered in interpretation of a series of visual fields.

Discrete scotomas may be preceded by variable threshold responses to repeated testing in the same area (17,207,208). This fluctuation has also been referred to as scatter (209), or localized minor disturbances. Studies show that patients with glaucoma have substantially greater short-term fluctuation, and to a lesser degree, long-term fluctuation (145,210,211). Although scatter is not a definitive sign of glaucomatous visual field damage, it should be looked on with suspicion as an early warning sign of impending absolute field loss.

Cluster Analysis

The global indices for localized loss are insensitive to the location of the defects. For example, three abnormal locations could either be randomly distributed or clustered. Attempts to improve the interpretation of data have led to the strategy of cluster analysis, or spatial correction. With this strategy, contiguous clusters of test locations, which have an increased probability of appearing together in typical glaucomatous field loss, are considered together in evaluating the visual field. They can be used in calculating local indices, which should be more sensitive than global indices are, and may help to dampen long-term fluctuation. In several studies, by using different cluster patterns, they have provided an enhanced probability of distinguishing normal from glaucomatous fields, as well as a stable glaucoma field from one that is deteriorating (212–215).

Glaucoma Hemifield Test

Another strategy to analyze the result of the visual field test is to compare sums of threshold values in corresponding areas of the superior and inferior hemispheres (216–218). In the Humphrey field analyzer Statpac (discussed later), this is called the glaucoma hemifield test (GHT) (Fig. 5.15D). The GHT performs analysis in five corresponding pairs of sectors that are based on the normal anatomy of the retinal NFL. It then looks at the distribution of changes in pattern deviation and analyzes the difference between upper and lower hemifields. It uses a large normal database to calculate the significance of differences between the two hemispheres and has been shown to significantly improve the ability to separate between normal and glaucoma fields (216,219). It has good sensitivity and specificity, although reproducibility is such that the use of two tests is recommended to improve specificity (220,221). This method allows a simple but clinically useful analysis of visual field changes in patients with glaucoma. The GHT provides five plain language messages about the results of the visual field test: within normal limits, outside normal limits, borderline, general reduction of sensitivity, and abnormally high sensitivity (216). One study evaluated the repeatability of the GHT and found that, although it was generally good on consecutive testing, there was enough disagreement to justify the use of a second test for improved specificity in a clinical trial setting (221). The GHT "outside normal limits," used together with the pattern deviation probability plot, has been shown to provide high sensitivity and specificity for detecting early glaucomatous visual field changes (222).

AGIS and CIGTS Scores

The Advanced Glaucoma Intervention Study (AGIS) investigators have developed a method of interpreting visual field results on the basis of the number and depth of clusters of adjacent depressed test sites in the upper and lower hemifields and in the nasal area of the total deviation plot, using the 24-2 threshold program of the Humphrey visual field analyzer (223). The Collaborative Initial Glaucoma Treatment Study (CIGTS) investigators used a similar scoring system with a modification to evaluate progression in patients with newly diagnosed glaucoma (224). Both AGIS and CIGTS scores range from 0 (no defect) to 20 (end-stage). Progression is defined as worsening of the score by 4 points in the AGIS system and by 3 points in the CIGTS system.

Trend Analysis

Statistical models are available with some automated perimeters to help the clinician determine the significance of visual field indices and variability. Those that have received several investigations are the Delta program with the Octopus perimeter (225) and the Statpac with the Humphrey field analyzer (226). With both systems, databases are used to calculate the probability of a measured value appearing in a given age-defined population. In the case of the Humphrey field analyzer, the Statpac uses a large normal database, and Statpac II uses a database of stable glaucoma patients. The Statpac printout includes the reliability and global indices, the GHT, and probability maps, which display the field results in terms of the frequency with which the measured findings are seen in the defined population (227,228). The Statpac II also includes linear regression analysis and glaucoma change probability.

The glaucoma progression analysis (GPA) (**Fig. 5.16**) replaces the glaucoma change probability that is used for full-threshold testing. The GPA defines progression as more than three test points in the same location on three consecutive tests.

A third statistical algorithm with the Humphrey field analyzer is the Progressor program for analysis of serial fields, which is downloaded to a personal computer (229). The Progressor uses the data from all visual fields in the series of examinations to perform pointwise linear regression analysis and to generate a color-coded graphic display for simultaneous interpretation of the spatial and temporal changes (230).

Although most statistical models provide better agreement than experienced clinical observers do regarding significant change over time, there is currently no generally accepted technique (231). One study, which compared the results of a threshold program on the Octopus perimeter to those from manual perimetry, demonstrated that indices used currently may not be clinically reliable in the assessment of changes in the visual field (232). A study evaluating the three commercially available computed statistical algorithms with serial Humphrey fields showed a high degree of variability among the three, with none correlating well with the clinical impression (229). A study comparing the Statpac II and Progressor showed that these two algorithms detected progression in the same patients, but Progressor detected progression earlier than Statpac II did (233). Until improved statistical algorithms are available, therefore, these data must be used with caution, and physicians should still rely primarily on their own clinical judgment.

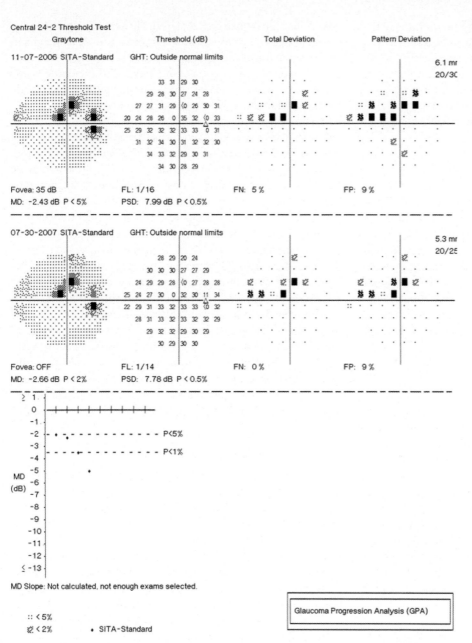

Figure 5.16 Example of the GPA, which plots the mean deviation of sequential visual fields over time.

Reversibility of Glaucomatous Field Defects

Although visual field loss from glaucoma has traditionally been thought to be irreversible, central visual acuity and the field of vision may improve if the IOP is reduced in the early stages of the disease (234–237). Visual field global indices with automated perimetry improved proportional to the amount of IOP reduction in two studies (238,239). Other investigators, however, could not demonstrate reversibility after pressure reduction was achieved by argon-laser trabeculoplasty (240, 241). These conflicting findings may indicate that a critical level of pressure reduction or intervention at a critical time in the disease process is needed to reverse field loss. Also, the ability to document improvement in visual fields after surgical reduction of IOP may be enhanced by focusing on subgroups of test points with lower baseline sensitivity (242).

Recording and Scoring Manual Visual Field Data

The complex nature of visual field data makes it difficult to reduce the information to simple descriptions or numbers. Therefore, storage of the data in its raw form—that is, as transferred directly from the testing screen—is usually the most practical means of record keeping. However, methods for conversion of visual fields from kinetic and static perimeter charts to computer use, for area calculations, graphic display, and storage in the patient's database, have been described (243,244).

Visual Impairment and Disability Assessment

When it is necessary to estimate the percentage of functional visual field loss, a system is available (the Esterman grids) in which the field is divided into 100 blocks of varying size according to functional value, with each representing 1% (245–247). The system has been adopted by the American Medical Association as a standard for rating visual field disability (248). Grids are available for scoring the tangent screen, perimeter, or the binocular field (245–247). In patients with severe visual loss from glaucoma, the binocular Esterman score of data generated by an automated perimeter correlated well with combined monocular visual field results (249).

Other Types of Perimetry

Glaucoma affects various components of the visual field, and subtle loss of central and peripheral vision can be demonstrated in some patients with glaucoma before visual field changes are detectable with standard techniques. Achromatic stimuli, used in standard automated perimetry, nonselectively stimulate ganglion cells involved in the magnocellular and parvocellular pathways, and therefore are not always sensitive enough to detect early glaucomatous damage. New strategies that are specifically designed to test subgroups of ganglion cells (250,251) are discussed next.

Short-Wavelength Automated Perimetry

Compared with white-on-white targets, color stimuli may influence the visual field results in one of two ways. Color targets typically have less luminance and a lower stimulus value than white targets do. More significantly, if the luminance is kept constant and the color saturation is varied, the stimulus value might be more sensitive to specific color vision defects, as in some patients with glaucoma (252). Early studies suggested that such a technique could reveal field defects that are larger than those obtained with conventional white-on-white perimetry (253,254), whereas other studies found color targets to be no more sensitive than white ones in detecting glaucomatous defects (255–257). These conflicting results may be related to the colors selected for the test. Continued study has led to the following observations with new test objects.

Testing one subgroup of small ganglion cells, called bistratified blue–yellow ganglion cells, that are sensitive to blue stimuli may detect loss of visual function at much earlier stage of glaucoma than with standard automated perimetry (258). Short-wavelength automated perimetry (SWAP) takes advantage of this glaucoma-induced color vision deficit by presenting standard Goldmann size V, short-wavelength blue targets on a bright yellow background (259,260). Studies indicate that SWAP deficits represent early glaucomatous damage and that the test may indicate significant change in visual function before it is apparent on standard white-on-white visual fields (261–265). Longitudinal studies have demonstrated the ability of blue-on-yellow perimetry to predict the development of glaucoma in patients with ocular hypertension, and in which patients early glaucomatous visual field loss is most likely to progress (266–268). Other studies have demonstrated a significant relationship between structural optic nerve damage and

SWAP visual field defects (263,269). However, the test is influenced by age and cataracts, and stringent statistical analysis in interpreting the results is necessary (270–273), but SWAP testing is unaffected by blue-blocking acrylic intraocular lens implants, compared with clear acrylic implants (274). One study investigated whether SWAP, using a screening program, can detect early glaucomatous damage before standard screening perimetric tests can, and found that the SWAP screening program is more advantageous than conventional tests in detecting early glaucomatous visual field defects (275). However, some patients with ocular hypertension and early glaucomatous structural abnormalities may have normal blue–yellow perimetry (276). The SWAP is available on the newer Humphrey field analyzer II. A new generation of SWAP techniques uses more efficient strategies, such as SITA. By using this approach, testing time has been reduced from 12 minutes to less than 4 minutes (277). SITA SWAP testing detects higher sensitivities than full-threshold SWAP does, and is equal to full-threshold SWAP in its ability to detect visual field abnormalities (278,279). The topography of the SWAP field is steeper than achromatic automated visual fields (280). SWAP testing is also subject to greater long-term fluctuation and more learning effect artifact, compared with achromatic automated visual fields. Thus, defects found by using this method should be interpreted cautiously, and confirmation with a repeated SWAP test is advisable (281,282).

Frequency Doubling Technology

Frequency doubling technology (FDT) perimetry is based on the frequency doubling illusion (283). Each test stimulus is a series of white and black bands flickering at 25 Hz (284). FDT perimetry is thought to be mediated by a subset of the large-diameter ganglion cells, called the M_y ganglion cells, that project to the magnocellular visual pathway (285). These cells are sensitive to motion and contrast and are thought to be more vulnerable to glaucomatous damage (85,286), although this view has been questioned by some authors (287–290). The FDT is a portable (**Fig. 5.17**) and relatively inexpensive tool with a short testing time (250,291), qualities that make it a useful screening device (250,291–294). When administered in a suprathreshold screening mode, FDT perimetry can be performed on a healthy eye in less than 90 seconds (284), and provide a higher detection rate for early glaucoma than with SAP (295). (A comparison of FDT and SAP readouts is shown in **Fig. 5.18**.) FDT showed greater than 96% sensitivity and specificity for detection of moderate and advanced glaucoma, and greater than 85% for early glaucoma, when compared with SAP in a prospective study (296). Because of its relatively quick acquisition times and high sensitivity, FDT is also advocated for use in children. Children older than 14 years have the same normal threshold limits as adults do; for children younger than 14 years, the mean deviations for normal decreased with decreasing age, with a linear best fit of mean deviation of -11 ± 1 dB for age down to 6 years (297). However, FDT perimetry was reported to be less sensitive to visual field

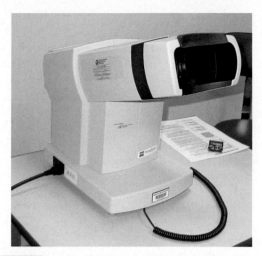

Figure 5.17 Frequency doubling technology perimeter.

damage associated with neurologic disorders, compared with SAP (298). Sensitivity to FDT was found to be reduced in the second tested eye if an opaque occluder was used, because of delayed postocclusion light adaptation; a translucent occluder eliminated this reduction in sensitivity in the second eye (299). The original FDT perimeter tested a maximum of 19 points over the central 20 (C-20) or 30 (N-30) degrees of the visual field with both screening and threshold strategies (300) (Fig. 5.18). A second-generation FDT (Humphrey Matrix, 2003) uses smaller stimuli to examine a larger number of test points, which may allow better early detection of glaucoma (300–302) and has the following testing strategies available: macula, 10-2; N30-F, 24-2, and 30-2. The GHT algorithm is available for the 24-2 and 30-2 testing strategies. FDT tests are also subject to learning and long-term fluctuation artifacts; thus, abnormal test results should be interpreted cautiously, and confirmation with a repeated test is advisable (303–305).

Contrast and Motion Sensitivity

As noted above, the eye with glaucomatous damage appears to have reduced ability to perceive motion and contrast, both centrally and peripherally (300,307,308). This may be related to preferential damage to larger retinal ganglion cells, and motion and contrast perception tests may prove useful in the detection of early glaucoma (306–308). The detection of vernier offsets is also affected in glaucoma, but it is not sensitive enough to distinguish patients with glaucoma from controls (309). Various perimetric tests measure contrast and motion sensitivity in glaucoma, including gratings tests for contrast sensitivity, vernier acuity, flickering stimuli, high-pass resolution perimetry, and random motion automated perimetry (309–315). (The application of these visual function tests in glaucoma is discussed in Chapter 6.)

High-Pass Resolution Perimetry

High-pass resolution perimetry, or ring perimetry, is presumed to selectively test the parvocellular system (314). The stimuli used in this test are rings of different size projected at different locations on the computer screen. The rings have dark borders and bright centers, creating average luminance of the stimulus equal to the luminance of the background. By also using high-pass spatial filtering, the targets can be detected and resolved at the same ring size, in an effect known as vanishing optotype, allowing rapid definition of the resolution threshold. The results of the test are presumed to correspond to the density of ganglion cells; this test is therefore essentially a peripheral visual acuity test (250). Healthy persons showed increased resolution threshold toward the periphery, a slight but significant decline in sensitivity with age, and high repeatability (316), as well as reliability indices comparable to SAP (317). Patients with glaucoma showed a significant reduction in overall resolution threshold (318), and the results were comparable to standard perimetry in sensitivity and specificity (319,320). Study findings suggest that high-pass resolution perimetry could identify

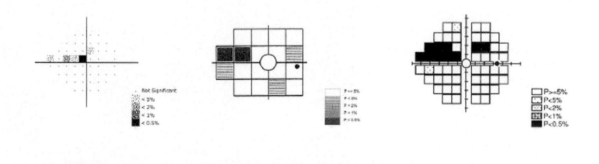

SAP-SITA   FDT N-30   FDT 24-2

Figure 5.18 Pattern deviation plots for SAP-SITA, FDT N-30, and FDT 24-2. Each plot shows the locations tested and the results expressed as a grayscale pattern (denser patterns indicate deeper defects). Probabilities are shown in the corresponding keys. (Reprinted from Racette L, Medeiros FA, Zangwill LM, et al., Diagnostic accuracy of the Matrix 24-2 and original N-30 frequency-doubling technology tests compared with standard automated perimetry. *Invest Ophthalmol Vis Sci.* 2008;49:954–960, with permission.)

glaucomatous visual field damage in early and moderate stages of the disease (321,322).

Random Dot Motion Automated Perimetry

Yet another technique, random dot motion automated perimetry, takes advantage of reduced motion sense in patients with glaucoma by presenting a shift in position of dots in a defined circular area against a background of fixed dots (306,323). The patient should tell the direction (up, down, left, right) in which the dots are moving. A preliminary study showed that patients with COAG manifest abnormal motion perception with the test, compared with healthy persons (315). Patients with glaucoma have demonstrated prolonged reaction time to the stimulus and less precise location of the stimuli (324). The test takes approximately 15 minutes to perform (250). Localized visual field loss detected by motion automated perimetry appeared to correspond to focal changes in optic disc topography, similar to those found by SWAP and SAP (325).

Combining results of functional tests with structural tests may identify different elements of glaucomatous damage and improve sensitivity and specificity of the tests (326).

Manual Perimetry

Although automated perimeters are being used with increasing frequency in clinical practice, the older, manual perimeters may still provide valuable information, especially when a skilled observer performs the test.

Tangent Screens

The tangent screen is a flat square of black felt or flannel with a central white fixation target on which 30 degrees of the visual field can be studied. The test is performed in mesopic lighting of approximately 7 foot-candles with the patient seated 1 or 2 m from the screen. Both kinetic and suprathreshold static techniques can be used with the tangent screen. With the kinetic approach, the examiner moves a test object from the periphery toward fixation until the patient indicates recognition of the target. The procedure is repeated at various intervals around fixation until the isopter has been mapped. The stimulus value of the test objects can be changed by varying the size and color. The corresponding isopter is designated by the ratio of target diameter to the distance between patient and target, with both expressed in millimeters, for example, "2/1000 white" for a 2-mm white test object at 1 m (when the color is not indicated it is understood to be white).

Suprathreshold static perimetry can be performed by turning the disc-shaped test object from the black to the white side or by using a self-illuminating target with an on–off switch. Specific locations at which the patient fails to see the target are then evaluated further with kinetic techniques.

The tangent screen has the advantages of low cost and simplicity of operation. However, reproducibility of the fields, which is essential in managing patients with glaucoma, is limited by variations in background lighting and stimulus value of the targets, and by difficulty in monitoring fixation. Furthermore, it does not include the peripheral field, where early glaucomatous defects may appear.

Arc and Bowl Perimeters

With these instruments, both the central and peripheral fields of vision can be examined. The screen of the perimeter may be a curved ribbon of metal (arc perimeter) or bowl shaped. The latter is preferable for glaucoma examinations, and the prototype is the Goldmann perimeter (**Fig. 5.19**) (327). Other similar instruments have been compared with the Goldmann unit,

Figure 5.19 Goldmann manual perimeter. **A:** Patient's side, showing headrest (*H*), fixation target (*F*), and projection device for test objects (*P*). **B:** Operator's side, showing telescope for fixation monitoring (*T*) and visual field chart (*C*) for locating and recording position of test objects.

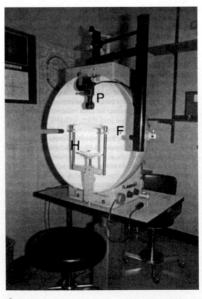

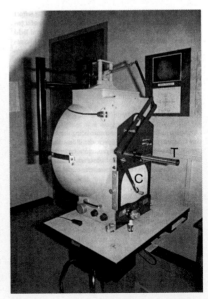

A   B

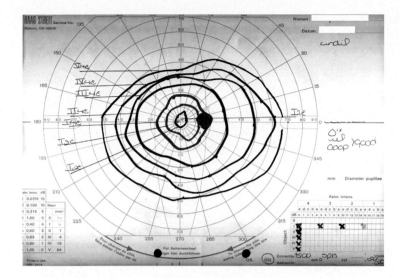

Figure 5.20 In-depth technique with Goldmann-type perimeter in which the visual field has been plotted with five targets. The size and stimulus of the corresponding isopters are shown in the table in the lower right of the figure. This demonstrates a normal visual field.

with variable results (328). The bowl of the Goldmann perimeter has a radius of 300 mm and extends 95% to each side of fixation. The target is projected onto the bowl, and the stimulus value of the test object can be varied by changing the size or the intensity. Arbitrary designations for each value variable are usually printed on the visual field chart, with O–V for size, and 1–4 for intensity. An isopter, therefore, might be designated as "I2e," which indicates a test object size of 0.25 mm^2 and an intensity of 10 millilamberts. The examiner can monitor the patient's fixation through a telescope in the center of the bowl. The Goldmann perimeter can be used for both kinetic and static visual field testing. The Tübingen perimeter has been designed exclusively for the measurement of static threshold (profile) fields and consists of a bowl-type screen and stationary test objects with variable light intensity (329,330).

Specific Techniques for Manual Perimetry

In the context of glaucoma detection and management, manual kinetic visual field testing has two basic aspects: (a) screening techniques to detect the presence of glaucomatous field loss, and (b) in-depth techniques to more accurately determine the extent of the damage and to follow the fields for evidence of progressive change.

Screening Techniques

Armaly developed a method of visual field screening for glaucoma that was modified by Drance and associates and is commonly referred to as selective perimetry, or the Armaly–Drance technique (331–334). The basic concept is to test those areas in the visual field that have the highest probability of showing glaucomatous defects. The technique uses Goldmann-type perimeter with suprathreshold static perimetry to test for central field defects and both suprathreshold static and kinetic perimetry to examine the peripheral field, with emphasis on the nasal and temporal periphery. This technique revealed a high sensitivity and specificity, which made it suitable for clinical and survey screening (332,334). An additional modification

is to use the V4e isopter nasally to rule out crowding of the peripheral nasal isopters (45).

Another technique for use with Goldmann-type perimeters uses three suprathreshold targets in three concentric zones from fixation in accordance with the normal physiologic sensitivity gradient (335). Other investigators have developed protocols to significantly reduce the number of test points without sacrificing sensitivity or specificity by concentrating the testing in those portions of the field where a defect is most likely to be found (336,337).

In-Depth Techniques

When a glaucomatous field defect is suspected by use of a screening technique, the physician has two choices. The patient can be asked to return another day for a repeated screening field or an in-depth study. In many cases, however, it is more practical to proceed with the in-depth test at the time the defect is detected. The principle of in-depth field testing is to map out the size and shape of all scotomas and complete isopters by using the central threshold target and two or more additional targets of greater stimulus value (**Fig. 5.20**). However, automated static perimetry has certainly more value in studying areas of known loss for the depth and shape of the scotoma and for subtle evidence of progressive damage in serial fields.

KEY POINTS

- The normal visual field may be depicted as a three-dimensional contour, representing areas of relative retinal sensitivity and characterized by a peak at the point of fixation, an absolute depression corresponding to the optic nerve head (blind spot), and a sloping of the remaining areas to the boundaries of the field.

- Early glaucomatous damage may produce a generalized depression of this contour, which can be demonstrated with several psychophysical tests.

- The more specific visual field changes of glaucoma, however, are localized defects that correspond to loss of retinal nerve fiber bundles, and include paracentral and arcuate scotomas above and below fixation and steplike defects along the nasal midline (nasal step).

- Instruments used to measure the field of vision (perimeters) may have static or kinetic targets, which can be controlled automatically or manually. The targets are presented against a background that is bowl shaped or flat (tangent screen), with the former units providing more reliable measurements.

- Comparative studies indicate that automated static perimeters, particularly those using new enhanced testing algorithms, are more sensitive than manual perimeters are at detecting and following glaucomatous visual field loss.

REFERENCES

1. Anderson DR, Patella VM. *Automated Static Perimetry.* St. Louis: Mosby; 1999.
2. Hart WM Jr, Burde RM. Three-dimensional topography of the central visual field. Sparing of foveal sensitivity in macular disease. *Ophthalmology.* 1983;90(8):1028–1038.
3. Armaly MF. The size and location of the normal blind spot. *Arch Ophthalmol.* 1969;81(2):192–201.
4. Jonas JB, Gusek GC, Fernandez MC. Correlation of the blind spot size to the area of the optic disk and parapapillary atrophy. *Am J Ophthalmol.* 1991;111(5):559–565.
5. LeBlanc EP, Becker B. Peripheral nasal field defects. *Am J Ophthalmol.* 1971;72(2):415–419.
6. Werner EB, Beraskow J. Peripheral nasal field defects in glaucoma. *Ophthalmology.* 1979;86(10):1875–1878.
7. Armaly MF. Visual field defects in early open angle glaucoma. *Trans Am Ophthalmol Soc.* 1971;69:147–162.
8. Armaly MF. Selective perimetry for glaucomatous defects in ocular hypertension. *Arch Ophthalmol.* 1972;87(5):518–524.
9. Schulzer M, Mikelberg FS, Drance SM. A study of the value of the central and peripheral isoptres in assessing visual field progression in the presence of paracentral scotoma measurements. *Br J Ophthalmol.* 1987; 71(6):422–427.
10. Caprioli J, Spaeth GL. Static threshold examination of the peripheral nasal visual field in glaucoma. *Arch Ophthalmol.* 1985;103(8):1150–1154.
11. Stewart WC, Shields MB, Ollie AR. Peripheral visual field testing by automated kinetic perimetry in glaucoma. *Arch Ophthalmol.* 1988; 106(2):202–206.
12. Miller KN, Shields MB, Ollie AR. Automated kinetic perimetry with two peripheral isopters in glaucoma. *Arch Ophthalmol.* 1989;107(9):1316–1320.
13. Ballon BJ, Echelman DA, Shields MB, et al. Peripheral visual field testing in glaucoma by automated kinetic perimetry with the Humphrey Field Analyzer. *Arch Ophthalmol.* 1992;110(12):1730–1732.
14. Harrington DO. The Bjerrum Scotoma. *Am J Ophthalmol.* 1965;59: 646–656.
15. Gramer E, Gerlach R, Krieglstein GK, et al. Topography of early glaucomatous visual field defects in computerized perimetry [in German]. *Klin Monatsbl Augenheilkd.* 1982;180(6):515–523.
16. Mikelberg FS, Drance SM. The mode of progression of visual field defects in glaucoma. *Am J Ophthalmol.* 1984;98(4):443–445.
17. Hart WM Jr, Becker B. The onset and evolution of glaucomatous visual field defects. *Ophthalmology.* 1982;89(3):268–279.
18. Drance SM. The glaucomatous visual field. *Br J Ophthalmol.* 1972; 56(3):186–200.
19. Haefliger IO, Flammer J. Fluctuation of the differential light threshold at the border of absolute scotomas. Comparison between glaucomatous visual field defects and blind spots. *Ophthalmology.* 1991;98(10): 1529–1532.
20. Mikelberg FS, Schulzer M, Drance SM, et al. The rate of progression of scotomas in glaucoma. *Am J Ophthalmol.* 1986;101(1):1–6.
21. Harrington DO. Differential diagnosis of the arcuate scotoma. *Invest Ophthalmol Vis Sci.* 1969;8(1):96–105.
22. Kitazawa Y, Yamamoto T. Glaucomatous visual field defects: their characteristics and how to detect them. *Clin Neurosci.* 1997;4(5): 279–283.
23. Trobe JD. Chromophobe adenoma presenting with a hemianopic temporal arcuate scotoma. *Am J Ophthalmol.* 1974;77(3):388–392.
24. Drance SM. The glaucomatous visual field. *Invest Ophthalmol Vis Sci.* 1972;11(2):85–96.
25. Lau LI, Liu CJ, Chou JC, et al. Patterns of visual field defects in chronic angle-closure glaucoma with different disease severity. *Ophthalmology.* 2003;110(10):1890–1894.
26. Bonomi L, Marraffa M, Marchini G, et al. Perimetric defects after a single acute angle-closure glaucoma attack. *Graefes Arch Clin Exp Ophthalmol.* 1999;237(11):908–914.
27. Lynn JR. Correlation of pathogenesis, anatomy, and patterns of visual loss in glaucoma. In: *Symposium on Glaucoma.* St. Louis: Mosby; 1975:151.
28. Gilpin LB, Stewart WC, Shields MB, et al. Hemianopic offsets in the visual field of patients with glaucoma. *Graefes Arch Clin Exp Ophthalmol.* 1990;228(5):450–453.
29. Damgaard-Jensen L. Demonstration of peripheral hemiopic border steps by static perimetry. *Acta Ophthalmol.* 1977;55(5):815–817.
30. Anctil JL, Anderson DR. Early foveal involvement and generalized depression of the visual field in glaucoma. *Arch Ophthalmol.* 1984; 102(3):363–370.
31. Stamper RL. The effect of glaucoma on central visual function. *Trans Am Ophthalmol Soc.* 1984;82:792–826.
32. Drance SM. Diffuse visual field loss in open-angle glaucoma. *Ophthalmology.* 1991;98(10):1533–1538.
33. Lachenmayr BJ, Drance SM, Chauhan BC, et al. Diffuse and localized glaucomatous field loss in light-sense, flicker and resolution perimetry. *Graefes Arch Clin Exp Ophthalmol.* 1991;229(3):267–273.
34. Lachenmayr BJ, Drance SM, Airaksinen PJ. Diffuse field loss and diffuse retinal nerve-fiber loss in glaucoma. *Ger J Ophthalmol.* 1992;1(1):22–25.
35. Polo V, Larrosa JM, Pinilla I, et al. Glaucomatous damage patterns by short-wavelength automated perimetry (SWAP) in glaucoma suspects. *Eur J Ophthalmol.* 2002;12(1):49–54.
36. Samuelson TW, Spaeth GL. Focal and diffuse visual field defects: their relationship to intraocular pressure. *Ophthalmic Surg.* 1993;24(8): 519–525.
37. Lachenmayr BJ, Drance SM. Diffuse field loss and central visual function in glaucoma. *Ger J Ophthalmol.* 1992;1(2):67–73.
38. Chauhan BC, LeBlanc RP, Shaw AM, et al. Repeatable diffuse visual field loss in open-angle glaucoma. *Ophthalmology.* 1997;104(3):532–538.
39. Henson DB, Artes PH, Chauhan BC. Diffuse loss of sensitivity in early glaucoma. *Invest Ophthalmol Vis Sci.* 1999;40(13):3147–3151.
40. Heijl A. Lack of diffuse loss of differential light sensitivity in early glaucoma. *Acta Ophthalmol.* 1989;67(4):353–360.
41. Asman P, Heijl A. Diffuse visual field loss and glaucoma. *Acta Ophthalmol.* 1994;72(3):303–308.
42. Langerhorst CT, van den Berg TJ, Greve EL. Is there general reduction of sensitivity in glaucoma? *Int Ophthalmol.* 1989;13(1–2):31–35.
43. Hart WM Jr, Yablonski M, Kass MA, et al. Quantitative visual field and optic disc correlates early in glaucoma. *Arch Ophthalmol.* 1978; 96(12):2209–2211.
44. Flammer J, Eppler E, Niesel P. Quantitative perimetry in the glaucoma patient without local visual field defects [in German]. *Graefes Arch Clin Exp Ophthalmol.* 1982;219(2):92–94.
45. de Oliveira Rassi M, Shields MB. Crowding of the peripheral nasal isopters in glaucoma. *Am J Ophthalmol.* 1982;94(1):4–10.
46. Singh K, de Frank MP, Shults WT, et al. Acute idiopathic blind spot enlargement. A spectrum of disease. *Ophthalmology.* 1991;98(4):497–502.
47. Khorram KD, Jampol LM, Rosenberg MA. Blind spot enlargement as a manifestation of multifocal choroiditis. *Arch Ophthalmol.* 1991; 109(10):1403–1407.
48. Watzke RC, Shults WT. Clinical features and natural history of the acute idiopathic enlarged blind spot syndrome. *Ophthalmology.* 2002;109(7): 1326–1335.
49. Drance SM. The early field defects in glaucoma. *Invest Ophthalmol Vis Sci.* 1969;8(1):84–91.
50. Horton JC, Adams DL. The cortical representation of shadows cast by retinal blood vessels. *Trans Am Ophthalmol. Soc* 2000;98:33–38.
51. Colenbrander MC. The early diagnosis of glaucoma. *Ophthalmologica.* 1971;162(4):276–280.
52. Schiefer U, Benda N, Dietrich TJ, et al. Angioscotoma detection with fundus-oriented perimetry. A study with dark and bright stimuli of different sizes. *Vision Res.* 1999;39(10):1897–1909.

53. Benda N, Dietrich T, Schiefer U. Models for the description of angioscotomas. *Vision Res.* 1999;39(10):1889–1896.

54. Safran AB, Halfon A, Safran E, et al. Angioscotomata and morphological features of related vessels in automated perimetry. *Br J Ophthalmol.* 1995;79(2):118–124.

55. Brais P, Drance SM. The temporal field in chronic simple glaucoma. *Arch Ophthalmol.* 1972;88(5):518–522.

56. Pennebaker GE, Stewart WC. Temporal visual field in glaucoma: a re-evaluation in the automated perimetry era. *Graefes Arch Clin Exp Ophthalmol.* 1992;230(2):111–114.

57. Boden C, Sample PA, Boehm AG, et al. The structure-function relationship in eyes with glaucomatous visual field loss that crosses the horizontal meridian. *Arch Ophthalmol.* 2002;120(7):907–912.

58. Lichter PR, Ravin JG. Risks of sudden visual loss after glaucoma surgery. *Am J Ophthalmol.* 1974;78(6):1009–1013.

59. Caprioli J, Sears M, Miller JM. Patterns of early visual field loss in open-angle glaucoma. *Am J Ophthalmol.* 1987;103(4):512–517.

60. Hitchings RA, Anderton SA. A comparative study of visual field defects seen in patients with low-tension glaucoma and chronic simple glaucoma. *Br J Ophthalmol.* 1983;67(12):818–821.

61. Caprioli J, Spaeth GL. Comparison of visual field defects in the low-tension glaucomas with those in the high-tension glaucomas. *Am J Ophthalmol.* 1984;97(6):730–737.

62. Drance SM. The visual field of low tension glaucoma and shock-induced optic neuropathy. *Arch Ophthalmol.* 1977;95(8):1359–1361.

63. Motolko M, Drance SM, Douglas GR. Visual field defects in low-tension glaucoma. Comparison of defects in low-tension glaucoma and chronic open angle glaucoma. *Arch Ophthalmol.* 1982;100(7):1074–1077.

64. Zeiter JH, Shin DH, Juzych MS, et al. Visual field defects in patients with normal-tension glaucoma and patients with high-tension glaucoma. *Am J Ophthalmol.* 1992;114(6):758–763.

65. Bhandari A, Crabb DP, Poinoosawmy D, et al. Effect of surgery on visual field progression in normal-tension glaucoma. *Ophthalmology.* 1997; 104(7):1131–1137.

66. Collaborative Normal-Tension Glaucoma Study Group. Comparison of glaucomatous progression between untreated patients with normal-tension glaucoma and patients with therapeutically reduced intraocular pressures. *Am J Ophthalmol.* 1998;126(4):487–497.

67. Radius RL, Maumenee AE. Visual field changes following acute elevation of intraocular pressure. *Trans Sect Ophthalmol Am Acad Ophthalmol Otolaryngol.* 1977;83(1):61–68.

68. McNaught EI, Rennie A, McClure E, et al. Pattern of visual damage after acute angle-closure glaucoma. *Trans Ophthalmol Soc UK.* 1974; 94(2):406–415.

69. Drance SM. Studies in the susceptibility of the eye to raised intraocular pressure. *Arch Ophthalmol.* 1962;68:478–485.

70. Tsamparlakis JC. Effects of transient induced elevation of the intraocular pressure on the visual field. *Br J Ophthalmol.* 1964;48:237–249.

71. Scott AB, Morris A. Visual field changes produced by artificially elevated intraocular pressure. *Am J Ophthalmol.* 1967;63(2):308–312.

72. Armaly MF. Effect of corticosteroids on intraocular pressure and fluid dynamics. III. Changes in visual function and pupil size during topical dexamethasone application. *Arch Ophthalmol.* 1964;71: 636–644.

73. Kolker AE, Becker B, Mills DW. Intraocular pressure and visual fields: effects of corticosteroids. *Arch Ophthalmol.* 1964;72:772–782.

74. LeBlanc RP, Stewart RH, Becker B. Corticosteroid provocative testing. *Invest Ophthalmol Vis Sci.* 1970;9(12):946–948.

75. Hart WM Jr, Becker B. Visual field changes in ocular hypertension. A computer-based analysis. *Arch Ophthalmol.* 1977;95(7):1176–1179.

76. Trible JR, Anderson DR. Factors associated with intraocular pressure-induced acute visual field depression. *Arch Ophthalmol.* 1997;115(12): 1523–1527.

77. Drance SM. The disc and the field in glaucoma. *Ophthalmology.* 1978; 85(3):209–214.

78. Zeyen TG, Caprioli J. Progression of disc and field damage in early glaucoma. *Arch Ophthalmol.* 1993;111(1):62–65.

79. Hoskins HD Jr, Gelber EC. Optic disk topography and visual field defects in patients with increased intraocular pressure. *Am J Ophthalmol.* 1975;80(2):284–290.

80. Shutt HK, Boyd TA, Salter AB. The relationship of visual fields, optic disc appearances and age in non-glaucomatous and glaucomatous eyes. *Can J Ophthalmol.* 1967;2(2):83–90.

81. Drance SM. Correlation between optic disc changes and visual field defects in chronic open-angle glaucoma. *Trans Sect Ophthalmol Am Acad Ophthalmol Otolaryngol.* 1976;81(2):224–226.

82. Hitchings RA, Spaeth GL. The optic disc in glaucoma II: correlation of the appearance of the optic disc with the visual field. *Br J Ophthalmol.* 1977;61(2):107–113.

83. Quigley HA, Addicks EM, Green WR. Optic nerve damage in human glaucoma. III. Quantitative correlation of nerve fiber loss and visual field defect in glaucoma, ischemic neuropathy, papilledema, and toxic neuropathy. *Arch Ophthalmol.* 1982;100(1):135–146.

84. Quigley HA, Dunkelberger GR, Green WR. Retinal ganglion cell atrophy correlated with automated perimetry in human eyes with glaucoma. *Am J Ophthalmol.* 1989;107(5):453–464.

85. Kerrigan-Baumrind LA, Quigley HA, Pease ME, et al. Number of ganglion cells in glaucoma eyes compared with threshold visual field tests in the same persons. *Invest Ophthalmol Vis Sci.* 2000;41(3):741–748.

86. Read RM, Spaeth GL. The practical clinical appraisal of the optic disc in glaucoma: the natural history of cup progression and some specific disc-field correlations. *Trans Am Acad Ophthalmol Otolaryngol.* 1974; 78(2):OP255–OP274.

87. Gloster J. Quantitative relationship between cupping of the optic disc and visual field loss in chronic simple glaucoma. *Br J Ophthalmol.* 1978;62(10):665–669.

88. Hitchings RA, Anderton S. Identification of glaucomatous visual field defects from examination of monocular photographs of the optic disc. *Br J Ophthalmol.* 1983;67(12):822–825.

89. Nyman K, Tomita G, Raitta C, et al. Correlation of asymmetry of visual field loss with optic disc topography in normal-tension glaucoma. *Arch Ophthalmol.* 1994;112(3):349–353.

90. Weinreb RN, Shakiba S, Sample PA, et al. Association between quantitative nerve fiber layer measurement and visual field loss in glaucoma. *Am J Ophthalmol.* 1995;120(6):732–738.

91. Airaksinen PJ, Drance SM, Douglas GR, et al. Neuroretinal rim areas and visual field indices in glaucoma. *Am J Ophthalmol.* 1985;99(2):107–110.

92. Guthauser U, Flammer J, Niesel P. The relationship between the visual field and the optic nerve head in glaucomas. *Graefes Arch Clin Exp Ophthalmol.* 1987;225(2):129–132.

93. Caprioli J, Miller JM. Correlation of structure and function in glaucoma. Quantitative measurements of disc and field. *Ophthalmology.* 1988; 95(6):723–727.

94. Jonas JB, Gusek GC, Naumann GO. Optic disc morphometry in chronic primary open-angle glaucoma. II. Correlation of the intrapapillary morphometric data to visual field indices. *Graefes Arch Clin Exp Ophthalmol.* 1988;226(6):531–538.

95. Sommer A, Miller NR, Pollack I, et al. The nerve fiber layer in the diagnosis of glaucoma. *Arch Ophthalmol.* 1977;95(12):2149–2156.

96. Sommer A, Pollack I, Maumenee AE. Optic disc parameters and onset of glaucomatous field loss. II. Static screening criteria. *Arch Ophthalmol.* 1979;97(8):1449–1454.

97. Airaksinen PJ, Drance SM, Douglas GR, et al. Visual field and retinal nerve fiber layer comparisons in glaucoma. *Arch Ophthalmol.* 1985; 103(2):205–207.

98. Drance SM, Airaksinen PJ, Price M, et al. The correlation of functional and structural measurements in glaucoma patients and normal subjects. *Am J Ophthalmol.* 1986;102(5):612–616.

99. Okado K, Minato T, Miyaji S. A method for contrasting control visual fields in the Humphrey Field Analyzer and monochromatic turned-over fundus photographs. *Jpn J Ophthalmol.* 1988;30:925.

100. Airaksinen PJ, Heijl A. Visual field and retinal nerve fibre layer in early glaucoma after optic disc haemorrhage. *Acta Ophthalmol.* 1983; 61(2):186–194.

101. Katz J, Sommer A. Similarities between the visual fields of ocular hypertensive and normal eyes. *Arch Ophthalmol.* 1986;104(11):1648–1651.

102. Armaly MF. The correlation between appearance of the optic disc and optic function. *Trans Am Acad Ophthalmol Otolaryngol.* 1969;73(5):898–913.

103. Funk J, Bornscheuer C, Grehn F. Neuroretinal rim area and visual field in glaucoma. *Graefes Arch Clin Exp Ophthalmol.* 1988;226(5):431–434.

104. Choplin NT, Sherwood MB, Spaeth GL. The effect of stimulus size on the measured threshold values in automated perimetry. *Ophthalmology.* 1990;97(3):371–374.

105. Johnson CA, Keltner JL. Optimal rates of movement for kinetic perimetry. *Arch Ophthalmol.* 1987;105(1):73–75.

106. Schiefer U, Strasburger H, Becker ST, et al. Reaction time in automated kinetic perimetry: effects of stimulus luminance, eccentricity, and movement direction. *Vision Res.* 2001;41(16):2157–2164.

107. Portney GL, Krohn MA. The limitations of kinetic perimetry in early scotoma detection. *Ophthalmology.* 1978;85(3):287–293.

108. Agarwal HC, Gulati V, Sihota R. Visual field assessment in glaucoma: comparative evaluation of manual kinetic Goldmann perimetry

and automated static perimetry. *Indian J Ophthalmol*. 2000;48(4): 301–306.

109. Ourgaud M. Static circular perimetry in open-angle glaucoma [in French]. *J Fr Ophtalmol*. 1982;5(6–7):387–391.

110. Katz J, Tielsch JM, Quigley HA, et al. Automated perimetry detects visual field loss before manual Goldmann perimetry. *Ophthalmology*. 1995; 102(1):21–26.

111. McLean IM, Mueller E, Buttery RG, et al. Visual field assessment and the Austroads driving standard. *Clin Experiment Ophthalmol*. 2002;30(1):3–7.

112. Klewin KM, Radius RL. Background illumination and automated perimetry. *Arch Ophthalmol*. 1986;104(3):395–397.

113. Drum B, Armaly MF, Huppert W. Scotopic sensitivity loss in glaucoma. *Arch Ophthalmol*. 1986;104(5):712–717.

114. Stirling RJ, Pawson P, Brimlow GM, et al. Patients with ocular hypertension have abnormal point scotopic thresholds in the superior hemifield. *Invest Ophthalmol Vis Sci*. 1996;37(8):1608–1617.

115. Lindenmuth KA, Skuta GL, Rabbani R, et al. Effects of pupillary constriction on automated perimetry in normal eyes. *Ophthalmology*. 1989;96(9):1298–1301.

116. McCluskey DJ, Douglas JP, O'Connor PS, et al. The effect of pilocarpine on the visual field in normals. *Ophthalmology*. 1986;93(6): 843–846.

117. Heuer DK, Anderson DR, Feuer WJ, et al. The influence of decreased retinal illumination on automated perimetric threshold measurements. *Am J Ophthalmol*. 1989;108(6):643–650.

118. Edgar DF, Crabb DP, Rudnicka AR, et al. Effects of dipivefrin and pilocarpine on pupil diameter, automated perimetry and LogMAR acuity. *Graefes Arch Clin Exp Ophthalmol*. 1999;237(2):117–124.

119. Lindenmuth KA, Skuta GL, Rabbani R, et al. Effects of pupillary dilation on automated perimetry in normal patients. *Ophthalmology*. 1990; 97(3):367–370.

120. Spry PG, Johnson CA. Senescent changes of the normal visual field: an age-old problem. *Optom Vis Sci*. 2001;78(6):436–441.

121. Haas A, Flammer J, Schneider U. Influence of age on the visual fields of normal subjects. *Am J Ophthalmol*. 1986;101(2):199–203.

122. Jaffe GJ, Alvarado JA, Juster RP. Age-related changes of the normal visual field. *Arch Ophthalmol*. 1986;104(7):1021–1025.

123. Johnson CA, Adams AJ, Lewis RA. Evidence for a neural basis of age-related visual field loss in normal observers. *Invest Ophthalmol Vis Sci*. 1989;30(9):2056–2064.

124. Heuer DK, Anderson DR, Knighton RW, et al. The influence of simulated light scattering on automated perimetric threshold measurements. *Arch Ophthalmol*. 1988;106(9):1247–1251.

125. Chen PP, Budenz DL. The effects of cataract extraction on the visual field of eyes with chronic open-angle glaucoma. *Am J Ophthalmol*. 1998; 125(3):325–333.

126. The AGIS Investigators. The advanced glaucoma intervention study, 6: effect of cataract on visual field and visual acuity. *Arch Ophthalmol*. 2000;118(12):1639–1652.

127. Bigger JF, Becker B. Cataracts and open-angle glaucoma. The effect of cataract extraction on visual fields. *Am J Ophthalmol*. 1971;1(1 pt 2): 335–340.

128. Smith SD, Katz J, Quigley HA. Effect of cataract extraction on the results of automated perimetry in glaucoma. *Arch Ophthalmol*. 1997;115(12): 1515–1519.

129. Hayashi K, Hayashi H, Nakao F, et al. Influence of cataract surgery on automated perimetry in patients with glaucoma. *Am J Ophthalmol*. 2001;132(1):41–46.

130. Wood JM, Wild JM, Smerdon DL, et al. Alterations in the shape of the automated perimetric profile arising from cataract. *Graefes Arch Clin Exp Ophthalmol*. 1989;227(2):157–161.

131. Guthauser U, Flammer J. Quantifying visual field damage caused by cataract. *Am J Ophthalmol*. 1988;106(4):480–484.

132. Radius RL. Perimetry in cataract patients. *Arch Ophthalmol*. 1978; 96(9):1574–1579.

133. Ruben JB, Lewis RA, Johnson CA, et al. The effect of Goldmann applanation tonometry on automated static threshold perimetry. *Ophthalmology*. 1988;95(2):267–270.

134. Weinreb RN, Perlman JP. The effect of refractive correction on automated perimetric thresholds. *Am J Ophthalmol*. 1986;101(6):706–709.

135. Heuer DK, Anderson DR, Feuer WJ, et al. The influence of refraction accuracy on automated perimetric threshold measurements. *Ophthalmology*. 1987;94(12):1550–1553.

136. Goldstick BJ, Weinreb RN. The effect of refractive error on automated global analysis program G-1. *Am J Ophthalmol*. 1987;104(3):229–232.

137. Koller G, Haas A, Zulauf M, et al. Influence of refractive correction on peripheral visual field in static perimetry. *Graefes Arch Clin Exp Ophthalmol*. 2001;239(10):759–762.

138. Drance SM, Berry V, Hughes A. Studies in the reproducibility of visual field areas in normal and glaucomatous subjects. *Can J Ophthalmol*. 1966;1(1):14–23.

139. Heijl A, Lindgren G, Olsson J. The effect of perimetric experience in normal subjects. *Arch Ophthalmol*. 1989;107(1):81–86.

140. Werner EB, Krupin T, Adelson A, et al. Effect of patient experience on the results of automated perimetry in glaucoma suspect patients. *Ophthalmology*. 1990;97(1):44–48.

141. Wild JM, Dengler-Harles M, Searle AE, et al. The influence of the learning effect on automated perimetry in patients with suspected glaucoma. *Acta Ophthalmol*. 1989;67(5):537–545.

142. Marra G, Flammer J. The learning and fatigue effect in automated perimetry. *Graefes Arch Clin Exp Ophthalmol*. 1991;229(6):501–504.

143. Zulauf M, Flammer J, Signer C. The influence of alcohol on the outcome of automated static perimetry. *Graefes Arch Clin Exp Ophthalmol*. 1986;224(6):525–528.

144. Trobe JD, Acosta PC, Shuster JJ, et al. An evaluation of the accuracy of community-based perimetry. *Am J Ophthalmol*. 1980;90(5):654–660.

145. Heijl A, Drance SM. Changes in differential threshold in patients with glaucoma during prolonged perimetry. *Br J Ophthalmol*. 1983; 67(8):512–516.

146. Fujimoto N, Adachi-Usami E. Fatigue effect within 10 degrees visual field in automated perimetry. *Ann Ophthalmol*. 1993;25(4):142–144.

147. Hudson C, Wild JM, O'Neill EC. Fatigue effects during a single session of automated static threshold perimetry. *Invest Ophthalmol Vis Sci*. 1994;35(1):268–280.

148. Asman P, Fingeret M, Robin A, et al. Kinetic and static fixation methods in automated threshold perimetry. *J Glaucoma*. 1999;8(5):290–296.

149. Wabbels B, Kolling G. Automated kinetic perimetry using different stimulus velocities [in German]. *Ophthalmologe*. 2001;98(2):168–173.

150. Britt JM, Mills RP. The black hole effect in perimetry. *Invest Ophthalmol Vis Sci*. 1988;29(5):795–801.

151. Desjardins D, Anderson DR. Threshold variability with an automated LED perimeter. *Invest Ophthalmol Vis Sci*. 1988;29(6):915–921.

152. Wilensky JT, Mermelstein JR, Siegel HG. The use of different-sized stimuli in automated perimetry. *Am J Ophthalmol*. 1986;101(6):710–713.

153. Zalta AH. Use of a central 10 degrees field and size V stimulus to evaluate and monitor small central islands of vision in end stage glaucoma. *Br J Ophthalmol*. 1991;75(3):151–154.

154. Li SG, Spaeth GL, Scimeca HA, et al. Clinical experiences with the use of an automated perimeter (Octopus) in the diagnosis and management of patients with glaucoma and neurologic diseases. *Ophthalmology*. 1979; 86(7):1302–1316.

155. Schmied U. Automatic (Octopus) and manual (Goldmann) perimetry in glaucoma. *Graefes Arch Clin Exp Ophthalmol*. 1980;213(4): 239–244.

156. Wilensky JT, Joondeph BC. Variation in visual field measurements with an automated perimeter. *Am J Ophthalmol*. 1984;97(3):328–331.

157. Beck RW, Bergstrom TJ, Lichter PR. A clinical comparison of visual field testing with a new automated perimeter, the Humphrey Field Analyzer, and the Goldmann perimeter. *Ophthalmology*. 1985;92(1):77–82.

158. Trope GE, Britton R. A comparison of Goldmann and Humphrey automated perimetry in patients with glaucoma. *Br J Ophthalmol*. 1987; 71(7):489–493.

159. Brenton RS, Argus WA. Fluctuations on the Humphrey and Octopus perimeters. *Invest Ophthalmol Vis Sci*. 1987;28(5):767–771.

160. Mills RP, Hopp RH, Drance SM. Comparison of quantitative testing with the Octopus, Humphrey, and Tubingen perimeters. *Am J Ophthalmol*. 1986;102(4):496–504.

161. King D, Drance SM, Douglas GR, et al. The detection of paracentral scotomas with varying grids in computed perimetry. *Arch Ophthalmol*. 1986;104(4):524–525.

162. Weber J, Dobek K. What is the most suitable grid for computer perimetry in glaucoma patients? *Ophthalmologica*. 1986;192(2):88–96.

163. Gramer E, Althaus G, Leydhecker W. The importance of grid density in automatic perimetry: a clinical study. *Z Prakt Augenheilkd*. 1986; 7:197.

164. Seamone C, LeBlanc R, Rubillowicz M, et al. The value of indices in the central and peripheral visual fields for the detection of glaucoma. *Am J Ophthalmol*. 1988;106(2):180–185.

165. Henson DB, Artes PH. New developments in supra-threshold perimetry. *Ophthalmic Physiol Opt*. 2002;22(5):463–468.

166. Artes PH, McLeod D, Henson DB. Response time as a discriminator between true- and false-positive responses in suprathreshold perimetry. *Invest Ophthalmol Vis Sci.* 2002;43(1):129–132.

167. Fankhauser F, Funkhouser A, Kwasniewska S. Evaluating the applications of the spatially adaptive program (SAPRO) in clinical perimetry: part I. *Ophthalmic Surg.* 1986;17(6):338–342.

168. Asman P, Britt JM, Mills RP, et al. Evaluation of adaptive spatial enhancement in suprathreshold visual field screening. *Ophthalmology.* 1988;95(12):1656–1662.

169. Stewart WC, Shields MB, Ollie AR. Full threshold versus quantification of defects for visual field testing in glaucoma. *Graefes Arch Clin Exp Ophthalmol.* 1989;227(1):51–54.

170. Araujo ML, Feuer WJ, Anderson DR. Evaluation of baseline-related suprathreshold testing for quick determination of visual field nonprogression. *Arch Ophthalmol.* 1993;111(3):365–369.

171. Flanagan JG, Wild JM, Trope GE. Evaluation of FASTPAC, a new strategy for threshold estimation with the Humphrey Field Analyzer, in a glaucomatous population. *Ophthalmology.* 1993;100(6):949–954.

172. Mills RP, Barnebey HS, Migliazzo CV, et al. Does saving time using FASTPAC or suprathreshold testing reduce quality of visual fields? *Ophthalmology.* 1994;101(9):1596–1603.

173. O'Brien C, Poinoosawmy D, Wu J, et al. Evaluation of the Humphrey FASTPAC threshold program in glaucoma. *Br J Ophthalmol.* 1994;78(7):516–519.

174. Glass E, Schaumberger M, Lachenmayr BJ. Simulations for FASTPAC and the standard 4-2 dB full-threshold strategy of the Humphrey Field Analyzer. *Invest Ophthalmol Vis Sci.* 1995;36(9):1847–1854.

175. Bengtsson B, Olsson J, Heijl A, et al. A new generation of algorithms for computerized threshold perimetry, SITA. *Acta Ophthalmol Scand.* 1997;75(4):368–375.

176. Bengtsson B, Heijl A. SITA Fast, a new rapid perimetric threshold test. Description of methods and evaluation in patients with manifest and suspect glaucoma. *Acta Ophthalmol Scand.* 1998;76(4):431–437.

177. Bengtsson B, Heijl A. Evaluation of a new perimetric threshold strategy, SITA, in patients with manifest and suspect glaucoma. *Acta Ophthalmol Scand.* 1998;76(3):268–272.

178. Wild JM, Pacey IE, O'Neill EC, et al. The SITA perimetric threshold algorithms in glaucoma. *Invest Ophthalmol Vis Sci.* 1999;40(9):1998–2009.

179. Bengtsson B, Heijl A. Comparing significance and magnitude of glaucomatous visual field defects using the SITA and Full Threshold strategies. *Acta Ophthalmol Scand.* 1999;77(2):143–146.

180. Sharma AK, Goldberg I, Graham SL, et al. Comparison of the Humphrey Swedish interactive thresholding algorithm (SITA) and full threshold strategies. *J Glaucoma.* 2000;9(1):20–27.

181. Budenz DL, Rhee P, Feuer WJ, et al. Sensitivity and specificity of the Swedish interactive threshold algorithm for glaucomatous visual field defects. *Ophthalmology.* 2002;109(6):1052–1058.

182. Budenz DL, Rhee P, Feuer WJ, et al. Comparison of glaucomatous visual field defects using standard full threshold and Swedish interactive threshold algorithms. *Arch Ophthalmol.* 2002;120(9):1136–1141.

183. Remky A, Arend O. Clinical experiences with the "Swedish interactive threshold algorithm" (SITA) [in German]. *Klin Monatsbl Augenheilkd.* 2000;216(3):143–147.

184. Lachkar Y, Barrault O, Lefrancois A, et al. Rapid Tendency Oriented Perimeter (TOP) with the Octopus visual field analyzer [in French]. *J Fr Ophtalmol.* 1998;21(3):180–184.

185. Maeda H, Nakaura M, Negi A. New perimetric threshold test algorithm with dynamic strategy and tendency oriented perimetry (TOP) in glaucomatous eyes. *Eye.* 2000;14(pt 5):747–751.

186. King AJ, Taguri A, Wadood AC, et al. Comparison of two fast strategies, SITA Fast and TOP, for the assessment of visual fields in glaucoma patients. *Graefes Arch Clin Exp Ophthalmol.* 2002;240(6):481–487.

187. Anderson AJ. Spatial resolution of the tendency-oriented perimetry algorithm. *Invest Ophthalmol Vis Sci.* 2003;44(5):1962–1968.

188. Demirel S, Vingrys AJ. Eye movements during perimetry and the effect that fixational instability has on perimetric outcomes. *J Glaucoma.* 1994;3(1):28–35.

189. Li Y, Mills RP. Kinetic fixation improves threshold sensitivity in the central visual field. *J Glaucoma.* 1992;1(2):108–116.

190. Katz J, Sommer A. Reliability indexes of automated perimetric tests. *Arch Ophthalmol.* 1988;106(9):1252–1254.

191. Bickler-Bluth M, Trick GL, Kolker AE, et al. Assessing the utility of reliability indices for automated visual fields. Testing ocular hypertensives. *Ophthalmology.* 1989;96(5):616–619.

192. Nelson-Quigg JM, Twelker JD, Johnson CA. Response properties of normal observers and patients during automated perimetry. *Arch Ophthalmol.* 1989;107(11):1612–1615.

193. Schulzer M, Mills RP, Hopp RH, et al. Estimation of the short-term fluctuation from a single determination of the visual field. *Invest Ophthalmol Vis Sci.* 1990;31(4):730–735.

194. Johnson LN, Aminlari A, Sassani JW. Effect of intermittent versus continuous patient monitoring on reliability indices during automated perimetry. *Ophthalmology.* 1993;100(1):76–84.

195. Lee M, Zulauf M, Caprioli J. A new reliability parameter for automated perimetry: inconsistent responses. *J Glaucoma.* 1993;2(4):279–284.

196. Jacobs NA, Patterson IH. Variability of the hill of vision and its significance in automated perimetry. *Br J Ophthalmol.* 1985;69(11):824–826.

197. Katz J, Sommer A. Asymmetry and variation in the normal hill of vision. *Arch Ophthalmol.* 1986;104(1):65–68.

198. Heijl A, Lindgren G, Olsson J. Normal variability of static perimetric threshold values across the central visual field. *Arch Ophthalmol.* 1987;105(11):1544–1549.

199. Werner EB, Petrig B, Krupin T, et al. Variability of automated visual fields in clinically stable glaucoma patients. *Invest Ophthalmol Vis Sci.* 1989;30(6):1083–1089.

200. Heijl A, Lindgren A, Lindgren G. Test-retest variability in glaucomatous visual fields. *Am J Ophthalmol.* 1989;108(2):130–135.

201. Haefliger IO, Flammer J. Increase of the short-term fluctuation of the differential light threshold around a physiologic scotoma. *Am J Ophthalmol.* 1989;107(4):417–420.

202. Diestelhorst M, Kullenberg C, Krieglstein GK. Short-term fluctuation of light discrimination sensitivity at the borders of glaucomatous visual field defects [in German]. *Klin Monatsbl Augenheilkd.* 1987;191(6):439–442.

203. Katz J, Sommer A. A longitudinal study of the age-adjusted variability of automated visual fields. *Arch Ophthalmol.* 1987;105(8):1083–1086.

204. Werner EB, Adelson A, Krupin T. Effect of patient experience on the results of automated perimetry in clinically stable glaucoma patients. *Ophthalmology.* 1988;95(6):764–767.

205. Hoskins HD, Magee SD, Drake MV, et al. Confidence intervals for change in automated visual fields. *Br J Ophthalmol.* 1988;72(8):591–597.

206. Weber J, Krieglstein GK, Papoulis C. Graphic analysis of topographic trends in perimetry follow-up of glaucoma [in German]. *Klin Monatsbl Augenheilkd.* 1989;195(5):319–322.

207. Werner EB, Drance SM. Early visual field disturbances in glaucoma. *Arch Ophthalmol.* 1977;95(7):1173–1175.

208. Werner EB, Saheb N, Thomas D. Variability of static visual threshold responses in patients with elevated IOPs. *Arch Ophthalmol.* 1982;100(10):1627–1631.

209. Werner EB, Drance SM. Increased scatter of responses as a precursor of visual field changes in glaucoma. *Can J Ophthalmol.* 1977;12(2):140–142.

210. Flammer J, Drance SM, Zulauf M. Differential light threshold. Short- and long-term fluctuation in patients with glaucoma, normal controls, and patients with suspected glaucoma. *Arch Ophthalmol.* 1984;102(5):704–706.

211. Flammer J, Drance SM, Fankhauser F, et al. Differential light threshold in automated static perimetry. Factors influencing short-term fluctuation. *Arch Ophthalmol.* 1984;102(6):876–879.

212. Chauhan BC, Drance SM, Lai C. A cluster analysis for threshold perimetry. *Graefes Arch Clin Exp Ophthalmol.* 1989;227(3):216–220.

213. Mandava S, Zulauf M, Zeyen T, et al. An evaluation of clusters in the glaucomatous visual field. *Am J Ophthalmol.* 1993;116(6):684–691.

214. Fankhauser F, Fankhauser F 2nd, Giger H. A cluster and scotoma analysis based on empiric criteria. *Graefes Arch Clin Exp Ophthalmol.* 1993;231(12):697–703.

215. Asman P, Heijl A, Olsson J, et al. Spatial analyses of glaucomatous visual fields; a comparison with traditional visual field indices. *Acta Ophthalmol.* 1992;70(5):679–686.

216. Asman P, Heijl A. Glaucoma Hemifield Test. Automated visual field evaluation. *Arch Ophthalmol.* 1992;110(6):812–819.

217. Duggan C, Sommer A, Auer C, et al. Automated differential threshold perimetry for detecting glaucomatous visual field loss. *Am J Ophthalmol.* 1985;100(3):420–423.

218. Sommer A, Enger C, Witt K. Screening for glaucomatous visual field loss with automated threshold perimetry. *Am J Ophthalmol.* 1987;103(5):681–684.

219. Asman P, Heijl A. Evaluation of methods for automated Hemifield analysis in perimetry. *Arch Ophthalmol.* 1992;110(6):820–826.

220. Susanna R Jr, Nicolela MT, Soriano DS, et al. Automated perimetry: a study of the glaucoma hemifield test for the detection of early glaucomatous visual field loss. *J Glaucoma.* 1994;3(1):12–16.

221. Katz J, Quigley HA, Sommer A. Repeatability of the Glaucoma Hemifield Test in automated perimetry. *Invest Ophthalmol Vis Sci.* 1995;36(8):1658–1664.

222. Johnson CA, Sample PA, Cioffi GA, et al. Structure and function evaluation (SAFE): I. criteria for glaucomatous visual field loss using standard automated perimetry (SAP) and short wavelength automated perimetry (SWAP). *Am J Ophthalmol.* 2002;134(2):177–185.

223. The AGIS Investigators. The advanced glaucoma intervention study, 2: visual field test scoring and reliability. *Ophthalmology.* 1994;101(8):1445–1455.

224. Musch DC, Lichter PR, Guire KE, et al. The Collaborative Initial Glaucoma Treatment Study: study design, methods, and baseline characteristics of enrolled patients. *Ophthalmology.* 1999;106(4):653–662.

225. Hills JF, Johnson CA. Evaluation of the *t* test as a method of detecting visual field changes. *Ophthalmology.* 1988;95(2):261–266.

226. Enger C, Sommer A. Recognizing glaucomatous field loss with the Humphrey STATPAC. *Arch Ophthalmol.* 1987;105(10):1355–1357.

227. Heijl A, Lindgren G, Olsson J, et al. Visual field interpretation with empiric probability maps. *Arch Ophthalmol.* 1989;107(2):204–208.

228. Heijl A, Asman P. A clinical study of perimetric probability maps. *Arch Ophthalmol.* 1989;107(2):199–203.

229. Birch MK, Wishart PK, O'Donnell NP. Determining progressive visual field loss in serial Humphrey visual fields. *Ophthalmology.* 1995;102(8):1227–1234; discussion 34–35.

230. Fitzke FW, Hitchings RA, Poinoosawmy D, et al. Analysis of visual field progression in glaucoma. *Br J Ophthalmol.* 1996;80(1):40–48.

231. Werner EB, Bishop KI, Koelle J, et al. A comparison of experienced clinical observers and statistical tests in detection of progressive visual field loss in glaucoma using automated perimetry. *Arch Ophthalmol.* 1988;106(5):619–623.

232. Chauhan BC, Drance SM, Douglas GR. The use of visual field indices in detecting changes in the visual field in glaucoma. *Invest Ophthalmol Vis Sci.* 1990;31(3):512–520.

233. Viswanathan AC, Fitzke FW, Hitchings RA. Early detection of visual field progression in glaucoma: a comparison of PROGRESSOR and STATPAC 2. *Br J Ophthalmol.* 1997;81(12):1037–1042.

234. Armaly MF. The visual field defect and ocular pressure level in open angle glaucoma. *Invest Ophthalmol Vis Sci.* 1969;8(1):105–1024.

235. Heilmann K. On the reversibility of visual field defects in glaucomas. *Trans Am Acad Ophthalmol Otolaryngol.* 1974;78(2):OP304–OP308.

236. Flammer J, Drance SM. Reversibility of a glaucomatous visual field defect after acetazolamide therapy. *Can J Ophthalmol.* 1983;18(3):139–141.

237. Katz LJ, Spaeth GL, Cantor LB, et al. Reversible optic disk cupping and visual field improvement in adults with glaucoma. *Am J Ophthalmol.* 1989;107(5):485–492.

238. Tsai CS, Shin DH, Wan JY, et al. Visual field global indices in patients with reversal of glaucomatous cupping after intraocular pressure reduction. *Ophthalmology.* 1991;98(9):1412–1419.

239. Gandolfi SA. Improvement of visual field indices after surgical reduction of intraocular pressure. *Ophthalmic Surg.* 1995;26(2):121–126.

240. Heijl A, Bengtsson B. The short-term effect of laser trabeculoplasty on the glaucomatous visual field. A prospective study using computerized perimetry. *Acta Ophthalmol.* 1984;62(5):705–714.

241. Holmin C, Krakau CE. Trabeculoplasty and visual field decay: a follow-up study using computerized perimetry. *Curr Eye Res.* 1984;3(9):1101–1105.

242. Salim S, Paranhos A, Lima M, et al. Influence of surgical reduction of intraocular pressure on regions of the visual field with different levels of sensitivity. *Am J Ophthalmol.* 2001;132(4):496–500.

243. Hart WM Jr. Computer processing of visual data. II. Automated pattern analysis of glaucomatous visual fields. *Arch Ophthalmol.* 1981;99(1):133–136.

244. Weleber RG, Tobler WR. Computerized quantitative analysis of kinetic visual fields. *Am J Ophthalmol.* 1986;101(4):461–468.

245. Esterman B. Grid for scoring visual fields. I. Tangent screen. *Arch Ophthalmol.* 1967;77(6):780–786.

246. Esterman B. Grid for scoring visual fields. II. Perimeter. *Arch Ophthalmol.* 1968;79(4):400–406.

247. Esterman B. Functional scoring of the binocular field. *Ophthalmology.* 1982;89(11):1226–1234.

248. American Medical Association. Impairment of visual field. In: Cocchiarella L, Andersson G, eds. *Guides to the Evaluation of Permanent Impairment.* 5th ed. Chicago: American Medical Association; 2000:287–295.

249. Mills RP, Drance SM. Esterman disability rating in severe glaucoma. *Ophthalmology.* 1986;93(3):371–378.

250. Delgado MF, Nguyen NT, Cox TA, et al. Automated perimetry: a report by the American Academy of Ophthalmology. *Ophthalmology.* 2002;109(12):2362–2374.

251. Johnson CA. Recent developments in automated perimetry in glaucoma diagnosis and management. *Curr Opin Ophthalmol.* 2002;13(2):77–84.

252. Hart WM, Jr., Hartz RK, Hagen RW, et al. Color contrast perimetry. *Invest Ophthalmol Vis Sci.* 1984;25(4):400–413.

253. Hart WM Jr, Gordon MO. Color perimetry of glaucomatous visual field defects. *Ophthalmology.* 1984;91(4):338–346.

254. Hart WM Jr, Silverman SE, Trick GL, et al. Glaucomatous visual field damage. Luminance and color-contrast sensitivities. *Invest Ophthalmol Vis Sci.* 1990;31(2):359–367.

255. Logan N, Anderson DR. Detecting early glaucomatous visual field changes with a blue stimulus. *Am J Ophthalmol.* 1983;95(4):432–434.

256. Mindel JS, Safir A, Schare PW. Visual field testing with red targets. *Arch Ophthalmol.* 1983;101(6):927–929.

257. Hart WM Jr, Burde RM. Color contrast perimetry. The spatial distribution of color defects in optic nerve and retinal diseases. *Ophthalmology.* 1985;92(6):768–776.

258. Sample PA. Short-wavelength automated perimetry: it's role in the clinic and for understanding ganglion cell function. *Prog Retin Eye Res.* 2000;19(4):369–383.

259. Sample PA, Weinreb RN. Color perimetry for assessment of primary open-angle glaucoma. *Invest Ophthalmol Vis Sci.* 1990;31(9):1869–1875.

260. Wild JM. Short wavelength automated perimetry. *Acta Ophthalmol Scand.* 2001;79(6):546–559.

261. Lewis RA, Johnson CA, Adams AJ. Automated perimetry and short wavelength sensitivity in patients with asymmetric intraocular pressures. *Graefes Arch Clin Exp Ophthalmol.* 1993;231(5):274–278.

262. Johnson CA, Brandt JD, Khong AM, et al. Short-wavelength automated perimetry in low-, medium-, and high-risk ocular hypertensive eyes. Initial baseline results. *Arch Ophthalmol.* 1995;113(1):70–76.

263. Girkin CA, Emdadi A, Sample PA, et al. Short-wavelength automated perimetry and standard perimetry in the detection of progressive optic disc cupping. *Arch Ophthalmol.* 2000;118(9):1231–1236.

264. Demirel S, Johnson CA. Incidence and prevalence of short wavelength automated perimetry deficits in ocular hypertensive patients. *Am J Ophthalmol.* 2001;131(6):709–715.

265. Sample PA, Weinreb RN. Progressive color visual field loss in glaucoma. *Invest Ophthalmol Vis Sci.* 1992;33(6):2068–2071.

266. Johnson CA, Adams AJ, Casson EJ, et al. Blue-on-yellow perimetry can predict the development of glaucomatous visual field loss. *Arch Ophthalmol.* 1993;111(5):645–650.

267. Sample PA, Taylor JD, Martinez GA, et al. Short-wavelength color visual fields in glaucoma suspects at risk. *Am J Ophthalmol.* 1993;115(2):225–233.

268. Johnson CA, Adams AJ, Casson EJ, et al. Progression of early glaucomatous visual field loss as detected by blue-on-yellow and standard white-on-white automated perimetry. *Arch Ophthalmol.* 1993;111(5):651–656.

269. Johnson CA, Sample PA, Zangwill LM, et al. Structure and function evaluation (SAFE): II. Comparison of optic disk and visual field characteristics. *Am J Ophthalmol.* 2003;135(2):148–154.

270. Moss ID, Wild JM, Whitaker DJ. The influence of age-related cataract on blue-on-yellow perimetry. *Invest Ophthalmol Vis Sci.* 1995;36(5):764–773.

271. Wild JM, Moss ID, Whitaker D, et al. The statistical interpretation of blue-on-yellow visual field loss. *Invest Ophthalmol Vis Sci.* 1995;36(7):1398–1410.

272. Sample PA, Martinez GA, Weinreb RN. Short-wavelength automated perimetry without lens density testing. *Am J Ophthalmol.* 1994;118(5):632–641.

273. Kim YY, Kim JS, Shin DH, et al. Effect of cataract extraction on blue-on-yellow visual field. *Am J Ophthalmol.* 2001;132(2):217–220.

274. Kara-Junior N, Jardim JL, de Oliveira Leme E, et al. Effect of the AcrySof Natural intraocular lens on blue-yellow perimetry. *J Cataract Refract Surg* 2006;32(8):1328–1330.

275. Maeda H, Tanaka Y, Nakamura M, et al. Blue-on-yellow perimetry using an Armaly glaucoma screening program. *Ophthalmologica.* 1999;213(2):71–75.

276. Ugurlu S, Hoffman D, Garway-Heath DF, et al. Relationship between structural abnormalities and short-wavelength perimetric defects in eyes at risk of glaucoma. *Am J Ophthalmol.* 2000;129(5):592–598.

277. Bengtsson B. A new rapid threshold algorithm for short-wavelength automated perimetry. *Invest Ophthalmol Vis Sci.* 2003;44(3):1388–1394.

278. Bengtsson B, Heijl A. Normal intersubject threshold variability and normal limits of the SITA SWAP and full threshold SWAP perimetric programs. *Invest Ophthalmol Vis Sci.* 2003;44(11):5029–5034.

279. Bengtsson B, Heijl A. Diagnostic sensitivity of fast blue-yellow and standard automated perimetry in early glaucoma: a comparison between different test programs. *Ophthalmology.* 2006;113(7):1092–1097.

280. Landers J, Sharma A, Goldberg I, et al. Topography of the frequency doubling perimetry visual field compared with that of short wavelength and achromatic automated perimetry visual fields. *Br J Ophthalmol.* 2006;90(1):70–74.

281. Rossetti L, Fogagnolo P, Miglior S, et al. Learning effect of short-wavelength automated perimetry in patients with ocular hypertension. *J Glaucoma.* 2006;15(5):399–404.

282. Hutchings N, Hosking SL, Wild JM, et al. Long-term fluctuation in short-wavelength automated perimetry in glaucoma suspects and glaucoma patients. *Invest Ophthalmol Vis Sci.* 2001;42(10):2332–2337.

283. Rosli Y, Maddess T, Dawel A, et al. Multifocal frequency-doubling pattern visual evoked responses to dichoptic stimulation. *Clin Neurophysiol.* 2009;120(12):2100–2108.

284. Alward WL. Frequency doubling technology perimetry for the detection of glaucomatous visual field loss. *Am J Ophthalmol.* 2000;129(3):376–378.

285. Maddess T, Goldberg I, Dobinson J, et al. Testing for glaucoma with the spatial frequency doubling illusion. *Vision Res.* 1999;39(25):4258–4273.

286. Quigley HA. Neuronal death in glaucoma. *Prog Retin Eye Res.* 1999;18(1):39–57.

287. Harwerth RS, Crawford ML, Frishman LJ, et al. Visual field defects and neural losses from experimental glaucoma. *Prog Retin Eye Res.* 2002;21(1):91–125.

288. Morgan JE. Retinal ganglion cell shrinkage in glaucoma. *J Glaucoma.* 2002;11(4):365–370.

289. Morgan JE. Selective cell death in glaucoma: does it really occur? *Br J Ophthalmol.* 1994;78(11):875–879; discussion 9–80.

290. Martin L, Wanger P, Vancea L, et al. Concordance of high-pass resolution perimetry and frequency-doubling technology perimetry results in glaucoma: no support for selective ganglion cell damage. *J Glaucoma.* 2003;12(1):40–44.

291. Quigley HA. Identification of glaucoma-related visual field abnormality with the screening protocol of frequency doubling technology. *Am J Ophthalmol.* 1998;125(6):819–829.

292. Johnson CA, Samuels SJ. Screening for glaucomatous visual field loss with frequency-doubling perimetry. *Invest Ophthalmol Vis Sci.* 1997;38(2):413–425.

293. Cioffi GA, Mansberger S, Spry P, et al. Frequency doubling perimetry and the detection of eye disease in the community. *Trans Am Ophthalmol Soc.* 2000;98:195–199; discussion 9–202.

294. Tatemichi M, Nakano T, Tanaka K, et al. Performance of glaucoma mass screening with only a visual field test using frequency-doubling technology perimetry. *Am J Ophthalmol.* 2002;134(4):529–537.

295. Sample PA, Bosworth CF, Blumenthal EZ, et al. Visual function-specific perimetry for indirect comparison of different ganglion cell populations in glaucoma. *Invest Ophthalmol Vis Sci.* 2000;41(7):1783–1790.

296. Cello KE, Nelson-Quigg JM, Johnson CA. Frequency doubling technology perimetry for detection of glaucomatous visual field loss. *Am J Ophthalmol.* 2000;129(3):314–322.

297. Quinn LM, Gardiner SK, Wheeler DT, et al. Frequency doubling technology perimetry in normal children. *Am J Ophthalmol.* 2006;142(6):983–989.

298. Wall M, Neahring RK, Woodward KR. Sensitivity and specificity of frequency doubling perimetry in neuro-ophthalmic disorders: a comparison with conventional automated perimetry. *Invest Ophthalmol Vis Sci.* 2002;43(4):1277–1283.

299. Anderson AJ, Johnson CA. Effect of dichoptic adaptation on frequency-doubling perimetry. *Optom Vis Sci.* 2002;79(2):88–92.

300. Johnson CA, Cioffi GA, Van Buskirk EM. Frequency doubling technology perimetry using a 24-2 stimulus presentation pattern. *Optom Vis Sci.* 1999;76(8):571–581.

301. Spry PG, Johnson CA. Within-test variability of frequency-doubling perimetry using a 24-2 test pattern. *J Glaucoma.* 2002;11(4):315–320.

302. Racette L, Medeiros FA, Zangwill LM, et al. Diagnostic accuracy of the Matrix 24-2 and original N-30 frequency-doubling technology tests compared with standard automated perimetry. *Invest Ophthalmol Vis Sci.* 2008;49(3):954–960.

303. Centofanti M, Fogagnolo P, Oddone F, et al. Learning effect of Humphrey matrix frequency doubling technology perimetry in patients with ocular hypertension. *J Glaucoma.* 2008;17(6):436–441.

304. Gonzalez-Hernandez M, de la Rosa MG, de la Vega RR, et al. Long-term fluctuation of standard automatic perimetry, pulsar perimetry and frequency-doubling technology in early glaucoma diagnosis. *Ophthalmic Res.* 2007;39(6):338–343.

305. Iester M, Capris P, Pandolfo A, et al. Learning effect, short-term fluctuation, and long-term fluctuation in frequency doubling technique. *Am J Ophthalmol.* 2000;130(2):160–164.

306. Bullimore MA, Wood JM, Swenson K. Motion perception in glaucoma. *Invest Ophthalmol Vis Sci.* 1993;34(13):3526–3533.

307. Fahle M, Wehrhahn C. Motion perception in the peripheral visual field. *Graefes Arch Clin Exp Ophthalmol.* 1991;229(5):430–436.

308. Ruben S, Fitzke F. Correlation of peripheral displacement thresholds and optic disc parameters in ocular hypertension. *Br J Ophthalmol.* 1994;78(4):291–294.

309. Piltz JR, Swindale NV, Drance SM. Vernier thresholds and alignment bias in control, suspect, and glaucomatous eyes. *J Glaucoma.* 1993;2(2):87–95.

310. Arden GB, Jacobson JJ. A simple grating test for contrast sensitivity: preliminary results indicate value in screening for glaucoma. *Invest Ophthalmol Vis Sci.* 1978;17(1):23–32.

311. McKendrick AM, Johnson CA, Anderson AJ, et al. Elevated vernier acuity thresholds in glaucoma. *Invest Ophthalmol Vis Sci.* 2002;43(5):1393–1399.

312. Anderson AJ, Vingrys AJ. Multiple processes mediate flicker sensitivity. *Vision Res.* 2001;41(19):2449–2455.

313. Rota-Bartelink A. The diagnostic value of automated flicker threshold perimetry. *Curr Opin Ophthalmol.* 1999;10(2):135–139.

314. Frisen L. High-pass resolution perimetry. A clinical review. *Doc Ophthalmol.* 1993;83(1):1–25.

315. Wall M, Ketoff KM. Random dot motion perimetry in patients with glaucoma and in normal subjects. *Am J Ophthalmol.* 1995;120(5):587–596.

316. House P, Schulzer M, Drance S, et al. Characteristics of the normal central visual field measured with resolution perimetry. *Graefes Arch Clin Exp Ophthalmol.* 1991;229(1):8–12.

317. Chauhan BC, Mohandas RN, Whelan JH, et al. Comparison of reliability indices in conventional and high-pass resolution perimetry. *Ophthalmology.* 1993;100(7):1089–1094.

318. Sample PA, Ahn DS, Lee PC, et al. High-pass resolution perimetry in eyes with ocular hypertension and primary open-angle glaucoma. *Am J Ophthalmol.* 1992;113(3):309–316.

319. Martinez GA, Sample PA, Weinreb RN. Comparison of high-pass resolution perimetry and standard automated perimetry in glaucoma. *Am J Ophthalmol.* 1995;119(2):195–201.

320. Chauhan BC, LeBlanc RP, McCormick TA, et al. Comparison of high-pass resolution perimetry and pattern discrimination perimetry to conventional perimetry in glaucoma. *Can J Ophthalmol.* 1993;28(7):306–311.

321. Chauhan BC. The value of high-pass resolution perimetry in glaucoma. *Curr Opin Ophthalmol.* 2000;11(2):85–89.

322. Iester M, Altieri M, Vittone P, et al. Detection of glaucomatous visual field defect by nonconventional perimetry. *Am J Ophthalmol.* 2003;135(1):35–39.

323. Silverman SE, Trick GL, Hart WM Jr. Motion perception is abnormal in primary open-angle glaucoma and ocular hypertension. *Invest Ophthalmol Vis Sci.* 1990;31(4):722–729.

324. Bosworth CF, Sample PA, Gupta N, et al. Motion automated perimetry identifies early glaucomatous field defects. *Arch Ophthalmol.* 1998;116(9):1153–1158.

325. Bosworth CF, Sample PA, Williams JM, et al. Spatial relationship of motion automated perimetry and optic disc topography in patients with glaucomatous optic neuropathy. *J Glaucoma.* 1999;8(5):281–289.

326. Bowd C, Zangwill LM, Berry CC, et al. Detecting early glaucoma by assessment of retinal nerve fiber layer thickness and visual function. *Invest Ophthalmol Vis Sci.* 2001;42(9):1993–2003.

327. Goldmann H. Fundamentals of exact perimetry. 1945. *Optom Vis Sci.* 1999;76(8):599–604.

328. Portney GL, Hanible JE. A comparison of four projection perimeters. *Am J Ophthalmol.* 1976;81(5):678–681.

329. Wohlrab TM, Erb C, Rohrbach JM, et al. Age-adjusted normal values with the Tubingen Automatic Perimeter TAP 2000 CC [in German]. *Ophthalmologe.* 1996;93(4):428–432.

330. Harms H. Entwicklungsmoglichkeiten der Perimetrie [in German]. *Graefes Arch Clin Exp Ophthalmol.* 1950;150:28–57.

331. Armaly MF. Ocular pressure and visual fields. A ten-year follow-up study. *Arch Ophthalmol.* 1969;81(1):25–40.

332. Rock WJ, Drance SM, Morgan RW. Visual field screening in glaucoma. An evaluation of the Armaly technique for screening glaucomatous visual fields. *Arch Ophthalmol.* 1973;89(4):287–290.

333. Drance SM, Brais P, Fairclough M, et al. A screening method for temporal visual defects in chronic simple glaucoma. *Can J Ophthalmol.* 1972;7(4): 428–429.

334. Rock WJ, Drance SM, Morgan RW. A modification of the Armaly visual field screening technique for glaucoma. *Can J Ophthalmol.* 1971;6(4): 283–292.

335. Fischer FW. Threshold-adjusted supraliminal pattern perimetry with the Goldmann perimeter [in German]. *Klin Monbl Augenheilkd.* 1984; 185(3):204–211.

336. Rabin S, Kolesar P, Podos SM, et al. A visual field screening protocol for glaucoma. *Am J Ophthalmol.* 1981;92(4):630–635.

337. Stepanik J. Diagnosis of glaucoma with the Goldmann perimeter [in German]. *Klin Monatsbl Augenheilkd.* 1983;183:330–332.

Glaucomatous Influence on Visual Function

In addition to the previously discussed visual field changes in glaucoma (see Chapter 5), other visual function tests may have abnormal results early in glaucoma. Some of these tests may one day prove useful in detecting the presence and progression of glaucoma and in judging the efficacy of glaucoma therapy.

BRIGHTNESS SENSITIVITY

Patients with glaucomatous optic atrophy have decreased light sensitivity when dark adapted, which correlates with the degree of nerve damage (1), and dark adaptation, tested with chromatic stimuli, has been reported to be abnormal in patients with ocular hypertension (2). The results of some studies provided little evidence for photoreceptor abnormalities in glaucoma (3,4), but other studies suggested that the photoreceptors may be involved in glaucomatous damage (5,6). Light sensitivity can also be evaluated with a brightness ratio test, in which the patient discriminates the difference in sensitivity of the two eyes to light, and it has been suggested that tests of this type may be useful in glaucoma screening (7,8). In preliminary studies, patients with open-angle glaucoma had abnormal responses on dichoptic testing, in which one half of a test object is presented to one eye, and the other half to the fellow eye, to help determine the location of a defect in the visual pathway (9).

COLOR VISION

Reduced sensitivity to colors has been described in patients with ocular hypertension, tilted discs, and various forms of glaucoma, and may precede any detectable loss of peripheral or central vision by standard acuity or visual field testing (10). Compared with achromatic sensitivity, color sensitivity was found to be more affected in glaucoma (11). Most studies agree that the color vision deficit is associated primarily with blue-sensitive pathways (12–25). This is consistent with the observation that blue signals are detected by the short-wavelength cones, and then processed by the blue–yellow bistratified ganglion cells, which are different from the midget ganglion cells (26,27). These cells project their axons to the interlaminar koniocellular layers of the lateral geniculate nucleus (28). Blue cones contribute little to the sensation of brightness or to visual acuity, which may account for why standard visual

acuity tests, perimetry, or contrast sensitivity studies might miss an associated visual deficit. The color visual dysfunction is strongly related to elevated intraocular pressure (IOP) levels (22,23), suggesting that the damage is pressure induced. Selective loss of red–green sensitivity has been observed in some patients with glaucoma (29). However, chromatic visual-evoked potential (VEP), which utilizes red–green flicker, was found to be altered in nonglaucomatous optic neuropathies, but not glaucoma (30).

It is unclear whether the loss of color vision and the visual field changes associated with nerve fiber bundle loss share the same mechanism. Ocular hypertensive eyes with yellow–blue and blue–green defects were found to have diffuse early changes in visual field sensitivity (17) and an increased risk of glaucomatous visual field loss, compared with similar eyes that did not have these color vision disturbances (14). The same color abnormalities in patients with early glaucoma correlated significantly with diffuse retinal nerve fiber loss (24). However, no significant correlation between color vision scores and visual field performance was found among patients with ocular hypertension when age correction was applied to the color variable (31), and another study revealed no clear association between early glaucomatous cupping and color vision anomalies (18). Specificity is limited by the fact that the tritan deficit is also the one most frequently seen with age-related changes. When study populations were matched for age and lens density, however, color vision loss in glaucoma was still attributable in part to the disease process (21).

In most reported studies, the color vision testing was performed with the Farnsworth–Munsell 100-hue test, dichotomous (D-15) tests, or variants of these, all of which are laborious and of questionable precision. One study has shown that halogen lighting is preferable for the Farnsworth–Munsell 100-hue test in glaucoma and confirmed the presence of blue–yellow pathway deficiency in glaucoma (32). Another study has shown that although the error scores on the Farnsworth–Munsell 100-hue test were elevated in glaucomatous eyes, the test did not always discriminate well and seemed to lack a high diagnostic value (33).

Various tests have been devised to overcome limitations of the Farnsworth–Munsell test, including computer-driven monitors that present flickering color contrasts or peripheral color contrasts, an automatic anomaloscope, a color contrast sensitivity test in which the target and surround have the same luminance but different chromaticity, and a personal computer (34–38). Even with the most sensitive, precise system, however, glaucoma is not always detected, suggesting that some patients with glaucoma have true preservation of color vision (37,39,40).

As discussed in Chapter 5, short-wavelength automated perimetry (SWAP), which projects a blue target on a yellow background, has been shown to detect glaucoma damage earlier than conventional white-on-white perimetry (41–44). SWAP has also been found to be more sensitive to progression of visual field loss and to progression of glaucomatous disc cupping (45,46).

Contrast Sensitivity

Subtle loss of both central and peripheral vision can be demonstrated in some patients with glaucoma, before visual field changes are detectable with standard techniques, by measuring the amount of contrast required for a patient to discriminate between adjacent visual stimuli (47–52). In some studies, the contrast sensitivity impairment correlates with visual field (48–50,53), especially with the central visual field and optic nerve head (50,54) damage. The yield of detecting glaucoma may be increased by measuring peripheral contrast sensitivity, 20 to 25 degrees eccentrically (55,56). Tests to measure contrast sensitivity may use spatial or temporal strategies. Although spatial contrast sensitivity may be a useful adjunct, caution has been advised in interpreting the results without considering additional clinical data (52). The overlap with other causes of reduced spatial contrast sensitivity, including age, creates high false-negative and false-positive rates (50,51,57,58). Spatial contrast sensitivity has been shown to decrease in persons with healthy eyes after 50 years of age, which appears to be independent of the crystalline lens (59,60). Although spatial summation properties differ between M- and P-mediated pathways, the underlying spatial summation properties associated with these pathways are similar in control patients and those with glaucoma (61). In a study comparing the decrease in contrast sensitivity between normal aging and glaucoma, aging decreased low-spatial frequency-sensitive components of both the M and P pathways. Glaucoma results in a further reduction of sensitivity that does not seem to be selective for M or P functions, which the investigators presumed were mediated by cells with larger receptive fields (62). For reference, frequency doubling technology (FDT) measures the contrast threshold to low spatial frequency, high temporal frequency sinusoidal luminance profile bars (63).

Sine-wave gratings of parallel light and dark bands (Arden gratings), in which the patient must detect the striped pattern at various levels of contrast and spatial frequencies, have been evaluated extensively in this group of psychophysical tests (47). The original Arden gratings were limited by the subjectivity of the required responses (64,65). A modification, in which the patient must indicate the orientation of the gratings, has been reported to minimize this limitation (65). The testing methods include computer-controlled video displays and photographically reproduced grating patterns, both of which have given good approximations of the spatial contrast sensitivity function (66). One of these tests uses sine-wave gratings of low spatial frequency and laser interference fringes to increase sensitivity to peripheral defects (67–69).

Performing these techniques, including sinusoidal grating targets, is difficult and time consuming. An effort to minimize these limitations has led to the development of high-pass resolution perimetry (discussed in Chapter 5).

Temporal contrast sensitivity, in which the patient must detect a visual stimulus flickering at various frequencies, provides another measure of contrast sensitivity and appears to be more useful than spatial contrast sensitivity in patients with glaucoma. The stimulus may be presented as a homogeneous flickering field (flicker fusion frequency) or as a counterphase flickering grating of low spatial frequency (spatiotemporal contrast sensitivity) (59,70,71). Patients with glaucoma may have reduced function with either method, although the latter appears to be a more sensitive test (71,72). Spatiotemporal contrast sensitivity was also found to be more useful in detecting glaucoma than spatial contrast sensitivity testing of the central retina was, although, again, the usefulness of the test is limited to those younger than 50 years (59). Other studies have found age to be a less significant factor in sensitivity loss, although one study suggested that cardiovascular disease may be associated with foveal dysfunction (73–75). There is also a question as to whether temporal contrast sensitivity loss among patients with ocular hypertension represents early glaucomatous damage or a transient effect of raised IOP. One study suggested that either mechanism may be found within subsets of this population (76). Reducing the IOP in patients with glaucoma may improve contrast sensitivity at high frequencies of 18 cycles/degree (77).

Several techniques have been evaluated to improve the usefulness of contrast sensitivity testing. One study suggested that the determination of a ratio between spatial contrast sensitivity and flicker sensitivity measures visual pathology more precisely than the absolute value of either test does (78). Another test of temporal contrast sensitivity, in which the patient must discriminate two rapidly successive pulses of light from a single pulse, is reported to be highly sensitive and specific in distinguishing glaucomatous eyes from healthy ones (79). Another test, the whole-field scotopic retinal sensitivity test, uses a flashlight-sized device in which the patient views a white light in the entire visual field and is asked to detect alternating illuminated and dark fields at 1-second intervals (80). This test may be useful as a screening tool (80,81), although one study found too much overlap between healthy persons and individuals with ocular hypertension (82).

Another attempt to use a temporal contrast or flickering target has been called temporal modulation perimetry or flicker perimetry (83–85). In healthy eyes there is an age-related loss of temporal modulation sensitivity (83). It appears to be less affected by visual acuity or retinal degradation than either light-sense or resolution perimetry, and it is more sensitive than light-sense perimetry to increasing IOP (84–86).

Different target shapes and patterns, which the patient must distinguish, are also reported to be of particular value in detecting optic nerve disease (87). In one study with pattern discrimination perimetry, long-term and short-term fluctuations were clinically significant but did not prevent adequate separation between normal and abnormal measurements (88). Visual function in glaucomatous eyes, as measured by contrast sensitivity, has been shown to improve after β-blocker therapy (89).

ELECTROPHYSIOLOGIC STUDIES

Most measures of visual fields and other visual functions are dependent on the patient's subjective response. A significant amount of work is also being done on alternative, objective methods of evaluating the visual field. The pattern electroretinogram, the photopic negative response of the electroretinogram, and the multifocal VEP (mfVEP) appear to have the most potential to detect early glaucomatous damage that may not be detected by standard automated perimetry (90–96). Of the currently available electrophysiologic tests, the mfVEP is the only one that can provide topographic information about the visual field defects. The relation between electrophysiologic tests and the underlying damage to ganglion cells is still not completely understood, but it has been suggested that the signal in the mfVEP response may be linearly related to the ganglion cells loss (93). Patients with glaucoma were also found in one study to have increased baseline values with electro-oculography (97), but a subsequent study did not confirm that finding (98).

Electroretinograms

Electroretinograms (ERGs) evoked by reversing checkerboard or grating patterns, referred to as pattern ERGs (PERGs), are sensitive to retinal ganglion cell and optic nerve dysfunction and have reduced amplitudes in patients with glaucoma (92,99–106). PERG may detect early damage to ganglion cells (91), which may explain why reduced PERG amplitudes appear in the early stages of glaucoma and in some eyes with ocular hypertension, especially those at elevated risk for glaucoma (101,105–110). These findings suggest that PERG may be useful in discriminating between those patients with ocular hypertension who will develop visual field loss and those who will not.

Studies differ on whether PERG correlates with IOP and disc topography, with one study showing no correlation and others showing an association with IOP control, computed optic nerve head analysis, or the retinal nerve fiber layer thickness (108,111–113). The PERG has been shown to correlate with visual field indices (114), and visual field defects are associated with PERG reduction in the corresponding hemisphere (115). However, no precise correlation was found with color vision deficits (116). Decreased amplitude and an increase in peak latency were found to correlate with increasing age (104), paralleling the estimated normal loss of ganglion cells. Indeed, reduction in PERG was directly related to

histologically defined optic nerve damage in a monkey model (117). PERG in combination with SWAP was shown in one study to improve the power to predict progression of visual field loss (118).

The ERG evoked by a flash of light (flash ERG) is affected more by outer retinal elements and is not typically abnormal in glaucoma. Acute IOP elevation in cats, however, caused a reduction in both pattern and flash ERG, proportional to the reduction in perfusion pressure and regardless of the absolute IOP, suggesting a vascular mechanism to which the ganglion cells are less likely to recover (119). Patients with glaucoma in one study had reduced ERG amplitudes in response to a flickering stimulus (flicker ERG) (106). One study suggested that the flash and pattern ERG changes in glaucoma cannot be attributed simply to optic atrophy, suggesting additional outer retinal damage in glaucoma (120).

Multifocal ERG (mfERG) (**Fig. 6.1**) permits simultaneous recording of multiple spatially localized ERG (121,122). It consists of the same components as a standard ERG (123). Preliminary studies suggest that it does not appear to correlate well with glaucomatous damage and may be able to detect abnormalities before automated achromatic visual fields can (124–129).

Visual-Evoked Potentials

VEPs may also be abnormal in patients with chronic or acute glaucoma, although this is more variable than the PERG response (15,99,102,103,117,130–133). However, larger diameter axons of the magnocellular pathway, which may be preferentially damaged in glaucoma (134), correlate with fast, transiently responding retinal ganglion cells, and a reduced response to high-frequency flicker VEP (greater than 13 Hz) has been shown to correlate with the degree of glaucomatous damage (135–138). Blue-on-yellow VEP may be useful in glaucoma research and may be an objective electrophysiologic test for monitoring patients with glaucoma (139,140).

mfVEPs (**Fig. 6.2**) can be recorded simultaneously from many regions of the visual field and appear to provide objective measures of glaucomatous damage (94,141–145). The amplitude and waveform of the mfVEP responses vary across individual patients and within the visual field of an individual. Methods for analyzing the responses and for displaying the results of mfVEP compare the monocular responses from the two eyes of an individual and produce a map of the defects in the form of a probability plot, similar to the one used to display visual field defects measured with standard automated perimetry. It is hypothesized that both the signal in the mfVEP and the sensitivity of the Humphrey visual field perimeter are linearly related to ganglion cell loss (94).

New approaches will allow a direct comparison of the efficacy of the mfVEP and standard automated perimetry in detecting glaucomatous damage. For example, one study evaluated the reliability of VEPs, obtained with chromatic and achromatic patterns in healthy persons and patients

Figure 6.1 The multifocal electroretinogram (mfERG) display. **A,** *top:* The mfERG display with circles drawn to indicate radii of 5 degrees (*thick, solid, dark gray*), 15 degrees (*thinner solid*), and 25 degrees (*dashed light gray*). **A,** *middle:* A schematic of the eye illustrates where the image of the display falls. **A,** *bottom:* The three-dimensional mfERG density plot of the responses (E) from a normal subject. **B:** The mfERG display at one moment in time. **C:** The stimulation sequence of two sectors in. **D:** The single continuous ERG record generated by the display. **E:** The 103 mfERG responses (first-order kernel) extracted by correlating the stimulus sequence (C) with the continuous ERG record (D). (From Hood DC, Odel JG, Chen CS, et al. The multifocal electroretinogram. *J Neuroophthalmol.* 2003;23:225.)

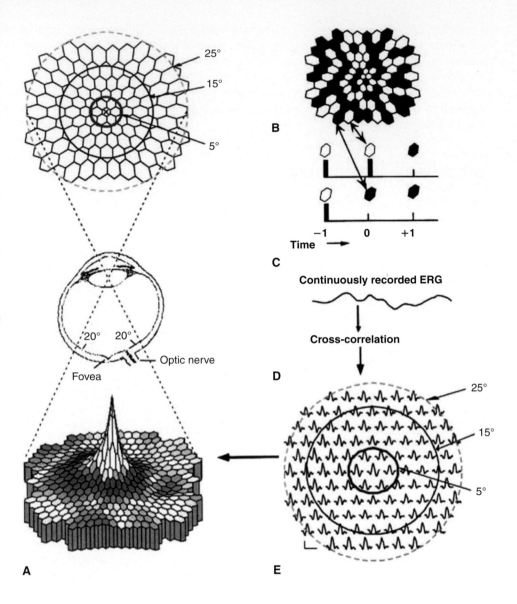

with suspected glaucoma without subjective visual field defects, and found that patients with suspected glaucoma had greater impairment of VEPs to blue–black checkerboards (146). The mfVEP may develop a significant role in the clinical management of glaucoma (145), although it is unlikely to replace static automated achromatic perimetry in the near future (142).

Steady-state VEP may be able to detect glaucomatous loss earlier than automatic achromatic perimetry can (63).

AFFERENT PUPILLARY DEFECT

A relative afferent pupillary defect offers yet another measure of visual pathway disturbance in glaucoma (147). It has been shown to be proportional to the amount of visual field loss and may precede detectable field loss by static automated perimetry (148–150). When pupillary status, such as marked miosis, prevents determination of relative afferent pupillary defect, bright-

ness comparison testing has been shown to correctly predict the presence of a relative afferent pupillary defect in 92% of patients with glaucoma (151). Pupillary evaluation by using pupillometry and testing relative sensitivity between stimuli present in superior and inferior visual fields was able to correctly identify visual field defects in 70% of patients with glaucoma (152).

KEY POINTS

- Some patients with glaucoma may have abnormal responses to brightness and contrast sensitivity (especially temporal) and color vision (especially blue sensitivity), although these findings are insufficiently consistent to have clinical value at this time.
- Objective measures of visual function, including ERG and VEP, may also be abnormal in glaucoma patients and may one day provide useful clinical tools.

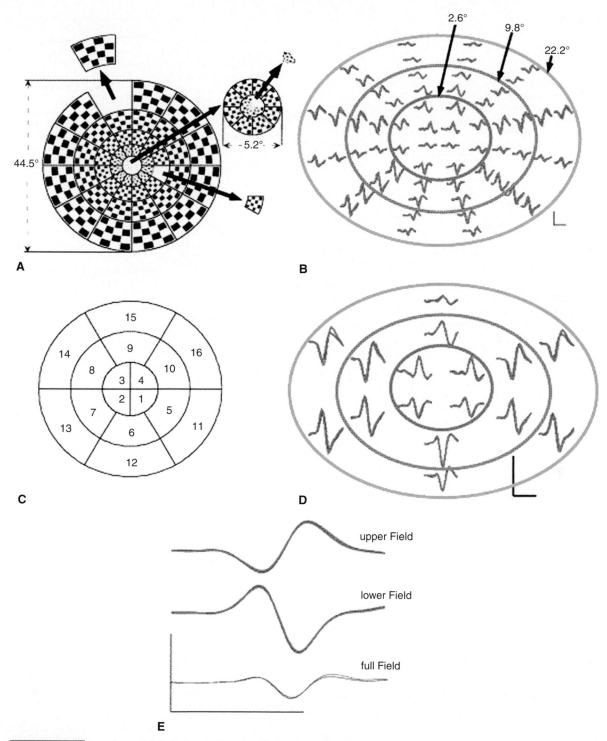

Figure 6.2 **A:** The mfVEP display with 60 scaled sectors. **B:** The averaged mfVEP responses from the right and left eyes of 30 control subjects for 60 sectors. The circles on the right have radii of 2.6 degrees (*inside*), 9.8 degrees (*middle*), and 22.2 degrees (*outside*). **C:** The mfVEP display divided into 16 groups. Each group includes four sectors, except for the (center four groups, which include three sectors. **D:** The averaged mfVEP responses from the 30 control subjects summed by the 16 groups shown in panel C. **E:** The responses from panel B summed and averaged separately for the upper and lower field and summed and averaged for the entire field. The calibration bars in panels B, D, and E indicate 200 nV and 100 ms. (Reprinted from Hood DC, Greenstein VC. Multifocal VEP and ganglion cell damage: applications and limitations for the study of glaucoma. *Prog Retin Eye Res.* 2003;22:201–251, with permission.)

REFERENCES

1. Jonas JB, Zach FM, Naumann GO. Dark adaptation in glaucomatous and nonglaucomatous optic nerve atrophy. *Graefes Arch Clin Exp Ophthalmol.* 1990;228:321–325.
2. Goldthwaite D, Lakowski R, Drance SM. A study of dark adaptation in ocular hypertensives. *Can J Ophthalmol.* 1976;11:55–60.
3. Holopigian K, Greenstein VC, Seiple W, et al. Electrophysiologic assessment of photoreceptor function in patients with primary open-angle glaucoma. *J Glaucoma.* 2000;9:163–168.
4. Kendell KR, Quigley HA, Kerrigan LA, et al. Primary open-angle glaucoma is not associated with photoreceptor loss. *Invest Ophthalmol Vis Sci.* 1995;36:200–205.
5. Velten IM, Korth M, Horn FK. The a-wave of the dark adapted electroretinogram in glaucomas: are photoreceptors affected? *Br J Ophthalmol.* 2001;85:397–402.
6. Nork TM, Ver Hoeve JN, Poulsen GL, et al. Swelling and loss of photoreceptors in chronic human and experimental glaucomas. *Arch Ophthalmol.* 2000;118:235–245.
7. Teoh SL, Allan D, Dutton GN, et al. Brightness discrimination and contrast sensitivity in chronic glaucoma—a clinical study. *Br J Ophthalmol.* 1990;74:215–219.
8. Cummins D, MacMillan ES, Heron G, et al. Simultaneous interocular brightness sense testing in ocular hypertension and glaucoma. *Arch Ophthalmol.* 1994;112:1198–1203.
9. Enoch JM. Quantitative layer-by-layer perimetry. *Invest Ophthalmol Vis Sci.* 1978;17:208–257.
10. Vuori ML, Mantyjarvi M. Tilted disc syndrome and colour vision. *Acta Ophthalmol Scan.* 2007;85:648–652.
11. Pearson P, Swanson WH, Fellman RL. Chromatic and achromatic defects in patients with progressing glaucoma. *Vision Res.* 2001;41:1215–1227.
12. Smith VC, Pokorny J. Spectral sensitivity of the foveal cone photopigments between 400 and 500 nm. *Vision Res.* 1975;15:161–171.
13. Stamper RL. The effect of glaucoma on central visual function. *Trans Am Ophthalmol Soc.* 1984;82:792–826.
14. Drance SM, Lakowski R, Schulzer M, et al. Acquired color vision changes in glaucoma: use of 100-hue test and Pickford anomaloscope as predictors of glaucomatous field change. *Arch Ophthalmol.* 1981;99:829–831.
15. Motolko M, Drance SM, Douglas GR. The early psychophysical disturbances in chronic open-angle glaucoma: a study of visual functions with asymmetric disc cupping. *Arch Ophthalmol.* 1982;100:1632–1634.
16. Adams AJ, Rodic R, Husted R, et al. Spectral sensitivity and color discrimination changes in glaucoma and glaucoma-suspect patients. *Invest Ophthalmol Vis Sci.* 1982;23:516–524.
17. Flammer J, Drance SM. Correlation between color vision scores and quantitative perimetry in suspected glaucoma. *Arch Ophthalmol.* 1984;102:38–39.
18. Hamill TR, Post RB, Johnson CA, et al. Correlation of color vision deficits and observable changes in the optic disc in a population of ocular hypertensives. *Arch Ophthalmol.* 1984;102:1637–1639.
19. Heron G, Adams AJ, Husted R. Central visual fields for short wavelength sensitive pathways in glaucoma and ocular hypertension. *Invest Ophthalmol Vis Sci.* 1988;29:64–72.
20. Adams AJ, Heron G, Husted R. Clinical measures of central vision function in glaucoma and ocular hypertension. *Arch Ophthalmol.* 1987;105:782–787.
21. Sample PA, Boynton RM, Weinreb RN. Isolating the color vision loss in primary open-angle glaucoma. *Am J Ophthalmol.* 1988;106:686–691.
22. Yamazaki Y, Lakowski R, Drance SM. A comparison of the blue color mechanism in high- and low-tension glaucoma. *Ophthalmology.* 1989;96:12–15.
23. Yamazaki Y, Drance SM, Lakowski R, et al. Correlation between color vision and highest intraocular pressure in glaucoma patients. *Am J Ophthalmol.* 1988;106:397–399.
24. Airaksinen PJ, Lakowski R, Drance SM, et al. Color vision and retinal nerve fiber layer in early glaucoma. *Am J Ophthalmol.* 1986;101:208–213.
25. Yamagami J, Koseki N, Araie M. Color vision deficit in normal-tension glaucoma eyes. *Jpn J Ophthalmol.* 1995;39:384–389.
26. Dacey DM, Lee BB. The 'blue-on' opponent pathway in primate retina originates from a distinct bistratified ganglion cell type. *Nature.* 1994;367:731–735.
27. Dacey DM. Morphology of a small-field bistratified ganglion cell type in the macaque and human retina. *Vis Neurosci.* 1993;10:1081–1098.
28. Martin PR, White AJ, Goodchild AK, et al. Evidence that blue-on cells are part of the third geniculocortical pathway in primates. *Eur J Neurosci.* 1997;9:1536–1541.
29. Alvarez SL, Pierce GE, Vingrys AJ, et al. Comparison of red-green, blue-yellow and achromatic losses in glaucoma. *Vision Res.* 1997;37:2295–2301.
30. Accornero N, Gregori B, Pro S, et al. Chromatic modulation of luminance visual evoked potential latencies in healthy subjects and patients with mild vision disorders. *Clin Neurophysiol.* 2008;119:1683–1688.
31. Breton ME, Krupin T. Age covariance between 100-hue color scores and quantitative perimetry in primary open-angle glaucoma. *Arch Ophthalmol.* 1987;105:642–645.
32. Nuzzi R, Bellan A, Boles-Carenini B. Glaucoma, lighting, and color vision: an investigation into their interrelationship. *Ophthalmologica.* 1997;211:25–31.
33. Budde WM, Junemann A, Korth M. Color axis evaluation of the Farnsworth Munsell 100-hue test in primary open-angle glaucoma and normal-pressure glaucoma. *Graefes Arch Clin Exp Ophthalmol.* 1996;234(suppl 1):S180–S186.
34. Gunduz K, Arden GB, Perry S, et al. Color vision defects in ocular hypertension and glaucoma: quantification with a computer-driven color television system. *Arch Ophthalmol.* 1988;106:929–935.
35. Yu TC, Falcao-Reis F, Spileers W, et al. Peripheral color contrast: a new screening test for preglaucomatous visual loss. *Invest Ophthalmol Vis Sci.* 1991;32:2779–2789.
36. Nguyen NX, Korth M, Wisse M, et al. Use of a new anomaloscope test in diagnosis of glaucoma [in German]. *Klin Monatsbl Augenheilkd.* 1994;204:149–154.
37. Falcao-Reis FM, O'Sullivan F, Spileers W, et al. Macular colour contrast sensitivity in ocular hypertension and glaucoma: evidence for two types of defect. *Br J Ophthalmol.* 1991;75:598–602.
38. Accornero N, Capozza M, Rinalduzzi S, et al. Color perimetry with personal computer. *Stud Health Technol Inform.* 1997;43(pt A):89–93.
39. Fristrom B. Peripheral colour contrast thresholds in ocular hypertension and glaucoma. *Acta Ophthalmol Scand.* 1997;75:376–382.
40. Fristrom B. Colour contrast sensitivity in ocular hypertension: a five-year prospective study. *Acta Ophthalmol Scand.* 2002;80:155–162.
41. Sample PA, Weinreb RN. Progressive color visual field loss in glaucoma. *Invest Ophthalmol Vis Sci.* 1992;33:2068–2071.
42. Johnson CA, Adams AJ, Casson EJ, et al. Blue-on-yellow perimetry can predict the development of glaucomatous visual field loss. *Arch Ophthalmol.* 1993;111:645–650.
43. Sample PA, Taylor JD, Martinez GA, et al. Short-wavelength color visual fields in glaucoma suspects at risk. *Am J Ophthalmol.* 1993;115:225–233.
44. Demirel S, Johnson CA. Short wavelength automated perimetry (SWAP) in ophthalmic practice. *J Am Optom Assoc.* 1996;67:451–456.
45. Johnson CA, Adams AJ, Casson EJ, et al. Progression of early glaucomatous visual field loss as detected by blue-on-yellow and standard white-on-white automated perimetry. *Arch Ophthalmol.* 1993;111:651–656.
46. Girkin CA, Emdadi A, Sample PA, et al. Short-wavelength automated perimetry and standard perimetry in the detection of progressive optic disc cupping. *Arch Ophthalmol.* 2000;118:1231–1236.
47. Arden GB, Jacobson JJ. A simple grating test for contrast sensitivity: preliminary results indicate value in screening for glaucoma. *Invest Ophthalmol Vis Sci.* 1978;17:23–32.
48. Lundh BL, Lennerstrand G. Eccentric contrast sensitivity loss in glaucoma. *Acta Ophthalmol (Copenh).* 1981;59:21–24.
49. Motolko MA, Phelps CD. Contrast sensitivity in asymmetric glaucoma. *Int Ophthalmol.* 1984;7:45–59.
50. Hitchings RA, Powell DJ, Arden GB, et al. Contrast sensitivity gratings in glaucoma family screening. *Br J Ophthalmol.* 1981;65:515–517.
51. Stamper RL, Hsu-Winges C, Sopher M. Arden contrast sensitivity testing in glaucoma. *Arch Ophthalmol.* 1982;100:947–950.
52. Sample PA, Juang PS, Weinreb RN. Isolating the effects of primary open-angle glaucoma on the contrast sensitivity function. *Am J Ophthalmol.* 1991;112:308–316.
53. Wilensky JT, Hawkins A. Comparison of contrast sensitivity, visual acuity, and Humphrey visual field testing in patients with glaucoma. *Trans Am Ophthalmol Soc.* 2001;99:213–218.
54. Zulauf M, Flammer J. Correlation of spatial contrast sensitivity and visual fields in glaucoma. *Graefes Arch Clin Exp Ophthalmol.* 1993;231:146–150.
55. Velten IM, Korth M, Horn FK, et al. Temporal contrast sensitivity with peripheral and central stimulation in glaucoma diagnosis. *Br J Ophthalmol.* 1999;83:199–205.
56. Falcão-Reis F, O'Donoghue E, Buceti R, et al. Peripheral contrast sensitivity in glaucoma and ocular hypertension. *Br J Ophthalmol.* 1990;74:712–716.
57. Sokol S, Domar A, Moskowitz A. Utility of the Arden grating test in glaucoma screening: high false-positive rate in normals over 50 years of age. *Invest Ophthalmol Vis Sci.* 1980;19:1529–1533.

58. Sponsel WE, DePaul KL, Martone JF, et al. Association of Vistech contrast sensitivity and visual field findings in glaucoma. *Br J Ophthalmol.* 1991;75:558–560.

59. Korth M, Horn F, Storck B, et al. Spatial and spatiotemporal contrast sensitivity of normal and glaucoma eyes. *Graefes Arch Clin Exp Ophthalmol.* 1989;227:428–435.

60. Owsley C, Gardner T, Sekuler R, et al. Role of the crystalline lens in the spatial vision loss of the elderly. *Invest Ophthalmol Vis Sci.* 1985;26:1165–1170.

61. Battista J, Badcock DR, McKendrick AM. Spatial summation properties for magnocellular and parvocellular pathways in glaucoma. *Invest Ophthalmol Vis Sci.* 2009;50:1221–1226.

62. McKendrick AM, Sapson GP, Walland MJ, et al. Contrast sensitivity changes due to glaucoma and normal aging: low-spatial-frequency losses in both magnocellular and parvocellular pathways. *Invest Ophthalmol Vis Sci.* 2007;48:2115–2122.

63. Vaegan, Rahman AM, Sanderson GF. Glaucoma affects steady state VEP contrast thresholds before psychophysics. *Optom Vis Sci.* 2008;85:547–558.

64. Higgins KE, Jaffe MJ, Coletta NJ, et al. Spatial contrast sensitivity. Importance of controlling the patient's visibility criterion. *Arch Ophthalmol.* 1984;102:1035–1041.

65. Vaegan BL, Halliday BL. A forced-choice test improves clinical contrast sensitivity testing. *Br J Ophthalmol.* 1982; 66:477–491.

66. Tweten S, Wall M, Schwartz BD. A comparison of three clinical methods of spatial contrast-sensitivity testing in normal subjects. *Graefes Arch Clin Exp Ophthalmol.* 1990;228:24–27.

67. Regan D, Beverley KI. Visual fields described by contrast sensitivity, by acuity, and by relative sensitivity to different orientations. *Invest Ophthalmol Vis Sci.* 1983;24:754–759.

68. Neima D, LeBlanc R, Regan D. Visual field defects in ocular hypertension and glaucoma. *Arch Ophthalmol.* 1984; 102:1042–1045.

69. Phelps CD. Acuity perimetry and glaucoma [review]. *Trans Am Ophthalmol Soc.* 1984;82:753–791.

70. Yoshiyama KK, Johnson CA. Which method of flicker perimetry is most effective for detection of glaucomatous visual field loss? *Invest Ophthalmol Vis Sci.* 1997;38:2270–2277.

71. Atkin A, Bodis-Wollner I, Wolkstein M, et al. Abnormalities of central contrast sensitivity in glaucoma. *Am J Ophthalmol.* 1979;88:205–211.

72. Tyler CW. Specific deficits of flicker sensitivity in glaucoma and ocular hypertension. *Invest Ophthalmol Vis Sci.* 1981; 20:204–212.

73. Breton ME, Wilson TW, Wilson R, et al. Temporal contrast sensitivity loss in primary open-angle glaucoma and glaucoma suspects. *Invest Ophthalmol Vis Sci.* 1991;32:2931–2941.

74. Lachenmayr BJ, Kojetinsky S, Ostermaier N, et al. The different effects of aging on normal sensitivity in flicker and light-sense perimetry. *Invest Ophthalmol Vis Sci.* 1994;35:2741–2748.

75. Eisner A, Samples JR. Flicker sensitivity and cardiovascular function in healthy middle-aged people. *Arch Ophthalmol.* 2000;118:1049–1055.

76. Tytla ME, Trope GE, Buncic JR. Flicker sensitivity in treated ocular hypertension. *Ophthalmology.* 1990;97:36–43.

77. Prata TS, Piassi MV, Melo LA Jr. Changes in visual function after intraocular pressure reduction using antiglaucoma medications. *Eye.* 2009;23:1081–1085.

78. Regan D, Neima D. Balance between pattern and flicker sensitivities in the visual fields of ophthalmological patients. *Br J Ophthalmol.* 1984;68:310–315.

79. Stelmach LB, Drance SM, Di Lollo V. Two-pulse temporal resolution in patients with glaucoma, suspected glaucoma, and in normal observers. *Am J Ophthalmol.* 1986;102:617–620.

80. Glovinsky Y, Quigley HA, Drum B, et al. A whole-field scotopic retinal sensitivity test for the detection of early glaucoma damage. *Arch Ophthalmol.* 1992;110:486–490.

81. Quigley HA, West SK, Munoz B, et al. Examination methods for glaucoma prevalence surveys. *Arch Ophthalmol.* 1993; 111:1409–1415.

82. Stewart WC, Chorak RP, Murrel HP. Evaluation of the whole-field scotopic retinal sensitivity tester in clinical glaucoma practice. *J Glaucoma.* 1994;3:280–285.

83. Casson EJ, Johnson CA, Nelson-Quigg JM. Temporal modulation perimetry: the effects of aging and eccentricity on sensitivity in normals. *Invest Ophthalmol Vis Sci.* 1993;34:3096–3102.

84. Lachenmayr BJ, Drance SM, Douglas GR, et al. Light-sense, flicker and resolution perimetry in glaucoma: a comparative study. *Graefes Arch Clin Exp Ophthalmol.* 1991;229:246–251.

85. Lachenmayr BJ, Gleissner M. Flicker perimetry resists retinal image degradation. *Invest Ophthalmol Vis Sci.* 1992; 33:3539–3542.

86. Lachenmayr BJ, Drance SM. The selective effects of elevated intraocular pressure on temporal resolution. *Ger J Ophthalmol.* 1992;1:26–31.

87. Johnson CA, Keltner JL, Balestrery FG. Acuity profile perimetry: description of technique and preliminary clinical trials. *Arch Ophthalmol.* 1979;97:684–689.

88. Nutaitis MJ, Stewart WC, Kelly DM, et al. Pattern discrimination perimetry in patients with glaucoma and ocular hypertension. *Am J Ophthalmol.* 1992;114:297–301.

89. Pomerance GN, Evans DW. Test-retest reliability of the CSV-1000 contrast test and its relationship to glaucoma therapy. *Invest Ophthalmol Vis Sci.* 1994;35:3357–3361.

90. Colotto A, Falsini B, Salgarello T, et al. Photopic negative response of the human ERG: losses associated with glaucomatous damage. *Invest Ophthalmol Vis Sci.* 2000;41:2205–2211.

91. Bach M. Electrophysiological approaches for early detection of glaucoma. *Eur J Ophthalmol.* 2001;11(suppl 2):S41–S49.

92. Drasdo N, Aldebasi YH, Chiti Z, et al. The s-cone PHNR and pattern ERG in primary open-angle glaucoma. *Invest Ophthalmol Vis Sci.* 2001;42:1266–1272.

93. Hood DC. Objective measurement of visual function in glaucoma. *Curr Opin Ophthalmol.* 2003;14:78–82.

94. Hood DC, Greenstein VC, Odel JG, et al. Visual field defects and multifocal visual evoked potentials: evidence of a linear relationship. *Arch Ophthalmol.* 2002;120:1672–1681.

95. Hood DC, Zhang X, Hong JE, et al. Quantifying the benefits of additional channels of multifocal VEP recording. *Doc Ophthalmol.* 2002;104:303–320.

96. Johnson CA. Recent developments in automated perimetry in glaucoma diagnosis and management. *Curr Opin Ophthalmol.* 2002;13:77–84.

97. Saraux H, Grall Y, Keller J, et al. Electro-oculography and the glaucomatous eye [in French (author's translation)]. *J Fr Ophtalmol.* 1982;5:243–247.

98. Mulak M, Misiuk-Hojlo M, Kaczmarek R. The role of electrooculographic examinations in the glaucoma diagnosis [in Polish]. *Klin Oczna.* 2000;102:41–43.

99. Bobak P, Bodis-Wollner I, Harnois C, et al. Pattern electroretinograms and visual-evoked potentials in glaucoma and multiple sclerosis. *Am J Ophthalmol.* 1983;96:72–83.

100. Wanger P, Persson HE. Pattern-reversal electroretinograms in unilateral glaucoma. *Invest Ophthalmol Vis Sci.* 1983;24:749–753.

101. Wanger P, Persson HE. Pattern-reversal electroretinograms and high-pass resolution perimetry in suspected or early glaucoma. *Ophthalmology.* 1987;94:1098–1103.

102. Papst N, Bopp M, Schnaudigel OE. Pattern electroretinogram and visually evoked cortical potentials in glaucoma. *Graefes Arch Clin Exp Ophthalmol.* 1984;222:29–33.

103. Price MJ, Drance SM, Price M, et al. The pattern electroretinogram and visual-evoked potential in glaucoma. *Graefes Arch Clin Exp Ophthalmol.* 1988;226:542–547.

104. Korth M, Horn F, Storck B, et al. The pattern-evoked electroretinogram (PERG): age-related alterations and changes in glaucoma. *Graefes Arch Clin Exp Ophthalmol.* 1989;227:123–130.

105. Watanabe I, Iijima H, Tsukahara S. The pattern electroretinogram in glaucoma: an evaluation by relative amplitude from the Bjerrum area. *Br J Ophthalmol.* 1989;73:131–135.

106. Odom JV, Feghali JG, Jin JC, et al. Visual function deficits in glaucoma: electroretinogram pattern and luminance nonlinearities. *Arch Ophthalmol.* 1990;108:222–227.

107. Weinstein GW, Arden GB, Hitchings RA, et al. The pattern electroretinogram (PERG) in ocular hypertension and glaucoma. *Arch Ophthalmol.* 1988;106:923–928.

108. Trick GL, Bickler-Bluth M, Cooper DG, et al. Pattern reversal electroretinogram (PRERG) abnormalities in ocular hypertension: correlation with glaucoma risk factors. *Curr Eye Res.* 1988;7:201–206.

109. Trick GL. PRRP abnormalities in glaucoma and ocular hypertension. *Invest Ophthalmol Vis Sci.* 1986;27:1730–1736.

110. O'Donaghue E, Arden GB, O'Sullivan F, et al. The pattern electroretinogram in glaucoma and ocular hypertension. *Br J Ophthalmol.* 1992;76:387–394.

111. Colotto A, Salgarello T, Giudiceandrea A, et al. Pattern electroretinogram in treated ocular hypertension: a cross-sectional study after timolol maleate therapy. *Ophthalmic Res.* 1995;27:168–177.

112. Bach M, Funk J. Pattern electroretinogram and computerized optic nerve-head analysis in glaucoma suspects. *Ger J Ophthalmol.* 1993;2:178–181.

113. Toffoli G, Vattovani O, Cecchini P, et al. Correlation between the retinal nerve fiber layer thickness and the pattern electroretinogram amplitude. *Ophthalmologica.* 2002;216:159–163.

114. Neoh C, Kaye SB, Brown M, et al. Pattern electroretinogram and automated perimetry in patients with glaucoma and ocular hypertension. *Br J Ophthalmol.* 1994;78:359–362.

115. Graham SL, Wong VA, Drance SM, et al. Pattern electroretinograms from hemifields in normal subjects and patients with glaucoma. *Invest Ophthalmol Vis Sci.* 1994;35:3347–3356.

116. Trick GL, Nesher R, Cooper DG, et al. Dissociation of visual deficits in ocular hypertension. *Invest Ophthalmol Vis Sci.* 1988;29:1486–1491.

117. Johnson MA, Drum BA, Quigley HA, et al. Pattern-evoked potentials and optic nerve fiber loss in monocular laser-induced glaucoma. *Invest Ophthalmol Vis Sci.* 1989;30:897–907.

118. Bayer AU, Erb C. Short wavelength automated perimetry, frequency doubling technology perimetry, and pattern electroretinography for prediction of progressive glaucomatous standard visual field defects. *Ophthalmology.* 2002;109:1009–1017.

119. Siliprandi R, Bucci MG, Canella R, et al. Flash and pattern electroretinograms during and after acute intraocular pressure elevation in cats. *Invest Ophthalmol Vis Sci.* 1988;29:558–565.

120. Vaegan BL, Graham SL, Goldberg I, et al. Flash and pattern electroretinogram changes with optic atrophy and glaucoma. *Exp Eye Res.* 1995; 60:697–706.

121. Sutter EE. Imaging visual function with the multifocal m-sequence technique. *Vision Res.* 2001;41:1241–1255.

122. Hood DC. Assessing retinal function with the multifocal technique. *Prog Retin Eye Res.* 2000;19:607–646.

123. Hood DC, Frishman LJ, Saszik S, et al. Retinal origins of the primate multifocal ERG: implications for the human response. *Invest Ophthalmol Vis Sci.* 2002;43:1673–1685.

124. Klistorner AI, Graham SL, Martins A. Multifocal pattern electroretinogram does not demonstrate localised field defects in glaucoma. *Doc Ophthalmol.* 2000;100:155–165.

125. Fortune B, Johnson CA, Cioffi GA. The topographic relationship between multifocal electroretinographic and behavioral perimetric measures of function in glaucoma. *Optom Vis Sci.* 2001;78:206–214.

126. Fortune B, Bearse MA Jr, Cioffi GA, et al. Selective loss of an oscillatory component from temporal retinal multifocal ERG responses in glaucoma. *Invest Ophthalmol Vis Sci.* 2002;43:2638–2647.

127. Palmowski AM, Allgayer R, Heinemann-Vernaleken B, et al. Multifocal electroretinogram with a multiflash stimulation technique in open-angle glaucoma. *Ophthalmic Res.* 2002; 34:83–89.

128. Hood DC, Odel JG, Chen CS, et al. The multifocal electroretinogram. *J Neuroophthalmol.* 2003;23:225–235.

129. Chu PH, Chan HH, Brown B. Luminance-modulated adaptation of global flash mfERG: fellow eye losses in asymmetric glaucoma. *Invest Ophthalmol Vis Sci.* 2007;48:2626–633.

130. Cappin JM, Nissim S. Visual evoked responses in the assessment of field defects in glaucoma. *Arch Ophthalmol.* 1975;93:9–18.

131. Towle VL, Moskowitz A, Sokol S, et al. The visual evoked potential in glaucoma and ocular hypertension: effects of check size, field size, and stimulation rate. *Invest Ophthalmol Vis Sci.* 1983;24:175–183.

132. Howe JW, Mitchell KW. The objective assessment of contrast sensitivity function by electrophysiological means. *Br J Ophthalmol.* 1984;68:626–638.

133. Mitchell KW, Wood CM, Howe JW, et al. The visual evoked potential in acute primary angle closure glaucoma. *Br J Ophthalmol.* 1989;73:448–456.

134. Quigley HA, Dunkelberger GR, Green WR. Chronic human glaucoma causing selectively greater loss of large optic nerve fibers. *Ophthalmology.* 1988;95:357–363.

135. Schmeisser ET, Smith TJ. High-frequency flicker visual-evoked potential losses in glaucoma. *Ophthalmology.* 1989;96:620–623.

136. Holopigian K, Seiple W, Mayron C, et al. Electrophysiological and psychophysical flicker sensitivity in patients with primary open-angle glaucoma and ocular hypertension. *Invest Ophthalmol Vis Sci.* 1990; 31:1863–1868.

137. Bray LC, Mitchell KW, Howe JW. Prognostic significance of the pattern visual evoked potential in ocular hypertension. *Br J Ophthalmol.* 1991; 75:79–83.

138. Klistorner AI, Graham SL. Early magnocellular loss in glaucoma demonstrated using the pseudorandomly stimulated flash visual evoked potential. *J Glaucoma.* 1999;8:140–148.

139. Korth M, Nguyen NX, Junemann A, et al. VEP test of the blue-sensitive pathway in glaucoma. *Invest Ophthalmol Vis Sci.* 1994;35:2599–2610.

140. Horn FK, Jonas JB, Budde WM, et al. Monitoring glaucoma progression with visual evoked potentials of the blue-sensitive pathway. *Invest Ophthalmol Vis Sci.* 2002;43:1828–1834.

141. Baseler HA, Sutter EE, Klein SA, et al. The topography of visual evoked response properties across the visual field. *Electroencephalogr Clin Neurophysiol.* 1994;90:65–81.

142. Hood DC, Greenstein VC. Multifocal VEP and ganglion cell damage: applications and limitations for the study of glaucoma. *Prog Retin Eye Res.* 2003;22:201–251.

143. Klistorner AI, Graham SL, Grigg JR, et al. Multifocal topographic visual evoked potential: improving objective detection of local visual field defects. *Invest Ophthalmol Vis Sci.* 1998;39:937–950.

144. Klistorner A, Graham SL. Objective perimetry in glaucoma. *Ophthalmology.* 2000;107:2283–2299.

145. Goldberg I, Graham SL, Klistorner AI. Multifocal objective perimetry in the detection of glaucomatous field loss. *Am J Ophthalmol.* 2002;133:29–39.

146. Accornero N, Gregori B, Galie E, et al. A new color VEP procedure discloses asymptomatic visual impairments in optic neuritis and glaucoma suspects. *Acta Neurol Scand.* 2000; 102:258–263.

147. Kohn AN, Moss AP, Podos SM. Relative afferent pupillary defects in glaucoma without characteristic field loss. *Arch Ophthalmol.* 1979;97: 294–296.

148. Thompson HS, Montague P, Cox TA, et al. The relationship between visual acuity, pupillary defect, and visual field loss. *Am J Ophthalmol.* 1982;93:681–688.

149. Brown RH, Zilis JD, Lynch MG, et al. The afferent pupillary defect in asymmetric glaucoma. *Arch Ophthalmol.* 1987; 105:1540–1543.

150. Johnson LN, Hill RA, Bartholomew MJ. Correlation of afferent pupillary defect with visual field loss on automated perimetry. *Ophthalmology.* 1988;95:1649–1655.

151. Browning DJ, Buckley EG. Reliability of brightness comparison testing in predicting afferent pupillary defects. *Arch Ophthalmol.* 1988;106: 341–343.

152. Chen Y, Wyatt HJ, Swanson WH, et al. Rapid pupil-based assessment of glaucomatous damage. *Optom Vis Sci.* 2008;85:471–481.

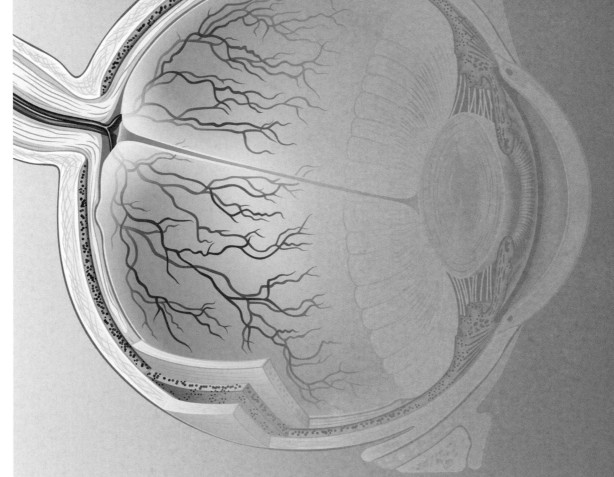

SECTION

II

The Clinical Forms
of Glaucoma

Classification of the Glaucomas

7

APPROACHES TO CLASSIFICATION OF GLAUCOMA

There are several systems by which the glaucomas have been classified. The most commonly used ones are based on (a) etiology—that is, the underlying disorder that leads to an alteration in aqueous humor dynamics or retinal ganglion cell loss or (b) mechanism—that is, the specific alteration in the anterior chamber angle that leads to a rise in intraocular pressure (IOP). One disadvantage of both systems is that they incorrectly suggest that elevated IOP is the primary risk factor in the glaucomas. A second disadvantage is that neither system incorporates the underlying genetic architecture that contributes to the majority of glaucomas. However, until we understand the causes and mechanisms of the glaucomas more completely, these systems provide the most useful ways to classify the glaucomas.

CLASSIFICATION BASED ON ETIOLOGY

The glaucomas have traditionally been divided on the basis of primary and secondary forms. This division is arbitrary and artificial, however, in that all glaucomas are secondary to some abnormality, whether inherited or environmental. The historical basis for this division was the assumption that the initial events leading to outflow obstruction and IOP elevation in those glaucomas called primary (e.g., open-angle, angle-closure, and congenital) are confined to the anterior chamber angle or conventional outflow pathway, with no apparent contribution from other ocular or systemic disorders. These conditions typically are bilateral and probably have a genetic basis. In contrast, other glaucomas have been classified as secondary because of a partial understanding of underlying, predisposing ocular or systemic events. These latter glaucomas may be unilateral or bilateral, and some may have a genetic basis, whereas others are acquired.

In reality, the concept of primary and secondary glaucomas largely reflects our incomplete understanding of the pathophysiologic events that ultimately lead to glaucomatous optic atrophy and visual field loss. As our knowledge of the mechanisms underlying the causes of the glaucomas continues to expand, the primary and secondary classifications become increasingly artificial and inadequate. Furthermore, glaucomas caused by developmental anomalies of the anterior chamber angle do not fit neatly into either category. For these reasons, we recommend replacing traditional concepts with a new scheme that provides a better working foundation for the concepts of mechanism, diagnosis, and therapy that will shape the management of the

glaucomas for the foreseeable future. This classification is used in this text for the discussion of the various forms of glaucoma.

Stages of Glaucoma

Glaucomas can be considered to consist of five stages:

Stage 1—initiating events
Stage 2—structural alterations
Stage 3—functional alterations
Stage 4—retinal ganglion cell and optic nerve damage
Stage 5—visual loss

The initiating events (stage 1) include the condition or series of conditions that set in motion the chain of events that may eventually lead to optic nerve damage and visual loss, but which precede any pathologic or physiologic alterations related to aqueous humor dynamics or optic nerve function. Structural alterations (stage 2) are those tissue changes that precede, but may eventually lead to, alterations of aqueous humor dynamics or optic nerve function. Functional alterations (stage 3) are those physiologic abnormalities that may lead indirectly or directly to optic nerve damage. Optic nerve damage (stage 4) represents the loss of retinal ganglion cells and their associated axons as a result of the events in stage 3, which eventually leads to progressive loss of vision (stage 5). The first three stages can be further subdivided into events that are pressure related and those that are pressure independent (**Table 7.1**).

In the pressure-related subdivision, the initiating events (stage 1) are the conditions that may lead to structural alterations in the aqueous outflow system. In some glaucomas, this could be a genetic defect with an associated protein abnormality; in other glaucomas, this may be due to acquired events, such as trauma, inflammation, or a retinal vascular disorder, some of which may also have a genetic predisposition or may be indirectly influenced by genetic disorders. The structural alterations (stage 2) are tissue changes in the outflow system, which may lead to increased resistance to aqueous outflow and subsequent elevation of the IOP. Such changes might be subtle alterations in the endothelial cells or extracellular matrix of the trabecular meshwork or more obvious obstructive mechanisms, such as membranes over the anterior chamber angle, scar tissue in the meshwork, intertrabecular debris, or developmental anomalies. These changes can sometimes be detected by gonioscopy. The functional alterations (stage 3) include obstruction to aqueous outflow that is sufficient to increase the IOP, which (in pressure-related glaucoma mechanisms) may lead to the glaucomatous optic neuropathy (stage 4) and eventually to progressive loss of visual field (stage 5). Another

Table 7.1	A Staging System for Glaucoma	
Stage	**Defining Aspect**	**Events**
1. Initiating events	The series of events that may lead to stages 2–5	Pressure-related: genetic, acquired Pressure-independent: genetic, toxic, or acquired susceptibility to apoptosis or ganglion cell death
2. Early structural alterations	Tissue changes	Pressure-related: alterations in aqueous outflow system Pressure-independent: alterations related to ganglion cells or optic nerve head (e.g., vascular, structural, or physiologic)
3. Functional alterations	Physiologic changes	Pressure-related: elevated IOP Pressure-independent: reduced axonal conduction, vascular perfusion, laminar deformity, others
4. Optic nerve damage	Retinal ganglion cell and axon loss	Glaucomatous optic neuropathy and visual field loss
5. Visual loss	Progressive loss of visual field	Glaucomatous optic neuropathy and visual field loss

emerging possibility is that cerebrospinal fluid pressure may be abnormally low or high, thus affecting the translamina cribrosa pressure gradient, weakening structural support to axons (as described in Chapter 4).

The specific events in the pressure-independent subdivision are not as well understood and are, in large part, only speculative. The initiating events (stage 1) probably have a genetic basis, however, with alterations in proteins that may lead to structural changes directly related to the ganglion cells or optic nerve head. The structural alterations (stage 2) may be subtle tissue changes in blood vessels supplying the optic nerve head or in supportive elements of the lamina cribrosa or, likely, in additional ways that are not yet understood. The functional alterations (stage 3) may be reduced axonal conduction, vascular perfusion to axons in the optic nerve head, or a progressive deformity of the lamina cribrosa that may lead (alone or in conjunction with a relative IOP elevation) to glaucomatous optic neuropathy (stage 4) and subsequent loss of visual field (stage 5).

Although our knowledge of the first three stages that lead to optic nerve damage and our ability to detect and treat these events are incomplete for most glaucomas, there are some glaucomas for which we have not only a partial knowledge of the events in each stage but also treatments for early intervention at stage 1. In neovascular glaucoma, for example, an initiating event (stage 1) may be a central retinal vein occlusion, which can lead to release of vascular endothelial growth factor and other cytokines that may lead to a structural alteration (stage 2) in the form of a fibrovascular membrane over the anterior chamber angle, which may eventually cause a functional alteration (stage 3) by obstructing aqueous outflow with a rise in IOP, which usually leads to optic nerve damage (stage 4) and eventual loss of visual field (stage 5). An understanding of this sequence provides a rational basis for early intervention with panretinal photocoagulation at stage 1 in selected patients. Such an approach to diagnosis and management should be the

ultimate goal for all forms of glaucoma. As the initial events for an increasing number of the glaucomas become known, a complete classification scheme may eventually be developed on the basis of these initial events. However, until continued research provides the answers to these gaps in our knowledge, the etiologic classification scheme shown in **Table 7.2** can be developed only partially.

Chronic Open-Angle Glaucomas

This category of glaucomas constitutes at least half of all the glaucomas and has been referred to by various names, including primary open-angle glaucoma, chronic open-angle glaucoma, and chronic simple glaucoma. To de-emphasize use of the "primary" and "secondary" terminology in glaucoma, the term chronic open-angle glaucoma is used in this text. A more appropriate term, however, might be idiopathic open-angle glaucoma, because our failure to provide more precise terminology stems from our lack of knowledge regarding the related mechanisms.

Although the initial events leading to chronic open-angle glaucoma are unknown, there is mounting evidence that inherited susceptibilities lead to increased resistance to aqueous outflow and increased vulnerability of the optic nerve head to a particular IOP level.

Pupillary Block Glaucoma

Among the so-called primary angle-closure glaucomas, the most common variation is pupillary block glaucoma. The term pupillary block glaucoma is best reserved for situations with evidence of optic nerve damage related to the angle-closure mechanism. A considerable amount of information is available regarding the initial events and mechanisms of outflow obstruction in pupillary block glaucoma. Therefore, there is no

Table 7.2	Classification of the Glaucomas Based on Initial Events

A. Open-angle glaucomas without other known ocular or systemic disorders
   1. Chronic open-angle glaucoma
   2. Normal-tension glaucoma

B. Angle-closure glaucomas without other known ocular or systemic disorders
   1. Pupillary block glaucomas
   2. Combined mechanism glaucoma

C. Developmental glaucomas
   1. Congenital glaucoma
   2. Juvenile open-angle glaucoma (overlap with chronic open-angle glaucoma)
   3. Axenfeld–Rieger syndrome
   4. Peters anomaly
   5. Aniridia
   6. Other developmental anomalies

D. Glaucomas associated with other ocular and systemic disorders
   1. Glaucomas associated with disorders of the corneal endothelium
      a. Iridocorneal endothelial syndrome
      b. Posterior polymorphous dystrophy
      c. Fuchs endothelial corneal dystrophy
   2. Glaucomas associated with disorders of the iris and ciliary body
      a. Pigmentary glaucoma
      b. Iridoschisis
      c. Plateau iris
      d. Iris and ciliary body cysts
   3. Glaucoma associated with disorders of the lens
      a. Exfoliation syndrome
      b. Glaucomas associated with cataracts
      c. Glaucomas associated with lens dislocation
   4. Glaucomas associated with disorders of the retina, choroid, and vitreous
      a. Neovascular glaucoma
      b. Glaucomas associated with retinal detachment and vitreoretinal abnormalities
   5. Glaucomas associated with intraocular tumors
      a. Malignant melanoma
      b. Retinoblastoma
      c. Metastatic carcinoma
      d. Leukemias and lymphomas
      e. Benign tumors
   6. Glaucomas associated with elevated episcleral venous pressure
   7. Glaucomas associated with inflammation
      a. Glaucomas associated with uveitis
      b. Glaucomas associated with keratitis, episcleritis, and scleritis
   8. Steroid-induced glaucoma
   9. Glaucomas associated with ocular trauma
   10. Glaucomas associated with hemorrhage
   11. Glaucomas after intraocular surgery
      a. Ciliary block (malignant) glaucoma
      b. Glaucomas in pseudophakia and aphakia
      c. Epithelial, fibrous, and endothelial proliferation
      d. Glaucomas associated with corneal surgery
      e. Glaucomas associated with vitreoretinal surgery

basis for distinguishing this condition—considered a primary glaucoma—from other disorders previously classified as secondary glaucomas. Pupillary block glaucoma may be divided into acute and subacute forms, although these forms merely represent different clinical manifestations, which can both occur at different times in the same patient. A third form, called chronic angle-closure glaucoma, is characterized by the presence of peripheral anterior synechiae. With a subset of chronic angle-closure glaucomas called creeping angle-closure glaucoma, peripheral anterior synechiae slowly advance forward circumferentially, making the iris insertion appear to become more and more anterior. With another form called combined mechanism glaucoma, IOP elevation persists after peripheral iridotomy for the angle-closure component, despite an open, normal-appearing anterior chamber angle. Some classification schemes have included the plateau iris syndrome with primary angle-closure glaucomas, although recent studies of the mechanism suggest that it might more appropriately be included with glaucomas associated with disorders of the iris and ciliary body (1).

Developmental Anomalies of the Anterior Chamber Angle

Numerous developmental disorders associated with anomalies of the anterior chamber angle can lead to IOP elevation. The initial event is probably a genetic defect in most cases, although some cases may stem from an acquired, intrauterine insult. The developmental anomaly may be a high insertion of the anterior uvea in the trabecular meshwork, incomplete development of the meshwork or Schlemm canal, or broad iridocorneal adhesions. One group of developmental glaucomas was previously classified with the primary glaucomas because it has no apparent consistent association with other ocular or systemic anomalies. This group includes congenital, or infantile, glaucoma and juvenile open-angle glaucoma, which differ primarily by the age of onset. Other conditions in this category have a wide range of associated ocular and systemic developmental abnormalities. Additional developmental disorders, such as those associated with the vitreous and retina, may lead to glaucoma, usually by an angle-closure mechanism; in the present scheme, these disorders are classified as glaucomas associated with abnormalities of a particular ocular structure (e.g., persistent hyperplastic primary vitreous).

Glaucomas Associated with Other Ocular Disorders

It is this large group of glaucomas that was previously classified as secondary glaucomas. In some cases, the initial events involve an abnormality of a specific ocular structure, such as the corneal endothelium, iris, ciliary body, lens, retina, choroid, or vitreous. In other cases, the initial events may involve a tumor, inflammation, hemorrhage, or accidental or surgical trauma. Many of these initial events are influenced by an inherited susceptibility, whereas others are acquired. Each of these broad categories of glaucoma usually contains subdivisions, based on different series of events that eventually lead to outflow obstruction.

A Note on Molecular Etiology

Now that several genes have been localized for various glaucomas, the hope of being able to reclassify these disorders on the basis of molecular etiology is being realized (2). Although separating patients with adult-onset chronic open-angle glaucoma on the basis of phenotype is difficult, the molecular classification has already allowed us to recognize several genetic forms of glaucoma. Characterizing additional genes and mutations will be extremely helpful in classifying disease in individual patients, with a view to being able to provide tailored prognostic and therapeutic information (as discussed in Chapter 8). Some glaucomas may be associated with more than one gene, such as the Axenfeld–Rieger syndrome, which appears to be caused by at least three different genes located on chromosomes 4, 6, and 13, once again underscoring genetic heterogeneity (3–6). Others are non-Mendelian or complex, and probably involve more than one gene plus environmental factors. An example is exfoliative glaucoma, in which polymorphisms of the *LOXL1* gene are strongly associated with this condition in multiple populations (see Chapter 15).

In addition, molecular genetics is helping to associate seemingly disparate diseases. For example, Rieger syndrome and iris hypoplasia can arise from mutations in the same gene on 4q25 (*PITX2*) (7). Similarly, juvenile open-angle glaucoma and iridogoniodysgenesis can be caused by mutations in the *FKHL7* gene on 6p25 (8,9). Improved understanding of the molecular etiology of various glaucomas will permit detailed reclassification of these disorders.

CLASSIFICATION BASED ON MECHANISM

An understanding of the initial events in each form of glaucoma will eventually allow for an improved classification system and a rationale for early glaucoma intervention. Until that information becomes available, however, most treatment strategies will continue to focus on IOP and depend on an understanding of the mechanisms of aqueous outflow obstruction.

As noted previously, one disadvantage of a classification based on the mechanism of aqueous outflow obstruction is that it ignores the causes unrelated to pressure. In addition, many of the glaucomas have more than one mechanism of outflow obstruction at different times in the course of the disease. As a result, some glaucomas must be classified under more than one mechanistic heading. It is for this reason that a classification based on initial events, rather than mechanisms of outflow obstruction, is used for organizing the chapters on clinical forms of glaucoma in this text.

On the other hand, the mechanistic classification has distinct advantages. First, our understanding of the mechanisms of aqueous outflow obstruction is in many cases more complete than our knowledge of the initial events. Second, because most current treatment strategies are directed at reducing IOP, an understanding of the mechanism that leads to aqueous outflow obstruction is important in developing a rationale for controlling the pressure in each form of glaucoma.

Barkan (10) first recognized the distinction between open-angle and closed-angle forms of glaucoma, which led to the basis for the mechanistic classification of the glaucomas (**Fig. 7.1**). A third group of glaucomas that does not fit well into either the open- or closed-angle mechanisms is the developmental glaucomas. The mechanistic classification, therefore, can be divided into three categories: (a) open-angle glaucoma mechanisms, (b) angle-closure glaucoma

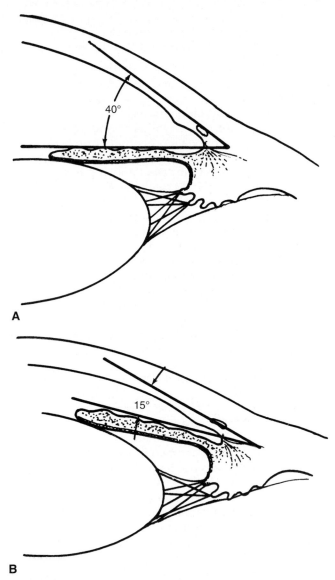

A

B

Figure 7.1 The angle of the anterior chamber is formed by the cornea and iris. **A:** The typical configuration in open-angle forms of glaucoma. **B:** The narrow angle that typically precedes most forms of angle-closure glaucoma.

mechanisms, and (c) developmental anomalies of the anterior chamber angle (**Table 7.3** and **Fig. 7.2**).

Open-Angle Glaucoma Mechanisms

The open-angle mechanisms are those in which the anterior chamber angle structures (i.e., trabecular meshwork, scleral spur, and ciliary body band) are visible by gonioscopy. The elements obstructing aqueous outflow may be located on the anterior chamber side of the trabecular meshwork (pretrabecular mechanisms); in the trabeculum (trabecular mechanisms); or distal to the meshwork, in the Schlemm canal, or further along the aqueous drainage system (posttrabecular mechanisms).

In the pretrabecular mechanisms, a translucent membrane extends across the open iridocorneal angle, leading to the obstruction of aqueous outflow. This obstructive element may be a fibrovascular membrane, an endothelial layer with a Descemet-like membrane, an epithelial membrane, a connective tissue membrane, or an inflammatory-related membrane.

With the trabecular mechanisms, the obstruction to aqueous outflow is located in the trabecular meshwork. The chronic open-angle glaucomas are included in this category, although the precise mechanisms of the obstruction are unknown. As previously noted, this category of the glaucomas likely represents distinct entities with differing mechanisms of outflow obstruction. In other glaucomas with a trabecular mechanism, there may be a "clogging" of the meshwork with red blood cells, macrophages, neoplastic cells, pigment particles, protein, lens zonules, viscoelastic agents, or vitreous. In still other cases, obstruction to outflow may result from acquired alterations of the trabecular meshwork tissue such as obstruction associated with inflammatory conditions, trauma with subsequent scarring, and toxic reactions associated with intraocular foreign bodies. Steroid-induced glaucoma and certain glaucomas associated with systemic diseases can lead to obstruction of aqueous outflow in the trabecular meshwork.

With the posttrabecular mechanisms, obstruction to aqueous outflow may result from increased resistance in the Schlemm canal due to collapse or absence of the canal, or, in patients with sickle cell anemia, from obstruction of the canal itself with sickled red blood cells. The role of collector channel obstruction remains a largely unexplored possibility. Perhaps the most common cause of the posttrabecular cases is elevated episcleral venous pressure.

Angle-Closure Glaucoma Mechanisms

The angle-closure mechanisms include situations in which the peripheral iris is in apposition to the trabecular meshwork or peripheral cornea. The peripheral iris may either be "pulled" (anterior mechanisms) or "pushed" (posterior mechanisms) into this position.

In the anterior mechanisms of angle-closure glaucoma, an abnormal tissue bridges the anterior chamber angle and subsequently undergoes contraction, pulling the peripheral iris into the iridocorneal angle. Examples of the contracting tissue include a fibrovascular membrane, an endothelial layer with a Descemet-like membrane, and inflammatory precipitates.

With the posterior mechanisms, pressure behind the iris, lens, or vitreous causes the peripheral iris to be pushed into the anterior chamber angle. This may occur with or without pupillary block.

Posterior mechanisms with pupillary block include pupillary block glaucoma (as previously described). Functional apposition between the peripupillary iris and lens in this condition increases resistance of aqueous humor flow into the anterior chamber, resulting in a relative increase in posterior chamber pressure and forward bowing of the peripheral iris. The functional apposition in these patients is due to a genetically influenced configuration of the anterior ocular segment. In other conditions, the same functional apposition may result from an acquired forward shift of the lens (e.g., intumescent cataract or subluxed lens). In still other cases, a pupillary block

OPEN-ANGLE GLAUCOMA MECHANISMS

A. Pretrabecular (membrane overgrowth)
   1. Fibrovascular membrane (neovascular glaucoma)
   2. Endothelial layer, often with Descemet-like membrane
      a. Iridocorneal endothelial syndrome
      b. Posterior polymorphous dystrophy
      c. Penetrating and nonpenetrating trauma
   3. Epithelial downgrowth
   4. Fibrous ingrowth
   5. Inflammatory membrane
      a. Fuchs heterochromic iridocyclitis
      b. Luetic interstitial keratitis
B. Trabecular (occlusion of intertrabecular spaces)
   1. Idiopathic
      a. Chronic open-angle glaucoma
      b. Steroid-induced glaucoma
   2. Obstruction of trabecular meshwork
      a. Red blood cells
         (1) Hemorrhagic glaucoma
         (2) Ghost cell glaucoma
      b. Macrophages
         (1) Hemolytic glaucoma
         (2) Phacolytic glaucoma
         (3) Melanomalytic glaucoma
      c. Neoplastic cells
         (1) Malignant tumors
         (2) Neurofibromatosis
         (3) Nevus of Ota
         (4) Juvenile xanthogranuloma
      d. Pigment particles
         (1) Pigmentary glaucoma
         (2) Exfoliation syndrome
         (3) Uveitis
         (4) Malignant melanoma
      e. Protein
         (1) Uveitis
         (2) Lens-induced glaucoma
      f. Viscoelastic agents
      g. α-Chymotrypsin–induced glaucoma
      h. Vitreous
   3. Alterations of the trabecular meshwork
      a. Edema
         (1) Uveitis (trabeculitis)
         (2) Scleritis and episcleritis
         (3) Alkali burns
      b. Trauma (angle recession)
      c. Intraocular foreign bodies (hemosiderosis, chalcosis)
C. Posttrabecular
   1. Obstruction of Schlemm canal
      a. Collapse of canal
      b. Obstruction of Schlemm canal (e.g., sickled red blood cells)
   2. Elevated episcleral venous pressure
      a. Carotid-cavernous fistula
      b. Cavernous sinus thrombosis
      c. Retrobulbar tumors
      d. Thyrotropic exophthalmos
      e. Superior vena cava obstruction
      f. Mediastinal tumors
      g. Sturge–Weber syndrome
      h. Elevated episcleral venous pressure

ANGLE-CLOSURE GLAUCOMA MECHANISMS

A. Anterior ("pulling" mechanism)
   1. Contracture of membranes
      a. Neovascular glaucoma
      b. Iridocorneal endothelial syndrome
      c. Posterior polymorphous dystrophy
      d. Penetrating and nonpenetrating trauma
   2. Contracture of inflammatory precipitates
B. Posterior ("pushing" mechanism)
   1. With pupillary block
      a. Pupillary block glaucoma
      b. Lens-induced mechanisms
         (1) Intumescent lens
         (2) Subluxation of lens
         (3) Mobile lens syndrome
      c. Posterior synechiae
         (1) Iris–intraocular lens block in pseudophakia
         (2) Uveitis with posterior synechiae
         (3) Iris–vitreous block in aphakia
   2. Without pupillary block
      a. Plateau iris syndrome
      b. Ciliary block (malignant) glaucoma
      c. Lens-induced mechanisms
         (1) Intumescent lens
         (2) Subluxation of lens
         (3) Mobile lens syndrome
      d. After lens extraction (forward vitreous shift)
      e. Secondary to scleral buckling surgery
      f. Secondary to panretinal photocoagulation
      g. Central retinal vein occlusion
      h. Intraocular tumors
         (1) Malignant melanoma
         (2) Retinoblastoma
      i. Cysts of the iris and ciliary body
      j. Retrolenticular tissue contracture
         (1) Retinopathy of prematurity (retrolental fibroplasia)
         (2) Persistent hyperplastic primary vitreous

DEVELOPMENTAL ANOMALIES OF THE ANTERIOR CHAMBER ANGLE

A. High insertion of anterior uvea
   1. Congenital (infantile) glaucoma
   2. Juvenile glaucoma
   3. Glaucomas associated with other developmental anomalies
B. Incomplete development of trabecular meshwork/Schlemm canal
   1. Axenfeld–Rieger syndrome
   2. Peters anomaly
   3. Glaucomas associated with other developmental anomalies
C. Iridocorneal adhesions
   1. Broad strands (Axenfeld–Rieger syndrome)
   2. Fine strands that contract to close angle (aniridia)

[a]Clinical examples cited in this table do not represent an all-inclusive list of the glaucomas.

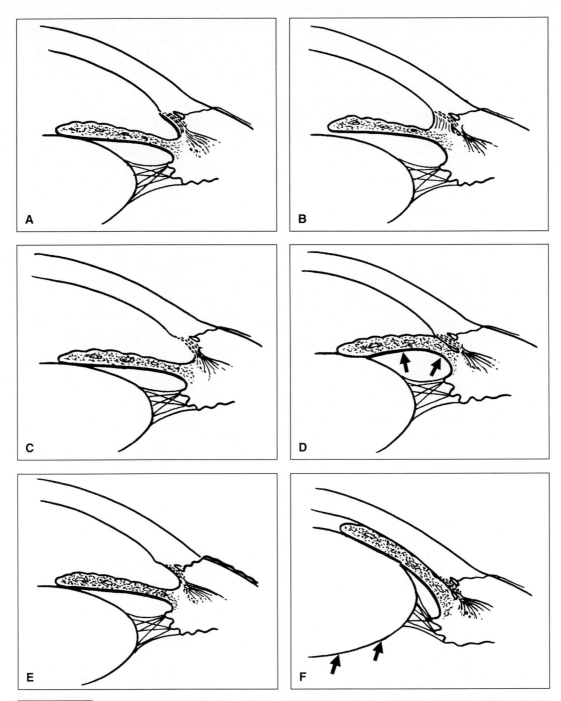

Figure 7.2 Open-angle forms of glaucoma may be of the pretrabecular (**A**), trabecular (**B**), or post-trabecular (**C**) type. Angle-closure forms of glaucoma may be of the anterior "pulling" type (**D**) or the posterior "pushing" type. The latter may occur with (**E**) or without (**F**) pupillary block. *Arrows* indicate location of force pushing the iris or lens–iris diaphragm forward. A third basic mechanism is developmental abnormalities of the anterior chamber angle.

may be due to posterior synechia associated with inflammation of the anterior ocular segment. In each of these conditions, apposition between the iris and the lens, intraocular lens, or vitreous obstructs the flow of aqueous humor into the anterior chamber, resulting in increased pressure in the posterior chamber and forward bowing of the peripheral iris into the anterior chamber angle.

In the posterior mechanisms of angle-closure glaucoma without pupillary block, increased pressure in the posterior portion of the eye pushes the lens–iris or vitreous–iris diaphragm forward. Examples include malignant (ciliary block) glaucoma, plateau iris syndrome, intraocular tumors, cysts of the iris and ciliary body, and contracture of retrolenticular tissue.

Developmental Anomalies of the Anterior Chamber Angle

These glaucomas are not readily separated into open-angle and angle-closure mechanisms, but typically represent incomplete development of structures in the conventional aqueous outflow pathway. Clinically recognized developmental defects include a high insertion of the anterior uvea, as in congenital (infantile) glaucoma, and many of the glaucomas associated with other developmental abnormalities. In other cases, the defect may manifest as an incompletely developed trabecular meshwork or Schlemm canal (e.g., Peters anomaly) or as iridocorneal adhesions (e.g., Axenfeld–Rieger syndrome).

KEY POINTS

- The many clinical forms of glaucoma are commonly classified by (a) cause or (b) mechanism. The former is based on the underlying disorder that leads through a multistage pathway to alterations in aqueous humor dynamics or optic neuropathy with subsequent visual field loss.

- The mechanistic classification is based on alterations in the anterior chamber angle, which may result from the underlying initiating abnormality and lead to the elevated IOP. The mechanistic classification is divided into open-angle and angle-closure mechanisms and developmental anomalies of the anterior chamber angle. These groups are then subdivided according to the underlying cause and specific structural alterations.

- The ongoing revolution in molecular genetics will likely change our current understanding of disease. This new knowledge will increasingly guide the classification of many types of glaucoma (as discussed in Chapter 8).

REFERENCES

1. Pavlin CJ, Ritch R, Foster FS. Ultrasound biomicroscopy in plateau iris syndrome. *Am J Ophthalmol.* 1992;113:390–395.
2. Alward WLM. Molecular genetics of glaucoma: effects on the future of disease classification. In: Van Buskirk EM, Shields MB, eds. *100 Years of Progress in Glaucoma.* Philadelphia, PA: Lippincott-Raven; 1997:143.
3. Semina EV, Reiter R, Leysens NJ, et al. Cloning and characterization of a novel bicoid-related homeobox transcription factor gene, RIEG, involved in Rieger syndrome. *Nat Genet.* 1996;14:392–399.
4. Mirzayans F, Gould DB, Heon E, et al. Axenfeld-Rieger syndrome resulting from mutation of the FKHL7 gene on chromosome 6p25. *Eur J Hum Genet.* 2000;8(1):71–74.
5. Phillips JC, del Bono EA, Haines JL, et al. A second locus for Rieger syndrome maps to chromosome 13q14. *Am J Hum Genet.* 1996;59(3):613–619.
6. Allingham RR, Liu Y, Rhee DJ. The genetics of primary open-angle glaucoma: a review. *Exp Eye Res.* 2009;88:837–844.
7. Héon E, Sheth BP, Kalenak JW, et al. Linkage of autosomal dominant iris hypoplasia to the region of the Rieger syndrome locus. *Hum Mol Genet.* 1995;4:1435–1439.
8. Nishimura D, Swiderski R, Alward W, et al. The forkhead transcription factor gene FKHL7 is responsible for glaucoma phenotypes which map to 6p25. *Nat Genet.* 1998;19:140–147.
9. Mears AJ, Jordan T, Mirzayans F, et al. Mutations of the forkhead/winged-helix gene, FKHL7, in patients with Axenfeld-Rieger anomaly. *Am J Hum Genet.* 1998;63:1316–1328.
10. Barkan O. Glaucoma: classification, causes, and surgical control—results of microgonioscopic research. *Am J Ophthalmol.* 1938;21:1099–1117.

Molecular Genetics and Pharmacogenomics of the Glaucomas

8

This chapter introduces the reader to the shift from a "single gene, rare disease" concept to a "complex and multiple gene disease" model. By reading this chapter, you will learn about the expectations of how genomic testing will pave the way to individualized treatment for patients with various forms of glaucoma. It begins with highlighting the difference between single genes, which when mutated may result in striking clinical phenotypes (e.g., Axenfeld–Rieger syndrome), versus genes that may have DNA sequence variants (known as polymorphisms) that, with or without environmental contributions, can be associated with more common forms of glaucoma (e.g., exfoliation syndrome). Insights into the etiology and pathogenesis of various forms of glaucoma gleaned from analysis of DNA, RNA, or protein are then described. These insights will likely lead to new targets for glaucoma therapy that are beyond simply lowering intraocular pressure (IOP). The chapter ends with a discussion of pharmacogenomics and how genomic testing may help clinicians develop more rational, personalized treatment for their patients.

This chapter begins with three cases to illustrate the promising application of molecular medicine in the clinical context.

CASES

Please review each of these clinical scenarios and keep them in mind as you go through this chapter. Comments will be made on each of these cases later in the chapter.

Case 1

A 17-year-old female patient presents to your office reporting blurred and gradually decreasing vision. On examination, her visual acuity is 20/20 OU and the IOP is 30 mm Hg OU. Her angles are open and normal by gonioscopy. Central corneal thicknesses measure 503 μm OD and 498 μm OS. She has near-total cupping of both optic nerves (**Fig. 8.1A**). Visual field testing demonstrates defects within 10 degrees of fixation OU (**Fig. 8.1B**).

On inquiring further, you learn that her mother and sister also have glaucoma that developed relatively early in life. The mother is blind in one eye, and the sister's eyes are stable after having glaucoma surgery in both eyes.

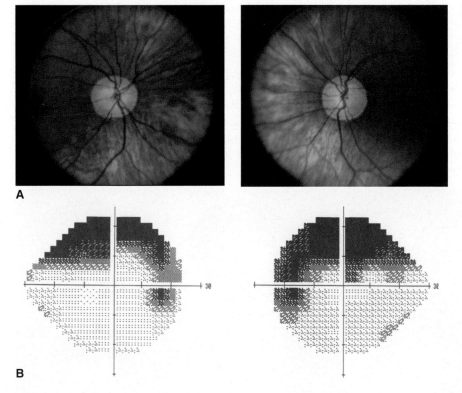

A

B

Figure 8.1 Optic disc photos (**A**) showing very thin neuroretinal rim in each eye. Visual fields (**B**) showing advanced nerve fiber bundle defects encroaching on fixation in the left visual field and within 10 degrees in the right visual field.

The authors gratefully acknowledge David Murrel and David M. Reed for their assistance with artwork in Chapters 8 and 27

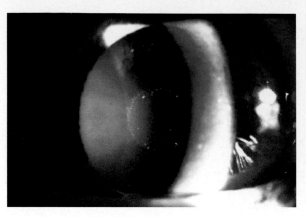
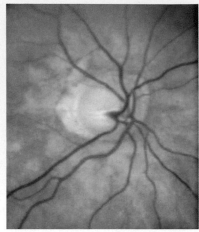

The patient asks several insightful questions:
1. What do I have?
2. Will I go blind if I don't receive treatment, and what is my best treatment option?
3. What are the chances that any future biological children of mine would also get this disease?
4. Can anything be done other than medications and surgery to treat my condition?

Case 2

A 40-year-old Scandinavian man has a mother with advanced exfoliative glaucoma (**Fig. 8.2**). He wants to know his chances of developing the same condition.

Case 3

A 68-year-old woman presents for advice about her glaucoma diagnosis and its impact on her children. She brings along her personal "smart card" that contains her medical history, past visual fields, optic disc imaging, and genomic sequence.

At diagnosis, her IOPs measured 33 mm Hg in both eyes, and her central corneal thickness measurements were 584 μm OD and 566 μm OS. She was otherwise asymptomatic, and she

was treated for glaucoma on the basis of the appearance of the neuroretinal rim of her optic disc (**Fig. 8.3**).

Over the following 18 years, her IOPs fluctuated between 7 mm Hg and 13 mm Hg with medical and surgical treatments. Despite this management, she developed progressive cupping of the optic disc and visual field loss (Fig. 8.3, *center* and *right*) over time. She asks: "Will the same thing happen to my children?"

THE HUMAN GENOME

Genes for glaucoma are found throughout the human genome (**Fig. 8.4**). There are approximately 20,500 genes encoded in the 6 billion base pairs that make up human DNA distributed on 46 chromosomes (1). In addition, 37 "mitochondrial" genes are encoded in the circular mitochondrial DNA that is inherited through the mother. An offshoot of the Human Genome Project (http://www.genome.gov/10001772) was the International HapMap project (http://www.hapmap.org/), which permitted the identification and cataloguing of genetic sequence variants among individuals across diverse populations. These variants are known as single-nucleotide polymorphisms, or SNPs (pronounced "snips"). These SNPs are recognized as markers for

Figure 8.3 Case demonstrating progression of glaucoma based on right optic disc photos (**A**) and right visual fields (**B**) over 18 years despite medical and surgical treatments with IOP reduction and fluctuation between 7 and 13 mm Hg. (Modified from Moroi SE, Richards JE. Glaucoma and genomic medicine. *Glaucoma Today.* 2008;1:16–24, with permission.)

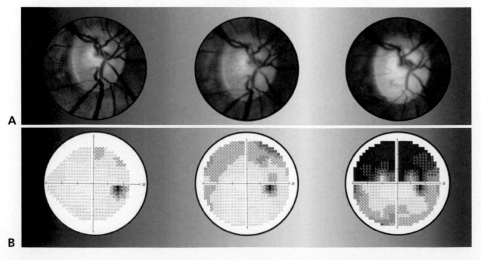

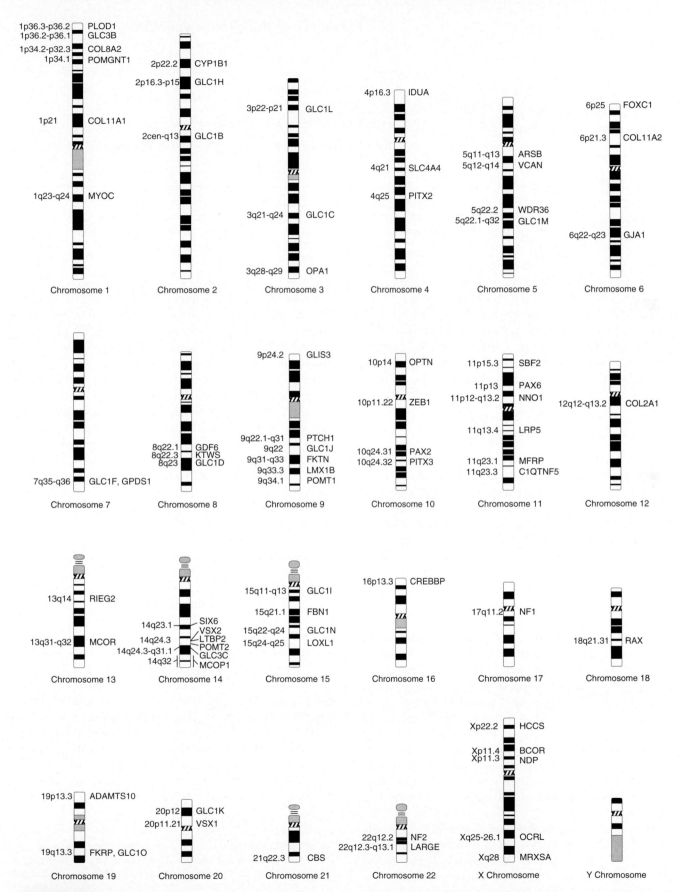

Figure 8.4 Chromosomal location of genes and loci for various forms of open- or closed-angle glaucoma are found throughout the human genome. Only the Y chromosome is believed not to harbor a gene or locus for glaucoma.

Frequency of the genetic variation

		High	Low
Penetrance of the genetic variation	High	Linkage and association approaches	Linkage approach
	Low	Association approach	Remains a challenge

Figure 8.5 Overview of application of linkage and association approaches to identify genes as markers for complex diseases and quantitative traits. The appropriate approach selected for a study depends on the frequency of the genetic variant and the penetrance of the disease mutation. (Modified from Moroi SM, Raoof DA, Reed DM, et al. Progress toward personalized medicine for glaucoma. *Expert Rev Ophthalmol.* 2009;4(2):145–161.)

chromosomal regions where genetic variants are shared among individuals of a given ethnic group. By taking advantage of these conserved DNA blocks marked by these SNPs, early successes have shown promise to identify certain SNPs as potential markers for disease. Future research may shed further insight on disease onset, disease severity, and treatment response, thus paving the way toward the advent of "personalized medicine."

Mendelian ("Single Gene") versus Non-Mendelian (Complex) Diseases

Mendelian disorders are typically rare diseases that follow Mendelian patterns of inheritance—the laws of segregation of alleles and the law of independent assortment. Common examples of Mendelian patterns of inheritance include autosomal-dominant, autosomal-recessive, and X-linked inheritance. Clinicians are familiar with these rare or uncommon clinical disorders because of the striking clinical phenotypes, such as juvenile open-angle glaucoma (JOAG), illustrated in Case 1, and others involving anterior segment dysgenesis, such as Axenfeld–Rieger syndrome. The genetics of such cases represent the "single gene—single disease" model.

In contrast, non-Mendelian, or complex, disorders do not follow the classical rules of Mendelian inheritance. Examples include quantitative traits that result from the additive effects of many genetic or environmental effects, polygenic traits that happen only if defects are present in more than one gene, traits displaying incomplete penetrance, codominant inheritance in which each of the three genotypic combinations for an allele have a different phenotype, imprinting effects caused by chemical modifications to the DNA, or mitochondrial inheritance. Representative conditions and diseases include exfoliation, normal-tension glaucoma, and chronic open-angle glaucoma (COAG).

There are various approaches used to identify a single gene or multiple genes that are involved in inherited disorders. These approaches can also be applied to the discovery of genes underlying treatment outcomes in the field of pharmacogenetics (how an individual's genes affect the way the individual's body responds to a medication or treatment) and pharmacogenomics (the study of drug responses in the context of the entire genome).

(The topic of pharmacogenetics and pharmacogenomics is addressed later in this chapter.) The selection of a particular approach or method depends on the frequency of the disease mutation and the penetrance of the mutation (the frequency with which the presence of a particular genotype in an organism results in the corresponding phenotype) (**Fig. 8.5**).

Two common approaches used to identify genetic variants that contribute to inherited diseases are termed linkage analysis and association analysis. Linkage studies involve genetic mapping based on the cotransmission of genetic markers and phenotypes from one generation to the next in one or more families. Association studies involve comparison of cases to controls to assess the relative contribution of genetic variants or environmental effects to the trait being studied. In addition, association studies may also be designed to study a quantitative trait, such as IOP, in a single large cohort.

Primary Glaucomas

Primary Congenital Glaucoma

Primary congenital glaucoma (PCG) is an uncommon disease with a frequency ranging from 1 in 1250 (among the Roma population of Slovakia) to 1 in 10,000 (2). The anterior segment often reveals an anteriorly inserted iris, with a maldeveloped angle and trabecular meshwork. Most cases of PCG are sporadic; in familial cases, autosomal-recessive inheritance is most common. Most of these patients require surgical management because current glaucoma medications and lasers are generally ineffective for this form of glaucoma. Two loci have been identified for the infantile form of congenital glaucoma: 2p21[1] and 1p36. The gene within the 2p21 locus, which accounts for the majority of familial cases, was identified in 1997 and encodes the protein cytochrome P4501B1 (CYP4501B1).

---

[1]Chromosomal location is numbered according to the following convention: The first number indicates the chromosome number, the letter "q" indicates long arm and "p" the short arm (*petit* in French), and the final number (with or without decimal point) indicates the band number on the chromosome; the banding is numbered according to distance from the centromere and morphologic features consistently found on the chromosome, such as Giemsa-staining band pattern.

Although the ocular substrate for cytochrome P450B1 remains unknown, this enzyme is likely to play an important role in ocular development (3). Libby and colleagues have shown that mutant $Cyp1b1^{-/-}$ mice deficient in cytochrome P450B1, where both copies of the $Cyp1b1$ gene are nonfunctional, develop focal defects in the anterior chamber angle, including an increase in basal lamina of the trabecular meshwork and a small or absent Schlemm canal. Other experiments testing for genes that enhance or suppress angle abnormalities in $Cyp1b1$ identified the tyrosinase gene (Tyr) as a modifier whose deficiency exacerbates defects in $Cyp1b1$ mutant mice (3). Eyes lacking cytochrome P450B1 and tyrosinase demonstrated severe dysgenesis that was alleviated by the administration of L-DOPA, a normal product of tyrosinase. Thus, a pathway involving tyrosinase appears to be important in anterior chamber angle development.

Juvenile-Onset Open-Angle Glaucoma

JOAG is an autosomal-dominant form of COAG with an early age of onset. It is characterized by extremely high IOP with subsequent damage to the optic nerve and visual field. Affected eyes are often myopic. This disease usually begins between the ages of 4 and 35 years, often in individuals with a strong family history. In patients with JOAG, response to drug or laser treatment is generally poor and surgical intervention is often required.

JOAG was first linked to chromosome 1q21–31 by Sheffield and colleagues in 1993. Four years later, mutations were found in the responsible gene, the trabecular meshwork glucocorticoid response gene ($TIGR$, later renamed myocilin (4)). At least five loci are now mapped for JOAG. Of all cases of JOAG, approximately 10% to 20% are caused by mutations in the myocilin gene (5).

Revisiting Case 1

The phenotype is classic for JOAG. A mutation in the myocilin gene was suspected, and hence the gene was sequenced. A single base change, C → T (Pro370Leu) in exon 3, was found (6). This missense mutation was found in the mother and the two affected daughters, but not in the father. Armed with this information, one can now respond to the patient's queries:

1. What do I have?
   JOAG
2. Will I go blind if I don't receive treatment, and what is my best treatment option?
   The Pro370Leu mutation is aggressive and leads to blindness if the pressure elevation is not treated. The best treatment option at present is aggressive IOP lowering with medication initially, and then surgery (e.g., trabeculectomy with an antimetabolite) if medical treatment does not lower the IOP to an appropriate target range.
3. What are the chances that any future biologic children of mine would also get this disease?
   JOAG is autosomal dominant with high penetrance, so the risk is approximately 50%.

4. Can anything be done other than medications and surgery to treat my condition?
   Not at present, but additional strategies may become possible in the future, including gene replacement and alteration of the trabecular meshwork cellular and extracellular milieu to enhance outflow facility.

Adult-Onset Chronic Open-Angle Glaucoma

The high prevalence of COAG, variability in age of onset, and nonpenetrance (lack of phenotypic expression of a disease despite carrying the genetic mutation) in some pedigrees indicate that most cases of COAG are not inherited as a single-gene defect but as a "complex" trait that does not demonstrate simple Mendelian inheritance. Interplay among various environmental and genetic factors, or among multiple genes, results in a high degree of variability in phenotypic expression and disease severity that makes linkage analysis extremely challenging. To date, linkage studies on families with COAG provide strong evidence for genetic heterogeneity. At least 11 loci have been identified, along with three genes (myocilin, optineurin, and $WDR36$) (**Table 8.1**).

Additional evidence for genetic susceptibility comes from polymorphisms of genes suspected of playing a role in glaucoma. Polymorphisms in the genes coding for the β-adrenergic receptors $ADRB1$ and $ADRB2$ expressed in the trabecular meshwork and ciliary body have been examined and may influence the pathophysiology of COAG in both COAG and normal-tension glaucoma in Japanese patients (7). However, the $ADRB2$ gene does not appear to be a "causative" COAG genetic risk, as shown in an appropriately powered study comparing controls and COAG cases among white individuals and persons of African ancestry (8). There may also be susceptibility genes that are essential to permit other genes or environmental factors to lead to glaucoma. For example, the $OPA1$ gene and *apolipoprotein E* gene have been associated with normal-tension glaucoma and COAG, respectively (9,10). It remains to be seen what role these disease-associated polymorphisms will play in patients with glaucoma.

Angle-Closure Glaucoma

There have been a growing number of investigators who have explored the familial basis of angle-closure glaucoma using both traditional Mendelian study design approaches and application of ocular biometry for quantitative trait design approach. In certain regions of the world, angle-closure glaucoma is the most common form of glaucoma, so it is important to understand the genetic mechanisms involved in this condition, which can be amenable to treatment with laser approaches.

Using a combination of a genetic approach applied to an epidemiology study, Hu found a sixfold-increased risk for angle-closure glaucoma among persons with any family history of angle-closure glaucoma in his population-based survey in Shunyi County, Beijing, which supports a genetic factor (11). Using a quantitative trait approach, a study of axial anterior chamber depth in twins (without angle-closure glaucoma) indicated that about 70% of the variance in dizygotic twins could be attributable to a genetic component (12). A biometric study showed a relatively shallow anterior chamber depth in siblings, children, nephews, nieces, and grandchildren of angle-closure

Table 8.1	Summary of Genes and Loci Associated with Glaucoma[a]	
Chromosome	**Symbol[b]**	**Phenotype**
1	PLOD1	Ehlers–Danlos syndrome, type VI
1	(GLC3B)	PCG, type B
1	COL8A2	Posterior polymorphous corneal dystrophy 2, Fuchs endothelial corneal dystrophy
1	POMGNT1	Muscle–eye–brain disease
1	COL11A1	Marshall syndrome, Stickler syndrome II
1	MYOC	JOAG
2	CYP1B1	PCG, Peters anomaly, COAG, JOAG
2	(GLC1H)	High-tension open-angle glaucoma
2	(GLC1B)	High-tension open-angle glaucoma
3	(GLC1L)	Open-angle glaucoma
3	(GLC1C)	High-tension open-angle glaucoma
3	OPA1	Optic nerve atrophy, normal-tension open-angle glaucoma
4	IDUA	Hurler syndrome, Hurler–Scheie syndrome, Scheie syndrome
4	SLC4A4	Renal tubular acidosis, mental retardation, glaucoma
4	PITX2	Iridogoniodysgenesis, type 2; Rieger type 1; Peters anomaly; ring dermoid of cornea
5	ARSB	Mucopolysaccharidosis VI, Maroteaux–Lamy syndrome
5	VCAN	Wagner syndrome 1
5	(GLC1M)	Open-angle glaucoma
5	WDR36	Open-angle glaucoma
6	COL11A2	Stickler syndrome III, Weissenbacher–Zweymuller syndrome
6	FOXC1	Iridogoniodysgenesis 1, anterior segment mesenchymal dysgenesis, Rieger anomaly, Axenfeld anomaly, iris hypoplasia, juvenile glaucoma
6	GJA1	Oculodentodigital dysplasia, microphthalmia
7	(GLC1F)	High-tension open-angle glaucoma
7	(GPDS1)	Pigment dispersion 1
8	KTWS	Klippel-Trenaunay–Weber syndrome
8	(GLC1D)	High-tension open-angle glaucoma
8	GDF6	Microphthalmia, isolated 4
9	GLIS3	Neonatal diabetes mellitus and hypothyroidism, PCG
9	(GLC1J)	JOAG
9	PTCH1	Basal cell nevus syndrome
9	FKTN	Walker–Warburg syndrome
9	LMX1B	Nail–Patella syndrome
9	POMT1	Walker–Warburg syndrome
10	OPTN	Normal-tension and high-tension open-angle glaucoma
10	ZEB1	Posterior polymorphous corneal dystrophy 3
10	PAX2	Renal-coloboma or papillorenal syndrome, "morning glory" optic nerve
10	PITX3	Anterior segment dysgenesis
11	PAX6	Aniridia II, Peters anomaly, "morning glory" optic nerve, coloboma
11	SBF2	Charcot–Marie–Tooth disease type 4B2
11	(NNO1)	Nanophthalmos 1
11	MFRP	Nanophthalmos 2
11	C1QTNF5	Late-onset retinal degeneration and long anterior zonules
11	LRP5	Osteogenesis imperfecta, ocular form
12	COL2A1	Stickler syndrome I
13	RIEG2	Rieger syndrome 2
13	MCOR[c]	Congenital microcoria
14	SIX6	Microphthalmia with cataract 2
14	POMT2	Walker–Warburg syndrome
14	LTBP2	PCG
14	VSX2	Microphthalmos
14	MCOP[c]	Microphthalmos
14	(GLC3D)	PCG

Table 8.1 *(Continued)*

Chromosome	Symbol[b]	Phenotype
15	(GLC1I)	High-tension open-angle glaucoma
15	FBN1	Weill–Marchesani syndrome, ectopia lentis, Marfan syndrome
15	LOXL1	Risk allele for exfoliation glaucoma
15	(GLC1N)	JOAG
16	CREBBP	Rubinstein–Taybi syndrome
17	NF1	Neurofibromatosis 1
18	RAX	Microphthalmos
19	ADAMTS10	Weill–Marchesani syndrome
19	FKRP	Walker–Warburg syndrome
19	(GLC1O)	COAG
20	(GLC1K)	JOAG, 3
20	VSX1	Posterior polymorphous corneal dystrophy 1
21	CBS	Homocystinuria, ectopia lentis
22	NF2	Neurofibromatosis 2
22	LARGE	Walker–Warburg syndrome
X	NDP	Coats disease, uveitis, secondary glaucoma, Norrie disease
X	BCOR	Microphthalmia, syndromic 2
X	HCCS	Microphthalmia, syndromic 7
X	OCRL	Lowe oculocerebrorenal syndrome
X	MRXSA[c]	Armfield X-linked mental retardation syndrome

[a]HUGO symbols are used (www.hugo-international.org); information cross-checked with GeneCards, version 2.39 (www.genecards.org, cross-referenced to HUGO, Entrez Gene, UniProt/Swiss-Prot, UniProt/TrEMBL, OMIM, GeneLoc, Ensembl).
[b]Symbols in parentheses are locus symbols. Unless otherwise noted, all other symbols are HUGO-approved gene symbols.
[c]The symbol is based on Entrez Gene because there is no approved symbol in HUGO.
COAG, chronic open-angle glaucoma; JOAG, juvenile open-angle glaucoma; PCG, primary congenital glaucoma.

glaucoma probands (13). A heritability of 70% was found in this study, indicating that about two thirds of the age- and sex-independent variation of anterior chamber depth is inherited. Furthermore, Lowe has suggested that inheritance of a shallow anterior chamber is polygenic with a threshold effect so that the action of a large number of grouped or independently inherited genes results in varying degrees of anterior chamber shallowing (14). A Chinese study of families with angle-closure glaucoma and shallow anterior chambers concluded that the inheritance of a shallow anterior chamber may be a genetically heterogeneous trait and influenced by sex with autosomal-dominant inheritance in subgroups (15).

In a rare phenotype on the spectrum of angle-closure glaucoma is nanophthalmos, which represents an ocular phenotype characterized by a biometrically small eye with relatively normal lens volume. Such individuals are at increased risk for angle-closure glaucoma due to a crowded anterior segment, uveal effusions due to thickened sclera, and aqueous misdirection (see Chapter 26). In a large family with 22 affected family members with highly penetrant nanophthalmos (16), a locus called NNO1 was mapped to chromosome 11. The gene has not yet been identified.

Using a molecular approach, a study quantifying SPARC protein (secreted protein, acidic, and rich in cysteine) in iridectomy specimens of eyes with chronic angle closure found that these irides had a significantly higher SPARC and collagen 1 protein content compared with nonglaucomatous eyes and eyes with COAG (17). The data suggest that SPARC could play a role in the development of angle-closure glaucoma by influencing the biomechanical properties of the iris through a change in extracellular matrix organization.

It has also been suggested that environmental triggers may alter anterior chamber depth or degree of pupillary block. These are associated with angle-closure glaucoma, including neural or humoral response to fatigue, mental stress, infection, and trauma (18).

Secondary Glaucomas

Developmental Glaucomas

Developmental glaucomas are secondary to morphologic malformations of the anterior segment and are relatively rare. Importantly, however, developmental abnormalities of the ocular drainage structures are not always clinically detectable, and abnormal development may affect the metabolism and function of the drainage structures without disturbing morphology. Glaucomas and known genes associated with developmental disorders are listed as part of Table 8.1. It is important to note that clinical findings overlap considerably, even within families, and mutations in the same gene can cause a range of phenotypes. The primary causative genes that have been identified are transcription factor–related genes: *PITX2*, *PITX3*, and *FOXC1*.

Pigmentary Glaucoma

Several investigators have demonstrated autosomal-dominant inheritance for the pigment dispersion syndrome (PDS) (19–21). In 1997, Andersen and colleagues described four autosomal-dominant PDS families and reported localization of a gene to chromosome 7q35–36 (22). The disorder is genetically heterogeneous, and further studies are under way to determine whether additional loci exist and to find the gene (or genes) involved. *DBA/2J* mice appear to develop a form of pigmentary glaucoma caused by mutations in the glycoprotein (transmembrane) *nmb* gene, *Gpnmb*, and the tyrosinase-related protein 1 gene, *Tyrp1*. As both genes encode melanosomal proteins, it has been hypothesized that these mutations permit toxic intermediates of pigment production to leak from melanosomes (23). A study examining glaucoma patients with PDS for DNA sequence variants in *TYRP1* did not find an association (24).

Exfoliation Syndrome

Evidence supports the concept that exfoliation is an inherited microfibrillopathy involving transforming growth factor-1, oxidative stress, and impaired cellular protection mechanisms as key factors (Fig. 15.12). In a study in the Icelandic and Swedish populations, a common genetic variant was identified as a major risk factor for exfoliation syndrome and glaucoma (25). Polymorphisms in the coding region of the gene lysyl oxidase-like 1 (*LOXL1*), located on chromosome 15q24, are associated with exfoliation and exfoliative glaucoma in these and other populations. The disease-associated polymorphisms are found in virtually all individuals with exfoliation within populations studied to date.

LOXL1 is one of many enzymes essential for the formation of elastin fibers: It plays a role in modifying tropoelastin, the basic building block of elastin, and catalyzes the process for monomers to cross-link and form elastin. Although *LOXL1* is a major risk factor for exfoliation syndrome and exfoliative glaucoma, evidence suggests that additional genetic or environmental factors will be identified that influence disease expression and severity. One example is a study of white persons in Australia with a ninefold-lower lifetime incidence of exfoliative glaucoma compared with Scandinavian populations that demonstrated a similar allelic architecture at the *LOXL1* locus (26). This suggests that unidentified genetic or environmental factors independent of *LOXL1* strongly influence the phenotypic expression of the syndrome.

The disease-associated *LOXL1* variant is extremely common and is found in up to 90% of affected and unaffected individuals worldwide. For this reason, genetic testing is of limited clinical value at this time (27).

Revisiting Case 2

The discovery of the variants in the *LOXL1* gene has the potential to lead to more exact diagnosis, better monitoring of glaucoma suspects, improved knowledge of pathogenesis, and eventually more effective treatment. Despite the importance of the identification of *LOXL1* as a major contributor to exfoliation syndrome and exfoliative glaucoma, given the high frequency of disease-associated polymorphisms in the population, DNA testing is not clinically useful at this time.

Systemic Diseases Associated with Glaucoma

A number of ocular disorders that have been linked are associated with open-angle forms of glaucoma as part of their phenotype. These are listed in Table 8.1. In addition, a number of systemic disorders are associated with open-angle forms of glaucoma (e.g., nail–patella syndrome and Marfan syndrome), and those for which the gene has been localized or identified are listed in Table 8.1.

GENETICS AND INSIGHTS INTO DISEASE MECHANISMS

After identifying genes that are causative for glaucoma and genes that contribute to risk factors for glaucoma, we will elucidate disease mechanisms for glaucoma. This will also involve well-established mouse-model systems for glaucoma that will allow studies on specific biochemical pathways that ultimately cause glaucoma (28). To reach an in-depth understanding of role of these genes among these pathways, however, it will be essential to combine the tools of genomics, molecular biology, developmental biology, bioinformatics, and computational biology. This should ultimately lead to a better understanding of the normal physiology of the trabecular meshwork, optic nerve, ganglion cells, and other glaucoma-relevant tissues. Improved understanding of the state of the eye in disease and health will facilitate the rational development of drugs tailored to specific subtypes of glaucoma.

PHARMACOGENETICS, PHARMACOGENOMICS, AND THE PROMISE OF "PERSONALIZED MEDICINE"

Although all this information on genetics may appear daunting to the clinician, it is important to put this genomic technology in perspective. All of this genomic information, and the anticipated proteomic and metabolomic information, will not substitute for solid clinical history-taking skills, observation, assessment, and development of a treatment plan for the individual patient. However, at present, using our clinical acumen, our treatment approach is a trial-and-error approach by recommending a medication, laser, or surgery with an expected optimal treatment outcome. There is great optimism that genetic profiling will help target patients with glaucoma to individualized treatments on the basis of validated disease-risk alleles, validated pharmacogenetic markers, and specific behavioral modification. Thus, one may view these newer technology advances to take the guesswork out of the treatment plan, with the expectation of improved efficacy because the optimal treatment is specified for certain individual profiles and for decreased adverse events to treatment because it will not be recommended in a susceptible individual.

It is important to remember, however, that genes merely represent the blueprint to uncover genetic variants in common diseases, and they will not provide "the answer" to the question "What causes glaucoma?" Considerable strides are needed to fully understand factors that affect gene expression, such as DNA methylation, gene repair, copy-number variation, and telomerase action. In addition, proteomics is arguably just as crucial to genomics when looking at normal physiology and disease. For instance, posttranslational modifications, such as glycosylation, adenosine diphosphate–ribosylation, and phosphorylation, that affect cell function may also contribute to differences in an individual's disease manifestation and response to treatment.

Pharmacogenomic studies could reveal genetic factors that predispose to poor IOP response (**Fig. 8.6**) as well as to higher-than-average risk for an adverse response—for example, the development of elevated IOP in response to corticosteroid therapy.

The new challenges of genomics, and for the expected technological advances with proteomics and metabolomics, are to determine whether we can predict disease risk, disease progression, and treatment outcome. Despite the intricate biological and physiologic interactions among expression of drug target genes, drug-metabolizing enzymes, and disease genes, an approach to identify genetic markers of "poor IOP responders" has the potential to target patients with disease to more appropriate treatment, such as surgery, to lower IOP more effectively, thus minimizing progressive optic nerve damage and visual field loss.

The promise of personalized medicine is new abilities to improve on clinical decision making regarding individualized treatment regimens based on the patient's genetic profile. It is equally as important to consider health behaviors—that is, adherence with treatments—while conducting appropriately designed studies. Lifestyle factors, such as diet, exercise, cigarette smoking, and alcohol use, are all included in the individual health behaviors but have not been extensively studied for glaucoma. The genetic profile would enable the assessment of risk for disease, protective genetic factors, disease progression, and variations in treatment responses of both efficacy and toxicity.

Revisiting Case 3

Our current knowledge can only begin to answer the patient's question. As our understanding grows about applying genomic results to this potentially blinding disease, clinicians will be expected to be informed about treatments that can be personalized for their patients. These treatments will be based on a patient's genetic profile and will incorporate information on disease risk, disease progression, and the likelihood of individual drug safety and efficacy.

Privacy and Counseling

The fear of genetic discrimination has presented an impediment to the widespread application of personalized medicine. Legislation to protect patients against this risk is essential. An example is the Genetic Information Nondiscrimination Act (GINA), was signed into law in the United States and which offers protection against discrimination based on genetic information when it comes to health insurance and employment (29).

As more widespread genetic testing becomes available, clinicians will need to safeguard these data and also ensure that appropriate genetic counseling is available. The role of the counselor is to be an informer, not an advisor. It will be important to provide the necessary facts and options, so that an informed decision can be made by the patient and his or her caregivers.

Concluding Remarks

Personalized medicine will become a reality through identification of disease and pharmacogenetic markers followed by careful study of how to employ this information for improving

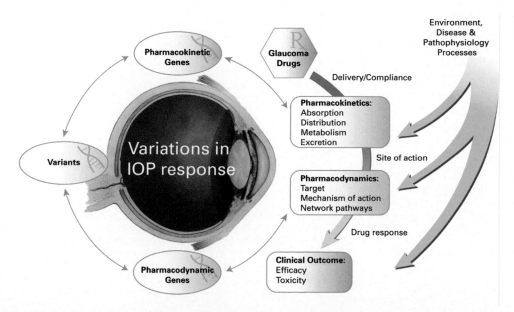

Figure 8.6 Variations in IOP response to glaucoma medical therapy are determined by pharmacokinetic and pharmacodynamic processes *(blue arrow)* and interaction with the environment, disease, and pathophysiologic processes. The sequence variants among pharmacokinetic and pharmacodynamic genes are predicted to have functional consequences that contribute to the genetic component of variance in IOP response. (Modified from pharmgkb.org, with permission of PharmGKB and Stanford University.)

treatment outcomes. With advances in genomic technologies, research has shifted from the simple monogenic disease model to a complex multigenic and environmental disease model. Our challenges lie in developing risk models incorporating gene–gene interactions, gene copy-number variations, environmental interactions, treatment effects, and clinical covariates.

Future approaches to glaucoma therapeutics encompass identification of genetic markers for "non-IOP responders"; problematic wound healing, which affects surgical outcomes; and incorporation of the utility of growth factors, stem cells, and other non–pressure-based mechanisms to decrease glaucoma neuropathy.

KEY POINTS

- Genetic studies have the ability to
  - identify risk alleles for disease and predict the chance of developing disease,
  - identify genetic modifiers of age of onset,
  - identify genetic modifiers for disease progression,
  - identify genetic markers of treatment response to glaucoma medications, and
  - assist with disease classification.
- The glaucomas are a complex group of diseases with considerable genetic heterogeneity. Genetic variations have been found that cause glaucoma or are associated with syndromes that include glaucoma, and loci have been identified that affect an individual's potential susceptibility to glaucoma.
- There are a large number of mapped locations for COAG, and three genes have been identified (*MYOC*, *OPTN*, and *WDR36*). However, the vast majority of the genetic contribution to this form of glaucoma and angle-closure glaucoma remains to be determined.
- The identification of *CYP1B1* gene for PCG, responsible for up to half of cases, is a major improvement in our understanding of this devastating disorder.
- Future studies in humans will provide an opportunity to correlate genotype to phenotype, while animal studies will continue to unravel the complexity of biochemical networks that cause glaucoma in its various manifestations. This may enable earlier detection, a better understanding of the pathophysiology, and thus natural history of disease, and eventually the institution of more rational, targeted therapy.
- Given the five different main classes of drugs for glaucoma therapy, it is important to recognize that genetic variability among the pharmacokinetic and pharmacodynamic pathways may influence responses to these drugs.

REFERENCES

1. Clamp M, Fry B, Kamal M, et al. Distinguishing protein-coding and noncoding genes in the human genome. *Proc Natl Acad Sci USA.* 2007; 104(49):19428–19433.
2. Ho CL, Walton DS. Primary congenital glaucoma: 2004 update. *J Pediatr Ophthalmol Strabismus.* 2004;41(5): 271–288.
3. Libby RT, Smith RS, Savinova OV, et al. Modification of ocular defects in mouse developmental glaucoma models by tyrosinase. *Science.* 2003; 299:1578–1581.
4. Stone EM, Fingert JH, Alward WL, et al. Identification of a gene that causes primary open angle glaucoma. *Science.* 1997;275:668–670.
5. Sud A, Del Bono EA, Haines JL, et al. Fine mapping of the GLC1K juvenile primary open-angle glaucoma locus and exclusion of candidate genes. *Mol Vis.* 2008;14:1319–1326.
6. Damji KF, Song X, Gupta SK, et al. Childhood-onset primary open angle glaucoma in a Canadian kindred: clinical and molecular genetic features. *Ophthalmic Genet.* 1999;20(4):211–218.
7. Inagaki Y, Mashima Y, Fuse N, et al. Polymorphism of beta-adrenergic receptors and susceptibility to open-angle glaucoma. *Mol Vis.* 2006;12: 673–680.
8. McLaren N, Reed DM, Musch DC, et al. Evaluation of the beta2-adrenergic receptor gene as a candidate glaucoma gene in 2 ancestral populations. *Arch Ophthalmol.* 2007;125(1):105–111.
9. Aung T, Ocaka L, Ebenezer ND, et al. A major marker for normal tension glaucoma: association with polymorphisms in the OPA1 gene. *Hum Genet.* 2002;110:52–56.
10. Copin B, Brezin AP, Valtot F, et al. Apolipoprotein E-promoter single-nucleotide polymorphisms affect the phenotype of primary open-angle glaucoma and demonstrate interaction with the myocilin gene. *Am J Hum Genet.* 2002;70:1575–1581.
11. Hu CN. An epidemiologic study of glaucoma in Shunyi County, Beijing. *Chung Hua Yen Ko Tsa Chih.* 1989;25:115–119.
12. Tornquist R. Shallow anterior chambers in acute glaucoma. *Acta Ophthalmol.* 1953;31:1–74.
13. Alsbirk PH. Anterior chamber depth and primary angle-closure glaucoma. II. A genetic study. *Acta Ophthalmol (Copenh).* 1975;53:436–449.
14. Lowe RF. Primary angle-closure glaucoma. Inheritance and environment. *Br J Ophthalmol.* 1972;56:13–19.
15. Tu YS, Yin ZQ, Pen HM, et al. Genetic heritability of a shallow anterior chamber in Chinese families with primary angle closure glaucoma. *Ophthalmic Genet.* 2008;29(4):171–176.
16. Othman MI, Sullivan SA, Skuta GL, et al. Autosomal dominant nanophthalmos (NNO1) with high hyperopia and angle-closure glaucoma maps to chromosome 11. *Am J Hum Genet.* 1998;63(5):1411–1418.
17. Chua J, Seet LF, Jiang Y, et al. Increased SPARC expression in primary angle closure glaucoma iris. *Mol Vis.* 2008;14:1886–1892.
18. Damji KF, Allingham RR. Genetics and glaucoma susceptibility. In: Tombran-Tink J, Shields MB, Barnstable CJ, eds. *Mechanisms of the Glaucomas: Disease Processes and Therapeutic Modalities.* Totowa, NJ: Humana Pr; 2008:191–204.
19. Becker B, Podos SM. Krukenberg's spindles and primary open-angle glaucoma. *Arch Ophthalmol.* 1966;76: 635–647.
20. McDermott JA, Ritch R, Berger A, et al. Inheritance of pigment dispersion syndrome. *Invest Ophthalmol Vis Sci.* 1978;28(suppl):153.
21. Mandelkorn R, Hoffman M, Olander K, et al. Inheritance of the pigmentary dispersion syndrome. *Ann Ophthalmol.* 1983;15:577–582.
22. Andersen J, Pralea A, Delbono A, et al. A gene responsible for the pigment dispersion syndrome maps to Chromosome 7q35-q36. *Arch Ophthalmol.* 1997;115:384–388.
23. Anderson MG, Smith RS, Hawes NL, et al. Mutations in genes encoding melanosomal proteins cause pigmentary glaucoma in DBA/2J mice. *Nat Genet.* 2002;30(1):81–85.
24. Lynch S, Yanagi G, DelBono E, et al. DNA sequence variants in the tyrosinase-related protein 1 (*TYRP1*) gene are not associated with human pigmentary glaucoma. *Mol Vis.* 2002;8:127–129.
25. Thorleifsson G, Magnusson KP, Sulem P, et al. Common sequence variants in the *LOXL1* gene confer susceptibility to exfoliation glaucoma. *Science.* 2007;736–737.
26. Hewitt AW, Sharma S, Burdon KP, et al. Ancestral *LOXL1* variants are associated with exfoliation in Caucasian Australians but with markedly lower penetrance than in Nordic people. *Hum Mol Genet.* 2008;17(5):710–716.
27. Challa P, Schmidt S, Liu Y, et al. Analysis of LOXL1 polymorphisms in a United States population with exfoliation glaucoma. *Mol Vis.* 2008;14: 146–149.
28. John SW. Mechanistic insights into glaucoma provided by experimental genetics: the Cogan lecture. *Invest Ophthalmol Vis Sci.* 2005;6:2649–2661.
29. Hudson KL, Holohan MK, Collins FS. Keeping pace with the times—the Genetic Information Nondiscrimination Act of 2008. *N Engl J Med.* 2008;358(25):2661–2663.

Clinical Epidemiology of Glaucoma

9

Glaucoma affects more than 67 million persons worldwide, of whom about 10%, or 6.6 million, are estimated to be blind (1). Glaucoma is the leading cause of irreversible blindness worldwide and is second only to cataracts as the most common cause of blindness overall (1). Glaucoma is responsible for 14% of all blindness (2). In the United States, chronic open-angle glaucoma (COAG) affects more than 2.2 million persons, and this number is projected to increase to 3.4 million by 2020 (3). Over the same time period in the developing world, the prevalence of glaucoma is expected to rise even more dramatically as the population of adults older than 60 years more than doubles (2).

The social and economic impact of glaucoma is enormous but difficult to quantify. Economic data on the cost of glaucoma are also limited. The total direct cost per case of treating newly diagnosed COAG or ocular hypertension for 2 years was estimated to average $2109 in the United States and $2160 in Sweden in 1998 (4). Costs have been shown to be greater for more advanced cases and uncontrolled disease and to increase following trabeculectomy (5,6). The annual direct costs of glaucoma and ocular hypertension in the United States were estimated at $3.9 billion in 2001 (7); a separate estimate from 1991 put the direct costs of glaucoma (excluding ocular hypertension) at $1.9 billion (8). National per capita estimates are similar for Canada but lower for Sweden and the United Kingdom (5,9,10).

FUNCTIONAL LIMITATIONS ASSOCIATED WITH GLAUCOMATOUS VISION LOSS

From the perspective of those whose visual function has been severely affected by glaucoma, the impact of the disease can be profound and may include difficulty with reading and writing, activities of daily living (cooking and eating, dressing and bathing, medication management, money management), mobility with increased risk of falls, ability to drive, vocational challenges, social isolation, and depression (11–16). As individuals age, the impact of visual dysfunction can be amplified if comorbidities are present. These include hearing loss, arthritis, head tremors, and cognitive impairment. The impact of glaucoma can be quantified by using various vision-targeted and generic health-related quality-of-life measures, but is difficult to predict on the basis of visual function measurements alone. Many factors such as physical health, psychological state, visual demands of daily living, values, adaptability, and social and cultural milieu shape the changing impact of glaucoma on individuals (17). This may explain in part the low correlation between visual field loss in glaucoma and vision-targeted and generic measurements of health-related quality of life (18,19). Vision-targeted measures of health-related quality of life have found lower scores in glaucoma suspects than in healthy controls and have been successively lower in those with early and moderate and advanced visual field changes (20–24); general health-related quality-of-life scores also have been shown to be decreased in persons with glaucoma (20–22,25). In general, these findings support the notion that glaucoma, as the "sneak thief" of vision, causes subtle symptoms and modestly affects health-related quality of life until the disease is advanced. Interestingly, visual changes associated with glaucoma are often not interpreted as symptoms of a visual problem until after a diagnosis has been made (17). An important consideration in the treatment of glaucoma is that therapy can itself adversely affect quality of life (26,27). Therapies may be inconvenient or expensive, cause discomfort, or lead to significant ocular and systemic complications.

It has been suggested that strategies aimed at improving an individual's function be tied to socially meaningful outcomes (28). Examples include maintaining functional independence; sustaining meaningful relationships; enhancing one's psychosocial well-being; and being able to access transportation, pursue leisurely activities, and maintain employment and economic productivity.

PREVALENCE, INCIDENCE, AND GEOGRAPHIC DISTRIBUTION OF GLAUCOMA

The prevalence of glaucoma has been studied extensively (**Table 9.1**), but the case definition of glaucoma has varied widely and clinical classification has been inconsistent among studies (52). Intraocular pressure (IOP), the appearance of the optic nerve head, and visual field abnormalities have all been used in varying combinations to define glaucoma; the status of the iridocorneal angle and the presence or absence of secondary causes are typically used to determine the clinical classification of glaucoma. These differences make it difficult to directly compare the prevalence findings of different studies. There is, however, growing acceptance of the concept that glaucoma is a progressive optic neuropathy characterized by a typical damage to the optic nerve head (cupping) and associated visual dysfunction. Glaucomatous damage to the optic nerve appears to be the final common pathway to a diverse assortment of etiologic factors and clinical subtypes.

There is some discussion in the literature about the value of distinguishing between normal-tension glaucoma and

Table 9.1	Prevalence of Glaucoma in Selected Population-Based Studies						
Racial/Ethnic Group and Location[a]	**Age-Group, y**	**Participants, n**	**Prevalence, by Type of Glaucoma, %**				
			Any	**COAG**	**ACG**	**SG**	
BLACK							
Baltimore, USA, 1991 (29)	>40	2396	4.7	4.7	—[b]	—[b]	
Barbados, 1994 (30)	40–84	4709	6.6	6.6	—[b]	—[b]	
Kongwa, Tanzania, 2000 (31)	>40	3268	4.2	3.1	0.6	0.5	
St. Lucia, 1989 (32)	30–86	1679	8.8	8.8	—[b]	—[b]	
Temba, South Africa, 2003 (33)	>40	839	5.3	2.9	0.5	2.0	
HISPANIC							
ARIZONA, USA, 2001 (34)	>40	4774	2.1	2.0	0.1	—[b]	
ASIAN							
Alaska, USA, 1987 (35)	>40	1923	2.7	—[b]	2.7	—[b]	
Andhra Pradesh, India, 2000 (36,37)	>40	1399	3.7	2.6	1.1	0.1	
Japan, 1991 (38)	>40	8126	3.5	2.6	0.3	0.6	
Hovsgol, Mongolia, 1996 (39)	>40	1000	2.2	0.5	1.4	0.3	
Singapore, 2000 (40)	40–79	1717	4.7	2.4	1.5	0.8	
Tamil Nadu, India, 2003 (41)	>40	5150	2.5	1.7	0.5	0.3	
WHITE							
Baltimore, USA, 1991 (29)	>40	2913	1.3	1.3	—[b]	—[b]	
Beaver Dam, USA, 1992 (42)	43–84	4926	2.1	2.1	—[b]	—[b]	
Bedford, UK, 1968 (43)	>30	5941	0.9	0.7	0.2	—[b]	
Blue Mountains, Australia, 1996 (44)	>49	3654	3.5	3	0.3	0.2	
Egna–Neumarket, Italy, 1998 (45)	>40	5816	2.1	1.4	0.6	0.1	
Framingham, USA, 1977 (46)	52–85	2477	1.2	1.2	—[b]	—[b]	
Melbourne, Australia, 1998 (47)	40–98	3271	2.0	1.7	0.1	0.2	
Rhonda Valley, UK, 1966 (48)	40–74	4231	0.7	0.3	0.1	0.3	
Roscommon, Ireland, 1993 (49)	>50	2186	1.9	1.9	—[b]	—[b]	
Rotterdam, Netherlands, 1994 (50)	>55	3062	3.1	3.1	—[b]	—[b]	
Reykjavik, Iceland, 2003 (51)	>50	1045	4.0	4.0	—[b]	—[b]	

[a]Numbers in parentheses are reference numbers.
[b]Data on glaucoma subtypes incomplete.
ACG, angle-closure glaucoma; COAG, chronic open-angle glaucoma; SG, secondary glaucoma.

COAG on the basis of IOP at presentation. In population-based studies, normal-tension glaucoma has been far more common than expected, accounting for between 40% and 75% of individuals with newly diagnosed COAG based on screening IOP (44,50,53). These entities are likely part of a spectrum of disease in which IOP plays an important role, and other factors such as vascular, apoptotic, or connective tissue factors are increasingly important at lower IOP levels (54); they less likely represent distinct varieties of glaucoma.

The prevalence of open-angle glaucoma varies greatly among racial and ethnic groups (Table 9.1). In the Baltimore Eye Survey, the prevalence of COAG in persons 40 years and older was found to be significantly higher among blacks than whites (4.7% vs. 1.3%). Hispanics in the United States have been found to have a prevalence of 2.0% for those 40 years of age and older, similar to findings of other studies for whites in the same age range. The prevalence of COAG in Asian populations varies

widely, with many populations having similar prevalence levels to whites (Chinese in Singapore, 2.4%; Japanese, 2.6%; Indians in Tamil Nadu, 1.7%), whereas other populations (Mongolian, 0.5%; Alaskan Inuit, 0.1%) appear to have rates that are considerably lower. This summary is limited by differences in definitions and classifications of glaucoma and different age distributions. However, the variation in the prevalence of COAG in blacks and angle-closure glaucoma and COAG in Asians probably also reflects the wide genetic heterogeneity within these broad racial and ethnic categories (55).

Age has an even more powerful influence on the prevalence of COAG than racial and ethnic grouping does (**Fig. 9.1** and **Table 9.2**). The age-specific prevalence of COAG (by race) is a useful starting point for clinicians to estimate the probability of COAG when beginning an initial assessment. COAG is uncommon before 40 years of age. In a pooled analysis of population-based surveys, the prevalence of COAG in whites increased from

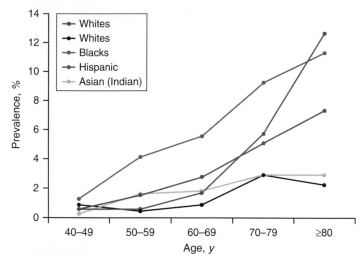

Figure 9.1 Age-specific prevalence of COAG from selected surveys. Data are from the Eye Diseases Prevalence Research Group, Aravind Comprehensive Eye Survey, Baltimore Eye Survey, and Proyecto VER.

0.6% for age 40 to 49 years to 1.5% for 50 to 59 years, to 2.7% for 60 to 69 years, to 5.1% for 70 to 79 years, and finally to 7.3% in the 80 years and older age-group, a greater than 10-fold increase from the 40- to 49-year age-group (Table 9.2) (3). In the Baltimore Eye Survey, the prevalence of COAG among blacks in the same survey was threefold to fourfold higher than in whites at almost every age interval (Table 9.2). In U.S. Hispanics, the age-specific prevalence of COAG was similar to that of whites but was significantly higher in the oldest age-group, equaling or exceeding the prevalence observed in blacks. Similar to overall prevalence, the age-specific prevalence of COAG in some Asian populations (in Tamil Nadu, India; Chinese in Singapore) is similar to that in whites, whereas in others (in Mongolia), it appears to be considerably lower. In almost all of these studies, roughly a 10-fold increase in prevalence occurs between the 40- to 49-year-old age-group and the oldest age bracket.

Another useful clinical perspective on the geographic distribution of glaucoma is the relative frequency of COAG, angle-closure glaucoma, and secondary glaucoma in different populations. In black and white populations, COAG usually accounts for 85% to 90% of all glaucomas. In contrast, angle-closure glaucoma predominates in some Asian populations, such as in Mongolia, where it accounts for 64% of glaucoma cases. Angle-closure glaucoma has been estimated to account for half of all cases of glaucoma worldwide (1). In other Asian populations, angle-closure glaucoma is less common than COAG, such as in a Chinese population in Singapore (angle-closure glaucoma, 32%; COAG, 42%) and an Indian population in Tamil Nadu (angle-closure glaucoma, 19%; COAG, 65%), whereas among Japanese patients, angle-closure glaucoma accounts for 9% of glaucoma, similar to rates in whites. It is easy to see how profoundly geographic location and the population being treated may affect an ophthalmologist's perspective on glaucoma. Secondary forms of glaucoma collectively account for between 5% and 20% of glaucoma cases in studies where this is specified (Table 9.1).

Whereas the prevalence of glaucoma is the proportion of a population with the disease at a given time point, incidence is the rate at which new cases occur during a specified period. The incidence of glaucoma is also strongly influenced by age and race. For the clinician, incidence serves as a point of reference to estimate the risk for glaucoma over a period of time (**Table 9.3**). The best estimates of the incidence of glaucoma come from a handful of population-based cohort studies (56–58). In the Melbourne Visual Impairment Project, the overall incidence of open-angle glaucoma in whites aged 40 years and older was 0.5% over 5 years, or roughly 1/1000 per year; in blacks of the same age in the Barbados Eye Study, the incidence was 2.2% over 4 years, or about 5.5/1000 per year. In both populations, the incidence increased steadily with age (Table 9.3). This comparison also suggests that the incidence of COAG in blacks increases at an earlier age than in whites and is much greater than in whites in the fourth and fifth decades of life, but is similar in the oldest age-group (80 years or older). However, differences in how progression was determined in these studies mean that direct comparisons may not be valid (59,60).

Table 9.2	Prevalence of Chronic Open-Angle Glaucoma (COAG), by Age, According to Race/Ethnicity and Study Location[a]				
Age–Group	**Prevalence of COAG, %**				
	White		**Black**	**Hispanic**	**Indian**
	United States	**Baltimore**	**Baltimore**	**Arizona**	**Tamil Nadu**
40–49 y	0.6	0.9	1.2	0.5	0.3
50–59 y	1.5	0.4	4.1	0.6	1.6
60–69 y	2.7	0.9	5.5	1.7	1.8
70–79 y	5.1	2.9	9.2	5.7	2.9
≥80 y	7.3	2.2	11.3	12.6	
All		1.3	4.7	2	1.2

[a]Study sources, by location: USA—Eye Diseases Prevalence Research Group (3); Baltimore (USA)—Baltimore Eye Survey (29); Arizona (USA)—Proyecto VER (34); Tamil Nadu (India)—Aravind Comprehensive Eye Survey (41).

Table 9.3	Incidence of Chronic Open-Angle (COAG), by Age, According to Race/Ethnicity, Study Location, and Incidence Period[a]				
Age–Group	**Incidence of COAG, %**				
	White			**Black**	
	Australia		**Sweden**	**Barbados**	
	5 y	**1 y**	**1 y**	**4 y**	**1 y**
40–49 y	0	—	—	1.2	0.3
50–59 y	0.1	0.02	—	1.5	0.38
60–69 y	0.6	0.12	—	3.2	0.8
70–79 y	1.4	0.28	—	—	—
≥80 y	4.1	0.82	—	4.2	1.05
All	0.5	0.1	0.24	2.2	0.55

[a]Study sources, by location: Melbourne, Australia—Melbourne Visual Impairment Project (VIP) (56); Dalby, Sweden—(57); Barbados—Barbados Eye Studies (58).

Several clinical trials have reported the risk of progression of established COAG without treatment. These estimates offer a benchmark to clinicians and patients against which to weigh the risks of treatment, bearing in mind that progression rates may vary widely depending on how progression is determined (59,60). In the Early Manifest Glaucoma Trial (EMGT), the rate of progression at 6 years was 62% without treatment and was decreased to 45%, with an average IOP lowering of 25%, with treatment (61,62). The Collaborative Normal Tension Glaucoma Study (CNTGS) followed a group with more advanced glaucoma and lower IOPs and observed progression in 60% at 5 years without treatment (63). This percentage fell to 20% with treatment targeting greater than 30% IOP lowering.

NATURAL HISTORY OF GLAUCOMA

The natural history of COAG can be divided into three phases of chronic disease to illustrate several important concepts relevant to clinical care (**Fig. 9.2**).

The first of these phases is called the latency phase. It begins with the onset of glaucomatous optic nerve damage and extends up to the detection threshold. The etiology of glaucomatous optic nerve damage is not well understood but is thought to result from a disturbance in the delicate balance of vascular, connective tissue, mechanical, and neural components that keep the optic nerve head healthy and functioning. An imbalance such as a rise in IOP and increased pressure gradient across the optic nerve head may, in some individuals, be intolerable to some axons and lead to cell death by apoptosis (64). However, many individuals with elevated IOP do not have glaucoma, and many persons with glaucoma have non elevated IOP (53). Clearly, other factors are also involved in glaucomatous optic nerve damage, and evidence continues to build in support

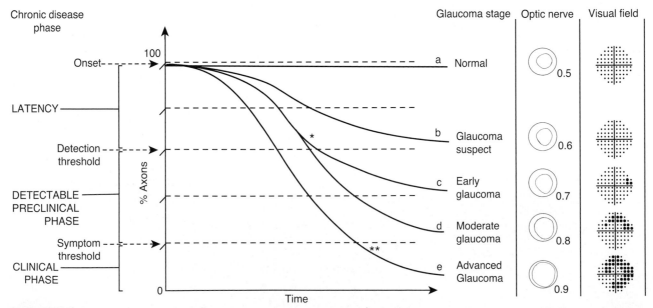

Figure 9.2 Natural history of COAG. Schematic depiction of the natural history of COAG showing loss of axons over time for selected patients with glaucoma. **a:** An individual without glaucoma. **b:** Subthreshold axonal loss from glaucoma that does not progress beyond the suspect category. **c:** Axonal loss from glaucoma that responds to treatment (*) compared with **d**, glaucoma that remains untreated because of a delay in diagnosis. **e:** Aggressive axonal loss from glaucoma that is detected only after the onset of symptoms and progresses to blindness despite treatment (**). The phases of chronic disease and clinical stages of glaucoma with fields and disc findings have been added to the graph along the left and right margins. The optic nerve drawings depict typical neural rim changes of glaucoma in a patient with a baseline cup-to-disc ratio of 0.5 before axonal loss; patients with a larger or smaller cup-to-disc ratio at baseline would have different neural rim findings at intermediate stages but would converge in advanced disease.

of vascular tissue, connective tissue, and neural causes, including variations in cerebrospinal fluid (CSF) pressure (see Chapter 4). It appears that low-level axonal loss may occur with aging in healthy individuals (65–68), but it is unclear how this relates to glaucomatous optic nerve damage.

The detection threshold for glaucoma is defined as the point at which glaucomatous optic nerve damage can be accurately detected by diagnostic testing. This marks the beginning of the lengthy asymptomatic phase during which glaucoma is detectable, the so-called detectable preclinical phase that continues until glaucomatous optic nerve damage leads to symptoms. The detection of early glaucomatous optic nerve damage is challenging. In terms of visual field testing, considerable glaucomatous optic nerve damage can occur before the threshold of detection is reached. It has been reported that up to 40% of axons can be lost before white-on-white Humphrey perimetry will show an abnormality (69,70), a finding supported by subsequent experimental studies in monkeys (71) (**Fig. 9.3**). Tests such as the frequency doubling technology and short-wavelength automated perimetry (SWAP) may be able to detect glaucomatous optic nerve damage before conventional white-on-white perimetry can, but they may have similar inherent psychophysical limitations. The detection of early glaucomatous optic nerve damage by optic nerve examination at a single visit is also difficult, but for different reasons, there is a large overlap between the appearance of healthy and glaucomatous optic nerves. Nerve fiber layer imaging techniques are helpful in distinguishing some normal variants from glaucomatous optic nerve damage. Careful documentation of optic nerve appearance, preferably by using stereoscopic disc photography or another form of imaging, permits earlier diagnosis and earlier detection of progression by allowing detection of subtle changes from glaucomatous

optic nerve damage on subsequent assessments that would otherwise be missed (see Chapter 4).

Finally, the clinical phase begins with the onset of symptoms; in COAG, this seldom occurs before the disease is advanced. However, chronic glaucoma is generally slowly progressive and may never reach this stage or may take decades to do so. As a result of the lengthy asymptomatic phase, glaucoma is often diagnosed in the course of periodic eye examinations before the clinical phase, but many cases are not. COAG may also behave aggressively and become symptomatic within several years of presumed onset. Ultimately, some patients with chronic glaucoma eventually go blind.

The natural histories of a patient with a healthy optic nerve and four other patients with COAG are shown in Figure 9.2. Using a "rule of tens," we can roughly approximate the distribution of a white or black population into the categories of COAG shown in this figure. For every 1000 persons aged 40 years and older, 100 are suspected of having COAG on the basis of field, disc, IOP findings, or dense risk factors; 10 have COAG, and approximately 1 will be blind as a result of COAG.

CLINICAL RISK FACTORS FOR CHRONIC OPEN-ANGLE GLAUCOMA

Risk factors are clinically useful to assess the risk for glaucoma based on the characteristics of the individual patient. To use this knowledge most effectively, it is helpful to understand the relative importance and magnitude of clinical risk factors. Although many risk factors have been identified for COAG, a much smaller number is well supported by evidence. Most of the evidence for COAG risk factors has been obtained from prevalence surveys or case–control studies. These have been complemented, especially in recent years, by high-quality clinical trials and cohort studies. In general, there is good agreement on risk-factor information based on prevalence and that based on incidence. Some risk factors for COAG are also risk factors for progression. Clinical risk factors may be divided into general risk factors, ocular risk factors, and systemic risk factors. (Risk factors for the conversion of suspected glaucoma with elevated IOP to COAG are discussed in Chapter 10.)

General Risk Factors

Age

As described previously, population-based studies of prevalence and incidence consistently show a steady rise in rates with increasing age. As a rule of thumb, prevalence tends to roughly double for each decade over 40 (i.e., relative risk [RR] of 2 per decade) and is about 10-fold higher in the 80 years and older group compared with the 40- to 49-year-old group (Table 9.2). In blacks, the RRs for incidence by decade are lower than in whites (because of the higher incidence seen in the 40- to 49-year-old reference group) (Table 9.3). In the EMGT, the RR of progression of early glaucoma was 1.5 for those 68 years of age and older, compared with younger persons (72).

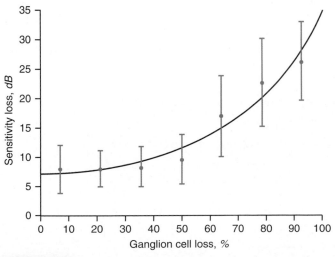

Figure 9.3 Loss of visual sensitivity as a function of loss of ganglion cells caused by experimental glaucoma in macaque monkeys, compared with the contralateral control eye. Mean values (± standard deviation [bars]) are shown for each of seven levels of ganglion cell loss with a fitted curve. Visual field defects greater than 15 dB are almost always caused by ganglion cell losses of more than 70% (71).

Race

In general, the prevalence of COAG is highest in black populations; intermediate in whites, Hispanics, and southern Asian populations (Singapore Chinese, Indian); and lowest in northern Asian populations (Mongolia, Inuit) (Table 9.1). The Baltimore Eye Survey found the prevalence of COAG in blacks to be four times greater than that in whites (29). A similar difference in the overall incidence of COAG for those aged 40 years and older has been observed between recent population-based cohorts of blacks and whites (56,73) (Table 9.3). In the Advanced Glaucoma Intervention Study (AGIS) (74), black race was not shown to be a risk factor for progression, in contrast to an earlier cohort study (75). In the CNTGS (76), Chinese patients had a significantly lower risk of progression than white patients.

Family History

A family history of COAG is an important risk factor for COAG. Having a first-degree relative (parent, sibling, or child) with glaucoma has been consistently associated with an increased risk for COAG in prevalence surveys (77–81). The odds ratio (OR) of COAG for a family history of glaucoma is higher if based on patients with previously diagnosed glaucoma (Baltimore OR, 4.7; Blue Mountains Eye Study OR, 4.2) than if based on newly detected cases (Baltimore OR, 2.8; Blue Mountain Eye Study OR, 2.4). This suggests that having a diagnosis of COAG leads to a greater awareness of glaucoma in the family. The association between COAG and family history may be stronger when the affected relative is a sibling (OR, 3.7) rather than a parent (OR, 2.2) or child (OR, 1.1) (78). In one population-based survey, researchers directly examined 497 siblings and offspring of patients with glaucoma and of control participants (80). For first-degree relatives of patients with definite glaucoma, the estimated lifetime RR for glaucoma was 9.2, albeit with very wide confidence intervals (CIs) (95% CI, 1.2 to 73.9). Family history was a risk factor for glaucoma in one prospective population-based study (RR, 2.1) (82), although no such association was found in the Ocular Hypertension Treatment Study (OHTS). In prospective studies of established glaucoma, family history has not been shown to be a significant predictor of progression (72,76).

Ocular Risk Factors

Intraocular Pressure

The evidence that IOP is a risk factor for glaucoma has recently become so strong that, unlike any other risk factor for glaucoma, it satisfies criteria commonly used to assess causality (83,84). A strong dose–response relationship between IOP and glaucoma has consistently been shown in prevalence surveys (Table 9.1) and in longitudinal studies of incidence and progression (73,82,85,86). The most decisive new evidence in recent years was the finding in randomized clinical trials that IOP lowering decreased the incidence and progression of glaucoma compared with no treatment (61,63,85). In addition, there is support for plausible biologic mechanisms that link elevated IOP to apoptosis of ganglion cell neurons through blockage of retrograde axonal transport (87,88). In short, IOP is best considered both a risk factor for and a cause of glaucoma. A good analogy is the relationship between smoking and lung cancer, in which smoking is both a strong risk factor for lung cancer and one of several causes.

In the Baltimore Eye Survey, the prevalence of COAG rose with increasing IOP (**Table 9.4**). The prevalence of COAG in persons with an IOP of 35 mm Hg or greater was more than 40 times as high as that in persons with an IOP less than 15 mm Hg. The incidence of COAG was found to increase steadily with IOP in the Barbados Eye Study to an RR of 25 for an IOP of more than 25 mm Hg, compared with a reference group with an IOP less than 17 mm Hg (Table 9.4). In the population of the Melbourne Visual Impairment Project, it was estimated that for every 1 mm Hg, the risk for glaucoma increased by 10%. Importantly, the OHTS also demonstrated that reducing the IOP by an average of 23% decreased the incidence of COAG by 60% (85). In the EMGT and the CNTGS, an IOP reduction of 25% and greater than 30% cut the risk of progression by 33% and 50%, respectively, compared with no treatment

Table 9.4	Intraocular Pressure (IOP) and the Rates of and Relative Risk for Chronic Open-Angle Glaucoma, by Study				
Baltimore Eye Survey[a]			**Barbados Eye Study**[b]		
IOP Level, *mm Hg*	Prevalence, %	Relative Risk	IOP Level, *mm Hg*	4-Year Incidence, %	Relative Risk
<15	0.7	1.0	<17	0.7	1.0
16–18	1.3	2.0	>17–19	1.1	1.6
19–21	1.8	2.8	>19–21	2.7	4.0
22–24	8.3	12.8	>21–23	3.6	4.8
25–29	8.3	12.8	>23–25	6.9	10.5
30–34	25.4	39	>25	18.3	24.7
≥35	26.1	40.1			

[a]Data shown are for black and white participants combined (53).
[b]Estimates adjusted for age, sex, hypertension, and IOP lowering (58).

(61,63). Other clinical trials of COAG report that greater pressure lowering results in less progression (86,89,90).

An important implication of these population-based data and the CNTGS findings is that IOP may contribute to the onset of glaucoma even in patients with untreated IOP in the low-normal range and that some of these patients will benefit from IOP reduction. An intriguing finding from AGIS was that persons with the greatest IOP reduction (mean IOP, 12.3 mm Hg with treatment vs. 23.3 mm Hg before treatment) had stable visual fields (based on mean field defect score; risk of progression in the group was 14.4%) in contrast to groups with higher levels of IOP that showed progressive field loss over the 8-year follow-up period (86). This suggests that, at least in hypertensive COAG, an IOP level exists below which progression of glaucoma is stopped or at least suppressed to subclinical levels in most patients. High diurnal variation in IOP may also be a risk factor for progression in addition to the risk related to mean IOP.

Optic Nerve Head and Peripapillary Features

When the parameters used to define glaucoma, such as cup-to-disc ratio, are also treated as risk factors, a problem with circular reasoning may result. One population-based study reported that the incidence of COAG for persons with a baseline cup-to-disc ratio of more than 0.7 was 8.6-fold higher than for those with a cup-to-disc ratio of less than 0.7 (56). However, this estimate may be inflated because one of the criteria for defining COAG was having a cup-to-disc ratio of more than 0.7. Another feature of the optic nerve head that may be associated with glaucoma is the vertical disc diameter and the disc area (91–93), possibly because of greater susceptibility to glaucomatous nerve damage (94,95). However, the reported associations may have occurred in part because larger discs have larger cup-to-disc ratios (96–99), which in turn were part of the diagnostic criteria in most of these studies.

Optic disc hemorrhages were first recognized as a precursor to glaucomatous optic nerve damage by Bjerrum in 1889. This somehow fell out of clinical lore until it was rediscovered in 1977, when Drance and colleagues provided the first longitudinal findings (100), subsequently confirmed by others (101,102), that eyes with a disc hemorrhage had an elevated risk for progressive visual field loss (62,103,104). Additional support has been provided by both the EMGT (RR, 1.02 per percentage of visits with disc hemorrhage present) and the CNTGS (RR, 2.72) (76). Population surveys that have specifically reported on optic disc hemorrhage have found prevalences in adults ranging from 0.9% to 1.4%, of which only 2% and 30%, respectively, were in persons with glaucoma (42,105). In the second of these two studies, the prevalence of glaucoma was found to be increased 10-fold in those with disc hemorrhages, and disc hemorrhages were much more common in normal-tension glaucoma (25%) than in high-tension glaucoma (8%) (105). Interestingly, in another population-based series of adults with disc hemorrhages but without glaucoma on screening, 5 of 12 patients followed up for more than 6 years developed visual field loss by year 7 (106). However, particularly in individuals with no other risk factors for glaucoma, an optic disc hemorrhage may be due to other causes, including microvascular disease from diabetes mellitus or hypertension or from a posterior vitreous detachment, Valsalva maneuver, or anticoagulation.

Atrophy of the neurosensory retina and retinal pigment epithelium about the optic nerve head is known as peripapillary atrophy and has been shown to correlate with the presence of glaucoma (96,107,108). Peripapillary atrophy may also worsen along with glaucoma progression (109), although this has not been a consistent finding. Zone alpha peripapillary atrophy has been found in 58% of a white population older than 55 years, rendering it of little diagnostic value; zone beta peripapillary atrophy has been reported to be three times as common in patients with COAG as in controls (96), but it is associated with myopia and is also quite common, with a prevalence of 13%. Peripapillary atrophy does not appear to be specific to glaucoma, and its role in the diagnosis and management of COAG remains unclear.

Myopia

An association between myopia, particularly high myopia, and open-angle glaucoma has long been recognized and is supported by numerous case series and case-control studies (110–114). This association is also supported by large population-based prevalence surveys that reported an elevation of prevalence of COAG in those with any myopia of 48%, 60%, and 70% after adjustment for age and sex (93,115–117). Another survey reported a twofold- to threefold-increased prevalence of glaucoma in individuals with myopia (118). However, individuals with myopia were not found to have a higher incidence or progression of glaucoma in the OHTS or the EMGT, respectively (72). Other longitudinal studies have previously shown high myopia to be a risk factor for progression (119,120).

Other

In EMGT, having exfoliation syndrome and having a relatively thin central corneal thickness were associated with an increased risk for progression (62).

Systemic Risk Factors

Diabetes Mellitus

The prevalence of COAG appears to be higher in the diabetic population by a factor of about 2 in the majority of population-based surveys (121–124), although an association was not found in others (125,126). Most of these studies did not use IOP in their criteria for defining COAG, and one of them showed that the association of diabetes and glaucoma persisted after adjustment for IOP (124). Findings from numerous clinical studies on the association of diabetes and glaucoma are inconsistent and are subject to greater methodological limitations than population-based surveys, particularly selection bias (127,128). IOP is an important confounder of the association between diabetes and glaucoma because persons with diabetes appear to have a slightly higher IOP and have been reported to have a higher prevalence of ocular hypertension and incidence of IOP elevation, compared with persons who do not have diabetes (72,123,124,128). Diabetes has not yet been shown to increase the incidence of glaucoma. Although the weight of available evidence suggests that diabetes is probably a risk factor for glaucoma, this has not been a consistent finding. Self-reported diabetes was associated with COAG progression in the AGIS and the CIGTS (Collaborative Initial Glaucoma Treatment Study) but not in the CNTGS or the EMGT (129).

Blood Pressure

The most meaningful blood pressure variable related to glaucoma appears to be diastolic ocular perfusion pressure or the difference between diastolic arterial pressure and IOP. Diastolic ocular perfusion pressure has consistently been associated with COAG in several large population-based surveys that reported a severalfold increase in the prevalence of COAG among those with lower perfusion pressures (128,130). These surveys suggest that a steep increase in the prevalence of glaucoma occurs when diastolic ocular perfusion pressure falls below 55 mm Hg. This is supported by a large population-based cohort study that showed a strong dose–response gradient between the incidence of glaucoma and diastolic perfusion pressure, with an RR for glaucoma of 3.2 for those with the lowest diastolic perfusion pressure (<55 mm Hg) (73).

The literature on the association between systolic or diastolic blood pressure and glaucoma is confusing, with some population-based studies showing an association and others not (46,122,128,130,131). Similarly, some clinical studies on risk factors link higher blood pressures to glaucoma, and others report that lower blood pressure is more common in those with COAG and those with progression of glaucoma (114,132–138). The best evidence comes from a large population-based cohort study that showed a 51%-decreased risk for COAG in persons with systolic hypertension at baseline and that this protective effect was greater at higher levels of blood pressure (73). One study also described an increased prevalence of glaucoma at both very low and very high levels of systolic blood pressure, with the lowest prevalence in the midrange (130). It may be that high and low blood pressures are linked to glaucomatous optic nerve damage by different mechanisms. This may explain, in part, the apparently contradictory literature on the association between blood pressure and glaucoma.

Lower blood pressure has been reported as a risk factor for progression of COAG in EMGT (129). Numerous large surveys have consistently found that IOP elevation is associated with increased systolic and diastolic blood pressure (122,128, 130). However, the associated change in IOP is not clinically significant. For example, in the Baltimore Eye Survey, a 10–mm Hg increase in systolic or diastolic blood pressure was associated with an increase in IOP of 0.25 and 0.19 mm Hg, respectively (128).

There has been considerable attention paid to the role of episodic decreases in blood pressure in glaucoma, particularly in normal-tension glaucoma. Nocturnal arterial hypotension, which has also been implicated in anterior ischemic optic neuropathy, has been linked to the presence of COAG and normal-tension glaucoma and the progression of normal-tension glaucoma and COAG (137,139–144). Several clinical studies also suggest that nocturnal arterial hypotension is more common in normal-tension glaucoma than in COAG with elevated IOP (139,145). There are several reports of a hemodynamic crisis precipitating optic nerve damage in patients with COAG, but it has not been shown to occur more frequently than in individuals without COAG (146,147). Individuals with glaucoma and diastolic perfusion pressures less than 55 mm Hg may be most at risk due to episodes of decreased blood pressure, such as from nocturnal arterial hypotension, general anesthesia, and overmedication for systemic hypertension; however, this remains to be established.

Migraine

Some evidence supports an association between migraine headaches and normal-tension glaucoma. Two case-control studies reported an association between a history of typical migraine headaches and normal-tension glaucoma but not COAG with elevated IOP (148). A third case-control study had similar findings for stringent definitions of migraine, but the results did not reach statistical significance. The CNTGS found that a history of migraine increased the risk of progression by a factor of 2.6. Vasospasm is thought to play a central role in the pathogenesis of migraine, and other studies have found a predisposition to vasospasm in patients with normal-tension glaucoma (149–153). Although a fair and growing amount of evidence links normal-tension glaucoma with migraine or vasospasm, this does not appear to be the case for all COAG in the general population, according to two large, population-based studies (154,155).

Cerebrospinal Fluid Pressure

A growing body of evidence suggests that lower CSF pressure may increase the risk for open-angle glaucoma in a similar manner to elevated IOP (see Chapter 4). Studies show that patients with COAG have lower CSF pressures, which increases translaminar pressure differences (156,157). Conversely, higher CSF pressures are found in persons with ocular hypertension, which would seemingly have the opposite effect. In prospectively conducted research, Ren and coworkers found that blood pressure was correlated with IOP and CSF pressure. Studying the role of CSF pressure in patients with glaucoma presents unusual challenges but may help clarify the relationships among IOP, blood pressure, and the risk for glaucoma.

Other Systemic Risk Factors

There is equivocal evidence linking several thyroid disorders to COAG. In two case series, hypothyroidism was more common among patients with glaucoma than among persons without glaucoma (158,159), and treating hypothyroidism has been shown to lower IOP and increase outflow facility (160). However, a case series of 100 consecutive patients with newly diagnosed hypothyroidism detected no glaucoma and found no association between thyroid function and IOP (161). An older case series also found no abnormalities in thyroid function in COAG (162). Graves disease has been associated with an increased prevalence of ocular hypertension and glaucoma (163,164), possibly secondary to orbital changes and raised episcleral venous pressure.

Other endocrine disorders have not been associated with COAG but may affect the IOP. Cushing syndrome may lead to elevated IOP, which normalizes with control of the disease (165,166). Pituitary dysfunction may be associated with IOP fluctuations (167). Elevated levels of progesterone or estrogen may lower eye pressure (168), whereas testosterone may raise it (167).

Sleep apnea is characterized by recurrent complete or partial upper airway obstruction during sleep, leading to episodes of transient hypoxia. The condition is amenable to treatment and is typically seen in overweight men with thickset necks, a history of loud snoring, and self-report of morning hypersomnolence. Two case series have described a higher-than-expected prevalence of sleep apnea in patients with COAG and normal-tension glaucoma (169,170).

Infectious and autoimmune risk factors have been associated with COAG (171–174). COAG does not appear to be associated with elevated cholesterol or high-density lipoprotein level or obesity (175,176).

PROGNOSIS FOR BLINDNESS

Risk for Blindness from COAG

The primary goal of glaucoma treatment is to minimize the lifetime risk for significant loss of vision-related quality of life due to glaucoma. However, there is limited information to help the clinician to quantify the lifetime risk for blindness for a particular patient. One source of useful data comes from the proportion of individuals with glaucoma who were bilaterally blind (from glaucoma) in population-based surveys. This ranges from 2.5% to 6.2% in whites and appears to be higher in blacks, at 7.9% (29,42,49,177). However, these figures include all individuals with glaucoma regardless of the duration of disease and consequently underestimate the risk for blindness from glaucoma at the end of life.

Outcomes from the long-term follow-up of cases are also helpful to estimate prognosis but must be used with caution because of limitations with generalizing from these studies to current patient care. In a community clinical practice in Olmstead County, Minnesota, the 20-year risk for blindness in individuals with newly diagnosed open-angle glaucoma between 1965 and 1980 was 22% in both eyes and 54% in one eye (178). In patients receiving treatment for ocular hypertension, the 20-year risk for blindness was 4% in both eyes and 14% in one eye. A more recent clinical series of patients from a subspecialty glaucoma clinic who received a diagnosis of COAG after 1975 showed a 15-year risk for blindness due to glaucoma of 6.4% in both eyes and 14.6% in one eye (179) (**Table 9.5**). One of the difficulties in using these findings is that a patient with newly diagnosed disease today would be expected to do much better because of improvements in glaucoma care over the past three or four decades. Perhaps, the greatest difficulty in applying these figures to the care of a particular patient is that these clinical studies lump together newly diagnosed COAG of all levels of severity at the time of diagnosis. Consequently, patients with early glaucoma should fare much better overall, whereas those with advanced glaucoma should have an even poorer prognosis (Table 9.5).

Risk Factors for Blindness from COAG

Advanced Stage

Rough general estimates of prognosis in glaucoma can be refined somewhat by the presence or absence of risk factors for glaucoma blindness, including advanced stage, young age, inadequate IOP control, and ongoing progression. Not only are more advanced stages of glaucoma further along in the process leading to blindness, but some evidence also suggests that more advanced glaucoma is more likely to progress than earlier stages of the disease and may require greater IOP lowering to halt

Table 9.5	Long-Term Estimated Risk for Blindness Due to Chronic Open-Angle Glaucoma in Selected Studies	
Study (Reference) and Description	**Type of Blindness Evaluated, and Timing**	**Risk for Blindness, %**
Hattenhauer et al., 1998 (178)[a]		
100 Patients followed up after receiving a diagnosis of COAG in 1965–1980	Monocular, at 20 y after COAG diagnosis	54
	Binocular, at 20 y after COAG diagnosis	22
191 Patients followed up and treated for OHT after diagnosis in 1965–1980	Monocular, at 20 y after OHT diagnosis	14
	Binocular, at 20 y after OHT diagnosis	4
Chen, 2003 (179)[a,b]		
186 Patients followed up at a glaucoma specialty clinic since receiving a diagnosis of COAG after 1975	Monocular, at 15 y after COAG diagnosis	15
	Binocular, at 15 y after COAG diagnosis	6
Kwon et al., 2001 (180)		
40 Eyes followed up at a glaucoma subspecialty clinic after trabeculectomy surgery done in or after 1972	In study eye, at 22 y after surgery	19

[a]Study sample included persons with exfoliation.
[b]Study sample included persons with pigment dispersion.
COAG, chronic open-angle glaucoma; OHT, ocular hypertension.

progression (181–184). However, other longitudinal studies have not found a more rapid progression in those with worse initial visual field scores (101,180,185).

Young Age

Onset of glaucoma at a younger age is another risk factor for blindness because the glaucoma is expected to have longer to progress. The median estimated duration of COAG in the United States is 13 years in whites, with 25% of cases beginning by age 64 and 50% by age 72 (1). In blacks, the median duration is estimated to be 16 years, with 25% of cases beginning by age 54 years and 50% by age 65 years (1). The onset of COAG before the median age of onset portends a longer duration of disease and a higher lifetime risk for blindness than the median; the onset of COAG in the earliest 25th percentile portends a considerably longer duration and higher level of risk. Furthermore, significant comorbidities may curtail life expectancy. The earlier onset and longer duration of COAG in black patients, compared with other patients, may largely account for the higher risk for glaucoma-related blindness among blacks in the United States (1), although other factors, such as decreased access to health care, may contribute (186–190).

Inadequate Intraocular Pressure Control

It has long been standard clinical practice to treat glaucoma by safely lowering IOP below the level at which optic nerve damage occurred. Recent clinical trials have conclusively shown that failure to do so forfeits the benefit of IOP lowering and results in a higher risk of progression to blindness. Patient nonadherence to glaucoma-treatment regimens is one cause of inadequate IOP lowering and has been shown to increase the risk for blindness by a factor of 1.8 (179). Several studies have noted marked differences in individual susceptibility to IOP and have stressed the importance of additional IOP lowering in the face of ongoing progression (182,191). This is supported by numerous studies showing that greater IOP reduction results in less progression (86,192–196). However, in blinding glaucoma, patients commonly progress to blindness despite IOP lowering to the mid to low teens (179,191). It may be that heightened susceptibility to IOP damage or non–IOP-dependent mechanisms of damage may be more prominent in patients with blinding glaucoma, at least in the last stages of the disease.

High Rate of Progression Despite Treatment

A high rate of progression despite treatment is itself another risk factor for glaucoma blindness. The rate of visual field progression has been found to be 3 to 10 times more rapid in those eventually progressing to blindness than in age- and initial field-matched controls, although the IOP was actually lowered further in those progressing to blindness (191). Clinically, time to definite progression is often used as a practical indicator of progression rate. As one reference point, the median time to definite progression in treated COAG (mean initial IOP, 15.5 mm Hg after 25% IOP reduction) was about 6 years in the EMGT with the simple endpoint of significant progression of the same three or more points on a glaucoma change

probability map (Humphrey 24-2) on three consecutive fields. However, even patients who take this long to show definite progression may eventually be blinded by glaucoma if they have advanced glaucoma; also, even slow progression may eventually lead to blindness in those with a long life expectancy or whose progression accelerates. COAG is often an asymmetric disease, and an aggressive clinical course in one eye may foreshadow the clinical course of the fellow eye (182,197,198). A strong family history of aggressive COAG may also put a patient at higher risk for significant vision loss.

Prognosis for Blindness for Angle-Closure and Secondary Glaucomas

Although the foregoing discussion on risk factors for blindness in glaucoma relates to COAG, most of the risk factors discussed also apply to angle-closure glaucoma and secondary glaucoma. Prevalence surveys suggest that blindness is more common with angle-closure glaucoma and secondary glaucoma than with COAG. In cases of angle-closure glaucoma, estimates of glaucoma blindness in at least one eye range from 10% to 50% in Inuit and Chinese patients, and bilateral blindness in angle-closure glaucoma has been reported in 21% of cases in blacks in East Africa (31,35,40,199). The corresponding figures for secondary glaucoma (neovascular, lens related, posttraumatic, and uveitic) with blindness in at least one eye were 71% in Chinese patients and for bilateral blindness were 25% in East Africans (31,40). In each setting, the estimates given were higher than those for blindness due to COAG.

Undiagnosed Glaucoma

Prevalence surveys in primarily white populations from established market economies have consistently shown that about 50% of cases of COAG in the population had not yet been diagnosed (46,47,49,200). Among Chinese patients in Singapore, this percentage is 91% for COAG but only 29% for angle-closure glaucoma (40), presumably because the clinical course of angle-closure glaucoma is more likely to cause symptoms. Diagnosis of glaucoma has been found to be more likely in those with a history of other eye disease, a first-degree family history of glaucoma, and the use of one or more general medications.

A number of lines of evidence suggest that it is not just early glaucoma that is undiagnosed in the population. A series of 220 consecutive cases of newly diagnosed glaucoma from a hospital-based ophthalmology clinic in the United Kingdom reported that 50% had a visual field defect within 5 degrees of fixation (201,202). Among patients with newly diagnosed COAG, between 6% and 10% were reported to be blind in at least one eye (178). In addition, 45% of new cases of glaucoma blindness registered on the Massachusetts Blindness registry between 1970 and 1980 were blind due to glaucoma in one or both eyes at the time of their glaucoma diagnosis, similar to earlier reports from the United Kingdom (203,204). Risk factors for late presentation include lower socioeconomic status and time since last ocular examination (201).

Missed Opportunities for Diagnosing Glaucoma

Although delayed diagnosis may be due to a lack of ocular assessment, missed opportunities for diagnosis may also play an important role. In Sweden, a 5-year program ending in 1997 screened for glaucoma by using tonometry and fundus photography as an initial examination and identified 402 cases of undiagnosed open-angle glaucoma. Of these newly diagnosed cases, 67% of patients had previously seen an ophthalmologist and 17% had seen an ophthalmologist in the preceding 2 years (205). In Australia, 51% (36 of 70) of patients with undiagnosed glaucoma in the Melbourne Visual Impairment Project had seen an ophthalmologist, optometrist, or both in the preceding year (206). Some missed cases of COAG may have resulted from differing diagnostic criteria or from progression of disease between assessments. More probably, missed cases arose from less accurate assessment for glaucoma.

In Sweden, among persons with newly identified open-angle glaucoma after screening, 21% of those with an IOP less than 21 mm Hg had seen an ophthalmologist in the preceding 2 years, compared with 12% of those with a screening IOP of 21 mm Hg or greater ($P < 0.001$) (205). Similar findings have been reported from the Tierp Glaucoma Survey, also in Sweden. These reports suggest that the finding of a normal IOP decreases detection of COAG in routine eye care.

The nature of opportunities to improve diagnosis for glaucoma varies widely from setting to setting. In the United Kingdom, one study assessed practice patterns for glaucoma assessment and found that four of five optometrists could improve their detection of glaucoma by at least 50% by performing ophthalmoscopy and tonometry in all patients and perimetry in persons belonging to high-risk groups (207).

Nonadherence and Undertreatment

Suboptimal treatment may also significantly hamper efforts at preventing blindness due to glaucoma. Nonadherence to treatment and follow-up are a particular concern. In patients older than 65 years in the New Jersey Medicaid Program who were initiated on topical agent for the treatment of glaucoma, 23% never filled their prescription and the remainder missed an average of 30% of treatment days (208). In a managed care setting in Massachusetts, 25% of patients newly initiated on glaucoma therapy missed at least 20% of patient days of treatment (209). Adherence to treatment is notoriously difficult to predict but has been found to be several times more frequent in those seen only once in the 12 months after initiation of new treatment (209,210). Models of care that focus on patient education in a supportive environment have the potential to enhance patient adherence (211).

Suboptimal treatment may also result from a failure to incorporate advances in management of glaucoma into practice. Currently, the data on quality of care for COAG are sparse. One study of U.S. working-age patients with COAG enrolled in managed care plans found that care was consistent with guidelines (212). However, one significant deficiency was that only 53% of patients with COAG received an optic nerve drawing or photograph on initial examination (212). Given the expected delays in adopting new innovations, IOP may be undertreated in the United States and elsewhere in light of recent clinical trials.

CHALLENGES FROM GLAUCOMA IN THE DEVELOPING WORLD

In much of the developing world, the situation with glaucoma is entirely different. Eye-care services are limited, often severely so, and the amount of glaucoma in the general population that has been diagnosed is small; reports of 7% of COAG in India and 2% in Tanzania are typical (41). Glaucoma usually presents symptomatically with severe vision loss in one or both eyes, or a painful acute attack. Surgical trabeculectomy with or without antimetabolites is the treatment of choice except in cases of angle-closure glaucoma amenable to peripheral iridotomy or iridectomy. Ongoing follow-up is typically a hardship for patients and is often not possible. For most people with glaucoma in the developing world, the disease simply follows its natural course without detection or intervention, at least until symptoms develop and blindness encroaches.

Challenges to Preventing Blindness: A Population Perspective

As the leading cause of irreversible blindness worldwide, affecting more than 6.6 million people, blindness due to glaucoma is a mounting problem of global public health importance. Glaucoma-related blindness is also largely preventable through timely diagnosis, effective treatment, and ongoing monitoring. Although this seems attainable in the developed world, glaucoma has proven itself a difficult adversary. The nature of most glaucomas is such that it typically evades detection until its final stages unless ocular assessment is done periodically to detect the disease early in its course; glaucoma is also unrelenting and takes advantage of any delays, lapses, or insufficiencies in treatment to destroy remaining axons. Consequently, a health services response sufficient to prevent blindness from glaucoma is resource intensive. Successful management of glaucoma typically requires long-term active involvement of the patient, except in the prevention of angle-closure glaucoma with iridotomy. From a clinical standpoint, determined efforts to detect glaucoma early and treat it effectively regularly meet with success in many patients, but even so, glaucoma has yet to be dislodged as a major cause of blindness in any country. Major deficiencies in the detection and treatment of glaucoma remain, even in developed countries.

STRATEGIES FOR PREVENTING BLINDNESS: IMPROVED EARLY DETECTION

There are numerous avenues to improve the prevention of blindness from glaucoma, but improved early detection offers the most potential. Undiagnosed glaucoma is probably the largest reservoir of preventable blindness in the developed world and is second only to cataract overall in the developing world. The strategies for the identification of asymptomatic individuals at increased risk for glaucoma run the gamut from population screening to case finding. Population screening is the presumptive identification of individuals who might benefit from further diagnostic assessment of glaucoma by an ophthalmologist or optometrist; case finding involves testing for glaucoma as opportunities arise in the course of clinical care, such as during periodic eye evaluations. A blend of approaches for detecting glaucoma from this spectrum can complement one another and may offer the best hope of minimizing undiagnosed glaucoma.

Improving Coverage of Case Finding

In most developed countries, periodic comprehensive ocular assessments form the backbone of primary eye care and provide as one of their chief benefits an excellent vehicle for glaucoma case finding. In fact, rates of coverage are surprisingly good in some settings. In Australia, 81% of those 40 years and older had had an examination by an ophthalmologist or optometrist within the previous 5 years (206). An identical level of 5-year coverage was reported among persons without diabetes in a Canadian population aged 30 years and older (213). Eye examinations in both these populations occurred least frequently in younger men of lower socioeconomic status or without private insurance, and Australians in rural areas were less likely to undergo eye examinations (206,213).

Coverage may be increased further by improving the provision of services to underserved segments of the population and targeting health promotion efforts to increase uptake of periodic ocular examinations in these groups (214). Changing population-wide use of preventive eye examinations is not an easy task, but even small percentage increases translate into a benefit to large numbers of individuals. An intensive use of this strategy in Australia, including targeted mailings and print and broadcast media announcements, successfully increased the use of retinal screening examinations in persons with diabetes from 55% to 70%. However, a targeted mailing campaign in the United States with the same objectives produced no sustained increase in retinal screening examinations (215).

Improving Accuracy of Case Finding

In clinical practice, the effectiveness of case finding for glaucoma in primary eye care may not be optimal (205,206). This may be due to the limited extent of examination carried out and undue reliance on elevated IOP to trigger a complete evaluation for glaucoma (205,207). In the U.S. context, the American Academy of Ophthalmology (AAO) has recommended the following elements for a comprehensive eye examination that pertain to improved detection of glaucoma (216): IOP, gonioscopy, slitlamp examination of the anterior segment, optic disc and nerve fiber layer evaluation with documentation of optic nerve appearance, and visual field examination. Alternatively, others suggest selective performance of visual field tests depending on risk factors and clinical findings (217). Similarly,

routine gonioscopy may not be necessary in those who, on examination, have normal peripheral anterior chamber depth and normal IOP. Careful documentation of the optic nerve appearance at baseline examination, preferably with stereoscopic photos or other suitable imaging (such as optical coherence tomography or scanning laser ophthalmoscopy), is important to permit glaucomatous changes to be identified on follow-up. A good baseline evaluation for glaucoma is of particular importance in following higher-risk patients, such as glaucoma suspects and patients with ocular hypertension, but it is worth remembering that almost any patient can develop glaucoma. In one large population-based cohort study, 28% of persons with newly diagnosed glaucoma were not considered to be glaucoma suspects or to have ocular hypertension when examined 4 years earlier (58).

To maximize cost-effective glaucoma case finding, the frequency of periodic assessment should be adjusted to a patient's level of risk for glaucoma. One recommendation for the frequency of comprehensive eye examinations that reflects the risk for glaucoma comes from the AAO (**Table 9.6**): every 1 to 2 years for those 65 years and older, every 1 to 3 years for those 55 to 64 years of age, every 2 to 4 years for those between the ages of 40 and 54 years, and 5 to 10 years for those before 40 years of age. For persons with a first-degree relative with glaucoma or those who are of African descent (or who have other risk factors supported by good evidence [**Table 9.7**]), the frequency may be increased and should be at least every 6 months to a year for patients 65 or older, every 1 to 2 years for those aged 55 to 64, every 1 to 3 years for those aged 40 to 54, and every 2 to 4 years for those younger than 40 years (216). Patient referral by primary care physicians to an eye specialist for periodic comprehensive eye examination is supported by the U.S. Preventive Services Task Force for those at increased risk for glaucoma (223).

Table 9.6	Recommended Frequency of Comprehensive Medical Eye Examinations, according to Risk-Factor Status for Chronic Open-Angle Glaucoma	
Age–Group	**Frequency of Examinations**	
	Adults with No Risk Factors	**Adults with ≥1 COAG Risk Factor**
<40 y	5–10 y	Every 2–4 y
40–54 y	Every 2–4 y	Every 1–3 y
55–64 y	Every 1–3 y	Every 1–2 y
≥65 y	Every 1–2 y	Every 6–12 mo

[a]Individuals are considered to have a risk factor for COAG if they have elevated intraocular pressure or a family history of glaucoma, or are of African or Latino/Hispanic descent.
COAG, chronic open-angle glaucoma.
Data from American Academy of Ophthalmology (AAO) Preferred Practice Patterns Committee. Preferred Practice Pattern Guidelines. Comprehensive Adult Medical Eye Evaluation. San Francisco, CA: AAO; 2005. Available at: http://www.aao.org/ppp.

Table 9.7	Variables with Good Evidence of Being Clinical Risk Factors for Chronic Open-Angle Glaucoma[a]	
Variable	**RR for COAG**	**Best Evidence: References**
Age (per decade >40 y)	2	3, 42, 50, 53
Black (white, referent)	4	29
Family history (first-degree relative)	2–4	78, 80, 82, 218
IOP (<15 mm Hg, referent)[b]		58, 72, 82, 102
19–21 mm Hg	3	
22–29 mm Hg	13	
≥30 mm Hg	40	
Myopia	1.5–3	116–118, 219
Exfoliation	5–10	82, 102, 118
Diastolic perfusion pressure (<55 mm Hg)	3	72, 126, 130, 218
Central corneal thickness	1.4	129
Pigment dispersion syndrome	—[c]	220

[a]Table shows only those variables meeting the standard of "good"-level evidence, as graded according to method of the U.S. Preventive Services Task Force (221). Display of risk-factor information modeled after Ref. 222.
[b]Relative risk data are from Ref. 53. For best evidence, see also Table 9.4.
[c]The estimated proportion of patients with pigment dispersion syndrome is 6% to 43%.
COAG, chronic open-angle glaucoma; IOP, intraocular pressure; RR, relative risk

Screening for Chronic Open-Angle Glaucoma

Screening for undiagnosed glaucoma in high-risk populations (e.g., blacks, older adults, socioeconomically disadvantaged persons) may complement periodic ocular examination, particularly when targeting individuals who cannot or have not accessed care (224). In some respects, COAG is an ideal disease for population screening: It is of public health importance; detectable during its prolonged asymptomatic phase; and amenable to effective therapy to prevent blindness, particularly when diagnosed early. However, many obstacles to large-scale screening for COAG remain, including the lack of an entirely satisfactory screening test and the weakness of the economic argument to justify the resources required compared with other preventive interventions. Currently, population screening for COAG is, for the most part, carried out sporadically and on a modest scale by community and research groups (205).

The specifications for a suitable test for population screening for glaucoma are more exacting than the criteria for clinical use. One set of criteria for screening devices for COAG from Prevent Blindness America illustrates the difficult balance of specifications required: high accuracy (sensitivity, 85% for moderate to advanced glaucoma; specificity, 95%); ease of administration and transport, set up by minimally trained personnel; low cost and low maintenance; short testing and process time; and ease of understanding and conduct for the patient. These criteria emphasize high specificity to reduce the large costs associated with false-positive referrals. For example, consider tonometry, the traditional screening modality for glaucoma. In the Baltimore Eye Survey, a screening IOP of more than 21 mm Hg detected only 47% of persons with COAG (i.e., sensitivity); using a criterion of IOP less than 21 mm Hg correctly identified 92% of persons without COAG (i.e., specificity) (29). For a prevalence of about 2%, such as in whites older than 39 years (Table 9.1), 9 of 100 persons would have a screening IOP greater than 21 mm Hg, of whom one would have COAG and eight would have false-positive results. If a different test were used with the same sensitivity but a higher specificity of 98%, then the number referred for definitive testing would be reduced to only 3 in 100, consisting of one person with COAG and two with false-positive results. This example illustrates the importance of high specificity in glaucoma screening. The fact that an IOP greater than 21 mm Hg detects only 50% of COAG also underlines the need for good sensitivity to avoid falsely reassuring those tested.

For varying reasons, none of the many useful diagnostic tests for glaucoma are completely satisfactory for population screening. Tonometry is now discouraged as a standalone method for screening because there is no IOP level that gives a reasonable balance between sensitivity and specificity (29). COAG screening by evaluation of the optic nerve head is limited by the cost of a highly trained clinician or of a suitable imaging device. The practicality of full threshold or threshold-related suprathreshold automated perimetry is limited by learning effects, the need for skilled interpretation, and relatively high costs. Frequency doubling perimetry may be one of the most promising psychophysical tests for population screening for glaucoma, although the cost remains significant and the specificity may be suboptimal unless adequate criteria are used to define an abnormal test (225).

Cost-Effectiveness of Screening for COAG

Population screening for COAG, although highly desirable, does not appear to be cost competitive with other preventive health care interventions (226,227). The cost per year of vision saved by glaucoma screening appears to be many times the cost per year of life saved from such interventions as screening for breast cancer (226). In contrast, a 1983 analysis suggested that population screening for glaucoma would probably be cost-effective if subgroups at known higher risk for glaucoma were targeted (228). Glaucoma screening programs have typically also screened for visual impairment, leading causes of which include refractive error and cataracts, which are amenable to treatment. This major benefit of glaucoma screening has not been built in to cost-effectiveness analyses. In fact, it is probably more accurate to think of glaucoma screening as a component of a vision screening examination. Further screening innovations and updated economic analyses will permit a stronger case to be made in the future for cost-effective screening for COAG, at least in high-risk segments of the population.

Screening for Angle-Closure Glaucoma

In Asian populations where angle-closure glaucoma is the predominant cause of morbidity from glaucoma, there is great potential for screening programs to prevent angle-closure glaucoma. In contrast to COAG, angle-closure glaucoma can be prevented by the bilateral laser iridotomies in individuals with occludable angles, a simple one-time intervention (229). Consequently, the cost of preventing angle-closure glaucoma is much less than that of providing long-term treatment for COAG. The risk for blindness is also much higher for angle-closure glaucoma than for COAG and therefore the benefit is greater for each case of angle-closure glaucoma prevented (31,39,40). As a result, population screening for angle-closure glaucoma in appropriate populations may be much more cost-effective than population screening for COAG.

Numerous modalities have been suggested for population screening for occludable angles, including anterior chamber depth measurement, Van Herick test (or peripheral anterior chamber depth measurement), and the oblique flashlight test. However, the accuracy of the tests is not completely satisfactory for population screening and varies with the biometric characteristics of the population (40). For an acceptable sensitivity of about 85%, both anterior chamber depth measurement ($\leq$2.22 mm by optical pachymetry) and Van Herick test (peripheral anterior chamber depth $\leq$15% peripheral corneal thickness) could achieve specificities of only 84% and 86%, respectively, for detecting occludable angles in a Mongolian population (40,230).

A clinical trial is under way in Mongolia to determine whether population screening and prophylactic iridotomies for occludable angles will reduce the incidence of angle-closure glaucoma (231). The screening criteria of an anterior chamber depth of less than 2.53 mm (by ultrasonography) or an IOP greater than 24 mm Hg tagged almost one third of the screening population for a definitive evaluation including gonioscopy; 24% had occludable angles. Although appropriate for the purposes of a clinical trial, more specific tests or criteria would greatly improve the feasibility of large-scale screening for angle-closure glaucoma.

Strategies for Prevention in the Developing World

In much of the developing world, the tremendous scarcity of resources for eye care greatly limits the feasible interventions to prevent blindness from glaucoma. It has been suggested that the best workable option in much of the developing world may be to integrate glaucoma case finding into other blindness prevention efforts, such as cataract surgical programs, and to offer inexpensive and high-quality filtering surgery for those cases of surgical glaucoma identified (232) and peripheral iridotomy for those with occludable angles.

Teleglaucoma: Using Distance Technology to Improve Access to Care

Given progress in information technology, it is possible to obtain high-quality digital photographs of the optic nerve and transmit compressed images for storage, retrieval, and evaluation via Web-based platforms. Such an approach, with or without recommendations on management of patients, is referred to as teleglaucoma.

Given that camera systems are portable, and assuming that a high-speed Internet link exists, it should be possible to set up mobile units or multiple fixed centers, which facilitate access to eye examinations so that patients do not need to travel a great deal unnecessarily (233). These images can be stored and read from a distance, and patients can be triaged into healthy, suspect, or definite categories. Referral and treatment decisions can be made as appropriate and conveyed to the patient via trained ophthalmic personnel (e.g., nurse or technician). Compression can take place without altering the quality of images significantly, and digital images appear to provide comparable information for the purposes of grading glaucomatous optic nerve involvement as traditional stereo slide film (234,235). More work is needed to assess whether two-dimensional images of the nerve convey adequate information, compared with stereoscopic images.

The deployment of advanced technologies can minimize the barriers of distance and geography to enhance access and facilitate the delivery of integrated health care (236). This is particularly important in areas with large underserved or rural populations or a limited number of ophthalmologists (237).

KEY POINT

- Glaucoma is the leading cause of irreversible blindness worldwide, and by 2020, the number of persons with glaucoma will almost double from the recent estimate of 67 million.
- The prevalence of COAG and angle-closure glaucoma varies across different populations: COAG accounts for about 90% of all glaucoma in blacks, whites, and some Asian populations (e.g., Japanese); angle-closure glaucoma predominates in certain Asian populations (e.g., Inuit, Mongolian) and has a similar prevalence to COAG in others (e.g., Chinese in Singapore).
- The age-specific prevalence of COAG (by population) is a useful starting point for clinicians to estimate the probability of COAG when beginning an initial assessment.
- Clinical risk factors are useful to assess the risk of COAG, but only a small number are well supported by evidence: age, race (black), elevated IOP, family history (first-degree relative), myopia, exfoliation syndrome, and diastolic ocular perfusion pressure (<55 mm Hg).
- The onset and progression of most glaucomas occur so slowly that careful documentation of baseline examination, including the optic nerve head appearance, is required to detect subtle changes.
- The lifetime risk for blindness from COAG probably exceeds 5% on average; risk factors for blindness from COAG include

early age of onset, advanced stage, inadequate IOP control, and a high rate of progression despite treatment.

- Undiagnosed COAG is probably the largest reservoir of preventable blindness in the world in that only 50% of COAG cases are identified, even in developed countries. A pressing need exists to complement this by developing cost-effective approaches for screening high-risk groups for COAG.

- In some Asian populations, screening and treatment of occludable angles with laser iridotomy to prevent angle-closure glaucoma may soon be demonstrated to be effective and feasible.

REFERENCES

1. Quigley HA. Number of people with glaucoma worldwide. *Br J Ophthalmol.* 1996;80(5):389–393.
2. Thylefors B, Negrel AD, Pararajasegaram R, et al. Global data on blindness. *Bull World Health Organ.* 1995;73(1):115–121.
3. Friedman DS, Wolfs RC, O'Colmain BJ, et al. Prevalence of open-angle glaucoma among adults in the United States. *Arch Ophthalmol.* 2004;122(4):532–538.
4. Kobelt-Nguyen G, Gerdtham UG, Alm A. Costs of treating primary open-angle glaucoma and ocular hypertension: a retrospective, observational two-year chart review of newly diagnosed patients in Sweden and the United States. *J Glaucoma.* 1998;7(2):95–104.
5. Iskedjian M, Walker J, Vicente C, et al. Cost of glaucoma in Canada: analyses based on visual field and physician's assessment. *J Glaucoma.* 2003;12(6):456–462.
6. Calissendorff BM. Costs of medical and surgical treatment of glaucoma. *Acta Ophthalmol Scand.* 2001;79(3):286–288.
7. Quigley HA. (Inter)National cost of glaucoma. *The Cost of Blindness Symposium.* Toronto; January 31–February 1, 2004. Available at: http://www.costofblindness.org/presentations/quigley/quigley.htm.
8. Tielsch JM. Therapy for glaucoma: costs and consequences. In: Ball SF, Franklin RM, eds. *Transactions of the New Orleans Academy of Ophthalmology.* Amsterdam, the Netherlands: Kugler; 1993:61–68.
9. Gerdtham UG, Hågå A, Karlsson G, et al. Observational costing study in open angle primary glaucoma in Sweden and the USA. *EPI research paper no. 65666.* Stockholm, Sweden: Stockholm School of Economics; 1996.
10. Coyle D, Drummond M. The economic burden of glaucoma in the UK. The need for a far-sighted policy. *Pharmacoeconomics.* 1995;7(6):484–489.
11. Glynn RJ, Seddon JM, Krug JH Jr, et al. Falls in elderly patients with glaucoma. *Arch Ophthalmol.* 1991;109(2):205–210.
12. Haymes SA, Leblanc RP, Nicolela MT, et al. Risk of falls and motor vehicle collisions in glaucoma. *Invest Ophthalmol Vis Sci.* 2007;48(3):1149–1155.
13. Haymes SA, LeBlanc RP, Nicolela MT, et al. Glaucoma and on-road driving performance. *Invest Ophthalmol Vis Sci.* 2008;49(7):3035–3041.
14. McGwin G Jr, Xie A, Mays A, et al. Visual field defects and the risk of motor vehicle collisions among patients with glaucoma. *Invest Ophthalmol Vis Sci.* 2005;46(12):4437–4441.
15. Jampel HD, Frick KD, Janz NK, et al. Depression and mood indicators in newly diagnosed glaucoma patients. *Am J Ophthalmol.* 2007;144(2):238–244.
16. Jayawant SS, Bhosle MJ, Anderson RT, et al. Depressive symptomatology, medication persistence, and associated healthcare costs in older adults with glaucoma. *J Glaucoma.* 2007;16(6):513–520.
17. Green J, Siddall H, Murdoch I. Learning to live with glaucoma: a qualitative study of diagnosis and the impact of sight loss. *Soc Sci Med.* 2002;55(2):257–267.
18. Mills RP, Janz NK, Wren PA, et al. Correlation of visual field with quality-of-life measures at diagnosis in the Collaborative Initial Glaucoma Treatment Study (CIGTS). *J Glaucoma.* 2001;10(3):192–198.
19. Jampel HD. Glaucoma patients' assessment of their visual function and quality of life. *Trans Am Ophthalmol Soc.* 2001;99:301–317.
20. Gutierrez P, Wilson MR, Johnson C, et al. Influence of glaucomatous visual field loss on health-related quality of life. *Arch Ophthalmol.* 1997;115(6):777–784.
21. Parrish RK II, Gedde SJ, Scott IU, et al. Visual function and quality of life among patients with glaucoma. *Arch Ophthalmol.* 1997;115(11):1447–1455.
22. Sherwood MB, Garcia-Siekavizza A, Meltzer MI, et al. Glaucoma's impact on quality of life and its relation to clinical indicators. A pilot study. *Ophthalmology.* 1998;105(3):561–566.
23. Viswanathan AC, McNaught AI, Poinoosawmy D, et al. Severity and stability of glaucoma: patient perception compared with objective measurement. *Arch Ophthalmol.* 1999;117(4):450–454.
24. Nelson P, Aspinall P, Papasouliotis O, et al. Quality of life in glaucoma and its relationship with visual function. *J Glaucoma.* 2003;12(2):139–150.
25. Wilson MR, Coleman AL, Yu F, et al. Functional status and well-being in patients with glaucoma as measured by the Medical Outcomes Study Short Form-36 questionnaire. *Ophthalmology.* 1998;105(11):2112–2116.
26. Barber BL, Strahlman ER, Laibovitz R, et al. Validation of a questionnaire for comparing the tolerability of ophthalmic medications. *Ophthalmology.* 1997;104(2):334–342.
27. Lee BL, Gutierrez P, Gordon M, et al. The Glaucoma Symptom Scale. A brief index of glaucoma-specific symptoms. *Arch Ophthalmol.* 1998;116(7):861–866.
28. Kennedy GJ. The geriatric syndrome of late-life depression. *Psychiatr Serv.* 1995;46(1):43–48.
29. Tielsch JM, Sommer A, Katz J, et al. Racial variations in the prevalence of primary open-angle glaucoma. The Baltimore Eye Survey. *JAMA.* 1991;266(3):369–374.
30. Leske MC, Connell AM, Schachat AP, et al. The Barbados Eye Study. Prevalence of open angle glaucoma. *Arch Ophthalmol.* 1994;112(6):821–829.
31. Buhrmann RR, Quigley HA, Barron Y, et al. Prevalence of glaucoma in a rural East African population. *Invest Ophthalmol Vis Sci.* 2000;41(1):40–48.
32. Mason RP, Kosoko O, Wilson MR, et al. National survey of the prevalence and risk factors of glaucoma in St. Lucia, West Indies. Part I. Prevalence findings. *Ophthalmology.* 1989;96(9):1363–1368.
33. Rotchford AP, Kirwan JF, Muller MA, et al. Temba glaucoma study: a population-based cross-sectional survey in urban South Africa. *Ophthalmology.* 2003;110(2):376–382.
34. Quigley HA, West SK, Rodriguez J, et al. The prevalence of glaucoma in a population-based study of Hispanic subjects: Proyecto VER. *Arch Ophthalmol.* 2001;119(12):1819–1826.
35. Arkell SM, Lightman DA, Sommer A, et al. The prevalence of glaucoma among Eskimos of northwest Alaska. *Arch Ophthalmol.* 1987;105(4):482–485.
36. Dandona L, Dandona R, Mandal P, et al. Angle-closure glaucoma in an urban population in southern India. The Andhra Pradesh eye disease study. *Ophthalmology.* 2000;107(9):1710–1716.
37. Dandona L, Dandona R, Srinivas M, et al. Open-angle glaucoma in an urban population in southern India: the Andhra Pradesh eye disease study. *Ophthalmology.* 2000;107(9):1702–1709.
38. Shiose Y, Kitazawa Y, Tsukahara S, et al. Epidemiology of glaucoma in Japan—a nationwide glaucoma survey. *Jpn J Ophthalmol.* 1991;35(2):133–155.
39. Foster PJ, Baasanhu J, Alsbirk PH, et al. Glaucoma in Mongolia. A population-based survey in Hovsgol province, northern Mongolia. *Arch Ophthalmol.* 1996;114(10):1235–1241.
40. Foster PJ, Oen FT, Machin D, et al. The prevalence of glaucoma in Chinese residents of Singapore: a cross-sectional population survey of the Tanjong Pagar district. *Arch Ophthalmol.* 2000;118(8):1105–1111.
41. Ramakrishnan R, Nirmalan PK, Krishnadas R, et al. Glaucoma in a rural population of southern India: the Aravind comprehensive eye survey. *Ophthalmology.* 2003;110(8):1484–1490.
42. Klein BE, Klein R, Sponsel WE, et al. Prevalence of glaucoma. The Beaver Dam Eye Study. *Ophthalmology.* 1992;99(10):1499–1504.
43. Bankes JL, Perkins ES, Tsolakis S, et al. Bedford glaucoma survey. *Br Med J.* 1968;1(5595):791–796.
44. Mitchell P, Smith W, Attebo K, et al. Prevalence of open-angle glaucoma in Australia. The Blue Mountains Eye Study. *Ophthalmology.* 1996;103(10):1661–1669.
45. Bonomi L, Marchini G, Marraffa M, et al. Prevalence of glaucoma and intraocular pressure distribution in a defined population. The Egna-Neumarkt Study. *Ophthalmology.* 1998;105(2):209–215.
46. Kahn HA, Leibowitz HM, Ganley JP, et al. The Framingham Eye Study. I. Outline and major prevalence findings. *Am J Epidemiol.* 1977;106(1):17–32.
47. Wensor MD, McCarty CA, Stanislavsky YL, et al. The prevalence of glaucoma in the Melbourne Visual Impairment Project. *Ophthalmology.* 1998;105(4):733–739.
48. Hollows FC, Graham PA. Intra-ocular pressure, glaucoma, and glaucoma suspects in a defined population. *Br J Ophthalmol.* 1966;50(10):570–586.
49. Coffey M, Reidy A, Wormald R, et al. Prevalence of glaucoma in the west of Ireland. *Br J Ophthalmol.* 1993;77(1):17–21.

50. Dielemans I, Vingerling JR, Wolfs RC, et al. The prevalence of primary open-angle glaucoma in a population-based study in The Netherlands. The Rotterdam Study. *Ophthalmology.* 1994;101(11):1851–1855.

51. Jonasson F, Damji KF, Arnarsson A, et al. Prevalence of open-angle glaucoma in Iceland: Reykjavik Eye Study. *Eye.* 2003;17(6):747–753.

52. Foster PJ, Buhrmann R, Quigley HA, et al. The definition and classification of glaucoma in prevalence surveys. *Br J Ophthalmol.* 2002;86(2): 238–242.

53. Sommer A, Tielsch JM, Katz J, et al. Relationship between intraocular pressure and primary open angle glaucoma among white and black Americans. The Baltimore Eye Survey. *Arch Ophthalmol.* 1991;109(8): 1090–1095.

54. Van Buskirk EM. The tale of normal-tension glaucoma. *J Glaucoma.* 1998;7(6):363–365.

55. Cavalli-Sforza LL, Menozzi P, Piazza A. *The History and Geography of Human Genes.* Princeton, NJ: Princeton University Press; 1994:158.

56. Mukesh BN, McCarty CA, Rait JL, et al. Five-year incidence of open-angle glaucoma: the visual impairment project. *Ophthalmology.* 2002; 109(6):1047–1051.

57. Bengtsson BO. Incidence of manifest glaucoma. *Br J Ophthalmol.* 1989; 73(7):483–487.

58. Leske MC, Connell AM, Wu SY, et al. Incidence of open-angle glaucoma: the Barbados Eye Studies. The Barbados Eye Studies Group. *Arch Ophthalmol.* 2001;119(1):89–95.

59. Katz J, Congdon N, Friedman DS. Methodological variations in estimating apparent progressive visual field loss in clinical trials of glaucoma treatment. *Arch Ophthalmol.* 1999;117(9):1137–1142.

60. Vesti E, Johnson CA, Chauhan BC. Comparison of different methods for detecting glaucomatous visual field progression. *Invest Ophthalmol Vis Sci.* 2003;44(9):3873–3879.

61. Heijl A, Leske MC, Bengtsson B, et al. Reduction of intraocular pressure and glaucoma progression: results from the Early Manifest Glaucoma Trial. *Arch Ophthalmol.* 2002;120(10):1268–1279.

62. Leske MC, Heijl A, Hyman L, et al. Predictors of long-term progression in the early manifest glaucoma trial. *Ophthalmology.* 2007;114(11): 1965–1972.

63. Collaborative Normal-Tension Glaucoma Study Group. The effectiveness of intraocular pressure reduction in the treatment of normal-tension glaucoma. *Am J Ophthalmol.* 1998;126(4):498–505.

64. Quigley HA, Nickells RW, Kerrigan LA, et al. Retinal ganglion cell death in experimental glaucoma and after axotomy occurs by apoptosis. *Invest Ophthalmol Vis Sci.* 1995;36(5):774–786.

65. Balazsi AG, Rootman J, Drance SM, et al. The effect of age on the nerve fiber population of the human optic nerve. *Am J Ophthalmol.* 1984;97(6): 760–766.

66. Repka MX, Quigley HA. The effect of age on normal human optic nerve fiber number and diameter. *Ophthalmology.* 1989;96(1):26–32.

67. Funaki S, Shirakashi M, Funaki H, et al. Relationship between age and the thickness of the retinal nerve fiber layer in normal subjects. *Jpn J Ophthalmol.* 1999;43(3):180–185.

68. Alamouti B, Funk J. Retinal thickness decreases with age: an OCT study. *Br J Ophthalmol.* 2003;87(7):899–901.

69. Kerrigan-Baumrind LA, Quigley HA, Pease ME, et al. Number of ganglion cells in glaucoma eyes compared with threshold visual field tests in the same persons. *Invest Ophthalmol Vis Sci.* 2000;41(3):741–748.

70. Quigley HA, Dunkelberger GR, Green WR. Retinal ganglion cell atrophy correlated with automated perimetry in human eyes with glaucoma. *Am J Ophthalmol.* 1989;107(5):453–464.

71. Harwerth RS, Carter-Dawson L, Shen F, et al. Ganglion cell losses underlying visual field defects from experimental glaucoma. *Invest Ophthalmol Vis Sci.* 1999;40(10):2242–2250.

72. Leske MC, Heijl A, Hussein M, et al. Factors for glaucoma progression and the effect of treatment: the early manifest glaucoma trial. *Arch Ophthalmol.* 2003;121(1):48–56.

73. Leske MC, Wu SY, Nemesure B, et al. Incident open-angle glaucoma and blood pressure. *Arch Ophthalmol.* 2002;120(7):954–959.

74. The Advanced Glaucoma Intervention Study (AGIS): 12. Baseline risk factors for sustained loss of visual field and visual acuity in patients with advanced glaucoma. *Am J Ophthalmol.* 2002;134(4):499–512.

75. Wilson R, Richardson TM, Hertzmark E, et al. Race as a risk factor for progressive glaucomatous damage. *Ann Ophthalmol.* 1985;17(10):653–659.

76. Drance S, Anderson DR, Schulzer M. Risk factors for progression of visual field abnormalities in normal-tension glaucoma. *Am J Ophthalmol.* 2001;131(6):699–708.

77. Rosenthal AR, Perkins ES. Family studies in glaucoma. *Br J Ophthalmol.* 1985;69(9):664–667.

78. Tielsch JM, Katz J, Sommer A, et al. Family history and risk of primary open angle glaucoma. The Baltimore Eye Survey. *Arch Ophthalmol.* 1994; 112(1):69–73.

79. Nemesure B, Leske MC, He Q, et al. Analyses of reported family history of glaucoma: a preliminary investigation. The Barbados Eye Study Group. *Ophthalmic Epidemiol.* 1996;3(3):135–141.

80. Wolfs RC, Klaver CC, Ramrattan RS, et al. Genetic risk of primary open-angle glaucoma. Population-based familial aggregation study. *Arch Ophthalmol.* 1998;116(12):1640–1645.

81. Mitchell P, Rochtchina E, Lee AJ, et al. Bias in self-reported family history and relationship to glaucoma: the Blue Mountains Eye Study. *Ophthalmic Epidemiol.* 2002;9(5):333–345.

82. Le A, Mukesh BN, McCarty CA, et al. Risk factors associated with the incidence of open-angle glaucoma: the visual impairment project. *Invest Ophthalmol Vis Sci.* 2003;44(9):3783–3789.

83. Hill AB. The Environment and disease: association or causation? *Proc R Soc Med.* 1965;58:295–300.

84. Rothman K, Greenland S. *Modern Epidemiology.* Philadelphia, PA: Lippincott-Raven; 1998:24.

85. Kass MA, Heuer DK, Higginbotham EJ, et al. The Ocular Hypertension Treatment Study: a randomized trial determines that topical ocular hypotensive medication delays or prevents the onset of primary open-angle glaucoma. *Arch Ophthalmol.* 2002;120(6):701–713; discussion 829–830.

86. The Advanced Glaucoma Intervention Study (AGIS): 7. The relationship between control of intraocular pressure and visual field deterioration. *Am J Ophthalmol.* 2000;130(4):429–440.

87. Kerrigan LA, Zack DJ, Quigley HA, et al. TUNEL-positive ganglion cells in human primary open-angle glaucoma. *Arch Ophthalmol.* 1997;115(8): 1031–1035.

88. Quigley HA, Addicks EM, Green WR, et al. Optic nerve damage in human glaucoma. II. The site of injury and susceptibility to damage. *Arch Ophthalmol.* 1981;99(4):635–649.

89. Jay JL, Allan D. The benefit of early trabeculectomy versus conventional management in primary open angle glaucoma relative to severity of disease. *Eye.* 1989;3(5):528–535.

90. Migdal C, Gregory W, Hitchings R. Long-term functional outcome after early surgery compared with laser and medicine in open-angle glaucoma. *Ophthalmology.* 1994;101(10):1651–1656; discussion 7.

91. Healey PR, Mitchell P. Optic disk size in open-angle glaucoma: the Blue Mountains Eye Study. *Am J Ophthalmol.* 1999;128(4):515–517.

92. Wang L, Damji KF, Munger R, et al. Increased disk size in glaucomatous eyes vs normal eyes in the Reykjavik eye study. *Am J Ophthalmol.* 2003; 135(2):226–228.

93. Quigley HA, Varma R, Tielsch JM, et al. The relationship between optic disc area and open-angle glaucoma: the Baltimore Eye Survey. *J Glaucoma.* 1999;8(6):347–352.

94. Quigley HA. Reappraisal of the mechanisms of glaucomatous optic nerve damage. *Eye.* 1987;1(2):318–322.

95. Cahane M, Bartov E. Axial length and scleral thickness effect on susceptibility to glaucomatous damage: a theoretical model implementing Laplace's law. *Ophthalmic Res.* 1992;24(5):280–284.

96. Jonas JB, Nguyen XN, Gusek GC, et al. Parapapillary chorioretinal atrophy in normal and glaucoma eyes. I. Morphometric data. *Invest Ophthalmol Vis Sci.* 1989;30(5):908–918.

97. Quigley HA, Brown AE, Morrison JD, et al. The size and shape of the optic disc in normal human eyes. *Arch Ophthalmol.* 1990;108(1):51–57.

98. Ramrattan RS, Wolfs RC, Jonas JB, et al. Determinants of optic disc characteristics in a general population: The Rotterdam Study. *Ophthalmology.* 1999;106(8):1588–1596.

99. Healey PR, Mitchell P, Smith W, et al. Relationship between cup-disc ratio and optic disc diameter: the Blue Mountains Eye Study. *Aust N Z J Ophthalmol.* 1997;25(suppl 1):S99–S101.

100. Drance SM, Fairclough M, Butler DM, et al. The importance of disc hemorrhage in the prognosis of chronic open angle glaucoma. *Arch Ophthalmol.* 1977;95(2):226–228.

101. Rasker MT, van den Enden A, Bakker D, et al. Rate of visual field loss in progressive glaucoma. *Arch Ophthalmol.* 2000;118(4):481–488.

102. Ekstrom C. Elevated intraocular pressure and exfoliation of the lens capsule as risk factors for chronic open-angle glaucoma. A population-based five-year follow-up study. *Acta Ophthalmol.* 1993;71(2): 189–195.

103. Kim SH, Park KH. The relationship between recurrent optic disc hemorrhage and glaucoma progression. *Ophthalmology.* 2006;113(4): 598–602.

104. Siegner SW, Netland PA. Optic disc hemorrhages and progression of glaucoma. *Ophthalmology.* 1996;103(7):1014–1024.

105. Healey PR, Mitchell P, Smith W, et al. Optic disc hemorrhages in a population with and without signs of glaucoma. *Ophthalmology*. 1998;105(2): 216–223.

106. Bengtsson B. Optic disc haemorrhages preceding manifest glaucoma. *Acta Ophthalmol*. 1990;68(4):450–454.

107. Primrose J. Early signs of the glaucomatous disc. *Br J Ophthalmol*. 1971; 55(12):820–825.

108. Wilensky JT, Kolker AE. Peripapillary changes in glaucoma. *Am J Ophthalmol*. 1976;81(3):341–345.

109. Uchida H, Ugurlu S, Caprioli J. Increasing peripapillary atrophy is associated with progressive glaucoma. *Ophthalmology*. 1998;105(8):1541–1545.

110. Fong DS, Epstein DL, Allingham RR. Glaucoma and myopia: are they related? *Int Ophthalmol Clin*. 1990;30(3):215–218.

111. Podos SM, Becker B, Morton WR. High myopia and primary open-angle glaucoma. *Am J Ophthalmol*. 1966;62(6):1038–1043.

112. Perkins ES, Phelps CD. Open angle glaucoma, ocular hypertension, low-tension glaucoma, and refraction. *Arch Ophthalmol*. 1982;100(9): 1464–1467.

113. Daubs JG, Crick RP. Effect of refractive error on the risk of ocular hypertension and open angle glaucoma. *Trans Ophthalmol Soc U K*. 1981; 101(1):121–126.

114. Wilson MR, Hertzmark E, Walker AM, et al. A case-control study of risk factors in open angle glaucoma. *Arch Ophthalmol*. 1987;105(8):1066–1071.

115. Mitchell P, Wang JJ, Hourihan F. The relationship between glaucoma and exfoliation: the Blue Mountains Eye Study. *Arch Ophthalmol*. 1999;117(10):1319–1324.

116. Weih LM, Nanjan M, McCarty CA, et al. Prevalence and predictors of open-angle glaucoma: results from the visual impairment project. *Ophthalmology*. 2001;108(11):1966–1972.

117. Wong TY, Klein BE, Klein R, et al. Refractive errors, intraocular pressure, and glaucoma in a white population. *Ophthalmology*. 2003;110(1):211–217.

118. Mitchell P, Hourihan F, Sandbach J, et al. The relationship between glaucoma and myopia: the Blue Mountains Eye Study. *Ophthalmology*. 1999; 106(10):2010–2015.

119. Phelps CD. Effect of myopia on prognosis in treated primary open-angle glaucoma. *Am J Ophthalmol*. 1982;93(5):622–628.

120. Chihara E, Liu X, Dong J, et al. Severe myopia as a risk factor for progressive visual field loss in primary open-angle glaucoma. *Ophthalmologica*. 1997;211(2):66–71.

121. Klein BE, Klein R, Jensen SC. Open-angle glaucoma and older-onset diabetes. The Beaver Dam Eye Study. *Ophthalmology*. 1994;101(7):1173–1177.

122. Leske MC, Connell AM, Wu SY, et al. Risk factors for open-angle glaucoma. The Barbados Eye Study. *Arch Ophthalmol*. 1995;113(7):918–924.

123. Dielemans I, de Jong PT, Stolk R, et al. Primary open-angle glaucoma, intraocular pressure, and diabetes mellitus in the general elderly population. The Rotterdam Study. *Ophthalmology*. 1996;103(8):1271–1275.

124. Mitchell P, Smith W, Chey T, et al. Open-angle glaucoma and diabetes: the Blue Mountains eye study, Australia. *Ophthalmology*. 1997;104(4): 712–718.

125. Kahn HA, Leibowitz HM, Ganley JP, et al. The Framingham Eye Study. II. Association of ophthalmic pathology with single variables previously measured in the Framingham Heart Study. *Am J Epidemiol*. 1977;106(1): 33–41.

126. Tielsch JM, Katz J, Sommer A, et al. Hypertension, perfusion pressure, and primary open-angle glaucoma. A population-based assessment. *Arch Ophthalmol*. 1995;113(2):216–221.

127. Armstrong JR, Daily RK, Dobson HL, et al. The incidence of glaucoma in diabetes mellitus. A comparison with the incidence of glaucoma in the general population. *Am J Ophthalmol*. 1960;50:55–63.

128. Tielsch JM, Katz J, Quigley HA, et al. Diabetes, intraocular pressure, and primary open-angle glaucoma in the Baltimore Eye Survey. *Ophthalmology*. 1995;102(1):48–53.

129. Coleman AL, Miglior S. Risk factors for glaucoma onset and progression. *Surv Ophthalmol*. 2008;53(suppl):S3–S10.

130. Bonomi L, Marchini G, Marraffa M, et al. Vascular risk factors for primary open angle glaucoma: the Egna-Neumarkt Study. *Ophthalmology*. 2000;107(7):1287–1293.

131. Bengtsson B. Findings associated with glaucomatous visual field defects. *Acta Ophthalmol*. 1980;58(1):20–32.

132. Leighton DA, Phillips CI. Systemic blood pressure in open-angle glaucoma, low tension glaucoma, and the normal eye. *Br J Ophthalmol*. 1972;56(6):447–453.

133. Drance SM. Some factors in the production of low tension glaucoma. *Br J Ophthalmol*. 1972;56(3):229–242.

134. Drance SM. Angle closure glaucoma among Canadian Eskimos. *Can J Ophthalmol*. 1973;8(2):252–254.

135. Goldberg I, Hollows FC, Kass MA, et al. Systemic factors in patients with low-tension glaucoma. *Br J Ophthalmol*. 1981;65(1):56–62.

136. Gramer E, Leydhecker W. Glaucoma without ocular hypertension. A clinical study (in German). *Klin Monbl Augenheilkd*. 1985;186(4):262–267.

137. Kaiser HJ, Flammer J, Graf T, et al. Systemic blood pressure in glaucoma patients. *Graefes Arch Clin Exp Ophthalmol*. 1993;231(12):677–680.

138. Richler M, Werner EB, Thomas D. Risk factors for progression of visual field defects in medically treated patients with glaucoma. *Can J Ophthalmol*. 1982;17(6):245–248.

139. Hayreh SS, Zimmerman MB, Podhajsky P, et al. Nocturnal arterial hypotension and its role in optic nerve head and ocular ischemic disorders. *Am J Ophthalmol*. 1994;117(5):603–624.

140. Landau K, Winterkorn JM, Mailloux LU, et al. 24-hour blood pressure monitoring in patients with anterior ischemic optic neuropathy. *Arch Ophthalmol*. 1996;114(5):570–575.

141. Follmann P, Palotas C, Suveges I, et al. Nocturnal blood pressure and intraocular pressure measurement in glaucoma patients and healthy controls. *Int Ophthalmol*. 1996;20(1-3):83–87.

142. Meyer JH, Brandi-Dohrn J, Funk J. Twenty four hour blood pressure monitoring in normal tension glaucoma. *Br J Ophthalmol*. 1996;80(10): 864–867.

143. Graham SL, Drance SM, Wijsman K, et al. Ambulatory blood pressure monitoring in glaucoma. The nocturnal dip. *Ophthalmology*. 1995;102(1): 61–69.

144. Bresson-Dumont H, Bechetoille A. Role of arterial blood pressure in the development of glaucomatous lesions (in French). *J Fr Ophthalmol*. 1996;19(6-7):435–442.

145. Bechetoille A, Bresson-Dumont H. Diurnal and nocturnal blood pressure drops in patients with focal ischemic glaucoma. *Graefes Arch Clin Exp Ophthalmol*. 1994;232(11):675–679.

146. Morgan RW, Drance SM. Chronic open-angle glaucoma and ocular hypertension. An epidemiological study. *Br J Ophthalmol*. 1975;59(4): 211–215.

147. Drance SM, Morgan RW, Sweeney VP. Shock-induced optic neuropathy: a cause of nonprogressive glaucoma. *N Engl J Med*. 1973;288(8):392–395.

148. Cursiefen C, Wisse M, Cursiefen S, et al. Migraine and tension headache in high-pressure and normal-pressure glaucoma. *Am J Ophthalmol*. 2000;129(1):102–104.

149. Drance SM, Douglas GR, Wijsman K, et al. Response of blood flow to warm and cold in normal and low-tension glaucoma patients. *Am J Ophthalmol*. 1988;105(1):35–39.

150. Gasser P, Flammer J, Guthauser U, et al. Do vasospasms provoke ocular diseases? *Angiology*. 1990;41(3):213–220.

151. Gasser P, Flammer J. Blood-cell velocity in the nailfold capillaries of patients with normal-tension and high-tension glaucoma. *Am J Ophthalmol*. 1991;111(5):585–588.

152. Buckley C, Hadoke PW, Henry E, et al. Systemic vascular endothelial cell dysfunction in normal pressure glaucoma. *Br J Ophthalmol*. 2002;86(2): 227–232.

153. O'Brien C, Butt Z. Blood flow velocity in the peripheral circulation of glaucoma patients. *Ophthalmologica*. 1999;213(3):150–153.

154. Klein BE, Klein R, Meuer SM, et al. Migraine headache and its association with open-angle glaucoma: the Beaver Dam Eye Study. *Invest Ophthalmol Vis Sci*. 1993;34(10):3024–3027.

155. Wang JJ, Mitchell P, Smith W. Is there an association between migraine headache and open-angle glaucoma? Findings from the Blue Mountains Eye Study. *Ophthalmology*. 1997;104(10):1714–1719.

156. Ren R, Jonas JB, Tian G, et al. Cerebrospinal fluid pressure in glaucoma: a prospective study. *Ophthalmology*. 2010;117(2):259–266.

157. Berdahl JP, Fautsch MP, Stinnett SS, et al. Intracranial pressure in primary open angle glaucoma, normal tension glaucoma, and ocular hypertension: a case-control study. *Invest Ophthalmol Vis Sci*. 2008;49(12):5412–5418.

158. McLenachan J, Davies DM. Glaucoma and the thyroid. *Br J Ophthalmol*. 1965;49(8):441–444.

159. Smith KD, Arthurs BP, Saheb N. An association between hypothyroidism and primary open-angle glaucoma. *Ophthalmology*. 1993;100(10): 1580–1584.

160. Smith KD, Tevaarwerk GJ, Allen LH. An ocular dynamic study supporting the hypothesis that hypothyroidism is a treatable cause of secondary open-angle glaucoma. *Can J Ophthalmol*. 1992;27(7):341–344.

161. Karadimas P, Bouzas EA, Topouzis F, et al. Hypothyroidism and glaucoma. A study of 100 hypothyroid patients. *Am J Ophthalmol*. 2001;131(1): 126–128.

162. Krupin T, Jacobs LS, Podos SM, et al. Thyroid function and the intraocular pressure response to topical corticosteroids. *Am J Ophthalmol*. 1977; 83(5):643–646.

163. Ohtsuka K, Nakamura Y. Open-angle glaucoma associated with Graves disease. *Am J Ophthalmol.* 2000;129(5):613–617.

164. Cockerham KP, Pal C, Jani B, et al. The prevalence and implications of ocular hypertension and glaucoma in thyroid-associated orbitopathy. *Ophthalmology.* 1997;104(6):914–917.

165. Neuner HP, Dardenne U. Ocular changes in Cushing's syndrome (in German). *Klin Monbl Augenheilkd.* 1968;152(4):570–574.

166. Haas JS, Nootens RH. Glaucoma secondary to benign adrenal adenoma. *Am J Ophthalmol.* 1974;78(3):497–500.

167. Abdel-Aziz M, Labib MA. The relationship of the intraocular pressure and the hormonal disturbance. II. The pituitary gland. *Bull Ophthalmol Soc Egypt.* 1969;62(66):61–72.

168. Treister G, Mannor S. Intraocular pressure and outflow facility. Effect of estrogen and combined estrogen-progestin treatment in normal human eyes. *Arch Ophthalmol.* 1970;83(3):311–318.

169. Mojon DS, Hess CW, Goldblum D, et al. High prevalence of glaucoma in patients with sleep apnea syndrome. *Ophthalmology.* 1999;106(5):1009–1012.

170. Marcus DM, Costarides AP, Gokhale P, et al. Sleep disorders: a risk factor for normal-tension glaucoma? *J Glaucoma.* 2001;10(3):177–183.

171. Kountouras J, Mylopoulos N, Boura P, et al. Relationship between Helicobacter pylori infection and glaucoma. *Ophthalmology.* 2001;108(3):599–604.

172. Tezel G, Seigel GM, Wax MB. Autoantibodies to small heat shock proteins in glaucoma. *Invest Ophthalmol Vis Sci.* 1998;39(12):2277–2287.

173. Tezel G, Edward DP, Wax MB. Serum autoantibodies to optic nerve head glycosaminoglycans in patients with glaucoma. *Arch Ophthalmol.* 1999;117(7):917–924.

174. Wax M, Yang J, Tezel G. Autoantibodies in glaucoma. *Curr Eye Res.* 2002;25(2):113–116.

175. Stewart WC, Sine C, Sutherland S, et al. Total cholesterol and high-density lipoprotein levels as risk factors for increased intraocular pressure. *Am J Ophthalmol.* 1996;122(4):575–577.

176. Gasser P, Stumpfig D, Schotzau A, et al. Body mass index in glaucoma. *J Glaucoma.* 1999;8(1):8–11.

177. Sommer A, Tielsch JM, Katz J, et al. Racial differences in the cause-specific prevalence of blindness in east Baltimore. *N Engl J Med.* 1991;325(20):1412–1417.

178. Hattenhauer MG, Johnson DH, Ing HH, et al. The probability of blindness from open-angle glaucoma. *Ophthalmology.* 1998;105(11):2099–2104.

179. Chen PP. Blindness in patients with treated open-angle glaucoma. *Ophthalmology.* 2003;110(4):726–733.

180. Kwon YH, Kim CS, Zimmerman MB, et al. Rate of visual field loss and long-term visual outcome in primary open-angle glaucoma. *Am J Ophthalmol.* 2001;132(1):47–56.

181. Fruhauf A, Groeschel W, Muller F. Glaucoma serial examinations 1964-65 in Dresden (in German). *Klin Monbl Augenheilkd.* 1967;151(3):403–415.

182. Grant WM, Burke JF Jr. Why do some people go blind from glaucoma? *Ophthalmology.* 1982;89(9):991–998.

183. Wilson R, Walker AM, Dueker DK, et al. Risk factors for rate of progression of glaucomatous visual field loss: a computer-based analysis. *Arch Ophthalmol.* 1982;100(5):737–741.

184. Mikelberg FS, Schulzer M, Drance SM, et al. The rate of progression of scotomas in glaucoma. *Am J Ophthalmol.* 1986;101(1):1–6.

185. Smith SD, Katz J, Quigley HA. Analysis of progressive change in automated visual fields in glaucoma. *Invest Ophthalmol Vis Sci.* 1996;37(7):1419–1428.

186. Glynn RJ, Gurwitz JH, Bohn RL, et al. Old age and race as determinants of initiation of glaucoma therapy. *Am J Epidemiol.* 1993;138(6):395–406.

187. Ontiveros JA, Black SA, Jakobi PL, et al. Ethnic variation in attitudes toward hypertension in adults ages 75 and older. *Prev Med.* 1999;29(6, pt 1):443–449.

188. Devgan U, Yu F, Kim E, et al. Surgical undertreatment of glaucoma in black beneficiaries of medicare. *Arch Ophthalmol.* 2000;118(2):253–256.

189. Wang F, Javitt JC, Tielsch JM. Racial variations in treatment for glaucoma and cataract among Medicare recipients. *Ophthalmic Epidemiol.* 1997;4(2):89–100.

190. Hiller R, Kahn HA. Blindness from glaucoma. *Am J Ophthalmol.* 1975;80(1):62–69.

191. Oliver JE, Hattenhauer MG, Herman D, et al. Blindness and glaucoma: a comparison of patients progressing to blindness from glaucoma with patients maintaining vision. *Am J Ophthalmol.* 2002;133(6):764–772.

192. Bergea B, Bodin L, Svedbergh B. Impact of intraocular pressure regulation on visual fields in open-angle glaucoma. *Ophthalmology.* 1999;106(5):997–1004; discussion 1004–1005.

193. Odberg T, Riise D. Early diagnosis of glaucoma. II. The value of the initial examination in ocular hypertension. *Acta Ophthalmol.* 1987;65(1):58–62.

194. Greve EL, Dake CL. Four year follow-up of a glaucoma operation. Prospective study of the double flap Scheie. *Int Ophthalmol.* 1979;1(3):139–145.

195. Werner EB, Drance SM, Schulzer M. Trabeculectomy and the progression of glaucomatous visual field loss. *Arch Ophthalmol.* 1977;95(8):1374–1377.

196. Mao LK, Stewart WC, Shields MB. Correlation between intraocular pressure control and progressive glaucomatous damage in primary open-angle glaucoma. *Am J Ophthalmol.* 1991;111(1):51–55.

197. Harbin TS Jr, Podos SM, Kolker AE, et al. Visual field progression in open-angle glaucoma patients presenting with monocular field loss. *Trans Sect Ophthalmol Am Acad Ophthalmol Otolaryngol.* 1976;81(2):253–257.

198. Kass MA, Kolker AE, Becker B. Prognostic factors in glaucomatous visual field loss. *Arch Ophthalmol.* 1976;94(8):1274–1276.

199. Drance SM, Sweeney VP, Morgan RW, et al. Studies of factors involved in the production of low tension glaucoma. *Arch Ophthalmol.* 1973;89(6):457–465.

200. Giuffre G, Giammanco R, Dardanoni G, et al. Prevalence of glaucoma and distribution of intraocular pressure in a population. The Casteldaccia Eye Study. *Acta Ophthalmol Scand.* 1995;73(3):222–225.

201. Fraser S, Bunce C, Wormald R, et al. Deprivation and late presentation of glaucoma: case-control study. *BMJ.* 2001;322(7287):639–643.

202. Fraser S, Bunce C, Wormald R. Risk factors for late presentation in chronic glaucoma. *Invest Ophthalmol Vis Sci.* 1999;40(10):2251–2257.

203. Miller SJ, Karseras AG. Blind registration and glaucoma simplex. *Br J Ophthalmol.* 1974;58(4):455–461.

204. Perkins ES. Blindness from glaucoma and the economics of prevention. *Trans Ophthalmol Soc U K.* 1978;98(2):293–295.

205. Grodum K, Heijl A, Bengtsson B. A comparison of glaucoma patients identified through mass screening and in routine clinical practice. *Acta Ophthalmol Scand.* 2002;80(6):627–631.

206. Keeffe JE, Weih LM, McCarty CA, et al. Utilisation of eye care services by urban and rural Australians. *Br J Ophthalmol.* 2002;86(1):24–27.

207. Tuck MW, Crick RP. The cost-effectiveness of various modes of screening for primary open angle glaucoma. *Ophthalmic Epidemiol.* 1997;4(1):3–17.

208. Gurwitz JH, Glynn RJ, Monane M, et al. Treatment for glaucoma: adherence by the elderly. *Am J Public Health.* 1993;83(5):711–716.

209. Gurwitz JH, Yeomans SM, Glynn RJ, et al. Patient noncompliance in the managed care setting. The case of medical therapy for glaucoma. *Med Care.* 1998;36(3):357–369.

210. Kass MA, Gordon M, Meltzer DW. Can ophthalmologists correctly identify patients defaulting from pilocarpine therapy? *Am J Ophthalmol.* 1986;101(5):524–530.

211. Blondeau P, Esper P, Mazerolle E. An information session for glaucoma patients. *Can J Ophthalmol.* 2007;42(6):816–820.

212. Fremont AM, Lee PP, Mangione CM, et al. Patterns of care for open-angle glaucoma in managed care. *Arch Ophthalmol.* 2003;121(6):777–783.

213. Buhrmann R, Assaad D, Hux JE, et al. Diabetes and the eye. In: Hux JE, Booth GL, Slaughter PM, et al., eds. *Diabetes in Ontario: An ICES Practice Atlas.* Canada: Institute for Clinical Evaluative Sciences; 2003:193–209.

214. Javitt JC. Preventing blindness in Americans: the need for eye health education. *Surv Ophthalmol.* 1995;40(1):41–44.

215. Prela CM, Smilie JG, McInerney MJ, et al. Direct mail intervention to increase retinal examination rates in Medicare beneficiaries with diabetes. *Am J Med Qual.* 2000;15(6):257–262.

216. American Academy of Ophthalmology (AAO) Preferred Practice Patterns Committee. Preferred Practice Pattern Guidelines. Comprehensive Adult Medical Eye Evaluation. San Francisco, CA: AAO; 2005. Available at: http://www.aao.org/ppp. Accessed June 10, 2010.

217. Tuck MW, Crick RP. Relative effectiveness of different modes of glaucoma screening in optometric practice. *Ophthalmic Physiol Opt.* 1993;13(3):227–232.

218. Leske MC, Wu SY, Hennis A, et al. Risk factors for incident open-angle glaucoma: the Barbados Eye Studies. *Ophthalmology.* 2008;115(1):85–93.

219. Wu SY, Nemesure B, Leske MC. Glaucoma and myopia. *Ophthalmology.* 2000;107(6):1026–1027.

220. Niyadurupola N, Broadway DC. Pigment dispersion syndrome and pigmentary glaucoma—a major review. *Clin Experiment Ophthalmol.* 2008;36:868–882.

221. Harris RP, Helfand M, Woolf SH, et al. Current methods of the US Preventive Services Task Force: a review of the process. *Am J Prev Med.* 2001;20(3, suppl):21–35.

222. Tuulonen A, Airaksinen PJ, Erola E, et al. The Finnish evidence-based guideline for open-angle glaucoma. *Acta Ophthalmol Scand.* 2003;81(1):3–18.

223. United States Preventive Services Task Force. Screening for Glaucoma. In: Diguiseppe C, ed. *Guide to Clinical Preventive Services*. Alexandria, VA: International Medical Publishing; 1996:383.

224. Ellish NJ, Higginbotham EJ. Differences between screening sites in a glaucoma screening program. *Ophthalmic Epidemiol*. 2002;9(4): 225–237.

225. Quigley HA. Identification of glaucoma-related visual field abnormality with the screening protocol of frequency doubling technology. *Am J Ophthalmol*. 1998;125(6):819–829.

226. Boivin JF, McGregor M, Archer C. Cost effectiveness of screening for primary open angle glaucoma. *J Med Screen*. 1996;3(3):154–163.

227. Eddy DM, Sanders LE, Eddy JF. The value of screening for glaucoma with tonometry. *Surv Ophthalmol*. 1983;28(3):194–205.

228. Gottlieb LK, Schwartz B, Pauker SG. Glaucoma screening. A cost-effectiveness analysis. *Surv Ophthalmol*. 1983;28(3):206–226.

229. Nolan WP, Foster PJ, Devereux JG, et al. YAG laser iridotomy treatment for primary angle closure in east Asian eyes. *Br J Ophthalmol*. 2000; 84(11):1255–1259.

230. Devereux JG, Foster PJ, Baasanhu J, et al. Anterior chamber depth measurement as a screening tool for primary angle-closure glaucoma in an East Asian population. *Arch Ophthalmol*. 2000;118(2):257–263.

231. Nolan WP, Baasanhu J, Undraa A, et al. Screening for primary angle closure in Mongolia: a randomised controlled trial to determine whether screening and prophylactic treatment will reduce the incidence of primary angle closure glaucoma in an east Asian population. *Br J Ophthalmol*. 2003;87(3):271–274.

232. Quigley HA, Vitale S. Models of open-angle glaucoma prevalence and incidence in the United States. *Invest Ophthalmol Vis Sci*. 1997;38(1):83–91.

233. Labiris G, Fanariotis M, Christoulakis C, et al. Tele-ophthalmology and conventional ophthalmology using a mobile medical unit in remote Greece. *J Telemed Telecare*. 2003;9(5):296–299.

234. Constable IJ, Yogesan K, Eikelboom R, et al. Fred Hollows lecture: digital screening for eye disease. *Clin Experiment Ophthalmol*. 2000;28(3):129–132.

235. Khouri AS, Szirth B, Realini T, et al. Comparison of digital and film stereo photography of the optic nerve in the evaluation of patients with glaucoma. *Telemed J E Health*. 2006;12(6):632–638.

236. Rheuban KS. The role of telemedicine in fostering health-care innovations to address problems of access, specialty shortages and changing patient care needs. *J Telemed Telecare*. 2006;12(suppl 2):S45–S50.

237. Tuulonen A, Ohinmaa T, Alanko HI, et al. The application of teleophthalmology in examining patients with glaucoma: a pilot study. *J Glaucoma*. 1999;8(6):367–373.

10

The Glaucoma Suspect: When to Treat?

Distinguishing healthy persons in the general population from those at considerably increased risk for chronic open-angle glaucoma (COAG) is important because patients in the latter group—commonly referred to as "glaucoma suspects"—need to be followed up more carefully to decide whether and how to begin prophylactic therapy. This chapter outlines the definition and prevalence of glaucoma suspect and reviews key diagnostic elements that need to be considered. The chapter also highlights challenges in management, summarizing the results of the Ocular Hypertension Treatment Study (OHTS), and addresses when it may be appropriate to initiate therapy. Practical guidelines for follow-up are also offered.

TERMINOLOGY

The term ocular hypertension was advocated in the 1970s to distinguish persons with "normal" intraocular pressure (IOP) (i.e., ≤21 mm Hg) from those with an IOP greater than 21 mm Hg, who were considered to be at increased risk for COAG (1,2). Chandler and Grant (3) suggested referring to this condition as early open-angle glaucoma without damage.

However, in addition to those with consistently elevated IOP, there are individuals who exhibit optic nerve features suggestive of early glaucoma or who have suspicious visual field defects. To include these categories and identify a subpopulation of individuals or eyes at increased risk for COAG glaucoma (**Table 10.1**) (4), the term "glaucoma suspect" was advocated by Shaffer (5). There are also patients at higher risk for angle-closure glaucoma—for example, those with an occludable angle as determined by gonioscopy. Given recent advances in molecular genetics, there are also patients who can be identified as having an elevated risk for glaucomatous optic nerve damage by virtue of harboring one or more disease-causing genetic mutations (see Chapter 8). In this chapter, we will use the term glaucoma suspect in the context of a patient at greater-than-average risk (compared with the general population) for COAG. (Individuals at increased risk for angle-closure glaucoma are discussed in Chapter 12, and those at increased risk by virtue of a genetic susceptibility are discussed in Chapter 8.)

PREVALENCE AND DEVELOPMENT OF CHRONIC OPEN-ANGLE GLAUCOMA

Studies that have used a definition of IOP greater than or equal to 21 mm Hg in one or both eyes (with normal visual fields and optic nerves) have reported a prevalence rate of 4% to 10% in persons older than 40 years (6–11).

Patients considered to be glaucoma suspects on the basis of elevated IOP have a rate of progression to COAG of approximately 1% per year over 5 to 15 years (**Table 10.2**) (12–25). In the OHTS (22), a randomized trial of topical ocular hypotensive treatment versus close observation in participants with "ocular hypertension," the cumulative probability of developing COAG over 5 years was about 1% per year in the medication group and about 2% per year in the observation group. In patients who are at higher risk for developing glaucomatous optic nerve damage (see risk factors in **Table 10.3**), the rate is approximately 3% to 5% per year (26–28).

Table 10.1	Definition of a Glaucoma Suspect

Open angle by gonioscopy and one of the following in at least one eye:

- IOP consistently >21 mm Hg by applanation tonometry
- Appearance of the optic disc or retinal nerve fiber layer suggestive of glaucomatous damage
- Diffuse or focal narrowing or sloping of the disc rim
- Diffuse or localized abnormalities of the nerve fiber layer, especially at superior and inferior poles
- Disc hemorrhage
- Asymmetric appearance of the disc or rim between fellow eyes (e.g., cup-to-disc ratio difference > 0.2), suggesting loss of neural tissue
- Visual fields suspicious for early glaucomatous damage

Adapted from American Academy of Ophthalmology. *Primary Open-Angle Glaucoma Suspect, Preferred Practice Pattern.* San Francisco, CA: American Academy of Ophthalmology, 2005. Available at: http://www.aao.org/ppp.

Table 10.2	Incidence of Chronic Open-Angle Glaucoma (COAG) among Persons with Ocular Hypertension		
Study[a]	**Patients with Ocular Hypertension, _n_**	**Observation Period, _y_**	**Patients Developing COAG, _n_ (%)**
Perkins, 1973 (12)	124	5–7	4 (3.2)
Walker, 1974 (13)	109	11	11 (10.1)
Wilensky et al., 1974 (14)	50	Mean, 6	3 (6.0)
Norskov, 1970 (15)	68	5	0
Linnér, 1976 (16)	92	10	0
Kitazawa et al., 1977 (17)	75	Mean, 9.5	7 (9.3)
David et al., 1977 (18)	61	Mean, 3.3 Range, 1–11	10 (16.4)
Hart et al., 1979 (19)	92	5	33 (35.9)
Armaly et al., 1980 (20)	5886	13	98 (1.7)
Lundberg et al., 1987 (21)	41	20	14 (34.1)
Kass et al., 2002 (22)	819[b]	5	89 (10.9)

[a]Numbers in parentheses are reference numbers.
[b]Control arm.

Although elevated IOP is a major risk factor for COAG, normotensive individuals can develop glaucoma. Some of these patients may have normal-tension glaucoma (see Chapter 11), whereas others may demonstrate elevated IOP at subsequent examinations (12,23).

SCREENING AND EARLY DETECTION

Screening is discussed in Chapter 9. In brief, if an IOP value of more than 21 mm Hg is used for screening, then there is a high rate of false-positive and false-negative results for COAG.

Skilled optic nerve examination is good but not always practical. Standard automated perimetry (SAP) can detect glaucomatous defects, but by the time a defect is detected, a substantial loss of axons has often occurred (29,30). A number of studies have demonstrated that defects on short-wavelength automated perimetry (SWAP) and frequency doubling technology (FDT) perimetry can precede development of SAP-detected defects in patients with elevated IOP. **Table 10.4** provides a comparative summary of these types of perimeters (31). Imaging devices may also be useful in the early detection of glaucoma. (These are covered in greater detail in Chapter 4 and below.)

Table 10.3	High-Risk Glaucoma Suspects

High-risk glaucoma suspects include patients who have one or more of the following:

- IOP consistently >30 mm Hg[a]
- Thin central corneal thickness (dependent on ethnicity)[a]
- Vertical cup-to-disc ratio >0.7[a]
- Older age[a]
- Abnormal visual field, e.g., increased pattern standard deviation on Humphrey Visual Field test[a]
- Presence of exfoliation or pigment dispersion syndrome
- Disc hemorrhage[a]
- Family history of glaucoma or known genetic predisposition
- Fellow eye of patient with severe unilateral glaucoma (excluding secondary unilateral glaucoma)
- Additional ocular (e.g., suspicious disc appearance, myopia, low optic nerve perfusion pressure, steroid responder) or systemic risk factors that might increase the likelihood of developing glaucomatous nerve damage (e.g., African ancestry, sleep apnea, diabetes mellitus, hypertension, cardiovascular disease, hypothyroidism, myopia, migraine headache, vasospasm)

[a]These factors were identified as significant risk factors for development of chronic open-angle glaucoma in the Ocular Hypertension Treatment Study and the European Glaucoma Prevention Study.

Table 10.4	Comparison of Advantages and Limitations of Manual Perimetry, SAP, SWAP, and FDT Perimetry	
Method	**Merits**	**Limitations**[a]
Manual (Goldmann) perimetry	Long track record Useful in patients who cannot perform automated perimetry (e.g., those with poor reliability, small field of vision, or unreliable SAP results, or who are much older adults)	Not standardized among different laboratories Not readily available in office Absence of statistical software analysis
SAP	Fully validated by long clinical experience and major clinical trials Screening and fast threshold techniques (e.g., SITA) available Long track record, stable technology Easy to read and intuitive printouts Diagnostic and progression statistical tools available High penetration in ophthalmology and optometry practices	Relatively difficult to perform, learning effect, artifacts possible, poor patient acceptance Difficult to apply in screening situations Not portable Relatively expensive
SWAP	Might detect changes earlier than SAP (still controversial) Fast threshold technique available Tested in long-term studies	More difficult to perform than SAP More affected by cataracts No progression software
FDT perimetry	Might detect changes earlier than SAP (still controversial) Relatively portable Screening and fast threshold techniques available Tested in screening situations Good test–retest variability profile Favorable patient acceptance	Limited evaluation in long-term studies Evolving technique, relatively short track record for Matrix device No progression software

[a]Some limitations to all techniques include a lack of consensus on what constitutes a defect or progression; relatively crude reliability indices; poor acceptance by patients; and relatively long duration for threshold tests, even with fast techniques.
FDT, frequency doubling technology; SAP, standard automated perimetry; SITA, Swedish interactive thresholding algorithm; SWAP, short-wavelength automated perimetry.
Modified from Canadian Ophthalmological Society evidence-based clinical practice guidelines for the management of glaucoma in the adult eye. *Can J Ophthalmol*. 2009;44(suppl 1):S7–S93.

According to the American Academy of Ophthalmology, the best method to detect early glaucoma is a comprehensive eye evaluation, which includes assessment of the IOP, optic nerve, and visual field (see Chapter 9). Guidelines for frequency of screening for glaucoma are listed in **Table 10.5** (4).

Intraocular Pressure and Pachymetry

To detect any change in IOP, optic nerve, or visual field status (i.e., early progression with structural or functional damage evident), it is essential to obtain good baseline documentation. In the case of IOP, it is worthwhile to measure central corneal thickness (CCT) with a pachymeter (**Fig. 10.1**). Patients classified as glaucoma suspects have been reported to have a higher CCT than individuals with COAG or healthy individuals (32–34), with 42% of glaucoma suspects having a CCT of greater than 585 μm (34). This is significant because the Goldmann

applanation tonometer was calibrated for a CCT of approximately 530 μm (35,36). Any significant deviation from this induces an artifact of measurement. It has been estimated that 30% to 57% of elevated IOPs in glaucoma suspects are actually artifacts of measurement (33,37,38).

There is no universally accepted formula, however, that can be applied to "correct" the IOP measurement for any given CCT. Based on a review of various correction-factor approaches, the range probably falls between 2.5 and 3.5 mm Hg per 50 μm of difference from normal (39). Hence, if a patient's CCT measured 650 μm (in the absence of any visible corneal pathology), then the "true" IOP would likely be several millimeters of mercury less than measured. To avoid confusion, however, when sharing patient information with other practitioners, it is recommended that IOP should always be communicated as the measured IOP rather than a "corrected" IOP.

Table 10.5	Recommended Guidelines for Follow-up of a Glaucoma Suspect, American Academy of Ophthalmology			
Treatment	Target IOP Achieved	High Risk	Follow-up Interval, *mo*	
			Examination	ONH/VF Evaluation
No	N/A	No	6–24	6–24
No	N/A	Yes	3–12	6–18
Yes	Yes	Yes	3–12	6–18
Yes	No	Yes	≤4	3–12

IOP, intraocular pressure; N/A, not applicable; ONH, optic nerve head; VF, visual field.
Modified from American Academy of Ophthalmology. *Primary Open-Angle Glaucoma Suspect, Preferred Practice Pattern.*
San Francisco, CA: American Academy of Ophthalmology, 2005. Available at: http://www.aao.org/ppp.

Slitlamp Biomicroscopy and Gonioscopy

Baseline documentation requires precise slitlamp examination and gonioscopy to exclude secondary causes of glaucoma. This includes angle closure and other secondary causes, such as angle recession, pigment dispersion, and inflammatory forms of glaucoma. After dilation, the anterior lens capsule should be examined for the presence of exfoliation.

Fundus Examination

In the posterior segment, it is important to document the appearance of the optic nerve head with careful drawings or stereo optic nerve head photos. Optic nerve head imaging devices (e.g., confocal laser scanning tomography) may also be

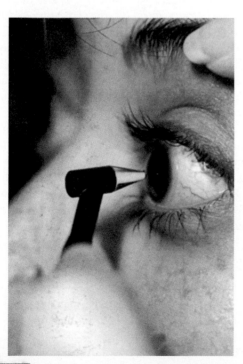

Figure 10.1 Proper technique for measuring CCT, with probe placed perpendicular to central cornea. A structurally thick cornea can artifactually raise measured applanation IOP.

useful. It is also worth studying the disc rim carefully for small hemorrhages, because these can precede visual field loss and future optic nerve damage. Similarly, the appearance of the nerve fiber layer (NFL) can be noted using red-free (green) light. It is important to document the presence or absence of NFL defects. Additional tools to document the NFL include laser polarimetry with the nerve fiber analyzer, scanning laser ophthalmoscopy, and optical coherence tomography (OCT) (see Chapter 4).

Visual Fields

An attempt should be made to obtain two or three baseline visual fields. Our preferred options include one or more of the following: (a) 24-2 Swedish interactive threshold algorithm (SITA) standard on Humphrey field analyzer II perimeter, (b) 24-2 full threshold white-on-white Humphrey perimetry or equivalent program on a different automated perimeter, (c) FDT (matrix preferred) or SWAP.

If an abnormality is found, it needs to be confirmed on repeated visual field examination. This was dramatically illustrated in OHTS (40). Over a 5-year period, 21,603 visual fields were obtained from 1637 OHTS participants. When follow-up visual field results were outside the normal limits on the Glaucoma Hemifield Test, the Corrected Pattern Standard Deviation, or both, follow-up visual fields were obtained to confirm the abnormality. Results of 748 visual fields were abnormal; of these, 703 (94%) were abnormal and reliable, and 45 (6%) were abnormal and unreliable. On retesting, abnormalities were not confirmed for 604 (85.9%) of the originally abnormal and reliable visual fields. Hence, most visual field abnormalities in OHTS participants were not verified on repeated testing and were probably due to the learning curve or long-term variability in the visual field.

Imaging of the Optic Nerve and Nerve Fiber Layer

Photographic assessment of the optic nerve head remains a mainstay in the diagnosis and management of glaucoma suspects. However, there are imaging tools capable of documenting the topographic features of the optic nerve head and measuring the thickness of the retinal NFL that can be useful adjuncts in the management of glaucoma suspects. These tools are reviewed in Chapter 4 and include the confocal scanning laser ophthalmoscope (manufactured as Heidelberg retinal tomography [HRT]), OCT, and scanning laser polarimetry (e.g., the GDx nerve fiber analyzer with variable corneal compensator [GDx-VCC]). Each of the technologies has good reproducibility and provides objective and quantitative analysis of ocular structure. An evidence-based medicine review of these technologies by the American Academy of Ophthalmology (41) came to the following conclusion:

> The [optic nerve head] and [retinal] NFL imaging devices provide quantitative information for the clinician. Based on studies that have compared the various available technologies directly, there is no single imaging device that outperforms the others in distinguishing patients with glaucoma from controls .... The information obtained from imaging devices is useful in clinical practice when analyzed in conjunction with other relevant parameters that define glaucoma diagnosis and progression.

Ocular Blood Flow

Whether blood flow to the optic nerve is reduced in glaucoma suspects and may be an early finding in the course of COAG remains to be proven. However, in one study using laser Doppler flowmetry, optic nerve head blood velocity, volume, and flow in four quadrants of the nerve were compared in patients with COAG, glaucoma suspects, and healthy participants (42). In the eyes of glaucoma suspects, flow was significantly lower in the superotemporal rim (16% lower), the cup (35% lower), and the inferotemporal neuroretinal rim (22% lower), compared with that in the controls. No significant difference between glaucoma suspect and control eyes was seen in the inferonasal rim or superonasal rim, and no significant difference was detected at any location between glaucoma suspect eyes and eyes with COAG. Further data are needed to clarify whether a reduction in blood flow to the optic nerve head plays a significant role in early damage to some optic nerves.

RISK FACTORS

The risk for glaucoma increases with the number and strength of risk factors. Studies that have evaluated risk factors in this context include longitudinal population studies and randomized, controlled trials comparing treatment with no treatment in persons with ocular hypertension (43).

Longitudinal population studies, such as the Barbados Incidence Study of Eye Diseases (BISED), the Melbourne Visual Impairment Project (Melbourne VIP) and the Rotterdam Eye Study (RES), provide information on risk factors that are involved in progression from normal to COAG. The most relevant risk factors consistently found in all three studies are older age at baseline and an approximately 1–mm Hg increase in IOP at

baseline. BISED and RES reported a 4% and 6% risk, respectively, of developing glaucoma for persons 1 year older versus baseline (baseline mean, 56.9 years in BISED and 65.7 years in RES). In all three studies, there was a 10% to 14% increased risk among persons with a baseline IOP 1 mm Hg or more higher than the average for the population of developing COAG over the following 5 to 9 years. Other risk factors in these studies include a family history of COAG, a thinner CCT, and lower ocular perfusion pressures (systemic blood pressure minus IOP) in BISED; the use of systemic calcium-channel blockers for the treatment of systemic hypertension in the RES; and exfoliation, large cup-to-disc ratios of the optic discs, or use of systemic α-agonist blockers in VIP.

High-quality studies examining the risk for progression from normal to glaucoma in those with ocular hypertension include the OHTS and the European Glaucoma Prevention Study (EGPS) (22,44). In OHTS, 1636 patients, aged 40 to 80 years, with no evidence of glaucomatous damage and with IOP between 24 and 32 mm Hg in one eye and between 21 and 32 mm Hg in the other eye were randomly assigned to either observation or treatment with topical medication. The goal in the medication group was to reduce the IOP by 20% or more and to reach an IOP of 24 mm Hg or less. In EGPS, 1081 patients aged 30 years or older with an IOP between 22 and 29 mm Hg were enrolled. Patients were randomly assigned to treatment with dorzolamide or placebo. Open-angle glaucoma in both studies was defined as the development of reproducible visual field abnormality or reproducible finding of optic nerve deterioration. Factors consistently identified in both studies as predictive of COAG development included elevated IOP, large cup-to-disc ratio, older age, thinner CCT, and higher pattern standard deviation values on the Humphrey automated perimeter. The EGPS also found vertical cup-to-disc asymmetry to be an important predictive factor (45). Other longitudinal studies have also shown suspicious disc appearance, myopia, and family history of glaucoma to be risk factors for the development of glaucomatous optic neuropathy and visual field loss (46–48). In OHTS and EGPS, predictive factors that occurred after baseline were a higher mean IOP during follow-up, a smaller IOP reduction from baseline, and optic disc hemorrhages (43). In addition, in EGPS the use of systemic diuretics to treat systemic hypertension during follow-up increased the risk for COAG. Interestingly, long-term fluctuation in IOP and diurnal fluctuation in IOP have not been associated with the development of COAG (44,46).

Risk Calculators

The risk for COAG in patients who are considered glaucoma suspects on the basis of elevated IOP can be estimated with risk calculators (49). The most recent risk calculators are available online and incorporate data from OHTS; EGPS; and another longitudinal study, the Diagnostic Innovations in Glaucoma Study (DIGS). This pooled analysis, which provides the 5-year risk for COAG in one eye in a patient aged 40 years with ocular hypertension, has narrowed the 95% confidence limits for prediction and strengthened the generalizability of the results.

Given the studies that risk calculators are based on, calculations may not apply to patients who are younger than 40 years, nonwhite or of African descent, and do not have an IOP of 22 mm Hg or higher.

Risk calculators also do not provide critical information that may guide therapy, such as life expectancy and psychological and social factors. The calculators may provide supplementary information for the physician and the patient, but caution needs to be exercised, as the clinical decision to treat is complex and involves taking the best available evidence and tailoring it to the individual patient.

WHEN TO TREAT

Whether to begin treatment in a glaucoma suspect is a complex decision that involves consideration of many factors, including visual, physical, medical, psychological, and social circumstances (50). Every attempt should be made to engage the patient in the decision-making process, because potentially exposing the patient to long-term therapy when there is no definite evidence of glaucomatous optic nerve damage is a major decision.

If the IOP is elevated, we suggest first stratifying the patient into low, moderate, or high risk for progression (Table 10.3 and **Table 10.6**). The OHTS and EGPS results should be kept in mind for identifying high-risk groups. In the OHTS, for those with a mean baseline IOP greater than 25.75 mm Hg, the risk for glaucomatous optic nerve damage at 5 years was 36% if the patient had a thin or average (555 μm) cornea, and 13% with a CCT of 565 to 588 μm. For a cup-to-disc ratio of more than 0.3, the risk for those with a thin or average cornea was 24%, and for those with a thickness of 565 to 588 μm was 16%.

Patients at high risk for progression warrant treatment to prevent optic nerve damage, whereas those at low risk can be observed at periodic intervals (51). If there is a moderate risk for progression, then a decision can be made to treat or observe at more frequent intervals than patients at low risk. If the IOP is not elevated and the disc or visual field is suspicious, there is no compelling evidence to guide clinicians regarding whether to treat or to simply observe.

The results of the OHTS indicate that reducing IOP by at least 20% (and to <24 mm Hg) in patients with elevated IOP and no evidence of glaucomatous damage can reduce the risk for COAG by more than half over a 5-year period (from 9.5% in the observation group to 4.4% in the medication group). However, although topical hypotensive medication was effective in delaying or preventing the onset of COAG in this group of patients, the results do not imply that all patients with borderline or elevated IOP should receive medication. In fact, most cases of elevated IOP did not progress to glaucoma over the 5-year follow-up. Furthermore, results of the EGPS suggest that patients treated with dorzolamide progressed at the same rate as patients receiving a placebo. However, this result is controversial and may relate to selective dropout of treated and untreated patients with higher IOPs and to the failure to achieve sufficient lowering of IOP (52).

If there is evidence of damage to or deterioration of the optic nerve or visual field in one or both eyes, then the patient's diagnosis changes to early COAG, and treatment should commence according to the principles outlined in Chapters 27 and 35. Kass (53) also suggests a lower threshold for treatment in patients with only one functional eye, where it is not possible to obtain reliable visual fields, or in patients in whom the optic disc cannot be visualized.

In its 2005 Preferred Practice Pattern, the American Academy of Ophthalmology recommends that, when deciding whether therapy is warranted, a risk–benefit analysis should be done, and the likelihood of development of glaucomatous optic nerve damage should be carefully weighed against the risks of treatment (4). The decision should be individualized, taking into account the rate at which glaucomatous optic nerve damage and visual impairment are likely to occur, the patient's life expectancy, and the patient's tolerance for effective treatment.

APPROACH TO TREATMENT

If a decision is made to treat, the choice of treatment should be governed by selecting a topical medication that will likely achieve the target IOP range (see discussion in Chapter 27)

Table 10.6	Making the Decision to Treat in Glaucoma Suspects with Elevated IOP

Stratify patients into low, moderate, or high risk for progression (based on best available evidence and clinical judgement):

- High risk: Suggest treatment be initiated
- Moderate risk: Can initiate treatment if appropriate, or monitor closely
- Low risk: Monitor IOP as well as optic nerve structure and function, and treat if evidence of progression

Carefully consider these factors when deciding whether to treat:

- Greater age and life expectancy
- Psychological factors
- Convictions (patient and physician)
- Social environment
- Availability for follow-up
- Pregnancy

with the least risk to ocular or systemic health and quality of life for the patient. Cost and convenience may also enter into this decision. Patients should be educated about the disease process and the rationale and goals of therapy, so that they can participate meaningfully in the development of an optimal treatment plan.

Whether laser trabeculoplasty has a role in early treatment of glaucoma suspects remains controversial. In our opinion, laser trabeculoplasty may be indicated, and it can be a useful adjunct in decreasing IOP by 20% to 25% if the target IOP range cannot be achieved with use of one or two medications.

Surgery is rarely, if ever, indicated as first-line therapy in a glaucoma suspect. However, trabeculectomy or other surgical approaches may be indicated if the patient has an extremely high, uncontrolled IOP (corrected for pachymetry) that the physician believes is certain to cause glaucomatous damage (i.e., 40 to 50 mm Hg). Additional factors such as poor adherence to medical therapy, inability to tolerate medical therapy (e.g., benzalkonium chloride sensitivity), quality of life, and longevity of the patient may need to be considered when deciding which IOP-lowering approach is best for the patient.

GUIDELINES FOR FOLLOW-UP

Follow-up of the glaucoma suspect is necessary to determine whether there is a change in the IOP, optic nerve head, or visual field status over time.

The frequency of follow-up visits depends on several factors: whether the patient is receiving medical therapy, whether the target IOP range has been achieved, and the number of risk factors for COAG the patient has. We believe that follow-up of glaucoma suspects should occur at least every 6 to 12 months, and more frequently in high-risk patients, especially those on treatment in whom the target IOP has not been achieved. There are no hard and fast rules on this subject, although the American Academy of Ophthalmology has developed some guidelines that represent the consensus of an expert panel and are listed in Table 10.5 (4).

At each visit, the IOP should be assessed, and the clinician should document whether the appearance of the optic nerve head has changed since baseline. Visual fields should be obtained once every 6 to 18 months and compared with the baseline measurement. Gonioscopy should be repeated if there is a suspicion of angle closure or other angle abnormality. Gonioscopy should also be considered if the patient is given a miotic agent, because this type of treatment can induce pupillary block and formation of peripheral anterior synechiae.

KEY POINTS

- The term "glaucoma suspect" is typically used when the patient has an IOP greater than 21 mm Hg with normal discs and visual fields, or an appearance of the optic nerve head, NFL, or visual field that is suggestive of but not definitive for

glaucoma. It can also be used when the optic nerve or visual field is suspicious for optic nerve damage.

- The physician should document good baseline data, including IOP, pachymetry, optic nerve head, NFL, and visual fields, so as to have a benchmark to assess whether progression has occurred on follow-up visits. The CCT should be measured routinely to assess the level of risk of these patients.

- Baseline factors that consistently predict the development of COAG in major prospective studies include older age, larger vertical or horizontal cup-to-disc ratio, higher IOP, greater pattern standard deviation, and thinner CCT. These criteria can be used to stage the glaucoma suspect into low, moderate, or high risk for progression.

- The decision to initiate therapy in a glaucoma suspect should be based on the patient's risk for developing visual loss; his or her systemic, psychological, and social health; and his or her preference.

REFERENCES

1. Kolker AE, Becker B. 'Ocular hypertension' vs. open-angle glaucoma: a different view. *Arch Ophthalmol.* 1977;95(4):586–587.
2. Phelps CD. Ocular hypertension: to treat or not to treat. *Arch Ophthalmol.* 1977;95(4):588–589.
3. Chandler PA, Grant WM. 'Ocular hypertension' vs. open-angle glaucoma. *Arch Ophthalmol.* 1977;95(4):585–586.
4. American Academy of Ophthalmology. *Primary Open-Angle Glaucoma Suspect, Preferred Practice Pattern.* San Francisco, CA: American Academy of Ophthalmology, 2005. Available at: http://www.aao.org/ppp. Accessed June 10, 2010.
5. Shaffer R. 'Glaucoma suspect' or 'ocular hypertension.' *Arch Ophthalmol.* 1977;95(4):588.
6. Bankes JL, Perkins ES, Tsolakis S, et al. Bedford glaucoma survey. *Br Med J.* 1968;1(5595):791–796.
7. Hollows FC, Graham PA. Intra-ocular pressure, glaucoma, and glaucoma suspects in a defined population. *Br J Ophthalmol.* 1966;50(10):570–586.
8. Leibowitz HM, Krueger DE, Maunder LR, et al. The Framingham Eye Study monograph: an ophthalmological and epidemiological study of cataract, glaucoma, diabetic retinopathy, macular degeneration, and visual acuity in a general population of 2631 adults, 1973–1975. *Surv Ophthalmol.* 1980;24(suppl):335–610.
9. Linnér E, Stromberg U. Ocular hypertension: a five-year study of the total population in a Swedish town, Skovde. In: Leydhecker W, ed. *International Congress of Ophthalmology, Tutzing Castle, Munich, 1966.* Basel, Switzerland: S Karger; 1967:187.
10. Norskov K. Routine tonometry in ophthalmic practice. I. Primary screening and further examinations for diagnostic purposes. *Acta Ophthalmol.* 1970;48(5):838–872.
11. Quigley HA, Vitale S. Models of open-angle glaucoma prevalence and incidence in the United States. *Invest Ophthalmol Vis Sci.* 1997;38(1):83–91.
12. Perkins ES. The Bedford glaucoma survey. I. Long-term follow-up of borderline cases. *Br J Ophthalmol.* 1973;57(3):179–185.
13. Walker WM. Ocular hypertension. Follow-up of 109 cases from 1963 to 1974. *Trans Ophthalmol Soc U K.* 1974;94(2):525–534.
14. Wilensky JT, Podos SM, Becker B. Prognostic indicators in ocular hypertension. *Arch Ophthalmol.* 1974;91(3):200–202.
15. Norskov K. Routine tonometry in ophthalmic practice. II. Five-year follow-up. *Acta Ophthalmol.* 1970;48(5):873–895.
16. Linnér E. Ocular hypertension. I. The clinical course during ten years without therapy. Aqueous humour dynamics. *Acta Ophthalmol.* 1976;54(6):707–720.
17. Kitazawa Y, Horie T, Aoki S, et al. Untreated ocular hypertension. A long-term prospective study. *Arch Ophthalmol.* 1977;95(7):1180–1184.
18. David R, Livingston DG, Luntz MH. Ocular hypertension—a long-term follow-up of treated and untreated patients. *Br J Ophthalmol.* 1977;61(11):668–674.
19. Hart WM Jr, Yablonski M, Kass MA, et al. Multivariate analysis of the risk of glaucomatous visual field loss. *Arch Ophthalmol.* 1979;97(8):1455–1458.

20. Armaly MF, Krueger DE, Maunder L, et al. Biostatistical analysis of the collaborative glaucoma study. I. Summary report of the risk factors for glaucomatous visual-field defects. *Arch Ophthalmol.* 1980;98(12): 2163–2171.

21. Lundberg L, Wettrell K, Linner E. Ocular hypertension. A prospective twenty-year follow-up study. *Acta Ophthalmol.* 1987;65(6):705–708.

22. Kass MA, Heuer DK, Higginbotham EJ, et al. The Ocular Hypertension Treatment Study: a randomized trial determines that topical ocular hypotensive medication delays or prevents the onset of primary open-angle glaucoma. *Arch Ophthalmol.* 2002;120(6):701–713.

23. Armaly MF. Ocular pressure and visual fields. A ten-year follow-up study. *Arch Ophthalmol.* 1969;81(1):25–40.

24. Graham PA. The definition of pre-glaucoma. A prospective study. *Trans Ophthalmol Soc U K.* 1969;88:153–165.

25. Leske MC. The epidemiology of open-angle glaucoma: a review. *Am J Epidemiol.* 1983;118(2):166–191.

26. Epstein DL, Krug JH Jr, Hertzmark E, et al. A long-term clinical trial of timolol therapy versus no treatment in the management of glaucoma suspects. *Ophthalmology.* 1989;96(10):1460–1467.

27. Kass MA, Gordon MO, Hoff MR, et al. Topical timolol administration reduces the incidence of glaucomatous damage in ocular hypertensive individuals. A randomized, double-masked, long-term clinical trial. *Arch Ophthalmol.* 1989;107(11):1590–1598.

28. Schulzer M, Drance SM, Douglas GR. A comparison of treated and untreated glaucoma suspects. *Ophthalmology.* 1991;98(3):301–307.

29. Quigley HA, Addicks EM, Green WR. Optic nerve damage in human glaucoma. III. Quantitative correlation of nerve fiber loss and visual field defect in glaucoma, ischemic neuropathy, papilledema, and toxic neuropathy. *Arch Ophthalmol.* 1982;100(1):135–146.

30. Kerrigan-Baumrind LA, Quigley HA, Pease ME, et al. Number of ganglion cells in glaucoma eyes compared with threshold visual field tests in the same persons. *Invest Ophthalmol Vis Sci.* 2000;41(3):741–748.

31. Canadian Ophthalmological Society Glaucoma Clinical Practice Guideline Expert Committee. Canadian Ophthalmological Society evidence-based clinical practice guidelines for the management of glaucoma in the adult eye. *Can J Ophthalmol.* 2009;44(suppl 1):S7–S93.

32. Argus WA. Ocular hypertension and central corneal thickness. *Ophthalmology.* 1995;102(12):1810–1812.

33. Herndon LW, Choudhri SA, Cox T, et al. Central corneal thickness in normal, glaucomatous, and ocular hypertensive eyes. *Arch Ophthalmol.* 1997;115(9):1137–1141.

34. Shah S, Chatterjee A, Mathai M, et al. Relationship between corneal thickness and measured intraocular pressure in a general ophthalmology clinic. *Ophthalmology.* 1999;106:2154–2160.

35. Goldmann H. Un nouveau tonometre a applanation [in French]. *Bull Mem Soc Fr Ophthalmol.* 1954;67:474–477.

36. Goldmann H, Schmidt T. Applanation tonometry [in German]. *Ophthalmologica.* 1957;134(4):221–242.

37. Copt RP, Thomas R, Mermoud A. Corneal thickness in ocular hypertension, primary open-angle glaucoma, and normal tension glaucoma. *Arch Ophthalmol.* 1999;117(1):14–16.

38. Brandt JD, Beiser JA, Kass MA, et al. Central corneal thickness in the Ocular Hypertension Treatment Study (OHTS). *Ophthalmology.* 2001;108(10):1779–1788.

39. Damji KF, Muni RH, Munger RM. Influence of corneal variables on accuracy of intraocular pressure measurement. *J Glaucoma.* 2003;12(1): 69–80.

40. Keltner JL, Johnson CA, Quigg JM, et al. Confirmation of visual field abnormalities in the Ocular Hypertension Treatment Study. Ocular Hypertension Treatment Study Group. *Arch Ophthalmol.* 2000;118(9): 1187–1194.

41. Lin SC, Singh K, Jampel HD, et al. Optic nerve head and retinal nerve fiber layer analysis: a report by the American Academy of Ophthalmology. *Ophthalmology.* 2007;114(10):1937–1949.

42. Piltz-seymour JR, Grunwald JE, Hariprasad SM, et al. Optic nerve blood flow is diminished in eyes of primary open-angle glaucoma suspects. *Am J Ophthalmol.* 2001;132(1):63–69.

43. Coleman AL, Miglior S. Risk factors for glaucoma onset and progression. *Surv Ophthalmol.* 2008;53(suppl 1):S3–S10.

44. Miglior S, Zeyen T, Pfeiffer N, et al. Results of the European Glaucoma Prevention Study. *Ophthalmology.* 2005;112(3):366–375.

45. Miglior S, Pfeiffer N, Torri V, et al. Predictive factors for open-angle glaucoma among patients with ocular hypertension in the European Glaucoma Prevention Study. *Ophthalmology.* 2007;114(1):3–9.

46. Bengtsson B, Heijl A. A long-term prospective study of risk factors for glaucomatous visual field loss in patients with ocular hypertension. *J Glaucoma.* 2005;14(2):135–138.

47. Kass MA, Hart WM Jr, Gordon M, et al. Risk factors favoring the development of glaucomatous visual field loss in ocular hypertension. *Surv Ophthalmol.* 1980;25(3):155–162.

48. Ponte F, Giuffre G, Giammanco R, et al. Risk factors of ocular hypertension and glaucoma. The Casteldaccia Eye Study. *Doc Ophthalmol.* 1994;85(3):203–210.

49. Mansberger SL, Medeiros FA, Gordon M. Diagnostic tools for calculation of glaucoma risk. *Surv Ophthalmol.* 2008;53(suppl 1):S11–S6.

50. Migdal C. Which therapy to use in glaucoma? In: Yanoff M, Duker JS, eds. *Ophthalmology.* London: Mosby; 1999;section 12:23. 1–4.

51. Higginbotham EJ. Treating ocular hypertension to reduce glaucoma risk: when to treat? *Drugs.* 2006;66(8):1033–1039.

52. Parrish RK II. The European Glaucoma Prevention Study and the Ocular Hypertension Treatment Study: Why do two studies have different results? [review]. *Curr Opin Ophthalmol.* 2006;17(2):138–141.

53. Kass MA. When to treat ocular hypertension. *Surv Ophthalmol.* 1983; 28(suppl):229–234.

11

Chronic Open-Angle Glaucoma and Normal-Tension Glaucoma

TERMINOLOGY

Chronic Open-Angle Glaucoma

As discussed in Chapter 7, the glaucomas have traditionally been classified according to primary and secondary forms. Within the former group, and indeed among all the glaucomas, by far the most prevalent condition has been commonly referred to as primary open-angle glaucoma. Continued research, however, has shown the concept of primary and secondary glaucomas to be arbitrary and one that should probably be abandoned. Research has also suggested that the view of primary open-angle glaucoma as a single entity is no longer valid. An alternative term, which we have elected to use in this text, is chronic open-angle glaucoma (COAG). Other synonymous terms that may also appear in the literature include chronic simple glaucoma, idiopathic open-angle glaucoma, and open-angle glaucoma. COAG is typically characterized by (a) an open, normal-appearing anterior chamber angle and increased intraocular pressure (IOP) without any apparent ocular or systemic abnormality that might account for the elevated IOP and (b) typical optic nerve head damage or glaucomatous visual field damage (as described in Chapters 4 and 5, respectively). A proposed definition of COAG (modified from the American Academy of Ophthalmology Preferred Practice Guidelines, 2005 (1)) is a multifactorial optic neuropathy in which there is characteristic atrophy of the optic nerve. Although abnormally elevated IOP had long been considered part of the definition, it is now considered a risk factor for COAG.

Ocular Hypertension or Glaucoma Suspect

Patients who have an IOP above 21 mm Hg for which there is no apparent cause but whose optic nerve heads and visual fields are normal are commonly said to have ocular hypertension (2,3). Chandler and Grant (4) suggested the term "early open-angle glaucoma without damage" for this condition, whereas Shaffer (5) preferred the term "glaucoma suspect" (see Chapter 10). The latter term may also include other factors that make the possibility of glaucoma more likely, such as suspicious optic nerve heads or visual fields. Whatever term one chooses to use for this condition, the most important point is that both physician and patient be fully aware of its potential consequences.

Normal-Tension Glaucoma

At the other end of the spectrum with regard to susceptibility to high IOP are patients with open, normal-appearing anterior chamber angles who have glaucomatous optic nerve head and visual field damage despite pressures that have never been documented above 21 mm Hg. These patients are said to have normal-tension glaucoma (NTG). The term "low-tension glaucoma" has also been used, although the IOP in these individuals is usually "normal" or "high normal" and is rarely "low normal." The criteria used to define NTG over the past 25 years have been highly variable (6). Some investigators believe that NTG is a variant of COAG, whereas others believe that the mechanism of optic atrophy in the two conditions is different (7). Although a number of differences between the two disorders have been described (see later text), COAG and NTG appear to represent a continuum of glaucomas in which the mechanism of the glaucomatous optic neuropathy shifts from predominantly elevated IOP in the former to additional IOP-independent factors in the latter, with considerable overlap of causative factors.

Chronic Open-Angle Glaucomas with Associated Abnormalities

Some forms of open-angle glaucoma, such as pigmentary glaucoma and the exfoliation syndrome, have been identified as distinct entities because of a partial understanding of associated, causative abnormalities and mechanisms of aqueous outflow obstruction. (These conditions are discussed in this section of the book.) Here, the focus is on those open-angle glaucomas for which laboratory and clinical findings have yet to clarify the glaucoma mechanisms and in which IOP plays a variable role. As the search continues into the causes and mechanisms of the open-angle glaucomas, especially in the field of molecular biology, an ever-increasing number of separate entities will likely be recognized within this spectrum of disorders.

EPIDEMIOLOGY

Significance of Intraocular Pressure

The commonly used IOP level of 21 mm Hg is based on the concept that two standard deviations above the mean within a Gaussian distribution for the white population represents the upper limit of "normal" for that biological parameter. However, because the distribution of IOP in the general population is skewed to the right, or to higher pressures, this principle provides only a rough approximation of the normal limits. More important, many eyes will not develop glaucomatous optic atrophy or visual field loss, at least not for long periods of time, despite having IOP well above 21 mm Hg, whereas others will have progressive glaucomatous damage at pressures that are never observed to exceed this level. These latter observations have brought into question the role of IOP in the mechanism of COAG. Even though many studies have confirmed a correlation between the level of IOP and the rate of visual field loss in some groups of patients with COAG, this correlation is not seen in all cases (8–10). Other causative factors figure into the formula for glaucomatous damage, which appears to explain the lack of absolute correlation between IOP and the development of COAG. In any case, this discrepancy between IOP level and glaucomatous damage has led to the use of additional terms within the general category of COAG, and these are reviewed hereunder.

Frequency among the Glaucomas

COAG is clearly the most common single form of glaucoma, although it is difficult to precisely establish the proportion of individuals with this disorder to the total number of patients with all forms of glaucoma. In a British survey of 4231 individuals between the ages of 40 and 75 years, one third of the glaucoma population and 0.28% of the general population had COAG (11). However, in a study of 8126 individuals in Japan who were at least 40 years of age, COAG accounted for 73% of the glaucomas detected (exclusive of patients with ocular hypertension), of which most were NTG (12). These epidemiologic surveys will obviously be influenced by the population being studied as well as the methods and criteria used to identify patients with glaucoma.

Prevalence in General Populations

Several large surveys have been conducted to determine the number of patients with ocular hypertension and COAG (or glaucoma in general) within a population at a given time (reviewed in Chapters 9 and 10). The prevalence of glaucoma in persons older than 40 years is between 1% and 2% in most studies, although reports again vary considerably according to the population studied and the diagnostic criteria and screening techniques used (13,14).

Natural History of Visual Field Loss in Chronic Open-Angle Glaucoma

Leydhecker (15) studied the distribution of IOP and glaucomatous visual field loss in a large population survey. When persons with pressures higher than 20 mm Hg and those with definite glaucomatous field defects were plotted against their age, the two slopes were parallel and separated horizontally by 18 years, which led to the notion that 10 to 20 years may elapse between the onset of ocular hypertension and the development of visual field loss. Lichter and Shaffer (16), however, found that field loss in a population of 378 patients with ocular hypertension, observed for an average of 12.75 years, occurred earlier than Leydhecker suggested, even though most were being treated during that time. The level of IOP appears to influence the rate of visual field loss. In one study of 177 untreated patients with COAG comparing the mean age of

presentation with the degree of field loss, it was estimated that untreated disease is likely to progress from early to end-stage visual field loss in 14.4 years at pressures of 21 to 25 mm Hg, in 6.5 years at pressures of 25 to 30 mm Hg, and in 2.9 years at pressures greater than 30 mm Hg (17). Furthermore, once field loss has occurred, further damage tends to progress more rapidly than in the fellow undamaged eye exposed to the same IOP, which appears to reflect the increased susceptibility of the damaged eye (18–20).

The "natural" course of NTG was evaluated in the Collaborative Normal-Tension Glaucoma Study (CNTGS) during the time before randomization and in patients assigned not to receive treatment (21). About one third of patients showed confirmed localized visual field progression at 3 years, and about one half showed further deterioration at 7 years. The change was typically small and slow, often insufficient to measurably affect the mean deviation index, and there was tremendous variability in progression rates, with women, older individuals, or those with a disc hemorrhage, or history of migraine having a greater risk for progression. In the Early Manifest Glaucoma Trial, 76% of patients demonstrated progression on specific optic nerve or visual field endpoints after an average 4 years of follow-up (22).

Identifying Patients and Those at Increased Risk

COAG has no associated symptoms or other warning signs before the development of advanced visual field loss. It is for this reason that public and family physician awareness programs are needed to ensure that high-risk patients receive glaucoma assessment examinations by eye care specialists. Such programs must use the systemic and ocular risk factors discussed in Chapter 9, which are commonly associated with the disease, to identify those segments of the population requiring the closest attention. In addition, once a patient has been found to have persistent IOP elevation (the most significant risk factor) but no apparent optic nerve head or visual field damage, the additional risk factors must be considered by the physician when trying to decide which of these individuals require closer observation or the initiation of therapy before definite damage occurs. (In Chapters 9 and 10, the risk factors for developing COAG and the use of these factors in determining the frequency of periodic eye examinations for detection of glaucoma are discussed.)

CLINICAL DIFFERENCES BETWEEN NTG AND COAG

Chronic Open-Angle Glaucoma

Intraocular Pressure

Measured IOP greater than 21 mm Hg before treatment is generally considered elevated. Even though an elevated IOP is only one of several risk factors for COAG, it is a causative risk factor, and most studies agree that it is the single most important risk factor.

Central Corneal Thickness

The cornea is typically normal in COAG. Measurement of central corneal thickness with ultrasonic or optical methods is helpful in interpreting the accuracy of applanation tonometry readings as well as in assisting with estimating the risk for progression. Published evidence regarding the value of central corneal thickness for prognostic information is strong in the case of patients with ocular hypertension but is considerably weaker in patients with established glaucoma (23). Hence, in patients with established COAG, a thinner cornea (if structurally normal) signifies that the "true" IOP is higher than measured but that the risk for progression may or may not be higher.

Anterior Chamber Angle

By traditional definition, the anterior chamber angle in eyes with COAG is open and grossly normal on gonioscopic examination (Chapter 3). Preliminary studies, however, suggest that these patients may have more iris processes, a higher insertion of the iris root, more trabecular meshwork pigmentation (24), and a greater-than-normal degree of segmentation in the pigmentation of the meshwork (25).

Optic Nerve Head

The appearance of the optic nerve head and peripapillary retina is the single most important clinical feature in establishing the presence of glaucomatous damage. A helpful early finding is defects in the retinal nerve fiber layer, which may be a sign of glaucomatous optic atrophy before apparent changes are seen in the nerve head (26). Other early findings include enlargement of the optic dose cup, thinning or saucerizing of the neural rim, disc hemorrhages, and peripapillary atrophy (as explained in Chapter 4).

Visual Abnormalities

Central visual acuity, as measured by standard clinical tests, typically remains normal until there is marked visual field loss within the central visual field. How little remaining central visual field is necessary to retain excellent visual acuity is often remarkable. Therefore, in cases where visual acuity is reduced while significant portions of the central 5 to 10 degrees are retained, other nonglaucomatous causes for visual acuity loss should be considered. Preliminary evidence, however, suggests that more subtle measures of vision dysfunction, such as contrast sensitivity, color vision, and motion perception (discussed in Chapter 6), may one day be useful as early indicators of visual dysfunction before the development of typical visual field loss. Once typical glaucomatous damage to the visual field has been documented in one eye, there is a high incidence of subsequent field loss in the fellow eye. The latter was reported to be 29% in 31 patients followed up for 3 to 7 years (27), and 25% of 104 individuals after 5 years of follow-up in another series (28).

Normal-Tension Glaucoma

As noted earlier, some investigators consider NTG to be clearly distinguishable from the high-tension form of COAG, but others do not. COAG likely is a spectrum of disorders in which elevated IOP is the most influential causative factor at one end, whereas other IOP-independent factors that influence glaucomatous optic atrophy predominate at the other end. In any case, clinical differences between NTG and COAG are considered here.

Optic Nerve Head

Some investigators have found the neural rim to be significantly thinner in patients with NTG, especially inferiorly and inferotemporally, than in other patients with COAG who have similar total visual field loss (7). Other studies have revealed less striking differences, with considerable overlap between high-tension glaucoma and NTG. A study of morphologic characteristics of the optic nerve head in high-tension glaucoma and NTG eyes showed no significant difference in any parameter as measured by laser scanning ophthalmoscopy (29).

Some studies have found that optic disc hemorrhages were more prevalent in the group with NTG, raising the possibility of vascular disease as another causative factor in these patients (7). The retinal nerve fiber layer has also been compared between patients with NTG and those with COAG, with the former having more localized defects, closer to the macula, and the latter more diffuse defects (30–32).

Visual Fields

Differences have also been reported in the nature of visual field loss between patients with NTG and those with COAG who have similar optic nerve damage. In general, patients with NTG appear to have deeper, more localized scotomas (33). There are also conflicting reports regarding the proximity of scotomas to fixation between the two groups, which may relate to the testing methods. One study found a significantly greater rate of progressive visual field loss in NTG (34), and another revealed a difference in the pattern of the progression, with the patients with high-tension glaucoma initially increasing mainly in area and later in depth, whereas the increases in area and depth remained in constant proportion in patients with NTG (35).

Intraocular Pressure

Although NTG, by definition, is distinguished from high-tension COAG by an IOP that is never recorded to exceed 21 mm Hg, the pressures do tend to be higher than those in the general healthy population (36). A number of studies have revealed a significant influence of IOP on the progression of visual field or neuroretinal rim damage in NTG (37,38), although another study showed no significant difference in IOP between patients with and those without field progression (39). In some studies of patients with NTG and asymmetric IOP, the visual field loss was typically worse in the eye with the higher pressure (40,41). However, a more rigorous, prospective evaluation of 190 patients with NTG in the Low-Pressure Glaucoma Treatment Study found IOP asymmetry to be unrelated to visual field asymmetry (42).

A randomized trial of treated versus untreated patients with NTG has convincingly shown that an IOP reduction of at least 30% is associated with protection of visual field and nerve status, thus validating the concept that IOP is a contributory factor in the optic neuropathy of NTG. The bulk of the evidence, therefore, suggests that IOP in the high-normal range is a causative factor in NTG, although other factors are also involved. In making the diagnosis of NTG and in the management of these patients, it is important to know the diurnal variation in IOP to confirm that their pressures are consistently below 21 mm Hg before therapy and are staying within the target level while on treatment. One study suggested that patients with NTG have wider diurnal fluctuations than the general healthy population (36), although other investigators found no significant difference in diurnal variation of IOP or of aqueous humor flow or resistance to outflow (43,44).

It is also important to note that IOP spikes may occur at night, and therefore IOPs measured during office hours may miss nocturnal spikes in many patients (7). The concomitant changes of nocturnal orbital blood pressure and IOP may affect blood perfusion to the optic nerve head differently in glaucomatous eyes, compared with healthy eyes, and this also might affect the susceptibility of the optic nerve to damage. When a patient has progressive visual field loss or optic disc or retinal nerve fiber layer damage in the presence of an apparently well-controlled IOP during the day, it is appropriate to consider that the nocturnal IOP (during sleep) may be elevated (45). Obtaining 24-hour IOP measurements is often difficult if not impossible. Furthermore, even if this were possible, whether the nighttime readings reflect the true IOP during sleep is unclear.

Ocular Vascular Abnormalities

As noted earlier in this section, additional causative factors may relate to the architecture of the lamina cribrosa and the vascular perfusion of the optic nerve head. Drance and coworkers (46,47) described two forms of NTG: (a) a nonprogressive form, which is usually associated with a transient episode of vascular shock, and (b) a more common progressive form, which is believed to result from chronic vascular insufficiency of the optic nerve head. Various cardiovascular and hematologic abnormalities have been described, which might account for both forms (48). Reported associated findings include hemodynamic crises, reduced diastolic ophthalmodynamometry levels and ocular pulse amplitudes, bilateral complete occlusion of the internal carotid artery with reversed ophthalmic artery flow, focal arteriolar narrowing around the optic nerve, and increased vascular resistance of the ophthalmic artery by color Doppler analysis (46,47,49–52). It is wise to consider untreated glaucomatous optic neuropathy to be a progressive rather than a quiescent process.

Systemic Vascular Abnormalities

Reports of alterations in systemic blood pressure are conflicting. However, patients with NTG have significantly greater nocturnal blood pressure drops than healthy persons (53), as well as elevated diastolic blood pressure (54). Twenty-four–hour electrocardiographic monitoring has shown significantly greater asymptomatic myocardial ischemia in patients with NTG (45%) than in healthy individuals (5%), with many ischemic episodes occurring during the night (55). Visual-evoked

responses during stepwise artificially increased IOP were significantly different between patients with NTG and those with high-tension COAG, suggesting a greater lack of autoregulation of optic nerve head circulation in the former group (56). In patients with NTG whose disease is progressing despite seemingly normal IOP, it may be appropriate to request 24-hour blood pressure monitoring, where available, to look for dips in nocturnal blood pressure and alterations of perfusion pressure to the optic nerve.

Patients with NTG were noted to have an increased frequency of headaches with or without migraine features (57). Another study failed to confirm this association (58), whereas a third investigation found that patients with NTG and headaches had significantly lower IOP than patients with NTG and no headaches, suggesting a subset within this group of patients (59). An abnormally reduced blood flow in the fingers, especially in response to exposure to cold, has also been reported (60,61). Other investigators again found two subsets of COAG: (a) a smaller one with vasospastic finger blood flow measurements and a highly positive correlation between visual field loss and IOP and (b) a larger group with disturbed coagulation and biochemical measurement, suggestive of vascular disease, with no correlation between field and highest IOP (62). A study of peripheral vascular endothelial function in patients with NTG found impaired acetylcholine-induced peripheral endothelium-mediated vasodilation in comparison with healthy age- and sex-matched controls (63), and a polymorphism of the endothelin receptor type A gene has been associated with NTG (64). The bulk of the observations, therefore, suggest that vasospastic events are involved in the mechanism of at least some forms of NTG. (The therapeutic implications of this are discussed at the end of this chapter.)

Hematologic abnormalities reported to be associated with NTG include increased blood and plasma viscosity and hypercoagulability (e.g., increased platelet adhesiveness and euglobulin lysis time) (41,46,65). Other studies, however, have revealed no statistically significant abnormalities in coagulation tests or in vascular or rheological profiles (66,67). Hypercholesterolemia is reported to be higher among patients with NTG (68). Magnetic resonance imaging in patients with NTG has revealed an increased incidence of diffuse cerebral ischemia, which may be further evidence for a vascular etiology (69,70).

There is also some evidence that immune mechanisms may play a role in the mechanism of NTG. In one study, 30% of the patients had one or more immune-related diseases, compared with 8% in a matched group of patients with ocular hypertension (71). Additional support for an immune mechanism includes the increased incidence of paraproteinemia and autoantibodies, such as antirhodopsin antibodies and anti–glutathione-S transferase (a retinal antigen) antibodies, in patients with NTG (72–74). There is also a report of postmortem histopathologic findings in a patient with NTG who had monoclonal gammopathy and serum immunoreactivity to retinal proteins. Immunoglobulin G and A deposition was noted in the ganglion cells and in inner and outer nuclear layers of the retina, and evidence of apoptotic cell death was noted in the ganglion cell and inner nuclear layers of the retina (75).

DIFFERENTIAL DIAGNOSIS OF NORMAL-TENSION GLAUCOMA

The differential diagnosis of NTG is summarized in **Table 11.1** and should include wide diurnal IOP fluctuations in which high pressures are occurring at times when they are not being recorded. Other patients may have once had high pressures that caused damage that have since spontaneously normalized. One example of this is pigmentary glaucoma, in which the IOP often improves with increasing age or where a significant exposure to steroid medications in the past was associated with undiagnosed secondary glaucoma–produced damage that stabilized once steroid use was stopped (76). Another situation to distinguish from NTG is the case of advanced optic atrophy and visual field loss, in which even mid-to-low pressures may be associated with or can cause further progressive damage. It is also important to rule out nonglaucomatous causes of disc and field changes (discussed in Chapters 4 and 5 and summarized in Table 11.1), and to consider the clinical scenarios when one may want to order neuroimaging (computed tomography or magnetic resonance imaging of the orbit and chiasm) or other studies (e.g., carotid Doppler, orbital B scan) to rule out these disorders (**Table 11.2**).

Adjunctive Tests

Numerous tests have been studied to find additional prognostic indicators of COAG. Although none of these has yet been clearly proven to be of clinical value, the physician should be familiar with some of the more frequently discussed adjunctive tests.

Tonography

This procedure and its limitations as a clinical tool in the diagnosis of COAG are discussed in Chapter 3.

Table 11.1	Differential Diagnosis of Normal-Tension Glaucoma

Congenital Disorders
Optic nerve anomalies, including coloboma, pits, oblique insertion
Autosomal dominant optic atrophy (Kjer type)

Acquired Disorders
History of steroid use by any route that may have led to elevated IOP
History of trauma or surgery that may have led to elevated IOP
Hemodynamic crisis
Methyl alcohol poisoning
Optic neuritis
Arteritic ischemic optic neuropathy
Nonarteritic ischemic optic neuropathy
Compressive lesions of the optic nerve and tract (e.g., meningioma, vascular lesion)
Trauma
Wide diurnal fluctuation in IOP

Table 11.2	Relative Indications to Perform Neuroimaging Evaluation in Normal-Tension Glaucoma

General
Age <50 y
New onset or increased severity of headaches
Localizing neurologic symptoms other than migraine
Neurologic visual abnormalities

Ocular
Color vision abnormalities
Pallor of the remaining neuroretinal rim
Highly asymmetric cupping
Lack of disc and visual field correlation
Visual field defect respecting the vertical (midline)

Provocative Tests

These tests are largely of historical value, and the interested reader is referred to the fourth edition of this text for a more detailed discussion with references.

Water Provocative Test

Drinking a large quantity of water in a short period of time will generally lead to a rise in the IOP. On the basis of the theory that glaucomatous eyes have a greater pressure response to water drinking, a "provocative" test was developed for the early detection of COAG. The test has little diagnostic value.

Dilatation Provocative Tests

These tests are used primarily in eyes suspected of having potentially occludable anterior chamber angles (see Chapter 12). However, cycloplegics and mydriatics have also been studied with regard to their influence on open-angle forms of glaucoma. These studies have not provided clinically useful diagnostic tests, but a few points can be gleaned from them. Patients with COAG are more likely to have a significant rise in IOP with strong cycloplegics (such as cyclopentolate, 1%; atropine, 1%; homatropine, 5%; or scopolamine, 0.25%) if they are undergoing long-term miotic therapy. The mechanism of the pressure response to strong cycloplegics is thought to include inhibition of the miotic effect and direct inhibitory action on the ciliary muscle. In some cases, the postdilation IOP spike can be marked.

The mydriatic action of cycloplegic–mydriatic agents or a mydriatic, such as phenylephrine, is also thought to be a cause of elevated IOP in some eyes with open anterior chamber angles that are not treated with miotics. This occurs only when an associated shower of pigment is in the anterior chamber. The mechanism is thought to be temporary obstruction of the trabecular meshwork by pigment granules. This occurs predominantly in eyes with the exfoliation syndrome or pigmentary glaucoma but may also occur in some cases of COAG with heavy pigmentation in the anterior chamber angle.

Other Adjunctive Tests

The tendency of patients with COAG, as well as a certain percentage of the general population, to respond to topical steroid therapy with an IOP rise has also been evaluated as a predictive test for COAG. However, steroid responsiveness has been found to correlate poorly with risk for COAG.

PROPOSED MECHANISM OF COAG

Mechanisms of Obstruction and Aqueous Outflow

As with virtually all forms of glaucoma, elevation of the IOP in COAG is due to obstruction of aqueous outflow. However, the precise mechanisms of outflow obstruction in this condition remain poorly understood despite having been studied intensively.

Histopathologic Observations

The most likely source for the eventual explanation of aqueous outflow obstruction in COAG lies in the study of histopathologic material and molecular biology (see Chapters 1 and 10). However, the interpretation of histopathologic findings must consider additional influences, such as age, the secondary effects of prolonged IOP elevation, the alterations that medical and surgical treatment of the glaucoma might have induced, and artifacts created by tissue processing.

Influence of Aqueous Humor

Growing evidence shows that abnormal constituents of the aqueous humor may adversely affect the outflow structures, increasing resistance to outflow. Transforming growth factors (TGFs) are a family of multifunctional polypeptides with several cellular regulatory properties, including inhibition of epithelial cell proliferation, induction of extracellular matrix protein synthesis, and stimulation of mesenchymal cell growth. The aqueous humor of patients with COAG has a significantly greater amount of TGF-β_2 than that of healthy individuals (77). Abnormal levels of TGF-β_2 in the aqueous of patients with COAG may decrease the cellularity of the trabecular meshwork and promote a buildup of excessive amounts of extracellular matrix materials with subsequent increased resistance to aqueous outflow.

Alterations of the Trabecular Meshwork

Grant demonstrated that the largest proportion of resistance to aqueous outflow in enucleated human eyes could be eliminated by incising the trabecular meshwork (78). Since then, a number of studies have demonstrated that the site of maximum resistance in the meshwork appears to be the juxtacanalicular tissue and inner wall of the Schlemm canal (79). The most characteristic structural change in the juxtacanalicular tissue is an increase in extracellular matrix and an accumulation of "plaque material." This material derives from thickened sheaths of elastic fibers, although the exact composition remains unknown (77).

Stress-Response Markers

Myocilin, the first gene to be identified as mutated in COAG, appears to be produced in the eye in greater amounts during times of stress. It is present in increased amounts in organ and cell culture experiments after undergoing dexamethasone treatment, oxidative stress, stretching, and treatment with TGF-β (80). Another class of stress-induced proteins studied is heat-shock proteins, such as αB-crystallin. A study of donor eyes with COAG demonstrated differences in staining of two potential stress-response markers, αB-crystallin and myocilin, in trabecular meshwork of glaucomatous eyes (COAG, exfoliative glaucoma, NTG) in comparison with age-matched controls (81). These proteins localized to many more regions of the meshwork and appeared more intense than in healthy eyes, regardless of the type or clinical severity of glaucoma.

Endothelial cells lining the trabeculae appear to be more active in COAG than in normotensive eyes and are reported to show proliferation with foamy degeneration and basement membrane thickening (82). The cellularity of the trabecular meshwork in eyes with COAG is lower than that in nonglaucomatous eyes, but the rate of decline with age is similar in the two groups (83). A reduced frequency of actin filaments (contractile proteins) in trabecular endothelium has also been demonstrated in eyes with COAG (84). Cross-linked actin networks, which alter the function of trabecular cells, were found in higher levels and increased more in response to dexamethasone in glaucoma eyes than in healthy control eyes in tissue culture (85).

Intertrabecular spaces, as might be anticipated from the general thickening of the trabeculae, are narrowed (86). In addition, they may contain red blood cells, pigment, and dense amorphous material (82). Glycosaminoglycans are reported to be more abundant in the meshwork of human eyes with COAG (87,88). However, hyaluronic acid has been shown to be decreased in the trabecular meshwork of eyes with COAG, and the loss of its surface-active properties may influence aqueous outflow resistance (89). Perfusion of cationized ferritin in enucleated eyes of patients with COAG suggests that the outflow obstruction is segmental (90).

Several observers have noted that juxtacanalicular connective tissue just beneath the inner wall endothelium of the Schlemm canal contains a layer of amorphous, osmophilic material (91). This has been described as moderately electron-dense, nonfibrillar material with characteristics of basement membrane and curly collagen and cytochemical properties of chondroitin sulfate protein complex (92,93). However, the concentration of electron-dense materials, although significantly higher than that of a healthy control participant, is not thought to be enough to account for the outflow reduction characteristic of COAG (91). Matrix vesicles, representing extracellular lysosomes, a sheath material from subendothelial elastic-like fibers, the extracellular glycoprotein fibronectin, and elastin have also been found in abnormal amounts in the juxtacanalicular connective tissue of eyes with COAG (94–97). These patients also differ from the healthy population in their collagen binding of plasma fibronectin (98). A study of glycosaminoglycan composition in the juxtacanalicular connective tissue of COAG eyes and age-matched healthy eyes demonstrated that the juxtacanalicular connective tissue in healthy eyes is stratified with hyaluronic acid as the predominant glycosaminoglycan in layers closest to the endothelium of the Schlemm canal (99). In COAG eyes, hyaluronic acid was depleted in all layers within the juxtacanalicular connective tissue, and accumulation of chondroitin sulfate was significantly higher in the juxtacanalicular connective tissue, possibly accounting for the increased outflow resistance in these eyes.

Pores and giant vacuoles are found in the inner wall endothelium of the Schlemm canal in healthy eyes and are thought to be related to aqueous transport. In eyes with COAG, the giant vacuoles have been found in most studies to be decreased or absent. Pore density has also been shown to be reduced and more unevenly distributed in COAG eyes than in healthy eyes (100). In addition, cul-de-sacs, which are described as terminations of aqueous channels, are markedly reduced in eyes with COAG (101).

In a study of the trabecular meshwork and optic nerve from 26 eyes of 14 donors, increasing severity of optic nerve damage (as quantitated by axon counts) was significantly correlated with an increase in the amount of sheath-derived plaque material in the juxtacanalicular connective tissue (102).

Collapse of the Schlemm Canal

Collapse of the Schlemm canal will also increase resistance to aqueous outflow and has been proposed as a mechanism of outflow obstruction in COAG. The collapse represents a bulge of trabecular meshwork into the canal, which might result from alterations in the meshwork or relaxation of the ciliary muscle. In support of this theory, some histopathologic studies have revealed a narrowed Schlemm canal with adhesions between the inner and outer walls (82). A mathematical model of the Schlemm canal, however, tentatively suggests that resistance to aqueous outflow is in the inner wall of the canal and is not caused by a weakening of the trabecular meshwork with a resultant collapse of the Schlemm canal alone (103).

In interpreting the histologic findings in the juxtacanalicular connective tissue and Schlemm canal, it is advisable to take into account a certain amount of segmental variability and to examine at least three quadrants per eye (104).

Alterations of the Intrascleral Channels

Alterations of the intrascleral channels could also be a mechanism of increased resistance to aqueous outflow in COAG. Histopathologic observations have revealed attenuation of the channels, which may be due to a swelling of glycosaminoglycans in the adjacent sclera (105). Krasnov (106) suggested that intrascleral blockage may be the mechanism of outflow obstruction in approximately half of the eyes with COAG. However, this theory was not supported by a study in which removal of tissue overlying the Schlemm canal failed to improve outflow facility until the canal was actually entered (107).

Corticosteroid Sensitivity

As previously noted, there is evidence that patients with COAG are unusually sensitive to corticosteroids and that this steroid sensitivity may be related to the abnormal resistance to aqueous outflow. This discussion first considers the evidence for the increased sensitivity and then looks at theories of how this may influence outflow.

Topical Corticosteroid Response

General population studies have been performed in which a potent topical corticosteroid, such as betamethasone, 0.1%, or dexamethasone, 0.1%, was given three to four times daily for 3 to 6 weeks. These studies found that a substantial proportion of individuals respond with variable degrees of IOP elevation. The studies have differed considerably, however, with regard to many important aspects of this pressure response. For example, the distribution of pressure responses in the general population was found in some studies to be trimodal, with approximately two thirds of participants having a low response (usually defined as an increase in IOP of less than 5 mm Hg), one third showing an intermediate response (increase of 6 to 15 mm Hg), and 4% to 5% having an increase greater than 15 mm Hg (108–110). Another study, however, could not confirm the trimodal concept (111), and when the topical corticosteroid test was repeated in the same population, individuals did not always have the same response each time (112).

COAG populations have more individuals with a high IOP response to topical corticosteroids. The actual reported percentage of high responders, however, varies according to the criteria used to define this group. Reports also differ as to whether patients with ocular hypertension do or do not have a greater incidence of high response than the general population (113,114). The topical corticosteroid response, however, has not been found to be a useful prognostic indicator for COAG (115,116).

Inheritance of the topical corticosteroid response and how this may relate to COAG have been matters of particular controversy. Becker postulated an autosomal recessive mode for the corticosteroid response and suggested that the gene is closely related or identical to that for COAG, which he thought had an autosomal recessive inheritance (108,117). Armaly agreed that the two conditions might be genetically related but proposed a polygenetic inheritance for COAG, with the gene for the topical corticosteroid response being one of the genes involved (110). Results of additional studies were consistent with a genetic basis for the topical corticosteroid response but could confirm neither the recessive mode nor even a relationship to glaucoma (114,118). Still other investigators could not even substantiate that the corticosteroid response was entirely genetic. A twin-heritability study of monozygotic and like-sex dizygotic twins revealed a low estimate of heritability that did not support a predominant role of inheritance in the response to corticosteroids and suggested that nongenetic factors play the major role (111,119–121). A study that further confuses the role of steroids in COAG found that eyes with unilateral angle-closure glaucoma or angle recession also respond to topical corticosteroids with a higher pressure rise in the involved eye than in the fellow eye, which had not had angle closure or trauma (122,123). These observations suggest that topical corticosteroid responsiveness is multifactorial.

Relationship of Intraocular Pressure to Corticosteroid Sensitivity

Investigators have tried to explain if or why patients with COAG are unusually sensitive to corticosteroids.

Hypothalamic–Pituitary–Adrenal Axis Theory

An abnormal response of the hypothalamic–pituitary–adrenal axis in patients with COAG, and possibly in other forms of glaucoma, may be related to alterations in aqueous humor dynamics in response to corticosteroids (124,125).

Cyclic–Adenosine Monophosphate Theory

It may be that corticosteroids influence the IOP by altering cyclic–adenosine monophosphate. Corticosteroids have a permissive effect on the β-adrenergic stimulation of adenyl cyclase, the enzyme responsible for the synthesis of cyclic–adenosine monophosphate (126). How this relates to aqueous humor dynamics is uncertain, although patients with COAG and high topical steroid responders appear to be unusually sensitive to cyclic–adenosine monophosphate.

Glycosaminoglycans Theory

It has also been proposed that IOP elevation associated with corticosteroid sensitivity may be related to glycosaminoglycans in the trabecular meshwork (127). When polymerized, glycosaminoglycans become hydrated, swell, and obstruct aqueous outflow. Catabolic enzymes, released from lysosomes in the trabecular cells, depolymerize the glycosaminoglycans. Corticosteroids stabilize the lysosome membrane, preventing release of these enzymes and thereby increasing the polymerized form of glycosaminoglycans and the resistance to aqueous outflow.

Phagocytosis Theory

The effect of steroids on IOP may be related to the phagocytic activity of endothelial cells lining the trabecular meshwork. These cells are normally phagocytic, and they may function to "clean" the aqueous of debris before it reaches the inner wall endothelium of the Schlemm canal. Failure to do so might result in a buildup of material that could account for the amorphous layer in the juxtacanalicular connective tissue (as previously described). Corticosteroids suppress phagocytosis, and it may be that the trabecular endothelium in patients with COAG is unusually sensitive, even to endogenous corticosteroids (128).

Mechanism of Optic Neuropathy

Histopathologic Observations

Axon loss in eyes with COAG has been reported to be associated with increasing connective tissue in the septa and surrounding the central retinal vessels, including increased amounts of types IV and VI collagen (129). The total number of capillaries and the density of capillaries decreased with loss of axons. Arteriosclerotic changes were more common in glaucomatous eyes than in age-matched control eyes.

Immunologic Studies

A number of reports suggest an immunoregulatory mechanism in the pathogenesis of COAG, at the level of the meshwork, ganglion cell bodies and optic nerve axons, retinal vessels, and lamina cribrosa. The roles of the immune system in glaucoma have been described as either neuroprotective or neurodestructive. It has been proposed that a critical balance between beneficial protective immunity and harmful sequelae of autoimmune neurodegenerative injury (such as heat-shock proteins) determines the ultimate fate of retinal ganglion cells in response to various stressors in patients with glaucoma. The Canadian Glaucoma Study reported that an elevated anticardiolipin antibody is associated with progression of COAG (130). Anticardiolipin antibody is one of the antiphospholipid antibodies found in elevated levels in patients with acquired thrombotic syndromes (131,132).

Blood Flow

Abnormalities of blood flow to the posterior segment of the eye in COAG have been shown by using color Doppler imaging, fluorescein angiography, laser Doppler flowmetry, and pulsatile ocular blood flow measurements (133–141). Rheological studies have also demonstrated differences in red cell aggregability, increased plasma viscosity, and activation of the clotting system in patients with COAG compared with controls (65,142,143). Altered autoregulation of blood flow in the optic nerve and retinal circulation has also been demonstrated (144,145).

Changes in the retrobulbar hemodynamics also appear to occur with age. Color Doppler imaging analysis of the ophthalmic, central retinal, and nasal and temporal posterior ciliary arteries in healthy men and women demonstrated age-related alterations in hemodynamics, similar to those seen in patients with glaucoma, suggesting that these age-related changes may contribute to an increased risk for glaucoma (146).

There is also evidence that the choroidal circulation is compromised in COAG (147,148), which is supported by electroretinographic data demonstrating outer retinal damage in eyes with glaucoma (149).

Apoptotic Susceptibility of Ganglion Cells

Ganglion cells appear to die by apoptosis in experimental glaucoma (150). This may relate to a multiplicity of factors (**Fig. 11.1**). Clinically, some evidence is related to excitotoxic cell death from accumulation of glutamate and an imbalance of proteases that modulate the extracellular matrix milieu in the retina (151,152).

Possible Infectious Susceptibility

In a study of 32 patients with COAG, 9 with exfoliative glaucoma, and 30 age-matched control patients with anemia, upper gastrointestinal endoscopy was performed to evaluate macroscopic abnormalities and gastric mucosal biopsy specimens were analyzed for the presence of *Helicobacter pylori* infection (153). Approximately 88% of the patients with COAG and exfoliative glaucoma had histologically confirmed *H. pylori* infection, compared with 47% among controls. Patients with

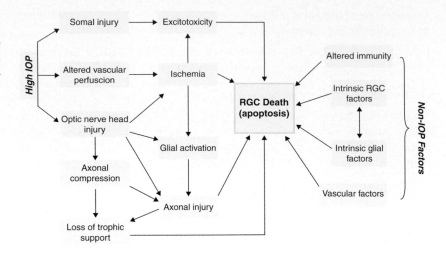

Figure 11.1 Diverse insults can lead to retinal ganglion cell death. These include IOP-related and non–IOP-related factors. (Reproduced from Libby RT et al. Complex genetics of glaucoma susceptibility. *Annu Rev Genomics Hum Genet.* 2005;6:15–44, with permission).

glaucoma also exhibited abnormal gastric mucosa, antral gastritis, and peptic ulcer disease. Not all studies have found this correlation (154).

Cerebrospinal Fluid Pressure

The lamina cribrosa is located between two pressurized compartments, intraocular space and the subarachnoid space posteriorly (see Chapter 4). The pressure difference between these two spaces has been termed the "translaminar pressure." In this context, a reduced cerebrospinal fluid (CSF) pressure would exert the same effect as an increase in IOP. Emerging evidence suggests that the translaminar pressure may play an important role in glaucomatous optic neuropathy (155–157). In these studies, the measured CSF pressure was significantly lower in participants with COAG compared with controls. In addition, CSF pressure was lower in participants with NTG, compared with those who had COAG associated with elevated IOP. These data, although preliminary, suggest that the dynamic interplay between these fluid spaces may play a role in glaucoma and may help explain why some individuals with normal IOP may develop glaucoma and others with elevated IOP may not.

MANAGEMENT

General Principles of Management

The principles of when and how to treat patients with COAG are discussed in Chapter 27. In brief, it is important to establish a target IOP range for both eyes of the patient—that is, an IOP range in which there will presumably be no further anticipated optic nerve damage. This begins with a detailed history, complete examination, and appropriate testing, after which the target IOP is set on the basis of stage of glaucomatous damage and risk factors for progression (as discussed here). The target is a dynamic concept that needs to be reevaluated at each visit. Once the target IOP range is set, it is achieved with topical medication in most cases. If the target IOP range cannot be

achieved despite maximum tolerable medical therapy, argon or selective laser trabeculoplasty is usually indicated, followed by glaucoma filtering surgery or other therapeutic maneuvers as deemed necessary. If optic nerve or visual field progression occurs despite achieving the target IOP range, it may be necessary to revise the target IOP downward and to consider IOP-independent mechanisms of the optic neuropathy.

Throughout the treatment course, the expense, inconvenience, and side effects of therapy should be considered and an effective treatment plan that includes patient education, efficacy and toxicity of therapy, and patient adherence should be established. A regimen of the least medication to achieve the desired therapeutic response should be chosen for each eye of the patient. Follow-up evaluation should be guided by the severity of the disease.

Treatment of Normal-Tension Glaucoma

Although damage to the optic nerve head and visual field may progress even at low-normal pressures in NTG, compelling evidence shows that IOP reduction from baseline values is effective. In the CNTGS, 57% of the patients achieved a 30% IOP reduction with topical medication, laser trabeculoplasty, or both (158). The remaining 43% required filtering surgery. Although filtering surgery did not help in one reported series (156), other surgeons have found that it may prevent progressive damage (159–162), and the CNTGS has confirmed the benefit of aggressive IOP reduction in these patients.

Despite the proven value of IOP reduction, some patients with NTG may have IOP-independent mechanisms of glaucomatous optic neuropathy, and this must especially be considered when damage is progressing with pressures in the single digits. An additional aspect of managing the patient with NTG may be the treatment of any cardiovascular abnormality, such as anemia, hypotension, congestive heart failure, transient ischemic attacks, and cardiac arrhythmias, to ensure maximum perfusion of the optic nerve head (163).

Ultimately, the treatment of choice may prove to be therapy that directly protects and improves the function of ganglion cells and the optic nerve head. A placebo-controlled 3-year study of the calcium-channel blocker nilvadipine on visual field and ocular circulation in 33 patients with NTG suggested that blood flow to the optic nerve and fovea was increased in the treated group. Furthermore, the mean negative slope in mean deviation of the visual field over time was also less in the treated group (164). Other studies involving patients with NTG receiving concurrent calcium-channel blocker therapy have demonstrated a significant reduction in the rate of disc and field progression, compared with similar NTG groups who were not receiving the concomitant therapy (165,166).

KEY POINTS

- COAG is the most common form of glaucoma worldwide. It has a familial tendency and is more prevalent with increasing age, black race, myopia, and certain systemic diseases, such as diabetes mellitus and cardiovascular abnormalities.

- COAG is typically asymptomatic until advanced visual field loss occurs and is characterized by an open, normal-appearing anterior chamber angle.

- A clinical subset of COAG, NTG, has similar disc and field changes but pressures that remain in the normal range without treatment. However, IOP is a contributing risk factor in both conditions, with an increasing influence of IOP-independent factors in NTG. NTG is a diagnosis of exclusion, and it is important to ensure that no atypical clinical features suggest nonglaucomatous causes of optic nerve cupping.

- The precise mechanism of increased resistance to aqueous outflow and to optic nerve damage in COAG remains unclear, although continued research, especially in molecular biology, is beginning to reveal answers to these complex processes.

REFERENCES

1. American Academy of Ophthalmology (AAO). Primary Open-Angle Glaucoma, Preferred Practice Pattern. San Francisco, CA: AAO; 2005. Available at: http://www.aao.org/ppp.
2. Kolker AE, Becker B. 'Ocular hypertension' vs open-angle glaucoma: a different view. *Arch Ophthalmol.* 1977;95(4):586–587.
3. Phelps CD. Ocular hypertension: to treat or not to treat. *Arch Ophthalmol.* 1977;95(4):588–589.
4. Chandler PA, Grant WM. 'Ocular hypertension' vs open-angle glaucoma. *Arch Ophthalmol.* 1977;95(4):585–586.
5. Shaffer R. 'Glaucoma suspect' or 'ocular hypertension'. *Arch Ophthalmol.* 1977;95(4):588.
6. Lee BL, Bathija R, Weinreb RN. The definition of normal-tension glaucoma. *J Glaucoma.* 1998;7(6):366–371.
7. Shields MB. Normal-tension glaucoma: is it different from primary open-angle glaucoma? *Curr Opin Ophthalmol.* 2008;19(2):85–88.
8. O'Brien C, Schwartz B, Takamoto T, et al. Intraocular pressure and the rate of visual field loss in chronic open-angle glaucoma. *Am J Ophthalmol.* 1991;111(4):491–500.
9. Weber J, Koll W, Krieglstein GK. Intraocular pressure and visual field decay in chronic glaucoma. *Ger J Ophthalmol.* 1993;2(3):165–169.
10. Chauhan BC, Drance SM. The relationship between intraocular pressure and visual field progression in glaucoma. *Graefes Arch Clin Exp Ophthalmol.* 1992;230(6):521–526.
11. Cedrone C, Mancino R, Cerulli A, et al. Epidemiology of primary glaucoma: prevalence, incidence, and blinding effects [review]. *Prog Brain Res.* 2008;173:3–14.
12. Leske MC. Open-angle glaucoma—an epidemiologic overview [review]. *Ophthalmic Epidemiol.* 2007;14(4):166–172.
13. Hollows FC, Graham PA. Intra-ocular pressure, glaucoma, and glaucoma suspects in a defined population. *Br J Ophthalmol.* 1966;50(10):570–586.
14. Shiose Y, Kitazawa Y, Tsukahara S, et al. Epidemiology of glaucoma in Japan—a nationwide glaucoma survey. *Jpn J Ophthalmol.* 1991; 35(2):133–155.
15. Leydhecker W. On the distribution of glaucoma simplex in apparently healthy population not treated by ophthalmologists [in German]. *Doc Ophthalmol.* 1959;13:359–388.
16. Lichter PR, Shaffer RN. Ocular hypertension and glaucoma. *Trans Pac Coast Otoophthalmol Soc.* 1973;54:63–75.
17. Jay JL, Murdoch JR. The rate of visual field loss in untreated primary open angle glaucoma. *Br J Ophthalmol.* 1993;77(3):176–178.
18. Harbin TS Jr, Podos SM, Kolker AE, et al. Visual field progression in open-angle glaucoma patients presenting with monocular field loss. *Trans Sect Ophthalmol Am Acad Ophthalmol Otolaryngol.* 1976;81(2): 253–257.
19. Grant WM, Burke JF Jr. Why do some people go blind from glaucoma? *Ophthalmology.* 1982;89(9):991–998.
20. Ekstrom C, Haglund B. Chronic open-angle glaucoma and advanced visual field defects in a defined population. *Acta Ophthalmol.* 1991; 69(5):574–580.
21. Anderson DR, Drance SM, Schulzer M. Natural history of normal-tension glaucoma. *Ophthalmology.* 2001;108(2):247–253.
22. Leske MC, Heijl A, Hyman L, et al. Predictors of long-term progression in the early manifest glaucoma trial. *Ophthalmology.* 2007;114(11): 1965–1972.
23. Behki R, Damji KF, Crichton A. Canadian perspectives in glaucoma management: the role of central corneal thickness [review]. *Can J Ophthalmol.* 2007;42(1):66–74.
24. Kimura R, Levene RZ. Gonioscopic differences between primary open-angle glaucoma and normal subjects over 40 years of age. *Am J Ophthalmol.* 1975;80(1):56–61.
25. Campbell DG, Boys-Smith JW, Woods WD. Variation of pigmentation and segmentation of pigmentation in primary open-angle glaucoma. *Invest Ophthalmol Vis Sci.* 1984;25(suppl):122.
26. Sommer A, Miller NR, Pollack I, et al. The nerve fiber layer in the diagnosis of glaucoma. *Arch Ophthalmol.* 1977;95(12):2149–2156.
27. Kass MA, Kolker AE, Becker B. Prognostic factors in glaucomatous visual field loss. *Arch Ophthalmol.* 1976;94(8):1274–1276.
28. Susanna R, Drance SM, Douglas GR. The visual prognosis of the fellow eye in uniocular chronic open-angle glaucoma. *Br J Ophthalmol.* 1978;62(5):327–329.
29. Iester M, Mikelberg FS. Optic nerve head morphologic characteristics in high-tension and normal-tension glaucoma. *Arch Ophthalmol.* 1999; 117(8):1010–1013.
30. Kim DM, Seo JH, Kim SH, et al. Comparison of localized retinal nerve fiber layer defects between a low-teen intraocular pressure group and a high-teen intraocular pressure group in normal-tension glaucoma patients. *J Glaucoma.* 2007;16(3):293–296.
31. Yamazaki Y, Koide C, Miyazawa T, et al. Comparison of retinal nerve-fiber layer in high- and normal-tension glaucoma. *Graefes Arch Clin Exp Ophthalmol.* 1991;229(6):517–520.
32. Kubota T, Khalil AK, Honda M, et al. Comparative study of retinal nerve fiber layer damage in Japanese patients with normal- and high-tension glaucoma. *J Glaucoma.* 1999;8(6):363–366.
33. Gramer E, Althaus G, Leydhecker W. Site and depth of glaucomatous visual field defects in relation to the size of the neuroretinal edge zone of the optic disk in glaucoma without hypertension, simple glaucoma, pigmentary glaucoma. A clinical study with the Octopus perimeter 201 and the optic nerve head analyzer [in German]. *Klin Monatsbl Augenheilkd.* 1986;189(3):190–198.
34. Gliklich RE, Steinmann WC, Spaeth GL. Visual field change in low-tension glaucoma over a five-year follow-up. *Ophthalmology.* 1989; 96(3):316–320.
35. Gramer E, Althaus G. Quantification and progression of the visual field defect in glaucoma without hypertension, glaucoma simplex and pigmentary glaucoma. A clinical study with the Delta Program of the 201 Octopus perimeter [in German]. *Klin Monatsbl Augenheilkd.* 1987; 191(3):184–198.
36. Gramer E, Leydhecker W. Glaucoma without ocular hypertension. A clinical study [in German]. Klin Monatsbl Augenheilkd. 1985;186(4):262–267.
37. Araie M, Sekine M, Suzuki Y, et al. Factors contributing to the progression of visual field damage in eyes with normal-tension glaucoma. *Ophthalmology.* 1994;101(8):1440–1444.

38. Jonas JB, Grundler AE, Gonzales-Cortes J. Pressure-dependent neuroretinal rim loss in normal-pressure glaucoma. *Am J Ophthalmol.* 1998;125(2):137–144.

39. Noureddin BN, Poinoosawmy D, Fietzke FW, et al. Regression analysis of visual field progression in low tension glaucoma. *Br J Ophthalmol.* 1991;75(8):493–495.

40. Cartwright MJ, Anderson DR. Correlation of asymmetric damage with asymmetric intraocular pressure in normal-tension glaucoma (low-tension glaucoma). *Arch Ophthalmol.* 1988;106(7):898–900.

41. Crichton A, Drance SM, Douglas GR, et al. Unequal intraocular pressure and its relation to asymmetric visual field defects in low-tension glaucoma. *Ophthalmology.* 1989;96(9):1312–1314.

42. Greenfield DS, Liebmann JM, Ritch R, et al. Visual field and intraocular pressure asymmetry in the low-pressure glaucoma treatment study. *Ophthalmology.* 2007;114(3):460–465.

43. Ido T, Tomita G, Kitazawa Y. Diurnal variation of intraocular pressure of normal-tension glaucoma. Influence of sleep and arousal. *Ophthalmology.* 1991;98(3):296–300.

44. Larsson LI, Rettig ES, Sheridan PT, et al. Aqueous humor dynamics in low-tension glaucoma. *Am J Ophthalmol.* 1993;116(5):590–593.

45. Weinreb RN, Liu JH. Nocturnal rhythms of intraocular pressure. *Arch Ophthalmol.* 2006;124(2):269–270.

46. Drance SM, Sweeney VP, Morgan RW, et al. Studies of factors involved in the production of low tension glaucoma. *Arch Ophthalmol.* 1973;89(6):457–465.

47. Drance SM, Morgan RW, Sweeney VP. Shock-induced optic neuropathy: a cause of nonprogressive glaucoma. *N Engl J Med.* 1973;288(8):392–395.

48. Goldberg I, Hollows FC, Kass MA, et al. Systemic factors in patients with low-tension glaucoma. *Br J Ophthalmol.* 1981;65(1):56–62.

49. James CB, Smith SE. Pulsatile ocular blood flow in patients with low tension glaucoma. *Br J Ophthalmol.* 1991;75(8):466–470.

50. Hashimoto M, Ohtsuka K, Ohtsuka H, et al. Normal-tension glaucoma with reversed ophthalmic artery flow. *Am J Ophthalmol.* 2000;130(5):670–672.

51. Rader J, Feuer WJ, Anderson DR. Peripapillary vasoconstriction in the glaucomas and the anterior ischemic optic neuropathies. *Am J Ophthalmol.* 1994;117(1):72–80.

52. Kondo Y, Niwa Y, Yamamoto T, et al. Retrobulbar hemodynamics in normal-tension glaucoma with asymmetric visual field change and asymmetric ocular perfusion pressure. *Am J Ophthalmol.* 2000;130(4):454–460.

53. Meyer JH, Brandi-Dohrn J, Funk J. Twenty four hour blood pressure monitoring in normal tension glaucoma. *Br J Ophthalmol.* 1996;80(10):864–867.

54. Hulsman CA, Vingerling JR, Hofman A, et al. Blood pressure, arterial stiffness, and open-angle glaucoma: the Rotterdam study. *Arch Ophthalmol.* 2007;125(6):805–812.

55. Waldmann E, Gasser P, Dubler B, et al. Silent myocardial ischemia in glaucoma and cataract patients. *Graefes Arch Clin Exp Ophthalmol.* 1996;234(10):595–598.

56. Pillunat LE, Stodtmeister R, Wilmanns I. Pressure compliance of the optic nerve head in low tension glaucoma. *Br J Ophthalmol.* 1987;71(3):181–187.

57. Phelps CD, Corbett JJ. Migraine and low-tension glaucoma. A case-control study. *Invest Ophthalmol Vis Sci.* 1985;26(8):1105–1108.

58. Usui T, Iwata K, Shirakashi M, et al. Prevalence of migraine in low-tension glaucoma and primary open-angle glaucoma in Japanese. *Br J Ophthalmol.* 1991;75(4):224–226.

59. Orgul S, Flammer J. Headache in normal-tension glaucoma patients. *J Glaucoma.* 1994;3(4):292–295.

60. Drance SM, Douglas GR, Wijsman K, et al. Response of blood flow to warm and cold in normal and low-tension glaucoma patients. *Am J Ophthalmol.* 1988;105(1):35–39.

61. Gasser P, Flammer J. Blood-cell velocity in the nailfold capillaries of patients with normal-tension and high-tension glaucoma. *Am J Ophthalmol.* 1991;111(5):585–588.

62. Schulzer M, Drance SM, Carter CJ, et al. Biostatistical evidence for two distinct chronic open angle glaucoma populations. *Br J Ophthalmol.* 1990;74(4):196–200.

63. Henry E, Newby DE, Webb DJ, et al. Peripheral endothelial dysfunction in normal pressure glaucoma. *Invest Ophthalmol Vis Sci.* 1999;40(8):1710–1714.

64. Kim SH, Kim JY, Kim DM, et al. Investigations on the association between normal tension glaucoma and single nucleotide polymorphisms of the endothelin-1 and endothelin receptor genes. *Mol Vis.* 2006;12:1016–1021.

65. Klaver JH, Greve EL, Goslinga H, et al. Blood and plasma viscosity measurements in patients with glaucoma. *Br J Ophthalmol.* 1985;69(10):765–770.

66. Joist JH, Lichtenfeld P, Mandell AI, et al. Platelet function, blood coagulability, and fibrinolysis in patients with low tension glaucoma. *Arch Ophthalmol.* 1976;94(11):1893–1895.

67. Carter CJ, Brooks DE, Doyle DL, et al. Investigations into a vascular etiology for low-tension glaucoma. *Ophthalmology.* 1990;97(1):49–55.

68. Winder AF. Circulating lipoprotein and blood glucose levels in association with low-tension and chronic simple glaucoma. *Br J Ophthalmol.* 1977;61(10):641–645.

69. Stroman GA, Stewart WC, Golnik KC, et al. Magnetic resonance imaging in patients with low-tension glaucoma. *Arch Ophthalmol.* 1995;113(2):168–172.

70. Ong K, Farinelli A, Billson F, et al. Comparative study of brain magnetic resonance imaging findings in patients with low-tension glaucoma and control subjects. *Ophthalmology.* 1995;102(11):1632–1638.

71. Cartwright MJ, Grajewski AL, Friedberg ML, et al. Immune-related disease and normal-tension glaucoma. A case-control study. *Arch Ophthalmol.* 1992;110(4):500–502.

72. Wax MB, Barrett DA, Pestronk A. Increased incidence of paraproteinemia and autoantibodies in patients with normal-pressure glaucoma. *Am J Ophthalmol.* 1994;117(5):561–568.

73. Romano C, Barrett DA, Li Z, et al. Anti-rhodopsin antibodies in sera from patients with normal-pressure glaucoma. *Invest Ophthalmol Vis Sci.* 1995;36(10):1968–1975.

74. Yang J, Tezel G, Patil RV, et al. Serum autoantibody against glutathione S-transferase in patients with glaucoma. *Invest Ophthalmol Vis Sci.* 2001;42(6):1273–1276.

75. Wax MB, Tezel G, Saito I, et al. Anti-Ro/SS-A positivity and heat shock protein antibodies in patients with normal-pressure glaucoma. *Am J Ophthalmol.* 1998;125(2):145–157.

76. Ritch R. Nonprogressive low-tension glaucoma with pigmentary dispersion. *Am J Ophthalmol.* 1982;94(2):190–196.

77. Tamm ER, Fuchshofer R. What increases outflow resistance in primary open-angle glaucoma? *Surv Ophthalmol.* 2007;52(suppl 2):S101–S104.

78. Grant WM. Further studies on facility of flow through the trabecular meshwork. *Arch Ophthalmol.* 1958;60(4 pt 1):523–533.

79. Johnson M. What controls aqueous humour outflow resistance? *Exp Eye Res.* 2006;82(4):545–557.

80. Johnson DH. Myocilin and glaucoma: A TIGR by the tail? *Arch Ophthalmol.* 2000;118(7):974–978.

81. Lutjen-Drecoll E, May CA, Polansky JR, et al. Localization of the stress proteins alpha B-crystallin and trabecular meshwork inducible glucocorticoid response protein in normal and glaucomatous trabecular meshwork. *Invest Ophthalmol Vis Sci.* 1998;39(3):517–525.

82. Zatulina NI. Electron microscopy of trabecular tissue in the advanced stage of simple open-angle glaucoma [in Russian]. *Oftalmol Zh.* 1973;28(2):115–118.

83. Alvarado J, Murphy C, Juster R. Trabecular meshwork cellularity in primary open-angle glaucoma and nonglaucomatous normals. *Ophthalmology.* 1984;91(6):564–579.

84. Tripathi RC, Tripathi BJ. Contractile protein alteration in trabecular endothelium in primary open-angle glaucoma. *Exp Eye Res.* 1980;31(6):721–724.

85. Clark AF, Miggans ST, Wilson K, et al. Cytoskeletal changes in cultured human glaucoma trabecular meshwork cells. *J Glaucoma.* 1995;4(3):183–188.

86. Finkelstein I, Trope GE, Basu PK, et al. Quantitative analysis of collagen content and amino acids in trabecular meshwork. *Br J Ophthalmol.* 1990;74(5):280–282.

87. Li Y, Yi YZ. Histochemical and electron microscopic studies of the trabecular meshwork in primary open-angle glaucoma [in Chinese]. *Yan Ke Xue Bao.* 1985;1(1):17–22.

88. Armaly MF, Wang Y. Demonstration of acid mucopolysaccharides in the trabecular meshwork of the Rhesus monkey. *Invest Ophthalmol.* 1975;14(7):507–516.

89. Knepper PA, Covici S, Fadel JR, et al. Surface-tension properties of hyaluronic Acid. *J Glaucoma.* 1995;4(3):194–199.

90. de Kater AW, Melamed S, Epstein DL. Patterns of aqueous humor outflow in glaucomatous and nonglaucomatous human eyes. A tracer study using cationized ferritin. *Arch Ophthalmol.* 1989;107(4):572–576.

91. Alvarado JA, Yun AJ, Murphy CG. Juxtacanalicular tissue in primary open angle glaucoma and in nonglaucomatous normals. *Arch Ophthalmol.* 1986;104(10):1517–1528.
92. Rodrigues MM, Spaeth GL, Sivalingam E, et al. Value of trabeculectomy specimens in glaucoma. *Ophthalmic Surg.* 1978;9(2):29–38.
93. Segawa K. Electron microscopic changes of the trabecular tissue in primary open-angle glaucoma. *Ann Ophthalmol.* 1979;11(1):49–54.
94. Rohen JW. Presence of matrix vesicles in the trabecular meshwork of glaucomatous eyes. *Graefes Arch Clin Exp Ophthalmol.* 1982;218(4):171–176.
95. Rohen JW. Why is intraocular pressure elevated in chronic simple glaucoma? Anatomical considerations. *Ophthalmology.* 1983;90(7):758–765.
96. Babizhayev MA, Brodskaya MW. Fibronectin detection in drainage outflow system of human eyes in ageing and progression of open-angle glaucoma. *Mech Ageing Dev.* 1989;47(2):145–157.
97. Umihira J, Nagata S, Nohara M, et al. Localization of elastin in the normal and glaucomatous human trabecular meshwork. *Invest Ophthalmol Vis Sci.* 1994;35(2):486–494.
98. Worthen DM, Cleveland PH, Slight JR, et al. Selective binding affinity of human plasma fibronectin for the collagens I–IV. *Invest Ophthalmol Vis Sci.* 1985;26(12):1740–1744.
99. Knepper PA, Goossens W, Palmberg PF. Glycosaminoglycan stratification of the juxtacanalicular tissue in normal and primary open angle glaucoma. *Invest Ophthalmol Vis Sci.* 1996;37(12):2414–2425.
100. Allingham RR, de Kater AW, Ethier CR, et al. The relationship between pore density and outflow facility in human eyes. *Invest Ophthalmol Vis Sci.* 1992;33(5):1661–1669.
101. Alvarado JA, Murphy CG. Outflow obstruction in pigmentary and primary open angle glaucoma. *Arch Ophthalmol.* 1992;110(12):1769–1778.
102. Gottanka J, Johnson DH, Martus P, et al. Severity of optic nerve damage in eyes with POAG is correlated with changes in the trabecular meshwork. *J Glaucoma.* 1997;6(2):123–132.
103. Johnson MC, Kamm RD. The role of Schlemm's canal in aqueous outflow from the human eye. *Invest Ophthalmol Vis Sci.* 1983;24(3):320–325.
104. Buller C, Johnson D. Segmental variability of the trabecular meshwork in normal and glaucomatous eyes. *Invest Ophthalmol Vis Sci.* 1994;35(11):3841–3851.
105. Ashton N. The exit pathway of the aqueous. *Trans Ophthalmol Soc U K.* 1960;80:397–421.
106. Krasnov MM. Symposium: microsurgery of the outflow channels. Sinusotomy. Foundations, results, prospects. *Trans Am Acad Ophthalmol Otolaryngol.* 1972;76(2):368–374.
107. Nesterov AP, Batmanov YE. Trabecular wall of Schlemm's canal in the early stage of primary open-angle glaucoma. *Am J Ophthalmol.* 1974;78(4):639–647.
108. Becker B, Hahn KA. Topical corticosteroids and heredity in primary open-angle glaucoma. *Am J Ophthalmol.* 1964;57:543–551.
109. Armaly MF. The heritable nature of dexamethasone-induced ocular hypertension. *Arch Ophthalmol.* 1966;75(1):32–35.
110. Armaly MF. Inheritance of dexamethasone hypertension and glaucoma. *Arch Ophthalmol.* 1967;77(6):747–751.
111. Schwartz JT, Reuling FH, Feinleib M, et al. Twin study on ocular pressure after topical dexamethasone. 1. Frequency distribution of pressure response. *Am J Ophthalmol.* 1973;76(1):126–136.
112. Palmberg PF, Mandell A, Wilensky JT, et al. The reproducibility of the intraocular pressure response to dexamethasone. *Am J Ophthalmol.* 1975;80(5):844–856.
113. Dean GO Jr, Deutsch AR, Hiatt RL. The effect of dexamethasone on borderline ocular hypertension. *Ann Ophthalmol.* 1975;7(2):193–198.
114. Levene R, Wigdor A, Edelstein A, et al. Topical corticosteroid in normal patients and glaucoma suspects. *Arch Ophthalmol.* 1967;77(5):593–597.
115. Lewis JM, Priddy T, Judd J, et al. Intraocular pressure response to topical dexamethasone as a predictor for the development of primary open-angle glaucoma. *Am J Ophthalmol.* 1988;106(5):607–612.
116. Klemetti A. The dexamethasone provocative test: a predictive tool for glaucoma? *Acta Ophthalmol.* 1990;68(1):29–33.
117. Becker B. The genetic problem of chronic simple glaucoma. *Ann Ophthalmol.* 1971;3(4):351–354.
118. Francois J, Heintz-de Bree CH, Tripathi RC. The cortisone test and the heredity of primary open-angle glaucoma. *Am J Ophthalmol.* 1966;62(5):844–852.
119. Schwartz JT, Reuling FH, Feinleib M, et al. Twin heritability study of the effect of corticosteroids on intraocular pressure. *J Med Genet.* 1972;9(2):137–143.
120. Schwartz JT, Reuling FH Jr, Feinleib M, et al. Twin heritability study of the corticosteroid response. *Trans Am Acad Ophthalmol Otolaryngol.* 1973;77(2):OP126–OP136.
121. Schwartz JT, Reuling FH, Feinleib M, et al. Twin study on ocular pressure following topically applied dexamethasone. II. Inheritance of variation in pressure response. *Arch Ophthalmol.* 1973;90(4):281–286.
122. Akingbehin AO. Corticosteroid-induced ocular hypertension. II. An acquired form. *Br J Ophthalmol.* 1982;66(8):541–545.
123. Spaeth GL. Traumatic hyphema, angle recession, dexamethasone hypertension, and glaucoma. *Arch Ophthalmol.* 1967;78(6):714–721.
124. Schwartz B. The hypothalamo-hypophyseal-adrenal gland system and steroid glaucoma [in German]. *Klin Monatsbl Augenheilkd.* 1972;161(3):280–287.
125. Schwartz B, Golden MA, Wiznia RA, et al. Differences of adrenal stress control mechanisms in subjects with glaucoma and normal subjects. Effect of vasopressin and pyrogen. *Arch Ophthalmol.* 1981;99(10):1770–1777.
126. Kass MA, Shin DH, Cooper DG, et al. The ocular hypotensive effect of epinephrine in high and low corticosteroid responders. *Invest Ophthalmol Vis Sci.* 1977;16(6):530–531.
127. Francois F, Victoria-Troncoso V. Mucopolysaccharides and pathogenesis of cortisone glaucoma [in German]. *Klin Monatsbl Augenheilkd.* 1974;165(1):5–10.
128. Bill A. The drainage of aqueous humor [editorial]. *Invest Ophthalmol.* 1975;14(1):1–3.
129. Gottanka J, Kuhlmann A, Scholz M, et al. Pathophysiologic changes in the optic nerves of eyes with primary open angle and exfoliation glaucoma. *Invest Ophthalmol Vis Sci.* 2005;46(11):4170–4181.
130. Chauhan BC, Mikelberg FS, Balaszi AG, et al. Canadian Glaucoma Study: 2. Risk factors for the progression of open-angle glaucoma. *Arch Ophthalmol.* 2008;126(8):1030–1036.
131. Grus FH, Joachim SC, Wuenschig D, et al. Autoimmunity and glaucoma [review]. *J Glaucoma.* 2008;17(1):79–84.
132. Wax MB, Tezel G. Immunoregulation of retinal ganglion cell fate in glaucoma [review]. *Exp Eye Res.* 2009;88(4):825–830.
133. Rankin SJ, Walman BE, Buckley AR, et al. Color Doppler imaging and spectral analysis of the optic nerve vasculature in glaucoma. *Am J Ophthalmol.* 1995;119(6):685–693.
134. Rankin SJ, Drance SM. Peripapillary focal retinal arteriolar narrowing in open angle glaucoma. *J Glaucoma.* 1996;5(1):22–28.
135. Nicolela MT, Walman BE, Buckley AR, et al. Ocular hypertension and primary open-angle glaucoma: a comparative study of their retrobulbar blood flow velocity. *J Glaucoma.* 1996;5(5):308–310.
136. Butt Z, O'Brien C, McKillop G, et al. Color Doppler imaging in untreated high- and normal-pressure open-angle glaucoma. *Invest Ophthalmol Vis Sci.* 1997;38(3):690–696.
137. Kerr J, Nelson P, O'Brien C. A comparison of ocular blood flow in untreated primary open-angle glaucoma and ocular hypertension. *Am J Ophthalmol.* 1998;126(1):42–51.
138. Schwartz B, Rieser JC, Fishbein SL. Fluorescein angiographic defects of the optic disc in glaucoma. *Arch Ophthalmol.* 1977;95(11):1961–1974.
139. Michelson G, Langhans MJ, Groh MJ. Perfusion of the juxtapapillary retina and the neuroretinal rim area in primary open angle glaucoma. *J Glaucoma.* 1996;5(2):91–98.
140. Findl O, Rainer G, Dallinger S, et al. Assessment of optic disk blood flow in patients with open-angle glaucoma. *Am J Ophthalmol.* 2000;130(5):589–596.
141. Trew DR, Smith SE. Postural studies in pulsatile ocular blood flow: II. Chronic open angle glaucoma. *Br J Ophthalmol.* 1991;75(2):71–75.
142. Hamard P, Hamard H, Dufaux J, et al. Optic nerve head blood flow using a laser Doppler velocimeter and haemorheology in primary open angle glaucoma and normal pressure glaucoma. *Br J Ophthalmol.* 1994;78(6):449–453.
143. O'Brien C, Butt Z, Ludlam C, et al. Activation of the coagulation cascade in untreated primary open-angle glaucoma. *Ophthalmology.* 1997;104(4):725–729, discussion 9–30.
144. Pillunat LE, Stodtmeister R, Wilmanns I, et al. Autoregulation of ocular blood flow during changes in intraocular pressure. Preliminary results. *Graefes Arch Clin Exp Ophthalmol.* 1985;223(4):219–223.
145. Grunwald JE, Riva CE, Stone RA, et al. Retinal autoregulation in open-angle glaucoma. *Ophthalmology.* 1984;91(12):1690–1694.
146. Harris A, Harris M, Biller J, et al. Aging affects the retrobulbar circulation differently in women and men. Arch Ophthalmol. 2000;118(8):1076–1080.
147. Hayreh SS. Blood supply of the optic nerve head and its role in optic atrophy, glaucoma, and oedema of the optic disc. *Br J Ophthalmol.* 1969;53(11):721–748.

148. Hayreh SS. Pathogenesis of visual field defects. Role of the ciliary circulation. *Br J Ophthalmol.* 1970;54(5):289–311.

149. Vaegan BL. The locus of outer retinal change in glaucoma using Sutter multifocal flash and pattern ERG field tests. *Aust NZ J Ophthalmol.* 1996;24:28.

150. Quigley HA. Neuronal death in glaucoma. *Prog Retin Eye Res.* 1999; 18(1):39–57.

151. Chintala SK. The emerging role of proteases in retinal ganglion cell death. *Exp Eye Res.* 2006;82(1):5–12.

152. Dreyer EB, Zurakowski D, Schumer RA, et al. Elevated glutamate levels in the vitreous body of humans and monkeys with glaucoma. *Arch Ophthalmol.* 1996;114(3):299–305.

153. Kountouras J, Mylopoulos N, Boura P, et al. Relationship between Helicobacter pylori infection and glaucoma. *Ophthalmology.* 2001;108(3): 599–604.

154. Kurtz S, Regenbogen M, Goldiner I, et al. No association between Helicobacter pylori infection or CagA-bearing strains and glaucoma. *J Glaucoma.* 2008;17(3):223–226.

155. Berdahl JP, Allingham RR, Johnson DH. Cerebrospinal fluid pressure is decreased in primary open-angle glaucoma. *Ophthalmology.* 2008; 115(5):763–768.

156. Berdahl JP, Fautsch MP, Stinnett SS, et al. Intracranial pressure in primary open angle glaucoma, normal tension glaucoma, and ocular hypertension: a case-control study. *Invest Ophthalmol Vis Sci.* 2008;49(12):5412–5418.

157. Ren R, Jonas JB, Tian G, et al. Cerebrospinal fluid pressure in glaucoma: a prospective study. *Ophthalmology.* 2010;117(2):259–266.

158. Schulzer M. The Normal Tension Glaucoma Study Group. Intraocular pressure reduction in normal-tension glaucoma patients. *Ophthalmology.* 1992;99(9):1468–1470.

159. Bloomfield S. The results of surgery for low-tension glaucoma. *Am J Ophthalmol.* 1953;36(8):1067–1070.

160. Sugar HS. Low tension glaucoma: a practical approach. *Ann Ophthalmol.* 1979;11(8):1155–1171.

161. Abedin S, Simmons RJ, Grant WM. Progressive low-tension glaucoma: treatment to stop glaucomatous cupping and field loss when these progress despite normal intraocular pressure. *Ophthalmology.* 1982; 89(1):1–6.

162. Yamamoto T, Ichien M, Suemori-Matsushita H, et al. Trabeculectomy with mitomycin C for normal-tension glaucoma. *J Glaucoma.* 1995; 4(3):158–163.

163. Chumbley LC, Brubaker RF. Low-tension glaucoma. *Am J Ophthalmol.* 1976;81(6):761–767.

164. Koseki N, Araie M, Tomidokoro A, et al. A placebo-controlled 3-year study of a calcium blocker on visual field and ocular circulation in glaucoma with low-normal pressure. *Ophthalmology.* 2008;115(11): 2049–2057.

165. Netland PA, Chaturvedi N, Dreyer EB. Calcium channel blockers in the management of low-tension and open-angle glaucoma. *Am J Ophthalmol.* 1993;115(5):608–613.

166. Sawada A, Kitazawa Y, Yamamoto T, et al. Prevention of visual field defect progression with brovincamine in eyes with normal-tension glaucoma. *Ophthalmology.* 1996;103(2):283–288.

Pupillary Block Glaucomas

12

TERMINOLOGY

Primary versus Secondary Angle-Closure Glaucomas

Angle closure is characterized by apposition of the peripheral iris against the trabecular meshwork, resulting in obstruction of aqueous outflow (see Chapter 7). The term glaucoma is used if there is evidence of glaucomatous optic nerve damage. Traditionally, some forms of angle-closure glaucoma have been referred to as primary angle-closure glaucoma because the mechanisms of angle closure were not thought to be associated with other ocular or systemic abnormalities or because the mechanisms were not well understood. Conditions that have been included in this group are pupillary block glaucoma, plateau iris, and combined-mechanism glaucoma. Other forms of angle-closure glaucoma have been called secondary angle-closure glaucoma because of associated ocular or systemic abnormalities or because of more apparent mechanisms of angle closure, such as contracting membranes or inflammatory precipitates that pull the angle closed or space-occupying lesions that push it closed. As continued research has expanded our knowledge of the associated abnormalities and mechanisms of primary angle-closure glaucomas, the distinction between the primary and secondary forms has become increasingly artificial, and the concept should probably be abandoned.

One example of how increased knowledge has progressively blurred the distinction between primary and secondary glaucomas is seen in the condition called plateau iris (1–3). This condition has traditionally been included with the primary angle-closure glaucomas. However, because of information regarding the mechanism of plateau iris, it is now considered to belong with the glaucomas associated with disorders of the iris and ciliary body (see Chapter 17).

In this chapter, we consider several forms of glaucoma that share the common mechanism of pupillary block and that have traditionally been grouped as primary angle-closure glaucomas. The conditions that have been called secondary angle-closure glaucomas are considered in subsequent chapters in this section.

Pupillary Block Glaucoma

Pupillary block glaucoma is the most common form of angle-closure glaucoma. The initiating event is thought to result from increased resistance to flow of aqueous humor between the pupillary portion of the iris and the anterior lens surface (4), which is associated with mid-dilatation of the pupil (5). The functional block produces increased fluid pressure in the posterior chamber, causing a forward shift of the iris. Anterior movement of the peripheral iris can result in closure of the anterior chamber angle (4–6) (**Fig. 12.1**). Four forms of pupillary block glaucoma may be distinguished on the basis of symptoms and clinical findings (7): acute angle-closure glaucoma, subacute angle-closure glaucoma, chronic angle-closure glaucoma, and combined-mechanism glaucoma.

Acute Angle-Closure Glaucoma

In acute angle-closure glaucoma, the symptoms are sudden and severe, with marked pain, blurred vision, and a red eye. The patient may also have nausea and vomiting.

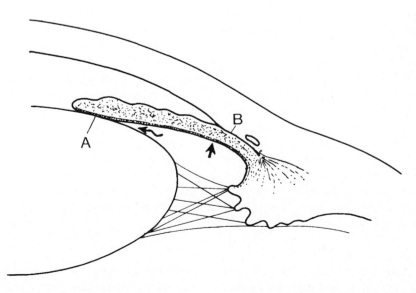

Figure 12.1 Pupillary block glaucoma. A functional block between the lens and iris (**A**) leads to increased pressure in the posterior chamber (*arrows*) with forward shift of the peripheral iris and closure of the anterior chamber angle (**B**).

Subacute Angle-Closure Glaucoma

Subacute angle-closure glaucoma is thought to have the same pupillary block mechanism as the acute form, but symptoms are mild or absent (8). The condition has also been called intermittent, prodromal, or subclinical (9). Patients with subacute angle-closure glaucoma may have repeated subacute or subclinical attacks before finally having an acute attack or developing peripheral anterior synechiae with chronic pressure elevation (8).

Chronic Angle-Closure Glaucoma

In chronic angle-closure glaucoma, portions of the anterior chamber angle are permanently closed by peripheral anterior synechiae, and the intraocular pressure (IOP) is chronically elevated (9,10). The synechial closure may result from a prolonged acute attack or repeated subacute attacks of angle-closure glaucoma. A variation of this condition has been called shortening of the angle or creeping angle-closure glaucoma (11,12). It is important to look carefully for evidence of exfoliation syndrome, because exfoliation can predispose to pupillary block in some patient populations (see Chapter 15).

Combined-Mechanism Glaucoma

In some eyes, the glaucoma appears to have open-angle and angle-closure mechanisms. The diagnosis is usually made after an acute angle-closure glaucoma attack in which the IOP remains elevated after a peripheral iridotomy, despite an open, normal-appearing angle.

EPIDEMIOLOGY

In most populations, pupillary block glaucoma is considerably less common than chronic open-angle glaucoma. However, there is a reversal in the ratio of angle-closure and open-angle glaucoma cases among Canadian, Alaskan, and Greenland Eskimos, with the former disorder occurring in approximately 0.5% of the general population and in 2% to 3% of those older than 40 years of age, with a predilection for women (13–16). A similar observation was made in population studies from China, Singapore, Mongolia, and South India and a mixed ethnic group in South Africa, in which the prevalence of angle-closure glaucoma was 2.3%, compared with 1.5% for chronic open-angle glaucoma (17–20). This prevalence of angle-closure glaucoma may be caused by a smaller corneal diameter and anterior chamber depth and a thicker, more anteriorly placed lens in affected individuals (21–23). A study among Alaskan Eskimos also showed a rapid increase in hyperopia after age 50, reaching 71.5% in persons older than 80 years (24).

Studies of the anterior chamber angle in various populations provide an impression of the prevalence of those at increased risk for pupillary block glaucoma. In two large studies, 5% to 6% of those screened had suspicious anterior chamber angles, but only 0.64% to 1.1% were considered to have critically narrow angles (25,26). In a Vietnamese population residing in the United States, 8.5% had critically narrow angles and were considered to be at high risk for occlusion (27).

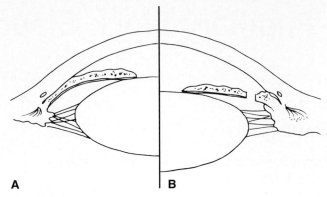

Figure 12.2   Pupillary block glaucoma (**A**) contrasted with the plateau iris syndrome (**B**). In the latter situation, notice the relatively deeper central anterior chamber, the flat iris plane, patent iridectomy, and bunching up of peripheral iris in the anterior chamber angle.

CLINICAL FEATURES

The diagnosis of pupillary block glaucoma has several facets. During the course of every ocular examination, the physician must consider general risk factors in the medical history and look for anatomic features that may predispose to angle closure. The gold standard examination is gonioscopy, which is essential in identifying eyes with some form of angle closure or those at increased risk for angle-closure glaucoma (i.e., occludable angles). In other situations, the patient may present with signs and symptoms suggesting angle-closure glaucoma, and the correct diagnosis will depend on an understanding of the symptoms, predisposing circumstances, physical findings of the disease, and the differential diagnosis (**Fig. 12.2**). The various aspects of diagnosing potential or manifest pupillary block glaucoma are considered in this chapter.

Risk Factors

General Features of Patients

Several factors influence the configuration of the anterior chamber angle and the risk for pupillary block glaucoma.

Age

The depth and volume of the anterior chamber diminish with age (28), which may result from thickening and forward displacement of the lens (29,30). Consequently, the percentage of individuals with critically narrow angles is higher in older age-groups. The prevalence of pupillary block glaucoma also increases with age, although it may peak earlier in life, compared with chronic open-angle glaucoma. One study found a bimodal pattern, with the first peak at ages 53 to 58 years and the second at 63 to 70 years (29). However, it can occur at any age, including rare cases in childhood (31).

Race

The relative prevalence of pupillary block glaucoma among all the glaucomas is increased in various populations of Inuit and individuals with Far Eastern Asian extraction (13–18). Acute angle-closure glaucoma is less common among blacks, but subacute or chronic angle-closure glaucoma is not uncommon and appears to be a regularly missed diagnosis (32–34). The explanation for this difference is uncertain. One study suggested that it might be caused by a thinner average lens thickness (33), although another investigation revealed the anterior chamber depth in Nigerian blacks to be equivalent to that of whites (35). The weaker response to mydriatics observed among African blacks could indicate that darker irides are less able to exert the force that may lead to acute pupillary block (36). Angle-closure glaucoma also has a reduced prevalence among American Indians and is often caused by a swollen lens when it does occur in this group (34).

Sex

There is a statistically significant predominance of females in populations with pupillary block glaucoma, which is probably because of the shallower anterior chamber among women in general (13,14,16,28).

Refractive Error

The depth and volume of the anterior chamber are related to the degree of ametropia, with smaller dimensions occurring in those with hyperopia (28). However, the presence of myopia does not eliminate the possibility of angle-closure glaucoma because rare cases have been reported in such patients (37), possibly indicting a spherical or anteriorly displaced lens or an increase in corneal curvature (38).

Family History

The potential for pupillary block glaucoma is generally believed to be inherited (see Chapter 8). In one study, 20% of 95 relatives of patients with angle-closure glaucoma were thought to have potentially occludable angles (39). However, aside from a few reported families in which many members developed angle-closure glaucoma, the family history is not very useful in predicting a future angle-closure attack (40).

Systemic Disorders

Researchers in one study found an inverse correlation between type 2 diabetes or an abnormal result on a glucose tolerance test and the anterior chamber depth (41). The same investigators also suggested that angle-closure glaucoma may be associated with an increased prevalence of denervation supersensitivity to autonomic agonists (42).

Findings on Routine Examination

Certain observations during the course of a routine ocular examination can help to establish the potential for angle closure.

Intraocular Pressure

Unless the patient has angle closure at the time of the examination, the IOP is usually normal. One study, however, found a larger-than-normal amplitude in the diurnal IOP curve, which the investigators thought might have prognostic value (43). Tonography also characteristically reveals normal outflow

facility before or between attacks, unless peripheral anterior synechiae are present (5).

Evaluation of Peripheral Anterior Chamber

Photogrammetric studies of all forms of angle-closure glaucoma have revealed anterior chamber depths, volumes, and diameters that are smaller than those of matched controls (44). Anterior chamber depth and volume have also been shown to have diurnal variation, with lower values in the evening (45), although a correlation between diurnal variations of chamber depth and IOP is not clear. In any case, the most important step in the diagnosis of potential or manifest angle-closure glaucoma is to evaluate the anterior chamber depth and especially the configuration of the anterior chamber angle. Although this is best accomplished by gonioscopy, there are preliminary screening measures that may be useful in some situations and techniques of quantifying the anterior chamber depth.

Penlight Examination

When a slitlamp and goniolens are not available, the anterior chamber depth can be estimated with oblique penlight illumination across the surface of the iris. With the light coming from the temporal side of the eye, a relatively flat iris is illuminated on the temporal and nasal sides of the pupil, whereas an iris that is bowed forward has a shadow on the nasal side (46) (**Fig. 12.3**).

Slitlamp Examination

The central anterior chamber depth may be estimated during examination with the slitlamp, and several techniques for quantitating this parameter have been proposed (47–49). However, the central anterior chamber depth only weakly correlates with the angle width (50), and the parameter of greater diagnostic value in the context of angle-closure glaucoma is the peripheral anterior chamber depth. van Herick and colleagues (51) developed a technique for making this estimation with the slitlamp by comparing the peripheral anterior chamber depth to the thickness of the adjacent cornea (**Figs. 12.4** and **12.5**). This is commonly referred to as the van Herick technique. When the peripheral anterior chamber depth is less than one fourth of the corneal thickness, the anterior chamber angle may be potentially occludable.

Gonioscopy

When the peripheral anterior chamber depth is thought to be shallow (i.e., less than one fourth of the corneal thickness by van Herick slitlamp examination), careful gonioscopic examination of the angle is required. This is best accomplished with a Zeiss four-mirror lens or similar goniolens. A 180-or-more–degree closure of the angle (i.e., trabecular meshwork is not visible) constitutes an occludable angle, and it is important to use compression gonioscopy to determine whether the closure is appositional or synechial. The patient should be examined in a dark room and with the use of a short, narrow slit-beam to avoid constricting the pupil and artifactually opening the angle. The examiner also should take care to avoid extra pressure on the cornea so that the angle does not deepen artifactually. If necessary, the goniomirror on the Goldmann three-mirror lens

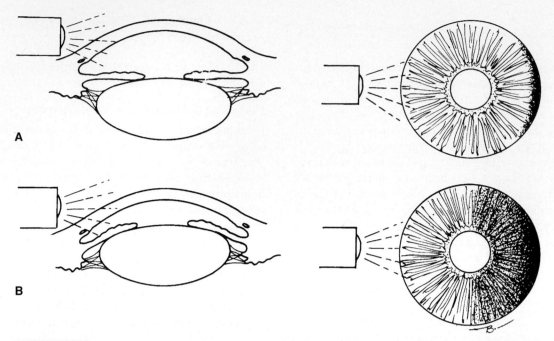

Figure 12.3 Oblique flashlight illumination as a screening measure for estimating the anterior chamber depth. **A:** With a deep chamber, nearly the entire iris is illuminated. **B:** When the iris is bowed forward, only the proximal portion is illuminated, and a shadow is seen in the distal half.

Figure 12.4 The slitlamp technique of van Herick and colleagues (51) is used for estimating the depth of the peripheral anterior chamber (PAC) by comparing it with the adjacent corneal thickness (CT). The PAC here is about 1 CT.

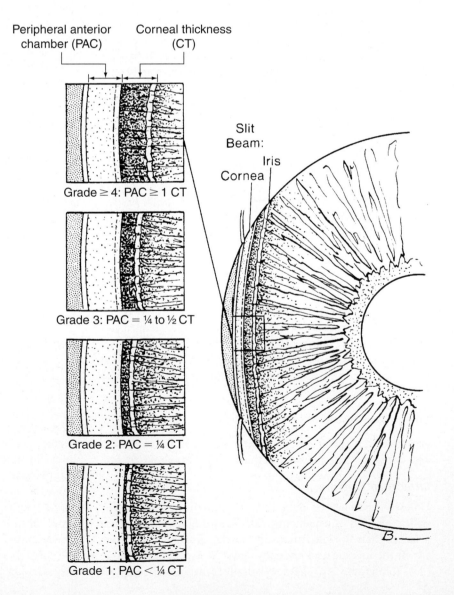

Peripheral anterior chamber (PAC)　　Corneal thickness (CT)

Grade ≥ 4: PAC ≥ 1 CT

Grade 3: PAC = ¼ to ½ CT

Grade 2: PAC = ¼ CT

Grade 1: PAC < ¼ CT

Slit Beam:
Iris
Cornea

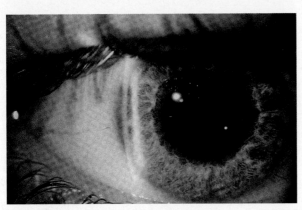

Figure 12.5 Slitlamp photograph of the van Herick technique for estimation of peripheral anterior chamber depth, showing the slit-beam on the cornea and iris.

can be used to avoid artifactual deepening of the chamber angle. If the peripheral iris is prominent, or the iris is very convex and it is difficult to see angle structures, it is often helpful to have the patient look in the direction of the mirror being viewed so that a more accurate assessment of what angle structures are visible can be made.

Numerous grading systems have been proposed to correlate gonioscopic appearance with the potential for angle closure. Scheie (52) proposed a system based on the extent of the

anterior chamber angle structures that can be visualized (**Fig. 12.6**). He observed a high risk of angle closure in eyes with grade III or IV angles. Shaffer (1) suggested using the angular width of the angle recess as the criterion for grading the angle and attempted to correlate this with the potential for angle closure (**Fig. 12.7**).

Other investigators think that any single criterion cannot fully describe the anterior chamber angle. Becker (53) proposed combining an estimation of the anterior chamber angle width and the height of the iris insertion, whereas Spaeth (26) suggested an evaluation of three variables: angular width of the angle recess, configuration of the peripheral iris, and apparent insertion of the iris root (**Fig. 12.8**). Whatever system the clinician prefers to use to document the appearance of the anterior chamber angle, it is important to pay close attention to these three aspects of the angle. One study proposed a relatively simple method for measurement of the distance from the iris insertion to the Schwalbe line using a reticule based in the slitlamp ocular during gonioscopy (54). The investigators called this technique biometric gonioscopy and found that it correlated well with other measures of anterior chamber angle, showing a higher degree of interobserver reliability than conventional gonioscopy. Additional features of the angle should also be studied and documented, such as peripheral anterior synechiae and degrees or abnormalities in pigmentation. One study found that patients with narrow angles may have a

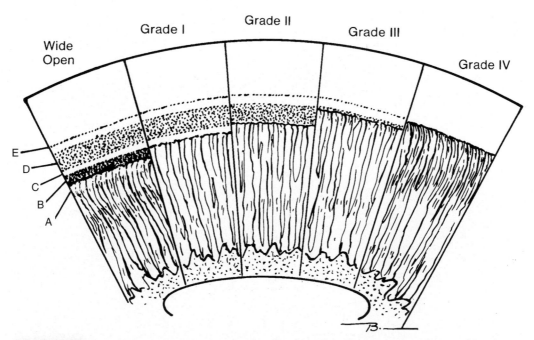

Figure 12.6 The Scheie gonioscopic classification of the anterior chamber angle, based on the extent of visible angle structures (52). **A:** Root of the iris. **B:** Ciliary body band. **C:** Scleral spur. **D:** Trabecular meshwork. **E:** Schwalbe line.

Classification	Gonioscopic Appearance
Wide open	All structures visible
Grade I narrow	Hard to see over iris root into recess
Grade II narrow	Ciliary body band obscured
Grade III narrow	Posterior trabecula obscured
Grade IV narrow (closed)	Only Schwalbe line visible

Figure 12.7 The Shaffer gonioscopic classification of the anterior chamber angle is based on the angular width of the angle recess (1). The angular width and clinical interpretation are given for each of the examples. **A:** Wide open (20 to 45 degrees): closure improbable. **B:** Moderately narrow (10 to 20 degrees): closure possible. **C:** Extremely narrow: closure possible. **D:** Partially or totally closed: closure present.

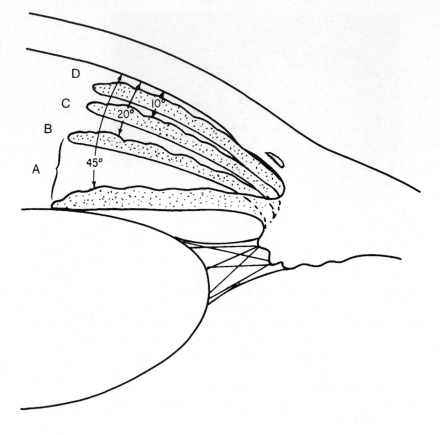

Figure 12.8 The Spaeth gonioscopic classification of the anterior chamber angle, based on three variables (26). **A:** Angular width of the angle recess. **B:** Configuration of the peripheral iris. **C:** Apparent insertion of the iris root.

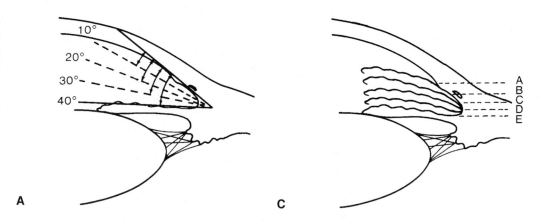

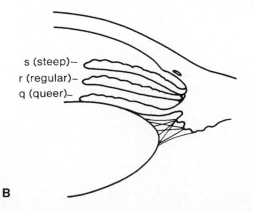

predominance of trabecular meshwork pigmentation in the superior quadrant, rather than the more common inferior location, which the investigators thought might be caused by rubbing between the peripheral iris and the meshwork (55).

Newer Techniques

Several newer forms of technology are being applied to evaluation of the anterior segment of the eye to more accurately quantify the anterior chamber depth and related dimensions. The use of high-frequency ultrasonography, referred to as ultrasound biomicroscopy, allows definition of the relationships of the iris, posterior chamber, lens, zonules, and ciliary body (see Chapter 3). This technique has potential value in understanding the mechanisms of glaucoma and in aiding the diagnosis of pupillary block glaucoma, especially when the media is not clear (56). It may also be of value in identifying eyes with potentially occludable anterior chamber angles. It has been suggested that anterior chamber depth measurement and the biometric calculation of the ratio of lens thickness to axial length can be used as a prognostic indicator of pupillary block glaucoma (57,58). Ultrasound biomicroscopy has also been used to image the dynamic changes in anterior ocular structures during provocative testing in a dark room (59,60).

Another technique that appears to be useful for assessing the relationship of the anterior chamber angle structures is optical coherence tomography (61) (see Chapter 3). Like ultrasound biomicroscopy, this technique is noninvasive and can provide a reasonable image of the anterior chamber angle. The main advantage is that it does not require the patient to have a probe with or without a gel or bath present on the eye; one drawback at present is that it does not appear to image structures posterior to the iris (e.g., ciliary body area) as well as ultrasound biomicroscopy does.

Specialized photographic techniques are also being used to better understand the anterior segment structures in angle-closure glaucomas. With one of these techniques, Scheimpflug video imaging, the iridocorneal angle can be quantitatively assessed and observed longitudinally (61).

When to Perform a Prophylactic Peripheral Iridotomy

Having decided that a patient has suspiciously narrow anterior chamber angles, the physician is faced with a difficult decision. If it could be predicted that the patient would eventually have an attack of angle-closure glaucoma, the appropriate course in most cases would be prophylactic peripheral iridotomies. The results of one study suggest that optic nerve damage occurs in the early period after IOP increases, supporting the value of detecting potentially occludable angles and performing prophylactic surgery before an attack (62).

If the angle is deemed occludable (i.e., 180 degrees or more of appositional angle closure), prophylactic peripheral iridotomy is warranted (see Chapter 35). The fellow eye should also be examined, and if deemed occludable, our recommendation is to proceed with iridotomy on both eyes at the same sitting.

Provocative Tests

Historically, some surgeons used tests to provoke pupillary block glaucoma when attempting to identify patients for whom treatment should be recommended. These tests included the prone test, the darkroom test, the prone darkroom test, and pharmacologic dilation of the pupil. The fourth edition of this textbook provides additional details on these tests.

Most ophthalmologists question the clinical value of any provocative test for angle-closure glaucoma because the false-positive and false-negative rates of such tests are high. In one study of 129 persons with suspected angle-closure glaucoma who underwent gonioscopy, refraction, anterior chamber pachymetry, ultrasound biomicroscopy, and an angle-closure provocative test, it was concluded that none of the test factors studied showed a high sensitivity or positive predictive accuracy in detecting eyes that later developed angle closure (63). Careful gonioscopic examination put into the context of available historical and clinical information has largely replaced the use of provocative tests to make management decisions about the development of angle-closure glaucoma (64).

Precipitating Factors

In an eye that is anatomically predisposed to develop angle closure, several factors may precipitate an attack.

Factors That Produce Mydriasis
Dim Illumination

A common history for the development of pupillary block glaucoma is the onset of an acute attack when the patient is in a dark room, such as a theater or restaurant. The incidence of angle closure is reported to increase in winter and autumn (65,66). In one study, however, there was a direct association with hours of sunshine and an inverse association with degree of cloudiness, which the investigators thought might be related to the contrast between day and evening levels of illumination (65).

Emotional Stress

Occasionally, an acute angle-closure attack follows severe emotional stress. This may be related to the mydriasis of increased sympathetic tone, although the exact mechanism is not understood.

Drugs

Use of mydriatic agents may precipitate an angle-closure attack in an anatomically predisposed eye. Use of anticholinergics (e.g., atropine, cyclopentolate, tropicamide) increases the risk for angle closure when administered topically (67). In one study, use of cyclopentolate, 0.5%, precipitated attacks in 9 (43%) of 21 high-risk eyes, and use of tropicamide, 0.5%, did the same in 19 (33%) of 58 eyes (68). However, in a population-based screening study of 4870 participants whose eyes were dilated with tropicamide, 1%, and phenylephrine, 2.5%, after penlight examination of the anterior chamber depth, none had an acute angle-closure attack (69). In another population-based study of 6760 persons, tropicamide, 0.5%, and phenylephrine, 5%, were used for diagnostic mydriasis (70). No persons were excluded on the basis of narrow angles, and only two participants (0.03%) experienced an attack of acute angle-closure glaucoma. Systemic atropine and other mydriatics can also create a hazard, especially when large doses are used in conjunction with spinal or general anesthesia during surgery (71). It has been suggested that high-risk eyes should be protected with topical pilocarpine before, during, and after surgery (72). However, miosis can also precipitate angle-closure attacks, and an alternative approach to managing the high-risk eye is close observation during the postoperative period or prophylactic peripheral iridotomy, depending on the degree of risk.

Other systemic drugs with weaker anticholinergic properties (e.g., antihistaminic, antiparkinsonian, antipsychotic, and gastrointestinal spasmolytic drugs) also present a risk proportional to their pupillary effect (68,73,74). The tricyclic antidepressants have the greatest anticholinergic properties of the various psychoactive drugs, and use of imipramine was believed to trigger pupillary block glaucoma in four reported cases (74). Botulinum toxin, used in the treatment of strabismus and blepharospasm, inhibits acetylcholine release with subsequent mydriasis, and it has been reported to cause acute angle-closure glaucoma (75).

Adrenergic agents (e.g., topical epinephrine) may precipitate an angle-closure attack in the predisposed eye. Phenylephrine can also precipitate an attack, although it was found to be safer than cyclopentolate or tropicamide for dilating high-risk eyes (71). Systemic drugs with adrenergic properties (e.g., vasoconstrictors, central nervous system stimulants, appetite depressants, bronchodilators, and hallucinogenic agents) may present a risk in the predisposed eye (67).

Factors That Produce Miosis

Miotic therapy may occasionally lead to an acute attack of pupillary block glaucoma. This has also been observed after the miosis induced by reading or bright lights. Possible mechanisms include an increase in the relative pupillary block due to a wider zone of contact between iris and lens and relaxation of the lens zonules, allowing a forward shift of the iris–lens diaphragm. With strong miotics, such as the cholinesterase inhibitors (e.g., di-isopropyl fluorophosphate, echothiophate iodide), the mechanism of angle closure may be the miosis or congestion of the uveal tract. Chandler (5) favored the former theory, because he observed that an acute increase in IOP after the use of a miotic did not occur in an eye with a peripheral iridectomy.

Symptoms of Angle-Closure Attack

Angle-closure glaucoma, in marked contrast to chronic open-angle glaucoma, is characterized by profound symptoms, although the severity of these symptoms varies considerably in different forms of the disorder.

Acute Angle-Closure Glaucoma

Acute angle-closure glaucoma is characterized by pain, redness, and blurred vision. The pain is typically a severe, deep ache that follows the trigeminal distribution and may be associated with nausea, vomiting, bradycardia, and profuse sweating. The marked conjunctival hyperemia usually consists of a ciliary flush and peripheral conjunctival congestion. The blurred vision, which is typically marked, may be caused by stretching of the corneal lamellae initially and later edema of the cornea, as well as a direct effect of the IOP on the optic nerve head. Rarely, the corneal decompensation may persist, requiring penetrating keratoplasty (76).

Subacute Angle-Closure Glaucoma

Subacute angle-closure glaucoma, a form of pupillary block glaucoma, may have no recognizable symptoms. In other cases, the patient may notice a dull ache behind the eye or slight blurring of vision. A symptom that is especially typical of the subacute attack is colored halos around lights. This is thought to result from corneal epithelial edema, which causes it to act as a diffraction grating, producing a blue–green central and yellow–red peripheral halo. These symptoms, which more often occur at night after the patient has been in a dark room, often spontaneously clear by the next morning, presumably because of the miosis of sleep.

Chronic Angle-Closure Glaucoma

Another form of pupillary block glaucoma, chronic angle-closure glaucoma, is typically asymptomatic until advanced visual field loss develops, although the patient may give a history suggestive of one or more episodes of subacute or acute angle-closure glaucoma.

Clinical Findings during an Acute Attack

The patient who presents during an acute angle-closure attack will typically have marked IOP elevation in the range of 40 mm Hg to greater than 60 mm Hg, with a profound reduction in central visual acuity. In the emergency room, digital palpation of the affected eye through a closed eyelid can be a helpful screening test, especially if a tonometer is not easily available. Digital palpation can reveal a very firm (i.e., rock-hard consistency) eye compared with the fellow eye, which feels much softer. The following additional findings help to confirm the diagnosis.

External Examination

Characteristic findings include conjunctival hyperemia, a cloudy cornea, and an irregular (usually vertically oval), mid-dilated, fixed pupil (**Fig. 12.9**). The pupillary change is thought to result from paralysis of the sphincter, which apparently is caused by a reduction in circulation induced by the elevated IOP and possibly by degeneration of the ciliary ganglion (77–80).

Slitlamp Examination

This step of the evaluation confirms the presence of the corneal edema, which frequently must be cleared by topical application of glycerin before the anterior chamber can be studied. The corneal edema usually clears after the pressure is normalized, although this is not always the case (76). Specular microscopic examination has revealed significant corneal endothelial cell

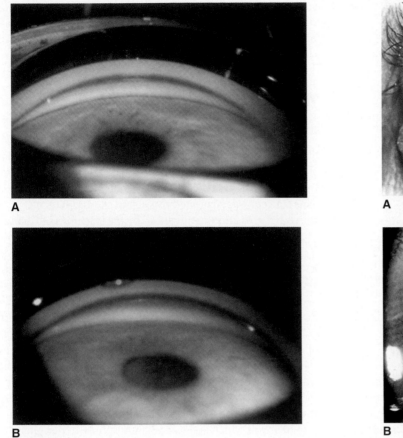

Figure 12.9 In these eyes with narrow angles, the iris is bowed forward in the periphery, as is typical of eyes with pupillary block. In (**A**), the anterior portion of the trabecular meshwork (*dark band*) is visible. In (**B**), the angle is even narrower, and only the Schwalbe line is visible, except for a possible thin rim of trabecular meshwork to the left of the view.

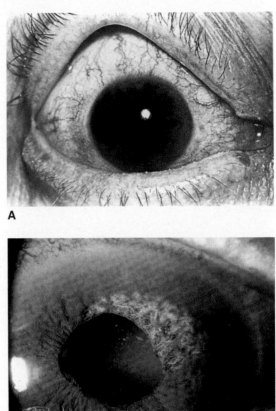

Figure 12.10 **A:** External appearance of eye during attack of acute angle-closure glaucoma, showing diffuse conjunctival hyperemia, cloudy cornea, and irregular, mid-dilated pupil. (Courtesy of H. Saul Sugar, MD.) **B:** Slitlamp photograph of eye after acute angle-closure glaucoma attack, showing glaukomflecken of the anterior lens capsule and sector iris atrophy.

loss in these cases, which correlates with the duration of IOP elevation (81), the degree of visual field loss, a large cup-to-disc ratio, and previous intraocular surgery (82).

The anterior chamber is shallow, but it typically is formed centrally with anterior bowing of the midperipheral iris, often making contact with peripheral cornea. Aqueous flare is often present. Other findings may include pigment dispersion, sector atrophy of the iris, posterior synechiae, and glaukomflecken, which are irregular white opacities in the anterior portion of the lens that correlate to areas of lens epithelial ischemia or necrosis (**Fig. 12.10**).

Gonioscopy

It is essential to confirm the diagnosis of angle-closure glaucoma by demonstrating a closed anterior chamber angle. If gonioscopy is not possible because of persistent corneal edema, gonioscopy of the fellow eye may provide useful information if it reveals an extremely narrow angle. In a study of 10 eyes with angle-closure glaucoma, the Koeppe lens was found to be more reliable than the Goldmann three-mirror or Zeiss four-mirror lenses in determining whether the angle was open or closed, because it caused no artifactual widening of the angle

and allowed the best view over a convex iris (83). From a practical perspective, the Goldmann three-mirror lens is more easily available than a Koeppe lens and provides a higher magnification view of the angle.

Peripheral anterior synechiae may also be present, and documenting the presence and extent of the synechiae is important in establishing the nature of the angle-closure glaucoma and in selecting the appropriate treatment (discussed later). Forbes (84,85) described compressive gonioscopy in which the degree of synechial closure is determined by indenting the central cornea with a Sussman or Zeiss goniolens. This forces aqueous into the peripheral portion of the anterior chamber, which deepens it and facilitates visualization of the angle (**Fig. 12.11**).

Fundus Examination

The optic nerve head may be hyperemic and edematous in the early stages of the attack. Monkeys exposed to high IOPs usually developed congestion of the optic nerve head within 12 to 15 hours, which persisted for 4 to 5 days (86). The disc then became pale, and glaucomatous cupping was observed after 9 to 10 days. In a study of human eyes with a history of angle-closure glaucoma, pallor without cupping was seen in eyes after acute

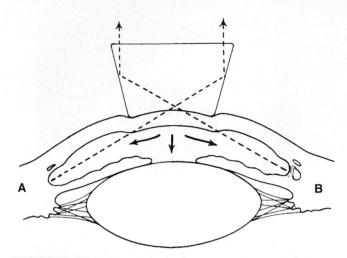

Figure 12.11 Compressive gonioscopy with a Zeiss four-mirror gonioprism deepens the peripheral anterior chamber by displacing aqueous from the central portion of the chamber (*arrows*). This facilitates gonioscopic examination of the anterior chamber angle before surgery by helping to distinguish between appositional (**A**) and synechial (**B**) closure of the angle (84,85).

attacks, but pallor and cupping occurred in chronic cases (87). Central retinal vein occlusion may also occur during acute angle-closure glaucoma (88). Conversely, central retinal vein occlusion may induce a secondary form of angle-closure glaucoma (see Chapter 19). There is also a case report of nonarteritic anterior ischemic optic neuropathy developing bilaterally about 2.5 weeks after the patient had an attack of angle closure in each eye (89).

Visual Fields

Visual field changes associated with an acute elevation of IOP most often show nonspecific constriction. In one study of 25 patients with acute angle-closure glaucoma that had been

surgically corrected, the most common field defect was constriction of the upper field (90), whereas another study revealed nerve fiber bundle defects in 7 of 18 acute cases and 9 of 11 chronic cases (87).

THEORIES OF MECHANISM

Relative Pupillary Block

The most common mechanism leading to angle-closure glaucoma appears to be increased resistance to aqueous flow from the posterior to the anterior chamber between the iris and lens. This concept was suggested by Curran (4) and Banziger (6) in the early 1920s and was advanced by the teachings of Chandler (5), who observed that an eye with a shallow anterior chamber has a wider zone of contact between the surfaces of the iris and lens. He postulated that the musculature of the iris exerts a backward pressure against the lens that increases the resistance to flow of aqueous into the anterior chamber. This increases the pressure in the posterior chamber, causing the thin peripheral iris to bulge into the anterior chamber angle. On the basis of gonioscopic studies, the angle closure may occur in two stages: iridocorneal contact anterior to the trabecular meshwork, followed by apposition of the iris to the meshwork as the pressure rises (91,92). Considerable clinical evidence strongly favors the basic concept of pupillary block, the most convincing of which is the excellent response to peripheral iridotomy, which presumably works by circumventing the block (5) (**Fig. 12.12**).

Anatomic Factors Predisposing to Pupillary Block

Several anatomic aspects of the eye combine to produce a shallow anterior chamber. These include a thicker, more anteriorly placed lens, a smaller diameter and shorter posterior

Figure 12.12 The strongest evidence in support of the pupillary block mechanism of angle-closure glaucoma is the excellent response to peripheral iridotomy, which circumvents the block (*arrow*).

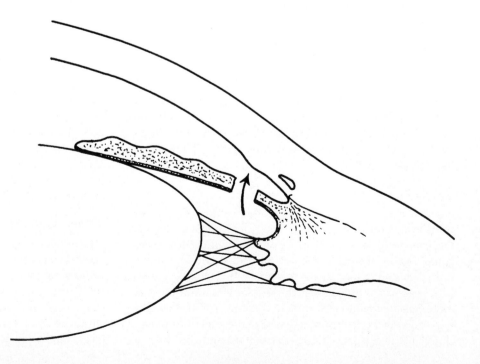

curvature of the cornea, and a shorter axial length of the globe (93–99). A study of patients of Asian or African ethnic background with chronic angle-closure glaucoma revealed an abnormal anterior lens position without an increase in lens thickness, suggesting an ethnic influence on these biometric parameters (100). The ratio of the lens thickness to the axial length appears to correlate best with the predisposition to angle closure (58). It has also been shown that the anterior chamber depth is not a static dimension; it can undergo rapid, transient change (101). Alsbirk (22) suggested that a shallow anterior chamber confers a survival advantage for populations living in extremely cold climates (e.g., Northern China, Mongolia, and Alaska). He suggested that the rich vascular plexus of the iris near the cornea might help to raise the temperature of the ocular surface and prevent the cornea from freezing. The narrow palpebral fissure typical of East Asians may offer a similar advantage.

Relatives of patients with pupillary block glaucoma have a more anterior insertion of the iris into the ciliary body, a narrower angular approach to the recess of the anterior chamber angle, and a more anterior peripheral convexity of the iris, compared with average eyes of persons in the general population (26). All of these parameters are variably influenced by hyperopia, increasing age, and genetics.

Another factor predisposing to a pupillary block mechanism may be a forward displacement to the lens due to loose zonules, which is worsened by miotic therapy and relieved with cycloplegia (David G. Campbell, MD, personal communication).

Significance of Pupillary Dilatation

Chandler (5) emphasized that a mid-dilated pupil of 3.5 to 6 mm is the critical degree of dilatation that seems to bring on the acute attack. He thought this might be caused by continued pupillary block combined with sufficient relaxation of peripheral iris to allow its forward displacement into the anterior chamber. Mapstone (102) proposed a mathematical model to explain the influence of a mid-dilated pupil, in which the combined pupil-blocking forces of the dilator and sphincter muscles and the stretching force of the iris were greatest with the iris in the mid-dilated position. Tiedeman (103), using basic physical principles, found that the Mapstone model involved incorrect use of the physical concepts of force and tension. He developed a model that can predict the profile of the iris by using the radii of the pupil and iris root and the anterior displacement of the pupil from the iris root. If the latter measurement were constant, the angle between the peripheral iris and trabecular meshwork would progressively narrow as the pupillary radius increased. However, because of the contour of the lens, the anterior displacement of the pupil decreases as the pupil dilates, resulting in the narrowest angle when the pupil is mid-dilated (103). Biometric photographs of eyes with narrow anterior chamber angles supported the validity of the Tiedeman model (104), whereas ultrasound biomicroscopic quantitative analysis of light–dark changes in eyes with pupillary block lends some support to the Mapstone model (105).

Chronic Angle-Closure Glaucoma

Peripheral anterior synechiae may eventually develop with prolonged or recurrent acute or subacute attacks, leading to chronic angle-closure glaucoma. The peripheral anterior synechiae in patients after acute angle-closure attacks tend to be broad based, are most commonly seen in the superior quadrant, and correlate with the duration of the acute attacks (106). A more insidious form has been recognized in which the angle slowly closes from the periphery toward the Schwalbe line (9–12). The synechial closure usually begins superiorly, where the angle is normally narrowest, and progresses inferiorly (10). This condition has been referred to as shortening of the angle or creeping angle closure (11,12). These cases are frequently cured by peripheral iridotomy in white patients if detected early enough, but may require additional medical therapy or filtering surgery (0% to 8%) (107,108). In Asian patients, however, filtering surgery may be required in 29% to 63% of eyes (109,110). Most eyes developing elevated IOP did so in the first 6 months in a study of Asian eyes, indicating the importance of close follow-up for this group (109,111).

One study evaluated the retrobulbar hemodynamics of patients with well-controlled chronic angle-closure glaucoma using color Doppler imaging. Patients were found to have decreased retrobulbar blood-flow velocities and increased vascular resistance in the central retinal artery and temporal short posterior ciliary artery, compared with age- and sex-matched healthy controls (112). The degree of hemodynamic impairment correlated well with the degree of glaucomatous visual field loss.

Plateau Iris

Plateau iris has traditionally been included among the primary angle-closure glaucomas largely because of an incomplete understanding of the mechanism of angle closure (1–3). Later evidence suggests that an anterior position of the ciliary body may cause the angle closure (113–115). (This condition is considered in more detail in Chapter 17.)

DIFFERENTIAL DIAGNOSIS

The sudden onset of pain, redness, and blurred vision, which characterizes the acute angle-closure attack, may also be seen with other forms of glaucoma, creating a differential diagnostic problem.

Open-Angle Glaucomas

Open-angle forms of glaucoma may occasionally manifest as an acute attack, especially when associated with events such as inflammation or hemorrhage. These cases are usually readily distinguished from acute forms of angle-closure glaucoma on the basis of the gonioscopic examination results and associated findings. However, in the eye with an elevated IOP and a narrow anterior chamber angle, it may be difficult to distinguish between pupillary block glaucoma and open-angle glaucoma with narrow angles. A thymoxamine test has been suggested for this situation (116). Unlike cholinergic miotics, which can lower IOP by opening a closed angle or by reducing resistance to trabecular outflow, thymoxamine, an α-adrenergic blocker, produces miosis by relaxation of the dilator muscle without effecting outflow through cyclotropia. As a result, topical thymoxamine, 0.5%, can often open a narrow or appositionally closed angle and lower the IOP in angle-closure glaucoma, but it cannot alter the pressure in an eye with open-angle glaucoma. Another approach to distinguishing between closed- and open-angle glaucoma is to perform a laser iridotomy, which relieves the pressure elevation in a pure angle-closure case, but additional measures will be required if an open-angle component is present.

Angle-Closure Glaucomas with Associated Abnormalities

There are many forms of angle-closure glaucoma with associated abnormalities, which may present even more difficult diagnostic problems, especially when the initiating event is posterior to the lens–iris diaphragm, where early detection can be difficult. The following are some of the ocular disorders that may lead to these forms of angle closure (details of these conditions are considered in subsequent chapters): plateau iris (see Chapter 17), central retinal vein occlusion (Chapter 19), ciliary body swelling, inflammation, or cysts (Chapter 17), ciliary block (malignant) glaucoma (Chapter 26), posterior segment tumors (Chapter 21), contracting retrolental tissue (Chapter 18), scleral buckling procedures and panretinal photocoagulation (Chapter 26), nanophthalmos (Chapter 14), corneal thickening and exfoliation syndrome (Chapter 15.)

MANAGEMENT

The details regarding drugs and surgical procedures used in the treatment of pupillary block glaucoma are considered in Section III of this textbook. The present discussion is limited to the general approach and basic concepts of management.

Medical Therapy

Although most eyes with acute, subacute, or chronic pupillary block glaucoma are managed surgically, it is desirable to first bring the glaucoma under medical control. An acute attack constitutes a medical emergency, and it should be approached in two stages: reduction of the IOP and relief of the angle closure.

Reduction of Intraocular Pressure

Miotic therapy is frequently ineffective when the IOP is high, presumably because of pressure-induced ischemia of the iris, which leads to paralysis of the sphincter muscle (77–79). For this reason, the first line of defense is to administer drugs that will promptly lower the IOP. In many cases, oral or intravenous carbonic anhydrase inhibitors, topical β-adrenergic blockers,

α$_2$-adrenergic agonists, and prostaglandin analogues can lower the pressure sufficiently to allow effective miotic therapy to open the angle (117–119). In especially difficult cases, hyperosmotic agents may be used to help in the initial pressure reduction. They may be given orally as glycerol or isosorbide, if available, or if the patient is too nauseated to tolerate oral medication, intravenous mannitol or urea may be given. Topical carbonic anhydrase inhibitors should probably be avoided because they can exacerbate or potentiate corneal edema, which may make laser treatment more challenging.

Relief of Angle-Closure Glaucoma

After the IOP has been reduced, a miotic is instilled to break the pupillary block and open the anterior chamber angle. A single drop of pilocarpine approximately 1 to 3 hours after administration of acetazolamide or timolol has been reported to effectively break the angle-closure attack (117,119). This is also safer than copious use of pilocarpine, because it reduces the chances of drug toxicity. The concentration of pilocarpine does not appear to be important in this situation, and a low dosage of a 1% to 2% solution is preferable. α-Adrenergic antagonists, such as thymoxamine, have theoretical advantages over pilocarpine, because the mechanism of miosis is relaxation of the dilator muscle, which may allow effective pupillary constriction even when the IOP is elevated (120,121). However, other investigators have not found thymoxamine alone to be effective in the treatment of angle-closure glaucoma (122).

Surgical Management

After the IOP has been brought under control medically or all efforts at medical control have been exhausted, the surgeon is faced with two decisions: when to operate and what procedure to use. These considerations have been influenced greatly by the replacement, in most cases, of incisional iridectomy with laser iridotomy.

When to Operate

In the days of incisional iridectomy when the elevated pressure could not be controlled medically, Chandler and Grant (123) advised considering surgery within the next few hours, especially if the vision was failing. However, the risks of incisional surgery are considerably higher under these circumstances, and mechanical techniques to lower the IOP before surgery may prove helpful. For example, indentation of the central cornea for several 30-second intervals, by using a blunt instrument such as a cotton-tipped applicator, may lower the pressure and occasionally break the attack by forcing aqueous from the central to the peripheral anterior chamber (**Fig. 12.13**) (124). Even with a laser iridotomy, it may be helpful to lower the IOP first to allow clearing of corneal edema. In any case, the safest approach to medically unresponsive cases is to proceed with the iridotomy. When an iridotomy cannot be achieved because of corneal edema, laser pupilloplasty or peripheral iridoplasty may break the attack (125,126). An alternative strategy is to use topical glycerin drops, to osmotically clear the cornea. This can work well but can be painful when applied to the ocular

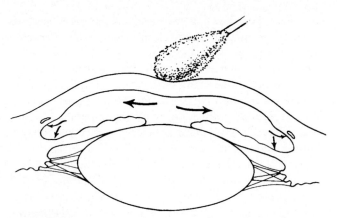

Figure 12.13 Corneal indentation with a soft instrument, such as a cotton-tipped applicator, may lower the IOP during an acute angle-closure attack by forcing aqueous from the central to the peripheral anterior chamber (*arrows*), thereby temporarily opening the chamber angle and reestablishing aqueous outflow (124).

surface; thus, before its instillation, a topical anesthetic should be applied. Yet another effective strategy to clear the cornea is to perform an anterior chamber paracentesis. This can be done by using a short 27-G or 30-G needle, with the bevel pointing anteriorly. The surgeon should enter the eye anterior to the limbus so that the needle tip will be between the iris and corneal endothelium, avoiding inadvertent damage to the iris or lens (127). A paracentesis typically results in rapid clearing of the cornea, and after the attack is broken laser iridotomy should be performed.

If the IOP does respond to medical therapy, the eye should be re-examined gonioscopically to determine the mechanism of the pressure reduction. An open anterior chamber angle without compressive gonioscopy suggests that the angle-closure attack has been broken. In this situation, there is less urgency about when surgical intervention should be performed. In the days of incisional surgical iridectomy, some surgeons preferred to wait 1 or 2 days for the inflammation to subside. With laser iridotomy, however, there is no advantage in waiting unless marked iritis or corneal edema is present. In one long-term study of 116 cases, a delay in treatment detrimentally affected the final outcome (128). If the gonioscopic examination reveals that the angle is still closed despite medical lowering of the IOP, the pressure reduction may be caused by the drug-induced reduction of aqueous production or vitreous volume, and the angle-closure might not have been relieved. Because the high pressure may recur as the effects of these medications begin to wear off, there is even more urgency in proceeding promptly with the laser iridotomy and, if necessary, incisional surgery (as detailed in the next section).

What Operation to Use

The eye with pupillary block glaucoma typically responds well to a peripheral iridotomy, and the initial procedure of choice in nearly every case is a laser iridotomy. One study compared 50 eyes treated with incisional iridectomy or laser iridotomy to 64 treated medically and found that the former group had a

greater number of improved anterior chamber configurations, a lower incidence of peripheral anterior synechiae, and a greater reduction in the need for glaucoma medications (129). Studies of anterior ocular segment configuration before and after iridotomy, using the Scheimpflug imaging technique, revealed a significant widening of the anterior chamber angle and a straightening of the iris contour, but found no significant change in the position of the anterior lens surface (130,131).

Follow-up studies indicate that many eyes treated with an iridotomy alone will eventually require medication to control chronic pressure elevation, and some will need filtering surgery (132–137). Factors associated with the need for additional treatment include the duration of the angle-closure attack and a history of intermittent, spontaneously resolved angle-closure episodes (132,137). These factors relate to the amount of permanent damage to the anterior chamber angle, which sometimes correlates with the extent of gonioscopically visible peripheral anterior synechiae.

Even if compressive gonioscopy reveals partial synechial closure of the anterior chamber angle, it is best to proceed first with the laser iridotomy, because this has been shown to control the pressure in many cases of chronic angle-closure glaucoma (107). If the iridotomy does not restore a normal IOP, the eye is then treated with medication or filtering surgery if required. Caution must be taken when performing filtering surgery (and an incisional surgical iridectomy) on eyes with angle-closure glaucoma because of the increased risk of malignant (ciliary block) glaucoma (138) (see Chapter 26). Care must also be taken with the prolonged use of topical corticosteroids after laser or incisional surgery in these patients, because a high percentage will have steroid-induced IOP elevation after an attack of angle-closure glaucoma (139,140).

Prophylactic peripheral iridotomy for the fellow eye is generally recommended at the same sitting or within a few days of an attack of pupillary block glaucoma. Several large studies have shown that approximately 50% to 75% of the patients who develop angle closure in one eye will have an attack in the fellow, unoperated eye within 5 to 10 years despite miotic prophylaxis (141,142), whereas such an attack is rare after an iridectomy. Because the attack in the fellow eye usually occurs in the first year after the initial event (143), the prophylactic procedure should be done promptly. Rare exceptions include a deeper anterior chamber in the fellow eye due to anisometropia, pseudophakia, aphakia, and a dislocated lens. Some surgeons have suggested that fellow eyes with negative provocative test results might be followed closely without surgery. However, with the relative safety of laser iridotomy, a prophylactic procedure in all high-risk fellow eyes appears to be prudent.

Lensectomy and implantation of a posterior chamber intraocular lens for patients with acute and chronic angle closure may offer successful IOP control and improve vision. One randomized trial compared early phacoemulsification cataract surgery with laser peripheral iridotomy in 62 Chinese patients with acute angle closure in whom the attack had been aborted with medical treatment (144). Early phacoemulsification was more effective than peripheral iridotomy in preventing IOP rise. After 18 months, mean IOP in the cataract surgery group was significantly lower (12.6 ± 1.9 mm Hg) than in the irido-tomy group (15.0 ± 3.4 mm Hg); the former group also required significantly fewer medications than the latter to maintain an IOP no higher than 21 mm Hg (0.03 ± 0.18 vs. 0.90 ± 1.14). High presenting IOP of greater than 55 mm Hg was an added risk factor for subsequent IOP rise. No eyes had significant (vision-threatening) complications. In another, nonrandomized trial comparing phacoemulsification cataract surgery with iridotomy in patients with acute or chronic angle-closure glaucoma, the cataract surgery group had significantly greater IOP lowering, compared with the laser iridotomy group, at 6 months postoperatively (145). Endothelial cell counts did not differ postoperatively between the groups.

Lensectomy, implantation of a posterior chamber intraocular lens, and trabeculectomy with use of an antimetabolite can also be helpful options in the management of patients with chronic angle-closure glaucoma and cataract. Two randomized trials found that phacotrabeculectomy with the use of mitomycin C provided superior IOP control compared with phacoemulsification alone, regardless of whether the IOP was medically controlled before surgery (146,147). However, in both trials, the phacotrabeculectomy group experienced more postoperative complications.

Lensectomy with lysis of peripheral anterior synechiae is yet another beneficial option in patients with chronic angle-closure glaucoma, provided that the procedure is performed within 6 to 12 months of an acute attack (148).

Cataract extraction appears to be helpful in each of the aforementioned scenarios by removing pupillary block and deepening the anterior segment, thus improving access to the peripheral angle. When after an acute attack lensectomy is most appropriate and whether the procedure should be combined with filtration surgery are currently unclear, however. An approach favored by many surgeons is to proceed with cataract surgery, with or without goniosynechialysis, in patients with a visually significant cataract or uncontrolled IOP. Phacotrabeculectomy with mitomycin C can be used when a patient has probably had peripheral anterior synechial closure for more than 1 year, or in the presence of moderate-to-advanced optic nerve damage. Further studies should help clarify how and when to use these approaches in the management of this challenging patient population.

KEY POINTS

- Angle-closure glaucoma is more common than chronic open-angle glaucoma in some Inuit and Asian populations.
- A predisposing factor to angle closure is a narrow anterior chamber angle, which has a familial tendency and is associated with increasing age and hyperopia.
- An angle-closure attack may be precipitated in a predisposed individual by factors that induce mydriasis, such as dim illumination, emotional stress, and drugs.
- The basic mechanism of pupillary block glaucoma is a functional block between the lens and iris, which obstructs aqueous flow from the posterior to the anterior chamber, resulting

in increased pressure in the posterior chamber, forward bowing of the peripheral iris, and closure of the anterior chamber angle.

- The clinical presentation of angle-closure glaucoma may be that of an acute attack with severe pain, marked conjunctival hyperemia, a cloudy cornea, and profound visual loss, or as a subacute attack with a dull ache, slight blurring of vision, and colored halos around lights. Still other cases may be chronic and typically asymptomatic.
- Patients at risk for angle-closure glaucoma should avoid taking over-the-counter decongestants, antihistamines, or other medications with warnings against use in glaucoma.
- Treatment usually begins with aggressive medical therapy to lower the IOP and relieve the angle closure, followed by a peripheral iridotomy to prevent future attacks. Argon laser iridoplasty or anterior chamber paracentesis can also help resolve an acute attack. The ideal role and optimal timing of cataract surgery in patients with angle-closure glaucoma remain to be determined.
- If IOP is still elevated after laser iridotomy, additional mechanisms should be considered, such as peripheral anterior synechiae formation, a combined mechanism (i.e., underlying open-angle or exfoliation glaucoma), or plateau iris.
- Lens extraction with IOL placement alone or in combination with surgical goniosynechialysis or trabeculectomy can be an effective treatment for chronic angle-closure glaucoma.

REFERENCES

1. Shaffer RN. Primary glaucomas. Gonioscopy, ophthalmoscopy and perimetry. *Trans Am Acad Ophthalmol Otolaryngol.* 1960;64:112–127.
2. Tornquist R. Angle-closure glaucoma in an eye with a plateau type of iris. *Acta Ophthalmol.* 1958;36(3):419–423.
3. Wand M, Grant WM, Simmons RJ, et al. Plateau iris syndrome. *Trans Sect Ophthalmol Am Acad Ophthalmol Otolaryngol.* 1977;83(1):122–130.
4. Curran EJ. A new operation for glaucoma involving a new principle in the aetiology and treatment of chronic primary glaucoma. *Arch Ophthalmol.* 1920;49:131–155.
5. Chandler PA. Narrow-angle glaucoma. *Arch Ophthalmol.* 1952;47(6):695–716.
6. Banziger T. The mechanism of acute glaucoma and the explanation for the effectiveness of iridectomy for the same [in German]. *Ber Dtsch Ophthalmol Ges.* 1922;43:43–48.
7. Barkan O. Glaucoma: classification, causes, and surgical control—results of microgonioscopic research. *Am J Ophthalmol.* 1938;21:1099–1117.
8. Chandler PA, Trotter RR. Angle-closure glaucoma: subacute types. *Arch Ophthalmol.* 1955;53(3):305–317.
9. Pollack IP. Chronic angle-closure glaucoma; diagnosis and treatment in patients with angles that appear open. *Arch Ophthalmol.* 1971;85(6):676–689.
10. Bhargava SK, Leighton DA, Phillips CI. Early angle-closure glaucoma. Distribution of iridotrabecular contact and response to pilocarpine. *Arch Ophthalmol.* 1973;89(5):369–372.
11. Gorin G. Shortening of the angle of the anterior chamber in angle-closure glaucoma. *Am J Ophthalmol.* 1960;49:141–146.
12. Lowe RF. Primary creeping angle-closure glaucoma. *Br J Ophthalmol.* 1964;48:544–550.
13. Drance SM. Angle closure glaucoma among Canadian Eskimos. *Can J Ophthalmol.* 1973;8(2):252–254.
14. Arkell SM, Lightman DA, Sommer A, et al. The prevalence of glaucoma among Eskimos of northwest Alaska. *Arch Ophthalmol.* 1987;105(4):482–485.
15. Alsbirk PH. Early detection of primary angle-closure glaucoma. Limbal and axial chamber depth screening in a high risk population (Greenland Eskimos). *Acta Ophthalmol.* 1988;66(5):556–564.

16. Clemmesen V, Alsbirk PH. Primary angle-closure glaucoma (a.c.g.) in Greenland. *Acta Ophthalmol.* 1971;49(1):47–58.
17. Aung T, Chew PT. Review of recent advancements in the understanding of primary angle-closure glaucoma. *Curr Opin Ophthalmol.* 2002;13(2):89–93.
18. Congdon N, Wang F, Tielsch JM. Issues in the epidemiology and population-based screening of primary angle-closure glaucoma. *Surv Ophthalmol.* 1992;36(6):411–423.
19. Dandona L, Dandona R, Mandal P, et al. Angle-closure glaucoma in an urban population in southern India. The Andhra Pradesh eye disease study. *Ophthalmology.* 2000;107(9):1710–1716.
20. Salmon JF, Mermoud A, Ivey A, et al. The prevalence of primary angle closure glaucoma and open angle glaucoma in Mamre, Western Cape, South Africa. *Arch Ophthalmol.* 1993;111(9):1263–1269.
21. Alsbirk PH. Corneal diameter in Greenland Eskimos. Anthropometric and genetic studies with special reference to primary angle-closure glaucoma. *Acta Ophthalmol.* 1975;53(4):635–646.
22. Alsbirk PH. Anterior chamber depth, genes and environment. A population study among long-term Greenland Eskimo immigrants in Copenhagen. *Acta Ophthalmol.* 1982;60(2):223–224.
23. Drance SM, Morgan RW, Bryett J, et al. Anterior chamber depth and gonioscopic findings among the Eskimos and Indians in the Canadian Arctic. *Can J Ophthalmol.* 1973;8(2):255–259.
24. van Rens GH, Arkell SM. Refractive errors and axial length among Alaskan Eskimos. *Acta Ophthalmol.* 1991;69(1):27–32.
25. Kolker A, Hetherington J Jr. *Becker-Shaffer's Diagnosis and Therapy of the Glaucomas.* 4th ed. St. Louis: CV Mosby; 1976:183–218.
26. Spaeth GL. The normal development of the human anterior chamber angle: a new system of descriptive grading. *Trans Ophthalmol Soc UK.* 1971;91:709–739.
27. Nguyen N, Mora JS, Gaffney MM, et al. A high prevalence of occludable angles in a Vietnamese population. *Ophthalmology.* 1996;103(9):1426–1431.
28. Fontana ST, Brubaker RF. Volume and depth of the anterior chamber in the normal aging human eye. *Arch Ophthalmol.* 1980;98(10):1803–1808.
29. Markowitz SN, Morin JD. Angle-closure glaucoma: relation between lens thickness, anterior chamber depth and age. *Can J Ophthalmol.* 1984;19(7):300–302.
30. Okabe I, Taniguchi T, Yamamoto T, et al. Age-related changes of the anterior chamber width. *J Glaucoma.* 1992;1(2):100–107.
31. Appleby RS Jr, Kinder RS. Bilateral angle-closure glaucoma in a 14-year-old boy. *Arch Ophthalmol.* 1971;86(4):449–450.
32. Alper MG, Laubach JL. Primary angle-closure glaucoma in the American Negro. *Arch Ophthalmol.* 1968;79(6):663–668.
33. Clemmesen V, Luntz MH. Lens thickness and angle-closure glaucoma. A comparative oculometric study in South African Negroes and Danes. *Acta Ophthalmol.* 1976;54(pt 2):193–197.
34. Wilensky JT, Gandhi N, Pan T. Racial influences in open-angle glaucoma. *Ann Ophthalmol.* 1978;10(10):1398–1402.
35. Olurin O. Anterior chamber depths of Nigerians. *Ann Ophthalmol.* 1977;9(3):315–326.
36. Emiru VP. Response to mydriatics in the African. *Br J Ophthalmol.* 1971;55(8):538–543.
37. Hagan JC III, Lederer CM Jr. Primary angle closure glaucoma in a myopic kinship. *Arch Ophthalmol.* 1985;103(3):363–365.
38. Cherny M, Brooks AM, Gillies WE. Progressive myopia in early onset chronic angle closure glaucoma. *Br J Ophthalmol.* 1992;76(12):758–759.
39. Spaeth GL. Gonioscopy: uses old and new. The inheritance of occludable angles. *Ophthalmology.* 1978;85(3):222–232.
40. Lichter PR, Anderson DR, eds. *Discussions on Glaucoma.* New York: Grune & Stratton; 1977:139.
41. Mapstone R, Clark CV. Prevalence of diabetes in glaucoma. *Br Med J.* 1985;291(6488):93–95.
42. Mapstone R, Clark CV. The prevalence of autonomic neuropathy in glaucoma. *Trans Ophthalmol Soc U K.* 1985;104(pt 3):265–269.
43. Shapiro A, Zauberman H. Diurnal changes of the intraocular pressure of patients with angle-closure glaucoma. *Br J Ophthalmol.* 1979;63(4):225–227.
44. Lee DA, Brubaker RF, Ilstrup DM. Anterior chamber dimensions in patients with narrow angles and angle-closure glaucoma. *Arch Ophthalmol.* 1984;102(1):46–50.
45. Mapstone R, Clark CV. Diurnal variation in the dimensions of the anterior chamber. *Arch Ophthalmol.* 1985;103(10):1485–1486.
46. Vargas E, Drance SM. Anterior chamber depth in angle-closure glaucoma. Clinical methods of depth determination in people with and without the disease. *Arch Ophthalmol.* 1973;90(6):438–439.
47. Douthwaite WA, Spence D. Slitlamp measurement of the anterior chamber depth. *Br J Ophthalmol.* 1986;70(3):205–208.
48. Jacobs IH. Anterior chamber depth measurement using the split-lamp microscope. *Am J Ophthalmol.* 1979;88(2):236–238.
49. Smith RJ. A new method of estimating the depth of the anterior chamber. *Br J Ophthalmol.* 1979;63(4):215–220.
50. Makabe R. Comparative studies of the width of the anterior chamber angle using echography and gonioscopy [in German]. *Klin Monatsbl ugenheilkd.* 1989;194(1):6–9.
51. van Herick W, Shaffer RN, Schwartz A. Estimation of width of angle of anterior chamber. Incidence and significance of the narrow angle. *Am J Ophthalmol.* 1969;68(4):626–629.
52. Scheie HG. Width and pigmentation of the angle of the anterior chamber; a system of grading by gonioscopy. *Arch Ophthalmol.* 1957;58(4):510–512.
53. Becker S. *Clinical Gonioscopy—A Test and Stereoscopic Atlas.* St. Louis: CV Mosby; 1972.
54. Congdon NG, Spaeth GL, Augsburger J, et al. A proposed simple method for measurement in the anterior chamber angle: biometric gonioscopy. *Ophthalmology.* 1999;106(11):2161–2167.
55. Desjardins D, Parrish RK II. Inversion of anterior chamber pigment as a possible prognostic sign in narrow angles. *Am J Ophthalmol.* 1985;100(3):480–481.
56. Aslanides IM, Libre PE, Silverman RH, et al. High frequency ultrasound imaging in pupillary block glaucoma. *Br J Ophthalmol.* 1995;79(11):972–976.
57. Devereux JG, Foster PJ, Baasanhu J, et al. Anterior chamber depth measurement as a screening tool for primary angle-closure glaucoma in an East Asian population. *Arch Ophthalmol.* 2000;118(2):257–263.
58. Panek WC, Christensen RE, Lee DA, et al. Biometric variables in patients with occludable anterior chamber angles. *Am J Ophthalmol.* 1990;110(2):185–188.
59. Ishikawa H, Esaki K, Liebmann JM, et al. Ultrasound biomicroscopy dark room provocative testing: a quantitative method for estimating anterior chamber angle width. *Jpn J Ophthalmol.* 1999;43(6):526–534.
60. Pavlin CJ, Harasiewicz K, Foster FS. An ultrasound biomicroscopic darkroom provocative test. *Ophthalmic Surg.* 1995;26(3):253–255.
61. Friedman DS, He M. Anterior chamber angle assessment techniques. *Surv Ophthalmol.* 2008;53(3):250–273.
62. Hillman JS. Acute closed-angle glaucoma: an investigation into the effect of delay in treatment. *Br J Ophthalmol.* 1979;63(12):817–821.
63. Wilensky JT, Kaufman PL, Frohlichstein D, et al. Follow-up of angle-closure glaucoma suspects. *Am J Ophthalmol.* 1993;115(3):338–346.
64. Lowe RF. Primary angle-closure glaucoma. A review of provocative tests. *Br J Ophthalmol.* 1967;51(11):727–732.
65. Hillman JS, Turner JD. Association between acute glaucoma and the weather and sunspot activity. *Br J Ophthalmol.* 1977;61(8):512–516.
66. Teikari J, Raivio I, Nurminen M. Incidence of acute glaucoma in Finland from 1973 to 1982. *Graefes Arch Clin Exp Ophthalmol.* 1987;225(5):357–360.
67. Grant WM. Ocular complications of drugs. Glaucoma. *JAMA.* 1969;207(11):2089–2091.
68. Mapstone R. Dilating dangerous pupils. *Br J Ophthalmol.* 1977;61(8):517–524.
69. Patel KH, Javitt JC, Tielsch JM, et al. Incidence of acute angle-closure glaucoma after pharmacologic mydriasis. *Am J Ophthalmol.* 1995;120(6):709–717.
70. Wolfs RC, Grobbee DE, Hofman A, et al. Risk of acute angle-closure glaucoma after diagnostic mydriasis in nonselected subjects: the Rotterdam Study. *Invest Ophthalmol Vis Sci.* 1997;38(12):2683–2687.
71. Fazio DT, Bateman JB, Christensen RE. Acute angle-closure glaucoma associated with surgical anesthesia. *Arch Ophthalmol.* 1985;103(3):360–362.
72. Schwartz H, Apt L. Mydriatic effect of anticholinergic drugs used during reversal of nondepolarizing muscle relaxants. *Am J Ophthalmol.* 1979;88(3 pt 2):609–612.
73. Potash SD, Ritch R. Acute angle-closure glaucoma secondary to chlor-trimeton. *J Glaucoma.* 1992;1(4):258–259.
74. Ritch R, Krupin T, Henry C, et al. Oral imipramine and acute angle closure glaucoma. *Arch Ophthalmol.* 1994;112(1):67–68.
75. Corridan P, Nightingale S, Mashoudi N, et al. Acute angle-closure glaucoma following botulinum toxin injection for blepharospasm. *Br J Ophthalmol.* 1990;74(5):309–310.
76. Krontz DP, Wood TO. Corneal decompensation following acute angle-closure glaucoma. *Ophthalmic Surg.* 1988;19(5):334–338.
77. Anderson DR, Davis EB. Sensitivities of ocular tissues to acute pressure-induced ischemia. *Arch Ophthalmol.* 1975;93(4):267–274.

78. Charles ST, Hamasaki DI. The effect of intraocular pressure on the pupil size. *Arch Ophthalmol.* 1970;83(6):729–733.

79. Rutkowski PC, Thompson HS. Mydriasis and increased intraocular pressure. I. Pupillographic studies. *Arch Ophthalmol.* 1972;87(1):21–24.

80. Kapoor S, Sood M. Glaucoma-induced changes in the ciliary ganglion. *Br J Ophthalmol.* 1975;59(10):573–576.

81. Bigar F, Witmer R. Corneal endothelial changes in primary acute angle-closure glaucoma. *Ophthalmology.* 1982;89(6):596–599.

82. Markowitz SN, Morin JD. The endothelium in primary angle-closure glaucoma. *Am J Ophthalmol.* 1984;98(1):103–104.

83. Campbell DG. A comparison of diagnostic techniques in angle-closure glaucoma. *Am J Ophthalmol.* 1979;88(2):197–204.

84. Forbes. Indentation gonioscopy and efficacy of iridectomy in angle-closure glaucoma. *Trans Am Ophthalmol Soc.* 1974;72:488–515.

85. Forbes M. Gonioscopy with corneal indentation. A method for distinguishing between appositional closure and synechial closure. *Arch Ophthalmol.* 1966;76(4):488–492.

86. Zimmerman LE, De Venecia G, Hamasaki DI. Pathology of the optic nerve in experimental acute glaucoma. *Invest Ophthalmol Vis Sci.* 1967;6(2):109–125.

87. Douglas GR, Drance SM, Schulzer M. The visual field and nerve head in angle-closure glaucoma. A comparison of the effects of acute and chronic angle closure. *Arch Ophthalmol.* 1975;93(6):409–411.

88. Sonty S, Schwartz B. Vascular accidents in acute angle closure glaucoma. *Ophthalmology.* 1981;88(3):225–228.

89. Slavin ML, Margulis M. Anterior ischemic optic neuropathy following acute angle-closure glaucoma. *Arch Ophthalmol.* 2001;119(8):1215.

90. McNaught EI, Rennie A, McClure E, et al. Pattern of visual damage after acute angle-closure glaucoma. *Trans Ophthalmol Soc U K.* 1974;94(2):406–415.

91. Mapstone R. One gonioscopic fallacy. *Br J Ophthalmol.* 1979;63(4):221–224.

92. Mapstone R. The mechanism and clinical significance of angle closure. *Glaucoma.* 1980;2:249.

93. Kerman BM, Christensen RE, Foos RY. Angle-closure glaucoma: a clinicopathologic correlation. *Am J Ophthalmol.* 1973;76(6):887–895.

94. Lowe RF. Causes of shallow anterior chamber in primary angle-closure glaucoma. Ultrasonic biometry of normal and angle-closure glaucoma eyes. *Am J Ophthalmol.* 1969;67(1):87–93.

95. Lowe RF, Clark BA. Posterior corneal curvature. Correlations in normal eyes and in eyes involved with primary angle-closure glaucoma. *Br J Ophthalmol.* 1973;57(7):464–470.

96. Markowitz SN, Morin JD. The ratio of lens thickness to axial length for biometric standardization in angle-closure glaucoma. *Am J Ophthalmol.* 1985;99(4):400–402.

97. Phillips CI. Aetiology of angle-closure glaucoma. *Br J Ophthalmol.* 1972;56(3):248–253.

98. Tomlinson A, Leighton DA. Ocular dimensions in the heredity of angle-closure glaucoma. *Br J Ophthalmol.* 1973;57(7):475–486.

99. Tornquist R. Corneal radius in primary acute glaucoma. *Br J Ophthalmol.* 1957;41(7):421–424.

100. Salmon JF, Swanevelder SA, Donald MA. The dimensions of eyes with chronic angle-closure glaucoma. *J Glaucoma.* 1994;3(3):237–243.

101. Mapstone R. Acute shallowing of the anterior chamber. *Br J Ophthalmol.* 1981;65(7):446–451.

102. Mapstone R. Mechanics of pupil block. *Br J Ophthalmol.* 1968;52(1):19–25.

103. Tiedeman JS. A physical analysis of the factors that determine the contour of the iris. *Am J Ophthalmol.* 1991;111(3):338–343.

104. Anderson DR, Jin JC, Wright MM. The physiologic characteristics of relative pupillary block. *Am J Ophthalmol.* 1991;111(3):344–350.

105. Woo EK, Pavlin CJ, Slomovic A, et al. Ultrasound biomicroscopic quantitative analysis of light-dark changes associated with pupillary block. *Am J Ophthalmol.* 1999;127(1):43–47.

106. Inoue T, Yamamoto T, Kitazawa Y. Distribution and morphology of peripheral anterior synechiae in primary angle-closure glaucoma. *J Glaucoma.* 1993;2(3):171–176.

107. Gieser DK, Wilensky JT. Laser iridectomy in the management of chronic angle-closure glaucoma. *Am J Ophthalmol.* 1984;98(4):446–450.

108. Robin AL, Pollack IP. Argon laser peripheral iridotomies in the treatment of primary angle closure glaucoma. Long-term follow-up. *Arch Ophthalmol.* 1982;100(6):919–923.

109. Alsagoff Z, Aung T, Ang LP, et al. Long-term clinical course of primary angle-closure glaucoma in an Asian population. *Ophthalmology.* 2000;107(12):2300–2304.

110. Salmon JF. Long-term intraocular pressure control after Nd-YAG laser iridotomy in chronic angle-closure glaucoma. *J Glaucoma.* 1993;2(4):291–296.

111. Aung T, Ang LP, Chan SP, et al. Acute primary angle-closure: long-term intraocular pressure outcome in Asian eyes. *Am J Ophthalmol.* 2001;131(1):7–12.

112. Cheng CY, Liu CJ, Chiou HJ, et al. Color Doppler imaging study of retrobulbar hemodynamics in chronic angle-closure glaucoma. *Ophthalmology.* 2001;108(8):1445–1451.

113. Pavlin CJ, Ritch R, Foster FS. Ultrasound biomicroscopy in plateau iris syndrome. *Am J Ophthalmol.* 1992;113(4):390–395.

114. Ritch R. Plateau iris is caused by abnormally positioned ciliary processes. *J Glaucoma.* 1992;1(1):23–26.

115. Wand M, Pavlin CJ, Foster FS. Plateau iris syndrome: ultrasound biomicroscopic and histologic study. *Ophthalmic Surg.* 1993;24(2):129–131.

116. Wand M, Grant WM. Thymoxamine test. Differentiating angle-closure glaucoma form open-angle glaucoma with narrow angles. *Arch Ophthalmol.* 1978;96(6):1009–1011.

117. Airaksinen PJ, Saari KM, Tiainen TJ, et al. Management of acute closed-angle glaucoma with miotics and timolol. *Br J Ophthalmol.* 1979;63(12):822–825.

118. Chew PT, Hung PT, Aung T. Efficacy of latanoprost in reducing intraocular pressure in patients with primary angle-closure glaucoma. *Surv Ophthalmol.* 2002;47(suppl 1):S125–S128.

119. Ganias F, Mapstone R. Miotics in closed-angle glaucoma. *Br J Ophthalmol.* 1975;59(4):205–206.

120. Halasa AH, Rutkowski PC. Thymoxamine therapy for angle-closure glaucoma. *Arch Ophthalmol.* 1973;90(3):177–179.

121. Rutkowski PC, Fernandez JL, Galin MA, et al. Alpha-adrenergic receptor blockade in the treatment of angle-closure glaucoma. *Trans Am Acad Ophthalmol Otolaryngol.* 1973;77(2):OP137–OP142.

122. Wand M, Grant WM. Thymoxamine hydrochloride: an alpha-adrenergic blocker. *Surv Ophthalmol.* 1980;25(2):75–84.

123. Chandler PA, Grant WM. *Glaucoma.* 2nd ed. Philadelphia: Lea & Febiger; 1979:140.

124. Anderson DR. Corneal indentation to relieve acute angle-closure glaucoma. *Am J Ophthalmol.* 1979;88(6):1091–1093.

125. Ritch R. Argon laser treatment for medically unresponsive attacks of angle-closure glaucoma. *Am J Ophthalmol.* 1982;94(2):197–204.

126. Shin DH. Argon laser treatment for relief of medically unresponsive angle-closure glaucoma attacks. *Am J Ophthalmol.* 1982;94(6):821–822.

127. Lam DS, Chua JK, Tham CC, et al. Efficacy and safety of immediate anterior chamber paracentesis in the treatment of acute primary angle-closure glaucoma: a pilot study. *Ophthalmology.* 2002;109(1):64–70.

128. David R, Tessler Z, Yassur Y. Long-term outcome of primary acute angle-closure glaucoma. *Br J Ophthalmol.* 1985;69(4):261–262.

129. Schwartz GF, Steinmann WC, Spaeth GL, et al. Surgical and medical management of patients with narrow anterior chamber angles: comparative results. *Ophthalmic Surg.* 1992;23(2):108–112.

130. Morsman CD, Lusky M, Bosem ME, et al. Anterior chamber angle configuration before and after iridotomy measured by Scheimpflug video imaging. *J Glaucoma.* 1994;3(2):114–116.

131. Jin JC, Anderson DR. The effect of iridotomy on iris contour. *Am J Ophthalmol.* 1990;110(3):260–263.

132. Buckley SA, Reeves B, Burdon M, et al. Acute angle closure glaucoma: relative failure of YAG iridotomy in affected eyes and factors influencing outcome. *Br J Ophthalmol.* 1994;78(7):529–533.

133. Hyams SW, Keroub C, Pokotilo E. Mixed glaucoma. *Br J Ophthalmol.* 1977;61(2):105–106.

134. Krupin T, Mitchell KB, Johnson MF, et al. The long-term effects of iridectomy for primary acute angle-closure glaucoma. *Am J Ophthalmol.* 1978;86(4):506–509.

135. Playfair TJ, Watson PG. Management of acute primary angle-closure glaucoma: a long-term follow-up of the results of peripheral iridectomy used as an initial procedure. *Br J Ophthalmol.* 1979;63(1):17–22.

136. Romano JH, Hitchings RA, Pooinasawmy D. Role of Nd:YAG peripheral iridectomy in the management of ocular hypertension with a narrow angle. *Ophthalmic Surg.* 1988;19(11):814–816.

137. Saunders DC. Acute closed-angle glaucoma and Nd-YAG laser iridotomy. *Br J Ophthalmol.* 1990;74(9):523–525.

138. Eltz H, Gloor B. Trabeculectomy in cases of angle closure glaucoma—successes and failures [in German]. *Klin Monatsbl Augenheilkd.* 1980;177(5):556–561.

139. Akingbehin AO. Corticosteroid-induced ocular hypertension. II. An acquired form. *Br J Ophthalmol.* 1982;66(8):541–545.

140. Akingbehin AO. Corticosteroid-induced ocular hypertension. I. Prevalence in closed-angle glaucoma. *Br J Ophthalmol.* 1982;66(8):536–540.

141. Benedikt O. Preventive iridectomy in the partner eye following angle block glaucoma [in German]. *Klin Monatsbl Augenheilkd.* 1970;156(1): 80–83.

142. Lowe RF. Acute angle-closure glaucoma: the second eye: an analysis of 200 cases. *Br J Ophthalmol.* 1962;46(11):641–650.

143. Edwards RS. Behaviour of the fellow eye in acute angle-closure glaucoma. *Br J Ophthalmol.* 1982;66(9):576–579.

144. Lam DS, Leung DY, Tham CC, et al. Randomized trial of early phacoemulsification versus peripheral iridotomy to prevent intraocular pressure rise after acute primary angle closure. *Ophthalmology.* 2008;115(7): 1134–1140.

145. Hata H, Yamane S, Hata S, et al. Preliminary outcomes of primary phacoemulsification plus intraocular lens implantation for primary angle-closure glaucoma. *J Med Invest.* 2008;55(3–4):287–291.

146. Tham CC, Kwong YY, Leung DY, et al. Phacoemulsification versus combined phacotrabeculectomy in medically controlled chronic angle closure glaucoma with cataract. *Ophthalmology.* 2008;115(12):2167–2173.

147. Tham CC, Kwong YY, Leung DY, et al. Phacoemulsification versus combined phacotrabeculectomy in medically uncontrolled chronic angle closure glaucoma with cataracts. *Ophthalmology.* 2009;116(4):725–731.

148. Campbell DG, Vela A. Modern goniosynechialysis for the treatment of synechial angle-closure glaucoma. *Ophthalmology.* 1984;91(9): 1052–1060.

13

Childhood Glaucomas: Classification and Examination

Childhood glaucomas constitute a rare, heterogeneous group of diseases. Often vision-threatening, these diseases present special challenges in diagnosis and optimal management. Parents and primary care providers usually first recognize the abnormalities that lead to the diagnosis of glaucoma in infants and young children, with devastating consequences when that correct diagnosis is substantially delayed. The clinical presentation of glaucoma varies with the age of onset and the severity of intraocular pressure (IOP) elevation. In addition, detailed ophthalmic examination of young children can be difficult, and management strategies for this rare condition are less familiar than those in adult patients. Pharmacologic, technological, and genetic advances in the diagnosis and treatment of glaucoma engender hope that children with this disease may face brighter visual futures.

CLASSIFICATION OF CHILDHOOD GLAUCOMAS

The glaucomas of childhood have been categorized in various ways, but one simple, commonly used system considers them as either primary or secondary in mechanism. Although this classification system is far from ideal (see Chapter 7), we use this terminology here because our somewhat limited insights today preclude a more meaningful conceptual framework for discussing childhood glaucomas.

The primary glaucomas, often genetic in origin, comprise those in which a developmental abnormality of the anterior chamber angle leads to obstruction of aqueous outflow. Within these primary glaucomas, congenital open-angle glaucoma—often termed primary congenital glaucoma (PCG)—and juvenile open-angle glaucoma present without consistently associated ocular or systemic developmental anomalies. By contrast, primary glaucomas associated with ocular abnormalities—often called developmental glaucomas—include primary glaucomas in which a developmental abnormality is responsible for the glaucoma, but in which additional ocular and systemic anomalies are typically present. Unlike the primary childhood glaucomas, secondary childhood glaucomas include glaucomas whose mechanism of outflow obstruction is acquired from other events, such as inflammation or neoplasia, rather than a primary anomaly of the angle. In a yearlong prospective study of all new childhood glaucoma cases in the United Kingdom and the Republic of Ireland, 99 cases were identified: 47 primary and 52 secondary in nature (1).

In this chapter, we consider the pediatric glaucoma patient and details of the examination specific to the child with known or suspected glaucoma. The following chapter, Chapter 14, addresses primary glaucomas of childhood, including PCG and the major developmental glaucomas. Because children are subject to many of the same secondary glaucomas as adults, these topics are discussed together in subsequent chapters of Section II, with special attention given to situations that apply only to children. One exception is the glaucoma occurring after removal of cataracts in infants and young children, as this "aphakic glaucoma" or "pseudophakic glaucoma" may well represent the second most commonly encountered single type of childhood glaucoma (after PCG) (1), and is therefore included in Chapter 14.

Table 13.1 (2) gives one scheme for considering childhood glaucomas (2). Some pediatric glaucomas may have both primary and secondary causes (e.g., infantile-onset glaucoma in Sturge–Weber syndrome, neurofibromatosis, and aniridia). Many of the primary and developmental glaucomas are genetic in origin (see Chapters 8 and 14). Continuing elucidation of the genetics behind many conditions associated with pediatric glaucoma will no doubt lead to replacement of the current phenotypically driven diagnostic labels, with names and categories based on underlying genetic abnormalities.

SIGNS AND SYMPTOMS OF GLAUCOMA IN CHILDHOOD

The signs and symptoms of glaucoma in children vary tremendously with the age of onset and the degree of IOP elevation. Infants and young children with glaucoma (usually with PCG, but occurring with early-onset glaucoma of any cause) usually present because the family or pediatrician has noticed something abnormal about the eyes or the infant's behavior. Corneal enlargement or opacification (resulting from stretching due to high IOP), or both, often signal glaucoma in the infant; both may progress rapidly over the first 2 years of life if IOP remains elevated (Figs. 13.1 and 13.2). Buphthalmos is a term to describe the abnormal enlargement of an infant's eye secondary to elevated IOP; in extreme cases, these eyes are vulnerable to lens subluxation and rupture with even minor trauma (Fig. 13.3). The classic triad of findings usually ascribed to PCG (see also Chapter 14)—epiphora, photophobia (Fig. 13.4), and blepharospasm (3)—results from corneal edema, often with associated breaks in the Descemet membrane called Haab striae. Descemet membrane breaks appear to occur only in the first 2 years of life; they leave permanent evidence of early-onset glaucoma and vary with respect to the

Table 13.1	Childhood Glaucomas: A Classification Scheme

I. Primary Glaucomas
 A. Congenital open-angle glaucoma[a]
  1. Newborn glaucoma (iridotrabeculodysgenesis)
  2. Infantile glaucoma (trabeculodysgenesis)
  3. Late-recognized
 B. Juvenile (open-angle) glaucoma
 C. Associated with ocular abnormalities (anterior segment dysgenesis)[a]
  1. Iridodysgenesis
   a. Aniridia[b]
   b. Congenital iris ectropion syndrome
   c. Iridotrabecular dysgenesis (iris hypoplasia)
  2. Corneodysgenesis (or iridocorneodysgenesis)
   a. Axenfeld–Rieger anomaly
   b. Peters anomaly
   c. Congenital microcornea with myopia
   d. Sclerocornea
   e. Congenital hereditary endothelial dystrophy
   f. Posterior polymorphous dystrophy
   g. Megalocornea
 D. Associated with systemic abnormalities
  1. Chromosomal disorders
   a. Trisomy 13–15 (trisomy D syndrome)
   b. Trisomy 18 (Edwards syndrome)
   c. Trisomy 21 (Down syndrome)
   d. Turner syndrome (XO)
  2. Connective tissue abnormalities
   a. Marfan syndrome[b]
   b. Stickler syndrome
   c. Others (see under secondary glaucomas)
  3. Metabolic disease
   a. Oculocerebrorenal syndrome (Lowe syndrome)
   b. Mucopolysaccharidosis (e.g., Hurler syndrome)
   c. Others (see under secondary glaucoma)[b]
  4. Phacomatoses
   a. Sturge–Weber syndrome (isolated vs. with CNS involvement)
   b. Neurofibromatosis type 1
   c. Nevus of Ota (ocular melanosis)
   d. von Hippel–Lindau syndrome
  5. Other
   a. Rieger syndrome (Axenfeld–Rieger syndrome)[a]
   b. Hepatocerebrorenal syndrome (Zellweger syndrome)
   c. Kniest dysplasia
   d. Hallermann–Streiff syndrome
   e. Michel syndrome
   f. Nail–Patella syndrome
   g. Oculodentodigital dysplasia
   h. Prader–Willi syndrome
   i. Rubinstein–Taybi syndrome
   j. Waardenburg syndrome
   k. Walker–Warburg syndrome
   l. Cutis marmorata telangiectasia congenita

II. Secondary Glaucomas
 A. Traumatic glaucoma
  1. Acute glaucoma
   a. Angle concussion
   b. Hyphema
   c. Ghost cell glaucoma
  2. Late-onset glaucoma with angle recession
  3. Arteriovenous fistula
 B. Secondary to intraocular neoplasm
  1. Retinoblastoma
  2. Juvenile xanthogranuloma
  3. Leukemia
  4. Melanoma
  5. Melanocytoma
  6. Iris rhabdomyosarcoma
  7. Aggressive nevi of the iris
 C. Secondary to uveitis
  1. Open-angle glaucoma
  2. Angle-blockage glaucoma
   a. Synechial angle closure
   b. Iris bombé with pupillary block
   c. Trabecular endothelialization
 D. Lens-induced glaucoma
  1. Subluxation–dislocation and pupillary block
   a. Marfan syndrome
   b. Homocystinuria
   c. Weill–Marchesani
  2. Spherophakia and pupillary block
  3. Phacolytic glaucoma
 E. After surgery for congenital cataract
  1. Lens tissue trabecular obstruction
  2. Pupillary block
  3. Chronic open-angle glaucoma associated with angle abnormalities
 F. Steroid-induced glaucoma
 G. Secondary to rubeosis
  1. Retinoblastoma
  2. Coats disease
  3. Medulloepithelioma
  4. Familial exudative vitreoretinopathy
  5. Chronic retinal detachment
 H. Secondary angle-closure glaucoma
  1. Retinopathy of prematurity
  2. Microphthalmos
  3. Nanophthalmos
  4. Retinoblastoma
  5. Persistent fetal vasculature
  6. Congenital pupillary iris–lens membrane
  7. Topiramate-induced
  8. Central retinal vein occlusion
  9. Iris stromal cysts
  10. Ciliary body cysts
  11. Cystinosis
 I. Malignant glaucoma

(Continued)

Table 13.1	Childhood Glaucomas: A Classification Scheme (*Continued*)

II. Secondary Glaucomas (*Continued*)
  J. Glaucoma associated with increased episcleral venus or venous pressure
    1. Sturge–Weber syndrome (isolated vs. CNS involvement)
    2. Cavernous or dural-venous fistula
    3. Orbital disease

K. Secondary to maternal rubella
L. Secondary to intraocular infection
    1. Acute recurrent toxoplasmosis
    2. Acute herpetic iritis
    3. Endogenous endophthalmitis

[a]These conditions are all considered anterior segment dysgeneses by some authorities, because of their genetic underpinnings and may be further classified as those of neural crest cell origin or non–neural crest cell origin (2).
[b]Glaucoma associated with these conditions may also be considered secondary in some cases.
CNS, central nervous system.

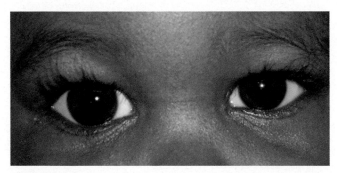

Figure 13.1 Infant with congenital glaucoma, showing buphthalmos and asymmetric enlargement of the corneas, right more than left. Corneal edema has resolved after successful angle surgery.

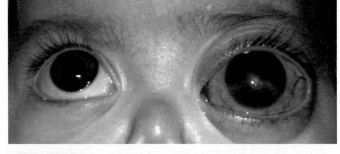

Figure 13.3 Severe buphthalmos in the left eye of a 6-month-old infant with congenital glaucoma and bilateral enlarged corneas and high myopia in the setting of Stickler–Marshall syndrome. This blind left eye was exposed and presumed painful and was subsequently enucleated.

associated corneal distortion and scarring (**Figs. 13.5** and **13.6**). Breaks with more vertical orientation may be seen after forceps delivery (**Fig. 13.7**) (4).

Additional nonspecific signs of glaucoma in early life include a deep anterior chamber and optic nerve cupping. In the absence of optic atrophy, the optic cup may decrease greatly in size with IOP reduction and will enlarge again if control of IOP is lost (3). Optic atrophy, which may result from chronic or severe IOP elevation, is irreversible.

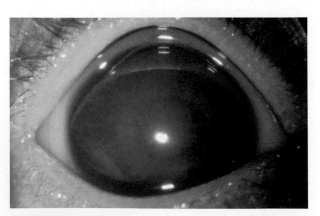

Figure 13.2 Right eye of a 3-month-old infant presenting with enlarged, cloudy cornea in the setting of newly diagnosed congenital glaucoma. IOP was 35 mm Hg.

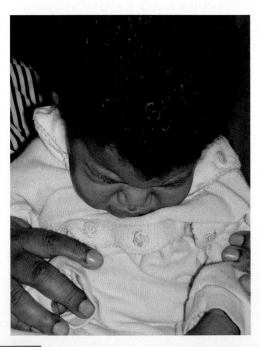

Figure 13.4 Extreme photophobia in an infant girl, 6 months of age, with PCG. Bilateral corneal edema and photophobia improved after surgical treatment.

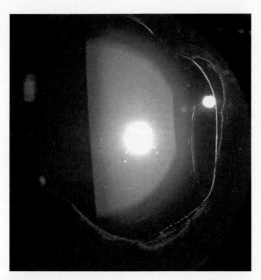

Figure 13.5 Slitlamp appearance of tears in Descemet membrane, or Haab striae, in a patient with congenital glaucoma.

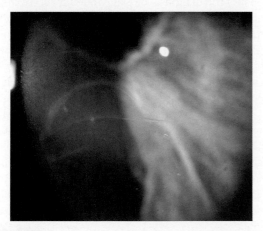

Figure 13.6 Haab striae in a patient with Axenfeld–Rieger glaucoma, viewed at the slitlamp under high magnification.

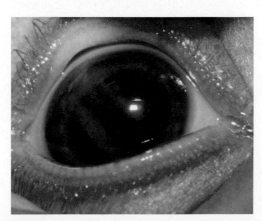

Figure 13.7 Forceps-related tears in Descemet membrane. Note the very straight Haab striae, oriented from superotemporal to inferonasal in the cornea of the right eye of this newborn infant boy. Permanent scarring and high astigmatism resulted in amblyopia in this eye.

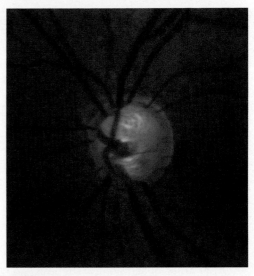

Figure 13.8 Severe optic nerve cupping in the left eye of an 8-year-old girl with juvenile-onset glaucoma.

In contrast to infants and very young children, older children with glaucoma typically present with decreased vision (usually from induced myopia, but occasionally from end-stage optic nerve damage) or because they are known glaucoma suspects (e.g., with Sturge–Weber syndrome, aniridia, or aphakia or pseudophakia). Although elevated IOP produces corneal enlargement limited to the first 3 years of life, scleral stretching persists for approximately 10 years, producing progressive myopia (and often astigmatism), usually seen in older children with glaucoma. While optic nerve cupping is not by itself a reliable indicator of glaucoma, its presence should prompt a thorough evaluation for possible glaucoma in a child of any age (**Fig. 13.8**). Older children infrequently present with symptoms of acute glaucoma, such as nausea associated with eye pain, headaches, and even colored haloes around lights (e.g., secondary to trauma or angle closure, as with cicatricial retinopathy of prematurity).

Visual loss from infant and childhood glaucoma most often results from pathologic changes in the eye, such as corneal opacification and optic nerve damage. Poor vision may also occur despite adequate IOP control, secondary to the development of anisometropia or strabismic amblyopia, especially in unilateral or asymmetric bilateral childhood glaucoma.

DIFFERENTIAL DIAGNOSIS

The clinical features of glaucoma in infancy and childhood overlap partly with those of other pediatric ophthalmic conditions, with the exception of elevated IOP (**Table 13.2**) (3,5). When faced with ocular signs or symptoms suggestive of possible glaucoma, the clinician must consider and rigorously exclude glaucoma, keeping in mind that identifying a coexisting nonglaucomatous disorder does not eliminate the possibility of glaucoma. For example, glaucoma may complicate uveitis, Peters anomaly, and megalocornea; glaucoma may even occur

Table 13.2	Differential Diagnosis of Features Commonly Found in Childhood Glaucomas

I. Disorders showing "red eye" and epiphora
   A. Congenital nasolacrimal duct obstruction
   B. Conjunctivitis (infectious, chemical exposure)
   C. Corneal epithelial defect/abrasion
   D. Keratitis (especially herpes simplex)
   E. Inflamed anterior segment (uveitis, trauma)
II. Disorders showing corneal edema or opacification
   A. Forceps-related birth trauma (with Descemet tears)
   B. Congenital malformation/anomaly
      1. Sclerocornea
      2. Peters anomaly
      3. Choristomas (dermoid-like)
      4. Other anterior segment dysgenesis
   C. Corneal dystrophy
      1. Congenital hereditary endothelial dystrophy
      2. Posterior polymorphous dystrophy
   D. Keratitis
      1. Herpetic
      2. Rubella[a]
      3. Phlyctenular
   E. Metabolic disease
      1. Mucopolysaccharidoses
      2. Mucolipidoses
      3. Cystinosis
      4. Oculocerebrorenal (Lowe) syndrome
III. Conditions showing corneal enlargement
   A. Axial myopia
   B. Megalocornea
   C. Megalophthalmos
IV. Conditions with actual or "pseudo" optic nerve cupping
   A. Physiologically large optic nerve cup
   B. Coloboma or pit of the optic nerve
   C. Atrophic optic nerve (with substance loss)
   D. Hypoplastic optic nerve
   E. Malformation of the optic nerve

[a]Rare in developed countries.
Adapted from Refs. 3 and 5.

coincident with the commonly encountered congenital naso-lacrimal duct obstruction (3).

THE DIAGNOSTIC EXAMINATION

Although any child with suspected glaucoma requires a detailed pediatric ophthalmic examination, there are specific goals of the glaucoma-related examination: (a) confirming or excluding the diagnosis of glaucoma, (b) determining the cause of the glaucoma (if present), and (c) gathering information (including any prior glaucoma interventions) vital to plan the optimal management. Examination under anesthesia may be avoided if the diagnosis of glaucoma can be confidently excluded (in an infant or young child) or if an older child would benefit from a medication trial. The examination under anesthesia, when it is indicated, provides a one-stop opportunity for more detailed gonioscopy and evaluation of the optic nerve head, as well as measurements of corneal diameter, central corneal thickness, and axial length, immediately followed by any needed surgical intervention.

Vision Testing (Acuity and Visual Fields)

Optimal vision-testing methods will vary with the patient's age and cognitive function. While central, maintained fixation behavior and absent nystagmus are encouraging in infants, older children should perform optotype testing with proper refractive correction. Visual loss in children with glaucoma often results from ocular changes related to glaucoma or from amblyopia in asymmetric cases; visual acuity loss resulting from optic nerve damage represents an unfortunate, often end-stage situation.

Visual field testing, especially quantitative automated static perimetry, often proves challenging for young children and for all children with nystagmus or poor vision. Hence, perimetry rarely makes the diagnosis of glaucoma but serves instead to assess adequacy of control in older children with glaucoma who can perform reliable baseline examination. Visual field assessment is nonetheless worthwhile in all children with glaucoma, because even confrontation visual fields can often verify suspected severe nasal field loss in children with severe glaucoma and poor vision. Children with associated neurologic conditions (e.g., Sturge–Weber syndrome) may have underlying homonymous hemifield loss independent of their glaucoma. Newer, faster testing algorithms may allow younger children to undergo automated (Humphrey) visual field testing more reliably (6) (**Fig. 13.9**). Frequency-doubling perimetry (see Chapter 5) may also hold promise for screening and following visual fields over time in children with known or suspected glaucoma (7,8).

External Examination

External examination helps identify evidence of associated abnormalities (e.g., neurofibromatosis, facial hemangioma), buphthalmos (especially asymmetry between the eyes), photophobia, or nasolacrimal obstruction. Overall assessment of the child's health and systemic features can also provide clues to a glaucoma diagnosis (e.g., facial features suggesting metabolic disorders, connective tissue disorders, chromosomal abnormalities). Occasionally, the ophthalmologist may be the first to suspect the systemic condition related to the ocular abnormality being examined (e.g., oculocerebrorenal or Lowe syndrome, neurofibromatosis).

Corneal Examination

This portion of the examination assesses the cornea for glaucoma-induced changes such as enlargement, edema, and scarring. Other abnormalities, if present, may also suggest coexisting ocular abnormalities (as with developmental glaucomas such as Axenfeld–Rieger or Peters, as discussed in Chapter 14).

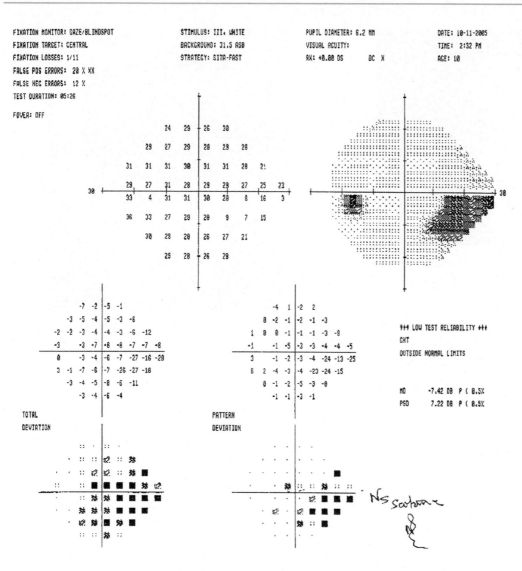

Figure 13.9 Humphrey visual field testing demonstrates an inferior arcuate scotoma in the left eye of this 11-year-old with juvenile open-angle glaucoma, who presented with severe optic nerve cupping and had successful control of glaucoma with mitomycin C–augmented trabeculectomy.

The healthy newborn's cornea has a horizontal diameter ranging from 9.5 to 10.5 mm, which enlarges by about 0.5 to 1.0 mm in the first year of life (9–11) (**Table 13.3**). Distention of the globe in response to elevated IOP (buphthalmos) leads to enlargement of the cornea, especially at the corneoscleral junction. A corneal diameter larger than 12 mm in the first year of life is a highly suspect finding. Asymmetry in diameter between the two corneas or a corneal diameter of 13 mm or more at any age strongly suggests abnormality (3). Corneal enlarge-

ment is more obvious in asymmetric cases (Fig. 13.1). Simple inspection of the corneas will often identify asymmetric corneal diameters of as little as 0.25 mm, likely because of the examiner's assessment of corneal area (rather than its diameter) by visual inspection. Corneal diameters can be measured by using a millimeter ruler held in the frontal plane in the office, or by calipers in the anesthetized state.

Acute, severe IOP elevation produces corneal enlargement in the newborn or infant, frequently accompanied by tears in the Descemet membrane (Haab striae). These often appear acutely as areas of increased corneal edema and clouding (3) (Figs. 13.5 and 13.6). In more advanced cases, dense opacification of the corneal stroma may persist despite IOP reduction (**Fig. 13.10**). In contrast, moderate IOP elevation insufficient to produce noticeable corneal opacity gradually enlarges the infant's corneas, sometimes proceeding unnoticed if symmetric, while concurrent optic nerve damage progresses to severe degrees (Fig. 13.8).

Tonometry (Intraocular Pressure Measurement)

Although IOP assessment in children with suspected or known glaucoma remains critical to their diagnosis and effective management, tonometry often presents challenges in the young

Table 13.3	Corneal Diameter in Children: Healthy and Glaucomatous Eyes[a]	
Age	**Corneal Diameter, *mm***	
	Normal	**Suspicious for Possible Glaucoma**
Birth–6 mo	9.5–11.5	>12
1–2 y	10–12	>12.5
>2 y	<12	>13

[a]Data are from Refs. 9 and 10.

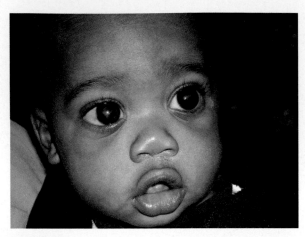

Figure 13.10 A 9-month-old boy with congenital glaucoma and residual corneal scarring from Haab striae, despite successful IOP control with angle surgery.

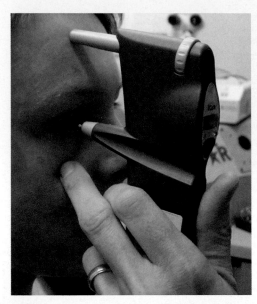

Figure 13.11 Icare tonometry being performed in the right eye of a 13-year-old boy 1 day after glaucoma drainage-device surgery for aphakic glaucoma.

patient. The best IOP measurements are those obtained in a calm child in the office setting, because IOP may be falsely elevated in a struggling patient and is often unpredictably altered by systemic sedatives and anesthetics (Table 13.5). A sleepy or hungry infant often permits tonometry while taking a bottle in his or her caregiver's arms.

Although various instruments have been used for IOP measurement in children, the Perkins applanation tonometer and the Tono-Pen (i.e., a handheld Mackay–Marg-type tonometer) rank highly in terms of accuracy and ease of use in these patients (12–15). Children as young as 3 or 4 years of age can often cooperate with Goldmann applanation tonometry (Freedman S, personal observation). The Icare tonometer (Icare Finland, Helsinki), a relatively new handheld device, records IOP in awake patients without requiring topical anesthetic and has a tiny tip that advances easily between the lids of a normally blinking child. Published reports of this rebound tonometer have shown the Icare similar in accuracy to the Tono-Pen and comparable with Goldmann tonometry for IOPs over a reasonable range in adults (Chapter 2) (**Fig. 13.11**). Icare was reported to be comfortable and highly reproducible for tonometry in healthy school-aged children (16). The Icare tonometer has already proven valuable as a screening tool in children and will probably allow IOP assessment in many infants and children previously requiring anesthetic examination. Home tonometry in children suspected of having large diurnal IOP variation is possible with this instrument (Freedman S, unpublished data).

The pneumatonometer (see also Chapter 2), although cumbersome to use on children in the office setting, often serves as a confirmatory technique to Tono-Pen or Perkins tonometry during examination under anesthesia. This tonometer may be particularly helpful in settings where an opaque or scarring corneal surface precludes useful measurement using handheld instruments; often the readings are several millimeters of mercury higher by pneumotonometry than by applanation. Schiötz indentation tonometry is not recommended for use in eyes with childhood glaucoma, even in the operating

room, because of its tendency to underestimate IOP in these eyes (David Walton, MD, personal communication).

The normal IOP in childhood, ranging from about 10 to 22 mm Hg depending on the tonometer and reported pediatric population (3), rises from infancy to reach normal adult levels by middle childhood (17) (**Table 13.4**).

IOP measurements are variably lowered by the use of sedatives, narcotics, and inhalation anesthetic agents (18–20), and elevated by endotracheal intubation (3) (**Table 13.5**). Ketamine anesthesia, previously reported to elevate IOP (21), has recently compared favorably with sevoflurane anesthesia in terms of

Table 13.4	Normal Intraocular Pressure by Age
Age, y	**Mean IOP, *mm Hg*[a]**
Birth	9.6
0–1	10.6
1–2	12.0
2–3	12.6
3–5	13.6
5–7	14.2
7–9	14.2
9–12	14.3
12–16	14.5

[a]Values obtained by using a noncontact tonometer (Keeler Pulsair, Keeler Ltd., Windsor, Berks, UK). IOP values for children vary widely, depending on the type of instrument used.
IOP, intraocular pressure.
Adapted from Ref. 17.

Table 13.5	Intraocular Pressure Effects of Selected Sedatives and Anesthetic Agents	
Effect on IOP	**Sedative/Anesthetic Agents/Related Events**	**Route of Administration**
Minimal effect	Chloral hydrate	Oral or rectal
Minimal to mild reduction	Methohexital (Brevital)	Rectal, intramuscular, intravenous
Minimal to mild reduction	Midazolam (Versed)	Rectal, intramuscular, intravenous
Minimal to mild reduction	Sevoflurance	Inhalation
Mild reduction	Oxygen	Inhalation
Mild reduction	Nitrous oxide/oxygen	Inhalation
Mild to significant reduction	Halothane	Inhalation
Minimal to mild increase	Ketamine	Intramuscular
Marked increase	Succinyl choline	Intravenous
Marked increase	Laryngospasm, Bell reflex	—
Marked increase	Endotracheal intubation	—

IOP, intraocular pressure.

minimally altering measured IOP over several minutes after induction (22). Chloral hydrate conscious sedation, effective only in small children and with careful monitoring, reportedly minimally affects awake IOP readings (23). Although IOP measurements taken in a sedated or anesthetic state are often less reliable than those recorded in a calm, awake child, high preoperative IOP measurements generally remain in an abnormal range, and asymmetric IOPs between the two eyes usually remain so and often signal abnormality. Special care must be taken to avoid spuriously high IOP measured in the anesthetized child who is in laryngospasm, or "light" with eyes rolled upward or downward compared with the midline.

Anterior Segment Examination (Biomicroscopy)

Anterior segment findings provide key information in the evaluation of the pediatric glaucoma patient. As noted earlier, simple inspection of the child's eyes often assists in overall assessment of the corneal size, symmetry, and clarity. Biomicroscopy (optimally with a handheld slitlamp) adds details of corneal architecture and affords improved examination of the corneal details, especially Haab striae. As the IOP is normalized and tears in the Descemet membrane are repaired by endothelial overgrowth, the corneal edema may clear; however, the linear opacities persist, and they are associated with reduced endothelial counts, as viewed by specular microscopy (24), and produce variable permanent scarring and refractive errors. Slitlamp biomicroscopy of the cornea may also demonstrate accompanying findings as clues to the underlying cause of the glaucoma (e.g., posterior embryotoxon in Axenfeld–Rieger syndrome, or central corneal opacity or corneal adhesions to the iris or lens in Peters anomaly).

The limbus may be dramatically stretched and thinned by ocular stretching in an infant eye with glaucoma, and the anterior chamber often deepens. Abnormalities of the iris and lens may signal primary anomalies or those secondary to other eye diseases (e.g., aniridia, Axenfeld–Rieger syndrome, ectropion uvea).

Gonioscopy

Gonioscopy, providing vital anatomic information about the mechanism of glaucoma in a given eye, can be performed in the office or under anesthesia. Indirect gonioscopy with a Zeiss or Sussman gonioprism proves simple to perform at the slit-lamp in the older child, whereas Koeppe (direct) gonioscopy is useful for infants and in the operating room, facilitating detailed inspection of the iris and angle structures (and optic nerve head, by using a direct ophthalmoscope) (**Fig. 13.12**). In contrast to the healthy adult angle, the healthy infant's angle demonstrates a trabecular meshwork that appears almost as a smooth, homogeneous membrane extending from the

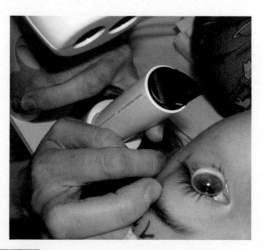

Figure 13.12 Technique of gonioscopy during examination under anesthesia, performed by using a Koeppe gonioscopy lens and portable slitlamp biomicroscope.

peripheral iris to the Schwalbe line. This trabecular meshwork becomes coarser and often increasingly pigmented over time (25,26). In darkly pigmented individuals, pigmentation of the uveal meshwork with increasing age enhances visibility of this lacy structure. Characteristic features of the child's angle structures help identify eyes with congenital glaucoma of varying severity (see below and Chapter 14). Additional abnormalities present in cases of anterior segment dysgenesis (e.g., aniridia, Axenfeld–Rieger, Peters), aphakic, and secondary glaucomas, for example (for additional details, see Chapter 14).

Taken together with other findings of anterior examination, the adequacy of the angle view and its findings are important guides to the appropriate surgical intervention that may be needed.

Optic Nerve and Fundus Examination

The appearance of the optic nerve head is usually the focus of the fundus examination in an eye with glaucoma, although associated fundus abnormalities may help confirm the glaucoma type (e.g., a stalk in persistent fetal vasculature, foveal hypoplasia in aniridia, or choroidal hemangioma in Sturge–Weber syndrome) or provide useful information for surgical planning (e.g., peripheral retinal pathology or vitreous stranding may suggest vitrectomy and peripheral laser, along with implantation of a glaucoma drainage device, in eyes with aphakia).

Evaluation of the optic nerve head is one of the most important methods for diagnosing childhood glaucoma and for assessing its response to therapy. Indirect ophthalmoscopy with a 28-diopter (D) or 30-D lens may minimize apparent optic nerve head cupping, better appreciated in the older child by using binocular viewing at the slitlamp, or with a 14-D indirect lens or direct ophthalmoscope through a Koeppe gonioscopy lens under anesthesia (which usually affords an adequate view, even with an undilated pupil).

The optic nerve head in healthy newborns is typically pink but may have slight pallor, and a small physiologic cup is usually present (27). The morphology of glaucomatous optic atrophy in childhood resembles that seen in adult eyes, with a preferential loss of neural tissue in the vertical poles (28). In contrast to the adult, however, the scleral canal in children enlarges in response to elevated IOP, especially in the horizontal meridian, causing further enlargement of the cup in addition to that resulting from the actual loss of neural tissue (28).

Cupping of the optic nerve head proceeds more rapidly in infants than in adults and is more likely to be reversible if the pressure is lowered early enough (15,17,29–34). The cupping appears to be caused by incomplete development of connective tissue in the lamina cribrosa, which allows compression or posterior movement of the optic disc tissue in response to elevated IOP, with an elastic return to normal when the pressure is lowered (32). Dramatic reversal of optic nerve cupping can even occur in older children with glaucoma on sustained lowering of IOP, although significant improvement of visual field loss does not necessarily occur (**Fig. 13.13**).

Significant optic nerve cup size and asymmetry of cupping between fellow eyes suggest, but do not confirm, glaucoma in

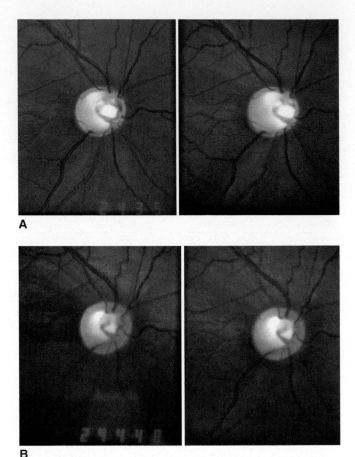

Figure 13.13 Reversal of cupping. This 14-year-old girl with end-stage juvenile open-angle glaucoma and total cupping of her right optic nerve (**A**) showed some reversal of cupping (**B**) (although no improvement in arcuate scotomas on visual field testing) 2 years after trabeculectomy with mitomycin C and a reduction in IOP from 30 mm Hg to about 10 mm Hg.

an infant. Possible explanations for cupping asymmetry in the absence of IOP-related changes include asymmetry in the size of the optic canal itself and significant differences in the axial lengths of the two eyes (e.g., in unilateral high myopia or hyperopia).

Other Useful Diagnostic Tests

Refraction

Refractive error determination cannot only suggest possible glaucoma (as when a myopic shift occurs rapidly after cataract removal, or asymmetric relative myopia occurs in the eye with higher IOP) but also serve a critical function in maximizing the visual function of the child with glaucoma, in whom high myopia, astigmatism, or anisometropia, singly or in combination, may result from IOP-induced corneal scarring or ocular enlargement.

The enlargement of the globe with elevated IOP in the first 3 years of life creates a myopic shift in the refractive error, which may lead to amblyopia if significant anisometropia is present. The presence of Haab striae often produces significant astigmatism, which also contributes to amblyopia, especially in unilateral or asymmetric cases. Children between 3 and 10 years of age with elevated IOP may develop progressive myopia and astigmatism, despite a stable corneal diameter. These refractive changes have been attributed to continued scleral stretching (3). Myopia is also commonly associated with forms of juvenile glaucoma (35), although it may be unclear whether glaucoma or myopia was the primary event.

Ultrasonography

Measurement of the axial length (by using ultrasonography, preferably by immersion technique, during examination under anesthesia) serves as an adjunct to serial corneal diameter determination for infants and young children being treated for glaucoma, because stabilization and even reduction in axial length can occur in the enlarged eye with stable IOP reduction (9). This axial length change may be evident within days after a significant IOP reduction, especially in aphakic eyes of infants after filtration surgery or implantation of a glaucoma drainage device (Freedman S, personal experience). Ultrasonography may also be helpful when glaucoma drainage-device surgery is being contemplated, because the size of the proposed implant reservoir may be limited by the globe size (see Chapter 40). B-scan ultrasonography helps confirm retinal status in eyes with opaque media and often aids in assessing the patency of a glaucoma drainage device when the bleb itself cannot be well seen (see Chapter 39). Anterior segment ultrasonography also plays a useful role in surgical management for selected patients in whom opaque media precludes adequate assessment of the anterior chamber and associated anterior segment structures (e.g., a demonstrated deep anterior chamber may allow glaucoma drainage-device placement, or congenital aphakia may allow endoscopic laser cycloablation; see also Chapter 40).

Central Corneal Thickness Measurement

Ultrasonic pachymetry (to measure the central corneal thickness) has become standard in the evaluation of adults with chronic open-angle glaucoma, because this variable seems to affect not only the accuracy of the measured IOP by applanation tonometry (elevated by an unusually thick central cornea, and vice versa) but also the potential susceptibility of an eye to glaucomatous vision loss at elevated IOP (36–39). In children, the reported central corneal thickness ranges from roughly 540 μm at 6 to 23 months of age to approximately 550 to 560 μm for older children, with thinner central corneal thickness reported in white compared with black children (40–46), and stable measurements over at least 1 year in healthy eyes and those controlled on glaucoma medication (47). Central corneal thickness is thinner in children with congenital glaucoma than in other children, and this is probably a function of the larger, stretched corneas in the eyes of many of the children with congenital glaucoma (41). By contrast, eyes with aniridia have thicker-than-average central corneas (48), as do eyes with aphakia and particularly those with aphakic glaucoma (47,49–52); this is perhaps an acquired rather than a congenital feature (49).

The importance of central corneal thickness in the evaluation and management of children with glaucoma currently remains undetermined, and although this feature is worthwhile to measure and consider when setting the target IOP, the clinician should avoid "adjusting" the measured IOP on the basis of the pachymetry results. It may be reasonable to make a downward adjustment in the target IOP for those eyes with thinner-than-normal central corneas.

Imaging Techniques: Fundus Photography, Optical Coherence Tomography

Fundus photography of the optic nerve head has long been a mainstay in the evaluation of adults with glaucoma over time and is useful in cooperative children with clear visual axes and without substantial nystagmus. Other imaging techniques that noninvasively image the optic nerve head (e.g., optical coherence tomography [OCT]) may be useful in older children with glaucoma, primarily to document changes over time, rather than to diagnose glaucoma.

OCT, a noninvasive imaging technique that can measure the thickness of the peripapillary nerve fiber layer and the macular area and volume in adults and in children (53–55), does correlate with the photographic evidence of glaucomatous optic nerve head damage and may prove valuable to evaluate the thinning of these parameters in children with glaucoma (54,56,57). At the present time, however, the utility of OCT is limited by the need for a clear visual axis and steady fixation, as well as a wide range of normal values, and lack in longitudinal data in children with glaucoma. Newly developed handheld spectral-domain OCT may prove useful for imaging in infants and young children who cannot currently be assessed by the standard technology (58).

DIAGNOSIS AND TREATMENT OF THE CHILD WITH GLAUCOMA

The clinician must decide whether the findings of the ophthalmic examination (in the office and under anesthesia, if needed) are sufficiently suspicious for glaucoma to proceed to treatment, or conversely, whether that diagnosis can safely be excluded. If the diagnosis of glaucoma has been established, appropriate treatment will depend on the type and severity of the particular glaucoma. Although the menu of medical and surgical options for pediatric glaucoma overlaps greatly with those options used in adults, therapeutic strategies in children often diverge significantly from those of their adult counterparts (see Chapters 14 and 40). The child with suspected glaucoma must be followed up at an interval appropriate to the level of concern for the diagnosis, so that the needed intervention may be initiated if circumstances change. Any child with an increased risk for or confirmed glaucoma should be followed up with complete ophthalmic examination periodically throughout life, even when the IOP has been controlled for years, as loss of glaucoma control can occur decades after successful treatment (as after angle surgery for congenital glaucoma; see Chapter 14). Providing optimal care for children with glaucoma requires a team approach, with collaboration between the child's family, ophthalmologist, and often others, such as teachers and counselors. As the patient grows into adulthood, he or she must ultimately become a key member of the team responsible for his or her ongoing treatment and follow-up.

KEY POINTS

- Childhood glaucomas represent an unusual but serious group of disorders that only partially overlap with glaucoma of adult onset.
- There are a variety of mechanisms responsible for pediatric glaucoma, many of which have a genetic underpinning.
- Often glaucoma accompanies other ocular or systemic abnormalities that also affect the child, and sometimes directly cause the glaucoma.
- The infant and young child with glaucoma experience consequences of high IOP and its effects on the expansile globe, while all children share the ultimate threat of optic nerve damage and visual loss from this disease.
- Recognizing the features of glaucoma unique to early childhood is critical to rapid diagnosis and effective treatment of most cases of PCG, as well as all types of glaucoma with early onset.
- Managing the young child with suspected or confirmed glaucoma includes familiar techniques such as tonometry and optic nerve examination, medical and surgical treatment modalities, and diligence to treat nonglaucomatous visual loss due to amblyopia and refractive issues.
- Successful care of the pediatric glaucoma patient requires a team approach including the ophthalmologist, family, patient, and members of the school and community.

REFERENCES

1. Papadopoulos M, Cable N, Rahi J, et al. The British Infantile and Childhood Glaucoma (BIG) Eye Study. *Invest Ophthalmol Vis Sci.* 2007;48(9): 4100–4106.
2. Idrees F, Vaideanu D, Fraser SG, et al. A review of anterior segment dysgeneses. *Surv Ophthalmol.* 2006;51(3):213–231.
3. DeLuise VP, Anderson DR. Primary infantile glaucoma (congenital glaucoma). *Surv Ophthalmol.* 1983;28(1):1–19.
4. Angell LK, Robb RM, Berson FG. Visual prognosis in patients with ruptures in Descemet's membrane due to forceps injuries. *Arch Ophthalmol.* 1981;99(12):2137–2139.
5. Raab EL. Congenital glaucoma. *Persp Ophthalmol.* 1978;2:35–41.
6. Donahue SP, Porter A. SITA visual field testing in children. *J AAPOS.* 2001;5(2):114–117.
7. Becker K, Semes L. The reliability of frequency-doubling technology (FDT) perimetry in a pediatric population. *Optometry.* 2003;74(3): 173–179.
8. Burnstein Y, Ellish NJ, Magbalon M, et al. Comparison of frequency doubling perimetry with humphrey visual field analysis in a glaucoma practice. *Am J Ophthalmol.* 2000;129(3):328–333.
9. Kiskis AA, Markowitz SN, Morin JD. Corneal diameter and axial length in congenital glaucoma. *Can J Ophthalmol.* 1985;20(3):93–97.
10. Becker B, Shaffer RN. *Diagnosis and therapy of the glaucomas.* St. Louis: CV Mosby; 1965.
11. Sampaolesi R, Caruso R. Ocular echometry in the diagnosis of congenital glaucoma. *Arch Ophthalmol.* 1982;100(4):574–577.
12. Minckler DS, Baerveldt G, Heuer DK, et al. Clinical evaluation of the Oculab Tono-Pen. *Am J Ophthalmol.* 1987;104(2):168–173.
13. Van Buskirk EM, Palmer EA. Office assessment of young children for glaucoma. *Ann Ophthalmol.* 1979;11(11):1749–1751.
14. Mendelsohn AD, Forster RK, Mendelsohn SL, et al. Comparative tonometric measurements of eye bank eyes. *Cornea.* 1987;6(3):219–225.
15. Armstrong TA. Evaluation of the Tono-Pen and the Pulsair tonometers. *Am J Ophthalmol.* 1990;109(6):716–720.
16. Sahin A, Basmak H, Niyaz L, et al. Reproducibility and tolerability of the ICare rebound tonometer in school children. *J Glaucoma.* 2007;16(2): 185–188.
17. Pensiero S, Da Pozzo S, Perissutti P, et al. Normal intraocular pressure in children. *J Pediatr Ophthalmol Strabismus.* 1992;29(2):79–84.
18. Murphy DF. Anesthesia and intraocular pressure. *Anesth Analg.* 1985; 64(5):520–530.
19. Watcha MF, Chu FC, Stevens JL, et al. Effects of halothane on intraocular pressure in anesthetized children. *Anesth Analg.* 1990;71(2):181–184.
20. Dominguez A, Banos S, Alvarez G, et al. Intraocular pressure measurement in infants under general anesthesia. *Am J Ophthalmol.* 1974;78(1): 110–116.
21. Ausinsch B, Rayburn RL, Munson ES, et al. Ketamine and intraocular pressure in children. *Anesth Analg.* 1976;55(6):773–775.
22. Blumberg D, Congdon N, Jampel H, et al. The effects of sevoflurane and ketamine on intraocular pressure in children during examination under anesthesia. *Am J Ophthalmol.* 2007;143(3):494–499.
23. Jaafar MS, Kazi GA. Effect of oral chloral hydrate sedation on the intraocular pressure measurement. *J Pediatr Ophthalmol Strabismus.* 1993;30(6):372–376.
24. Wenzel M, Krippendorff U, Hunold W, et al. Corneal endothelial damage in congenital and juvenile glaucoma [in German]. *Klin Monatsbl Augenheilkd.* 1989;195(6):344–348.
25. Walton DS. Primary congenital open angle glaucoma: a study of the anterior segment abnormalities. *Trans Am Ophthalmol Soc.* 1979;77:746–768.
26. Walton DS. Diagnosis and treatment of glaucoma in childhood. In: Epstein DL, ed. *Chandler and Grant's Glaucoma.* 3rd ed. Philadelphia, PA: Lea & Febiger; 1986.
27. Khodadoust AA, Ziai M, Biggs SL. Optic disc in normal newborns. *Am J Ophthalmol.* 1968;66(3):502–504.
28. Robin AL, Quigley HA, Pollack IP, et al. An analysis of visual acuity, visual fields, and disk cupping in childhood glaucoma. *Am J Ophthalmol.* 1979;88(5):847–858.
29. Spierer A, Huna R, Hirsh A, et al. Normal intraocular pressure in premature infants. *Am J Ophthalmol.* 1994;117(6):801–803.
30. Radtke ND, Cohan BE. Intraocular pressure measurement in the newborn. *Am J Ophthalmol.* 1974;78(3):501–504.
31. Shaffer RN, Hetherington J Jr. The glaucomatous disc in infants. A suggested hypothesis for disc cupping. *Trans Am Acad Ophthalmol Otolaryngol.* 1969;73(5):923–935.
32. Quigley HA. The pathogenesis of reversible cupping in congenital glaucoma. *Am J Ophthalmol.* 1977;84(3):358–370.
33. Quigley HA. Childhood glaucoma: results with trabeculotomy and study of reversible cupping. *Ophthalmology.* 1982;89(3):219–226.
34. Robin AL, Quigley HA. Transient reversible cupping in juvenile-onset glaucoma. *Am J Ophthalmol.* 1979;88(3 pt 2):580–584.
35. Lotufo D, Ritch R, Szmyd L Jr, et al. Juvenile glaucoma, race, and refraction. *JAMA.* 1989;261(2):249–252.
36. Argus WA. Ocular hypertension and central corneal thickness. *Ophthalmology.* 1995;102(12):1810–1812.
37. Herndon LW, Choudhri SA, Cox T, et al. Central corneal thickness in normal, glaucomatous, and ocular hypertensive eyes. *Arch Ophthalmol.* 1997;115(9):1137–1141.
38. Brandt JD. Central corneal thickness—tonometry artifact, or something more? *Ophthalmology.* 2007;114(11):1963–1964.
39. Leske MC, Heijl A, Hyman L, et al. Predictors of long-term progression in the early manifest glaucoma trial. *Ophthalmology.* 2007;114(11): 1965–1972.
40. Dai E, Gunderson CA. Pediatric central corneal thickness variation among major ethnic populations. *J AAPOS.* 2006;10(1):22–25.
41. Henriques MJ, Vessani RM, Reis FA, et al. Corneal thickness in congenital glaucoma. *J Glaucoma.* 2004;13(3):185–188.
42. Hussein MA, Paysse EA, Bell NP, et al. Corneal thickness in children. *Am J Ophthalmol.* 2004;138(5):744–748.
43. Muir KW, Jin J, Freedman SF. Central corneal thickness and its relationship to intraocular pressure in children. *Ophthalmology.* 2004;111(12): 2220–2223.
44. Herse P, Yao W. Variation of corneal thickness with age in young New Zealanders. *Acta Ophthalmol.* 1993;71(3):360–364.

45. Ehlers N, Sorensen T, Bramsen T, et al. Central corneal thickness in newborns and children. *Acta Ophthalmol.* 1976;54(3):285–290.
46. Copt RP, Thomas R, Mermoud A. Corneal thickness in ocular hypertension, primary open-angle glaucoma, and normal tension glaucoma. *Arch Ophthalmol.* 1999;117(1):14–16.
47. Muir KW, Duncan L, Enyedi LB, et al. Central corneal thickness in children: stability over time. *Am J Ophthalmol.* 2006;141(5):955–957.
48. Brandt JD, Casuso LA, Budenz DL. Markedly increased central corneal thickness: an unrecognized finding in congenital aniridia. *Am J Ophthalmol.* 2004;137(2):348–350.
49. Muir KW, Duncan L, Enyedi LB, et al. Central corneal thickness: congenital cataracts and aphakia. *Am J Ophthalmol.* 2007;144(4):502–506.
50. Simon JW, O'Malley MR, Gandham SB, et al. Central corneal thickness and glaucoma in aphakic and pseudophakic children. *J AAPOS.* 2005;9(4):326–329.
51. Simsek T, Mutluay AH, Elgin U, et al. Glaucoma and increased central corneal thickness in aphakic and pseudophakic patients after congenital cataract surgery. *Br J Ophthalmol.* 2006;90(9):1103–1106.
52. Tai TY, Mills MD, Beck AD, et al. Central corneal thickness and corneal diameter in patients with childhood glaucoma. *J Glaucoma.* 2006;15(6):524–528.
53. Ahn HC, Son HW, Kim JS, et al. Quantitative analysis of retinal nerve fiber layer thickness of normal children and adolescents. *Korean J Ophthalmol.* 2005;19(3):195–200.
54. Hess DB, Asrani SG, Bhide MG, et al. Macular and retinal nerve fiber layer analysis of normal and glaucomatous eyes in children using optical coherence tomography. *Am J Ophthalmol.* 2005;139(3):509–517.
55. Salchow DJ, Oleynikov YS, Chiang MF, et al. Retinal nerve fiber layer thickness in normal children measured with optical coherence tomography. *Ophthalmology.* 2006;113(5):786–791.
56. El-Dairi MA, Holgado S, Asrani SG, et al. Correlation between optical coherence tomography and glaucomatous optic nerve head damage in children. *Br J Ophthalmol.* 2009;93(10):1325–1330.
57. Mrugacz M, Bakunowicz-Lazarczyk A. Optical coherence tomography measurement of the retinal nerve fiber layer in normal and juvenile glaucomatous eyes. *Ophthalmologica.* 2005;219(2):80–85.
58. Scott AW, Farsiu S, Enyedi LB, et al. Imaging the infant retina with a hand-held spectral-domain optical coherence tomography device. *Am J Ophthalmol.* 2009;147(2):364–373.

14

Childhood Glaucomas: Clinical Presentation

Childhood glaucomas constitute a heterogenous group of disorders affecting the pediatric age-group. The previous chapter (Chapter 13) considered the general classification of these diseases, and provided a general approach to the infant or child with glaucoma. In this chapter, we highlight important features of the more common types of primary, and a few of the secondary, pediatric glaucomas, with attention to those features specific to children (since some of the secondary glaucomas also affect adults) (Table 13.1). Recall that the primary pediatric glaucomas can be broadly divided into (a) those with an isolated aqueous outflow abnormality and (b) those with associated ocular abnormalities, systemic abnormalities, or both. The former group can be further divided into (a) those presenting in the first 3 years of life (primary congenital/infantile glaucoma [PCG]) and (b) those presenting after that period but before adulthood (juvenile open-angle glaucoma [JOAG]). The latter group, often termed developmental glaucomas, comprises many different disorders, a few of which will be included in more detail in this chapter.

The secondary pediatric glaucomas are caused by a preceding process in the eye, and many are common to both adults and children, although some seem specific to children (such as glaucoma after removal of congenital cataracts). In addition, the mechanism of glaucoma in selected developmental cases (see Table 13.1) may be secondary rather than strictly primary.

PRIMARY CONGENITAL GLAUCOMAS

Classification

When they occur without a consistent association with other ocular or systemic anomalies (in other words, they seem primary), congenital glaucomas have traditionally been called PCG or primary congenital open-angle glaucoma (1). In this chapter, we will refrain from referring to other birth- or infancy-onset childhood glaucomas as PCG unless the outflow pathway defect and resultant elevated intraocular pressure (IOP) occur in apparent isolation. Newborn glaucoma, the most severe form of PCG, is apparent at birth, whereas infantile glaucoma refers to cases of PCG with clinical onset after birth but in the first 3 years of life (2). In general, the terms PCG and primary infantile glaucoma may be used interchangeably. Although PCG has also been called buphthalmos (i.e., cow's eye) or hydrophthalmia, referring to the enlargement of the eye that may occur with this condition (3), these terms should not be used as synonyms for PCG because enlargement of the globe is seen with other childhood glaucomas if they occur early enough in life.

Primary congenital glaucoma has also been referred to as isolated trabeculodysgenesis or goniodysgenesis, to indicate that the iris and cornea are morphologically normal. Newborn glaucoma, a severe variant of PCG present at birth, is also considered by some as iridotrabeculodysgenesis (Table 13.1). PCG can therefore be considered as one form of anterior segment dysgenesis.

When primary glaucoma appears later in childhood or early adulthood, it is sometimes referred to as juvenile glaucoma (also JOAG) (4). Three years of age is generally taken as the division between PCG and JOAG, because it is at approximately this age that the eye no longer expands in response to elevated IOP (1,4). Others prefer a broader definition for juvenile glaucoma that includes all forms of open-angle glaucoma diagnosed between the ages of 10 and 35 years (5) (see JOAG, Chapter 11).

General Features

Demographic Features

The most common of the primary pediatric glaucomas, PCG has an estimated incidence of 1 in 10,000 to 20,000 live births in Western countries, while it presents more frequently in the Middle East and among the Roma population of Slovakia, where parental consanguinity may play a role in the increased incidence (6). Lacking clear sex or racial–ethnic predilection (except where consanguinity or small population may play a role), most PCG cases (65% to 80%) are bilateral, and greater than 75% present in the first year of life. About 25% of patients with PCG present initially as newborns, and more than 60% of PCG diagnoses are made in infants younger than 6 months of age (7). Nonetheless, this condition occurs much less frequently than the open-angle and angle-closure glaucomas seen in adults, and it has been estimated that the average ophthalmic practice encounters one new case of congenital glaucoma every 5 years.

Heredity

PCG occurs in both sporadic and familial patterns. Inheritance is usually autosomal recessive in familial cases, and hence, there is increased incidence with consanguinity. Three genetic loci—GLC3A, GLC3B, and GLC3C (Table 8.1)—have been identified by linkage analysis in large pedigrees with multiple affected individuals (8,9). The presence of additional loci has also been suggested (10). Thus far, two main causative genes have been reported—the *CYP1B1* gene, on the GLC3A locus, and the *LTBP2* gene, possibly on the GLC3C locus (9–12). The *MYOC* gene has also been implicated in rare cases of PCG (13–15).

The *CYP1B1* gene (Online Mendelian Inheritance in Man [OMIM] number, 601771) was the first reported PCG-causing gene (9,16). It is located on chromosome 2p22–p21 on the GLC3A locus. It belongs to the cytochrome P450 superfamily of enzymes and oxidizes several compounds important to eye structure and function, including steroids, retinoids, arachidonate, and melatonin (17–22). The *CYP1B1* enzyme is thought to participate in the metabolism of an unknown molecule that is important to eye development and therefore plays an important role in the development of PCG. Studies have demonstrated its expression in fetal and adult ciliary body and neuroepithelium (23). Since the *CYP1B1* gene's discovery, many PCG cohorts have been screened for *CYP1B1* sequence variants. Several *CYP1B1* sequence variants have been determined to cause PCG (24). The proportion of PCG patients whose disease is due to *CYP1B1* mutations varies with ethnicity, ranging from 100% in the Roma population of Slovakia to 20% in Japan (25,26).

The *MYOC* gene (OMIM 601652) has been associated with juvenile and adult forms of open-angle glaucoma and a few rare cases of PCG (13,15,16). It is located on chromosome 1q24.3–q25.2 (27). MYOC or myocilin is also known as trabecular meshwork–induced glucocorticoid-response protein (TIGR). As its name implies, treatment of trabecular meshwork cells with glucocorticoids results in the induction of MYOC (28). It is speculated that MYOC obstructs trabecular meshwork outflow and thus causes increased IOP (27). Increased IOP may also be caused by changes in the ciliary body secondary to MYOC. Studies have revealed expression of *MYOC* in both the trabecular meshwork and ciliary body (29). Disease-causing *MYOC* sequence variants, both with and without *CYP1B1* alterations, have been reported in families with early-onset open-angle glaucoma, including PCG (13–15).

LTBP2 (OMIM 602091) is the most recent gene to be associated with PCG (11,12,16). LTBP2, or latent transforming growth factor beta binding protein 2, is located on chromosome 14q24 (30). Its location is 1.5 Mb from the GLC3C locus. Whether LTBP2 and GLC3C represent the same genetic component remains to be determined. In nonocular tissues, *LTBP2* functions in tissue repair and cell adhesion (31–34). The role *LTBP2* plays in PCG is still unknown. Ocular expression of *LTBP2* has been demonstrated in the trabecular meshwork and ciliary processes (35). Null mutations of *LTBP2* have been found in consanguineous Pakistani and Iranian families, as well as Slovakian Roma, with PCG (11,12).

All siblings of any child with PCG (or early-onset JOAG) should be examined carefully; infants should be followed up closely, especially during the first year of life, to exclude this disease. A discussion of the risk of having additional children with PCG should be carried out with parents, either with the ophthalmologist or a genetic counselor.

Clinical Features

PCG is bilateral in 65% to 80% of cases (3,36), although a significant IOP elevation may occur in only one eye in 25% to 30% of the cases. Several ocular features, with the possible exception of gonioscopic findings, are not unique to the PCG, but they may be a part of any childhood glaucoma during the

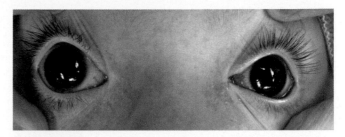

Figure 14.1 Infantile glaucoma, with asymmetric involvement. Note marked enlargement of the right, compared with the left, cornea. The IOP was higher in the right eye, where multiple Haab striae and corneal edema were present.

first few years of life. The neonatal globe is distensible and often greatly enlarges with exposure to elevated IOP. Stretching of the infant eye is not limited to the cornea and may involve the anterior chamber angle structures, sclera, optic nerve, scleral canal, and lamina cribrosa (7) (see also Chapter 13).

History

Infants with PCG usually present for ophthalmologic evaluation because the pediatrician or the parents have noticed something unusual about the appearance of the patient's eyes or behavior. Often, corneal opacification and enlargement (resulting from elevated IOP) are the signs that signal glaucoma in the infant (**Figs. 14.1, 13.2,** and **14.2**). In other cases, the child's glaucoma manifests as one or more of the classic triad of findings, any one of which should arouse suspicion of glaucoma in an infant or young child: (a) epiphora (i.e., excessive tearing); (b) photophobia (i.e., hypersensitivity to light), which results from corneal edema and is manifested by the child hiding his or her face in bright lighting or even in ordinary lighting in severe cases; and (c) blepharospasm (i.e., squeezing the eyelids), which may be another manifestation of photophobia.

The severity of presenting signs and symptoms varies among infants with PCG, probably because of differences in

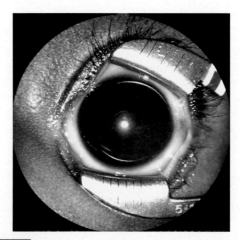

Figure 14.2 Corneal edema with a central Haab striae in the eye of a 5-month-old infant girl with PCG. IOP was 28 mm Hg on maximal tolerated medications at examination under anesthesia, several weeks after trabeculotomy was performed from the temporal limbus. Further angle surgery was planned. (See also Fig. 13.2.)

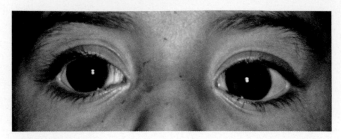

Figure 14.3 A child whose diagnosis of congenital glaucoma was delayed until 2.5 years of age. Corneal diameters were 15 mm OU. The IOP was 40 mm Hg, and the optic nerves showed total cupping; best vision was less than 20/400 OU. IOP control was achieved by using goniotomy and medications for 6 years; the patient then required trabeculectomy with use of mitomycin C for glaucoma control.

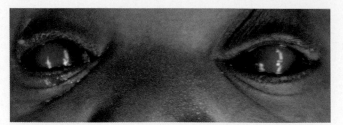

Figure 14.4 Newborn-onset congenital glaucoma with severe bilateral corneal edema and opacification. Despite IOP reduction after surgery, central corneal opacification did not clear completely.

the magnitude and duration of the IOP elevation. For example, newborn infants presenting with enlarged, very cloudy corneas presumably had elevated IOP in utero, whereas those with milder signs and symptoms might have experienced the IOP elevation beginning sometime after birth. Parents and healthcare providers have occasionally failed to recognize glaucoma in infants with clear but enlarged corneas (37) (**Fig. 14.3**). Some bilateral cases may manifest with such asymmetric signs and symptoms that glaucoma is initially suspected only in the more severely affected eye. In children with glaucoma onset after 1 year of age, fewer overt signs and symptoms may occur because of the decreased expansibility of the eye.

External Examination

The infant with PCG presents as an otherwise healthy child, without any systemic or facial features to suggest a different diagnosis. Often the examiner notes that the child is unusually photophobic and fussy, and parents frequently relate a history of eye rubbing.

Corneal Features

Corneal Diameter

The healthy newborn's cornea has a horizontal diameter ranging from 9.5 to 10.5 mm, which enlarges about 0.5 to 1.0 mm in the first year of life (38–40) (Table 13.2). Distention of the globe in response to elevated IOP (buphthalmos) leads to additional enlargement of the cornea, especially at the corneoscleral junction. A corneal diameter larger than 12 mm in the first year of life is a highly suspect finding. Asymmetry in diameter between the two corneas or a corneal diameter of 13 mm or more at any age strongly suggests abnormality (7). Corneal enlargement is more obvious in asymmetric cases (Fig. 14.1). In one study, corneal diameter was found to be a more reliable guide than axial length in the assessment of congenital glaucoma (38).

Corneal Edema

Initially, corneal edema may be a direct result of the elevated IOP, producing a corneal haze that clears with normalization of the pressure. Often, there are underlying breaks in the

Descemet membrane (Haab striae) that occur as the cornea stretches because of elevated IOP. These often appear acutely as areas of increased corneal edema and clouding; clinical onset may take only a matter of hours (7) (see Slitlamp section). In more advanced cases, a dense opacification of the corneal stroma may persist despite reduction of the IOP (**Fig. 14.4**). Results of one study suggest that the latter may result from reduced aqueous production with poor corneal nutrition (41).

Refractive Error

The enlargement of the globe with elevated IOP in the first 3 years of life creates a myopic shift in the refractive error, which may lead to amblyopia if significant anisometropia is present. The presence of Haab striae often produces significant astigmatism, which also contributes to amblyopia, especially in unilateral or asymmetric cases. Children between 3 and 10 years of age with elevated IOP may develop progressive myopia and astigmatism, despite a stable corneal diameter. These refractive changes have been attributed to continued scleral stretching (7).

Tonometry

Measurement of the IOP in an infant or child suspected of having PCG should ideally be performed in the office, with the child as calm as possible. Useful handheld devices include the Perkins, Tono-Pen, and ICare tonometers, while the cooperative patient older than about 3 years (and without nystagmus) can often sit for Goldmann applanation. It is important to avoid traumatizing a child to obtain the IOP, because tonometry performed in a struggling child will invariably produce falsely elevated readings, which will be useless in diagnosing PCG or assessing control of known PCG. Infants with PCG commonly present with unanesthetized IOPs in the range of 30 to 40 mm Hg, although occasionally values above or below this range occur (42). Target pressures for children with PCG depend entirely on the details of the particular case; while IOPs in the low 20-mm Hg range may be adequate for a child with healthy optic nerves and stable refraction, others with more severe disease may progress at these same IOPs and require lower target IOP (see also Chapters 13 and 40).

Measuring the IOP under anesthesia is sometimes necessary, but should be coupled with an assessment of the overall status of the eye (or eyes), together with subsequent surgical intervention when necessary. When the IOP in infants and young children is measured during general anesthesia, the possible influence of the anesthesia on IOP must be considered (see Table 13.4), with the IOP measurement taken as soon as the airway is secure. A pressure of 20 mm Hg or greater should arouse suspicion (43). In cases of unilateral PCG, asymmetry of IOP measured under anesthesia may be very helpful, even if the true IOP has been altered in this setting.

Slitlamp Examination

This portion of the examination is best performed with a portable slitlamp, with or without general anesthesia. Tears in the Descemet membrane (i.e., Haab striae) are classic findings of PCG; they may be single or multiple, and are characteristically oriented horizontally or concentric to the limbus (**Fig. 14.5**). They are typically associated with corneal edema in the early phases of glaucoma. Haab striae are found in about 25% of eyes with a diagnosis of PCG at birth and in more than

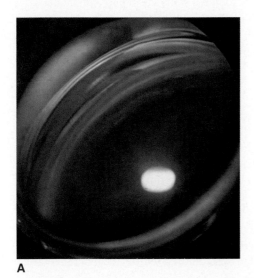

A

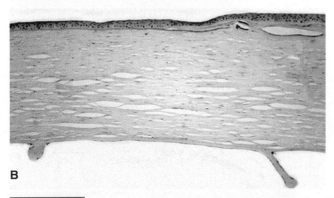

B

Figure 14.5 **A:** Haab striae in the peripheral cornea of a 10-year-old child with congenital glaucoma. IOP was controlled with angle surgery and medications, but the scar remains. (See also Figs. 13.5 and 13.6.) **B:** Healed breaks in Descemet membrane (Haab striae) are seen in the cornea with congenital glaucoma. The Bowman layer contains basophilic deposits (band keratopathy) as a degenerative change (stain, hematoxylin–eosin). (From Milman T. Congenital anomalies. In: Tasman W, Jaeger EA, eds. *Duane's Foundations of Clinical Ophthalmology.* Vol. 3. Philadelphia, PA: Lippincott Williams & Wilkins; 2008:chap 2.)

60% of those with that diagnosis at 6 months of age (44). These Haab striae remain as a testament to the early onset of the IOP elevation, even in late-diagnosed cases, or those rare cases with spontaneous resolution of the IOP elevation. As the IOP is normalized and the tears are repaired by endothelial overgrowth, the corneal edema may clear, but the linear opacities persist. Specular microscopy has shown that these patients also have a significantly reduced corneal endothelial cell count.

The anterior chamber is characteristically deep, especially when the globe is distended. The iris is typically normal, although it may have stromal hypoplasia with loss of the crypts.

Gonioscopy

Evaluation of the anterior chamber angle is essential for the accurate diagnosis of PCG. (The instruments and techniques of gonioscopy are discussed in Chapter 3.) In performing gonioscopy on infants and children under anesthesia, an infant Koeppe goniolens is recommended, together with a portable slitlamp for illumination and magnification. (See Chapter 13 for description of normal childhood gonioscopy findings.)

The anterior chamber angle has a characteristic, although slightly variable, appearance in PCG (**Fig. 14.6**). Usually, the iris has an insertion more anterior than that of the healthy infant, with altered translucency of the angle face rendering rather indistinct ciliary body band, trabecular mesh, and scleral spur. This translucent tissue has historically been referred to as Barkan membrane (45,46). The scalloped border of the iris pigment epithelium and the trabecular meshwork itself, often prominent in PCG, may appear through the translucent peripheral iris stroma as if viewed through a morning mist.

Although the angle is usually avascular, loops of vessels from the major arterial circle may be seen above the iris root, which has been called the Loch Ness monster phenomenon (45). The clinical features of PCG seem to merge with other forms of developmental glaucoma. A gonioscopic assessment of more than 100 eyes with developmental glaucoma revealed a spectrum ranging from the common form described earlier, through a more cicatrized, vascularized condition, to the gross anomalies of the Axenfeld–Rieger syndrome (47).

Funduscopy

Evaluation of the optic nerve head is one of the most important methods for diagnosing PCG and for assessing the response to therapy. This is usually done with the child anesthetized or sedated, often with an undilated pupil, in which case visualization of the disc may be facilitated by using a direct ophthalmoscope with a Koeppe gonioscopy lens on the cornea or a lens designed for vitrectomy surgery (48).

Cupping of the optic nerve head proceeds more rapidly in infants than in adults and is more likely to be reversible if the pressure is lowered early enough (49–56).

Significant optic nerve cup size and asymmetry of cupping between fellow eyes suggest, but do not confirm, glaucoma in an infant. The cup-to-disc ratio exceeded 0.3 in 68% of 126 eyes with PCG examined by Shaffer and Hetherington (53), but did so in only 2.6% of 936 healthy newborn eyes examined by Richardson (57). Marked optic cup asymmetry was observed

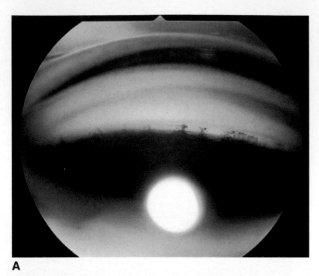

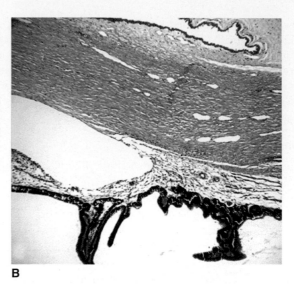

A

B

Figure 14.6 **A:** Gonioscopic appearance of infantile glaucoma. Note the relatively high iris insertion, with indistinct angle landmarks and fine iris processes. The angle appears wider on the right side of the photograph, at the site of prior goniotomy surgery. **B:** Fetal angle manifests anterior insertion of the iris root and anterior displacement of the ciliary processes. The scleral spur is poorly developed. Trabecular meshwork and Schlemm canal are poorly defined; mesenchymal tissue is present in the anterior chamber angle. (From Milman T. Congenital anomalies. In: Tasman W, Jaeger EA, eds. *Duane's Foundations of Clinical Ophthalmology.* Vol. 3. Philadelphia, PA: Lippincott Williams & Wilkins; 2008:chap 2.)

in only 0.6% of healthy eyes in the latter study, in contrast to 89% for infants with monocular glaucoma.

Visual Fields

When tested after the child becomes old enough for a reliable study (typically about 8 to 9 years of age for a child without cognitive impairment and nystagmus), the visual fields are similar to those in adult-onset glaucoma, with an initial predilection for loss in the arcuate areas (56).

Visual Acuity

Good vision may be achieved if the IOP is controlled before optic atrophy occurs. Occasionally, however, the acuity is poor despite adequate pressure control. In some cases, this is caused by optic nerve damage, corneal opacity from breaks in the Descemet membrane or persistent stromal haze, or irregular astigmatism (44,58). Other children may have normal-appearing optic nerve heads and clear media but develop amblyopia from anisometropia or strabismus (59). Retinal detachment is also an occasional cause of poor visual results (60).

Ultrasonography

Ultrasonography may be helpful in documenting progression of infantile glaucoma by recording changes in the axial length of the globe (40,61,62). It has also been reported that the axial length may decrease by as much as 0.8 mm after surgical reduction of the IOP (62). This change in axial length may be evident within days after a significant IOP reduction, especially in aphakic eyes of infants after filtration surgery or implantation of a glaucoma drainage device (Freedman SF, personal experience). Ultrasonography may also be helpful when glaucoma drainage-device surgery is being contemplated, because the size

of the proposed implant reservoir may be limited by the globe size (see Chapter 40). After such surgery, ultrasonography can be helpful in confirming the presence of fluid around the device's reservoir, especially in patients in whom the bleb cannot easily be visualized in the office setting (**Fig. 14.7**).

Other Testing Techniques

Corneal pachymetry to measure central corneal thickness may prove useful after corneal edema has cleared, to help set a target IOP for a particular eye. Children with PCG generally have a

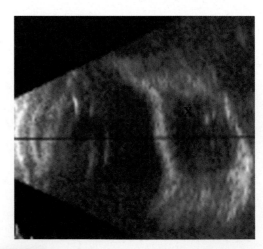

Figure 14.7 In an eye with a functional Ahmed glaucoma drainage device, B-scan ultrasonography reveals fluid-filled space surrounding the implant reservoir in the superotemporal quadrant (indicated by an *x*), indenting the sclera. In the office setting, the bleb was difficult to visualize but its presence was confirmed easily by using ultrasonography.

relatively low central corneal thickness, presumably because of the enlargement of their corneas in early infancy (63) (see Chapter 13). Care should be taken not to "adjust" the measured IOP based on central corneal thickness readings, but rather to guide the determination of the eye's target IOP.

Other technologies, such as optical coherence tomography (OCT) (64) (Chapter 4), may prove useful in assessing nerve fiber layer loss in children too young to perform reliable visual field testing.

Etiology

Normal Development of the Anterior Ocular Segment

A basic understanding of the normal development of the anterior ocular segment is necessary before considering the theories of mechanism for congenital glaucoma or for any of the developmental glaucomas with associated anomalies.

General Development

The lens vesicle begins to develop as an invagination of surface ectoderm during the third week of gestation and separates from the latter structure by the sixth week (65). A study of 53 human embryos showed that the adhesion between the lens vesicle and presumptive corneal epithelium at the 8-mm stage is replaced by a "clear zone" at the 12.5-mm stage (66). The same study suggested that the formation of the eye is influenced by signals from neural and pigmented layers and that the lens, with its relatively large size and high mitosis, participates in the early embryogenesis of the rudimentary anterior chamber.

At the same time that the lens vesicle is separating from surface ectoderm, the optic cup, which arises from neural ectoderm, has reached the periphery of the lens, and a triangular mass of undifferentiated cells overrides the rim of the cup and surrounds the anterior periphery of the lens. From this tissue mass will arise portions of the cornea, iris, and the anterior chamber angle structures.

Neural Crest Cell Contribution

The undifferentiated cell mass destined to become the cornea, iris, and anterior chamber angle was originally thought to be derived from mesoderm. Subsequent studies, however, indicated that the tissue is of cranial neural crest cell origin. Johnston and colleagues (67) studied orofacial development in chick embryos. By using these models, it was determined that corneal endothelium and the stroma, iris, ciliary body, and sclera are of neural crest origin, except for the associated vascular endothelium, which is derived from mesodermal mesenchyme. Immunohistochemical studies have provided support for the concept that cells of human trabecular meshwork are also of neural crest origin by showing evidence of neuronal cell–specific enolase (68,69). These cells were found in the anterior region of the meshwork and in the inner uveal beams (68,69), whereas the cells lining the Schlemm canal were found to share many immunophenotypical features with vascular endothelial cells (69).

Development of Cornea and Iris

From the mass of undifferentiated cells, three waves of tissue come forward between the surface ectoderm and lens. The first of these layers differentiates into the primordial corneal endothelium by the eighth week and subsequently produces Descemet membrane, and the second wave grows between the corneal endothelium and epithelium to produce the stroma of the cornea (70,71). The third wave insinuates between the primordia of the cornea and the lens and gives rise to the pupillary membrane and the stroma of the iris. In later months, the pigment epithelial layer of the iris develops from neural ectoderm.

Development of Anterior Chamber Angle

The aqueous outflow structures in the anterior chamber angle appear to arise from the mesenchymal mass of neural crest cell origin. The precise details of this development are not fully understood. Theories have included atrophy or resorption (i.e., progressive disappearance of portions of fetal tissue), cleavage (i.e., separation of two pre-existing tissue layers due to differential growth rates), and rarefaction (i.e., mechanical distention due to growth of the anterior ocular segment) (46,65,72,73). Subsequent work suggests that none of these concepts is completely correct.

Anderson (74) studied 40 healthy fetal and infant eyes by light and electron microscopy and found that the anterior surface of the iris at 5 months' gestation inserts at the edge of the corneal endothelium, covering the cells that are destined to become trabecular meshwork. This appears to be what Worst (45) called the fetal pectinate ligament, separating the corneoscleral meshwork primordium from the anterior chamber angle. Anderson observed a posterior repositioning of the anterior uveal structures in relation to the cornea and sclera in progressively older tissue specimens, presumably because of the differential growth rates. At birth, the insertion of the iris and ciliary body is near the level of the scleral spur, and the posterior migration of these structures continues for about the first year of life.

There is some difference of interpretation regarding the innermost layer of the trabecular meshwork primordium, as it is uncovered by the posteriorly receding iris. Anderson (74) thought that the smooth surface represents multilayered mesenchymal tissue, which begins to cavitate by the seventh fetal month. Others have suggested that a true endothelial layer covers the meshwork during gestation (45,75). Hansson and Jerndal (75) observed that the anterior chamber angle portion of the endothelial layer begins to flatten, with loss of clear-cut cell borders, by the seventh fetal month. During the final weeks of gestation and the first weeks after birth, the endothelial layer undergoes fenestration with migration of cells into the underlying uveal meshwork. Van Buskirk (76) observed a similar endothelial layer and its progressive fenestration in macaque monkey eyes. He noticed that fenestration and gradual retraction of this tissue occurred in the third trimester and progressed in a posterior-to-anterior direction. McMenamin (77), however, in a scanning electron microscopic study of 32 human fetal eyes, found that the endothelial layer in the iridocorneal angle was perforated by discrete intercellular gaps by 12 to 14 weeks and that the gaps between the inner uveal trabecular

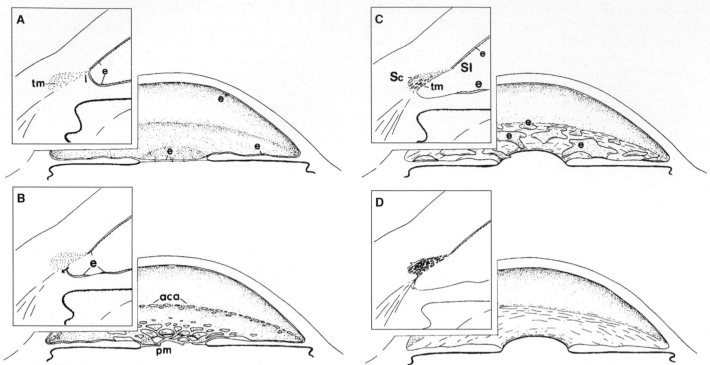

Figure 14.8 A concept of anterior chamber angle development (*insets* show cross-sectional views of the chamber angle). **A:** At 5 months' gestation, a continuous layer of endothelium (*e*) creates a closed cavity of the anterior chamber (according to most studies), and the anterior surface of the iris (*i*) inserts in front of the primordial trabecular meshwork (*tm*). **B:** In the third trimester, the endothelial layer progressively disappears from the pupillary membrane (*pm*) and iris and cavitates over the anterior chamber angle (*aca*), possibly becoming incorporated in the trabecular meshwork. At the same time, the peripheral uveal tissue begins to slide posteriorly in relation to the chamber angle structures (*arrow*). **C:** Development of the trabecular lamellae and intertrabecular spaces begins in the inner, posterior aspect of the primordial tissue and progresses toward the Schlemm canal (*Sc*) and Schwalbe line (*Sl*). **D:** The normal anterior chamber angle is not fully developed until 1 year of age. (From Shields MB. Axenfeld–Rieger syndrome: a theory of mechanism and distinctions from the iridocorneal endothelial syndrome. *Trans Am Ophthalmol Soc.* 1983;81:736, Republished with permission of the American Ophthalmological Society.)

endothelial cells were sufficiently developed by 18 to 20 weeks to allow a route of communication between the fetal anterior chamber and primitive trabecular tissue.

McMenamin (78) also showed, in light and electron microscopic studies of human fetal eyes between 12 and 22 weeks' gestation, that the trabecular anlage doubles in cross-sectional area, cell density decreases but the absolute number of cells increases twofold to threefold, extracellular matrix increases in a predictable fashion by 360%, and the intertrabecular spaces increase in a more variable manner by 200%. It appears that the trabecular meshwork develops by a simple process of growth and differentiation. These observations have been combined in a concept of anterior chamber angle development (79), which is depicted in **Figure 14.8**.

Theories of Abnormal Development in Congenital Glaucoma

Although it is generally agreed that the IOP elevation in congenital glaucoma is caused by an abnormal development of the anterior chamber angle that leads to obstruction of aqueous outflow, there is no universal agreement on the nature of the developmental alteration. Theories of pathogenesis parallel the

basic concepts regarding the normal development of the anterior chamber angle, most of which are no longer accepted as being entirely correct. We first review the major theories that have been proposed in the past and then consider how they fit with our current understanding of the developmental abnormality of congenital glaucoma.

In 1928, Mann (80) postulated that incomplete atrophy of anterior chamber mesoderm resulted in retention of abnormal tissue that blocked aqueous outflow. In 1955, Barkan (46) suggested that incomplete resorption of the mesodermal cells by adjacent tissue led to the formation of a membrane across the anterior chamber angle. This structure became known as the Barkan membrane, although its existence has not been proved histologically. Electron microscopic studies by Anderson (46,81) revealed no membrane, despite the appearance of such a structure by gonioscopy and the dissecting microscope. In 1955, Allen and colleagues (72) postulated that incomplete cleavage of mesoderm in the anterior chamber angle resulted in the congenital defect. In 1966, Worst (45) proposed a combined theory that included elements of the atrophy and resorption concepts but rejected the cleavage theory. However, all of the theories for normal development of the anterior chamber angle, on which each of the previous theories of pathogenesis was based, are no longer thought to be correct.

In 1959, Maumenee (82,83) observed an abnormal anterior insertion of the ciliary musculature into the trabecular meshwork and reasoned that this might compress the scleral spur forward and externally, narrowing the Schlemm canal. Anderson (74) and others (84) provided further histopathologic support for the high insertion of the anterior uvea into the trabecular meshwork, suggesting that it is caused by a developmental arrest in the normal migration of the uvea across the meshwork in the third trimester of gestation. Maumenee (83) also noticed the absence of Schlemm canal in some histopathologic specimens and suggested that this might be a cause of aqueous outflow obstruction in congenital glaucoma, although Anderson (81) thought it might be a secondary change.

In 1971, Smelser and Ozanics (73) explained congenital glaucoma as a failure of anterior chamber angle anlage to become properly rearranged into the normal trabecular meshwork. Subsequent light and electron microscopic studies favored this theory by showing structural changes of the uveal meshwork and, in some cases of infantile and juvenile glaucoma, a thick layer of amorphous material beneath the internal endothelium of the Schlemm canal (81,85–89). Kupfer and colleagues (90,91) emphasized the contribution of the cranial neural crest cells in the development of the anterior chamber angle and suggested that abnormal development of structures derived from these cells may result in the defects of the various forms of congenital glaucoma.

In summary, most forms of congenital glaucoma appear to result from a developmental arrest of anterior chamber angle tissue derived from neural crest cells, leading to aqueous outflow obstruction by one or more of several mechanisms. The high insertion of ciliary body and iris into the posterior portion of the trabecular meshwork may compress the trabecular beams. There may be primary developmental defects at various levels of the meshwork and, in some cases, the Schlemm canal. However, a true membrane over the meshwork does not appear to be a feature of this disorder.

Differential Diagnosis

Some of the clinical features of PCG are also found in other conditions, and these must be considered in the differential diagnosis (Table 13.2).

Excessive Tearing

In the infant, excessive tearing is most commonly caused by obstruction of the lacrimal drainage system. The epiphora of nasolacrimal duct obstruction is distinguished from that of PCG (or any infantile-onset glaucoma) in that the former condition may be associated with fullness of the lacrimal sac and often has a purulent discharge. The epiphora of PCG (and any infantile glaucoma) is frequently associated with photophobia and blepharospasm, although these three findings can also result from various external ocular disorders. Any of the several types of conjunctivitis in the infant may manifest with epiphora and a "red eye," but photophobia is usually absent. When epiphora,

photophobia, or blepharospasm accompanies a red eye, ocular inflammation (i.e., uveitis) and corneal injury or keratitis (e.g., abrasion, herpetic dendrite) should be considered.

Corneal Disorders

Large Corneas

Large corneas may represent congenital megalocornea without glaucoma or an enlarged globe due to high myopia. However, PCG (and any infantile-onset glaucoma) also typically causes progressive myopia resulting from enlargement of the globe. Infants with megalocornea often present with symmetrically enlarged, clear corneas with diameters larger than 14 mm, with deep anterior chambers, and with iridodonesis, but without elevated IOP or optic nerve cupping. Megalocornea is a rare, X-linked recessive disorder; families have been described in which some individuals have megalocornea alone, whereas others present with primary infantile glaucoma (58,92). A pedigree has been described with autosomal dominant megalocornea and congenital glaucoma in which the inheritance pattern is thought to represent germ-line mosaicism (93).

Eyes with axial myopia often show enlargement of the globe and cornea, but without elevated IOP; posterior segment examination usually demonstrates an oblique optic nerve head insertion and scleral crescent, often with suggestive chorioretinal findings. Any infant with corneal enlargement should be followed up over time for the development of elevated IOP.

Tears in Descemet Membrane

Tears in the Descemet membrane may result from forceps injury during birth (94). These tears are usually vertical or oblique, in contrast to those of congenital glaucoma (i.e., Haab striae) (Fig. 13.7), which tend to be horizontal or concentric with the limbus. Tears in the Descemet membrane may also be confused with band-like structures in posterior polymorphous dystrophy and posterior corneal vesicles (95,96). Haab striae may be distinguished from these disorders by thin, smooth areas between thickened, curled edges, contrasting with the central thickening in posterior polymorphous dystrophy and posterior corneal vesicles (95).

Corneal Opacification

Corneal opacification in infancy may be associated with various disorders (97): developmental anomalies (i.e., Peters anomaly and sclerocornea), dystrophies (i.e., congenital hereditary corneal dystrophy and posterior polymorphous dystrophy), choristomas (i.e., dermoid and dermis-like choristoma), edema due to birth trauma, intrauterine inflammation or keratitis (i.e., congenital syphilis, rubella, and herpetic infection), and inborn errors of metabolism (i.e., mucopolysaccharidoses [MPS] and cystinosis).

Other Glaucomas of Childhood

The differential diagnosis of PCG should include developmental glaucomas with associated anomalies and the childhood glaucomas associated with other ocular and systemic disorders (many of which are discussed later in this chapter).

Although other nonglaucomatous eye conditions may share one or more findings with PCG, care must be taken to rule out other types of childhood glaucoma in each of these cases. For example, glaucoma may complicate uveitis and has been reported in the setting of MPS; corneal dystrophy; congenital anomalies, such as Peters anomaly; and megalocornea. Glaucoma has occurred coincidentally with congenital nasolacrimal duct obstruction (98).

Management

Medical Therapy

Definitive treatment of PCG is surgical in nature, with medical therapy playing an adjunctive role. Preoperatively, medications may help clear the cornea to facilitate angle surgery (especially goniotomy), and postoperatively, they may help control IOP until the adequacy of the surgical procedure has been verified. Medical therapy is also indicated in managing difficult cases in which surgery poses life-threatening risks or has incompletely controlled the glaucoma (7). In general, the same basic principles of medical therapy apply to the treatment of PCG as to adult glaucomas. One possible exception is the use of miotics, which paradoxically may increase the IOP by collapse of the trabecular meshwork because of the high insertion of uveal tissue into the posterior meshwork. (Dosages for children and special precautions are discussed in Chapter 40.) Many obstacles conspire against the success of chronic medical therapy for PCG, including inadequate IOP control, difficulties with long-term adherence, and the potential adverse systemic effects of protracted therapy.

Surgical Therapy

The primary surgical techniques are designed to eliminate the resistance to aqueous outflow created by the structural abnormalities in the anterior chamber angle. This "angle surgery" may be achieved with incisional surgery, by using an internal (goniotomy) or external (trabeculotomy) approach. Some surgeons prefer to perform a combined angle and filtration surgery (i.e., trabeculotomy and trabeculectomy) as the initial procedure; others use this technique after initial angle surgery has failed; and still others always perform filtration surgery only after angle surgery has failed (99–101). This discussion is limited to the concepts of management. (Details of the operative procedures are considered in Chapter 40.)

Goniotomy

Barkan (102) described a technique in which abnormal tissue (originally thought to be Barkan membrane) is incised under direct visualization with the aid of a goniolens. It is now believed that the incision is not through a membrane, but rather through the inner portion of the trabecular meshwork. This presumably relieves the compressive traction of the anterior uvea on the meshwork and eliminates any resistance imposed by incompletely developed inner meshwork.

Trabeculotomy

Harms and Dannheim (103) described a technique in which the Schlemm canal is identified by external dissection, and the trabecular meshwork is incised by passing a probe into the canal and then rotating it into the anterior chamber. One advantage of this procedure is that it can be performed in eyes with cloudy corneas, whereas goniotomy surgery requires visualization of the angle. Although some surgeons use the technique only in cases with corneal opacification, or when multiple goniotomies have failed, others prefer it as the initial procedure in PCG. In a modification of the earlier techniques, the Schlemm canal is cannulated for its entire circumference with a suture or an illuminated endoscopic probe, and then the encircling suture or endoscope is pulled, achieving a 360-degree trabeculotomy (104) (see also Chapter 40).

Goniotomy and trabeculotomy each have their advocates, and reported success rates vary considerably, with neither procedure having clear-cut superiority. Although goniotomy spares conjunctival tissues for possible later surgery, trabeculotomy can proceed even when corneal opacity precludes an angle view. (A more detailed comparison of the two operations is presented in Chapter 40.) With both procedures, success is related to the severity and duration of the glaucoma. The worst prognosis occurs for infants with elevated pressures and cloudy corneas at birth (primary newborn glaucoma). The most favorable outcomes are seen in infants who undergo surgery between the second and eighth month of life (primary infantile glaucoma), and the surgery then becomes less effective with increasing age (105). One study of long-term surgical outcome after trabeculotomy divided 71 children into groups of congenital glaucoma (i.e., existing before 2 months of age), infantile glaucoma (i.e., occurring between 2 months and 2 years), and juvenile glaucoma (i.e., after 2 years) and reported success rates with one or more trabeculotomies of 60.3% ± 5.9%, 96.3% ± 3.6%, and 76.4% ± 7.5%, respectively (106). Future studies may someday allow genetic identification of the patients with PCG who are more likely than others to benefit from angle surgery (107).

Other Glaucoma Procedures

When incisional angle surgery (e.g., goniotomies, trabeculotomies) has failed, alternatives include filtration surgery, glaucoma drainage-device surgery, and cyclodestruction, usually in that order. (Chapter 40 includes detailed review of published series using trabeculectomy with and without the use of antimetabolites, such as mitomycin C, to treat children with glaucoma.) Although older children with phakic eyes often achieve successful glaucoma control with this surgery (108), trabeculectomy is less likely to successfully control glaucoma in young infants because of their exuberant healing and scarring response. In addition, trabeculectomy in any child carries with it a lifetime risk for endophthalmitis (109–112).

Glaucoma drainage-device surgery also has a role in the management of infants and other children refractory to angle surgery and trabeculectomy. (Detailed discussion of implant surgery in children can be found in Chapter 40.) The Molteno, Baerveldt, and Ahmed implants have been used in children, with widely varying rates of success—from about 50% to greater than 90% (113–122). Glaucoma drainage-device surgery can successfully control glaucoma in children, although many patients need postoperative glaucoma medication therapy and repeated surgery. In one retrospective study, glaucoma drainage-device surgery had 5- and 10-year success rates of approximately 60% and 45%, respectively, in children with refractory PCG (123).

In contrast to trabeculectomy and glaucoma drainage-device surgeries, cyclodestructive procedures reduce the rate of aqueous production by injuring the ciliary processes; success is only modest (about 50%), results are often unpredictable, and complications occur frequently. Cyclodestruction nonetheless constitutes a valid means of attempting control of especially refractory cases of PCG after medical and other surgical means have been exhausted or have proved inadequate to the task. This modality may be reasonable to decrease aqueous production in eyes with elevated IOP despite patent glaucoma drainage-device surgery (Freedman SF, unpublished data). Cyclocryotherapy has been used to treat difficult childhood glaucomas for many years. Unfortunately, overall success (i.e., pressure control without severe visual loss or phthisis) has been poor (i.e., 30% success in a large series of children with advanced congenital glaucoma), and retreatment has been the rule (124). Transscleral cyclophotocoagulation with the contact Nd:YAG and diode lasers has reduced IOP in a fashion at least comparable to cyclocryotherapy in children with refractory glaucomas, and with a lower reported incidence of phthisis and hypotony (125–128). The endoscopic use of the diode laser for cycloablation has been applied to children (mostly with glaucoma in aphakia), with modestly encouraging results (129,130).

Penetrating Keratoplasty

Corneal cloudiness due to permanent scarring may persist after normalization of the IOP in some severe cases, prompting consideration of penetrating keratoplasty. Penetrating keratoplasty in young children is difficult, especially when the case is complicated by glaucoma and buphthalmos (131–134). These patients often do not fare well, with only 25% of eyes achieving 20/40 or better vision in one series (131). The most common postoperative complications are IOP elevation and graft failure. Although significant visual improvement can be achieved with penetrating keratoplasty (135), it is suggested that it be reserved for patients with severe visual disability whose glaucoma is well controlled (131). Optical iridectomy may be a less risky surgical compromise in eyes with central corneal opacity.

Postoperative Care, Prognosis, and Follow-up

The follow-up care of patients with PCG has several important facets. In the early postoperative period, close observation is required to maximize proper healing and odds of surgical success. In addition to IOP reduction, other clinical indicators of successful glaucoma control include clearing of corneal edema, reversal of optic nerve cupping, and even reduction in myopia in some cases (136). The IOP has also been related to postoperative visual capacity, with substantially better vision reported among those whose IOP remained no higher than 19 mm Hg in one series (105).

As with older patients, the target IOP for children with PCG should be guided by the severity of the optic nerve damage, with lower targets set for those eyes with lower central corneal thickness. In infants with healthy-appearing optic nerves (e.g., cup-to-disc ratio <0.5), a target pressure of about 20 mm Hg is often adequate; the stability of the optic nerve, corneal diameter, and refraction help confirm the adequacy of the IOP. Conversely, target pressures in the mid-teens are usually set for infants and children with severe pre-existing optic nerve damage. In selected cases, eyes can remain stable despite IOPs in the low- to mid-20s when optic nerve cupping and ocular expansion have been minimal. Medications should be used to further reduce the IOP after surgery if the target IOP is not met. As with adults, auxiliary techniques such as visual fields and serial optic nerve examination should be used and the target IOP altered if progression occurs despite IOP control at the previously set target level.

Even when the IOP is well controlled, a substantial number of children never achieve good vision. In previous studies, approximately one half of the patients had visual acuities of less than 20/50 (105,136,137). This reduction may result from persistent corneal changes or from irreversible optic nerve damage. A high percentage of patients, however, suffer amblyopia from the induced anisometropia, and it is critical that this condition be diagnosed early and managed appropriately.

Patients with PCG constitute a heterogeneous group, with overall IOP control achievable in more than 80% of cases. Although in rare cases primary infantile glaucoma has seemed to spontaneously remit (138,139), most untreated cases result in buphthalmos and blindness (3). The prognosis for control of PCG varies with the patient's age at initial presentation and at surgery. Most favorable for IOP control with angle surgery are patients presenting after the first 2 months and within the first year of life (90%). Children presenting with glaucoma at birth or after the first year have a poorer prognosis for IOP control with angle surgery (50%) (7,140). Even children whose glaucoma is well controlled after surgical therapy (with or without adjunctive medical therapy) deserve lifelong follow-up. Loss of IOP control (reported in as many as approximately one third of cases (7)) may occur months or even decades after initial success with surgery and may be asymptomatic in the older child or young adult.

Congenital glaucoma is usually managed surgically, initially with a goniotomy or trabeculotomy. Visual loss due to amblyopia is common and should be aggressively treated. Lifelong follow-up is needed to guard against late loss of IOP control and to detect associated ocular problems such as corneal decompensation, cataract, and progressive optic nerve injury from inadequate IOP.

PRIMARY GLAUCOMAS WITH ASSOCIATED ABNORMALITIES (DEVELOPMENTAL GLAUCOMAS)

General Terminology

There have been considerable discussion and confusion regarding the lumping, splitting, and classifying of this large number of disorders. As the molecular genetics of anterior segment dysgenesis is further elucidated, the genetic classification of many of these disorders may supersede our current phenotypic descriptions. Nonetheless, the historical basis of our current classification system is worthy of further description here because management of many of these cases still rests firmly on their phenotypic presentation.

For simplicity, we consider all of the primary glaucomas that have associated ocular abnormalities to be forms of anterior segment dysgenesis. Based on the observation that most of the ocular and facial structures involved in these developmental disorders are of neural crest origin (67,141), the term neurocristopathies has been used as a unifying concept for diseases arising from neural crest maldevelopment (142,143). Hoskins and colleagues (144) advocated a shift away from eponyms and syndrome names for individual disorders and toward an emphasis on descriptive terminology. Noting that the trabecular meshwork, iris, and cornea are the three major structures involved in these conditions, they suggested using the terms trabeculodysgenesis, iridodysgenesis, and corneodysgenesis, or combinations thereof, to classify the developmental defects. In a recent review, Idrees and colleagues (145) consider the anterior segment dysgenesis to include not only Axenfeld–Rieger syndrome, iridogoniodysgenesis–iris hypoplasia, and Peters anomaly, but also PCG, sclerocornea, megalocornea, congenital hereditary endothelial dystrophy, and aniridia. Although most of these anterior segment dysgeneses are attributed to defects in neural crest migration or differentiation, aniridia is considered to be of non–neural crest origin. Many of the anterior segment dysgeneses also may occur with associated systemic abnormalities, further blurring the distinction between primary glaucomas with associated ocular abnormalities and those with associated systemic abnormalities (Table 13.1).

Although there is value in categorizing disorders on the basis of anatomic descriptions and mechanisms, the overlapping of manifestations and limited understanding of disease mechanisms make it difficult to apply such a system in all cases of developmental glaucomas with associated anomalies. There is often great phenotypic variability between individuals with the identical genetic cause for a disease; variation may even occur among members of the same family, making tissue classification inaccurate. For these reasons, traditional eponyms and syndrome names are retained with some suggested modifications for the purpose of discussion in this chapter. (For additional genetic information related to these conditions, see Table 8.1.)

Axenfeld–Rieger Syndrome

Terminology

In 1920, Axenfeld (146) described a patient with a white line in the posterior aspect of the cornea, near the limbus, and tissue strands extending from peripheral iris to this prominent line. Beginning in the mid-1930s, Rieger (147–149) reported cases with similar anterior segment anomalies, but with additional changes in the iris, including corectopia, atrophy, and hole formation. Some of these patients also had associated systemic developmental defects, especially of the teeth and facial bones

(150,151). Axenfeld referred to his case as posterior embryotoxon of the cornea (146), and Rieger used the term mesodermal dysgenesis of the cornea and iris (149). Traditionally, these conditions have been designated by three eponyms: (a) Axenfeld anomaly (i.e., limited to peripheral anterior segment defects), (b) Rieger anomaly (i.e., peripheral abnormalities with additional changes in the iris), and (c) Rieger syndrome (i.e., ocular anomalies plus systemic developmental defects).

The similarity of anterior chamber angle abnormalities in the Axenfeld anomaly and the Rieger anomaly and syndrome led most investigators to agree that these three arbitrary categories represent a spectrum of developmental disorders (79,152,153). The overlap of ocular and systemic anomalies is such that the traditional classification is difficult to apply in all cases. Various collective terms have been applied to this spectrum of disorders, such as anterior chamber cleavage syndrome and mesodermal dysgenesis of the cornea and iris (149,152). As discussed earlier, the theories of normal development on which these names are based are no longer believed to be correct. The former collective term included the central ocular defects of Peters anomaly (discussed later in this chapter). Although some patients may have the combined defects of the Axenfeld anomaly or the Rieger anomaly and the Peters anomaly, the association is rare and the mechanisms of the two disorders differ in most cases.

The alternative term, Axenfeld–Rieger syndrome, was proposed for all clinical variations within this spectrum of developmental disorders and is now commonly used in the literature (79,154). This name retains reference to the original eponyms and does not depend on any theory of normal development, the understanding of which is still incomplete, nor does it require arbitrary subclassification of the clinical variations.

General Features

All patients with the Axenfeld–Rieger syndrome, irrespective of ocular manifestations, share the same general features: a bilateral, developmental disorder of the eyes; a frequent family history of the disorder, with an autosomal dominant mode of inheritance; no sex predilection; frequent systemic developmental defects; and a high incidence of associated glaucoma. The age at which the Axenfeld–Rieger syndrome is diagnosed ranges from birth to adulthood, with most cases recognized in infancy or childhood. The diagnosis may result from the discovery of an abnormal iris or other ocular anomaly, signs of congenital glaucoma, reduced vision in older patients, or systemic anomalies. In other cases, the condition is diagnosed during a routine examination, which might have been prompted by a family history of the disorder.

Ocular Features

Ocular defects in the Axenfeld–Rieger syndrome are typically bilateral. The structures most commonly involved are the peripheral cornea, anterior chamber angle, and iris.

Cornea

The characteristic abnormality of the cornea is a prominent, anteriorly displaced Schwalbe line. This appears on slitlamp

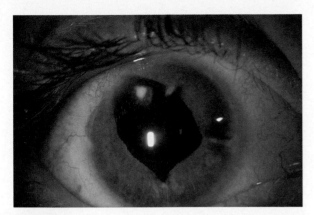

Figure 14.9 Right eye of a 6-year-old girl with Axenfeld–Rieger syndrome and congenital glaucoma. Note the prominent anteriorly displaced Schwalbe line, visible for almost 360 degrees. Ectropion uveae is also prominent. The pupil peaks toward the 11-o'clock position as a result of a glaucoma drainage device placed at 2 months of age. The tube also caused a focal cataract and an endothelial scar (before tube-shortening procedure). IOP is controlled and vision corrected to 20/40.

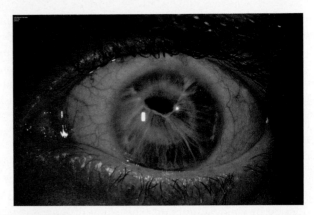

Figure 14.10 Left eye of a 16-year-old patient with Axenfeld–Rieger syndrome and congenital glaucoma. Note the corectopia, with the pupil displaced toward prominent peripheral tissue strands superiorly.

examination as a white line on the posterior cornea near the limbus. The prominent line may be incomplete, usually limited to the temporal quadrant; in other patients, it may be seen for 360 degrees (**Fig. 14.9**). In some cases, the line can only be seen by gonioscopy, although rare cases with other ocular and systemic features of the syndrome may have grossly normal Schwalbe lines (155).

It is not uncommon for an individual to have a prominent Schwalbe line with no other evidence of Axenfeld–Rieger syndrome. This isolated defect is often referred to as posterior embryotoxon, the term originally used by Axenfeld (146), and it reportedly occurs in 8% to 15% of the general population (156,157). Although it may represent a forme fruste of the Axenfeld–Rieger syndrome in some cases, it is not usually included in this spectrum of anomalies. A prominent Schwalbe line may only rarely be associated with other disorders, including congenital glaucoma and the iridocorneal endothelial (ICE) syndrome (83,158) (Chapter 16).

The cornea is otherwise normal in the typical patient with the Axenfeld–Rieger syndrome, with the exception of occasional variation in the overall size (i.e., megalocornea or, less often, microcornea) or shape of the cornea (156). Congenital opacities of the central cornea have also been observed in a few cases. The corneal endothelium is typically normal. By specular microscopy, the cells have distinct margins, although mild-to-moderate variations in the size and shape are commonly observed, especially in older patients and those with long-standing glaucoma or previous intraocular surgery (79).

Anterior Chamber Angle

Gonioscopic examination typically reveals a prominent Schwalbe line, although the extent of enlargement and anterior displacement of the Schwalbe line varies considerably among patients. Occasionally, the line is suspended from the cornea in some areas by a thin membrane (79,159). Tissue strands bridge

the anterior chamber angle from the peripheral iris to the prominent ridge. These iridocorneal adhesions are typically similar in color and texture to the adjacent iris. The strands range in size from threadlike structures to broad bands extending for a clock-hour or more of the circumference. In some eyes, only one to two tissue strands are seen, whereas others have several per quadrant. Beyond the tissue strands, the anterior chamber angle is open and the trabecular meshwork is visible, but the scleral spur is typically obscured by peripheral iris, which inserts into the posterior portion of the meshwork (79,156,160).

Iris

Aside from the peripheral abnormalities, the iris may be normal in some patients with the Axenfeld–Rieger syndrome. In other cases, defects of the iris range from mild stromal thinning to marked atrophy with hole formation, corectopia, and ectropion uveae. When corectopia is present, the pupil is usually displaced toward a prominent peripheral tissue strand, which is often visible by slitlamp biomicroscopy (**Fig. 14.10**). The atrophy and hole formation typically occur in the quadrant away from the direction of the corectopia.

In a small number of patients with the Axenfeld–Rieger syndrome, abnormalities of the central iris have been observed to progress (79,161). This is more often seen in the first years of life, but may also occur in older patients. The progressive changes usually consist of displacement or distortion of the pupil and occasional thinning or hole formation of the iris. In some cases, these progressive iris changes may be confused with those of ICE syndrome. Abnormalities of the peripheral iris or anterior chamber angle do not appear to progress after birth, except for occasional thickening of iridocorneal tissue strands (79).

Additional Ocular Abnormalities

Many additional ocular abnormalities have been reported in one or more cases or pedigrees. Although none occurs with sufficient frequency to be included as a typical feature of the Axenfeld–Rieger syndrome and they may represent separate entities, these patients can have a wide range of ocular anomalies—including strabismus, limbal dermoids, corneal pannus, cataracts, congenital ectropion uveae, congenital pupillary–iris–lens membrane, peripheral spokelike transillumination defects of the iris, retinal detachment, macular degeneration, chorioretinal colobomas, choroidal hypoplasia, and hypoplasia of the optic nerve heads (79,156,162–166).

Glaucoma

Slightly more than one half of the patients with the Axenfeld–Rieger syndrome develop glaucoma. The glaucoma may manifest in infancy, although it more commonly appears in childhood or young adulthood. The extent of the iris defects and iridocorneal strands does not correlate precisely with the presence or severity of the glaucoma. However, the high insertion of peripheral iris into the trabecular meshwork, which is present to some degree in all cases, appears to be more pronounced in those eyes with glaucoma (79). The proposed mechanism of glaucoma in these cases relates to abnormalities of the trabecular meshwork and Schlemm canal (discussed in the Histopathologic Features and Theories of Mechanism section).

Systemic Features

The systemic anomalies most commonly associated with the Axenfeld–Rieger syndrome are developmental defects of the teeth and facial bones. The dental abnormalities include a reduced crown size (i.e., microdontia), a decreased but evenly spaced number of teeth (i.e., hypodontia), and a focal absence of teeth (i.e., oligodontia or anodontia) (150,151,167). The teeth most commonly missing are anterior maxillary primary and permanent central incisors. Facial anomalies include maxillary hypoplasia with flattening of the midface and a receding upper lip and prominent lower lip, especially in association with dental hypoplasia. Hypertelorism, telecanthus, a broad flat nose, micrognathia, and mandibular prognathism have also been described (156,162).

Anomalies in the region of the pituitary gland are a less common but more serious finding associated with the Axenfeld–Rieger syndrome. A primary empty sella syndrome has been documented in several patients (154,168), and in one case of congenital parasellar, an arachnoid cyst was reported (154). Growth hormone deficiency and short stature have also been described in association with the entity (169,170). Other associated abnormalities include redundant periumbilical skin and hypospadias, oculocutaneous albinism, heart defects, middle-ear deafness, mental deficiency, and various neurologic, dermatologic, and skeletal disorders (156,171–173).

Histopathologic Features and Theories of Mechanism

The central cornea is typically normal, but the peripheral cornea has the characteristic prominent, anteriorly displaced Schwalbe line. The latter structure is composed of dense collagen and ground substance covered by a monolayer of spindle-shaped cells with a basement membrane (79,157,159) (**Fig. 14.11**). The peripheral iris is attached in some areas to the corneoscleral junction by tissue strands, which usually connect

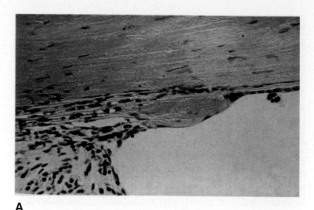

A

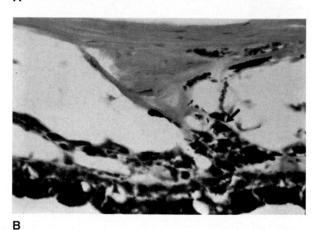

B

Figure 14.11 Light microscopic view of an eye with Axenfeld–Rieger syndrome shows a prominent Schwalbe line, composed of dense collagen and ground substance covered by a monolayer of spindle-shaped cells with a basement membrane. **A:** Anterior insertion of the iris is present; this may be seen in several forms of developmental glaucoma. (Courtesy of Ramesh C. Tripathi, MD, PhD.) **B:** An iridocorneal adhesion (*arrow*) extending from the peripheral iris to the prominent Schwalbe line.

with the prominent Schwalbe line. Occasionally, however, the adhesions insert anterior or posterior to the Schwalbe line or on both sides of the ridge (79). The strands consist of iris stroma, a membrane composed of a monolayer of spindle-shaped cells or a basement membrane-like layer, or both.

A membrane, similar to that associated with the iridocorneal tissue strands, has been observed on the iris, usually on the portion toward which the pupil is distorted (79,156,174). In the quadrants away from the direction of pupillary displacement, the stroma of the iris is often thin or absent, exposing pigment epithelium, which may also contain holes.

The iris peripheral to the iridocorneal adhesions inserts into the posterior aspect of the trabecular meshwork. The meshwork may be composed of a scant number of attenuated lamellae, which extend from beneath peripheral iris to the prominent Schwalbe line and are often compressed, especially in the outer layers. Transmission electron microscopic study suggests that the apparent compression may be caused by incomplete development of the trabecular meshwork (79). The Schlemm canal is rudimentary or absent.

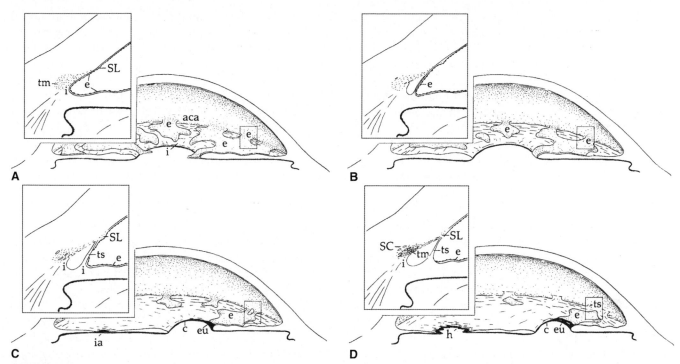

Figure 14.12 Theory of the mechanism for ocular abnormalities of Axenfeld–Rieger syndrome; *insets* show cross-sectional views of anterior chamber angle corresponding to area within the rectangle. **A:** Partial retention of the primordial endothelium (*e*) on the iris (*i*) and anterior chamber angle (*aca*); incomplete posterior recession of peripheral uvea from trabecular meshwork (*tm*); and abnormal differentiation between corneal and chamber angle endothelium with a prominent, anteriorly displaced Schwalbe line (*SL*). **B:** Development of tissue strands from retained endothelium crossing the anterior chamber angle. **C:** Contraction of retained endothelium with iris changes of corectopia (*c*), ectropion uvea (*eu*), and iris atrophy (*ia*), which may continue after birth; a tissue strand (*ts*) can also be seen. **D:** Incomplete development of trabecular meshwork and Schlemm canal (*SC*); continued traction on the iris with possible secondary ischemia leads to hole formation (*h*). (From Shields MB. Axenfeld–Rieger syndrome: a theory of mechanism and distinctions from the iridocorneal endothelial syndrome. *Trans Am Ophthalmol Soc.* 1983;81:736–784. Republished with permission of the American Ophthalmological Society.)

On the basis of clinical and histopathologic observations and the current concepts of normal anterior segment development, a developmental arrest, occurring late in gestation, of certain anterior segment structures derived from neural crest cells has been postulated as the mechanism of the Axenfeld–Rieger syndrome (79). This leads to the abnormal retention of the primordial endothelial layer on portions of the iris and anterior chamber angle and alterations in the aqueous outflow structures (**Fig. 14.12**). The retained endothelium with associated basement membrane is believed to create the iridocorneal strands, whereas contraction of this tissue layer on the iris leads to the iris changes, which sometimes continue to progress after birth. The developmental arrest also accounts for the high insertion of anterior uvea into the posterior trabecular meshwork, similar to the alterations seen in congenital glaucoma. This results in the incomplete maturation of the trabecular meshwork and Schlemm canal, and these defects are thought to be responsible for the associated glaucoma.

The neural crest cells also give rise to most of the mesenchyme related to the forebrain and pituitary gland, bones and cartilages of the upper face, and dental papillae (142,143). This may explain the developmental anomalies involving the pituitary gland, the facial bones, and the teeth. Neural crest cells also contribute to many other structures, including the walls of the aortic arches, genitalia, spinal ganglia, long bones, and melanocytes (172,173), which appears to explain the wide range of systemic anomalies that may be seen in some patients with the Axenfeld–Rieger syndrome.

Genetic Linkage

The Axenfeld–Rieger syndrome is thought to have a genetic basis, with an autosomal dominant pattern of inheritance. Tremendous advances have been made in the understanding of the molecular genetics of Axenfeld–Rieger malformations (175–185) (Table 8.2). Three chromosomal loci have been demonstrated to link to the Axenfeld–Rieger syndrome and related phenotypes. These loci are on chromosomes 4q25, 6p25, and 13q14. The genes at chromosomes 4q25 and 6p25 have been identified as *PITX2* and *FOXC1*, respectively (182). Mutations in these genes can cause a wide variety of phenotypes that share features with the Axenfeld–Rieger syndrome, Axenfeld anomaly, Rieger anomaly, Rieger syndrome, iridogoniodysgenesis anomaly, iridogoniodysgenesis syndrome, iris hypoplasia, and familial glaucoma iridogoniodysplasia; these conditions all have sufficient genotypic and phenotypic overlap to be considered one disorder (16,182). Genetically, the

Axenfeld–Rieger syndromes can be considered in three types. Axenfeld–Rieger syndrome type 1 is caused by mutation in a homeobox transcription factor gene, *PITX2* (OMIM 601542) (16). Linkage studies indicate that a second type of Axenfeld–Rieger syndrome maps to chromosome 13q14 (RIEG2; OMIM 601499). A third form of Axenfeld–Rieger syndrome (RIEG3; OMIM 602482) is caused by mutation in the *FOXC1* gene (OMIM 601090) on chromosome 6p25 (16).

In a clinical series of patients with Axenfeld–Rieger syndrome and mutations in the *PITX2* or *FOXC1* genes (186), 75% of the patients had glaucoma that developed in adolescence or early adulthood, and patients with *PITX2* defects or *FOXC1* duplications had a more severe prognosis for glaucoma development than patients with *FOXC1* mutations did (186). This complex genetic disorder has overlap with other anterior segment dysgeneses, and future studies may someday help predict how phenotype–genotype classification may assist in genetic counseling, as well as prognosis for glaucoma treatment and vision preservation in affected individuals.

Differential Diagnosis

Molecular genetic studies may ultimately make the differentiation among the following phenotypic entities less relevant. The following items are nonetheless useful for phenotypic classification of these disorders.

Iridocorneal Endothelial (ICE) Syndrome

The iris and anterior chamber angle abnormalities in this spectrum of disease (Chapter 16) resemble those of Axenfeld–Rieger syndrome clinically and histopathologically. This has led some investigators to suggest that the two syndromes are parts of a common spectrum of disorders (174,187). However, clinical features that distinguish the ICE syndrome from the Axenfeld–Rieger syndrome include corneal endothelial abnormalities, unilaterality, absence of family history, and onset in young adulthood. Both conditions are characterized histopathologically by a membrane over the angle and iris, which is associated with many of the alterations in each disorder. Although the membrane in the Axenfeld–Rieger syndrome represents a primordial remnant, that of the ICE syndrome results from proliferation of the abnormal corneal endothelium.

Posterior Polymorphous Corneal Dystrophy

One variation of this developmental disorder of the corneal endothelium (Chapter 16) has changes of the iris and anterior chamber angle similar to those of the Axenfeld–Rieger syndrome. However, differentiation can be made on the basis of the typical corneal endothelial abnormality.

Peters Anomaly

The spectrum of disorders that constitutes Peters anomaly involves the central portion of the cornea, the iris, and the lens. Similar changes have been reported in association with the peripheral defects of the Axenfeld–Rieger syndrome, and the two conditions were once included in a single category of developmental disorders (153). However, this association is rare, and the mechanisms for the two groups of disorders are distinctly different. Nonetheless, families with known mutation in the *FOXC1* gene have been reported with Axenfeld–Rieger syndrome in most members but Peters anomaly in others (177,188).

Aniridia

The rudimentary iris and anterior chamber abnormalities with associated glaucoma in this developmental disorder (discussed later) may lead to confusion with the Axenfeld–Rieger syndrome in some cases. Mutations in the *PITX2* gene may manifest with a wide variation in anterior segment anomalies, including those phenotypically similar to aniridia (185).

Iridogoniodysgenesis: Congenital Hypoplasia of the Iris

Patients may have congenital hypoplasia of the iris without the anterior chamber angle defects of the Axenfeld–Rieger syndrome. Autosomal dominant iridogoniodysgenesis anomaly type I (gene map locus 6p26) is caused by mutations in the *FOXC1* gene and is characterized by iris hypoplasia, goniodysgenesis, and juvenile glaucoma. A distinct form of this condition also includes nonocular features and is referred to as iridogoniodysgenesis syndrome or iridogoniodysgenesis type 2. It maps to 4q25, is caused by mutations in the gene *PITX2* (OMIM 601631, 137600), and may be allelic with Axenfeld–Rieger syndrome (16).

Oculodentodigital Dysplasia

The dental anomalies in oculodentodigital dysplasia are similar to those seen in the Axenfeld–Rieger syndrome. These patients occasionally have mild stromal hypoplasia of the iris, anterior chamber angle defects, microphthalmia, and glaucoma (189). This condition is caused by mutation in the connexin-43 gene (*GJA1*, gene map locus 6q21–q23.2, OMIM 164200) (16).

Ectopia Lentis et Pupillae

Ectopia lentis et pupillae is an autosomal recessive condition characterized by bilateral displacement of the lens and pupil (190), with the two typically displaced in opposite directions. The corectopia in this disorder may resemble that of the Axenfeld–Rieger syndrome, but the absence of anterior chamber angle defects is a differential feature (see Chapter 18).

Congenital Ectropion Uveae

Congenital ectropion uveae is a rare, nonprogressive anomaly characterized by the presence of pigment epithelium on the stroma of the iris (191,192). It may be an isolated finding or appear in association with systemic anomalies, including neurofibromatosis, facial hemiatrophy, and the Prader–Willi syndrome (191). Glaucoma is present in a high percentage of cases, and the ectropion uvea may be confused with that found in some patients with the Axenfeld–Rieger syndrome.

Congenital Microcoria and Myopia

The condition of congenital microcoria and myopia, characterized by bilateral small pupils and myopia, results from an underdevelopment of the dilator pupillae muscle of the iris. Transmitted as an autosomal dominant trait, this disorder has been associated with goniodysgenesis and glaucoma

(193–195). Congenital microcoria has been linked to gene map locus 13q31–q32 (EntrezGene symbol *MCOR*, OMIM 156600) (16).

Patients with the Axenfeld–Rieger syndrome may have a wide variety of associated ocular and systemic developmental abnormalities, and it has not yet been established in many of these cases whether the patient has a variation of the Axenfeld–Rieger syndrome or whether the findings should be considered a separate entity.

Management

The primary concern about the management of ocular defects in a patient with the Axenfeld–Rieger syndrome is detection and control of the associated glaucoma. IOP elevation most often develops between childhood and early adulthood, but it may appear in infancy or, in rare cases, not until late adulthood (79,154). Patients with the Axenfeld–Rieger syndrome must be followed to detect glaucoma throughout their lives.

With the exception of infantile cases, medical therapy should usually be initiated before surgical intervention is recommended. Drugs that reduce aqueous production, such as β-adrenergic blockers, carbonic anhydrase inhibitors, and α₂-adrenergic agonists, are most likely to be beneficial. Initial surgical options include goniotomy, trabeculotomy, and trabeculectomy. Goniotomy and trabeculotomy have been used in infantile cases with limited success. Trabeculectomy is the surgical procedure of choice for most patients with glaucoma associated with the Axenfeld–Rieger syndrome; the success rate in older children has been about 75%, but with the same risks of late bleb leak and infection as seen in other children after trabeculectomy, especially if mitomycin C has been used (Freedman SF, unpublished data) (see Chapter 40). In infants and in cases refractory to medication and trabeculectomy, glaucoma drainage-device surgery and cycloablation remain options for treatment. In a retrospective clinical series of 126 patients with Axenfeld–Rieger syndrome attributable to mutations in *PITX2* and *FOXC1*, Strungaru and colleagues noted that glaucoma in only 18% of the patients with *PITX2* or *FOXC1* genetic defects responded to medical or surgical treatment (used solely or in combination) (186).

Peters Anomaly

In 1897, von Hippel (196) reported a case of buphthalmos with bilateral central corneal opacities and adhesions from these defects to the iris. Peters, beginning in 1906 (197), described similar patients with what has become generally known as Peters anomaly.

General Features

Peters anomaly is present at birth and is usually bilateral. Most cases are sporadic, although there are reported cases of autosomal recessive inheritance and, less commonly, autosomal dominant transmission (198,199). Peters anomaly occurs in the absence of additional abnormalities, although associations with a wide range of systemic and other ocular anomalies have been reported, including defects of the ear and auditory system,

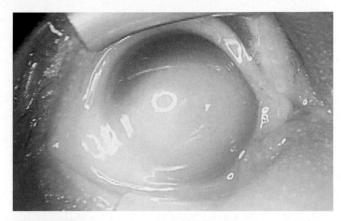

Figure 14.13 External appearance of the right eye of a 10-day-old infant with unilateral Peters anomaly. The IOP is normal, but a dense central corneal opacity covers the pupil. Anterior segment ultrasonography demonstrated a formed anterior chamber centrally, without apparent corneal-lens contact.

orofacial system, heart, genitourinary system, spine, and musculoskeletal system (200–202). Because of the varied genetic and nongenetic patterns and the spectrum of ocular and systemic abnormalities, Peters anomaly is probably a morphologic finding rather than a distinct entity (200). Peters anomaly can be caused by mutation in the *PAX6*, *PITX2*, *CYP1B1*, or *FOXC1* gene (OMIM 607108, 601542, 601771, and 601090, respectively) (16) (Table 8.2).

Clinicopathologic Features

The hallmark of Peters anomaly is a central corneal abnormality—a defect in the Descemet membrane and corneal endothelium with thinning and opacification of the corresponding area of corneal stroma (203–206) (**Fig. 14.13**). Iris adhesions may extend to the borders of this corneal defect. Bowman layer may also be absent centrally (205,206). Immunohistochemical studies of the cornea suggest that extracellular matrix elements, such as fibronectin, may be important in the pathogenesis of Peters anomaly (207). The disorder has been subdivided into three groups (**Fig. 14.14**), each of which may have more than one pathogenetic mechanism (204).

In Peters anomaly not associated with keratolenticular contact or cataract, the defect in the Descemet membrane may represent primary failure of corneal endothelial development (205). However, rare cases may result from intrauterine inflammation (208), which was originally postulated by von Hippel (196) and gave rise to the term von Hippel internal corneal ulcer.

In eyes with Peters anomaly associated with keratolenticular contact or cataract, histopathologic studies suggest that the lens developed normally and was then secondarily pushed forward against the cornea by one of several mechanisms, causing the loss of Descemet membrane (204,205,209). Some cases may result from incomplete separation of the lens vesicle from surface ectoderm.

Peters anomaly may rarely be associated with Axenfeld–Rieger syndrome (see above).

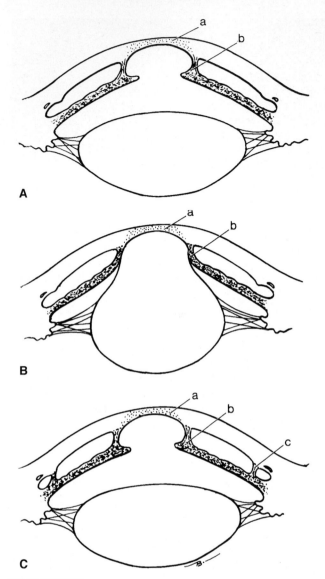

Figure 14.14 Peters anomaly with a central corneal defect (*a*) and adhesions (*b*) from a corneal defect to the central iris. Shown are three forms described by Townsend and colleagues (70). **A:** Without keratolenticular contact or cataract. **B:** With keratolenticular contact or cataract. **C:** With peripheral defects of Axenfeld–Rieger syndrome (*c*).

Associated Glaucoma

Approximately one half of the patients with Peters anomaly will develop glaucoma, which is frequently present at birth. The mechanism of the glaucoma is uncertain, because the anterior chamber angle is usually grossly normal by clinical examination. Histopathologic studies have revealed peripheral anterior synechiae in some cases (204), whereas ultrastructural studies of two young patients with Peters anomaly and open angles revealed changes in the trabecular meshwork that are characteristic of aging (209,210). In cases of Peters anomaly associated with the anterior chamber angle abnormalities of the Axenfeld–Rieger syndrome, the mechanism of glaucoma is presumably the same as in the latter condition (discussed earlier in this chapter). Some cases of Peters anomaly demonstrate a shallow

or flat anterior chamber, which may also play a role in the manifestation of glaucoma.

Differential Diagnosis

Other Causes of Central Corneal Opacities in Infants

The corneal clouding of Peters anomaly must be distinguished from that of PCG, birth trauma, the MPS, and congenital hereditary endothelial dystrophy.

Posterior Keratoconus

This rare disorder is characterized by a thinning of the central corneal stroma, with excessive curvature of the posterior corneal surface and variable overlying stromal haze (153,211). An ultrastructural study revealed a multilaminar Descemet membrane with abnormal anterior banding and localized posterior excrescences (212). Glaucoma is rarely associated with posterior keratoconus (153).

Congenital Corneal Leukomas and Staphylomas

These cases represent the more severe forms of central dysgenesis of the anterior segment and are frequently associated with glaucoma (156).

Management

All infants and children with cloudy corneas must be examined carefully for the possibility of associated glaucoma. The glaucoma associated with Peters anomaly usually requires surgical intervention, although some mild cases may be managed medically (Freedman SF, unpublished data). Although trabeculotomy or trabeculectomy may be reasonable in milder cases with adequate anterior chamber depth, glaucoma drainage-device surgery or cyclodestructive surgery is often needed in refractory or more severely affected cases.

Penetrating keratoplasty is also frequently necessary, although the results are typically poor, which probably is caused partly by the associated glaucoma and its surgical treatment. A study of 47 children reported on 144 penetrating keratoplasty procedures; 29% of eyes had visual acuity better than 20/400, while 38% had light perception or no light perception. This series included only 14 eyes with glaucoma (213). Although Zaidman and colleagues reported more favorable visual outcomes after corneal transplantation in patients with mild Peters anomaly (i.e., no lens involvement), the eyes with glaucoma in that series had poorer outcomes (214).

Diode endocyclophotocoagulation has been applied in patients after corneal transplantation with uncontrolled glaucoma; limited success and high rates of corneal graft failure have occurred (215,216; Freedman SF, unpublished data). The uniformly poor prognosis for long-term corneal graft survival in patients with Peters anomaly (especially in the presence of glaucoma) suggests that partially clear corneas be considered for initial conservative management or that alternatives to corneal transplantation, such as sector iridectomy, be used in hopes of attaining some useful visual function (217,218) (**Fig. 14.15**). Although endoscopic diode laser has limited success when used as the sole treatment for refractory glaucoma associated with Peters anomaly, glaucoma drainage-device

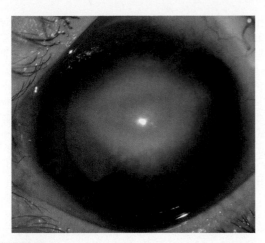

Figure 14.15 Left eye of a 3-year-old child with bilateral Peters anomaly and severe congenital glaucoma. The other eye has a failed penetrating keratoplasty. This eye has undergone implantation of an Ahmed glaucoma drainage device and optical iridectomy; IOP is controlled without the use of medications, and the child has ambulatory vision.

surgery may be a reasonable surgical option in selected cases, often combined with careful vitrectomy in aphakic eyes (219).

Aniridia

General Features

Aniridia is a bilateral developmental disorder characterized by the congenital absence of a normal iris. The name aniridia is a misnomer because the iris is only partially absent, with a rudimentary stump of variable width. Aniridia is associated with multiple ocular defects, some of which are present at birth, whereas others may become manifest later in childhood or early adulthood. Some forms of aniridia may have associated systemic abnormalities.

Four phenotypes of aniridia have been identified on the basis of associated ocular and systemic abnormalities (220): associated with foveal hypoplasia, nystagmus, corneal pannus, glaucoma, and reduced vision; predominant iris changes and normal visual acuity; associated with Wilms tumor (i.e., the aniridia–Wilms tumor syndrome) or other genitourinary anomalies; and associated with mental retardation.

Aniridia is inherited in an autosomal dominant fashion with almost complete penetrance but variable expression in about two thirds of cases. The remaining one third of cases are sporadic. Aniridia has been shown to be associated with mutations in the *PAX6* gene, located on chromosome 11p13 (locus symbol AN2), telomeric to the Wilms tumor predisposition gene (*WT1*) (OMIM 106210) (16) (Table 8.2).

Approximately 68% of patients with a deletion of chromosome 11 and aniridia will develop Wilms tumor before the age of 3 years (221). Patients with the 11p13 deletion, aniridia, and Wilms tumor also have a wide range of other ocular and nonocular developmental disorders (221).

Aniridia is caused by a reduction in the activity of *PAX6*, a paired-box transcription factor, located on the short arm of

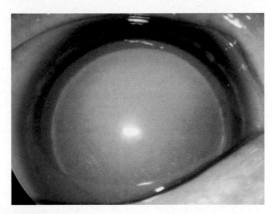

Figure 14.16 Aniridia in a 6-month-old patient. Note the peripheral iris rim and the clear view of the lens equator.

chromosome 11 (11p13) (222). This can occur by heterozygous null mutations in *PAX6*, by cytogenetic deletions of chromosome 11p13 that encompass *PAX6*, or even by chromosomal rearrangements that disrupt 11p13 remote from *PAX6*. Lauderdale and colleagues (223) provide further support for haploinsufficiency as the basis of aniridia rather than a dominant-negative mechanism. A high frequency of chromosomal rearrangements was associated with sporadic and familial aniridia in a cohort of 77 patients with aniridia (224). The *PAX6* gene on chromosome 11p13 is located telomeric to the Wilms tumor predisposition gene, *WT1* (225). Phenotypic aniridia (along with Peters anomaly) has been reported in association with *PITX2* mutations, occurring in families where most members have Axenfeld–Rieger syndrome (185).

Clinicopathologic Features

Iris

In some cases, the iris is so rudimentary that it can only be seen by gonioscopy (**Fig. 14.16**), whereas other eyes may have enough peripheral iris to be visible by external and slitlamp examination. In some cases, the iris involvement is so minimal that other features of the disorder must be used to make the diagnosis (226). Iris and retinal fluorescein angiography have also been shown to help in identifying these patients by showing abnormal iris vascular remodeling that resulted in incomplete iris collarettes and decreased retinal foveal avascular zones (227).

Cornea

In a high percentage of cases, corneal pannus and opacity begin in the peripheral cornea in early life and advance toward the center of the cornea with increasing age. A study of ocular surface abnormalities in nine patients with nearly total aniridia and superficial corneal opacification and vascularization of the peripheral or entire cornea revealed a complete absence of the palisades of Vogt and an increase in goblet cell density, suggesting that the conjunctival epithelium had invaded the cornea (228). Microcornea and iridocorneal and keratolenticular adhesions have also been reported (229–232). Aniridic eyes have a high central corneal thickness, compared with healthy eyes, which has been attributed to thicker stroma (233), although certainly corneal edema must be considered in advanced cases with corneal decompensation.

Lens

Localized congenital opacities of the lens are common but usually insignificant. However, progressive cataracts may lead to significant visual impairment by approximately the third decade of life. The lens may also be subluxated or congenitally absent, or it may be reabsorbed (229,230,234).

Foveal Hypoplasia

Poor visual acuity and nystagmus are typical findings in patients with aniridia. The absence of a pupillary effect was once thought to cause the visual impairment, although some patients with aniridia have reasonably good vision and no nystagmus despite significant hypoplasia of the iris (220). Foveal hypoplasia is a frequent finding in aniridia and presumably accounts for the poor visual acuity and nystagmus. Spectral-domain OCT can be used to confirm the presence of foveal hypoplasia in eyes with aniridia, and this correlates well with visual acuity independent of the iris rim width (Freedman SF, unpublished data).

Other Ocular and Systemic Defects

Aniridia has been associated with a wide range of other ocular and nonocular developmental anomalies. These anomalies include choroidal colobomas, persistent pupillary membranes, sclerocornea and the Hallermann–Streiff syndrome, small optic nerve heads, strabismus, ptosis, Marfan syndrome with cervical ribs and dental anomalies, tracheomalacia and delayed closure of the anterior fontanelle, and retinoblastoma (231,234–238).

Associated Glaucoma

Glaucoma occurs in 50% to 75% of patients with aniridia, but it usually does not appear before late childhood or adolescence (239), although congenital onset has been reported and carries a poor prognosis (Freedman SF, unpublished data). The development of the glaucoma appears to correlate with the gonioscopic appearance of the anterior chamber angle. In infancy, the angle is usually open and unobstructed, although some eyes may have strands of tissue with occasional fine blood vessels extending from the iris root to the trabecular meshwork or higher (239). Some patients have congenital anomalies in the filtration angle, which may lead to glaucoma early in life (240).

During the first 5 to 15 years of life, many eyes with aniridia undergo progressive change in the anterior chamber angle as the rudimentary stump of iris comes to lie over the trabecular meshwork. The progressive obstruction of the anterior chamber angle may be caused by contracture of the tissue strands between the peripheral iris and angle wall (239).

Management
Glaucoma

Conventional medical therapy, especially with agents to reduce aqueous production, may control the IOP initially, but this approach eventually proves to be inadequate in most cases. Goniotomy is of no value in advanced cases, but published experience suggests that early goniotomy to separate the strands between the iris and the trabecular meshwork in high-risk cases of aniridia may prevent the development of glaucoma (239,241). Others have reported that trabeculotomy can effectively reduce IOP after glaucoma has developed in eyes with aniridia; in one series, IOP was controlled in 10 of 12 eyes after one or two trabeculotomy procedures (mean follow-up, 9.5 years) (242).

Trabeculectomy is often used as the first surgical procedure in cases of aniridic glaucoma refractory to medical treatment, but the postoperative period is made difficult by the propensity to develop a flat anterior chamber (Freedman SF, unpublished data). Trabeculectomy in infants and very young children carries with it the same difficulties and poor success rates found in those with other refractory glaucoma (see Chapter 40). In one small series of 10 eyes in patients younger than 40 who had aniridia, the investigators reported a 14.6-month "mean good IOP control period" after trabeculectomy, with no serious complications (243).

Glaucoma drainage devices may offer a reasonable alternative to trabeculectomy, especially in infants and patients with aphakia. In a retrospective series of eight eyes, investigators reported favorable success with glaucoma drainage-device surgery for aniridic glaucoma, citing success of 88% at 1 year, according to Kaplan–Meier analysis (244). Care must be taken to place the tube of the glaucoma drainage device far from the corneal endothelium, because corneal decompensation often ensues in cases of tube–corneal proximity (**Fig. 14.17**). Cyclocryotherapy and transscleral cyclophotocoagulation are reasonable options in cases refractory to trabeculectomy or glaucoma drainage-device surgery, but aniridic eyes may be more prone than others to phthisis after cyclocryotherapy (245).

Cataracts and Corneal Opacities

Cataract surgery is often difficult in the aniridic eye because of reduced corneal clarity, limited iris support, and poor zonular integrity. The remaining anterior capsule often opacifies, which can create a "pseudoiris"(**Fig. 14.18**). Other attempts to compensate for the missing iris (which would not be expected to improve visual acuity but may reduce photophobia) include

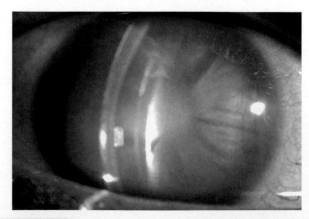

Figure 14.17 Right eye of a 10-year-old girl with aniridia, glaucoma, and acute progression of a developmental cataract. Note the corneal edema overlying the Baerveldt glaucoma drainage device in the superotemporal anterior chamber.

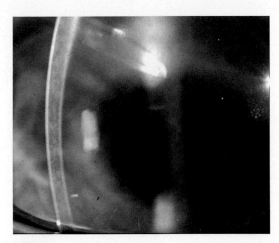

Figure 14.18   Same eye as in Figure 14.17, now pseudophakic. Note the proximity of the glaucoma drainage-device tube to the cornea, with resultant overlying edema. Note also the pseudoiris where the peripheral capsule has opacified.

insertion of an intraocular lens with a peripheral black diaphragm or a frosted surface (246,247).

Penetrating keratoplasty is also difficult in these patients, likely because of the high incidence of corneal vascularization as well as peripheral corneal pannus. In a series of 8 patients who underwent keratoplasty in 11 eyes, graft rejection occurred in 7 eyes, and the glaucoma became more difficult to control in 5 of 9 eyes (248). Another series reported a high incidence of graft failure and limited visual improvement after corneal transplantations in one large family with aniridia (249).

OTHER SYNDROMES WITH ASSOCIATED GLAUCOMA

In addition to the disorders already considered in this chapter, glaucoma may be a feature of many other congenital syndromes. This discussion is limited to syndromes that represent multisystem, developmental anomalies and represents only a partial list of this extensive group of developmental disorders. (Further information on the loci and genes for systemic diseases associated with glaucoma can be found in Table 8.1.)

Chromosomal Anomalies

Trisomy 21: Down Syndrome

This condition is characterized by mental retardation and atypical facies. Ocular findings include epicanthus, blepharitis, nystagmus, strabismus, light-colored and spotted irides, keratoconus, cataracts, and congenital glaucoma (250). The glaucoma, although not commonly reported in series on the ocular features of Down syndrome (251), usually appears in infancy, with the typical findings of PCG (252).

Trisomy 13–15: Trisomy D Syndrome

The principal systemic features of trisomy D syndrome include mental retardation, deafness, heart disease, and motor seizures. The condition is usually not compatible with life, although milder forms have been reported (253). Ocular findings include microphthalmia, coloboma with cartilage, congenital cataracts, retinal dysplasia, persistent fetal vasculature, and dysembryogenesis of the anterior chamber angle (254). Glaucoma may be a result of several of these developmental defects.

Trisomy 18: Edwards Syndrome

The ocular histopathologic findings in one infant with trisomy 18 included an anterior position of the iris obstructing the anterior chamber angle (255).

XO: Turner Syndrome

Patients with Turner syndrome are typically short stature, postadolescent females with sexual infantilism and multiple systemic anomalies. Ocular findings include ptosis, epicanthus, cataract, strabismus, blue sclera, corneal nebulae, and color blindness (256). Developmental glaucoma is rarely associated (257).

Cystinosis

Cystinosis is a rare autosomal recessive metabolic disorder characterized by widespread accumulation of cystine crystals in ocular and nonocular tissues. The disorder is caused by mutation in the gene encoding cystinosin (*CTNS*, gene map locus 17p13, OMIM 219800) (16). Pupillary block glaucoma in one patient was thought to be caused by the cystine accumulation in the iris stroma (258).

Fetal Alcohol Syndrome

Fetal alcohol syndrome presumably results from a teratogenic effect of alcohol during a critical period of gestation, possibly influenced by a genetic background. The anterior ocular segment may be involved, with developmental abnormalities resembling those of the Axenfeld–Rieger syndrome and Peters anomaly (201,259). Mouse studies suggest that the ocular abnormalities result from an acute insult to the optic primordia during a specific period that corresponds to the third week after fertilization in the human (260).

Hepatocerebrorenal Syndrome: Zellweger Syndrome

Zellweger syndrome, or the hepatocerebrorenal syndrome, is a multisystem congenital disorder characterized by central nervous system abnormalities, hepatic interstitial fibrosis, and renal cysts. Ocular findings include nystagmus, corneal clouding, cataracts, retinal vascular and pigmentary abnormalities, optic nerve head lesions, and congenital glaucoma (261). Iridocorneal adhesions may be the mechanism of the glaucoma (262). This disease is a peroxisomal biogenesis disorder, inherited in an autosomal recessive manner and resulting from mutations in any of at least 12 genes associated with exfoliation syndrome that encode peroxins. Affected individuals rarely live beyond the first year of life (263,264).

Hallermann–Streiff Syndrome

Micrognathia and dwarfism in persons with Hallermann–Streiff syndrome may be associated with ocular findings, including cataracts and microphthalmos. Glaucoma may also occur because of absorption of lens material or associated aniridia or after cataract surgery (236,265). This condition has been reported only in isolated cases, with no pattern of inheritance demonstrated.

Kniest Dysplasia

Kniest dysplasia resembles classic metatropic dwarfism, but it has an autosomal dominant inheritance pattern and is caused by mutations in the *COL2A1* gene (gene map locus 12q13.11–q13.2, OMIM 156550) (16). Congenital glaucoma has been described in a patient with presumed Kniest syndrome (266).

Lowe Syndrome

Lowe syndrome (i.e., oculocerebrorenal syndrome) is an autosomal recessive, X-linked disorder characterized by mental retardation, renal rickets, aminoaciduria, hypotonia, acidemia, and irritability. The two principal ocular abnormalities are cataracts, which are usually bilateral and occur in nearly all cases, and glaucoma, which is seen in approximately two thirds of patients. Other ocular findings include microphthalmia, strabismus, nystagmus, miosis, and iris atrophy. Female carriers may be identified by cortical lens opacities and genetic studies (267). Lowe syndrome (OMIM 309000) can be caused by mutation in the *OCRL1* gene, locus Xq26.1 (OMIM 300535), mutations that also cause Dent disease (OMIM 300009) (16,268).

Glaucoma in Lowe syndrome results from a primary filtration-angle anomaly, likely with additional abnormalities secondary to removal of concurrent congenital cataracts. In a small retrospective gonioscopic study of eyes in patients with Lowe syndrome, anterior insertion of the iris, narrowing of the ciliary body band, and decreased visibility of the scleral spur were observed. Goniotomy surgery was uniformly unsuccessful in controlling the glaucoma, perhaps because of the superimposed adverse effects of cataract surgery on the filtration-angle structures. Nonangle surgical interventions are needed to control most cases, although selected milder cases of glaucoma have been managed medically (269) (**Fig. 14.19**).

Michel Syndrome

Michel syndrome is characterized by congenital anomalies of the anterior ocular segment, eyelids, and skeletal system and has an apparent autosomal recessive pattern of transmission (270,271). This condition can be caused by mutations in the *FGF3* gene, locus 11q13 (OMIM 610706) (16). Tekin (272) proposed that this syndrome be called deafness with labyrinthine aplasia, microtia, and microdontia (LAMM). Ocular findings include corneal opacities, conjunctival telangiectasia, and iridocorneal adhesions with blepharoptosis, blepharophimosis, and telecanthus; systemic findings include oromandibular anomalies, short stature, clinodactyly, subnormal intelligence,

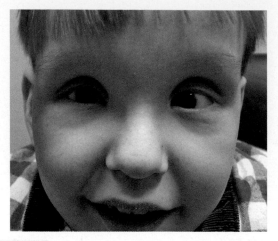

Figure 14.19 A 13-year-old boy with Lowe syndrome and glaucoma controlled with medication use. He has aphakia in both eyes after removal of congenital cataracts, and has small stature, developmental delay, and esotropia.

and hearing loss. Glaucoma may occur in eyes with extensive anterior segment anomalies (270).

Mucopolysaccharidoses

The MPS constitute a group of inherited disorders caused by deficiency of specific lysosomal enzymes needed for the degradation of glycosaminoglycans, or mucopolysaccharides. The accumulation of partially degraded glycosaminoglycans causes interference with cell, tissue, and organ function.

Deficiency of alpha-L-iduronidase (from mutations in the *IDUA* gene, locus 4p16.3) can result in a wide range of phenotypic involvement with three major recognized clinical entities: Hurler (MPS IH; OMIM 607014), Scheie (MPS IS; OMIM 607016), and Hurler–Scheie (MPS IH/S) syndromes. The Hurler and Scheie syndromes represent phenotypes at the severe and mild ends of the MPS I clinical spectrum, respectively, and the Hurler–Scheie syndrome is intermediate in phenotypic expression (16).

The prototype, Hurler syndrome, is an autosomal recessive disease with central nervous system, skeletal, and visceral abnormalities. The typical ocular finding is corneal clouding. Glaucoma has also been reported in Hurler syndrome and was thought to result from mucopolysaccharide-containing cells in the aqueous outflow system (273). In a 3-year-old child with Hurler syndrome and open-angle glaucoma, the IOP returned to normal after bone marrow transplantation (274). Medications and angle surgery are reasonable options to treat this glaucoma (Freedman SF, unpublished data).

Angle-closure glaucoma has occurred in Hurler–Scheie syndrome, responding initially to peripheral iridectomy and medications, but ultimately requiring clear lens extraction and then glaucoma drainage-device implantation; the mechanism of angle closure remains elusive (Freedman SF, unpublished data).

Patients with mucopolysaccharidosis type VI, the Maroteaux–Lamy syndrome, may have acute or chronic angle-closure glaucoma, which appears to be associated more with increased thickness of the peripheral cornea than with pupillary block (264,275). This autosomal recessive disorder results from deficiency of the enzyme *N*-acetylgalactosamine-4-sulfatase, due to mutations in the gene *ARSB* (arylsulfatase B, locus 5q11–q13, OMIM 253200) (16).

Glaucoma (apparently with open angles) was also described in two siblings with mucopolysaccharidosis type IV, the Morquio syndrome (276). Two types of MPS IV are now recognized: (a) Morquio syndrome A, resulting from mutations in the gene encoding the enzyme galactosamine-6-sulfate sulfatase (GALNS; OMIM 612222; locus 16p24.3, OMIM 612222) and (b) Morquio syndrome B (OMIM 253010), a genetically distinct disorder with overlapping clinical features caused by mutation in the beta-galactosidase gene (*GLB1*; OMIM 611458) (16).

Nail–Patella Syndrome

The nail–patella syndrome, which includes dysplasia of the nails and absent or hypoplastic patella as cardinal features, has been associated with open-angle glaucoma. Two groups have reported cosegregation of primary open-angle glaucoma and nail–patella syndrome as the result of a pleiotropic effect of the gene causing nail–patella syndrome (*LMX1B*, gene map locus 9q34.1, OMIM 161200) (16,277,278).

Oculodentodigital Dysplasia

The systemic features of oculodentodigital dysplasia are hypoplastic dental enamel, microdontia, bilateral syndactyly, and a characteristic thin nose. Multiple ocular anomalies have been described, including glaucoma. There are probably several mechanisms of glaucoma in this syndrome, with reported cases of mild developmental abnormalities of the anterior chamber angle, gonioscopic changes resembling infantile glaucoma, and one case of chronic angle-closure glaucoma associated with bilateral microcornea (189,279,280). This autosomal dominant disorder is caused by mutation in the connexin-43 gene (*CJA1*, gene locus 6q21–q23.2, OMIM 164200) (16).

Prader–Willi Syndrome

Prader–Willi syndrome, characterized by muscular hypotonia, hypogonadism, obesity, and mental retardation, is frequently caused by an abnormality of chromosome 15. This syndrome may be a contiguous gene syndrome due to deletion of the paternal copies of the imprinted SNRPN gene (OMIM 182279), the necdin gene (OMIM 602117), and possible other genes in the region 15q11–q13 (OMIM 176270) (16). Ocular findings include oculocutaneous albinism and congenital ectropion uveae, which may be associated with open-angle glaucoma (281). One patient with Prader–Willi syndrome, congenital ectropion uvea, and glaucoma had factor XI deficiency and the suggestion of a primary hypothalamic defect (282).

Rubinstein–Taybi Syndrome

Individuals with Rubinstein–Taybi (broad thumb) syndrome have mental and motor retardation and typical congenital skeletal deformities with characteristically large, broad thumbs

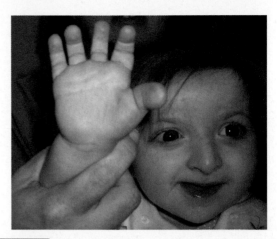

Figure 14.20 A 3-year-old girl with Rubinstein–Taybi (broad thumb) syndrome. She has 13.5-mm corneas and is followed up for suspected glaucoma, but IOPs and optic nerves have been normal thus far.

and first toes. Ocular findings include bushy brows, hypertelorism, epicanthus, antimongoloid slant of eyelids, and hyperopia. Infantile or juvenile glaucoma has also been observed in several patients (283–285). This autosomal dominant disorder is caused by mutation in the gene encoding the transcriptional coactivator CREB-binding protein (gene locus 16p13.3, OMIM 180849) (16) (**Fig. 14.20**).

Stickler Syndrome and Similar Syndromes

Stickler syndrome, or hereditary progressive arthroophthalmopathy, is an autosomal dominant connective tissue dysplasia, characterized by ocular, orofacial, and generalized skeletal abnormalities (286). The Pierre Robin anomaly of mandibular hypoplasia, glossoptosis, and cleft palate may be seen in some patients. The most common ocular manifestations are high myopia, open-angle glaucoma, cataracts, vitreoretinal degeneration, and retinal detachment (287,288). In one study of 39 patients from 12 families, 10% had ocular hypertension, which may be associated with numerous iris processes, suggestive of a developmental abnormality of the angle (288). Neovascular glaucoma has also been reported in association with Stickler syndrome (289). The open-angle glaucoma can usually be controlled medically, although miotics should be avoided if possible because of the potential for retinal detachment.

Three forms of Stickler syndrome have been recognized genetically and involve abnormalities in collagen genes. The Stickler syndrome type I results from a mutation in the *COL2A1* gene (OMIM 120140, locus 12q13.11–q13.2) and includes glaucoma among its ocular clinical features. The Stickler syndrome type II results from a mutation in the α_1-polypeptide of collagen XI (*COL11A1*, OMIM 121280, locus 6p21.3) and includes reported glaucoma (16). The Stickler syndrome type III is caused by mutations in the collagen, type XI, alpha 2 gene (*COL11A2*, OMIM 120290, locus 1p21) and does not have reported ocular features (16). There is evidence for at least one more Stickler syndrome locus. Although the above-described forms of Stickler syndrome have an autosomal dominant in-

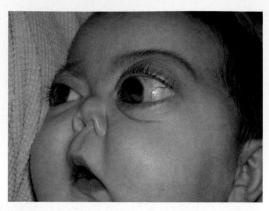

Figure 14.21 A 4-month-old infant girl with bilateral glaucoma, and buphthalmic left eye. The eye was blind with corneal exposure and highly elevated IOP, and enucleation was elected.

heritance pattern, an autosomal recessive form of this syndrome can be attributed to mutations in the *COL9A1* gene (OMIM 120210.0002).

Wagner syndrome can be caused by mutation in the gene encoding chondroitin sulfate proteoglycan-2 (*CSPG2*; OMIM 118661, 5q13–q14) (16), also called versican, a proteoglycan found in the vitreous. Wagner syndrome and Marshall syndrome (which can result from mutations in the *COL11A1* gene [OMIM 120280], as can Stickler type II) show some clinical overlap with one another and with Stickler syndrome, but they may be distinct disorders (290), and all can be associated with glaucoma (**Figs. 14.21** and **14.22**).

Weissengacher–Zweymuller syndrome (OMIM 277610), also called Pierre Robin syndrome with fetal chondrodysplasia, links to gene map locus 6p21.3 and is caused by a mutation in the *COL11A2* gene (as in Stickler syndrome type III). Congenital glaucoma has been reported in a baby with this disorder (291).

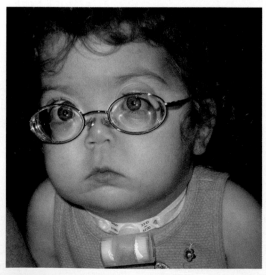

Figure 14.22 Same child as in Figure 14.21, now 3 years of age, after enucleation of the left eye with prosthesis fitting. The right eye has medically controlled glaucoma but has a large, clear cornea, with very high myopia. Note the trachestomy due to coexisting Pierre Robin syndrome.

Waardenburg Syndrome

Waardenburg syndrome is an autosomal dominant disorder characterized by lateral displacement of the medial canthi; hyperplasia of the medial brows; a prominent, broad root of the nose; sectorial or complete iris heterochromia; congenital deafness; and a white forelock (292,293). It is thought to represent a defect of neural crest–derived tissues and is caused by a mutation in the *PAX3* gene (gene map locus 2q35, OMIM 193500) (16). Open-angle glaucoma is an uncommon finding, although it was present in one of Waardenburg's original cases, and it may be caused by a developmental abnormality of neural crest–derived tissues in the angle (293).

Walker–Warburg Syndrome

The Walker–Warburg syndrome, also known as the HARD±E syndrome, maps to gene locus 9q34.1 (OMIM 236670) (16). It is a congenital syndrome characterized by hydrocephalus (H), agyria (A), retinal dysplasia (RD), with or without encephalocele (±E), and it is usually fatal in the first year of life. Multiple eye abnormalities have been reported, including congenital glaucoma (294).

Cockayne Syndrome

Cockayne syndrome is an autosomal recessive disorder that is characterized by dwarfism and birdlike facies. Ocular manifestations include "salt and pepper" retinopathy, cataracts, corneal ulcers or opacities, nystagmus, hypoplastic irides, and irregular pupils. Although glaucoma has not been an associated condition, histopathologic examination of one case revealed a high insertion of the anterior uvea into the posterior aspect of the trabecular meshwork (295), similar to that seen in congenital glaucoma and the Axenfeld–Rieger syndrome.

SECONDARY CHILDHOOD GLAUCOMAS

Pediatric glaucoma may occur secondary to a wide variety of ophthalmic conditions (see Table 13.1). While secondary glaucoma is a consequence of another eye disease rather than a primary disorder of the aqueous humor filtration mechanism, the true mechanism of glaucoma in some conditions may be both primary and secondary. The distinction between primary glaucoma and secondary glaucoma has been largely abandoned in considering adult glaucomas, but continues to prove useful in the general classification of childhood glaucomas.

Trauma

Trauma-associated glaucoma in the pediatric population usually relates to an acute or secondary anterior chamber hemorrhage (hyphema). Rather than occurring acutely, the elevation of IOP elevation more commonly begins several days after acute blunt trauma, accompanied by a large initial hyphema or rebleeding. Clinical treatment of hyphema with moderately frequent administration of topical steroid, use of cycloplegics, and bedrest may decrease the risk of rebleeding. Children with sickle-cell hemoglobinopathies are especially susceptible to optic nerve damage with moderate IOP elevation, and should be followed up, as should all patients with hyphema, with serial examination and IOP measurement. Children presenting with elevated IOP in the setting of a hyphema can usually be managed with medications, and with gentle anterior chamber irrigation in refractory cases, because IOP often normalizes after the hyphema resolves, even in cases with angle recession. Patients showing angle recession on gonioscopic examination should be followed up long term, because the onset of chronic glaucoma may be delayed by years to decades (see Chapter 25).

Intraocular Neoplasm

Neoplasms infrequently produce childhood glaucoma (see also Chapter 21). Advanced retinoblastoma is the most common cause of such glaucoma, usually due to neovascular glaucoma and angle dysfunction or closure rather than tumor cells in the anterior chamber (296). Medulloepithelioma, a neoplasm of the ciliary epithelium, can also induce secondary neovascular glaucoma (297).

Juvenile xanthogranuloma, a rare systemic disorder sometimes associated with histiocytic infiltration of the iris, can present with glaucoma due to spontaneous hyphema or the accumulation of histiocytes blocking the trabecular meshwork. Although conservative treatment with glaucoma medications, along with use of topical and systemic steroids, usually suffices, refractory cases may require surgical intervention, made challenging by the tendency for continued iris bleeding whenever the IOP is lowered (298).

Inflammation and Steroid-Related Glaucoma

Pediatric glaucoma secondary to chronic inflammation often presents in association with chronic anterior uveitis (e.g., antinuclear antibody–associated idiopathic uveitis or arthritis) and less often with other inflammatory conditions (299) (see also Chapter 22). Uveitis-associated glaucoma occurs by various possible mechanisms in these children. IOP elevation may result acutely from trabeculitis, trabecular obstruction, iris bombé, and pupillary block, or chronically from peripheral anterior synechiae, trabecular scarring or dysfunction, and steroid-induced trabecular obstruction. The diagnosis of uveitis-related glaucoma is sometimes delayed in children, because the IOP rise is thought to be steroid induced, but inflammation-related aqueous outflow reduction masks the true glaucoma when inflammation increases from steroid reduction. Judicious use of systemic steroid-sparing therapy (best comanaged with pediatric rheumatologists) often proves vital to manage refractory uveitis cases (300).

Managing glaucoma secondary to uveitis requires control of the underlying inflammation, followed initially by medical management, provided the anterior chamber angle remains open. Angle surgery often controls the IOP when medication is insufficient, but success is reduced in those eyes with extensive peripheral anterior synechiae and after cataract removal (301,302); glaucoma drainage-device surgery has also been successful in refractory cases (303), whereas trabeculectomy surgery has a high incidence of complications in this population (304). Cycloablation should be used with extreme caution in patients with uveitic glaucoma, because of the risk of phthisis.

Lens-Induced Glaucoma

Acute glaucoma with pupillary block and angle closure may develop in any child with ectopia lentis (from various causes, e.g., homocystinuria, Weill–Marchesani syndrome, Marfan syndrome), because of forward shifting of the lens into the pupillary aperture (see also Chapter 18). The angle-closure attack can sometimes be broken by nonsurgical means, including supine patient positioning, manual displacement of the lens posteriorly in the eye, medication with aqueous suppressants, mydriatics, and analgesics, and subsequent miotic use. Iridectomy helps prevent repeated IOP elevation but not anterior lens displacement, and lensectomy may ultimately be needed (but is more safely performed in eyes with controlled IOP) (305).

Aphakic (Pseudophakic) Glaucoma

Glaucoma often occurs after removal of congenital or developmental cataracts, with reported incidence ranging from 3% to 41%. This aphakic or pseudophakic glaucoma represents a serious cause of late visual loss in eyes after cataract removal. Aphakic or pseudophakic glaucoma is usually of the open-angle type, asymptomatic, and delayed in onset for many years after cataract removal (median postsurgical onset, 5 years) (306,307). Factors associated with an increased risk for glaucoma after cataract extraction include cataract removal in the first year of life, microphthalmia, and coexistence of persistent fetal vasculature. The pathogenesis of open-angle glaucoma after cataract removal remains elusive; proposed theories include both mechanical (trabecular collapse due to loss of zonular tension on the scleral spur) and chemical (postoperative inflammatory trabecular damage or vitreous-derived toxic factors), with no proof of either (308).

When angle-closure glaucoma occurs in an aphakic or pseudophakic eye, prompt peripheral iridectomy (and sometimes synechialysis or anterior vitrectomy, or both) is mandatory, and often curative. By contrast, medical therapy is the first-line treatment in aphakic or pseudophakic eyes with open-angle glaucoma; the angle, albeit open, often has typical acquired angle abnormalities (309). When medical therapy has failed to control aphakic or pseudophakic glaucoma, angle surgery often has disappointing results, although 360-degree trabeculotomy sometimes temporizes in cases of early-onset glaucoma (Freedman SF, unpublished data). Trabeculectomy with antiproliferative agents should be used with extreme caution in aphakic or pseudophakic eyes because of the likelihood of bleb scarring and the high risk of endophthalmitis should postoperative bleb infection occur. Moderate success has been reported with glaucoma drainage-device surgery, and cycloablation in selected refractory cases (123,129). Intraocular lens implantation, either primary or secondary, does not protect against glaucoma after cataract removal (310).

Miscellaneous Causes

Children may develop glaucoma in response to topical steroid use (see Chapter 23) and because of various other reported causes (Table 13.1). Although there is no consensus on the optimal strategy for managing secondary pediatric glaucoma, determining the cause in each case assists the clinician in planning reasonable treatment options.

KEY POINTS

- Childhood glaucomas constitute a heterogenous group of serious conditions.
- Current classification systems are varied, but all fall short of complete consistency and consensus.
- Glaucoma disorders in children share clinical features often related to the age of onset and the magnitude of IOP elevation.
- Many of the developmental glaucomas have coexisting ocular and systemic abnormalities. These disorders, most of which have a genetic basis, are typically bilateral and are usually diagnosed at birth or in early childhood.
- Children may also develop glaucoma secondary to acquired outflow pathway defects, many of which are shared by adults (examples include uveitic and traumatic glaucoma). One notable exception is glaucoma occurring after surgical removal (in childhood) of congenital or developmental cataracts.
- Although genetic advances may assist in our understanding of the complex interplay between genotype and phenotype in developmental glaucomas, much future work awaits before visual loss from childhood glaucoma will be adequately curtailed.

REFERENCES

1. Walton DS. Primary congenital open-angle glaucoma. In: Chandler PA, Grant WM, eds. *Glaucoma.* Philadelphia, PA: Lea & Febiger; 1979:329–343.
2. Shaffer RN, Weiss DI. *Congenital and Pediatric Glaucomas.* St. Louis: CV Mosby; 1970.
3. Duke-Elder S. *Congenital Deformities. System of Ophthalmology.* Vol 3. (pt 2). St. Louis: CV Mosby; 1969.
4. Kwito ML. *Glaucoma in Infants and Children.* New York: Appleton-Century-Crofts; 1973.
5. Lotufo D, Ritch R, Szmyd L Jr, et al. Juvenile glaucoma, race, and refraction. *JAMA.* 1989;261(2):249–252.
6. Papadopoulos M, Cable N, Rahi J, et al. The British Infantile and Childhood Glaucoma (BIG) Eye Study. *Invest Ophthalmol Vis Sci.* 2007;48(9):4100–4106.
7. deLuise VP, Anderson DR. Primary infantile glaucoma (congenital glaucoma). *Surv Ophthalmol.* 1983;28(1):1–19.
8. Akarsu AN, Turacli ME, Aktan SG, et al. A second locus (GLC3B) for primary congenital glaucoma (Buphthalmos) maps to the 1p36 region. *Hum Mol Genet.* 1996;5(8):1199–203.
9. Stoilov I, Akarsu AN, Alozie I, et al. Sequence analysis and homology modeling suggest that primary congenital glaucoma on 2p21 results from mutations disrupting either the hinge region or the conserved core structures of cytochrome P4501B1. *Am J Hum Genet.* 1998;62(3):573–584.
10. Chitsazian F, Tusi BK, Elahi E, et al. CYP1B1 mutation profile of Iranian primary congenital glaucoma patients and associated haplotypes. *J Mol Diagn.* 2007;9(3):382–393.
11. Narooie-Nejad M, Paylakhi SH, Shojaee S, et al. Loss of function mutations in the gene encoding latent transforming growth factor beta binding protein 2, LTBP2, cause primary congenital glaucoma. *Hum Mol Genet.* 2009;18(20):3969–3977.
12. Ali M, McKibbin M, Booth A, et al. Null mutations in LTBP2 cause primary congenital glaucoma. *Am J Hum Genet.* 2009;84(5):664–671.
13. Kaur K, Reddy AB, Mukhopadhyay A, et al. Myocilin gene implicated in primary congenital glaucoma. *Clin Genet.* 2005;67(4):335–340.
14. Vincent AL, Billingsley G, Buys Y, et al. Digenic inheritance of early-onset glaucoma: CYP1B1, a potential modifier gene. *Am J Hum Genet.* 2002;70(2):448–460.
15. Zhuo YH, Wang M, Wei YT, et al. Analysis of MYOC gene mutation in a Chinese glaucoma family with primary open-angle glaucoma and primary congenital glaucoma. *Chin Med J.* 2006;119(14):1210–1214.
16. Online Mendelian Inheritance in Man, OMIM (TM). 2009. Available at: http://www.ncbi.nlm.nih.gov/omim/.
17. Sutter TR, Tang YM, Hayes CL, et al. Complete cDNA sequence of a human dioxin-inducible mRNA identifies a new gene subfamily of cytochrome P450 that maps to chromosome 2. *J Biol Chem.* 1994;269(18):13092–13099.
18. Tang YM, Wo YY, Stewart J, et al. Isolation and characterization of the human cytochrome P450 CYP1B1 gene. *J Biol Chem.* 1996;271(45):28324–28330.
19. Belous AR, Hachey DL, Dawling S, et al. Cytochrome P450 1B1-mediated estrogen metabolism results in estrogen-deoxyribonucleoside adduct formation. *Cancer Res.* 2007;67(2):812–817.
20. Choudhary D, Jansson I, Stoilov I, et al. Metabolism of retinoids and arachidonic acid by human and mouse cytochrome P450 1b1. *Drug Metab Dispos.* 2004;32(8):840–847.
21. Ma X, Idle JR, Krausz KW, et al. Metabolism of melatonin by human cytochromes p450. *Drug Metab Dispos.* 2005;33(4):489–494.
22. Shimada T, Gillam EM, Sutter TR, et al. Oxidation of xenobiotics by recombinant human cytochrome P450 1B1. *Drug Metab Dispos.* 1997;25(5):617–622.
23. Bejjani BA, Xu L, Armstrong D, et al. Expression patterns of cytochrome P4501B1 (Cyp1b1) in FVB/N mouse eyes. *Exp Eye Res.* 2002;75(3):249–257.
24. Vasiliou V, Gonzalez FJ. Role of CYP1B1 in glaucoma. *Annu Rev Pharmacol Toxicol.* 2008;48:333–358.
25. Plasilova M, Stoilov I, Sarfarazi M, et al. Identification of a single ancestral CYP1B1 mutation in Slovak Gypsies (Roms) affected with primary congenital glaucoma. *J Med Genet.* 1999;36(4):290–294.
26. Mashima Y, Suzuki Y, Sergeev Y, et al. Novel cytochrome P4501B1 (CYP1B1) gene mutations in Japanese patients with primary congenital glaucoma. *Invest Ophthalmol Vis Sci.* 2001;42(10):2211–2216.
27. Stone EM, Fingert JH, Alward WL, et al. Identification of a gene that causes primary open angle glaucoma. *Science.* 1997;275(5300):668–670.
28. Shepard AR, Jacobson N, Fingert JH, et al. Delayed secondary glucocorticoid responsiveness of MYOC in human trabecular meshwork cells. *Invest Ophthalmol Vis Sci.* 2001;42(13):3173–3181.
29. Takahashi H, Noda S, Mashima Y, et al. The myocilin (MYOC) gene expression in the human trabecular meshwork. *Curr Eye Res.* 2000;20(2):81–84.
30. Li X, Yin W, Perez-Jurado L, et al. Mapping of human and murine genes for latent TGF-beta binding protein-2 (LTBP2). *Mamm Genome.* 1995;6(1):42–45.
31. Hyytiainen M, Keski-Oja J. Latent TGF-beta binding protein LTBP-2 decreases fibroblast adhesion to fibronectin. *J Cell Biol.* 2003;163(6):1363–1374.
32. Hyytiainen M, Taipale J, Heldin CH, et al. Recombinant latent transforming growth factor beta-binding protein 2 assembles to fibroblast extracellular matrix and is susceptible to proteolytic processing and release. *J Biol Chem.* 1998;273(32):20669–20676.
33. Rifkin DB. Latent transforming growth factor-beta (TGF-beta) binding proteins: orchestrators of TGF-beta availability. *J Biol Chem.* 2005;280(9):7409–7412.
34. Sinha S, Heagerty AM, Shuttleworth CA, et al. Expression of latent TGF-beta binding proteins and association with TGF-beta 1 and fibrillin-1 following arterial injury. *Cardiovasc Res.* 2002;53(4):971–983.
35. Schlotzer-Schrehardt U, Zenkel M, Kuchle M, et al. Role of transforming growth factor-beta1 and its latent form binding protein in exfoliation syndrome. *Exp Eye Res.* 2001;73(6):765–780.
36. Hoskins HD, Shaffer RN. Evaluation techniques for congenital glaucomas. *J Pediatr Ophthalmol Strabismus.* 1971;8:81–87.
37. Seidman DJ, Nelson LB, Calhoun JH, et al. Signs and symptoms in the presentation of primary infantile glaucoma. *Pediatrics.* 1986;77(3):399–404.

38. Kiskis AA, Markowitz SN, Morin JD. Corneal diameter and axial length in congenital glaucoma. *Can J Ophthalmol.* 1985;20(3):93–97.

39. Becker B, Shaffer RN. *Diagnosis and Therapy of the Glaucomas.* St. Louis: CV Mosby; 1965.

40. Sampaolesi R, Caruso R. Ocular echometry in the diagnosis of congenital glaucoma. *Arch Ophthalmol.* 1982;100(4):574–577.

41. Imre G, Bogi J. Corneal edema in young glaucoma patients [in German]. *Klin Monbl Augenheilkd.* 1981;179(6):465–466.

42. Walton DS. Diagnosis and treatment of glaucoma in childhood. In: Epstein DL, ed. *Chandler and Grant's glaucoma.* 3rd ed. Philadelphia, PA: Lea & Febiger; 1986.

43. Dominguez A, Banos S, Alvarez G, et al. Intraocular pressure measurement in infants under general anesthesia. *Am J Ophthalmol.* 1974; 78(1):110–116.

44. Morin JD, Bryars JH. Causes of loss of vision in congenital glaucoma. *Arch Ophthalmol.* 1980;98(9):1575–1576.

45. Worst JGF. *The Pathogenesis of Congenital Glaucoma: An Embryological and Goniosurgical Study.* Springfield, IL: Charles C Thomas; 1966.

46. Barkan O. Pathogenesis of congenital glaucoma: gonioscopic and anatomic observation of the angle of the anterior chamber in the normal eye and in congenital glaucoma. *Am J Ophthalmol.* 1955;40(1):1–11.

47. Luntz MH. Congenital, infantile, and juvenile glaucoma. *Ophthalmology.* 1979;86(5):793–802.

48. Budenz DL, Hodapp E. Vitrectomy lens for examination of the optic disk in young children with glaucoma. *Am J Ophthalmol.* 1995;119(4): 523–524.

49. Armstrong TA. Evaluation of the Tono-Pen and the Pulsair tonometers. *Am J Ophthalmol.* 1990;109(6):716–720.

50. Spierer A, Huna R, Hirsh A, et al. Normal intraocular pressure in premature infants. *Am J Ophthalmol.* 1994;117(6):801–803.

51. Pensiero S, Da Pozzo S, Perissutti P, et al. Normal intraocular pressure in children. *J Pediatr Ophthalmol Strabismus.* 1992;29(2):79–84.

52. Radtke ND, Cohan BE. Intraocular pressure measurement in the newborn. *Am J Ophthalmol.* 1974;78(3):501–504.

53. Shaffer RN, Hetherington J Jr. The glaucomatous disc in infants. A suggested hypothesis for disc cupping. *Trans Am Acad Ophthalmol Otolaryngol.* 1969;73(5):923–935.

54. Quigley HA. The pathogenesis of reversible cupping in congenital glaucoma. *Am J Ophthalmol.* 1977;84(3):358–370.

55. Quigley HA. Childhood glaucoma: results with trabeculotomy and study of reversible cupping. *Ophthalmology.* 1982;89(3):219–226.

56. Robin AL, Quigley HA. Transient reversible cupping in juvenile-onset glaucoma. *Am J Ophthalmol.* 1979;88(3 pt 2):580–584.

57. Richardson KT. Optic cup symmetry in normal newborn infants. *Invest Ophthalmol.* 1968;7(2):137–140.

58. Robin AL, Quigley HA, Pollack IP, et al. An analysis of visual acuity, visual fields, and disk cupping in childhood glaucoma. *Am J Ophthalmol.* 1979;88(5):847–858.

59. Rice NS. Management of infantile glaucoma. *Br J Ophthalmol.* 1972; 56(3):294–298.

60. Cooling RJ, Rice NS, McLeod D. Retinal detachment in congenital glaucoma. *Br J Ophthalmol.* 1980;64(6):417–421.

61. Sampaolesi R. Corneal diameter and axial length in congenital glaucoma. *Can J Ophthalmol.* 1988;23(1):42–44.

62. Tarkkanen A, Uusitalo R, Mianowicz J. Ultrasonographic biometry in congenital glaucoma. *Acta Ophthalmol.* 1983;61(4):618–623.

63. Henriques MJ, Vessani RM, Reis FA, et al. Corneal thickness in congenital glaucoma. *J Glaucoma.* 2004;13(3):185–188.

64. Liu X, Ling Y, Luo R, et al. Optical coherence tomography in measuring retinal nerve fiber layer thickness in normal subjects and patients with open-angle glaucoma. *Chin Med J.* 2001;114(5):524–529.

65. Mann IC. *The Development of the Human Eye.* 3rd ed. New York: Grune & Stratton; 1964.

66. Kashani AA. Early formation of the anterior chamber of the eye in the human embryo. *Ital J Ophthalmol.* 1989;3:65–76.

67. Johnston MC, Noden DM, Hazelton RD, et al. Origins of avian ocular and periocular tissues. *Exp Eye Res.* 1979;29(1):27–43.

68. Tripathi BJ, Tripathi RC. Neural crest origin of human trabecular meshwork and its implications for the pathogenesis of glaucoma. *Am J Ophthalmol.* 1989;107(6):583–590.

69. Foets B, van den Oord J, Engelmann K, et al. A comparative immunohistochemical study of human corneotrabecular tissue. *Graefes Arch Clin Exp Ophthalmol.* 1992;230(3):269–274.

70. Wulle KG. Electron microscopy of the fetal development of the corneal endothelium and Descemet's membrane of the human eye. *Invest Ophthalmol.* 1972;11(11):897–904.

71. Hay ED. Development of the vertebrate cornea. *Int Rev Cytol.* 1979;63: 263–322.

72. Allen L, Burian HM, Braley AE. A new concept of the development of the anterior chamber angle; its relationship to developmental glaucoma and other structural anomalies. *Arch Ophthalmol.* 1955;53(6): 783–798.

73. Smelser GK, Ozanics V. The development of the trabecular meshwork in primate eyes. *Am J Ophthalmol.* 1971;1(1 pt 2):366–385.

74. Anderson DR. The development of the trabecular meshwork and its abnormality in primary infantile glaucoma. *Trans Am Ophthalmol Soc.* 1981;79:458–485.

75. Hansson HA, Jerndal T. Scanning electron microscopic studies on the development of the iridocorneal angle in human eyes. *Invest Ophthalmol.* 1971;10(4):252–265.

76. Van Buskirk EM. Clinical implications of iridocorneal angle development. *Ophthalmology.* 1981;88(4):361–367.

77. McMenamin PG. Human fetal iridocorneal angle: a light and scanning electron microscopic study. *Br J Ophthalmol.* 1989;73(11):871–879.

78. McMenamin PG. A quantitative study of the prenatal development of the aqueous outflow system in the human eye. *Exp Eye Res.* 1991; 53(4):507–517.

79. Shields MB. Axenfeld-Rieger syndrome: a theory of mechanism and distinctions from the iridocorneal endothelial syndrome. *Trans Am Ophthalmol Soc.* 1983;81:736–784.

80. Mann IC. *Development of the Human Eye.* Cambridge: Cambridge University Press; 1928.

81. Anderson DR. Pathology of the glaucomas. *Br J Ophthalmol.* 1972; 56(3):146–157.

82. Maumenee AE. The pathogenesis of congenital glaucoma: a new theory. *Am J Ophthalmol.* 1959;47(6):827–858.

83. Maumenee AE. Further observations on the pathogenesis of congenital glaucoma. *Am J Ophthalmol.* 1963;55:1163–1176.

84. Wright JD Jr, Robb RM, Dueker DK, et al. Congenital glaucoma unresponsive to conventional therapy: a clinicopathological case presentation. *J Pediatr Ophthalmol Strabismus.* 1983;20(5):172–179.

85. Sampaolesi R, Argento C. Scanning electron microscopy of the trabecular meshwork in normal and glucomatous eyes. *Invest Ophthalmol Vis Sci.* 1977;16(4):302–314.

86. Maul E, Strozzi L, Munoz C, et al. The outflow pathway in congenital glaucoma. *Am J Ophthalmol.* 1980;89(5):667–673.

87. Rodrigues MM, Spaeth GL, Weinreb S. Juvenile glaucoma associated with goniodysgenesis. *Am J Ophthalmol.* 1976;81(6):786–796.

88. Tawara A, Inomata H. Developmental immaturity of the trabecular meshwork in congenital glaucoma. *Am J Ophthalmol.* 1981;92(4):508–525.

89. Tawara A, Inomata H. Developmental immaturity of the trabecular meshwork in juvenile glaucoma. *Am J Ophthalmol.* 1984;98(1):82–97.

90. Kupfer C, Ross K. The development of outflow facility in human eyes. *Invest Ophthalmol.* 1971;10(7):513–517.

91. Kupfer C, Kaiser-Kupfer MI. Observations on the development of the anterior chamber angle with reference to the pathogenesis of congenital glaucomas. *Am J Ophthalmol.* 1979;88(3 pt 1):424–426.

92. Kolker AE, Hetherington J Jr. *Becker-Shaffer's Diagnosis and Therapy of the Glaucomas.* St. Louis: CV Mosby; 1976.

93. Pearce WG. Autosomal dominant megalocornea with congenital glaucoma: evidence for germ-line mosaicism. *Can J Ophthalmol.* 1991;26(1):21–26.

94. Angell LK, Robb RM, Berson FG. Visual prognosis in patients with ruptures in Descemet's membrane due to forceps injuries. *Arch Ophthalmol.* 1981;99(12):2137–2139.

95. Cibis GW, Tripathi RC. The differential diagnosis of Descemet's tears (Haab's striae) and posterior polymorpous dystrophy bands. A clinicopathologic study. *Ophthalmology.* 1982;89(6):614–620.

96. Pardos GJ, Krachmer JH, Mannis MJ. Posterior corneal vesicles. *Arch Ophthalmol.* 1981;99(9):1573–1577.

97. Ching FC. Corneal opacification in infancy. *Med Coll Va Q.* 1972;8:230.

98. Walton DS. Glaucoma in infants and children. In: Nelson L, Calhoun JH, Harley RD, eds. *Pediatric Ophthalmology.* 3rd ed. Philadelphia, PA: WB Saunders; 1991:258.

99. Elder MJ. Combined trabeculotomy-trabeculectomy compared with primary trabeculectomy for congenital glaucoma. *Br J Ophthalmol.* 1994; 78(10):745–748.

100. Mandal AK, Bhatia PG, Gothwal VK, et al. Safety and efficacy of simultaneous bilateral primary combined trabeculotomy-trabeculectomy for developmental glaucoma. *Indian J Ophthalmol.* 2002;50(1):13–19.

101. Mullaney PB, Selleck C, Al-Awad A, et al. Combined trabeculotomy and trabeculectomy as an initial procedure in uncomplicated congenital glaucoma. *Arch Ophthalmol.* 1999;117(4):457–460.

102. Barkan O. Goniotomy for the relief of congenital glaucoma. *Br J Ophthalmol.* 1948;32(9):701–728.

103. Harms H, Dannheim R. In: MacKenson G, ed. *Microsurgery in Glaucoma.* Basel: Karger; 1970.

104. Beck AD, Lynch MG. 360 degrees trabeculotomy for primary congenital glaucoma. *Arch Ophthalmol.* 1995;113(9):1200–1202.

105. Dannheim R, Haas H. Visual acuity and intraocular pressure after surgery in congenital glaucoma [in German]. *Klin Monbl Augenheilkd.* 1980; 177(3):296–303.

106. Akimoto M, Tanihara H, Negi A, et al. Surgical results of trabeculotomy ab externo for developmental glaucoma. *Arch Ophthalmol.* 1994;112(12): 1540–1544.

107. Hollander DA, Sarfarazi M, Stoilov I, et al. Genotype and phenotype correlations in congenital glaucoma: CYP1B1 mutations, goniodysgenesis, and clinical characteristics. *Am J Ophthalmol.* 2006;142(6):993–1004.

108. Mandal AK, Bhatia PG, Bhaskar A, et al. Long-term surgical and visual outcomes in Indian children with developmental glaucoma operated on within 6 months of birth. *Ophthalmology.* 2004;111(2):283–290.

109. Freedman SF, McCormick K, Cox TA. Mitomycin C-augumented trabeculectomy with postoperative wound modulation in pediatric glaucoma. *J AAPOS.* 1999;3(2):117–124.

110. Sidoti PA, Lopez PF, Michon J, et al. Delayed-onset pneumococcal endophthalmitis after mitomycin-C trabeculectomy: association with cryptic nasolacrimal obstruction. *J Glaucoma.* 1995;4(1):11–15.

111. Waheed S, Ritterband DC, Greenfield DS, et al. Bleb-related ocular infection in children after trabeculectomy with mitomycin C. *Ophthalmology.* 1997;104(12):2117–2120.

112. Beck AD, Freedman SF. Trabeculectomy with mitomycin-C in pediatric glaucomas. *Ophthalmology.* 2001;108(5):835–837.

113. Billson F, Thomas R, Aylward W. The use of two-stage Molteno implants in developmental glaucoma. *J Pediatr Ophthalmol Strabismus.* 1989; 26(1):3–8.

114. Molteno AC, Ancker E, Van Biljon G. Surgical technique for advanced juvenile glaucoma. *Arch Ophthalmol.* 1984;102(1):51–57.

115. Lloyd MA, Sedlak T, Heuer DK, et al. Clinical experience with the single-plate Molteno implant in complicated glaucomas. Update of a pilot study. *Ophthalmology.* 1992;99(5):679–687.

116. Hill RA, Heuer DK, Baerveldt G, et al. Molteno implantation for glaucoma in young patients. *Ophthalmology.* 1991;98(7):1042–1046.

117. Fellenbaum PS, Sidoti PA, Heuer DK, et al. Experience with the baerveldt implant in young patients with complicated glaucomas. *J Glaucoma.* 1995;4(2):91–97.

118. Molteno AC. Children with advanced glaucoma treated by draining implants. *S Afr Arch Ophthalmol.* 1973;1:55–61.

119. Munoz M, Tomey KF, Traverso C, et al. Clinical experience with the Molteno implant in advanced infantile glaucoma. *J Pediatr Ophthalmol Strabismus.* 1991;28(2):68–72.

120. Coleman AL, Smyth RJ, Wilson MR, et al. Initial clinical experience with the Ahmed Glaucoma Valve implant in pediatric patients. *Arch Ophthalmol.* 1997;115(2):186–191.

121. Englert JA, Freedman SF, Cox TA. The Ahmed valve in refractory pediatric glaucoma. *Am J Ophthalmol.* 1999;127(1):34–42.

122. Eid TE, Katz LJ, Spaeth GL, et al. Long-term effects of tube-shunt procedures on management of refractory childhood glaucoma. *Ophthalmology.* 1997;104(6):1011–1016.

123. O'Malley Schotthoefer E, Yanovitch TL, Freedman SF. Aqueous drainage device surgery in refractory pediatric glaucomas: I. Long-term outcomes. *J AAPOS.* 2008;12(1):33–39.

124. al Faran MF, Tomey KF, al Mutlaq FA. Cyclocryotherapy in selected cases of congenital glaucoma. *Ophthalmic Surg.* 1990;21(11):794–798.

125. Phelan MJ, Higginbotham EJ. Contact transscleral Nd:YAG laser cyclophotocoagulation for the treatment of refractory pediatric glaucoma. *Ophthalmic Surg Lasers.* 1995;26(5):401–403.

126. Bock CJ, Freedman SF, Buckley EG, et al. Transscleral diode laser cyclophotocoagulation for refractory pediatric glaucomas. *J Pediatr Ophthalmol Strabismus.* 1997;34(4):235–239.

127. Izgi B, Demirci H, Demirci FY, et al. Diode laser cyclophotocoagulation in refractory glaucoma: comparison between pediatric and adult glaucomas. *Ophthalmic Surg Lasers.* 2001;32(2):100–107.

128. Kirwan JF, Shah P, Khaw PT. Diode laser cyclophotocoagulation: role in the management of refractory pediatric glaucomas. *Ophthalmology.* 2002;109(2):316–323.

129. Carter BC, Plager DA, Neely DE, et al. Endoscopic diode laser cyclophotocoagulation in the management of aphakic and pseudophakic glaucoma in children. *J AAPOS.* 2007;11(1):34–40.

130. Carter BC, Plager DA, Neely DE, et al. Endoscopic diode laser cyclophotocoagulation in the management of aphakic and pseudophakic glaucoma in children. *J AAPOS.* 2007;11(1):34–40.

131. Huang SC, Soong HK, Brenz RM, et al. Problems associated with penetrating keratoplasty for corneal edema in congenital glaucoma. *Ophthalmic Surg.* 1989;20(6):399–402.

132. Cowden JW. Penetrating keratoplasty in infants and children. *Ophthalmology.* 1990;97(3):324–328; discussion 8–9.

133. Erlich CM, Rootman DS, Morin JD. Corneal transplantation in infants, children and young adults: experience of the Toronto Hospital for Sick Children, 1979-88. *Can J Ophthalmol.* 1991;26(4):206–210.

134. Frueh BE, Brown SI. Transplantation of congenitally opaque corneas. *Br J Ophthalmol.* 1997;81(12):1064–1069.

135. Frucht-Pery J, Feldman ST, Brown SI. Transplantation of congenitally opaque corneas from eyes with exaggerated buphthalmos. *Am J Ophthalmol.* 1989;107(6):655–658.

136. Kargi SH, Koc F, Biglan AW, et al. Visual acuity in children with glaucoma. *Ophthalmology.* 2006;113(2):229–238.

137. Morgan KS, Black B, Ellis FD, et al. Treatment of congenital glaucoma. *Am J Ophthalmol.* 1981;92(6):799–803.

138. Barkan O. Goniotomy. *Trans Am Acad Ophthalmol Otolaryngol.* 1955; 59(3):322–332.

139. Scheie HG. Symposium on congential glaucoma: diagnosis, clinical course, and treatment other than goniotomy. *Trans Am Acad Ophthalmol Otolaryngol.* 1955;59(3):309–321.

140. Haas J. Principles and problems of therapy in congenital glaucoma. *Invest Ophthalmol.* 1968;7(2):140–146.

141. Le Douarin NM. The neural crest in the neck and other parts of the body. *Birth Defects Orig Artic Ser.* 1975;11(7):19–50.

142. Bolande RP. The neurocristopathies: a unifying concept of disease arising in neural crest maldevelopment. *Hum Pathol.* 1974;5:409–422.

143. Beauchamp GR, Knepper PA. Role of the neural crest in anterior segment development and disease. *J Pediatr Ophthalmol Strabismus.* 1984;21(6): 209–214.

144. Hoskins HD Jr, Shaffer RN, Hetherington J. Anatomical classification of the developmental glaucomas. *Arch Ophthalmol.* 1984;102(9):1331–1336.

145. Idrees F, Vaideanu D, Fraser SG, et al. A review of anterior segment dysgeneses. *Surv Ophthalmol.* 2006;51(3):213–231.

146. Axenfeld TH. Embryotoxon corneae posterius. *Ber Dtsch Ophthalmol Ges.* 1920;42:301–305.

147. Rieger H. Demonstration von zwei: Fallen von verlagerund und schlitzform der pupille mit hypoplasie des irisvorderblattes an beiden augen einer 10- und 25-jarhrigen patientin [in German]. *Z Augenheilk.* 1934;84:98–99.

148. Rieger H. Beitrage zur kenntnis seltener missbildungen der iris. II. Über hypoplasie der irisvorderblattes mit verlagerund und entrundung der pupille [in German]. *Graefes Arch Clin Exp Ophthalmol.* 1935;133:602–635.

149. Rieger H. Dysgenesis mesodermalis corneae et iridis [in German]. *Z Augenheilk.* 1935;86:333.

150. Mathis H. Zahnunterzahl und missbildungen der iris [in German]. *Z Stomatol.* 1936;34:895–909.

151. Rieger H. Erbfragen in der augenheilkunde [in German]. *Graefes Arch Clin Exp Ophthalmol.* 1941;143:277–299.

152. Reese AB, Ellsworth RM. The anterior chamber cleavage syndrome. *Arch Ophthalmol.* 1966;75(3):307–318.

153. Waring GO III, Rodrigues MM, Laibson PR. Anterior chamber cleavage syndrome. A stepladder classification. *Surv Ophthalmol.* 1975;20(1):3–27.

154. Shields MB, Buckley E, Klintworth GK, et al. Axenfeld–Rieger syndrome. A spectrum of developmental disorders. *Surv Ophthalmol.* 1985;29(6): 387–409.

155. Chisholm IA, Chudley AE. Autosomal dominant iridogoniodysgenesis with associated somatic anomalies: four-generation family with Rieger's syndrome. *Br J Ophthalmol.* 1983;67(8):529–534.

156. Alkemade PPH. *Dysgenesis Mesodermalis of the Iris and the Cornea: A Study of Rieger's Syndrome and Peters' Anomaly.* Assen, The Netherlands: Van Goreum; 1969.

157. Burian HM, Braley AE, Allen L. External and gonioscopic visibility of the ring of Schwalbe and the trabecular zone: an interpretation of the posterior corneal embryotoxon and the so-called congenital hyaline membranes on the posterior corneal surface. *Trans Am Ophthalmol Soc.* 1954;52:389–428.

158. Shields MB, Campbell DG, Simmons RJ. The essential iris atrophies. *Am J Ophthalmol.* 1978;85(6):749–759.

159. Wolter JR, Sandall GS, Fralick FB. Mesodermal dysgenesis of anterior eye with a partially separated posterior embryotoxon. *J Pediatr Opthalmol Strabismus.* 1967;4:41–46.

160. Burian HM. A case of Marfan's syndrome with bilateral glaucoma. With description of a new type of operation for developmental glaucoma (trabeculotomy ab externo). *Am J Ophthalmol.* 1960;50:1187–1192.

161. Cross HE, Maumenee AE. Progressive spontaneous dissolution of the iris. *Surv Ophthalmol.* 1973;18:186–199.

162. Piper HF, Schwinger E, von Domarus H. Dysplasia of the corneal limbus, the mesodermal iris layer and the jaw skeleton in a family [in German]. *Klin Monbl Augenheilkd.* 1985;186(4):287–293.

163. Henkind P, Friedman AH. Iridogoniodysgenesis with cataract. *Am J Ophthalmol.* 1971;72(5):949–954.

164. Dowling JL Jr, Albert DM, Nelson LB, et al. Primary glaucoma associated with iridotrabecular dysgenesis and ectropion uveae. *Ophthalmology.* 1985;92(7):912–921.

165. Cibis GW, Waeltermann JM, Hurst E, et al. Congenital pupillary-iris-lens membrane with goniodysgenesis (a new entity). *Ophthalmology.* 1986; 93(6):847–852.

166. Spallone A. Retinal detachment in Axenfeld–Rieger syndrome. *Br J Ophthalmol.* 1989;73(7):559–562.

167. Wesley RK, Baker JD, Golnick AL. Rieger's syndrome: (oligodontia and primary mesodermal dysgenesis of the iris) clinical features and report of an isolated case. *J Pediatr Ophthalmol Strabismus.* 1978;15(2):67–70.

168. Kleinmann RE, Kazarian EL, Raptopoulos V, et al. Primary empty sella and Rieger's anomaly of the anterior chamber of the eye: a familial syndrome. *N Engl J Med.* 1981;304(2):90–93.

169. Feingold M, Shiere F, Fogels HR, et al. Rieger's syndrome. *Pediatrics.* 1969;44(4):564–569.

170. Sadeghi-Nejad A, Senior B. Autosomal dominant transmission of isolated growth hormone deficiency in iris-dental dysplasia (Rieger's syndrome). *J Pediatr.* 1974;85(5):644–648.

171. Jorgenson RJ, Levin LS, Cross HE, et al. The Rieger syndrome. *Am J Med Genet.* 1978;2(3):307–318.

172. Lubin JR. Oculocutaneous albinism associated with corneal mesodermal dysgenesis. *Am J Ophthalmol.* 1981;91(3):347–350.

173. Steinsapir KD, Lehman E, Ernest JT, et al. Systemic neurocristopathy associated with Rieger's syndrome. *Am J Ophthalmol.* 1990;110(4):437–438.

174. Troeber R, Rochels R. Histological findings in dysgenesis mesodermalis iridis et corneae Rieger [in German]. *Albrecht Von Graefes Arch Klin Exp Ophthalmol.* 1980;213(3):169–174.

175. Lines MA, Kozlowski K, Walter MA. Molecular genetics of Axenfeld–Rieger malformations. *Hum Mol Genet.* 2002;11(10):1177–1184.

176. Quentien MH, Pitoia F, Gunz G, et al. Regulation of prolactin, GH, and Pit-1 gene expression in anterior pituitary by Pitx2: an approach using Pitx2 mutants. *Endocrinology.* 2002;143(8):2839–2851.

177. Honkanen RA, Nishimura DY, Swiderski RE, et al. A family with Axenfeld–Rieger syndrome and Peters Anomaly caused by a point mutation (Phe112Ser) in the FOXC1 gene. *Am J Ophthalmol.* 2003;135(3):368–375.

178. Komatireddy S, Chakrabarti S, Mandal AK, et al. Mutation spectrum of FOXC1 and clinical genetic heterogeneity of Axenfeld–Rieger anomaly in India. *Mol Vis.* 2003;9:43–48.

179. Kozlowski K, Walter MA. Variation in residual PITX2 activity underlies the phenotypic spectrum of anterior segment developmental disorders. *Hum Mol Genet.* 2000;9(14):2131–2139.

180. Kawase C, Kawase K, Taniguchi T, et al. Screening for mutations of Axenfeld–Rieger syndrome caused by FOXC1 gene in Japanese patients. *J Glaucoma.* 2001;10(6):477–482.

181. Suzuki T, Takahashi K, Kuwahara S, et al. A novel (Pro79Thr) mutation in the FKHL7 gene in a Japanese family with Axenfeld–Rieger syndrome. *Am J Ophthalmol.* 2001;132(4):572–575.

182. Alward WL. Axenfeld–Rieger syndrome in the age of molecular genetics. *Am J Ophthalmol.* 2000;130(1):107–115.

183. Amendt BA, Semina EV, Alward WL. Rieger syndrome: a clinical, molecular, and biochemical analysis. *Cell Mol Life Sci.* 2000;57(11): 1652–1666.

184. Saadi I, Kuburas A, Engle JJ, et al. Dominant negative dimerization of a mutant homeodomain protein in Axenfeld–Rieger syndrome. *Mol Cell Biol.* 2003;23(6):1968–1982.

185. Perveen R, Lloyd IC, Clayton-Smith J, et al. Phenotypic variability and asymmetry of Rieger syndrome associated with PITX2 mutations. *Invest Ophthalmol Vis Sci.* 2000;41(9):2456–2460.

186. Strungaru MH, Dinu I, Walter MA. Genotype-phenotype correlations in Axenfeld–Rieger malformation and glaucoma patients with FOXC1 and PITX2 mutations. *Invest Ophthalmol Vis Sci.* 2007;48(1):228–237.

187. Kupfer C, Kaiser-Kupfer MI, Datiles M, et al. The contralateral eye in the iridocorneal endothelial (ICE) syndrome. *Ophthalmology.* 1983;90(11): 1343–1350.

188. Weissschuh N, Wolf C, Wissinger B, et al. A novel mutation in the FOXC1 gene in a family with Axenfeld–Rieger syndrome and Peters' anomaly. *Clin Genet.* 2008;74(5):476–480.

189. Judisch GF, Martin-Casals A, Hanson JW, et al. Oculodentodigital dysplasia. Four new reports and a literature review. *Arch Ophthalmol.* 1979; 97(5):878–884.

190. Cross HE. Ectopia lentis et pupillae. *Am J Ophthalmol.* 1979;88(3 pt 1): 381–384.

191. Ritch R, Forbes M, Hetherington J Jr, et al. Congenital ectropion uveae with glaucoma. *Ophthalmology.* 1984;91(4):326–331.

192. Gramer E, Krieglstein GK. Infantile glaucoma in unilateral uveal ectropion. *Albrecht Von Graefes Arch Klin Exp Ophthalmol.* 1979;211(3):215–219.

193. Mazzeo V, Gaiba G, Rossi A. Hereditary cases of congenital microcoria and goniodysgenesis. *Ophthalmic Paediatr Genet.* 1986;7(2):121–125.

194. Tawara A, Inomata H. Familial cases of congenital microcoria associated with late onset congenital glaucoma and goniodysgenesis. *Jpn J Ophthalmol.* 1983;27(1):63–72.

195. Toulemont PJ, Urvoy M, Coscas G, et al. Association of congenital microcoria with myopia and glaucoma. A study of 23 patients with congenital microcoria. *Ophthalmology.* 1995;102(2):193–198.

196. von Hippel E. Uber hydophthalmus congenitus nebst Bemerkungen über die Verfarbung der Cornea durch Blutfarbstoff. Pathologisch-anatomische Untersuchung. *Graefes Arch Clin Exp Ophthalmol.* 1897;44:539.

197. Peters A. Uber angeborene Defektbildung der Descemetschen membran. *Klin Monatsbl Augenheilkd.* 1906;44:27–40.

198. DeRespinis PA, Wagner RS. Peters' anomaly in a father and son. *Am J Ophthalmol.* 1987;104(5):545–546.

199. Holmstrom GE, Reardon WP, Baraitser M, et al. Heterogeneity in dominant anterior segment malformations. *Br J Ophthalmol.* 1991;75(10):591–597.

200. Kivlin JD, Fineman RM, Crandall AS, et al. Peters' anomaly as a consequence of genetic and nongenetic syndromes. *Arch Ophthalmol.* 1986; 104(1):61–64.

201. Traboulsi EI, Maumenee IH. Peters' anomaly and associated congenital malformations. *Arch Ophthalmol.* 1992;110(12):1739–1742.

202. Sullivan TJ, Clarke MP, Heathcote JG, et al. Multiple congenital contractures (arthrogryposis) in association with Peters' anomaly and chorioretinal colobomata. *J Pediatr Ophthalmol Strabismus.* 1992;29(6): 370–373.

203. Townsend WM. Congenital corneal leukomas. 1. Central defect in Descemet's membrane. *Am J Ophthalmol.* 1974;77(1):80–86.

204. Townsend WM, Font RL, Zimmerman LE. Congenital corneal leukomas. 2. Histopathologic findings in 19 eyes with central defect in Descemet's membrane. *Am J Ophthalmol.* 1974;77(2):192–206.

205. Stone DL, Kenyon KR, Green WR, et al. Congenital central corneal leukoma (Peters' anomaly). *Am J Ophthalmol.* 1976;81(2):173–193.

206. Nakanishi I, Brown SI. The histopathology and ultrastructure of congenital, central corneal opacity (Peters' anomaly). *Am J Ophthalmol.* 1971;72(4):801–812.

207. Lee CF, Yue BY, Robin J, et al. Immunohistochemical studies of Peters' anomaly. *Ophthalmology.* 1989;96(7):958–964.

208. Polack FM, Graue EL. Scanning electron microscopy of congenital corneal leukomas (Peters' anomaly). *Am J Ophthalmol.* 1979;88(2):169–178.

209. Kuper C, Kuwabara T, Stark WJ. The histopathology of Peters' anomaly. *Am J Ophthalmol.* 1975;80(4):653–660.

210. Heath DH, Shields MB. Glaucoma and Peters' anomaly. A clinicopathologic case report. *Graefes Arch Clin Exp Ophthalmol.* 1991;229(3):277–280.

211. Wolter JR, Haney WP. Histopathology of keratoconus posticus circumscriptus. *Arch Ophthalmol.* 1963;69:357–362.

212. Krachmer JH, Rodrigues MM. Posterior keratoconus. *Arch Ophthalmol.* 1978;96(10):1867–1873.

213. Yang LL, Lambert SR, Drews-Botsch C, et al. Long-term visual outcome of penetrating keratoplasty in infants and children with Peters anomaly. *J AAPOS.* 2009;13(2):175–180.

214. Zaidman GW, Flanagan JK, Furey CC. Long-term visual prognosis in children after corneal transplant surgery for Peters anomaly type I. *Am J Ophthalmol.* 2007;144(1):104–108.

215. Neely DE, Plager DA. Endocyclophotocoagulation for management of difficult pediatric glaucomas. *J AAPOS.* 2001;5(4):221–229.

216. Yang LL, Lambert SR. Peters' anomaly. A synopsis of surgical management and visual outcome. *Ophthalmol Clin North Am.* 2001;14(3):467–477.

217. Althaus C, Sundmacher R. Keratoplasty in newborns with Peters' anomaly. *Ger J Ophthalmol.* 1996;5(1):31–35.

218. Junemann A, Gusek GC, Naumann GO. Optical sector iridectomy: an alternative to perforating keratoplasty in Peters' anomaly [in German]. *Klin Monbl Augenheilkd.* 1996;209(2-3):117–124.

219. Al-Haddad CE, Freedman SF. Endoscopic laser cyclophotocoagulation in pediatric glaucoma with corneal opacities. *J AAPOS*. 2007;11(1): 23–28.

220. Elsas FJ, Maumenee IH, Kenyon KR, et al. Familial aniridia with preserved ocular function. *Am J Ophthalmol*. 1977;83(5):718–724.

221. Turleau C, de Grouchy J, Tournade MF, et al. Del 11p/aniridia complex. Report of three patients and review of 37 observations from the literature. *Clin Genet*. 1984;26(4):356–362.

222. Hanson I, Jordan T, van Heyningen V. In: Wright AF, Jay B, eds. *Molecular Genetics of Inherited Eye Disorders*. Switzerland: Harwood Academic; 1994:445–467.

223. Lauderdale JD, Wilensky JS, Oliver ER, et al. 3' Deletions cause aniridia by preventing PAX6 gene expression. *Proc Natl Acad Sci U S A*. 2000; 97(25):13755–13759.

224. Crolla JA, van Heyningen V. Frequent chromosome aberrations revealed by molecular cytogenetic studies in patients with aniridia. *Am J Hum Genet*. 2002;71(5):1138–1149.

225. Wolf MT, Lorenz B, Winterpacht A, et al. Ten novel mutations found in Aniridia. *Hum Mutat*. 1998;12(5):304–313.

226. Pearce WG. Variability of iris defects in autosomal dominant aniridia. *Can J Ophthalmol*. 1994;29(1):25–29.

227. Mintz-Hittner HA, Ferrell RE, Lyons LA, et al. Criteria to detect minimal expressivity within families with autosomal dominant aniridia. *Am J Ophthalmol*. 1992;114(6):700–707.

228. Nishida K, Kinoshita S, Ohashi Y, et al. Ocular surface abnormalities in aniridia. *Am J Ophthalmol*. 1995;120(3):368–375.

229. David R, MacBeath L, Jenkins T. Aniridia associated with microcornea and subluxated lenses. *Br J Ophthalmol*. 1978;62(2):118–121.

230. Yamamoto Y, Hayasaka S, Setogawa T. Family with aniridia, microcornea, and spontaneously reabsorbed cataract. *Arch Ophthalmol*. 1988;106(4): 502–504.

231. Jotterand V, Boisjoly HM, Harnois C, et al. 11p13 deletion, Wilms' tumour, and aniridia: unusual genetic, non-ocular and ocular features of three cases. *Br J Ophthalmol*. 1990;74(9):568–570.

232. Beauchamp GR. Anterior segment dysgenesis keratolenticular adhesion and aniridia. *J Pediatr Ophthalmol Strabismus*. 1980;17(1):55–58.

233. Whitson JT, Liang C, Godfrey DG, et al. Central corneal thickness in patients with congenital aniridia. *Eye Contact Lens*. 2005;31(5):221–224.

234. Shields MB, Reed JW. Aniridia and congenital ptosis. *Ann Ophthalmol*. 1975;7(2):203–205.

235. Hamming N, Wilensky J. Persistent pupillary membrane associated with aniridia. *Am J Ophthalmol*. 1978;86(1):118–120.

236. Schanzlin DJ, Goldberg DB, Brown SI. Hallermann-Streiff syndrome associated with sclerocornea, aniridia, and a chromosomal abnormality. *Am J Ophthalmol*. 1980;90(3):411–415.

237. Sachdev MS, Sood NN, Kumar H, et al. Bilateral aniridia with Marfan's syndrome and dental anomalies—a new association. *Jpn J Ophthalmol*. 1986;30(4):360–366.

238. To KW, Mukai S, Friedman AH. Association and chance occurrence of aniridia and retinoblastoma. *Am J Ophthalmol*. 1994;118(6):820–822.

239. Grant WM, Walton DS. Progressive changes in the angle in congenital aniridia, with development of glaucoma. *Am J Ophthalmol*. 1974;78(5): 842–847.

240. Margo CE. Congenital aniridia: a histopathologic study of the anterior segment in children. *J Pediatr Ophthalmol Strabismus*. 1983;20(5):192–198.

241. Chen TC, Walton DS. Goniosurgery for prevention of aniridic glaucoma. *Arch Ophthalmol*. 1999;117(9):1144–1148.

242. Adachi M, Dickens CJ, Hetherington J Jr, et al. Clinical experience of trabeculotomy for the surgical treatment of aniridic glaucoma. *Ophthalmology*. 1997;104(12):2121–2125.

243. Okada K, Mishima HK, Masumoto M, et al. Results of filtering surgery in young patients with aniridia. *Hiroshima J Med Sci*. 2000;49(3):135–138.

244. Arroyave CP, Scott IU, Gedde SJ, et al. Use of glaucoma drainage devices in the management of glaucoma associated with aniridia. *Am J Ophthalmol*. 2003;135(2):155–159.

245. Wagle NS, Freedman SF, Buckley EG, et al. Long-term outcome of cyclocryotherapy for refractory pediatric glaucoma. *Ophthalmology*. 1998;105(10):1921–1926; discussion 6–7.

246. Reinhard T, Engelhardt S, Sundmacher R. Black diaphragm aniridia intraocular lens for congenital aniridia: long-term follow-up. *J Cataract Refract Surg*. 2000;26(3):375–381.

247. Vajpayee RB, Majji AB, Taherian K, et al. Frosted-iris intraocular lens for traumatic aniridia with cataract. *Ophthalmic Surg*. 1994;25(10):730–731.

248. Kremer I, Rajpal RK, Rapuano CJ, et al. Results of penetrating keratoplasty in aniridia. *Am J Ophthalmol*. 1993;115(3):317–320.

249. Tiller AM, Odenthal MT, Verbraak FD, et al. The influence of keratoplasty on visual prognosis in aniridia: a historical review of one large family. *Cornea*. 2003;22(2):105–110.

250. Shapiro MB, France TD. The ocular features of Down's syndrome. *Am J Ophthalmol*. 1985;99(6):659–663.

251. Creavin AL, Brown RD. Ophthalmic abnormalities in children with Down syndrome. *J Pediatr Ophthalmol Strabismus*. 2009;46(2):76–82.

252. Traboulsi EI, Levine E, Mets MB, et al. Infantile glaucoma in Down's syndrome (trisomy 21). *Am J Ophthalmol*. 1988;105(4):389–394.

253. Lichter PR, Schmickel RD. Posterior vortex vein and congenital glaucoma in a patient with trisomy 13 syndrome. *Am J Ophthalmol*. 1975;80(5): 939–942.

254. Hoepner J, Yanoff M. Ocular anomalies in trisomy 13–15: an analysis of 13 eyes with two new findings. *Am J Ophthalmol*. 1972;74(4):729–737.

255. Mayer UM, Grosse KP, Schwanitz G. Ophthalmologic findings in trisomy 18 (Morbus Edwards) [in German]. *Graefes Arch Clin Exp Ophthalmol*. 1982;218(1):46–50.

256. Lessell S, Forbes AP. Eye signs in Turner's syndrome. *Arch Ophthalmol*. 1966;76(2):211–213.

257. Rao VA, Kaliaperumal S, Subramanyan T, et al. Goldenhar's sequence with associated juvenile glaucoma in Turner's syndrome. *Indian J Ophthalmol*. 2005;53(4):267–268.

258. Wan WL, Minckler DS, Rao NA. Pupillary-block glaucoma associated with childhood cystinosis. *Am J Ophthalmol*. 1986;101(6):700–705.

259. Miller MT, Epstein RJ, Sugar J, et al. Anterior segment anomalies associated with the fetal alcohol syndrome. *J Pediatr Ophthalmol Strabismus*. 1984;21(1):8–18.

260. Cook CS, Nowotny AZ, Sulik KK. Fetal alcohol syndrome. Eye malformations in a mouse model. *Arch Ophthalmol*. 1987;105(11):1576–1581.

261. Cohen SM, Brown FR III, Martyn L, et al. Ocular histopathologic and biochemical studies of the cerebrohepatorenal syndrome (Zellweger's syndrome) and its relationship to neonatal adrenoleukodystrophy. *Am J Ophthalmol*. 1983;96(4):488–501.

262. Haddad R, Font RL, Friendly DS. Cerebro-hepato-renal syndrome of Zellweger. Ocular histopathologic findings. *Arch Ophthalmol*. 1976;94(11): 1927–1930.

263. Folz SJ, Trobe JD. The peroxisome and the eye. *Surv Ophthalmol*. 1991; 35(5):353–368.

264. Brosius U, Gartner J. Cellular and molecular aspects of Zellweger syndrome and other peroxisome biogenesis disorders. *Cell Mol Life Sci*. 2002;59(6):1058–1069.

265. Roulez FM, Schuil J, Meire FM. Corneal opacities in the Hallermann-Streiff syndrome. *Ophthalmic Genet*. 2008;29(2):61–66.

266. Mawn LA, O'Brien JE, Hedges TR III. Congenital glaucoma and skeletal dysplasia. *J Pediatr Ophthalmol Strabismus*. 1990;27(6):322–324.

267. Wadelius C, Fagerholm P, Pettersson U, et al. Lowe oculocerebrorenal syndrome: DNA-based linkage of the gene to Xq24-q26, using tightly linked flanking markers and the correlation to lens examination in carrier diagnosis. *Am J Hum Genet*. 1989;44(2):241–247.

268. Mueller OT, Hartsfield JK Jr, Gallardo LA, et al. Lowe oculocerebrorenal syndrome in a female with a balanced X;20 translocation: mapping of the X chromosome breakpoint. *Am J Hum Genet*. 1991;49(4): 804–810.

269. Walton DS, Katsavounidou G, Lowe CU. Glaucoma with the oculocerebrorenal syndrome of Lowe. *J Glaucoma*. 2005;14(3):181–185.

270. De La Paz MA, Lewis RA, Patrinely JR, et al. A sibship with unusual anomalies of the eye and skeleton (Michels' syndrome). *Am J Ophthalmol*. 1991;112(5):572–580.

271. Michels VV, Hittner HM, Beaudet AL. A clefting syndrome with ocular anterior chamber defect and lid anomalies. *J Pediatr*. 1978;93(3):444–446.

272. Tekin M, Ozturkmen Akay H, Fitoz S, et al. Homozygous FGF3 mutations result in congenital deafness with inner ear agenesis, microtia, and microdontia. *Clin Genet*. 2008;73(6):554–565.

273. Spellacy E, Bankes JL, Crow J, et al. Glaucoma in a case of Hurler disease. *Br J Ophthalmol*. 1980;64(10):773–778.

274. Christiansen SP, Smith TJ, Henslee-Downey PJ. Normal intraocular pressure after a bone marrow transplant in glaucoma associated with mucopolysaccharidosis type I-H. *Am J Ophthalmol*. 1990;109(2):230–231.

275. Cantor LB, Disseler JA, Wilson FM II. Glaucoma in the Maroteaux-Lamy syndrome. *Am J Ophthalmol*. 1989;108(4):426–430.

276. Cahane M, Treister G, Abraham FA, et al. Glaucoma in siblings with Morquio syndrome. *Br J Ophthalmol*. 1990;74(6):382–383.

277. Lichter PR, Richards JE, Downs CA, et al. Cosegregation of open-angle glaucoma and the nail-patella syndrome. *Am J Ophthalmol*. 1997;124(4): 506–515.

278. McIntosh I, Clough MV, Schaffer AA, et al. Fine mapping of the nail-patella syndrome locus at 9q34. *Am J Hum Genet.* 1997;60(1):133–142.

279. Traboulsi EI, Parks MM. Glaucoma in oculo-dento-osseous dysplasia. *Am J Ophthalmol.* 1990;109(3):310–313.

280. Sugar HS. Oculodentodigital dysplasia syndrome with angle-closure glaucoma. *Am J Ophthalmol.* 1978;86(1):36–38.

281. Hittner HM, King RA, Riccardi VM, et al. Oculocutaneous albinoidism as a manifestation of reduced neural crest derivatives in the Prader-Willi syndrome. *Am J Ophthalmol.* 1982;94(3):328–337.

282. Futterweit W, Ritch R, Teekhasaenee C, et al. Coexistence of Prader-Willi syndrome, congenital ectropion uveae with glaucoma, and factor XI deficiency. *JAMA.* 1986;255(23):3280–3282.

283. Mangitti E, Lavin JR. Le Glaucoma congenital dans le syndrome de Rubinstein–Taybi [in French]. *Ann Oculist.* 1972;205:1005.

284. Weber U, Bernsmeier H. Rubinstein–Taybi syndrome and juvenile glaucoma [in German]. *Klin Monbl Augenheilkd.* 1983;183(1):47–49.

285. Shihab ZM. Pediatric glaucoma in Rubinstein–Taybi syndrome. *Glaucoma.* 1984;3:288.

286. Stickler GB, Belau PG, Farrell FJ, et al. Hereditary Progressive Arthro-Ophthalmopathy. *Mayo Clin Proc.* 1965;40:433–455.

287. Blair NP, Albert DM, Liberfarb RM, et al. Hereditary progressive arthro-ophthalmopathy of Stickler. *Am J Ophthalmol.* 1979;88(5):876–888.

288. Spallone A. Stickler's syndrome: a study of 12 families. *Br J Ophthalmol.* 1987;71(7):504–509.

289. Young NJ, Hitchings RA, Sehmi K, et al. Stickler's syndrome and neovascular glaucoma. *Br J Ophthalmol.* 1979;63(12):826–831.

290. Ayme S, Preus M. The Marshall and Stickler syndromes: objective rejection of lumping. *J Med Genet.* 1984;21(1):34–38.

291. Scribanu N, O'Neill J, Rimoin D. The Weissenbacher–Zweymuller phenotype in the neonatal period as an expression in the continuum of manifestations of the hereditary arthro-ophthalmopathies. *Ophthalmic Paediatr Genet.* 1987;8(3):159–163.

292. Enright KA, Neelon FA. The eyes have it: Waardenburg's syndrome. *N C Med J.* 1986;47(12):592–596.

293. Nork TM, Shihab ZM, Young RS, et al. Pigment distribution in Waardenburg's syndrome: a new hypothesis. *Graefes Arch Clin Exp Ophthalmol.* 1986;224(6):487–492.

294. Gershoni-Baruch R, Mandel H, Miller B, et al. Walker–Warburg syndrome with microtia and absent auditory canals. *Am J Med Genet.* 1990;37(1):87–91.

295. Levin PS, Green WR, Victor DI, et al. Histopathology of the eye in Cockayne's syndrome. *Arch Ophthalmol.* 1983;101(7):1093–1097.

296. de Leon JM, Walton DS, Latina MA, et al. Glaucoma in retinoblastoma. *Semin Ophthalmol.* 2005;20(4):217–222.

297. Singh A, Singh AD, Shields CL, et al. Iris neovascularization in children as a manifestation of underlying medulloepithelioma. *J Pediatr Ophthalmol Strabismus.* 2001;38(4):224–228.

298. Vendal Z, Walton D, Chen T. Glaucoma in juvenile xanthogranuloma. *Semin Ophthalmol.* 2006;21(3):191–194.

299. Sabri K, Saurenmann RK, Silverman ED, et al. Course, complications, and outcome of juvenile arthritis-related uveitis. *J AAPOS.* 2008;12(6):539–545.

300. Holland GN, Stiehm ER. Special considerations in the evaluation and management of uveitis in children. *Am J Ophthalmol.* 2003;135(6):867–878.

301. Freedman SF, Rodriguez-Rosa RE, Rojas MC, et al. Goniotomy for glaucoma secondary to chronic childhood uveitis. *Am J Ophthalmol.* 2002;133(5):617–621.

302. Ho CL, Walton DS. Goniosurgery for glaucoma secondary to chronic anterior uveitis: prognostic factors and surgical technique. *J Glaucoma.* 2004;13(6):445–449.

303. Ozdal PC, Vianna RN, Deschenes J. Ahmed valve implantation in glaucoma secondary to chronic uveitis. *Eye.* 2006;20(2):178–183.

304. Wright MM, McGehee RF, Pederson JE. Intraoperative mitomycin-C for glaucoma associated with ocular inflammation. *Ophthalmic Surg Lasers.* 1997;28(5):370–376.

305. Harrison DA, Mullaney PB, Mesfer SA, et al. Management of ophthalmic complications of homocystinuria. *Ophthalmology.* 1998;105(10):1886–1890.

306. Egbert JE, Wright MM, Dahlhauser KF, et al. A prospective study of ocular hypertension and glaucoma after pediatric cataract surgery. *Ophthalmology.* 1995;102(7):1098–1101.

307. Parks MM, Johnson DA, Reed GW. Long-term visual results and complications in children with aphakia. A function of cataract type. *Ophthalmology.* 1993;100(6):826–840; discussion 40–41.

308. Kirwan C, O'Keefe M. Paediatric aphakic glaucoma. *Acta Ophthalmol Scand.* 2006;84(6):734–739.

309. Walton DS. Pediatric aphakic glaucoma: a study of 65 patients. *Trans Am Ophthalmol Soc.* 1995;93:403–413.

310. Levin AV. Aphakic glaucoma: a never-ending story? *Br J Ophthalmol.* 2007;91(12):1574–1575.

Exfoliation Syndrome and Exfoliative Glaucoma

Exfoliation syndrome is the most common identifiable cause of open-angle glaucoma worldwide (1). It is a systemic disorder with important eye manifestations, including development of open- and closed-angle glaucoma and of cataract with zonular instability (**Table 15.1, Fig. 15.1A,** and **Fig. 15.2**) (2). It may also be associated with increased systemic risk of cardiovascular disorders (3). In this chapter, we present an epidemiologic, clinical, and pathophysiologic overview of exfoliation syndrome and exfoliative glaucoma.

TERMINOLOGY

In 1917, Lindberg (4) described cases of chronic glaucoma in which flakes of whitish material adhered to the pupillary border of the iris. Subsequent study revealed that this material is derived from various sources in the anterior segment. Over the years, there has been some debate regarding nomenclature for this disorder. Given the rarity of true lens capsule delamination (sometimes referred to as exfoliation of the lens capsule) we have chosen to use the term exfoliation syndrome throughout this chapter; when exfoliation syndrome is accompanied by glaucoma, we use the term exfoliative glaucoma. However, readers should be aware that in the literature, the terms pseudoexfoliation syndrome and pseudoexfoliation glaucoma, as well as capsular glaucoma, continue to be used.

Capsular Delamination

In capsular delamination, superficial layers of lens capsule separate from the deeper capsular layers to form scroll-like margins and occasionally to float in the anterior chamber as thin, clear membranes (Fig. 15.1A). Elschnig (5) first described this condition in glassblowers, leading to the term glassblower cataracts, and it was subsequently found that extended exposure to infrared radiation in a variety of occupations was responsible. The condition is uncommon because of the widespread use of protective goggles by exposed workers, although clinically similar cases may be seen in association with trauma, intraocular inflammation, and idiopathically, usually with advanced age (6–10). Glaucoma is not a common feature of this disorder. The condition has been called capsular delamination or exfoliation of the lens capsule, prompting Dvorak-Theobald (11) to suggest the term true exfoliation of the lens capsule, to distinguish it from "exfoliation."

EPIDEMIOLOGY

The prevalence of exfoliation increases dramatically with age and varies considerably among populations worldwide (12). The tremendous variation in prevalence of exfoliation syndrome is caused by true differences in the populations studied, but it may also vary because of other factors such as differences

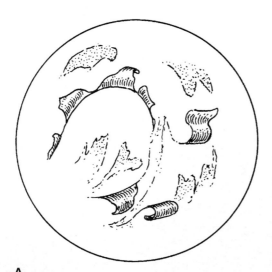

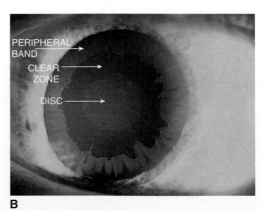

PERIPHERAL BAND
CLEAR ZONE
DISC

A

B

Figure 15.1 Anterior lens capsule delamination and exfoliation syndrome. **A:** Capsular delamination, also sometimes termed exfoliation of the lens capsule characterized by thin, clear membranes separating from the anterior lens capsule and often curling at the margins. **B:** Exfoliation syndrome is demonstrated by three distinct zones: a central, translucent disc; a clear zone; and a peripheral granular zone, often with radial striations. (Courtesy of Joseph A. Halabis, OD.)

Table 15.1	Early Signs, Clinical Complications, and Surgical Complications of Exfoliation Syndrome		
Ocular Tissue Involved	**Early Clinical Signs**	**Clinical Complications**	**Surgical Complications**
Lens, ciliary body, zonules	Diffuse precapsular layer Phacodonesis Exfoliation deposits on zonules on ultrasonographic biomicroscopy	Cataract (nuclear) Phacodonesis Lens subluxation	Zonular rupture/dialysis Vitreous loss Rupture of posterior capsule
		Angle-closure glaucoma due to papillary, ciliary block	Decentration of the lens implant Anterior capsule fibrosis Secondary cataract
Iris	Peripupillary atrophy, iris sphincter region transillumination	Melanin dispersion Poor mydriasis	Miosis/poor surgical access Intraoperative hyphema, postoperative hyphema
	Melanin dispersion associated with pupillary dilatation	Iris rigidity Capillary hemorrhage	Postoperative inflammation Prolonged blood–aqueous barrier breakdown
	Poor mydriasis, asymmetric pupil sizes	Blood–aqueous barrier defects, pseudouveitis Anterior chamber hypoxia Posterior synechiae	Posterior synechiae, pupillary block
Trabecular meshwork	Pigment deposition Markedly asymmetric IOPs Marked increase in IOP after pupillary dilatation	Intraocular hypertension Open-angle glaucoma	Postoperative increase in IOP
Cornea	Atypical cornea guttata	Endothelial decompensation Endothelial migration/ proliferation	Endothelial decompensation
Posterior segment		Retinal venous occlusion	

Adapted from Schlotzer-Schrehardt U, Naumann GOH. Ocular and systemic exfoliation syndrome. *Am J Ophthalmol.* 2006; 141(5):921–937.

in age, environmental influences, definition of exfoliation syndrome, and examination techniques. Exfoliation syndrome is more common in older age-groups, with most cases occurring in the late 60s and early 70s. The condition may be unilateral or bilateral, and over half of unilateral cases become bilateral over a 20-year period (13).

Geographic and ethnic differences appear to be important, with exfoliation syndrome prevalences worldwide varying from 0% in Inuit populations in Alaska, Greenland, and Canada to 38% in the Navajo population in the United States. Exfoliation syndrome is also widely prevalent in the Scandinavian countries, Europe, the United Kingdom, and the Middle East. Exfoliation syndrome has been found in East and South Africa, India, Southeast Asia, Australia, and many regions in South America.

Within countries, the prevalence can vary from region to region. Ringvold (14) reported rates of 10.2%, 19.6%, and 21.0% in three closely situated municipalities in central Norway. The influence of race differs among geographic populations. In South Africa, exfoliation syndrome was found in 20% of black patients with open-angle glaucoma, compared with 1.4% of whites (15), whereas a study in southern Louisiana revealed a prevalence of 0.3% in blacks and 2.0% in whites (16). Geographic distribution patterns may be explained by regional gene pools or by environmental influences. Differences in altitude and ultraviolet light exposure have been suggested, but the evidence to date for either factor is marginal (17). There is no clear relation between exfoliation syndrome prevalence and sex. The percentage of exfoliation syndrome patients

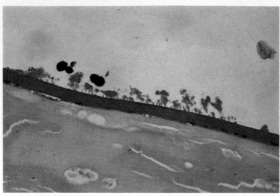

A

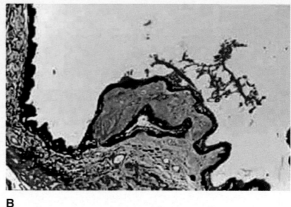

B

Figure 15.2 **A:** Exfoliation fibers on the lens capsule. The dark areas are pigment aggregates (PAS, ×146). (From Kincaid MC. Pathology of the lens. In: Tasman W, Jaeger EA, eds. *Duane's Foundations of Clinical Ophthalmology*. Vol. 3. Philadelphia, PA: Lippincott Williams & Wilkins; chap 12.) **B:** Light micrograph of exfoliative material overlying ciliary body process (PAS, ×100). (Courtesy of Marilyn C. Kincaid, MD, Armed Forces Institute of Pathology. From Khaimi MA, Skuta GL, Morgan RK. Exfoliation syndrome, pigment dispersion syndrome, and the associated glaucomas. In: Tasman W, Jaeger EA, eds. *Duane's Clinical Ophthalmology*. Vol. 3. Philadelphia, PA: Lippincott Williams & Wilkins; chap 54B: 2008.)

with glaucoma is different for every population. Overall, studies indicate about 40% of exfoliation syndrome patients will develop glaucoma (18). The reported prevalence of exfoliation syndrome among patients with open-angle glaucoma also shows considerable geographic variation, with 26% in Denmark, 75% in Sweden, 60% in Norway, 46.9% in the Mediterranean area of Turkey, and 44.5% in the northwest of Spain, compared with reports of 1% to 12% in the United States (16,19–24).

More large-scale, population-based studies need to be conducted with standardized classification criteria, particularly outside of Europe, to determine a more accurate worldwide distribution of exfoliation syndrome and exfoliative glaucoma.

CLINICAL AND PATHOLOGIC FEATURES

Corneal Changes

Flakes of exfoliative material and pigment accumulation may be seen on the corneal endothelium (**Fig. 15.3A**), scattered diffusely or in the form of a vertical spindle similar to the Krukenberg spindle in pigmentary glaucoma. Specular microscopy of the corneal endothelium has revealed a significantly lower-than-normal cell density in eyes with the exfoliation syndrome and changes in cell size and shape (25). These findings have also been observed in the unaffected eye of unilateral cases, leading the researchers to suggest that these corneal endothelial changes might serve as an early sign of the disorder (25). Ultrastructural studies have revealed clumps of exfoliative material adhering to the corneal endothelium and incorporated into the posterior Descemet membrane, which the investigators believe indicate that the

exfoliative material was formed by degenerative endothelial cells (26) (**Fig. 15.3B,C**).

It has been suggested that corneal endotheliopathy in exfoliation syndrome can give rise to an appearance of guttata but is distinct from Fuchs endothelial corneal dystrophy or pseudophakic or aphakic bullous keratopathy (27,28). Exfoliation syndrome endotheliopathy differs from Fuchs endothelial corneal dystrophy in that the former typically has less and more diffusely distributed guttata-like structures and is associated with more melanin dispersion in the anterior segment and peripupillary iris atrophy.

Lens, Zonule, and Ciliary Body Changes

The characteristic appearance of exfoliative material on the anterior lens capsule has three distinct zones (**Fig. 15.1B**): a translucent, central disc with occasional curled edges; a clear zone, probably corresponding to contact with the moving iris; and a peripheral granular zone, which may have radial striations (29). The central zone is absent in 20% of cases or more, but the peripheral defect is a consistent finding, and the pupil must be dilated before the lens changes can be seen in some cases.

A precapsular film has been noted on the anterior lens capsule of many older individuals, which has a ground-glass appearance and has been shown by ultrastructural studies to be a fibrillar layer similar to exfoliative material. The precapsular layer may be a precursor of the exfoliation syndrome (**Fig. 15.4**).

Cataracts occur frequently in eyes with exfoliation syndrome (24). Although this may be in part a function of the age of the patient population, cataracts in eyes with exfoliation syndrome have a higher percentage of nuclear opacities and smaller percentage of cortical and supranuclear opacities (30). In patients with uniocular exfoliation syndrome, the involved

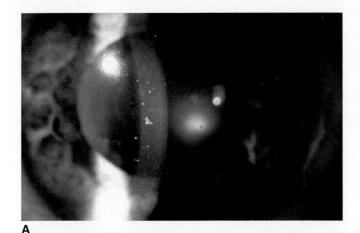

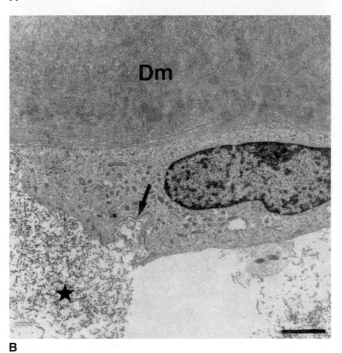

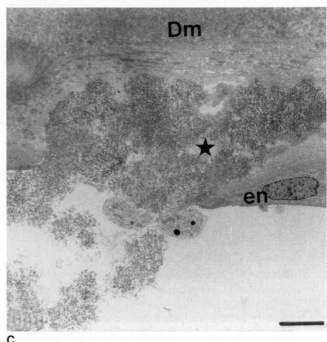

eye typically has the more advanced cataract. The Reykjavik Eye Study, however, found no association between cataract and exfoliation (31).

Exfoliative material may be detected earliest on the ciliary processes and zonules (**Fig. 15.5**). In patients with apparently unilateral exfoliation syndrome, cycloscopy reveals exfoliative material on the ciliary processes, zonules, or both in 77% of fellow eyes in which exfoliative material was not clinically visible on the lens surface or pupillary border (32). By using gonioscopy, exfoliative material can be observed on ciliary processes through a patent basal iridectomy.

Involvement of the zonules can lead to lens subluxation and phacodonesis (33). This instability of the zonules can be understood by examining exfoliation aggregates at the origin and anchorage of the zonules between nonpigmented ciliary epithelial cells and at the insertion of the zonules on the preequatorial region of the lens (**Fig. 15.6**). In these areas, exfoliation aggregates erupt through the basement membrane and involve the zonular lamellae, producing areas of weakness (34).

Proteolytic enzymes in the exfoliative material may facilitate zonular disintegration. These alterations, which can lead to lens instability, need to be kept in mind for all patients with exfoliation syndrome undergoing cataract surgery.

Iris Changes

Exfoliative material may also be seen as white flecks on the pupillary margin of the iris, with loss of pigment at the pupillary ruff (35) (**Fig. 15.7A**). Iris transillumination typically reveals a moth-eaten pattern near the pupillary sphincter (**Fig. 15.7B**), and many patients also have diffuse midperipheral transillumination defects (35,36). Light and scanning electron microscopy demonstrate exfoliative material on the posterior surface of the iris. Fluorescein angiographic studies of the iris have revealed hypoperfusion, peripupillary leakage, and neovascularization (37). These findings are more pronounced with increasing age of the patient, longer duration of the disease, and the presence of

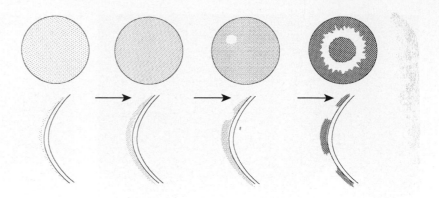

Figure 15.4 Clinical classification of exfoliation syndrome based on morphologic alterations of the anterior lens capsule. **A:** Preclinical stage. **B:** Suspected exfoliation syndrome. **C:** Mini-exfoliation syndrome. **D:** Classic exfoliation syndrome. (Modified from Naumann GO, Schlötzer-Schrehardt U, Kuchle M. Exfoliation syndrome for the comprehensive ophthalmologist: intraocular and systemic manifestations. *Ophthalmology.* 1998;105(6):951–968, with permission.)

A Preclinical Stage clinically invisible

B "Suspected Exfoliation Syndrome" precapsular layer

C "Mini-Exfoliation Syndrome" focal defect starts nasal-superiorly

D Classic Exfoliation Syndrome

glaucoma, and they may represent secondary features of the disease. Ultrastructural studies suggest that vascular abnormalities or abnormal extracellular matrix production causes tissue hypoxia (38). Conversely, it has been observed that eyes with transient ischemic attacks have an increased incidence of abnormal iris transillumination and exfoliative material, suggesting that hypoperfusion may be a contributory factor in the development of the exfoliation syndrome (39,40).

Whether a primary or secondary feature, the iris hypoxia is associated with atrophy of the iris pigment epithelium, stroma, and muscle cells (38). Atrophy of the pigment epithelium may be associated with anterior chamber melanin dispersion, which may be seen as a whorl-like pattern of pigment particles on the iris sphincter and pigment deposition on the peripheral iris (35), whereas atrophy of the muscle cells may account for the poor mydriasis, which is also a typical finding in the exfoliation syndrome (38).

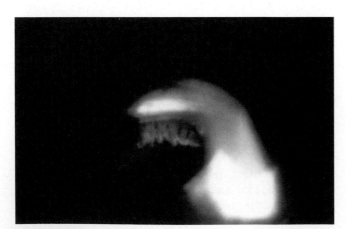

Figure 15.5 Exfoliative material on ciliary processes as seen through sector iridectomy in an aphakic eye. (From Khaimi MA, Skuta GL, Morgan RK. Exfoliation syndrome, pigment dispersion syndrome, and the associated glaucomas. In: Tasman W, Jaeger EA, eds. *Duane's Clinical Ophthalmology*, Vol. 3. Philadelphia, PA: Lippincott Williams & Wilkins; 2008:chap 54B.)

Gonioscopic Findings

The exfoliation syndrome is associated with excessive pigment dispersion, which leads to increased trabecular meshwork pigmentation. The pigmentation of the meshwork has a more variegated (uneven) distribution than that seen in pigmentary glaucoma and may be associated with flecks of exfoliative material (**Fig. 15.8**). An accumulation of pigment may also be seen along the Schwalbe line, which has been termed the Sampaolesi line (41). In eyes with marked asymmetry of meshwork pigmentation, glaucoma is more common in the more pigmented eye. However, increased pigmentation of the trabecular meshwork has also been observed in the fellow eye without apparent exfoliation syndrome, and it has been suggested that this may be the earliest detectable sign of exfoliation syndrome (42). Although the anterior chamber depth is normal in most eyes with the exfoliation syndrome, the anterior chamber angle is occludable in a high percentage of cases (43). The latter cases typically have a shallower central and peripheral anterior chamber depths (44). In studies of patients with the exfoliation syndrome, 9% to 18% had angles that were considered to be occludable (42,45), and 14% had evidence of angle closure on the basis of peripheral anterior synechiae (42).

Ultrastructural studies indicate that there is active exfoliation production in the trabecular meshwork, Schlemm canal, and collector channels, as well as passive deposition of exfoliative material within intertrabecular spaces (46) (**Fig. 15.9**). The progressive accumulation of the exfoliative material leads to swelling of the juxtacanalicular meshwork and gradual narrowing and disorganization of the Schlemm canal architecture in advanced cases. Occasionally, proliferating and migrating corneal endothelial cells produce a pretrabecular sheet of abnormal extracellular matrix that covers the inner surface of the uveal meshwork (46).

Other Slitlamp Findings

Exfoliative material may also be seen after cataract surgery on the anterior hyaloid in aphakic eyes (**Fig. 15.10**) and on a posterior chamber intraocular lens in pseudophakic eyes. Eyes

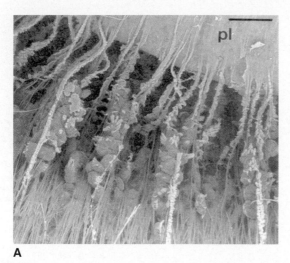

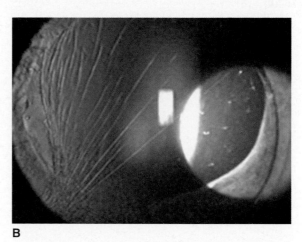

A   **B**

Figure 15.6 Exfoliation syndrome zonulopathy. **A:** Scanning electron micrograph shows an accumulation of exfoliation syndrome material on zonules in the region of the ciliary processes (pars plicata) and the posterior lens equator *(pl)*. Zonules appear to be loosened and, in some cases, broken. (From Naumann GO, Schlötzer-Schrehardt U, Kuchle M. Exfoliation syndrome for the comprehensive ophthalmologist: intraocular and systemic manifestations. *Ophthalmology.* 1998;105(6):951–968, with permission.) **B:** Exfoliation syndrome has created zonular tension so that the posterior capsule tension is flaccid, which makes cortex removal incomplete and capsular vacuuming impossible. As fibrosis progressed, substantial oblique striae developed with their apex at the area of retained cortex. (From Davison JA, et al. Intraocular lenses. In: Tasman W, Jaeger EA, eds. *Duane's Clinical Ophthalmology.* Vol. 6. Philadelphia, PA: Lippincott Williams & Wilkins; chap 11.)

with the exfoliation syndrome may also have increased aqueous flare and cells as quantitated by a laser flare-cell meter (47).

Ultrasound Biomicroscopic Findings

Ultrasonographic biomicroscopy can be a useful tool to look for the presence of exfoliation syndrome material on zonules or the peripheral lens capsule, particularly when the pupil cannot be easily dilated and the diagnosis of exfoliation syndrome is uncertain (**Fig. 15.11**) (48).

COURSE OF GLAUCOMA

The presence of exfoliative material in the eye is a major risk factor for conversion to glaucoma in patients with ocular hypertension. In the Early Manifest Glaucoma Trial (EMGT), patients with ocular hypertension and exfoliation syndrome were twice as likely as age- and sex-matched controls without exfoliation syndrome to convert to glaucoma (49). Exfoliation syndrome was also a risk factor for progression in patients with established glaucoma (50).

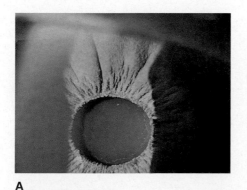

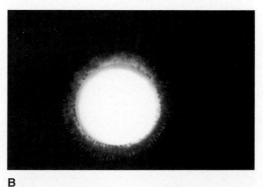

A   **B**

Figure 15.7 Exfoliation syndrome iridopathy. **A:** Exfoliative material at pupil border (called Fnock by Icelanders). (Courtesy of Joseph A. Halabis, OD.) **B:** "Moth-eaten" pattern of peripupillary transillumination defects from degeneration of the iris sphincter muscle. (From Khaimi MA, Skuta GL, Morgan RK. Exfoliation syndrome, pigment dispersion syndrome, and the associated glaucomas. In: Tasman W, Jaeger EA, eds. *Duane's Clinical Ophthalmology*, Vol. 3. Philadelphia, PA: Lippincott Williams & Wilkins; 2008:chap 54B.)

Figure 15.8 Gonioscopic view of an eye with exfoliation syndrome shows irregular pigmentation of trabecular meshwork and white flecks of exfoliative material.

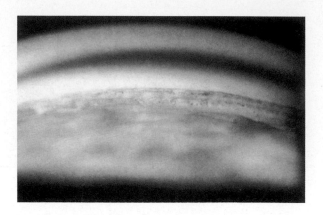

Figure 15.9 Exfoliation syndrome trabeculopathy. **A:** Schematic of the trabecular meshwork shows localization of exfoliation syndrome deposits of presumed endotrabecular and exotrabecular origin. **B:** Transmission electron micrograph shows an accumulation of exfoliation syndrome material (*star*) in the juxtacanalicular tissue along the inner wall of Schlemm canal (*Sc*) (bar = 3 μm). **C:** Scanning electron micrograph of the inner surface of the trabecular meshwork shows exfoliation syndrome deposits (*stars*) in the uveal pores (bar = 15 μm). (Modified from Naumann GO, Schlötzer-Schrehardt U, Kuchle M. Exfoliation syndrome for the comprehensive ophthalmologist: intraocular and systemic manifestations. *Ophthalmology.* 1998;105(6):951–968, with permission.)

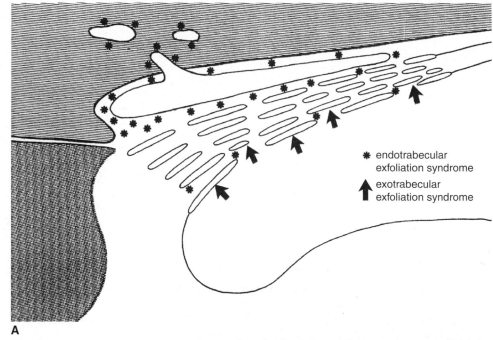

✳ endotrabecular
exfoliation syndrome

➤ exotrabecular
exfoliation syndrome

A

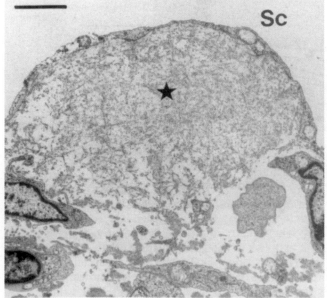

B

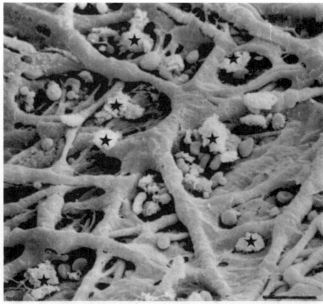

C

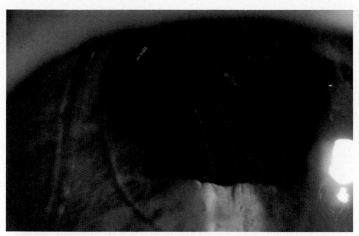

Figure 15.10 Exfoliative material on the anterior hyaloid face.

Not all patients with the exfoliation syndrome develop glaucoma, and reports vary considerably regarding the frequency of glaucoma in eyes with this condition. In one study of patients with the exfoliation syndrome but without glaucoma on the initial examination, one third developed glaucoma during a 1.5-year follow-up (51). Some patients with bilateral exfoliation syndrome have glaucoma in both eyes, but others have a pressure rise in only one of the eyes with exfoliation. Less commonly, a patient with unilateral exfoliation may have open-angle glaucoma in both eyes (20).

Open-Angle Glaucoma

Most eyes with exfoliative glaucoma have an open-angle mechanism, although acute angle-closure glaucoma also occurs in a small number of cases (24,29,52,53). It is not uncommon for patients with the exfoliation syndrome to have an acute onset of high intraocular pressure (IOP) in the presence of open angles.

The observation that glaucoma does not develop in all eyes with the exfoliation syndrome but may develop in both eyes of a patient with unilateral exfoliation has led to the theory that exfoliative glaucoma and chronic open-angle glaucoma (COAG) may share similar mechanisms of aqueous outflow obstruction (24,29,54,55). However, the much greater incidence of glaucoma in eyes with exfoliation syndrome is thought to indicate a causal relationship between the abnormal material and the elevated IOP (56). Patients with exfoliation syndrome do not have the same response to topical corticosteroids as patients with COAG do (57,58). Furthermore, although some lysyl oxidase-like 1 gene (*LOXL1*) variants predispose to exfoliative glaucoma, they do not appear to be associated with COAG (59). It therefore appears that exfoliative glaucoma represents a distinct form of glaucoma, but it may be superimposed on COAG in some patients. Mechanisms of IOP elevation in exfoliative glaucoma-associated open angles may include local production of exfoliative material, endothelial cell damage of the trabecular meshwork, and passive deposition of exfoliative material and pigment originating from elsewhere in the anterior segment.

Once open-angle glaucoma has developed in an eye with exfoliation, the IOP tends to run higher and may be more

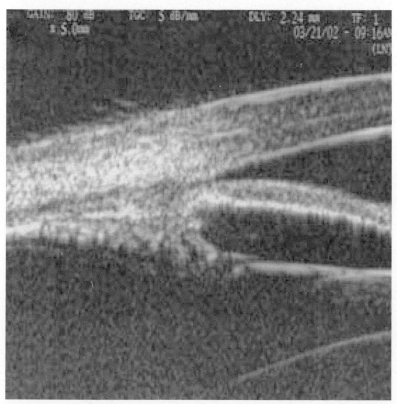

Figure 15.11 Value of ultrasonographic biomicroscopy in detecting exfoliation syndrome material and zonular weakness and breakage. **A:** Normal zonules.

A

Figure 15.11 (*Continued*) **B:** Uneven or disrupted zonules with peripheral lens accumulation of exfoliative material (*arrow*). **C:** Patchy deposits (*arrows*) on zonules characteristic of exfoliation syndrome. (Adapted from Ritch R, Vessani RM, Tran HV. Ultrasound biomicroscopic assessment of zonular appearance in exfoliation syndrome. *Acta Ophthalmol Scand.* 2007;85(5):495–499, with permission.)

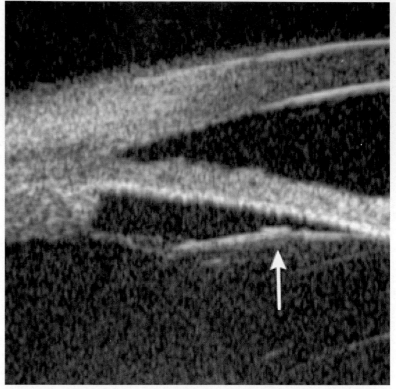

B

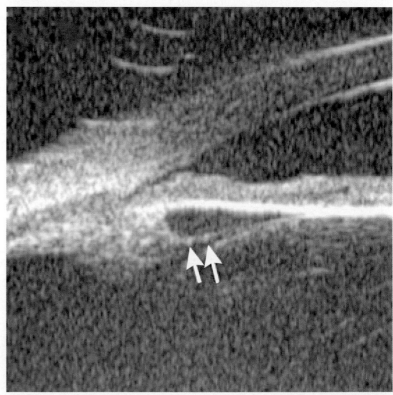

C

difficult to control than in cases of COAG (60–62). It has also been observed that the probability of developing glaucomatous optic neuropathy is higher in eyes with exfoliative glaucoma than in other forms of glaucoma at similar IOP levels (53), suggesting an intrinsic vulnerability in the optic nerve in the former group. Although disc area and other morphometric features of the optic nerve head do not differ between nonglaucomatous eyes with and without exfoliation (63), glaucomatous neuroretinal rim damage tends to be more diffuse with exfoliative glaucoma, as opposed to the sectorial preference in COAG (64). Immunoelectron microscopic studies of the lamina cribrosa have shown elastosis, suggesting abnormal regulation of elastin synthesis or degradation, or both, in the optic nerve head of patients with the exfoliation syndrome, consistent with the role of *LOXL1* (65).

Acute Increases in Intraocular Pressure

Patients with exfoliation syndrome and open angles may present with acute glaucoma mimicking angle-closure glaucoma (i.e. a red eye, corneal edema, and IOP often >50 mm Hg) (52,55,66). In a study of 139 cases of "acute" glaucoma, comprising 25% of a series of patients with exfoliation syndrome and glaucoma, 86 had open-angle glaucoma, 21 had neovascular glaucoma, and 18 had acute angle-closure glaucoma (53). In all the latter eyes, the anterior chamber depth was less than 2.2 mm.

Angle-Closure Glaucoma

A less-common mechanism of glaucoma in patients with the exfoliation syndrome is acute or chronic angle-closure glaucoma (24,29,42,52,53). A number of mechanisms may create a tendency toward pupillary block and angle closure, including zonular weakness, causing anterior movement of the lens; lens thickening from cataract formation; increased adhesiveness of the iris to the lens (occasionally with posterior synechiae) due to exfoliative material, sphincter muscle degeneration, and uveitis; and iris rigidity from hypoxia. Patients with exfoliation syndrome predisposed to angle closure may have a relatively small anterior segment despite normal axial length. Naumann coined the term relative anterior microphthalmos to describe eyes with normal axial lengths but disproportionately smaller anterior segment, as defined by a horizontal corneal diameter of 11 mm or less (67). Such patients tend to have a shallower central anterior chamber depth and a greater-than-average lens thickness.

ETIOLOGY AND PATHOGENESIS

The ultrastructural appearance of exfoliation syndrome is that of random 10 to 12 nm fibrils, arranged in a fibrillogranular matrix and occasionally coiled as spirals (68,69). Evidence supports the concept that exfoliation is an inherited microfibrillopathy involving transforming growth factor-1, oxidative stress, and impaired cellular protection mechanisms as key pathogenetic factors (**Fig. 15.12**). In a landmark study

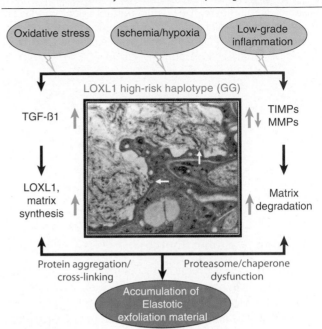

Exfoliation syndrome: Model of pathogenesis

Figure 15.12 Summary of current understanding of exfoliation syndrome pathogenesis. TIMP, tissue inhibitor of matrix metallo-proteinase *(MMP)*; TGF-β1, transforming growth factor beta 1. (Courtesy of Ursula Schlötzer-Schrehardt, PhD.)

in the Icelandic and Swedish populations, a common genetic variant was identified as a major risk factor for exfoliation syndrome and glaucoma (70). Polymorphisms in the coding region of *LOXL1* located on chromosome 15q24 are associated with exfoliation syndrome and exfoliative glaucoma in these and other populations. The disease-associated polymorphisms are found in virtually all individuals with exfoliation syndrome in the studied populations. *LOXL1* is one of many enzymes essential for the formation of elastin fibers: It plays a role in modifying tropoelastin, the basic building block of elastin, and catalyzes the process for monomers to cross-link and form elastin (**Fig.15.13**). Mice lacking *LOXL1* protein have diffuse elastic tissue changes associated with tropoelastin accumulation, including pelvic organ prolapse, enlarged airspaces of the lung, loose skin, and vascular abnormalities (71).

Although *LOXL1* is a major risk factor for exfoliation syndrome and exfoliative glaucoma, strong evidence suggests that additional genetic or environmental factors will be identified that influence disease expression and severity. For example, despite similar prevalences of *LOXL1* risk variants, the clinical prevalence of exfoliation syndrome is ninefold lower in a white population from Australia compared with whites in Iceland (72). Nevertheless, the finding of *LOXL1* involvement will provide critical insights into the pathophysiology of exfoliation syndrome, providing an opportunity for novel treatment approaches. Since the disease-associated *LOXL1* variant is commonly found in both affected and unaffected individuals, genetic testing is of limited clinical value at this time (73).

Figure 15.13 *LOXL1* is one of a family of lysyl oxidase enzymes essential for the formation of elastin fibers. It has an important role in modifying tropoelastin, the basic building block of elastin, and catalyzing process for monomers to cross-link and form elastin. TE, tropoelastin. (Reproduced from Liu X, Zhao Y, Gao J. Elastic fiber homeostasis requires lysyl oxidase-like 1 protein. *Nat Genet.* 2004;36(2):178–182, with permission.)

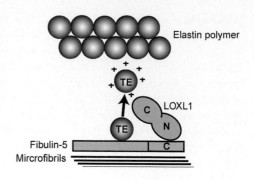

Ocular and Systemic Sources

Exfoliative material is produced by many cell types in the anterior segment, including lens capsule epithelium, iris epithelium, vascular endothelium, corneal endothelium, and Schlemm canal endothelium. The material has also been found in extrabulbar tissue, including the conjunctiva (67,74,75), which appears to be another independent source of the material. This has been demonstrated in conjunctival biopsies of eyes that did not have the typical clinical appearance of exfoliative material on the anterior lens capsule but were suspected on the basis of other signs, such as pigment dispersion and iris transillumination defects (76). Other extrabulbar sites where exfoliative material has been identified include extraocular muscles, orbital septa, posterior ciliary arteries, vortex veins, and central retinal vessels passing through the optic nerve sheaths (75).

The exfoliative material has also been demonstrated in tissues throughout the body of patients with the exfoliation syndrome, including lung, heart, liver, gallbladder, skin, kidney, and cerebral meninges (77,78), suggesting a systemic process involving generalized abnormal elastin metabolism.

DIFFERENTIAL DIAGNOSIS

The exfoliation syndrome must be distinguished from other forms of lens exfoliation and from other causes of pigment dispersion.

Capsular Delamination

Another group of disorders that involve exfoliation of the anterior lens capsule has been referred to as true exfoliation of the lens capsule or capsular delamination (8–11). These cases differ from the exfoliation syndrome in that an underlying precipitating factor, such as trauma, exposure to intense heat, or severe uveitis, is often, but not always, present (5–10). The nature of the lens exfoliation also differs, with thin, clear membrane-like material separating from the anterior lens capsule and often curling at the margins (8–10). Glaucoma occurs infrequently with capsular delamination.

Primary Amyloidosis

This generalized, systemic disease, which may be familial or nonfamilial (79,80), has numerous ocular manifestations, including glaucoma. The amyloid may be deposited as a white, flaky substance throughout the eye, including the pupillary margin of the iris, the anterior lens capsule, and the anterior chamber angle, creating a clinical picture that resembles the exfoliation syndrome (79,80). In the autosomal-dominant condition, familial amyloidotic polyneuropathy, glaucoma is the most common ocular manifestation, and an ultrastructural study revealed accumulations of amyloid fibrils and multilayered plaques of basement membrane-like material in the intertrabecular spaces (81).

Pigment Dispersion

Many conditions in addition to the exfoliation syndrome are characterized by increased pigmentation of the trabecular meshwork. They include the pigment dispersion syndrome and pigmentary glaucoma (see Chapter 17); some forms of anterior uveitis (see Chapter 22), melanosis and melanomas (see Chapter 21), and COAG; and otherwise normal eyes with unusually heavy pigment dispersion. These conditions can usually be distinguished from the exfoliation syndrome by observing the characteristic appearance of the anterior lens capsule and iris in the latter disorder. However, the exfoliation syndrome has developed in patients with the pigmentary dispersion syndrome (82).

MANAGEMENT

Glaucoma

Glaucoma associated with exfoliation syndrome can be particularly challenging to manage (61,62). IOP can fluctuate considerably, and care should be taken when setting the target pressure range. Because of higher IOP fluctuation, some choose to set a lower target IOP and follow up these patients more closely. Patients with exfoliative glaucoma typically have an excellent response to prostaglandin analogues and laser trabeculoplasty, particularly argon laser trabeculopexy (83–85). When incisional surgical intervention becomes necessary, filtering surgery is generally advocated. One study suggested that exfoliative glaucoma has a poorer response to medical therapy than COAG but that it has a better response to trabeculectomy (86). Cataract surgery may also decrease the IOP in patients with exfoliation syndrome and exfoliative glaucoma and open angles (87).

Cataract

Although lens extraction is not advocated for the management of exfoliative glaucoma, cataract extraction for improvement of visual acuity is frequently indicated and requires special consideration in these patients. With traditional extracapsular cataract surgery and with phacoemulsification, patients with the exfoliation syndrome have a higher-than-average risk of zonular and capsular breaks (88). This is most likely caused by degeneration of the zonular fibrils (33), but it may also be associated with a thin posterior lens capsule (89). Other factors that may complicate cataract surgery in these patients are poor pupillary dilatation and occasional synechiae between the iris pigment epithelium and the peripheral anterior lens capsule (90). Preoperatively, the surgeon should look for evidence of zonular dialysis, such as phacodonesis and asymmetric anterior chamber depth (33); the corneal endothelium should also be evaluated carefully for compromise. Ultrasonographic biomicroscopy can be very helpful when trying to decide if significant zonular dialysis is present, and also to detect the presence of stretched zonules.

Helpful tips for cataract surgery are to make the capsulorrhexis large so as to enable the nucleus or pieces of the nucleus to prolapse into the anterior chamber, thus minimizing zonular stress; a large capsulorrhexis also helps prevent capsular phimosis, which is common in eyes with exfoliation syndrome. During hydrodissection, care should be taken to tap on the center of the nucleus from time to time to decompress fluid pressure on a weak posterior capsule. If zonular weakness is evident intraoperatively, a capsule tension ring or capsule tension segments can be helpful. In addition to taking special care to minimize zonular stress during nucleus manipulation and removal of the cortex, if the pupil size is small, the surgeon should consider mechanically dilating and maintaining pupil dilatation. The use of a posterior chamber intraocular lenses is well tolerated in patients with the exfoliation syndrome, although there may be a greater risk for fibrinoid reaction in these patients (91).

KEY POINTS

■ Exfoliation syndrome is an inherited microfibrillopathy associated with polymorphisms in *LOXL1*. It is generally recognized by the typical appearance of exfoliative material on the anterior lens capsule and is a relatively common disorder in older individuals among many populations worldwide. It is characterized by a protein-like material on the lens, iris, and various other ocular and extraocular structures.

■ It is a major risk factor for development of open-angle glaucoma and, in some cases, angle-closure glaucoma. The condition may be unilateral or bilateral, and about 40% of patients with exfoliation syndrome may have associated glaucoma.

■ Early recognition and appropriate management are essential to good outcomes. Early signs of exfoliation syndrome include a light frosting of material on the lens capsule best seen with a dilated pupil, heavy (often irregular) pigment in the trabecular meshwork, and visualization of exfoliative material on the zonules or ciliary body. Ocular manifestations associated with exfoliation syndrome include glaucoma, cataract, zonular and lens capsule weakness, poor pupillary dilatation, blood–aqueous barrier breakdown, corneal endothelial decompensation, and retinal vein occlusion.

■ Any patient with exfoliation and a shallow peripheral and central anterior chamber depth should have gonioscopy and be evaluated for a prophylactic peripheral iridotomy.

■ When contemplating cataract surgery in a patient with exfoliation syndrome, check the status of the lens zonules (i.e., examine for presence of phacodonesis or lens subluxation).

■ Glaucoma is especially challenging to control in patients with exfoliation syndrome. Care should be taken to set the target pressure range and follow carefully, because there is greater diurnal IOP fluctuation in exfoliative glaucoma patients, and IOP can spike out of control in a short period. Patients may require aggressive treatment and frequent, close follow-up.

REFERENCES

1. Ritch R. Exfoliation syndrome: the most common identifiable cause of open-angle glaucoma. *J Glaucoma.* 1994;3(2):176–177.
2. Schlotzer-Schrehardt U, Naumann GOH. Ocular and systemic exfoliation syndrome. *Am J Ophthalmol.* 2006;141(5):921–937.
3. Mitchell P, Wang JJ, Smith W. Association of exfoliation syndrome with increased vascular risk. *Am J Ophthalmol.* 1997;124(5):685–687.
4. Lindberg JG. Clinical investigations on depigmentation of the pupillary border and translucency of the iris in cases of senile cataract and in normal eyes in elderly persons. *Acta Ophthalmol Suppl.* 1989;190:1–96.
5. Elschnig A. Detachment of the zonular lamellae in glass blowers [in German]. *Klin Monastsbl Augenheilkd.* 1922;69:732–734.
6. Kraupa E. Linsenkapselrisse ohne Wundstar [in German]. *Z Augenheilkd.* 1922;48:93.
7. Butler TH. Capsular glaucoma. *Trans Ophthalmol Soc U K.* 1938;68:575–589.
8. Radda TM, Klemen UM. True idiopathic exfoliation [in German]. *Klin Monbl Augenheilkd.* 1982;181(4):276–277.
9. Brodrick JD, Tate GW Jr. Capsular delamination (true exfoliation) of the lens. Report of a case. *Arch Ophthalmol.* 1979;97(9):1693–1698.
10. Cashwell LF Jr, Holleman IL, Weaver RG, et al. Idiopathic true exfoliation of the lens capsule. *Ophthalmology.* 1989;96(3):348–351.
11. Dvorak-Theobald G. Pseudo-exfoliation of the lens capsule: relation to true exfoliation of the lens capsule as reported in the literature and role in the production of glaucoma capsulocuticulare. *Am J Ophthalmol.* 1954;37(1):1–12.
12. Ringvold A. Epidemiology of the pseudo-exfoliation syndrome. *Acta Ophthalmol Scand.* 1999;77(4):371–375.
13. Astrom S, Stenlund H, Linden C. Incidence and prevalence of exfoliations and open-angle glaucoma in northern Sweden: II. Results after 21 years of follow-up. *Acta Ophthalmol Scand.* 2007;85(8):832–837.
14. Ringvold A, Blika S, Elsas T, et al. The prevalence of exfoliation in three separate municipalities of Middle-Norway. A preliminary report. *Acta Ophthalmol Suppl.* 1987;182:17–20.
15. Luntz MH. Prevalence of pseudo-exfoliation syndrome in an urban South African clinic population. *Am J Ophthalmol.* 1972;74(4):581–587.

16. Ball SF, Graham S, Thompson H. The racial prevalence and biomicroscopic signs of exfoliative syndrome in the glaucoma population of southern Louisiana. *Glaucoma.* 1989;11:169–175.

17. Damji KF, Bains HS, Amjadi K, et al. Familial occurrence of exfoliation in Canada. *Can J Ophthalmol.* 1999;34(5):257–265.

18. Ritch R, Schlotzer-Schrehardt U. Exfoliation syndrome. *Surv Ophthalmol.* 2001;45(4):265–315.

19. Ohrt V, Nehen JH. The incidence of glaucoma capsulare based on a Danish hospital material. *Acta Ophthalmol.* 1981;59:888–893.

20. Lindblom B, Thorburn W. Observed incidence of glaucoma in Halsingland, Sweden. *Acta Ophthalmol.* 1984;62(2):217–222.

21. Blika S, Ringvold A. The occurrence of simple and capsular glaucoma in Middle-Norway. *Acta Ophthalmol Suppl.* 1987;182:11–16.

22. Yalaz M, Othman I, Nas K, et al. The frequency of exfoliation syndrome in the eastern Mediterranean area of Turkey. *Acta Ophthalmol.* 1992;70(2):209–213.

23. Moreno-Montanes J, Alvarez Serna A, Alcolea Paredes A. Pseudoexfoliative glaucoma in patients with open-angle glaucoma in the northwest of Spain. *Acta Ophthalmol.* 1990;68(6):695–699.

24. Roth M, Epstein DL. Exfoliation syndrome. *Am J Ophthalmol.* 1980;89(4):477–481.

25. Miyake K, Matsuda M, Inaba M. Corneal endothelial changes in exfoliation syndrome. *Am J Ophthalmol.* 1989;108(1):49–52.

26. Schlotzer-Schrehardt UM, Dorfler S, Naumann GOH. Corneal endothelial involvement in exfoliation syndrome. *Arch Ophthalmol.* 1993;111(5):666–674.

27. Naumann GOH, Schlotzer-Schrehardt U. Keratopathy in exfoliation syndrome as a cause of corneal endothelial decompensation: a clinicopathologic study. *Ophthalmology.* 2000;107(6):1111–1124.

28. Naumann GOH, Schlotzer-Schrehardt U. Corneal endotheliopathy of exfoliation syndrome (letter). *Arch Ophthalmol.* 1994;112:297.

29. Layden WE, Shaffer RN. Exfoliation syndrome. *Am J Ophthalmol.* 1974;78(5):835–841.

30. Seland JH, Chylack LT Jr. Cataracts in the exfoliation syndrome (fibrillopathia epitheliocapsularis). *Trans Ophthalmol Soc UK.* 1982;102 Pt 3:375–379.

31. Arnarsson A, Jonasson F, Sasaki H, et al. Risk factors for nuclear lens opacification: the Reykjavik Eye Study. *Dev Ophthalmol.* 2002;35:12–20.

32. Mizuno K, Muroi S. Cycloscopy of exfoliation. *Am J Ophthalmol.* 1979;87(4):513–518.

33. Futa R, Furuyoshi N. Phakodonesis in capsular glaucoma: a clinical and electron microscopic study. *Jpn J Ophthalmol.* 1989;33(3):311–317.

34. Schlotzer-Schrehardt U, Naumann GOH. A histopathologic study of zonular instability in exfoliation syndrome. *Am J Ophthalmol.* 1994;118(6):730–743.

35. Prince AM, Ritch R. Clinical signs of the exfoliation syndrome. *Ophthalmology.* 1986;93(6):803–807.

36. Repo LP, Terasvirta ME, Tuovinen EJ. Generalized peripheral iris transluminance in the exfoliation syndrome. *Ophthalmology.* 1990;97(8):1027–1029.

37. Brooks AM, Gillies WE. The development of microneovascular changes in the iris in exfoliation of the lens capsule. *Ophthalmology.* 1987;94(9):1090–1097.

38. Asano N, Schlotzer-Schrehardt U, Naumann GOH. A histopathologic study of iris changes in exfoliation syndrome. *Ophthalmology.* 1995;102(9):1279–1290.

39. Repo LP, Terasvirta ME, Koivisto KJ. Generalized transluminance of the iris and the frequency of the exfoliation syndrome in the eyes of transient ischemic attack patients. *Ophthalmology.* 1993;100(3):352–355.

40. Repo LP, Suhonen MT, Terasvirta ME, et al. Color Doppler imaging of the ophthalmic artery blood flow spectra of patients who have had a transient ischemic attack. Correlations with generalized iris transluminance and exfoliation syndrome. *Ophthalmology.* 1995;102(8):1199–1205.

41. Sampaolesi R. Neue Untersuchungen über das Pseudo-Kapselhäutchen-Glaukom (Glaucoma Capsulare) [in German]. *Ber Deutsch Ophthal Ges.* 1959;62:177–183.

42. Wishart PK, Spaeth GL, Poryzees EM. Anterior chamber angle in the exfoliation syndrome. *Br J Ophthalmol.* 1985;69(2):103–107.

43. Ritch R. Exfoliation syndrome and occludable angles. *Trans Am Ophthalmol Soc.* 1994;92:845–944.

44. Shah KC, Damji KF, Chialant D, et al. Why do some patients with exfoliation syndrome develop angle closure glaucoma? *Invest Ophthalmol Vis Sci.* 1999;40:S80.

45. Gross FJ, Tingey D, Epstein DL. Increased prevalence of occludable angles and angle-closure glaucoma in patients with exfoliation. *Am J Ophthalmol.* 1994;117(3):333–336.

46. Schlotzer-Schrehardt U, Naumann GOH. Trabecular meshwork in exfoliation syndrome with and without open-angle glaucoma. A morphometric, ultrastructural study. *Invest Ophthalmol Vis Sci.* 1995;36(9):1750–1764.

47. Kuchle M, Nguyen NX, Horn F, et al. Quantitative assessment of aqueous flare and aqueous 'cells' in exfoliation syndrome. *Acta Ophthalmol.* 1992;70(2):201–208.

48. Ritch R, Vessani RM, Tran HV, et al. Ultrasound biomicroscopic assessment of zonular appearance in exfoliation syndrome. *Acta Ophthalmol Scand.* 2007;85(5):495–499.

49. Grodum K, Heijl A, Bengtsson B. Risk of glaucoma in ocular hypertension with and without exfoliation. *Ophthalmology.* 2005;112(3):386–390.

50. Leske MC, Heijl A, Hussein M, et al. Factors for glaucoma progression and the effect of treatment: the early manifest glaucoma trial. *Arch Ophthalmol.* 2003;121(1):48–56.

51. Slagsvold JE. The follow-up in patients with exfoliation of the lens capsule with and without glaucoma. 2. The development of glaucoma in persons with exfoliation. *Acta Ophthalmol.* 1986;64(3):241–245.

52. Brooks AM, Gillies WE. The presentation and prognosis of glaucoma in exfoliation of the lens capsule. *Ophthalmology.* 1988;95(2):271–276.

53. Gillies WE, Brooks AM. The presentation of acute glaucoma in exfoliation of the lens capsule. *Aust N Z J Ophthalmol.* 1988;16(2):101–106.

54. Sampaolesi R, Argento C. Scanning electron microscopy of the trabecular meshwork in normal and glucomatous eyes. *Invest Ophthalmol Vis Sci.* 1977;16(4):302–314.

55. Cebon L, Smith RJ. Exfoliation of lens capsule and glaucoma. Case report. *Br J Ophthalmol.* 1976;60(4):279–282.

56. Aasved H. Intraocular pressure in eyes with and without fibrilliopathia epitheliocapsularis (so-called senile exfoliation or exfoliation). *Acta Ophthalmol.* 1971;49(4):601–610.

57. Pohjola S, Horsmanheimo A. Topically applied corticosteroids in glaucoma capsulare. *Arch Ophthalmol.* 1971;85(2):150–153.

58. Gillies WE. Corticosteroid-induced ocular hypertension in pseudoexfoliation of lens capsule. *Am J Ophthalmol.* 1970;70(1):90–95.

59. Liu Y, Schmidt S, Qin X, et al. Lack of association between LOXL1 variants and primary open-angle glaucoma in three different populations. *Invest Ophthalmol Vis Sci.* 2008;49(8):3465–3468.

60. Lindblom B, Thorburn W. Functional damage at diagnosis of primary open angle glaucoma. *Acta Ophthalmol.* 1984;62(2):223–229.

61. Futa R, Shimizu T, Furuyoshi N, et al. Clinical features of capsular glaucoma in comparison with primary open-angle glaucoma in Japan. *Acta Ophthalmol.* 1992;70(2):214–219.

62. Olivius E, Thorburn W. Prognosis of glaucoma simplex and glaucoma capsulare. A comparative study. *Acta Ophthalmol.* 1978;56(6):921–934.

63. Puska P, Raitta C. Exfoliation syndrome as a risk factor for optic disc changes in nonglaucomatous eyes. *Graefes Arch Clin Exp Ophthalmol.* 1992;230(6):501–504.

64. Tezel G, Tezel TH. The comparative analysis of optic disc damage in exfoliative glaucoma. *Acta Ophthalmol.* 1993;71(6):744–750.

65. Netland PA, Ye H, Streeten BW, et al. Elastosis of the lamina cribrosa in exfoliation syndrome with glaucoma. *Ophthalmology.* 1995;102(6):878–886.

66. Gillies WE, West RH. Exfoliation of the lens capsule and glaucoma. *Aust J Ophthalmol.* 1977;5:18–20.

67. Naumann GOH. *Pathologie des Auges.* Vol 2. 2nd ed. Berlin: Springer; 1997:1264.

68. Dark AJ, Streeten BW, Cornwall CC. Pseudoexfoliative disease of the lens: a study in electron microscopy and histochemistry. *Br J Ophthalmol.* 1977;61(7):462–472.

69. Davanger M. The pseudo-exfoliation syndrome. A scanning electron microscopic study. I. The anterior lens surface. *Acta Ophthalmol.* 1975;53(6):809–820.

70. Thorleifsson G, Magnusson KP, Sulem P, et al. Common sequence variants in the LOXL1 gene confer susceptibility to exfoliation glaucoma. *Science.* 2007;317(5843):1397–1400.

71. Liu X, Zhao Y, Gao J, et al. Elastic fiber homeostasis requires lysyl oxidase-like 1 protein. *Nat Genet.* 2004;36(2):178–182.

72. Hewitt AW, Sharma S, Burdon KP, et al. Ancestral LOXL1 variants are associated with exfoliation in Caucasian Australians but with markedly

lower penetrance than in Nordic people. *Hum Mol Genet.* 2008;17(5):710–716.

73. Challa P, Schmidt S, Liu Y, et al. Analysis of LOXL1 polymorphisms in a United States population with exfoliation glaucoma. *Mol Vis.* 2008;14:146–149.

74. Streeten BW, Bookman L, Ritch R, et al. Pseudoexfoliative fibrillopathy in the conjunctiva. A relation to elastic fibers and elastosis. *Ophthalmology.* 1987;94(11):1439–1449.

75. Schlotzer-Schrehardt U, Kuchle M, Naumann GOH. Electron-microscopic identification of exfoliation material in extrabulbar tissue. *Arch Ophthalmol.* 1991;109(4):565–570.

76. Prince AM, Streeten BW, Ritch R, et al. Preclinical diagnosis of exfoliation syndrome. *Arch Ophthalmol.* 1987;105(8):1076–1082.

77. Schlotzer-Schrehardt UM, Koca MR, Naumann GOH, et al. Exfoliation syndrome. Ocular manifestation of a systemic disorder? *Arch Ophthalmol.* 1992;110(12):1752–1756.

78. Streeten BW, Li ZY, Wallace RN, et al. Pseudoexfoliative fibrillopathy in visceral organs of a patient with exfoliation syndrome. *Arch Ophthalmol.* 1992;110(12):1757–1762.

79. Tsukahara S, Matsuo T. Secondary glaucoma accompanied with primary familial amyloidosis. *Ophthalmologica.* 1977;175(5):250–262.

80. Schwartz MF, Green WR, Michels RG, et al. An unusual case of ocular involvement in primary systemic nonfamilial amyloidosis. *Ophthalmology.* 1982;89(4):394–401.

81. Silva-Araujo AC, Tavares MA, Cotta JS, et al. Aqueous outflow system in familial amyloidotic polyneuropathy, Portuguese type. *Graefes Arch Clin Exp Ophthalmol.* 1993;231(3):131–135.

82. Layden WE, Ritch R, King DG, et al. Combined exfoliation and pigment dispersion syndrome. *Am J Ophthalmol.* 1990;109(5):530–534.

83. Konstas AG, Hollo G, Irkec M, et al. Diurnal IOP control with bimatoprost versus latanoprost in exfoliative glaucoma: a crossover, observer-masked, three-centre study. *Br J Ophthalmol.* 2007;91(6):757–760.

84. Threlkeld AB, Hertzmark E, Sturm RT, et al. Comparative study of the efficacy of argon laser trabeculoplasty for exfoliation and primary open-angle glaucoma. *J Glaucoma.* 1996;5(5):311–316.

85. Damji KF, Bovell AM, Hodge WG, et al. Selective laser trabeculoplasty versus argon laser trabeculoplasty: results from a 1-year randomised clinical trial. *Br J Ophthalmol.* 2006;90(12):1490–1494.

86. Konstas AG, Jay JL, Marshall GE, et al. Prevalence, diagnostic features, and response to trabeculectomy in exfoliation glaucoma. *Ophthalmology.* 1993;100(5):619–627.

87. Damji KF, Konstas AG, Liebmann JM, et al. Intraocular pressure following phacoemulsification in patients with and without exfoliation syndrome: a 2 year prospective study. *Br J Ophthalmol.* 2006;90(8):1014–1018.

88. Skuta GL, Parrish RK II, Hodapp E, et al. Zonular dialysis during extracapsular cataract extraction in exfoliation syndrome. *Arch Ophthalmol.* 1987;105(5):632–634.

89. Ruotsalainen J, Tarkkanen A. Capsule thickness of cataractous lenses with and without exfoliation syndrome. *Acta Ophthalmol.* 1987;65(4):444–449.

90. Carpel EF. Pupillary dilation in eyes with exfoliation syndrome. *Am J Ophthalmol.* 1988;105(6):692–694.

91. Raitta C, Tarkkanen A. Posterior chamber lens implantation in capsular glaucoma. *Acta Ophthalmologica.* 1987;65(S182):24–26.

16

Glaucomas Associated with Disorders of the Corneal Endothelium

In the clinical setting of glaucoma and disorders of the cornea, it is helpful to consider two categories of conditions. In the first category, there are developmental anterior segment abnormalities, acquired conditions of the cornea, or primary disorders of the corneal endothelium that occur with glaucoma. In the second category, the cornea changes are secondary to the underlying glaucoma condition. **Table 16.1** summarizes these categories and the various clinical disease categories. The subject of this chapter is primary corneal endothelial disorders that are associated with glaucoma, which include iridocorneal endothelial (ICE) syndrome; posterior polymorphous corneal dystrophy (PPCD), also called posterior polymorphic dystrophy (of cornea) (PPMD); and Fuchs endothelial dystrophy. (The remaining clinical conditions are discussed in other chapters.)

IRIDOCORNEAL ENDOTHELIAL SYNDROME

General Clinical Features and Terminology

The ICE syndrome is characterized by a primary corneal endothelial abnormality (1). Historically, three clinical variants were distinguished on the basis of changes in the iris (**Table 16.2**), but it is now recognized that progressive iris atrophy, Chandler syndrome, and Cogan–Reese syndrome represent a spectrum of ICE syndrome rather than distinct clinical identities. During the lifetime of a patient with ICE syndrome, the difference in clinical features may reflect the time at which the patient is seen. For example, a patient with initial findings of Chandler syndrome may later develop iris hole formation or nodules, changing the diagnosis to progressive iris atrophy or the Cogan–Reese syndrome, respectively. In other cases, however, the disease does not progress. Among the three clinical variants of ICE syndrome, Chandler syndrome appears to be the most common (2).

In general, the clinical features include presentation in early to middle adulthood, predilection for women, reduced visual acuity, pain, abnormalities of the iris, unilateral occurrence with variable amount of cornea edema but with subclinical abnormalities of the corneal endothelium in the fellow eye, anterior chamber angle abnormalities, and glaucoma (3,4). Familial cases are rare, and there is no consistent association with systemic diseases. In

---

Table 16.1 Glaucoma and Corneal Disorders

DISORDERS OF THE CORNEA ASSOCIATED WITH GLAUCOMA

A. Developmental disorders (Chapter 14)
   1. Peters anomaly
   2. Sclerocornea
   3. Aniridia
   4. Axenfeld–Rieger syndrome
B. Acquired conditions
   1. Keratouveitis (Chapter 22)
   2. Trauma (Chapter 25)
   3. Full thickness or endothelial keratoplasty (Chapter 26)
C. Primary disorders of the cornea endothelium
   1. Iridocorneal endothelial syndrome
   2. Posterior polymorphous corneal dystrophy
   3. Fuchs endothelial dystrophy

GLAUCOMA WITH SECONDARY ABNORMALITIES OF THE CORNEA

A. Pressure-induced corneal changes
   1. Epithelial and stromal edema (acute or marked IOP elevation)
   2. Endothelial changes (chronic IOP elevation)
   3. Haab striae (childhood glaucoma) (Chapter 13)
B. Exfoliation-induced corneal endothelial changes (Chapter 15)
C. Drug-induced changes in the cornea
   1. Endothelial decompensation with topical carbonic anhydrase inhibitors (Chapter 31)
   2. Toxic effect to cornea epithelium (e.g., benzalkonium chloride, β-blockers [Chapter 29], miotics [Chapter 32])

Table 16.2 Iridocorneal Endothelial Syndrome

Major Clinical Variations	Characteristic Features
Progressive iris atrophy	Iris features predominate with marked corectopia, atrophy, and hole formation
Chandler syndrome	Changes in the iris are mild to absent, whereas corneal edema, often at normal IOP levels, is typical
Cogan–Reese syndrome	Nodular, pigmented lesions of the iris are the hallmark and may be seen with the entire spectrum of corneal and other iris defects

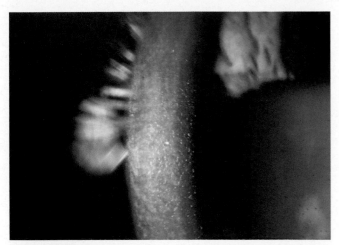

Figure 16.1 Slitlamp view shows the fine, beaten-silver appearance of a corneal endothelial abnormality in a patient with ICE syndrome.

some cases, the corneal edema may occur at intraocular pressure (IOP) levels that are normal or only slightly elevated.

In one study of 37 consecutive cases of the ICE syndrome in the United States, Chandler syndrome was the most common clinical variation, accounting for 21 cases (56%), and was characterized by more severe corneal edema despite less severe glaucoma than in the rest of the group (2). However, in a study

of 60 consecutive patients with ICE syndrome in Thailand, 38 patients had Cogan–Reese syndrome, 14 had Chandler syndrome, and 8 had progressive iris atrophy (5). In both studies, glaucoma occurred, most commonly in patients with progressive iris atrophy.

Pathologic Features

Changes in the Cornea

The common feature of the ICE syndrome is a corneal endothelial abnormality, which may be seen by slitlamp biomicroscopy as a "fine hammered silver" appearance of the posterior cornea, similar to that of Fuchs endothelial dystrophy (**Fig. 16.1**).

The findings seen on specular microscopy of the corneal endothelium are virtually pathognomonic of the ICE syndrome. The affected endothelial cells appear dark by specular microscopy except for a light central spot and a light peripheral zone with various degrees of pleomorphism in size and shape and loss of the clear hexagonal margins (**Fig. 16.2**) (4,6). As discussed earlier under the clinical features, most patients who have ICE syndrome are symptomatic in one eye; however, abnormalities in the contralateral asymptomatic eye can be identified by specular microscopy.

Light microscopy of the cornea of a patient with ICE syndrome has revealed a monolayer of reduced cell density with

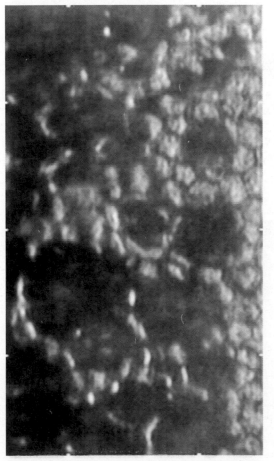

A

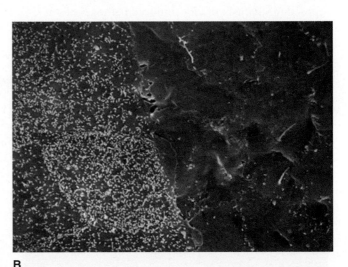

B

Figure 16.2 **A:** Specular microscopy of corneal endothelium in ICE syndrome. Cell borders are obscured, resulting in loss of the normal endothelial mosaic. Note dark areas within endothelial cells. Brighter reflections are believed to be from cell borders. **B:** Cornea, ICE syndrome. Scanning electron microscopy demonstrates sharp demarcation between abnormal (ICE) cells with microvilli and relatively unaffected endothelial cells. (From Cockerham GC, Kenyon KR. The corneal dystrophies. In: Tasman W, Jaeger EA, eds. *Duane's Clinical Ophthalmology.* Vol 4. Philadelphia, PA: Lippincott Williams & Wilkins; 2006:chap 16.)

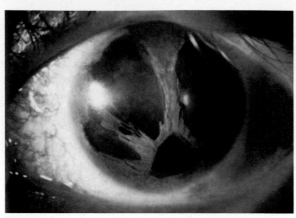

Figure 16.3 Eye of a patient with progressive iris atrophy, a variation of ICE syndrome, with extensive hole formation in the iris. Patients typically have more marked corectopia (the pupil is in the inferior quadrant in this eye).

occasional acellular zones and multiple endothelial layers, suggesting loss of contact inhibition (7). The ICE cells undergo metaplasia taking on morphologic features of epithelial cells, such as positive immunohistochemical staining for cytokeratins that are normally expressed by epithelium rather than endothelium (8). Some specimens have shown mononuclear inflammatory cells between the ICE cells (9), which support a proposed mechanism of viral-induced pathogenesis of ICE syndrome (as discussed later) (10).

This metaplasia is supported by scanning electron microscopy where the ICE cells showed numerous microvilli on the apical surface, in addition to cytoplasmic tonofilaments, and indentations on the basal surface containing clumps of fibrillar collagenous material (9). Other endothelial cells showed filopodium and cytoplasmic actin filaments suggesting migration (11). Another observation was a multilayered collagenous membrane posterior to the normal prenatal and postnatal layers of the collagenous structures of the Descemet membrane (12).

Changes in the Iris

The abnormalities of the iris constitute the primary basis for initially distinguishing clinical variations within the ICE syndrome, but as mentioned earlier, it is now recognized that these represent a spectrum the disease (3). In progressive iris atrophy, the hallmark is hole formation associated with corectopia and ectropion uvea that usually occur in the direction toward the quadrant with the most prominent area of peripheral anterior synechia (**Fig. 16.3**) (13). There appear to be two forms of atrophic iris holes. With stretch holes, the iris is markedly thinned in the quadrant away from the direction of pupillary distortion, and the holes develop within the area that is being stretched. In other eyes, melting holes develop without associated corectopia or thinning of the iris, which is thought to occur due to ischemia of the iris based on iris angiography (14).

In Chandler syndrome, there may be no clinically appreciated iris changes or there is minimal corectopia and mild atrophy of the stroma of the iris (**Fig. 16.4**). In the Cogan–Reese syndrome, the iris is distinguished by pigmented, pedunculated nodules on the surface (**Fig. 16.5**).

Light microscopy of the iris in ICE syndrome shows a cellular membrane on the anterior surface of the iris (**Fig. 16.6**), which is also referred to as a retrocorneal membrane that is continuous with that seen over the anterior chamber angle in the quadrant toward which the pupil is distorted (1,13). The nodular lesions that are characteristic of Cogan–Reese syndrome have an ultrastructure similar to that of the underlying stroma of the iris and are always surrounded by the previously described cellular membrane (15) (**Fig. 16.7**).

Changes in the Lens

In rare cases, the retrocorneal membrane of the ICE syndrome may grow over the anterior lens surface, simulating the anterior lens capsule, which can create confusion when performing a capsulorrhexis during cataract surgery (16). This retrocorneal membrane can also appear on the anterior surface of an intraocular lens implant (**Fig. 16.8**).

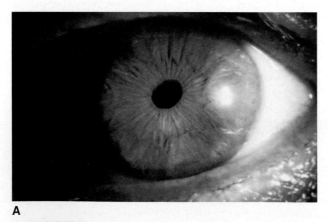

A

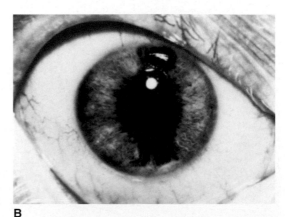

B

Figure 16.4 In patients with Chandler syndrome, a clinical variation of ICE syndrome, the eye may have a grossly normal-appearing iris or minimal corectopia and mild peripheral iris stromal atrophy (**A**), or more obvious iris changes, with a distorted, displaced pupil and variable degrees of iris stromal atrophy but no hole formation in the iris (**B**).

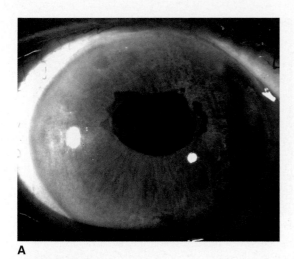

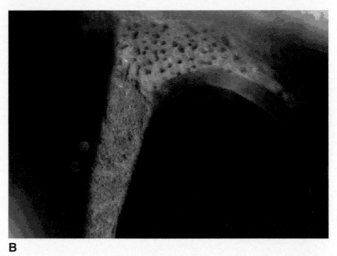

A   **B**

Figure 16.5   **A:** Cogan–Reese syndrome, a variation of ICE syndrome, shows ectropion uvea, some pupil distortion, and numerous dark nodules that are most prominent on the superior area of the iris stroma. **B:** ICE syndrome. Iris distortion and dark nodules (nevi) are present. Abnormal endothelium is often present on the iris surface. (From Cockerham GC, Kenyon KR. The corneal dystrophies. In: Tasman W, Jaeger EA, eds. *Duane's Clinical Ophthalmology.* Vol 4. Philadelphia, PA: Lippincott Williams & Wilkins; 2006:chap 16.)

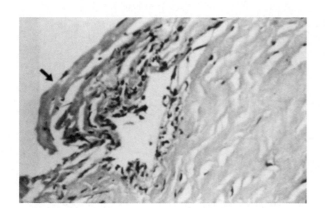

Figure 16.6   The glaucoma in ICE syndrome does not correlate precisely with the degree of synechial closure, and cases have been reported in which the angle was entirely open. In such cases, it is presumed that the trabecular meshwork is covered by a cellular membrane, consisting of a single layer of endothelial cells and Descemet-like membrane (*arrow*).

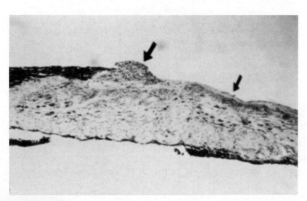

Figure 16.7   Light microscopic view of an iris specimen from an eye with Cogan–Reese syndrome.

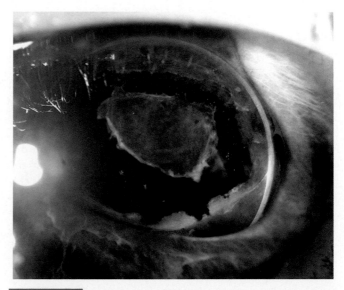

Figure 16.8   Retrocorneal membrane in ICE syndrome on the anterior surface of the intraocular lens, which was treated with an Nd:YAG anterior capsulotomy.

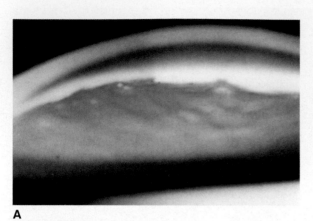
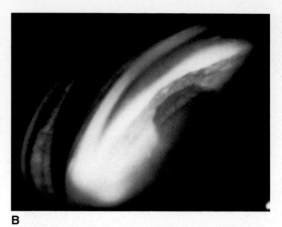

A   **B**

Figure 16.9 **A:** Glaucoma occurs in a large proportion of patients with the ICE syndrome. In most cases, the glaucoma is associated with peripheral anterior synechiae, which usually extend to or beyond the Schwalbe line. **B:** This gonioscopic image shows the high peripheral anterior synechiae, especially in the center of the view, which also reveals a broad area of ectropion uveae. (Courtesy of William A. MacIlwaine IV, MD.)

Gonioscopic Findings

Peripheral anterior synechia, usually extending to or beyond the Schwalbe line, is another clinical feature common to the ICE syndrome (**Fig. 16.9**). Elevated IOP usually begins as the synechiae progressively close the anterior chamber angle. However, the glaucoma does not correlate precisely with the degree of synechial closure and has been reported to occur when the entire angle was open but apparently covered by the cellular membrane (17,18).

These angle findings were confirmed in a histology study that revealed a Descemet-like membrane with a single layer of endothelial cells extending from the peripheral cornea and covering an open anterior chamber angle in some areas or synechial closure of the angle elsewhere in the same eye (1).

Theories of Mechanism

On the basis of the clinical and histopathologic evidence discussed earlier, Campbell and colleagues (13) proposed a "membrane theory" that a primary abnormality of the corneal endothelium was responsible for the findings in ICE syndrome (**Fig. 16.10**). The etiology that leads to the corneal endothelial changes is unknown. The absence of a positive family history and the presence of the postnatal layer of Descemet membrane suggest that it is an acquired disorder.

With evidence of inflammation in some cornea histopathology specimens, a virus-mediated mechanism has been proposed (7). Another study from this group supports this virus etiology for ICE syndrome based on the presence of DNA polymerase gene products for herpes simplex that was confirmed by sequencing the product (10). Specifically, among 31 cases (25 cornea specimens from patients with ICE syndrome and 6 from patients with chronic herpetic keratitis), 16 ICE syndrome (64%) and 4 herpetic keratitis (67%) were positive for herpes simplex virus DNA, which was localized to expression in the endothelium. Control corneas ($n = 15$) were negative for herpes simplex. In a smaller subset of nine ICE

syndrome cases, the specimens were negative for the Epstein–Barr and herpes zoster viruses. With this high (64%), specific expression of herpes simplex (i.e., negative for Epstein–Barr and zoster viruses) in the cornea endothelium of ICE syndrome specimens, it is conceivable to consider that a herpes simplex–mediated infection of the cornea endothelium transforms these cells to lose contact inhibition and to transform into an epithelial-like cell. These biologically transformed cells form a proliferative cellular membrane across the anterior chamber angle, which can obstruct the trabecular meshwork, and onto the surface of the iris, which can lead to formation of peripheral anterior synechiae and to the various iris changes observed in the spectrum of progressive iris atrophy, Cogan–Reese syndrome, and Chandler syndrome.

Differential Diagnosis

There are several disorders of the cornea or iris, many of which have associated glaucoma, which can be confused with ICE syndrome. It is helpful to think of these in the following three categories: (a) endothelial disorders, (b) dissolution of the iris, and (c) nodular lesions of the iris.

Among the other corneal endothelial disorders, PPMD may be associated with glaucoma and changes of the anterior chamber angle and iris that resemble the ICE syndrome. However, the corneal abnormalities and other clinical features clearly distinguish these two spectra of disease (discussed in the next section). Specular microscopy may be helpful in distinguishing between ICE syndrome and PPMD (19). Fuchs endothelial dystrophy has changes in the cornea endothelium that are very similar to those of the ICE syndrome but none of the chamber angle or iris features of the latter condition (discussed in the last section).

In the category of dissolution of the iris, the Axenfeld–Rieger syndrome has striking clinical and histopathologic similarities to the ICE syndrome, but the congenital nature, bilaterality, and other features described in Chapter 14 help to

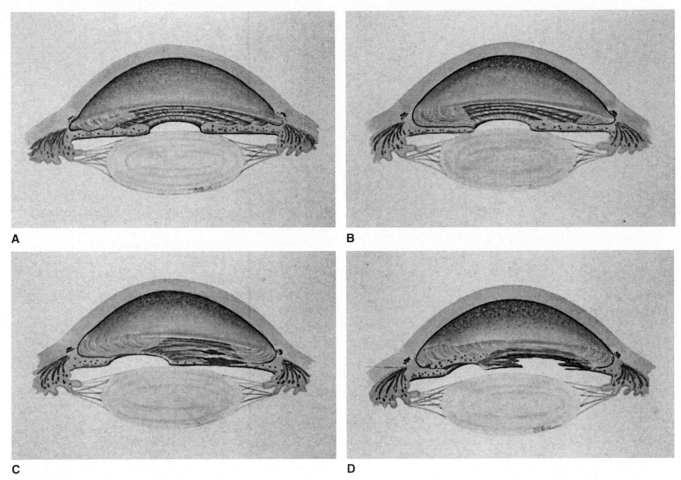

Figure 16.10 Membrane theory of Campbell for pathogenesis of ICE syndrome. **A:** Extension of the membrane from the corneal endothelium over the anterior chamber angle and onto the iris. **B:** Contraction of the membrane, creating peripheral anterior synechiae and corectopia. **C:** Thinning and atrophy of iris in quadrants away from the corectopia. **D:** Hole formation in an area of atrophy (in progressive iris atrophy), ectropion uvea in the direction of the corectopia, and nodules in the area of the membrane (in Cogan–Reese syndrome). (From Shields MB. Progressive essential iris atrophy, Chandler syndrome, and the iris nevus [Cogan–Reese] syndrome: a spectrum of disease. *Surv Ophthalmol.* 1979;24(1):3–20, with permission.)

separate the two conditions. Some advanced cases of progressive iris atrophy might resemble aniridia, but the bilaterality of the latter disorder is a helpful differential feature (Chapter 14). Iridoschisis is characterized by separation of superficial layers of iris stroma and may be associated with glaucoma, but it is typically a disease affecting older adults (Chapter 17).

Among the category of nodular lesions of the iris, melanomas of the iris (20); iris melanosis, which may be familial (21); Lisch nodules seen in neurofibromatosis type 1 (22); bilateral diffuse iris nodular nevi (23); and nodular inflammatory disorders, such as sarcoidosis, may also have pedunculated nodules strikingly similar to those of the Cogan–Reese syndrome.

Management

Patients with ICE syndrome may require treatment for corneal edema, the associated glaucoma, or both during the course of the disease. Given the unpredictable biological behavior of the abnormal corneal endothelium, patients with ICE syndrome should be monitored regularly based on signs and symptoms of

the disease. For instance, one case has been reported in which the pigmented nodules appeared on the iris 20 years after the initial diagnosis of ICE syndrome (24). Although specular microscopy can help to diagnose ICE syndrome, the findings do not correlate with the degree of corneal edema or decompensation or with the level of IOP elevation (25).

In the early stages, the glaucoma can often be controlled medically, especially with drugs that reduce aqueous production. When the IOP can no longer be controlled medically, surgical intervention is indicated, and a high percentage of patients with the ICE syndrome eventually require surgery. Given the membrane theory of this disease (Fig. 16.10), laser trabeculoplasty is not effective for this disease and is not recommended as treatment. In one study of 66 patients, glaucoma occurred in 33 (50%), and 22 (66%) of these underwent surgery; 45% of the patients who had a trabeculectomy required more than one procedure (26). Filtering surgery is reasonably successful, although late failures have occurred because of endothelialization of the filtering bleb (27). Adjunctive use of 5-fluorouracil did not improve the surgical outcomes (28). Adjunctive mitomycin C has been reported to offer reasonable intermediate-term success (29). Another surgical option is glaucoma drainage-device surgery (30). However, repeated filtering procedures, glaucoma drainage-device revision, and cyclodestructive laser may be additional options to lower IOP if previous surgical interventions have failed.

The corneal edema may be improved by lowering the IOP, although the additional use of hypertonic saline solutions may be required. However, in corneas with marked dysfunction of the endothelium, the edema will not clear, and penetrating keratoplasty is usually indicated for this situation after the glaucoma has been controlled (31). In one series of 14 patients who had ICE syndrome treated by penetrating keratoplasty, repeated corneal grafts were required in 6 (43%) over an average follow-up of 58 months (32). In the future, the development of therapies can be directed more specifically at the underlying disease process. For example, if the theory of a viral cause proves to be correct, it may allow treatment with antiviral agents. Another approach may be to prevent the growth of the endothelial membrane. An immunotoxin has been described that inhibits the proliferation of human corneal endothelium in tissue culture.

POSTERIOR POLYMORPHOUS CORNEAL DYSTROPHY

General Clinical Features and Terminology

Posterior polymorphous corneal dystrophy is a rare, bilateral, autosomal dominant familial disorder of the corneal endothelium. Presently, the three genes that have been identified for PPMD are *COL8A2* on chromosome 1p34.3 (33), *ZEB1* (formerly called *TCF8*) on chromosome 10p11.2 (34), and *VSX1* on chromosome 20p (35) (Chapter 8).

In general, the clinical features of PPMD include symptoms presenting in young adulthood and a clinical spectrum of characteristic corneal changes, peripheral iridocorneal adhesions, iris atrophy, and corectopia (discussed in detail later). Glaucoma occurs in approximately 15% of patients with PPMD (36).

Pathologic Features

Changes in the Cornea

By slitlamp biomicroscopy, the posterior cornea has the appearance of blisters or vesicles at the level of Descemet membrane (**Fig. 16.11A**). The vesicles may be linear (**Fig. 16.11B**) or in groups and may be surrounded by an aureole of gray haze (36). Band-like thickenings may also be seen at the level of Descemet membrane (37). On specular microscopy, several abnormal patterns have been described: either vesicles and band patterns at the level of Descemet membrane or a geographic pattern with associated haze of Descemet membrane and deep corneal stroma (38). An interesting observation was that 48 patients with PPMD, who had classic vesicles alone (42%) or vesicles with bands (48%) or diffuse abnormality of Descemet membrane (10%), had no other ocular abnormalities other than those of the cornea (39). In contrast, the latter specular pattern of prominent haze of Descemet membrane appears to be associated more with iridocorneal adhesions and glaucoma (38).

Ultrastructural studies reveal an unusually thin Descemet membrane covered by multiple layers of collagen and lined by cells that have been described as abnormal endothelium with epithelial-like and fibroblast-like features (40–42). In an unusually aggressive form of PPMD, a patient underwent 25 ocular procedures over 17 years for glaucoma, cataract, cornea, retina, and postoperative problems (43). Electron microscopy

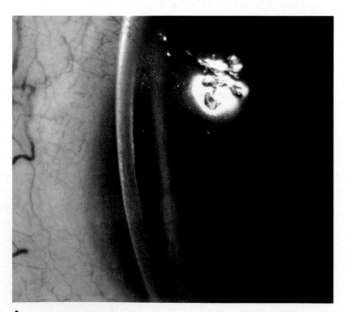
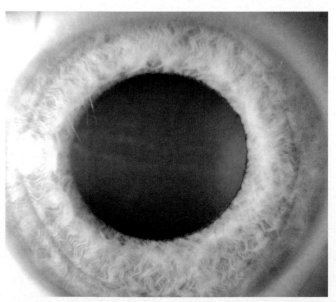

A   **B**

Figure 16.11 Slitlamp image of a patient with PPMD shows typical, irregular vesicular lesion of the posterior corneal surface (**A**) and subtle snail track across the central cornea (**B**).

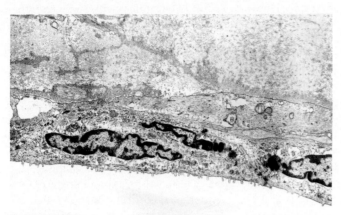

Figure 16.12 Transmission electron microscopy of left corneal button from a patient with PPMD showed stratified endothelial cells with nuclei, microvilli, and desmosomal attachments.

on the cornea revealed microvilli, tonofilaments, and desmosomes consistent with endothelial transformation (**Fig. 16.12**), which was confirmed by positive anticytokeratin AE1/AE3 and CAM 5.2 immunoreactivity. Negative immunoreactivity in epithelium and positive in endothelium with anticytokeratin 7 supported the diagnosis of PPMD rather than epithelial downgrowth.

Changes in the Iris, Angle, and Lens

A small number of patients may have broad peripheral anterior synechiae extending to or beyond the Schwalbe line, which may be associated with corectopia, ectropion uvea, and atrophy of the iris (**Fig. 16.13**) (36,44). The glaucoma may be

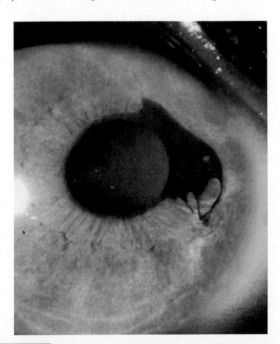

Figure 16.13 Slitlamp image showing corectopia, ectropion uvea, and focal iris atrophy of the right eye in a patient with PPMD. (Modified from Moroi SM, Gokhale PA, Schteingart MT, et al. Clinicopathologic correlation and genetic analysis in a case of posterior polymorphous corneal dystrophy. *Am J Ophthalmol.* 2003;135(4):461–470, with permission.)

caused by the iridocorneal adhesions in these cases. However, the extent of the iridocorneal adhesions does not correlate with the presence or severity of glaucoma, because the adhesions that bridge an otherwise open trabecular meshwork may not obstruct aqueous outflow (45). Histopathologic studies of such cases have revealed a membrane composed of epithelial-like cells and a Descemet-like membrane extending over the anterior chamber angle and onto the iris (43,44). Three types of peripheral anterior synechiae have been described: without an associated membrane, with iridotrabecular and iridocorneal apposition, and bridging open trabecular meshwork (45). The abnormal membrane is associated with the latter two configurations.

Glaucoma may be present in some of the cases with peripheral anterior synechiae, but it has also been observed in eyes with open angles (46). In the latter situation, gonioscopy may reveal a high insertion of the iris into the posterior aspect of the trabecular meshwork. An ultrastructural evaluation of such an eye confirmed the high insertion of anterior uvea into the meshwork with collapse of the trabecular beams.

In the particularly aggressive form of PPMD described earlier, a prominent retrocorneal membrane grew onto the crystalline lens and intraocular lens (43).

Theories of Mechanism

A membrane theory, similar to that for the ICE syndrome, has been proposed for cases of PPMD. It is postulated that a metaplastic endothelium shows features of epithelial cells, loses contact inhibition, produces a basement membrane–like material, extends across the anterior chamber angle and onto the iris, and leads to synechia formation and changes in the iris (36,47). The mechanism of glaucoma in eyes with PPMD may be due to either a closed-angle mechanism from the membrane alone or from the synechia formation (45), or the less common observation of open-angle mechanism with the high insertion of the anterior uvea that represents a developmental anomaly of the anterior chamber angle, as seen in several of the developmental glaucomas (46).

Among the three causative genes for PPMD—*VSX1*, *COL8A2*, and *ZEB1* (formerly called *TCF8*)—transcripts for all three genes have been demonstrated in the cornea (34). *ZEB1* (formerly called *TCF8*), accounts for about one third of PPMD familial cases (48). In the initial family used to identify *ZEB1* as the *PPCD3* gene, inguinal hernia, hydrocele, and possible bone anomalies in affected individuals were also reported (34). The association with hernias was also replicated in another study (48). A potential molecular mechanism was suggested by the ectopic expression of *COL4A3*, which is collagen type IV alpha 3, in corneal endothelium of the proband of the original *PPCD3* family. Mutations in the *COL4A3* gene cause Alport syndrome, and *ZEB1* has a complex binding site in the promoter of Alport syndrome gene *COL4A3*. It was proposed that the loss of function of *ZEB1* allowed for expression of *COL4A3*, a regulatory target for *ZEB1*, and contributes to the molecular mechanism for endothelial dysfunction in PPMD (34).

Differential Diagnosis

Conditions that may be confused with PPMD include other forms of posterior corneal dystrophy, such as Fuchs endothelial dystrophy, congenital hereditary corneal dystrophy, and posterior amorphous corneal dystrophy. The last condition is characterized by diffuse gray-white, sheet-like opacities of the posterior stroma, with occasional fine iris processes extending to the Schwalbe line for 360 degrees and various abnormalities of the iris but no glaucoma (49). When iridocorneal adhesions are present, Axenfeld–Rieger syndrome and ICE syndrome should be considered. The band-like thickenings of PPMD may be confused with the Haab striae of congenital glaucoma, although the latter are distinguished by the characteristic thinned areas with thickened edges (37).

Management

Most cases of PPMD are asymptomatic and do not require treatment. Corneal edema may require conservative management or penetrating keratoplasty. In one series of 21 keratoplasties for PPMD, 9 grafts failed, 6 of which were associated with iridocorneal adhesions and glaucoma, and it has been suggested that keratoplasty should be avoided in these patients until absolutely necessary (47). Recurrence of PPMD has been reported after penetrating keratoplasty. The glaucoma may respond to drugs that lower aqueous production. Laser trabeculoplasty is not likely to be successful in these cases, and filtering surgery, glaucoma drainage-device surgery, or laser cyclodestruction is indicated when medical therapy is no longer adequate. PPMD is a common feature of Alport syndrome, a basement membrane disorder with hereditary nephritis, sensorineural hearing loss, anterior lenticonus, and retinal flecks (50). Management of patients with PPMD should include an examination for renal abnormalities and hearing loss and hernias (34,50).

FUCHS ENDOTHELIAL CORNEAL DYSTROPHY

General Clinical Features and Terminology

Cornea guttata is a common and typically asymptomatic condition that increases significantly with age (51). Slitlamp biomicroscopy reveals a beaten-silver appearance of the central posterior cornea, similar to that seen in the ICE syndrome.

When patients who have the same posterior corneal changes as described earlier develop edema of the corneal stroma and endothelium, it is called Fuchs endothelial dystrophy (52). The condition may lead to severe visual reduction, often requiring penetrating keratoplasty. The disorder is bilateral with a predilection for women and an onset usually between the ages of 40 and 70 years (53). There is a strong familial tendency, and an autosomal dominant inheritance pattern has been described (54). The gene for Fuchs endothelial corneal dystrophy, *COL8A2*, was identified on chromosome 1p (see Chapter 8).

Reports are conflicting regarding the association of open-angle glaucoma with corneal guttata and Fuchs endothelial

dystrophy. However, a study of 64 families with Fuchs endothelial dystrophy revealed only one case of open-angle glaucoma (55). Acute elevations of IOP cause secondary changes in the corneal endothelium with edema in the stroma and epithelium. Reduced cell densities have been reported in association with ocular hypertension, angle-closure glaucoma, exfoliative glaucoma, and glaucomatocyclitic crisis (56–59). However, the degree of endothelial alteration does not always correlate with the height of IOP elevation, suggesting that other factors, such as aging and inflammation (60,61), also influence the association between glaucoma and corneal endothelial changes.

There is more evidence for an association of angle-closure glaucoma and Fuchs endothelial corneal dystrophy. Patients with Fuchs corneal endothelial dystrophy have a higher incidence of angle-closure glaucoma due to axial hypermetropia and shallow anterior chambers (62,63).

Pathologic Features

On specular microscopy, there is a characteristic pattern of enlarged corneal endothelial cells with dark areas that overlap the cell borders (64). The primary pathology is an alteration in the corneal endothelium that leads to a deposition of collagen on the posterior surface of Descemet membrane, which on histology appear as warts or excrescences in the pure form of cornea guttata or may be covered by additional basement membrane or there may be a uniform thickening of the posterior collagen layers (65).

Theories of Mechanism

Aqueous humor dynamic studies have shown that aqueous humor composition is normal (66). In a study using wide-field specular microscopy, the mean value for facility of outflow was similar between patients with cornea guttata and controls (67). Thus, the normal aqueous humor dynamic studies support that Fuchs endothelial dystrophy is a primary disorder of the corneal endothelium.

Differential Diagnosis

Clinically, the corneal endothelial changes in Fuchs endothelial dystrophy may resemble those in exfoliation keratopathy (Chapter 15). However, the latter typically has fewer guttata-like structures that are more diffusely distributed. Exfoliation syndrome is associated with more melanin dispersion in the anterior segment and peripupillary iris atrophy.

Management of Glaucoma

Although glaucoma is usually not present in eyes with Fuchs endothelial dystrophy, reducing IOP may sometimes help to minimize the corneal edema. The use of topical carbonic anhydrase inhibitors should be avoided, because cases of further compromise of the cornea with this class of glaucoma medications have been reported (68). When glaucoma is present, the open-angle form is managed in the same manner as chronic open-angle glaucoma, but the angle-closure form requires an iridotomy or filtering procedure.

KEY POINTS

- ICE syndrome is a primary disorder of the corneal endothelium, which manifests in young adulthood as a unilateral abnormality of the cornea, anterior chamber angle, and iris. It appears to be an acquired condition, possibly caused by a virus.

- The abnormal endothelium in ICE syndrome often causes corneal edema and proliferates over the angle and iris with subsequent contraction, leading to glaucoma and variable degrees of iris distortion. The latter changes are the basis for clinical variations, including Chandler syndrome, progressive iris atrophy, and the Cogan–Reese syndrome.

- PPMD is another spectrum of disease in which an endothelial abnormality is the fundamental disorder. Glaucoma is present in a small percentage of these cases, and in some patients, a proliferation of the abnormal endothelium causes changes of the anterior chamber angle and iris, resembling those in the ICE syndrome. The condition differs from the latter syndrome, however, in that it is inherited and bilateral and has a different clinical appearance of the posterior cornea.

- A third primary disorder of the corneal endothelium, Fuchs endothelial dystrophy, occasionally has associated glaucoma, usually with an angle-closure mechanism.

REFERENCES

1. Eagle RC Jr, Font RL, Yanoff M, et al. Proliferative endotheliopathy with iris abnormalities. The iridocorneal endothelial syndrome. *Arch Ophthalmol.* 1979;97(11):2104–2111.
2. Wilson MC, Shields MB. A comparison of the clinical variations of the iridocorneal endothelial syndrome. *Arch Ophthalmol.* 1989;107(10): 1465–1468.
3. Shields MB. Progressive essential iris atrophy, Chandler's syndrome, and the iris nevus (Cogan–Reese) syndrome: a spectrum of disease. *Surv Ophthalmol.* 1979;24(1):3–20.
4. Hirst LW, Quigley HA, Stark WJ, et al. Specular microscopy of iridocorneal endothelia syndrome. *Am J Ophthalmol.* 1980;89(1):11–21.
5. Teekhasaenee C, Ritch R. Iridocorneal endothelial syndrome in Thai patients: clinical variations. *Arch Ophthalmol.* 2000;118(2):187–192.
6. Sherrard ES, Frangoulis MA, Muir MG, et al. The posterior surface of the cornea in the irido-corneal endothelial syndrome: a specular microscopical study. *Trans Ophthalmol Soc U K.* 1985;104(pt 7):766–774.
7. Alvarado JA, Murphy CG, Maglio M, et al. Pathogenesis of Chandler's syndrome, essential iris atrophy and the Cogan–Reese syndrome. I. Alterations of the corneal endothelium. *Invest Ophthalmol Vis Sci.* 1986;27(6):853–872.
8. Hirst LW, Bancroft J, Yamauchi K, et al. Immunohistochemical pathology of the corneal endothelium in iridocorneal endothelial syndrome. *Invest Ophthalmol Vis Sci.* 1995;36(5):820–827.
9. Lee WR, Marshall GE, Kirkness CM. Corneal endothelial cell abnormalities in an early stage of the iridocorneal endothelial syndrome. *Br J Ophthalmol.* 1994;78(8):624–631.
10. Alvarado JA, Underwood JL, Green WR, et al. Detection of herpes simplex viral DNA in the iridocorneal endothelial syndrome [see comments]. *Arch Ophthalmol.* 1994;112(12):1601–1609.
11. Rodrigues MM, Stulting RD, Waring GO III. Clinical, electron microscopic, and immunohistochemical study of the corneal endothelium and Descemet's membrane in the iridocorneal endothelial syndrome. *Am J Ophthalmol.* 1986;101(1):16–27.
12. Shields MB, McCracken JS, Klintworth GK, et al. Corneal edema in essential iris atrophy. *Ophthalmology.* 1979;86(8):1533–1550.
13. Campbell DG, Shields MB, Smith TR. The corneal endothelium and the spectrum of essential iris atrophy. *Am J Ophthalmol.* 1978;86(3): 317–324.
14. Jampol LM, Rosser MJ, Sears ML. Unusual aspects of progressive essential iris atrophy. *Am J Ophthalmol.* 1974;77(3):353–357.
15. Eagle RC Jr, Font RL, Yanoff M, et al. The iris naevus (Cogan–Reese) syndrome: light and electron microscopic observations. *Br J Ophthalmol.* 1980;64(6):446–452.
16. Azuara-Blanco A, Wilson RP, Eagle RC Jr, et al. Pseudocapsulorrhexis in a patient with iridocorneal endothelial syndrome. *Arch Ophthalmol.* 1999;117(3):397–398.
17. Shields MB, Campbell DG, Simmons RJ. The essential iris atrophies. *Am J Ophthalmol.* 1978;85(6):749–759.
18. Weber PA, Gibb G. Iridocorneal endothelial syndrome glaucoma without peripheral anterior synechias. *Glaucoma.* 1984;6:128.
19. Laganowski HC, Sherrard ES, Muir MG, et al. Distinguishing features of the iridocorneal endothelial syndrome and posterior polymorphous dystrophy: value of endothelial specular microscopy. *Br J Ophthalmol.* 1991;75(4):212–216.
20. Henderson E, Margo CE. Iris melanoma. *Arch Pathol Lab Med.* 2008;132(2):268–272.
21. Joondeph BC, Goldberg MF. Familial iris melanosis—a misnomer? *Br J Ophthalmol.* 1989;73(4):289–293.
22. Jett K, Friedman JM. Clinical and genetic aspects of neurofibromatosis 1. *Genet Med.* 2010;12(1):1–11.
23. Ticho BH, Rosner M, Mets MB, et al. Bilateral diffuse iris nodular nevi. Clinical and histopathologic characterization. *Ophthalmology.* 1995; 102(3):419–425.
24. Daus W, Volcker HE, Steinbruck M, et al. Clinical aspects and histopathology of the Cogan–Reese syndrome. *Klin Monbl Augenheilkd.* 1990;197(2):150–155.
25. Bourne WM, Brubaker RF. Progression and regression of partial corneal involvement in the iridocorneal endothelial syndrome. *Am J Ophthalmol.* 1992;114(2):171–181.
26. Laganowski HC, Kerr Muir MG, Hitchings RA. Glaucoma and the iridocorneal endothelial syndrome. *Arch Ophthalmol.* 1992;110(3):346–350.
27. Kidd M, Hetherington J, Magee S. Surgical results in iridocorneal endothelial syndrome. *Arch Ophthalmol.* 1988;106(2):199–201.
28. Wright MM, Grajewski AL, Cristol SM, et al. 5-Fluorouracil after trabeculectomy and the iridocorneal endothelial syndrome. *Ophthalmology.* 1991;98(3):314–316.
29. Lanzl IM, Wilson RP, Dudley D, et al. Outcome of trabeculectomy with mitomycin-C in the iridocorneal endothelial syndrome. *Ophthalmology.* 2000;107(2):295–297.
30. Kim DK, Aslanides IM, Schmidt CM Jr, et al. Long-term outcome of aqueous shunt surgery in ten patients with iridocorneal endothelial syndrome. *Ophthalmology.* 1999;106(5):1030–1034.
31. Buxton JN, Lash RS. Results of penetrating keratoplasty in the iridocorneal endothelial syndrome. *Am J Ophthalmol.* 1984;98(3):297–301.
32. Alvim PT, Cohen EJ, Rapuano CJ, et al. Penetrating keratoplasty in iridocorneal endothelial syndrome. *Cornea.* 2001;20(2):134–140.
33. Biswas S, Munier FL, Yardley J, et al. Missense mutations in COL8A2, the gene encoding the alpha 2 chain of type VIII collagen, cause two forms of corneal endothelial dystrophy. *Hum Mol Genet.* 2001;10(21): 2415–2423.
34. Krafchak CM, Pawar H, Moroi SE, et al. Mutations in TCF8 cause posterior polymorphous corneal dystrophy and ectopic expression of COL4A3 by corneal endothelial cells. *Am J Hum Genet.* 2005;77(5):694–708.
35. Heon E, Greenberg A, Kopp KK, et al. VSX1: a gene for posterior polymorphous dystrophy and keratoconus. *Hum Mol Genet.* 2002;11(9): 1029–1036.
36. Cibis GW, Krachmer JA, Phelps CD, et al. The clinical spectrum of posterior polymorphous dystrophy. *Arch Ophthalmol.* 1977;95(9): 1529–1537.
37. Cibis GW, Tripathi RC. The differential diagnosis of Descemet's tears (Haab's striae) and posterior polymorphous dystrophy bands. A clinicopathologic study. *Ophthalmology.* 1982;89(6):614–620.
38. Hirst LW, Waring GO III. Clinical specular microscopy of posterior polymorphous endothelial dystrophy. *Am J Ophthalmol.* 1983;95(2):143–155.
39. Laganowski HC, Sherrard ES, Muir MG. The posterior corneal surface in posterior polymorphous dystrophy: a specular microscopical study. *Cornea.* 1991;10(3):224–232.
40. Johnson BL, Brown SI. Posterior polymorphous dystrophy: a light and electron microscopic study. *Br J Ophthalmol.* 1978;62(2):89–96.

41. Rodrigues MM, Sun TT, Krachmer J, et al. Epithelialization of the corneal endothelium in posterior polymorphous dystrophy. *Invest Ophthalmol Vis Sci.* 1980;19(7):832–835.

42. Henriquez AS, Kenyon KR, Dohlman CH, et al. Morphologic characteristics of posterior polymorphous dystrophy. A study of nine corneas and review of the literature. *Surv Ophthalmol.* 1984;29(2):139–147.

43. Moroi SE, Gokhale PA, Schteingart MT, et al. Clinicopathologic correlation and genetic analysis in a case of posterior polymorphous corneal dystrophy. *Am J Ophthalmol.* 2003;135(4):461–470.

44. Cibis GW, Krachmer JH, Phelps CD, et al. Iridocorneal adhesions in posterior polymorphous dystrophy. *Trans Am Acad Ophthalmol Otolaryngol.* 1976;81(5):770–777.

45. Threlkeld AB, Green WR, Quigley HA, et al. A clinicopathologic study of posterior polymorphous dystrophy: implications for pathogenetic mechanism of the associated glaucoma. *Trans Am Ophthalmol Soc.* 1994;92:133–165.

46. Bourgeois J, Shields MB, Thresher R. Open-angle glaucoma associated with posterior polymorphous dystrophy. A clinicopathologic study. *Ophthalmology.* 1984;91(4):420–423.

47. Krachmer JH. Posterior polymorphous corneal dystrophy: a disease characterized by epithelial-like endothelial cells which influence management and prognosis. *Trans Am Ophthalmol Soc.* 1985;83:413–475.

48. Aldave AJ, Yellore VS, Yu F, et al. Posterior polymorphous corneal dystrophy is associated with TCF8 gene mutations and abdominal hernia. *Am J Med Genet A.* 2007;143A(21):2549–2556.

49. Dunn SP, Krachmer JH, Ching SS. New findings in posterior amorphous corneal dystrophy. *Arch Ophthalmol.* 1984;102(2):236–239.

50. Teekhasaenee C, Nimmanit S, Wutthiphan S, et al. Posterior polymorphous dystrophy and Alport syndrome. *Ophthalmology.* 1991;98(8):1207–1215.

51. Lorenzetti DW, Uotila MH, Parikh N, et al. Central cornea guttata. Incidence in the general population. *Am J Ophthalmol.* 1967;64(6):1155–1158.

52. Fuchs E. Dystrophis epithelialis corneal. *Arch Ophthalmol.* 1910;76:478.

53. Afshari NA, Pittard AB, Siddiqui A, et al. Clinical study of Fuchs corneal endothelial dystrophy leading to penetrating keratoplasty: a 30-year experience. *Arch Ophthalmol.* 2006;124(6):777–780.

54. Klintworth GK. The molecular genetics of the corneal dystrophies—current status. *Front Biosci.* 2003;8:d687–d713.

55. Krachmer JH, Purcell Jr. Young CW, et al. Corneal endothelial dystrophy. A study of 64 families. *Arch Ophthalmol.* 1978;96(11):2036–2039.

56. Hong C, Kandori T, Kitazawa Y, et al. The corneal endothelial cells in ocular hypertension. *Jpn J Ophthalmol.* 1982;26(2):183–189.

57. Bigar F, Witmer R. Corneal endothelial changes in primary acute angle-closure glaucoma. *Ophthalmology.* 1982;89(6):596–599.

58. Vannas A, Setala K, Ruusuvaara P. Endothelial cells in capsular glaucoma. *Acta Ophthalmol.* 1977;55(6):951–958.

59. Setala K, Vannas A. Endothelial cells in the glaucomato-cyclitic crisis. *Adv Ophthalmol.* 1978;36:218–224.

60. Kaufman HE, Capella JA, Robbins JE. The human corneal endothelium. *Am J Ophthalmol.* 1966;61(5 pt 1):835–841.

61. Olsen T. Changes in the corneal endothelium after acute anterior uveitis as seen with the specular microscope. *Acta Ophthalmol.* 1980;58(2):250–256.

62. Pitts JF, Jay JL. The association of Fuchs's corneal endothelial dystrophy with axial hypermetropia, shallow anterior chamber, and angle closure glaucoma. *Br J Ophthalmol.* 1990;74(10):601–604.

63. Lowenstein A, Hourvitz D, Goldstein M, et al. Association of Fuchs' corneal endothelial dystrophy with angle-closure glaucoma. *J Glaucoma.* 1994;3:201–205.

64. Chiou AG, Kaufman SC, Beuerman RW, et al. Confocal microscopy in cornea guttata and Fuchs' endothelial dystrophy. *Br J Ophthalmol.* 1999;83(2):185–189.

65. Waring GO III, Rodrigues MM, Laibson PR. Corneal dystrophies. II. Endothelial dystrophies. *Surv Ophthalmol.* 1978;23(3):147–168.

66. Wilson SE, Bourne WM, Maguire LJ, et al. Aqueous humor composition in Fuchs' dystrophy. *Invest Ophthalmol Vis Sci.* 1989;30(3):449–453.

67. Roberts CW, Steinert RF, Thomas JV, et al. Endothelial guttata and facility of aqueous outflow. *Cornea.* 1984;3(1):5–9.

68. Konowal A, Morrison JC, Brown SV, et al. Irreversible corneal decompensation in patients treated with topical dorzolamide. *Am J Ophthalmol.* 1999;127(4):403–406.

Pigmentary and Other Glaucomas Associated with Disorders of the Iris and Ciliary Body

17

IRIS OR CILIARY BODY DISORDERS WITH ASSOCIATED GLAUCOMA

There are several conditions in which a disorder of the iris or ciliary body is believed to be involved in the initial events that eventually lead to various forms of glaucoma (**Table 17.1**). Most of these, such as developmental disorders, inflammatory conditions, and intraocular tumors, are considered in other chapters in Section II. In this chapter, we consider additional conditions—pigmentary glaucoma, iridoschisis, plateau iris, pseudoplateau iris, and swelling of the ciliary body—that do not fit precisely into any of these general systems of disease.

PIGMENTARY GLAUCOMA

Terminology

As a normal feature of maturation and aging, a variable amount of uveal pigment is chronically released and dispersed into the anterior ocular segment. This is best appreciated by observing the trabecular meshwork, which is nonpigmented in the infant eye but becomes progressively pigmented to various degrees with the passage of years because of the accumulation of the dispersed pigment in the aqueous outflow system. There is therefore a spectrum of ocular pigment dispersion in the general population. As can be anticipated, this spectrum of pigment dispersion is also found among individuals with various forms of glaucoma, although the pigment in most of these cases is not believed to be a major factor in the mechanism of the glaucoma. Several ocular conditions are associated with an unusually heavy dispersion of pigment, which may be significantly involved in the increased resistance to aqueous outflow. In 1940, Sugar (1) briefly described one such case with marked pigment dispersion and glaucoma. In 1949, Sugar and Barbour (2) reported the details of this entity, which differed from other forms of pigment dispersion by typical clinical and histopathologic features. They referred to the condition as pigmentary glaucoma (2). When the typical findings are encountered without associated glaucoma, the term pigment dispersion syndrome (PDS) has been advocated (3).

General Features

The typical patient is young, myopic, and male. The disorder appears most frequently in the third decade of life, and there is a tendency for it to decrease in severity or disappear in later life (4,5). Most studies agree that PDS is more common among men,

with a male-to-female ratio of approximately 2:1, although studies differ on the ratio of those converting to pigmentary glaucoma (3–11). The reason for the male predilection appears to be the sex difference in anterior chamber depth, which one study showed to be 3.22 ± 0.42 mm in men and 2.88 ± 0.38 mm in women (12). (The significance of chamber depth in the mechanism of pigment dispersion is discussed later in this chapter.)

Pigmentary glaucoma is seen predominantly in whites (3–11), although it may be more common among blacks than previously recognized (13). In black patients, signs of PDS may be overlooked because dark, thick iris stroma may obscure transillumination defects and pigment granules on the stroma; corneal endothelial pigmentation may be minimal or absent; and greater degrees of trabecular meshwork pigmentation may be interpreted as normal in black patients. It has been suggested that pigment accumulation on the lens zonules and equatorial or posterior lens regions may be particularly helpful in making the diagnosis of PDS in black patients (13). In one report, 20 black patients with presumed PDS had heavy pigment deposition on the corneal endothelium and trabecular meshwork. These patients differed clinically from that described in the

Table 17.1	Conditions with Iris or Ciliary Body Disorders and Associated Glaucoma[a]
Developmental defects [14]	
Axenfeld–Rieger syndrome	
Peters anomaly	
Aniridia	
Iris atrophy with corneal disease [13]	
Iridocorneal endothelial syndrome	
Posterior polymorphous corneal dystrophy	
Pigmentary glaucoma[b]	
Iridoschisis[b]	
Plateau iris[b]	
Exfoliation syndrome [15]	
Neovascular glaucoma [19]	
Iris tumors [21]	
Anterior uveitis [22]	
Trauma [25]	
Complications of intraocular surgery [26]	

[a]Numbers in brackets indicate the chapters in which the conditions are discussed.
[b]Discussed in the current chapter.

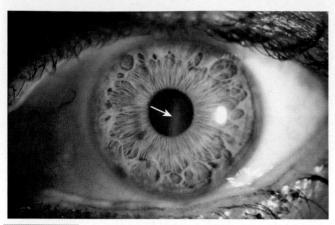

Figure 17.1 Krukenberg spindle (*arrow*) in a patient with pigmentary glaucoma. (Courtesy of Ralf R. Buhrmann, MD, PhD.)

white population in that their mean age was 73 years, and most were hyperopic and lacked iris transillumination defects on slit-lamp examination (14). One report described iridocorneal angle anomalies in a group of black probands with presumed PDS and among their first-degree relatives (15). A hereditary basis has been suggested for the classic form of PDS (see Chapter 8).

Clinical Features

Slitlamp Biomicroscopic Findings

Corneal Findings

Pigment dispersion occurs throughout the anterior ocular segment but is seen by slitlamp examination primarily on the cornea and iris. Krukenberg spindle is an accumulation of pigment on the posterior surface of the central cornea in a vertical, spindle-shaped pattern (**Fig. 17.1**). Dispersed pigment is deposited on the cornea in this pattern because of aqueous convection currents and is then phagocytosed by adjacent endothelial cells (3). This feature is commonly seen in eyes with pigmentary glaucoma, but it is neither invariable nor pathognomonic of the disorder. In one study, only 2 of 43 patients with Krukenberg spindles developed field loss during a follow-up that averaged 5.8 years (16). Krukenberg spindle is more

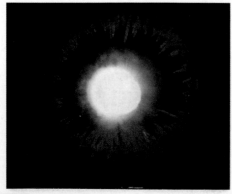

Figure 17.2 Transillumination of the iris in a patient with pigmentary glaucoma showing typical midperipheral spoke-like defects.

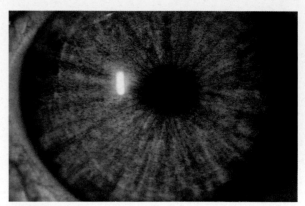

Figure 17.3 Pigment granules on iris stroma in a patient with pigmentary glaucoma.

common in women and may have a hormonal relationship (16,17). Specular microscopy of the corneal endothelium reveals distinct pleomorphism and polymegathism (i.e., abnormality in shape and size of cells); however, normal cell counts and central corneal thickness are found (18,19).

Iris Findings

Iris transillumination is a valuable diagnostic clinical feature of pigmentary glaucoma because it represents areas where pigment has been dispersed. The characteristic appearance is a radial spoke-like pattern in the midperiphery of the iris (20) (**Fig. 17.2**). This feature can be seen during slitlamp biomicroscopy by directing the light beam through the pupil perpendicular to the plane of the iris or by using scleral transillumination and observing the retinal light reflex through the defects in the iris. In some patients, however, a dark, thick iris stroma may prevent transillumination of the defects, and the absence of this finding therefore does not rule out the diagnosis of pigmentary glaucoma. This could explain the absence of iris transillumination in black patients with pigmentary glaucoma (14). An infrared videographic technique has been developed that allows visualization of discrete iris transillumination defects not visible by slitlamp examination (21).

Pigment granules are frequently dispersed on the stroma of the iris, which may give the iris a progressively darker appearance or create heterochromia in asymmetric cases (9) (**Fig. 17.3**). Asymmetric pigment dispersion has also been reported in association with unilateral cataract formation or extraction (22). Patients with PDS may also have anisocoria, in which the eye with the larger pupil is on the side with the greater iris transillumination. The iris heterochromia and anisocoria of PDS may mimic Horner syndrome (23).

Other anterior segment locations where pigment dispersion may be seen by slitlamp examination include the posterior lens capsule (**Fig. 17.4**), lens zonules, and the interior of a glaucoma filtering bleb (9).

Gonioscopic Findings

The principal gonioscopic feature of pigmentary glaucoma is a dense, homogeneous band of dark brown pigment in the full circumference of the trabecular meshwork (**Fig. 17.5A**). The

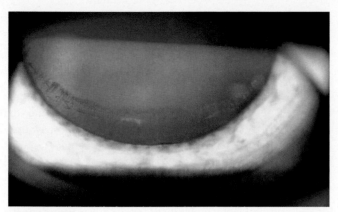

Figure 17.4 Pigmented line on posterior lens capsule at the insertion of zonules. This is termed the Zentmayer line or a Scheie stripe.

dispersed pigment may also accumulate along the Schwalbe line, especially inferiorly, creating a thin, dark band.

Fundus Findings

Retinal detachments are more common in patients with PDS or pigmentary glaucoma (24), occurring in 6.4% of patients in one study (11). A study of 60 patients with pigment dispersion or pigmentary glaucoma revealed lattice degeneration in 12 patients (20%) and full-thickness retinal breaks in 7 patients (12%) (25).

Clinical Course of the Glaucoma

Patients with PDS may go for years before developing pigmentary glaucoma or may never have a rise in intraocular pressure (IOP). In one study of 97 eyes with pigment dispersion

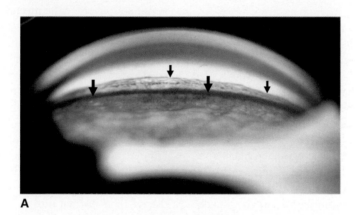

A

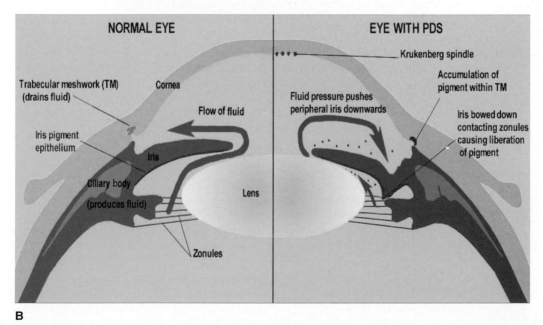

B

Figure 17.5 **A:** Gonioscopic view of patient with pigmentary glaucoma showing typical features of wide open angle with dense, homogenous pigmentation of trabecular meshwork (*large arrows*) and heavy pigment accumulation on the Schwalbe line (*small arrows*). **B:** Schematic diagram illustrating a cross section of a normal eye (*left half*) and an eye with PDS (*right half*). A normal anterior segment is shown on the left and illustrates normal flow of aqueous humor (*curved arrow*). Note the flat iris configuration and ample space between the iris and lens for fluid flow. On the right side, note that the iris is touching the lens near the pupil and only permits anterior flow of aqueous. This leads to a higher pressure anterior to the iris, causing backward bowing (concavity) of the peripheral iris. The iris pigment epithelium is thus brought into contact with the zonules and tips of the ciliary processes. This leads to cell damage and liberation of pigment that circulates with the aqueous humor into the anterior chamber, leading to the characteristic signs of PDS.

throughout the anterior ocular segment, glaucoma was present in 42 (26), whereas in another study of 407 patients with the dispersion syndrome, only one fourth had glaucoma (11). In a long-term study that spanned 5 to 35 years, 13 of 37 patients with PDS (35%) converted to pigmentary glaucoma (6). The glaucoma usually develops within 15 years of the presentation of the PDS, although some may take more than 20 years (6). In another study, with follow-up averaging 27 months, progression of the iris transillumination defects and pigment dispersion could be documented in 31 of 55 patients and correlated with worsening of the glaucoma in most of these (27). A study of 111 patients with PDS or pigmentary glaucoma identified male sex, black race, high myopia, and Krukenberg spindles as risk factors for the development and severity of glaucoma in this population (10). However, another study found that sex did not influence the development or severity of glaucoma among patients with PDS (6).

In some patients, strenuous exercise, such as jogging, or spontaneous changes in the pupillary diameter may be associated with marked pigment release into the anterior chamber, although this does not appear to significantly elevate the IOP in most cases (28). In patients in whom exercise-induced pigment dispersion causes a significant IOP rise, use of pilocarpine has effectively inhibited this phenomenon. Phenylephrine-induced mydriasis also causes a significant shower of pigment into the anterior chamber in some patients with pigmentary glaucoma or PDS, although this transient liberation of pigment is not consistently associated with IOP elevations (28).

After pigmentary glaucoma becomes established, it may be somewhat more difficult to control than chronic open-angle glaucoma (COAG) is. In one long-term follow-up study of 38 patients (75 eyes), 39 eyes were controlled medically, 15 required laser trabeculoplasty, and 20 underwent a trabeculectomy (29). However, 67 eyes (89%) retained normal vision during the study (mean follow-up, 10 years). With increasing age, there is a tendency for the glaucoma to become less severe, but the condition must be treated aggressively during the active years to avoid irreversible loss of vision in later life.

Theories of Mechanism

Two fundamental questions must be considered regarding the pathogenesis of PDS and the mechanism of pigmentary glaucoma. What are the factors leading to the pigment dispersion and how do the dispersed pigment and additional features cause the glaucoma?

Mechanism of Pigment Dispersion

An inherent weakness or degeneration in the iris pigment epithelium was first proposed as a cause of PDS by Scheie and Fleischauer in 1958 (26). Subsequently, histopathologic observations of the iris in eyes with the PDS or pigmentary glaucoma have revealed changes in the iris pigment epithelium, which include focal atrophy and hypopigmentation, an apparent delay in melanogenesis, and hyperplasia of the dilator muscle (26, 30–32). In contrast, eyes with COAG and various degrees of

pigment dispersion had minimal hypopigmentation of the iris epithelium with normal dilator muscle and melanogenesis (32). These observations have led some observers to think that a developmental abnormality of the iris pigment epithelium is the fundamental defect in PDS (30–32). The additional observation of retinal pigment epithelial dystrophy in two brothers with pigmentary glaucoma raises the possibility of an inherited defect of pigment epithelium in the anterior and posterior ocular segments (33). On the basis of fluorescein angiography of the iris, hypovascularity of the iris may also play a role in PDS (34,35).

Campbell (36) proposed an alternative mechanical theory for the mechanism of pigment liberation from the iris (**Fig. 17.5B**). He observed that the peripheral radial defects of the iris corresponded in location and number to anterior packets of lens zonules and suggested that a background bowing of the peripheral iris led to the mechanical rubbing of the lens zonules against the iris pigment epithelium with the subsequent dispersion of pigment. This hypothesis was supported by histologic studies showing a correlation between packets of zonules and deep groves in the iris pigment epithelium and posterior stroma (36,37). Sugar (7) suggested that the radial folds of iris pigment epithelium rubbing against the lens capsule itself might be an additional mechanism of pigment release.

The mechanical theory of Campbell is also supported by biometric and photogrammetric studies of anterior chamber dimensions, which revealed deeper anterior chambers and flatter lenses in the involved eyes of unilateral cases and a deeper-than-normal midperipheral chamber depth with corresponding concavity of the iris in eyes with the PDS (38,39). Further support for the mechanical theory comes from studies with ultrasonographic biomicroscopy indicating that the distance between the base of the trabecular meshwork and the point of insertion of the iris is greater in eyes with PDS than in healthy controls. Ultrasonographic biomicroscopy studies in patients with PDS have shown that the radial width of the iris compared with the size of the anterior segment is larger than normal (40). This larger size results in a floppier iris, which may predispose to iridozonular contact when combined with the posterior iris insertion. The mechanical theory is also consistent with clinical observations and helps to explain certain features of the disease. For example, the low incidence of the condition among nonwhite persons may be because of the heavy pigmentation and compactness of the iris stroma in these individuals, which prevents posterior sagging of the midperipheral iris (41). The tendency for the disease to ameliorate with increasing age may be attributed to the increasing axial length of the lens, which pulls the peripheral iris away from the zonules (5,36). A case has also been reported in which subluxation of the lens apparently caused remission of pigmentary glaucoma (42).

The mechanical theory must include an explanation of the mechanism by which the peripheral iris is bowed backward. This missing piece of the puzzle came with the observation that a laser iridotomy relieves the posterior bowing, which led to the concept of reverse pupillary block (43). This concept suggests that aqueous is moved into the anterior chamber against the normal pressure gradient, possibly by the movement of the peripheral iris in response to movement of the eye (e.g., blinking) or accommodation. Once in the anterior chamber, the aqueous is prevented from returning to the posterior chamber by a one-way valve effect between the iris and lens, resulting in a relatively greater pressure in the anterior chamber and subsequent backward bowing of the peripheral iris. The theory of reverse pupillary block has been supported by studies with ultrasound biomicroscopy and Scheimpflug photography, both of which demonstrate the posterior bowing of the iris in patients with PDS and pigmentary glaucoma (28). The posterior bowing is eliminated by a peripheral iridotomy, miotic therapy, or prevention of blinking. Exercise, however, increases the iris concavity (44). The observations regarding blinking and exercise appear to support the concept that eye movement is responsible for the pumping of aqueous into the anterior chamber. It has also been observed that accommodation in patients with PDS leads to increased posterior bowing of the iris, which the investigators explain by the forward movement of the lens, which reduces the volume, thereby increasing the pressure in the anterior chamber (45). Iridotomy abolishes the change in the iris profile that is

normally seen with accommodation in patients with PDS (46). The mechanical theory, however, does not fully explain why not all eyes with myopia are subject to PDS, and it may be that additional iris defects (as previously discussed) are necessary for development of this syndrome.

Another mechanism of pigment dispersion involves elongated anterior zonules that may be pigmented (**Fig. 17.6A,B**), encroaching in the central visual axis (47,48). Normally, the anterior zonular insertion leaves a zonule-free zone of 6.9 mm (49). The clinical appearance and electron microscopic appearance (**Fig. 17.6C**) of an anterior capsule specimen obtained during cataract surgery suggest a mechanism of pigment release from the pigmented epithelium located at the papillary ruff and the central iris, which are close to the elongated zonules (48). This mechanism appears to be distinct from PDS in which iridozonular contact occurs in the region of the posterior chamber between the midperipheral iris and anterior zonule bundles (36). The zonules appear normal, as standard phacoemulsification did not indicate fragility (48,50). Although subtle and easily missed on biomicroscopy, long anterior zonules may be more common than suspected but not previously recognized as a distinct entity associated with pigment dispersion.

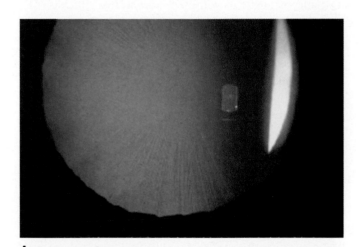

A

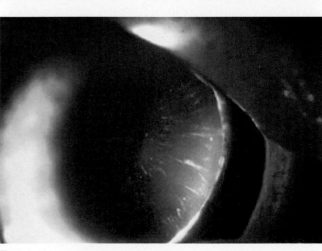

B

Figure 17.6 Variant of pigment dispersion syndrome in a patient with African ancestry and hyperopia illustrating a distinct mechanism of pigment dispersion. **A:** Long anterior zonules are visible on the anterior capsule surface following dilation with direct and retroillumination. **B:** Pigment is commonly noted with some of the long anterior zonules. **C:** Transmission electron microscopy shows central anterior lens capsule covered by an irregular zonule lamella with pigment granules and degenerative lens epithelium in pigmented long anterior zonules. (Courtesy of Ursula Schlötzer Schrehardt, PhD.)

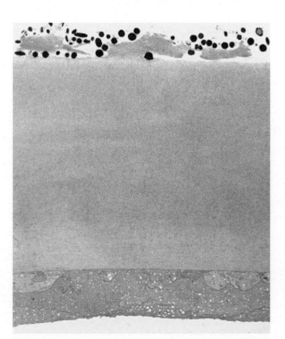

C

Mechanism of Intraocular Pressure Elevation

In 1963, Grant (51) demonstrated that pigment granules perfused in human autopsy eyes caused a significant obstruction to aqueous outflow. Clinical studies have also shown that pigment release caused by pharmacologically induced movement of the iris causes a transient pressure rise in some eyes and that the number of aqueous melanin granules (as quantified by the cell count mode of a laser flare-cell meter) is strongly correlated with high IOP and visual field loss (52–54). However, perfusion of living monkey eyes with uveal pigment particles caused only a transient obstruction to aqueous outflow (55), and histologic studies of human eyes with pigmentary glaucoma showed that only 3.5% of the pigment in the trabecular meshwork was in the juxtacanalicular tissue, which was thought to be insufficient to account for the outflow obstruction (56). It appears that other or additional factors must be involved in the mechanism of pigmentary glaucoma.

Although many histopathologic studies of eyes with pigmentary glaucoma have revealed excessive amounts of pigment granules and cell debris in the trabecular meshwork, it is the associated changes in the trabecular endothelial cells and collagen beams that are believed to lead to the glaucoma (28) (**Fig. 17.7**). On the basis of these observations, the following pathophysiologic sequence of events has been proposed for the development of pigmentary glaucoma (57). Trabecular cells engulf melanin, which eventually leads to cell injury and death from phagocytic overload. Because melanoprotein is only partially digested, it is retained in intracellular storage vacuoles, where it generates deleterious oxygen-free radicals. Macrophages migrate to the necrotic trabecular cells, possibly in response to cytokines released by the injured cells, and carry off the pigment and debris through the Schlemm canal and into the circulation. The trabecular cell loss leaves the collagen beams denuded and vulnerable to fusion, with obliteration of

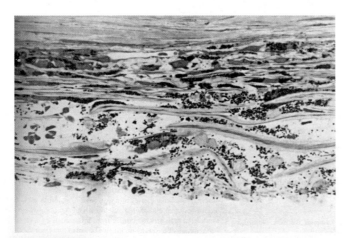

Figure 17.7 Light microscopic view of trabecular meshwork from a patient with pigmentary glaucoma showing free pigment granules primarily in the uveal meshwork and in the inner portion of the corneoscleral meshwork, with intracellular pigment in the deeper portions of the meshwork. (Reprinted with permission from Richardson TM. Pigmentary glaucoma. In: Ritch R, Shields MB, eds. *The Secondary Glaucomas.* St. Louis: CV Mosby; 1982.)

the aqueous channels. Histologic studies reveal that the cul-de-sacs, which normally terminate in aqueous channels, are markedly reduced in pigmentary glaucoma, accounting for a major portion of the increased resistance to aqueous outflow.

An alternative theory suggests that a primary developmental anomaly of the anterior chamber angle may lead to aqueous outflow obstruction (9). This concept is based on the previously described abundant iris processes that have been seen in some cases. However, this is not a consistent finding and probably plays little or no role in the mechanism of pigmentary glaucoma.

A third hypothesis is that pigmentary glaucoma represents a variation of COAG. This theory was derived from observations that COAG and pigmentary glaucoma could be seen in the same family. In one study, individuals with Krukenberg spindles had topical corticosteroid responses that were similar to those seen in close relatives of patients with COAG (58). However, patients with pigmentary glaucoma were not found to have the same corticosteroid sensitivity to in vitro inhibition of lymphocyte transformation as COAG patients (59). Human leukocyte antigen testing revealed differences between PDS, pigmentary glaucoma, and COAG (60), but another study showed no significant difference among patients with pigmentary glaucoma, patients with PDS, and healthy controls (61). The bulk of the current evidence suggests that pigmentary glaucoma and COAG are separate entities.

Differential Diagnosis

In several disorders, an excessive dispersion of pigment may be associated with glaucoma, with or without a cause-and-effect relationship. These conditions constitute the differential diagnosis for pigmentary glaucoma. One such condition is the exfoliation syndrome (see Chapter 15), in which rubbing between the midperipheral lens and peripupillary iris leads to the pigment dispersion. This condition is usually distinguished from pigmentary glaucoma by the typical lens appearance and older age of the patients, although the two conditions have occurred together (62). Other conditions associated with increased anterior segment pigmentation and glaucoma include some forms of uveitis (see Chapter 22), trauma (Chapter 25), ocular melanosis and melanoma (Chapter 21), ciliary body melanocytoma (63), complications of intraocular surgery (Chapter 26), and COAG with excessive pigment dispersion (Chapter 11). Unilateral PDS may be evident after implantation of posterior chamber phakic refractive intraocular lenses, after anterior rotation or displacement of posterior chamber intraocular lens, and in the case of unilateral angle recession (64–66).

Management

Medical Therapy

The mechanical theory of Campbell (36) suggests that taking measures to eliminate contact between the iris and lens zonules is the most appropriate way to prevent the progressive development of pigmentary glaucoma. Pilocarpine has the theoretical advantage of relieving this mechanism of pigment dispersion by creating miosis, while at the same time lowering the IOP by the direct effect on aqueous outflow. However, it is usually not tolerated by the young patient with myopia because of further induced myopia. Pilocarpine may provide the desired miosis and improved facility of outflow without excessive induced myopia in some patients with pigmentary glaucoma. When using cholinergic agonists in patients with pigmentary glaucoma, special attention must be given to the risk of retinal detachment, which is more common in this population (24). The α-adrenergic antagonist thymoxamine has been advocated because it produces miosis without cyclotropia (36); however, the drug is not available in most parts of the world. An alternative α-blocker, dapiprazole, was proposed for this use, but it was found to be less effective than pilocarpine, 1.6%, in constricting the pupil or relieving posterior iris bowing in patients with PDS (67). Dapiprazole is no longer commercially available for use in the United States.

Alternative medications to miotic therapy include prostaglandin analogues, β-adrenergic antagonists, and carbonic anhydrase inhibitors. With all of these nonmiotic drugs, the IOP may be reduced, but the mechanism of continued pigment dispersion is not eliminated.

Laser Surgery

In 1991, Campbell reported that a laser iridotomy (suggested initially by Dr. B. Kurwa) effectively relieved the posterior iris bowing in pigmentary glaucoma (Campbell DG, lecture honoring H. Saul Sugar, MD, American Glaucoma Society Fourth Annual Scientific Meeting, San Diego, CA, December 1991). This was confirmed by Karickhoff the following year in a report of six patients (43). This effect, however, has not been observed in all cases (68), and iridotomy did not completely eliminate exercise-induced pigment dispersion in a patient with PDS (69). An ultrasound biomicroscopic study of patients with PDS and peripheral iris concavity has shown that the iris flattens after peripheral iridotomy (70). In a study of 21 patients with PDS and IOP less than 18 mm Hg in both eyes, an Nd:YAG laser iridotomy was randomly performed in one eye, and the fellow eye was used as a control (71). After 2 years of follow-up, one treated eye (4.7%), compared with 11 untreated eyes (52.3%), demonstrated an IOP elevation of more than 5 mm Hg. This difference in IOP elevation was inversely related to patient age. A retrospective review of 46 patients with pigmentary glaucoma who underwent unilateral laser iridotomy and were followed up for 2 or more years found that the mean IOP decreased by 4 mm Hg, compared with 1.9 mm Hg in the fellow eye; however, a higher mean baseline IOP in the treated eye accounted for the apparent treatment effect, and the authors concede that their data are inconclusive regarding whether laser iridotomy is beneficial in this group of patients (72). If performing a laser iridotomy in patients with PDS, it may be prudent to use only dilute pilocarpine, because these patients are at increased risk for retinal detachment. An alternative involves avoiding pilocarpine and using a transilluminator light held up to the opposite eye to provide pupillary constriction by the consensual light reflex (73). Whether a prophylactic laser iridectomy can prevent the

development of glaucomatous optic neuropathy in patients with pigment dispersion or prevent progression in patients with pigmentary glaucoma awaits the results of long-term, multicenter trials.

When the glaucoma can no longer be controlled medically, argon or selective laser trabeculoplasty is usually indicated. Patients with pigmentary glaucoma respond well initially to the laser treatment, although the IOP control tends to decline with time and the surgery is less effective in patients who are older (e.g., patients in their 50s compared with those in their 30s) or who have had the glaucoma for a longer period of time (e.g., 10 years vs. 2 or 3 years) (74–76). In general, these patients do well with minimal laser energy per spot (e.g., starting with 300 mW per spot if using argon laser trabeculoplasty, and 0.4 mJ per spot with selective laser trabeculoplasty). Low-energy settings are particularly important in patients who have had pigmentary glaucoma for a prolonged period and have advanced glaucomatous nerve damage to minimize the risk of a sustained postoperative IOP spike (77).

Incisional Surgery

When medical therapy and laser trabeculoplasty have failed to adequately control the IOP, glaucoma filtering surgery is usually indicated. A higher percentage of patients with pigmentary glaucoma than of those with COAG require surgery, and men appear to require it at an earlier age than women do (10,11). Success rates are similar to that with other forms of open-angle glaucoma at comparable age levels.

Physical Activity

Exercise may increase pigmentary dispersion and elevate the IOP, which can be a concern in this population of young, active individuals (28). One approach to dealing with this question is to measure the IOP (and observe the amount of pigment in the anterior chamber) before and 30 minutes after the patient's typical exercise routine. If a significant pressure rise is observed, the use of pilocarpine, 0.5%, during exercise may be beneficial.

IRIDOSCHISIS

General Features

Iridoschisis is an uncommon condition, and in contrast to the young age of onset in pigmentary glaucoma, it usually appears in the sixth or seventh decade of life, although it may be seen in younger individuals. A case has been reported in a child with associated microphthalmos (78) and in a 30-year-old person with keratoconus (79). The hallmark is a bilateral separation of the layers of iris stroma, typically in the inferior quadrants. The disorder is complicated by glaucoma in approximately one-half of patients. Corneal edema is also an occasional sequela. Most cases are not associated with other ocular disorders, although concomitant conditions may be seen, including angle-closure glaucoma, angle-recession glaucoma, and syphilitic interstitial keratitis (in addition to those described earlier) (80–82).

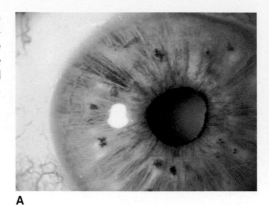
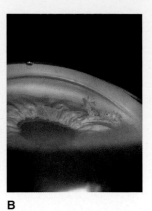

A   **B**

Figure 17.8 | **A:** Slitlamp view of a patient with iridoschisis. Note the regions of thinning, or "shredding," of the iris stroma, most noticeable at the 10 o'clock position. **B:** Gonioscopic image of an eye with iridoschisis. Note strands of iris extending toward the cornea. (Photographs courtesy of Joseph A. Halabis, OD.)

Clinicopathologic Features

Slitlamp biomicroscopic examination typically reveals sheets or strands of iris stroma that have partially separated from the rest of the iris (**Fig. 17.8A**), especially in the inferior quadrants. In some cases, the loose tissue may touch the corneal endothelium with adjacent edema of the cornea. By gonioscopy (**Fig. 17.8B**), the strands of iris tissue may obscure visualization of the anterior chamber angle.

Histopathologic studies of involved iris revealed marked atrophy of the iris stroma with scant or absent collagen fibrils in the area of separation, although there was no evidence of vascular or neural alterations (83). Specular microscopy of the corneal endothelium has revealed a marked decrease in cell density and a high degree of polymegathism in the area directly over the iridoschisis (84). Histopathology of a corneal button, removed because of bullous keratopathy, showed degeneration and focal loss of endothelial cells, patchy posterior banding (110 nm) of Descemet membrane with irregular connective tissue, and stromal and epithelial edema (83).

Mechanisms of Glaucoma

Some patients with iridoschisis and glaucoma have angle closure (60,83), and it is presumed that a pupillary block mechanism is present, because an iridotomy results in deepening of the anterior chamber (83). Iridoschisis may be an unusual manifestation of iris stromal atrophy resulting from the intermittent or acute IOP evaluation of pupillary block glaucoma (80). In other patients, the angle is open, in which case the meshwork is apparently obstructed by release of pigment from the iris or by the shredded iris stroma (83).

Differential Diagnosis

The main conditions that must be distinguished from iridoschisis are other causes of iris stromal dissolution, such as the iridocorneal endothelial syndrome and Axenfeld–Rieger syndrome, both of which differ from iridoschisis by a much younger age of onset. Trauma can lead to disruption of the iris, creating clinical findings that resemble iridoschisis, which may explain the relationship to angle-recession glaucoma (81). In one patient with iridoschisis, strands of iris floating in the anterior chamber after a trabeculectomy were mistaken for a fungal infection (85).

Management

Eyes with an angle-closure mechanism of glaucoma should be treated with a laser iridotomy, or with conventional surgical iridectomy if corneal edema prevents laser surgery. The open-angle form of glaucoma can be controlled medically in some patients by using an approach similar to that for COAG, but other patients require glaucoma filtering surgery.

PLATEAU IRIS

One mechanism leading to angle-closure glaucoma appears to result from an abnormal anatomic configuration of the anterior chamber angle without pupillary block (86,87). It is far less common than pupillary block glaucoma and is usually only recognized after a peripheral iridotomy for a presumed pupillary block mechanism has failed. Consequently, two variations of plateau iris have been described (88).

Plateau Iris Configuration

This diagnosis is made preoperatively on the basis of the gonioscopic findings of a closed anterior chamber angle but a flat iris plane (as opposed to the forward bowing of peripheral iris with the pupillary block mechanism) and a more normal central anterior chamber depth. Relative pupillary block plays a significant role in this situation, and most of these cases are cured by peripheral iridotomy.

Recently, plateau iris configuration (with an angle that is appositionally closed after iridotomy) was described in association with long anterior zonules (89).

Plateau Iris Syndrome

Plateau iris syndrome constitutes a small percentage of eyes with the plateau iris configuration and represents the true plateau iris mechanism. The peripheral iris is anteriorly displaced (**Fig. 17.9A**) so that, as the pupil is dilated, it bunches up and closes the anterior chamber angle despite a patent

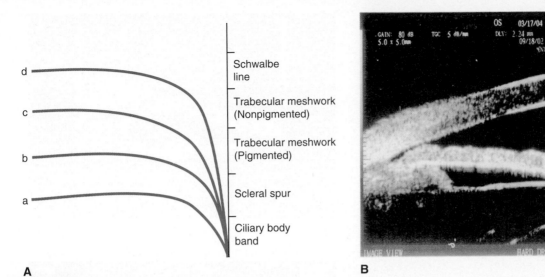

A   **B**

Figure 17.9   **A:** Schematic showing height of plateau and relationship to angle structures. When the height of the plateau is such that dilation of the pupil will result in occlusion of the trabecular meshwork (*c* and *d*), then angle closure is possible despite a patent peripheral iridotomy. **B:** Ultrasonographic biomicroscopy shows plateau iris with the ciliary body touching the posterior iris.

iridotomy. This was traditionally believed to be caused at least partly by an anterior insertion of the iris, although studies with ultrasonographic biomicroscopy suggest that an anterior position of the ciliary processes prevents the peripheral iris from falling posteriorly after an iridotomy (**Fig. 17.9B**) (90–92). Progressive anterior dislocation of the ciliary body with bolstering of the peripheral iris and formation of peripheral anterior synechiae (i.e., chronic angle closure) has been described in a case of plateau iris with long-term follow-up with use of ultrasonographic biomicroscopy (93).

Clinically, it is important to suspect this syndrome if the peripheral anterior chamber is shallow (i.e., van Herick technique, less than one fourth of the corneal thickness) despite a patent peripheral iridotomy or if there is a "high" plateau iris configuration on gonioscopy or an attack of angle-closure glaucoma despite a patent peripheral iridotomy. Additional tests that may help confirm the diagnosis include ultrasonographic biomicroscopy and provoking angle closure with phenylephrine (2.5% or 5%), ensuring that the pupil dilates to more than 7 mm and that the IOP increases after dilation. These cases are usually treated with dilute pilocarpine at bedtime or with peripheral iridoplasty (see Chapter 12).

Pseudoplateau Iris Due to Cysts of the Iris or Ciliary Body

Since the advent of ultrasonographic biomicroscopy, it has become evident that cysts of the iris or ciliary body epithelium can mimic the plateau iris syndrome (94). Clinically, this condition can be termed pseudoplateau iris and may be difficult to distinguish from true plateau iris. In a review of patients with plateau and pseudoplateau iris (with diagnosis based on results of ultrasound biomicroscopic examination), patients with pseudoplateau iris had a greater degree of trabecular meshwork pigmentation, had fewer clock-hours of gonioscopic angle

closure, and were more likely to be male and have a bumpy peripheral iris appearance (visualized by using a narrow slit beam [**Fig. 17.10A**]), compared with patients who had plateau iris. Spherical equivalent did not differ significantly between the two groups (95).

It is important to confirm the diagnosis and the extent of cysts by performing ultrasound biomicroscopic examination (**Fig. 17.10B,C**), because secondary cysts can result from traumatic implantation of epithelium, from metastatic or parasitic lesions, or after the long-term use of miotics (96). If significant angle closure is not present, the prognosis is generally good (97,98). In the case of significant angle closure, treatment may necessitate puncture of the cysts with a needle or with an Nd:YAG laser. Iridoplasty can also be helpful (99).

Swelling of the Ciliary Body

Any disorder giving rise to the swelling of the ciliary body or forward rotation of the ciliary body can create a plateau-like configuration of the iris.

Sulfa-based compounds may cause an idiosyncratic transient myopia, presumably produced by lens swelling and a forward movement of the lens–iris diaphragm associated with choroidal detachments and ciliary body swelling. Use of oral hydrochlorothiazide, oral acetazolamide, and topiramate, a new sulfa-derived antiepileptic medication, have all been reported to precipitate bilateral angle-closure glaucoma, presumably by this mechanism (100–102).

Supraciliary effusions and ciliary body thickening also appear to be common after scleral buckling procedures. They can produce conditions conducive to angle closure through a combination of direct anterior iris rotation and induced pupillary block (103).

Other conditions associated with ciliary body swelling include aqueous misdirection (see Chapter 26), acquired

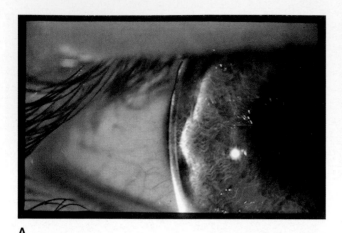

A

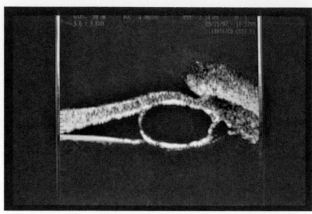

B

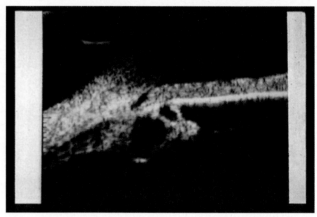

C

Figure 17.10 **A:** Slitlamp examination shows a "bump" on the peripheral iris. **B:** Ultrasonographic biomicroscopy reveals a large cyst in the iridociliary sulcus creating a "bump" in the peripheral iris. **C:** Ultrasonographic biomicroscopy reveals multiple cysts within the iridociliary sulcus, creating a plateau-like configuration to the iris.

immunodeficiency syndrome (AIDS) and other inflammatory disorders (see Chapter 22), and idiopathic uveal effusion syndrome.

KEY POINTS

- Pigmentary glaucoma is typically seen in young adults with myopia, with a predilection for men.
- Iridozonular and iridociliary contact in these individuals apparently leads to liberation of pigment granules from the iris pigment epithelium.
- Clinical findings include transillumination defects in the peripheral iris and deposition of the dispersed pigment on the corneal endothelium, iris stroma, trabecular meshwork, and other anterior ocular structures.
- The glaucoma associated with the pigment dispersion is related to the accumulation of pigment in the trabecular meshwork, with subsequent alteration of the trabecular beams, leading to elevated IOP and glaucomatous damage.
- Iridoschisis is an uncommon affliction of the elderly, characterized by a separation of layers of iris stroma with occasional associated glaucoma.
- Plateau iris is a form of angle-closure glaucoma in which an anterior position of the ciliary processes appears to be responsible for the angle closure.

- Pseudoplateau iris is a condition in which primary cysts in the iridociliary sulcus result in a plateau iris–like configuration with subsequent angle-closure glaucoma.
- Swelling of the ciliary body with angle closure can occur by various mechanisms, including use of sulfa-based oral medications and scleral buckling.

REFERENCES

1. Sugar HS. Concerning the chamber angle. I. Gonioscopy. *Am J Ophthalmol.* 1940;23:853–866.
2. Sugar HS, Barbour FA. Pigmentary glaucoma: a rare clinical entity. *Am J Ophthalmol.* 1949;32(1):90–92.
3. Sugar HS. Pigmentary glaucoma. A 25-year review. *Am J Ophthalmol.* 1966;62(3):499–507.
4. Speakman JS. Pigmentary dispersion. *Br J Ophthalmol.* 1981;65(4):249–251.
5. Ritch R. Nonprogressive low-tension glaucoma with pigmentary dispersion. *Am J Ophthalmol.* 1982;94(2):190–196.
6. Migliazzo CV, Shaffer RN, Nykin R, et al. Long-term analysis of pigmentary dispersion syndrome and pigmentary glaucoma. *Ophthalmology.* 1986;93(12):1528–1536.
7. Sugar S. Pigmentary glaucoma and the glaucoma associated with the exfoliation–exfoliation syndrome: update. Robert N. Shaffer lecture. *Ophthalmology.* 1984;91(4):307–310.
8. Lichter PR, Shaffer RN. Diagnostic and prognostic signs in pigmentary glaucoma. *Trans Am Acad Ophthalmol Otolaryngol.* 1970;74(5):984–998.
9. Lichter PR. Pigmentary glaucoma—current concepts. *Trans Am Acad Ophthalmol Otolaryngol.* 1974;78(2):OP309–OP313.

10. Farrar SM, Shields MB, Miller KN, et al. Risk factors for the development and severity of glaucoma in the pigment dispersion syndrome. *Am J Ophthalmol.* 1989;108(3):223–229.

11. Scheie HG, Cameron JD. Pigment dispersion syndrome: a clinical study. *Br J Ophthalmol.* 1981;65(4):264–269.

12. Orgul S, Hendrickson P, Flammer J. Anterior chamber depth and pigment dispersion syndrome. *Am J Ophthalmol.* 1994;117(5):575–577.

13. Roberts DK, Chaglasian MA, Meetz RE. Clinical signs of the pigment dispersion syndrome in blacks. *Optom Vis Sci.* 1997;74(12):993–1006.

14. Semple HC, Ball SF. Pigmentary glaucoma in the black population. *Am J Ophthalmol.* 1990;109(5):518–522.

15. Roberts DK, Flynn MF, Gable EM. Anterior chamber angle anomalies associated with signs of pigment dispersion in a group of black probands and their first-degree relatives. *Optom Vis Sci.* 2001;78(3):133–141.

16. Wilensky JT, Buerk KM, Podos SM. Krukenberg's spindles. *Am J Ophthalmol.* 1975;79(2):220–225.

17. Duncan TE. Krukenberg spindles in pregnancy. *Arch Ophthalmol.* 1974;91(5):355–358.

18. Lehto I, Ruusuvaara P, Setala K. Corneal endothelium in pigmentary glaucoma and pigment dispersion syndrome. *Acta Ophthalmol.* 1990;68(6):703–709.

19. Murrell WJ, Shihab Z, Lamberts DW, et al. The corneal endothelium and central corneal thickness in pigmentary dispersion syndrome. *Arch Ophthalmol.* 1986;104(6):845–846.

20. Donaldson DD. Transillumination of the iris. *Trans Am Ophthalmol Soc.* 1974;72:89–106.

21. Alward WL, Munden PM, Verdick RE, et al. Use of infrared videography to detect and record iris transillumination defects. *Arch Ophthalmol.* 1990;108(5):748–750.

22. Ritch R, Chaiwat T, Harbin TS Jr. Asymmetric pigmentary glaucoma resulting from cataract formation. *Am J Ophthalmol.* 1992;114(4):484–488.

23. Haynes WL, Thompson HS, Kardon RH et al. Asymmetric pigmentary dispersion syndrome mimicking Horner's syndrome. *Am J Ophthalmol.* 1991;112(4):463–464.

24. Delaney WV Jr. Equatorial lens pigmentation, myopia, and retinal detachment. *Am J Ophthalmol.* 1975;79(2):194–196.

25. Weseley P, Liebmann J, Walsh JB, et al. Lattice degeneration of the retina and the pigment dispersion syndrome. *Am J Ophthalmol.* 1992;114(5):539–543.

26. Scheie HG, Fleischhauer HW. Idiopathic atrophy of the epithelial layers of the iris and ciliary body: a clinical study. *Arch Ophthalmol.* 1958;59(2):216–228.

27. Richter CU, Richardson TM, Grant WM. Pigmentary dispersion syndrome and pigmentary glaucoma. A prospective study of the natural history. *Arch Ophthalmol.* 1986;104(2):211–215.

28. Niyadurupola N, Broadway DC. Pigment dispersion syndrome and pigmentary glaucoma—a major review. *Clin Experiment Ophthalmol.* 2008;36(9):868–882.

29. Lehto I. Long-term prognosis of pigmentary glaucoma. *Acta Ophthalmol.* 1991;69(4):437–443.

30. Brini A, Porte A, Roth A. Atrophy of the epithelial layers of the iris; study of a case of pigmentary glaucoma by light microscope and electron microscope [in French]. *Doc Ophthalmol.* 1969;26:403–423.

31. Kupfer C, Kuwabara T, Kaiser-Kupfer M. The histopathology of pigmentary dispersion syndrome with glaucoma. *Am J Ophthalmol.* 1975;80(5):857–862.

32. Rodrigues MM, Spaeth GL, Weinreb S, et al. Spectrum of trabecular pigmentation in open-angle glaucoma: a clinicopathologic study. *Trans Sect Ophthalmol Am Acad Ophthalmol Otolaryngol.* 1976;81(2):258–276.

33. Piccolino FC, Calabria G, Polizzi A, et al. Pigmentary retinal dystrophy associated with pigmentary glaucoma. *Graefes Arch Clin Exp Ophthalmol.* 1989;227(4):335–339.

34. Gillies WE, Tangas C. Fluorescein angiography of the iris in anterior segment pigment dispersal syndrome. *Br J Ophthalmol.* 1986;70(4):284–289.

35. Brooks AM, Gillies WE. Hypoperfusion of the iris and its consequences in anterior segment pigment dispersal syndrome. *Ophthalmic Surg.* 1994;25(5):307–310.

36. Campbell DG. Pigmentary dispersion and glaucoma. A new theory. *Arch Ophthalmol.* 1979;97(9):1667–1672.

37. Kampik A, Green WR, Quigley HA, et al. Scanning and transmission electron microscopic studies of two cases of pigment dispersion syndrome. *Am J Ophthalmol.* 1981;91(5):573–587.

38. Strasser G, Hauff W. Pigmentary dispersion syndrome. A biometric study. *Acta Ophthalmol.* 1985;63(6):721–722.

39. Davidson JA, Brubaker RF, Ilstrup DM. Dimensions of the anterior chamber in pigment dispersion syndrome. *Arch Ophthalmol.* 1983;101(1):81–83.

40. Ritch R. A unification hypothesis of pigment dispersion syndrome. *Trans Am Ophthalmol Soc.* 1996;94:381–405; discussion 9.

41. Richardson TM. Pigmentary glaucoma. In: Ritch R, Shields MB, eds. *The Secondary Glaucomas.* St. Louis: CV Mosby; 1982:84–98.

42. Ritch R, Manusow D, Podos SM. Remission of pigmentary glaucoma in a patient with subluxed lenses. *Am J Ophthalmol.* 1982;94(6):812–813.

43. Karickhoff JR. Pigmentary dispersion syndrome and pigmentary glaucoma: a new mechanism concept, a new treatment, and a new technique. *Ophthalmic Surg.* 1992;23(4):269–277.

44. Jensen PK, Nissen O, Kessing SV. Exercise and reversed pupillary block in pigmentary glaucoma. *Am J Ophthalmol.* 1995;120(1):110–112.

45. Pavlin CJ, Harasiewicz K, Foster FS. Posterior iris bowing in pigmentary dispersion syndrome caused by accommodation. *Am J Ophthalmol.* 1994;118(1):114–116.

46. Pavlin CJ, Macken P, Trope GE, et al. Accommodation and iridotomy in the pigment dispersion syndrome. *Ophthalmic Surg Lasers.* 1996;27(2):113–120.

47. Roberts DK, Lo PS, Winters JE, et al. Prevalence of pigmented lens striae in a black population: a potential indicator of age-related pigment dispersal in the anterior segment. *Optom Vis Sci.* 2002;79(11):681–687.

48. Moroi SE, Lark KK, Sieving PA, et al. Long anterior zonules and pigment dispersion. *Am J Ophthalmol.* 2003;136(6):1176–1178.

49. Sakabe I, Oshika T, Lim SJ, et al. Anterior shift of zonular insertion onto the anterior surface of human crystalline lens with age. *Ophthalmology.* 1998;105(2):295–299.

50. Koch DD, Liu JF. Zonular encroachment on the anterior capsular zonular-free zone. *Am J Ophthalmol.* 1988;106(4):491–492.

51. Grant WM. Experimental aqueous perfusion in enucleated human eyes. *Arch Ophthalmol.* 1963;69:783–801.

52. Epstein DL, Boger WP III, Grant WM. Phenylephrine provocative testing in the pigmentary dispersion syndrome. *Am J Ophthalmol.* 1978;85(1):43–50.

53. Mapstone R. Pigment release. *Br J Ophthalmol.* 1981;65(4):258–263.

54. Mardin CY, Kuchle M, Nguyen NX, et al. Quantification of aqueous melanin granules, intraocular pressure and glaucomatous damage in primary pigment dispersion syndrome. *Ophthalmology.* 2000;107(3):435–440.

55. Epstein DL, Freddo TF, Anderson PJ, et al. Experimental obstruction to aqueous outflow by pigment particles in living monkeys. *Invest Ophthalmol Vis Sci.* 1986;27(3):387–395.

56. Murphy CG, Johnson M, Alvarado JA. Juxtacanalicular tissue in pigmentary and primary open angle glaucoma. The hydrodynamic role of pigment and other constituents. *Arch Ophthalmol.* 1992;110(12):1779–1785.

57. Alvarado JA, Murphy CG. Outflow obstruction in pigmentary and primary open angle glaucoma. *Arch Ophthalmol.* 1992;110(12):1769–1778.

58. Becker B, Podos SM. Krukenberg's spindles and primary open-angle glaucoma. *Arch Ophthalmol.* 1966;76(5):635–639.

59. Zink HA, Palmberg PF, Sugar A, et al. Comparison of in vitro corticosteroid response in pigmentary glaucoma and primary open-angle glaucoma. *Am J Ophthalmol.* 1975;80(3 pt 1):478–484.

60. Becker B, Shin DH, Cooper DG, et al. The pigment dispersion syndrome. *Am J Ophthalmol.* 1977;83(2):161–166.

61. Kaiser-Kupfer MI, Mittal KK. The HLA and ABO antigens in pigment dispersion syndrome. *Am J Ophthalmol.* 1978;85(3):368–372.

62. Layden WE, Ritch R, King DG, et al. Combined exfoliation and pigment dispersion syndrome. *Am J Ophthalmol.* 1990;109(5):530–534.

63. Bhorade AM, Edward DP, Goldstein DA. Ciliary body melanocytoma with anterior segment pigment dispersion and elevated intraocular pressure. *J Glaucoma.* 1999;8(2):129–133.

64. Brandt JD, Mockovak ME, Chayet A. Pigmentary dispersion syndrome induced by a posterior chamber phakic refractive lens. *Am J Ophthalmol.* 2001;131(2):260–263.

65. Micheli T, Cheung LM, Sharma S, et al. Acute haptic-induced pigmentary glaucoma with an AcrySof intraocular lens. *J Cataract Refract Surg.* 2002;28(10):1869–1872.

66. Ritch R, Alward WL. Asymmetric pigmentary glaucoma caused by unilateral angle recession. *Am J Ophthalmol.* 1993;116(6):765–766.

67. Haynes WL, Thompson HS, Johnson AT, et al. Comparison of the miotic effects of dapiprazole and dilute pilocarpine in patients with the pigment dispersion syndrome. *J Glaucoma.* 1995;4(6):379–385.

68. Jampel HD. Lack of effect of peripheral laser iridotomy in pigment dispersion syndrome. *Arch Ophthalmol.* 1993;111(12):1606.

69. Haynes WL, Alward WL, Tello C, et al. Incomplete elimination of exercise-induced pigment dispersion by laser iridotomy in pigment dispersion syndrome. *Ophthalmic Surg Lasers.* 1995;26(5):484–486.

70. Breingan PJ, Esaki K, Ishikawa H, et al. Iridolenticular contact decreases following laser iridotomy for pigment dispersion syndrome. *Arch Ophthalmol.* 1999;117(3):325–328.

71. Gandolfi SA, Vecchi M. Effect of a YAG laser iridotomy on intraocular pressure in pigment dispersion syndrome. *Ophthalmology.* 1996;103(10):1693–1695.
72. Reistad CE, Shields MB, Campbell DG, et al. The influence of peripheral iridotomy on the intraocular pressure course in patients with pigmentary glaucoma. *J Glaucoma.* 2005;14(4):255–259.
73. Moster MR, George-Lomax KM. The use of the consensual light reflex as an aid to performing laser peripheral iridectomy in patients with pigment dispersion syndrome and pigmentary glaucoma. *J Glaucoma.* 1998;7(2):93–94.
74. Lunde MW. Argon laser trabeculoplasty in pigmentary dispersion syndrome with glaucoma. *Am J Ophthalmol.* 1983;96(6):721–725.
75. Lehto I. Long-term follow up of argon laser trabeculoplasty in pigmentary glaucoma. *Ophthalmic Surg.* 1992;23(9):614–617.
76. Ritch R, Liebmann J, Robin A, et al. Argon laser trabeculoplasty in pigmentary glaucoma. *Ophthalmology.* 1993;100(6):909–913.
77. Harasymowycz PJ, Papamatheakis DG, Latina M, et al. Selective laser trabeculoplasty (SLT) complicated by intraocular pressure elevation in eyes with heavily pigmented trabecular meshworks. *Am J Ophthalmol.* 2005;139(6):1110–1113.
78. Summers CG, Doughman DJ, Letson RD, et al. Juvenile iridoschisis and microphthalmos. *Am J Ophthalmol.* 1985;100(3):437–439.
79. Eiferman RA, Law M, Lane L. Iridoschisis and keratoconus. *Cornea.* 1994;13(1):78–79.
80. Salmon JF, Murray AD. The association of iridoschisis and primary angle-closure glaucoma. *Eye.* 1992;6:267–272.
81. Salmon JF. The association of iridoschisis and angle-recession glaucoma. *Am J Ophthalmol.* 1992;114(6):766–767.
82. Pearson PA, Amrien JM, Baldwin LB, et al. Iridoschisis associated with syphilitic interstitial keratitis. *Am J Ophthalmol.* 1989;107(1):88–90.
83. Rodrigues MC, Spaeth GL, Krachmer JH, et al. Iridoschisis associated with glaucoma and bullous keratopathy. *Am J Ophthalmol.* 1983;95(1):73–81.
84. Weseley AC, Freeman WR. Iridoschisis and the corneal endothelium. *Ann Ophthalmol.* 1983;15(10):955–959, 63–64.
85. Zimmerman TJ, Dabezies OH Jr, Kaufman HE. Iridoschisis: a case report. *Ann Ophthalmol.* 1981;13(3):297–298.
86. Tornquist R. Angle-closure glaucoma in an eye with a plateau type of iris. *Acta Ophthalmol.* 1958;36(3):419–423.
87. Shaffer RN. Primary glaucomas. Gonioscopy, ophthalmoscopy and perimetry. *Trans Am Acad Ophthalmol Otolaryngol.* 1960;64:112–127.
88. Wand M, Grant WM, Simmons RJ, et al. Plateau iris syndrome. *Trans Sect Ophthalmol Am Acad Ophthalmol Otolaryngol.* 1977;83(1):122–130.
89. Roberts DK, Ayyagari R, Moroi SE. Possible association between long anterior lens zonules and plateau iris configuration. *J Glaucoma.* 2008;17(5):393–396.
90. Pavlin CJ, Ritch R, Foster FS. Ultrasound biomicroscopy in plateau iris syndrome. *Am J Ophthalmol.* 1992;113(4):390–395.
91. Ritch R. Plateau iris is caused by abnormally positioned ciliary processes. *J Glaucoma.* 1992;1(1):23–26.
92. Wand M, Pavlin CJ, Foster FS. Plateau iris syndrome: ultrasound biomicroscopic and histologic study. *Ophthalmic Surg.* 1993;24(2):129–131.
93. Miki A, Otori Y, Morimura H, et al. Long-term follow-up of plateau iris syndrome using the ultrasound biomicroscope [in Japanese]. *Fol Ophthalmol Jpn.* 2001;52(5):404–408.
94. Azuara-Blanco A, Spaeth GL, Araujo SV, et al. Plateau iris syndrome associated with multiple ciliary body cysts. Report of three cases. *Arch Ophthalmol.* 1996;114(6):666–668.
95. Shukla S, Damji KF, Harasymowycz P, et al. Clinical features distinguishing angle closure from pseudoplateau versus plateau iris. *Br J Ophthalmol.* 2008;92(3):340–344.
96. Marigo FA, Esaki K, Finger PT, et al. Differential diagnosis of anterior segment cysts by ultrasound biomicroscopy. *Ophthalmology.* 1999;106(11):2131–2135.
97. Shields JA, Kline MW, Augsburger JJ. Primary iris cysts: a review of the literature and report of 62 cases. *Br J Ophthalmol.* 1984;68(3):152–166.
98. Fine N, Pavlin CJ. Primary cysts in the iridociliary sulcus: ultrasound biomicroscopic features of 210 cases. *Can J Ophthalmol.* 1999;34(6):325–329.
99. Crowston JG, Medeiros FA, Mosaed S, et al. Argon laser iridoplasty in the treatment of plateau-like iris configuration as result of numerous ciliary body cysts. *Am J Ophthalmol.* 2005;139(2):381–383.
100. Geanon JD, Perkins TW. Bilateral acute angle-closure glaucoma associated with drug sensitivity to hydrochlorothiazide. *Arch Ophthalmol.* 1995;113(10):1231–1232.
101. Banta JT, Hoffman K, Budenz DL, et al. Presumed topiramate-induced bilateral acute angle-closure glaucoma. *Am J Ophthalmol.* 2001;132(1):112–114.
102. Rhee DJ, Goldberg MJ, Parrish RK. Bilateral angle-closure glaucoma and ciliary body swelling from topiramate. *Arch Ophthalmol.* 2001;119(11):1721–1723.
103. Pavlin CJ, Rutnin SS, Devenyi R, et al. Supraciliary effusions and ciliary body thickening after scleral buckling procedures. *Ophthalmology.* 1997;104(3):433–438.

Glaucomas Associated with Disorders of the Lens

18

Several disorders of the crystalline lens are associated with various forms of glaucoma. In some cases, such as the exfoliation syndrome (see Chapter 15), a cause-and-effect relationship between the lenticular abnormality and the glaucoma is uncertain. In other situations, including some forms of dislocated lenses and cataracts, the glaucoma is more clearly a result of the alteration in the lens.

GLAUCOMAS ASSOCIATED WITH DISLOCATION OF THE LENS

Terminology

Several terms have been applied to the clinical situation in which the crystalline lens is displaced from its normal, central position behind the iris. Subluxation of the lens implies an incomplete dislocation in which the lens is still at least partially behind the iris but is tilted or displaced slightly in an anterior or a posterior direction or perpendicular to the optical axis. With complete dislocation, the entire lens may be in the anterior chamber or may have fallen posteriorly into the vitreous cavity. The term ectopia of the lens, or ectopia lentis, is also applied to cases of lens dislocation, but it is nonspecific with regard to the degree of lens displacement.

Subluxation or complete dislocation of the lens may be associated with a number of clinical conditions, all of which can lead to glaucoma by a variety of mechanisms. We first review the more common clinical forms of ectopia lentis and then consider the mechanisms by which these conditions may lead to intraocular pressure (IOP) elevation and how these glaucomas are managed.

Clinical Forms of Ectopia Lentis

Traumatic Dislocation

Trauma is the most common cause of a displaced lens (1,2) (**Fig. 18.1**). In one series of 166 cases, injury was reported to account for 53% of the total group (2).

Exfoliation Syndrome

The exfoliation syndrome can be associated with spontaneous or traumatic lens subluxation or dislocation (see Chapter 15).

Simple Ectopia Lentis

Dislocation of the lens may occur without associated ocular or systemic abnormalities as a congenital anomaly or as a spontaneous disorder later in life (3). Both forms are typically inherited by an autosomal dominant mode (3). The condition is usually bilateral and symmetrical, with lens dislocation generally upward and outward and occasionally into the anterior chamber. Associated problems include glaucoma and retinal detachment.

Ectopia Lentis et Pupillae

Ectopia lentis et pupillae is a rare, autosomal recessive condition characterized by small, subluxated lenses and by oval or slit-shaped pupils that are displaced, usually in the opposite direction from that of the lens (3) (**Fig. 18.2**). The condition is associated with a wide variety of other ocular abnormalities, including severe axial myopia with related fundus changes, enlarged corneal diameters, iris transillumination defects, poor pupillary dilation, persistent pupillary membranes, iridohyaloid adhesions, prominent iris processes, cataracts, retinal detachment, and glaucoma (4). The condition is usually bilateral, although marked variation may be seen between eyes of the same patient. The pathogenesis of this disorder is unknown, but an ultrasound biomicroscopic study of an affected patient demonstrated a lack of definition of the ciliary processes except in the quadrant toward which the pupil was displaced and a membrane-like structure extending from the proximal pupillary margin over the tips of the ciliary processes to a more posterior origin (5). The investigators proposed a localized abnormality of the secondary vitreous with persistence of the marginal bundle of Drualt, resulting in a mechanical tethering of the iris or pupil margin to the vitreous base or anterior vitreous face and localized zonular disruption. Others have suggested a neuroectodermal defect resulting in hypoplasia or absence of the posterior pigment epithelium layer and dilator

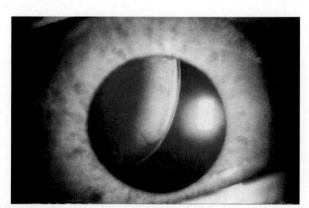

Figure 18.1 Dislocation or subluxation of the lens can result from various disorders that can lead to glaucoma. In this case, the lens is dislocated superotemporally in a patient with ectopia lentis et papillae, which is characterized by small, subluxed lenses and oval or slit-like pupils that are displaced in the opposite direction of the lens.

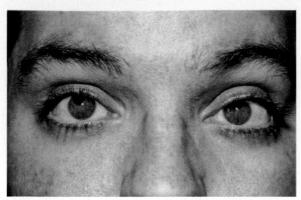

Figure 18.2 Patient with ectopia lentis et pupillae, showing typical displacement of pupils.

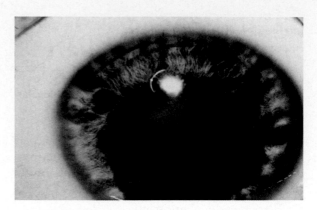

Figure 18.3 Upward lens subluxation in a patient with Marfan syndrome.

muscle of the iris or a mesodermal defect with persistence of the anterior and lateral elements of the tunica vasculosa lentis (4). The ultrasound biomicroscopy findings are consistent with histopathologic case reports in the German literature from the beginning of the past century (6–8).

It has been suggested that simple ectopia lentis may be an incomplete expression of ectopia lentis et pupillae, because both may occur in the same family and have peripheral iris transillumination (4). Some patients with ectopia lentis et pupillae may have mild systemic changes suggestive of Marfan syndrome.

Marfan Syndrome

This autosomal dominant disorder is characterized by a tall, slender individual with long, slender fingers and toes (i.e., arachnodactyly) and frequent cardiovascular disease (3). Marfan syndrome and ectopia lentis have been linked to a single fibrillin gene on chromosome 15, and arachnodactyly was linked to the fibrillin gene on chromosome 5 (9). In a review of 160 consecutive patients, the most striking ocular abnormality was enlargement of the globe, presumably caused by scleral stretching (10). The lens was dislocated in 193 of the eyes, and this correlated with increased ocular axial length, suggesting that stretching and rupture of the zonular fibers lead to the dislocation. The ectopia lentis typically appears in the fourth to fifth decade of life and is rarely complete, but it is usually seen as an upward subluxation (**Fig. 18.3**). Bilateral spontaneous lens dislocation has been described in early childhood with associated glaucoma (11). Glaucoma may result from the lens dislocation, but it is also associated with surgical aphakia or occurs as an anomaly of the anterior chamber angle. In one review of 573 patients, 29 (5%) had glaucoma, and the most common mechanisms were chronic open angle and glaucoma following lens extraction or scleral buckling procedure (12). Retinal detachment is also a common finding in the phakic or aphakic eye of a patient with Marfan syndrome.

Homocystinuria

Patients with homocystinuria may resemble those with Marfan syndrome in habitus and ocular problems, but they differ by having an autosomal recessive inheritance pattern and frequently having mental retardation (3,13). Homocystinuria may result from one of several enzyme deficiencies in homocysteine metabolism. The diagnosis can be confirmed by the demonstration of homocysteine in the urine. The differentiation between Marfan syndrome and homocystinuria is important because the patient with homocystinuria is subject to thromboembolic episodes, which can lead to death in early adulthood and creates a significant surgical risk. If the condition is diagnosed in a newborn, appropriate dietary treatment and vitamin supplementation can substantially reduce the risk for ocular complications (14). The lens dislocation occurs earlier in life than in the Marfan syndrome and is more often in a downward direction, and complete dislocation into the vitreous or anterior chamber is frequent. Glaucoma is more commonly related to the lens dislocation than is the case with Marfan syndrome. Retinal detachment is a common problem.

One article examined the results of medical versus surgical treatment for lens subluxation or dislocation in a retrospective case series of 45 patients (15). Medical therapy was attempted initially in all patients and was the sole therapy used for five patients. Eighty-two procedures were performed with the patients under general anesthesia, and two surgical complications and one postoperative complication occurred. Lens dislocation into the anterior chamber was the most frequent indication for surgery (50%), followed by pupillary block glaucoma (12%). Prophylactic peripheral iridectomy was not successful in preventing lens dislocation into the anterior chamber in five patients. The investigators recommend that surgical treatment should be considered, especially for cases of repeated lens dislocation into the anterior chamber or pupillary block glaucoma.

Weill–Marchesani Syndrome

Weill–Marchesani syndrome is the antithesis of the aforementioned conditions with respect to habitus; these patients are short and stocky (16,17). The principal features of the syndrome are short fingers (i.e., brachydactyly); muscular hypertrophy; and small, round lenses (i.e., microspherophakia) (**Fig. 18.4**). Lens dislocation in these patients occurs as frequently as in patients with Marfan syndrome and homocystinuria, and glaucoma is more common than in either of the latter two conditions (18). In his original publication, Marchesani (17) hypothesized that an overdevelopment or hyperplasia of the ciliary

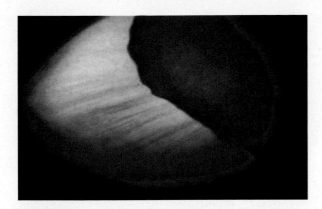

Figure 18.4 Partial lens dislocation in a patient with Weill–Marchesani syndrome. The loose zonules allow the lens to assume a typical, small round shape (i.e., microspherophakia).

Table 18.1	Conditions Associated with Ectopia Lentis
Trauma	
Simple ectopia lentis	
Ectopia lentis et pupillae	
Marfan syndrome	
Homocystinuria	
Weill–Marchesani syndrome	
High myopia	
Uveitis	
Buphthalmos	
Megalocornea	
Ehlers–Danlos syndrome	
Hyperlysinemia	
Sulfite oxidase deficiency	
Aniridia	
Scleroderma	
Alport syndrome	
Mandibulofacial dysostosis	
Klinefelter syndrome	
Retinitis pigmentosa	
Persistent pupillary membrane	
Axenfeld–Rieger syndrome	
Dominantly inherited blepharoptosis and high myopia	
Marfan-like syndrome with hyaloretinal degeneration	
Sturge–Weber syndrome	
Syphilis	
Crouzon disease	
Refsum syndrome	

Modified from Refs. 3 and 27.

body might be the reason for spherophakia. However, an ultrasonographic biomicroscopy study of three patients with this syndrome and normal axial lengths demonstrated that the ciliary body actually appeared smaller than normal (19). The investigators hypothesized that the small ciliary body represents the underlying reason for elongated zonules and that it may be exerting less force on the lens, giving rise to the spherical shape of the lens. An ultrastructural study of the lens from a patient with the Weill–Marchesani syndrome revealed degeneration and necrosis of the epithelial cells and destruction of cortical fibers, which was thought to result, in part, from the trauma and irritation of a highly mobile lens in close contact with the iris (20). The small, round lens in this condition also has loose zonules, and the glaucoma may be related to lens dislocation or a forward shift of the lens, causing pupillary block glaucoma (18), which can be precipitated or aggravated by miotic therapy. Bilateral angle-closure glaucoma has also been reported after mid-dilatation with cyclopentolate in a child with the Weill–Marchesani syndrome but without lens subluxation (21). Angle-closure glaucoma may be treated with laser iridectomy or peripheral iridoplasty depending on the relative proportion of pupillary block as the mechanism of the angle closure (22).

Spontaneous Dislocation

In some middle-aged or older individuals, dislocation of the lens may occur spontaneously, usually in association with cataract formation (1). Spontaneous dislocation has also been reported in eyes with high myopia, uveitis, buphthalmos, or megalocornea.

Other Conditions with Associated Ectopia Lentis

Other rare congenital disorders associated with lens dislocation include Ehlers–Danlos syndrome, hyperlysinemia, sulfite oxidase deficiency, and aniridia. Additional conditions associated with ectopia lentis are included in **Table 18.1**.

Examination and Investigation

Slitlamp examination may reveal lenticular subluxation and dislocation. If zonules are weak, then phacodonesis or iridodonesis may also be present. Even with these signs, the

nature of the accompanying zonular defect may be uncertain. Ultrasonographic biomicroscopy enables in vivo imaging of the zonules and can detect zonular loss and stretching directly (**Fig. 18.5**) (23). In a study of 18 eyes with clinically suspected zonular abnormalities, ultrasonographic biomicroscopy demonstrated evidence of missing zonules in 11 eyes and evidence of zonular stretch in 11 eyes. All of the eyes examined demonstrated increased lenticular sphericity in the area of the zonular disorder, and nine eyes showed ciliary body flattening.

Mechanisms of Glaucoma Associated with Subluxated or Dislocated Lens

Subluxation or complete dislocation of the lens in any of the aforementioned clinical conditions may lead to glaucoma by various mechanisms. In general, these mechanisms of glaucoma apply to all forms of ectopia lentis.

Figure 18.5 **A:** Ultrasonographic biomicroscopy showing stretched zonules. **B:** Ultrasonographic biomicroscopy showing broken zonules with rounding up of the ciliary body and adjacent lens equator.

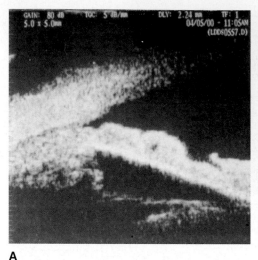 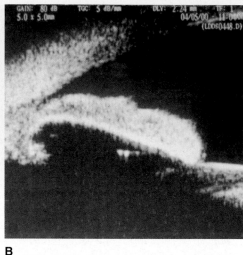

A B

Pupillary Block

The lens may block aqueous flow through the pupil if it is dislocated into the pupil or anterior chamber or subluxed or tilted forward against the iris without entering the anterior chamber. This mechanism is particularly common with microspherophakia, as in the Weill–Marchesani syndrome, because of loose zonules of the lens. Pupillary block in the latter condition is often worsened by miotic therapy, which allows further relaxation of zonular support, and cycloplegic agents may help by pulling the lens posteriorly. Pupillary block may also be associated with a dislocated lens due to herniation of vitreous into the pupil. Peripheral anterior synechiae may develop from a long-standing pupillary block and produce chronic IOP elevation.

Phacolytic Glaucoma

In some cases, the lens may dislocate completely into the vitreous cavity and later undergo degenerative changes with release of material that obstructs aqueous outflow (24). In one reported case, this condition was associated with retinal perivasculitis, which cleared along with the glaucoma after removal of the lens (25). (Phacolytic glaucoma without dislocation is discussed later in this chapter.)

Concomitant Trauma

In cases of traumatic dislocation of the lens, concomitant trauma to the anterior chamber angle from the initial injury may be the cause of the associated glaucoma (1,3). A transient pressure elevation of uncertain origin may persist for days or weeks after traumatic dislocation of the lens. (The mechanisms of glaucoma associated with trauma are considered in more detail in Chapter 25.)

Management

If the lens is displaced anteriorly in the anterior chamber or partially through the pupil, the condition may be relieved by dilating the pupil and allowing the lens to reposit back into the posterior chamber (26). A miotic agent may then be used to keep the lens behind the iris, but miotic therapy should be avoided when the pupillary block is caused by loose zonules, because contraction of the ciliary muscle further relaxes the zonular support, making the pupillary block worse (27). If the lens is completely dislocated in the anterior chamber, it is probably better to constrict the pupil and surgically remove the lens, rather than letting it fall back into the vitreous. Cycloplegic agents may help to break the attack by pulling the lens posteriorly. Hyperosmotic agents, carbonic anhydrase inhibitors, or topical β-blockers may also be useful in breaking the attack. The definitive treatment, however, is laser iridotomy (or incisional iridectomy, if necessary). The iridotomy should be placed peripherally to avoid subsequent obstruction by the lens. Prophylactic iridotomy in cases of microspherophakia has also been advocated to avoid pupillary block glaucoma (27). Laser peripheral iridoplasty may also be helpful in some cases of angle-closure glaucoma without a significant pupillary block component (22). The extraction of a subluxated lens is associated with increased surgical risk and should usually be avoided unless the lens is in the anterior chamber or lens extraction is needed to relieve the glaucoma or improve vision.

Phacolytic Glaucoma

Phacolytic glaucoma is the only situation in cases of lens dislocation in which cataract extraction is the procedure of choice (28). Subluxated lenses can be successfully removed through a pars plana approach with vitreous instruments (25).

Chronic Glaucomas

Chronic glaucoma due to peripheral anterior synechiae or concomitant trauma in eyes with dislocated lenses is generally managed by standard medical measures. Laser trabeculoplasty has a low success rate in eyes with open-angle glaucoma associated with trauma, although this approach is often reasonable to try when medical therapy is no longer adequate before recommending incisional surgical intervention.

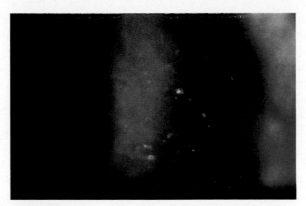

Figure 18.6 High-magnification slitlamp view showing iridescent particles in the aqueous in a patient with phacolytic glaucoma. The white, cloudy cornea is seen to the right, and the dark iris to the left, of the photograph. (Courtesy of L. Frank Cashwell Jr, MD.)

GLAUCOMAS ASSOCIATED WITH CATARACT FORMATION

It has long been recognized clinically that several forms of glaucoma may occur in association with the formation of cataracts. However, an incomplete understanding of the various mechanisms for these glaucomas has led to a plethora of terms and considerable controversy and confusion. Later observations have provided new explanations and terminology for several of the glaucomas associated with cataract formation.

Phacolytic (Lens Protein) Glaucoma

Terminology

In 1900, Gifford (29) described a form of open-angle glaucoma associated with a hypermature cataract. Among the terms subsequently suggested for this condition were phacogenic glaucoma and lens-induced uveitis (30,31). Flocks and colleagues (32) reported histologic findings suggesting that the glaucoma-inducing mechanism was a macrophagic response to lens material. They proposed that this condition be called phacolytic glaucoma, which is the term most often used today. However, Epstein and colleagues (33,34) have provided evidence that high-molecular-weight lens protein may be primarily responsible for the obstruction to aqueous outflow in this disorder, and the term lens protein glaucoma has been suggested (35).

Clinical Features

The typical patient presents with an acute onset of monocular pain and redness. There is usually a history of gradual reduction in visual acuity over the preceding months or years. Vision at the time of presentation may be reduced to light perception. The examination reveals a high IOP, conjunctival hyperemia, and diffuse corneal edema. The anterior chamber angle is open and usually grossly normal. A heavy flare is typically seen in the anterior chamber and is often associated with iridescent or hyperrefringent particles (**Fig. 18.6**). The latter have been variably reported to represent calcium oxalate or cholesterol crystals and are a helpful diagnostic sign in phacolytic glaucoma (36–38). Chunks of white material may also be seen in the aqueous and on the anterior lens capsule and corneal endothelium. In five cases, specular microscopy revealed regular, round cells, about three times the size of an erythrocyte, which were found by histologic study of aqueous aspirates to represent macrophages (37). Rare cases of vitreous opacification have been reported (39). The opacities were observed at the time of cataract surgery and resolved spontaneously over 12 weeks. The cataract is typically mature and opaque (**Fig. 18.7A**) or hypermature (i.e., liquid cortex), but it may, rarely, be immature. A less common variation of phacolytic glaucoma is the previously discussed situation in which the lens has dislocated into the vitreous and undergone phacolysis (**Fig. 18.7B**). The latter cases differ clinically in that the glaucoma tends to be more subacute.

Theories of Mechanism

It is generally accepted that part of the pathogenesis in phacolytic glaucoma is the release of soluble lens protein into the aqueous through microscopic defects in the lens capsule.

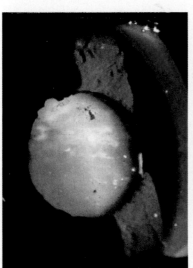

A

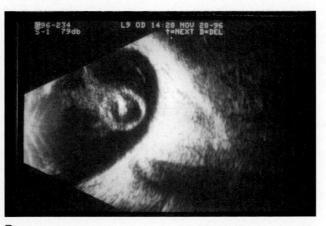

B

Figure 18.7 **A:** Mature cataract in a patient with phacolytic glaucoma. **B:** B-scan ultrasonography shows a lens dislocated in the vitreous cavity.

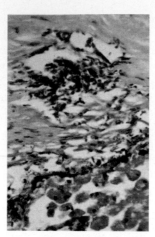

Figure 18.8 Light microscopic photograph of the trabecular meshwork area in a patient with phacolytic glaucoma demonstrates numerous macrophages in the anterior chamber angle (*bottom*) adjacent to the meshwork.

However, theories vary as to how this protein leads to the elevated IOP.

It has been postulated that macrophages, laden with phagocytosed lens material, block the trabecular meshwork to produce the acute glaucoma (**Fig. 18.8**) (33). This theory has been supported by the demonstration of macrophages in the aqueous and trabecular meshwork of eyes with phacolytic glaucoma (40,41). By electron microscopic study, these macrophages were found to have phagocytized, degenerated lens material (42). Electron microscopy has also demonstrated free-floating degenerated lens material in the aqueous and trabecular meshwork of an eye with phacolytic glaucoma (42). Against the macrophage theory is the observation that lens-laden macrophages in the anterior chamber do not invariably lead to elevated IOP. For example, a macrophagic cellular reaction has been found in the anterior chamber aspirate after needling and aspiration of a cataract but did not appear to obstruct aqueous outflow (43). However, the number of macrophages in the aqueous may be greater in phacolytic glaucoma.

An alternative theory is that high-molecular-weight soluble protein from the lens directly obstructs the outflow of aqueous (33–35). Such protein has been shown to cause a significant decrease in outflow when perfused in enucleated human eyes (33). High-molecular-weight soluble protein is known to increase in the cataractous lens and has been demonstrated in the aqueous of eyes with phacolytic glaucoma in quantities sufficient to obstruct aqueous outflow (34,44). High-molecular-weight protein is rare in childhood lenses, which may explain why phacolytic glaucoma rarely occurs in children.

Differential Diagnosis

Several forms of glaucoma manifest with the sudden onset of pain and redness, creating diagnostic confusion with phacolytic glaucoma. Acute angle-closure glaucoma must be ruled out on the basis of the gonioscopic examination. Open-angle glaucoma associated with uveitis may be more difficult to distinguish. In some cases, a paracentesis and microscopic examination of the aqueous may be helpful by demonstrating amorphous protein-like fluid and occasional macrophages in eyes with phacolytic glaucoma (38). A therapeutic trial of topical steroids can produce only temporary remission when phacolysis is the underlying problem, which may help to distinguish it from a primary uveitis. Other conditions, such as neovascular glaucoma, trauma, and rarely, an occult posterior segment tumor, may also present with a similar clinical picture. Usually, these causes can be readily distinguished on the basis of history or clinical findings. It is always wise to perform B-scan ultrasonography when the view of the posterior segment is obscured by media opacity.

Management

Phacolytic glaucoma should be handled as an emergency, ultimately by removal of the lens (45). It is desirable to first bring the IOP under medical control with hyperosmotics, carbonic anhydrase inhibitors, and topical β-blockers or α_2-agonists and possibly to minimize associated inflammation with topical steroid therapy (38). When the pressure cannot be lowered medically, it may be necessary to accomplish this at the time of surgery by gradual release of aqueous through a paracentesis incision. Phacoemulsification or traditional extracapsular cataract extraction with posterior chamber intraocular lens implantation can often be performed with good results. The anterior chamber should be thoroughly irrigated and all lens material removed to avoid postoperative IOP rise. After uncomplicated cataract surgery, the glaucoma usually clears, and there is often a return of good vision despite a significant preoperative reduction.

In a retrospective study of eyes with phacolytic glaucoma in which trabeculectomy was added to standard cataract surgery if symptoms endured for more than 7 days or if preoperative control of IOP with maximal medical treatment was inadequate, IOP was significantly lower in the combined-surgery group compared with the group receiving cataract surgery only (46). At 6 months, IOP and visual acuity did not differ between the two groups. Another study of patients with phacolytic glaucoma and cataract surgery found IOP was less than 21 mm Hg in all patients without use of any antiglaucoma medication (47). This included a group of eyes that underwent extracapsular cataract extraction with posterior chamber intraocular lens implantation and another group of eyes that underwent only extracapsular cataract extraction. Eighteen of the 45 patients initially presented with light perception without projection, and 44% of these patients regained a visual acuity of 20/40 or better. There were no significant intraoperative or postoperative complications. In view of the previously described studies, it seems reasonable to proceed with cataract extraction alone in patients with phacolytic glaucoma who have surgery within a week or so of symptom onset. If, however, symptoms have persisted for more than a week, combining trabeculectomy with cataract extraction to prevent a postoperative rise in IOP and to decrease the need for systemic hypotensive medications is reasonable to consider.

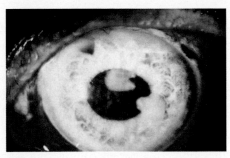

Figure 18.9 "Fluffed-up" lens cortical material is retained in the anterior chamber in this patient with lens particle glaucoma. (Courtesy of Brooks W. McCuen II, MD.)

Lens Particle Glaucoma

Terminology

It was once thought that a primary toxicity of cataractous lens material caused an inflammatory reaction called phacotoxic uveitis and that it led to glaucoma in some cases. Subsequent studies have not supported the concept that liberated lens material is toxic (48). Cases incorrectly given this diagnosis are actually caused by liberation of lens particles and debris after disruption of the lens capsule, and the term "lens particle glaucoma" has been proposed for this entity (35).

Clinical Features

Lens particle glaucoma is typically associated with disruption of the lens capsule by cataract extraction or a penetrating injury. The onset of IOP elevation usually occurs soon after the primary event and is generally proportional to the amount of "fluffed-up" lens cortical material in the anterior chamber (**Fig. 18.9**). Uncommon clinical variations include an onset of glaucoma many years after capsular disruption or after a spontaneous rupture in the lens capsule. The latter condition may be hard to distinguish from phacolytic glaucoma, although cases of lens particle glaucoma tend to have a greater inflammatory component, often associated with posterior and anterior synechiae and inflammatory pupillary membranes (35).

Theories of Mechanism

Perfusion studies with enucleated human eyes have demonstrated that small amounts of free particulate lens material significantly reduce outflow (33). This is presumed to be the principal mechanism of trabecular meshwork obstruction in cases of lens particle glaucoma. However, the associated inflammation, whether in response to the surgery, trauma, or retained lens material, may contribute to the glaucoma in this condition.

Differential Diagnosis

In its typical form, lens particle glaucoma is usually easy to diagnose on the basis of history and physical findings. In atypical forms, such as delayed onset or spontaneous capsule rupture, the condition might be confused with phacoanaphylaxis,

phacolytic glaucoma, or uveitic conditions with associated open-angle glaucoma. When doubt exists, microscopic examination of aqueous from an anterior chamber tap may help to diagnose lens particle glaucoma by demonstrating leukocytes and macrophages along with lens cortical material (35).

Management

In some cases, the IOP is possible to control medically with drugs that reduce aqueous production. Because inflammation is also present, the pupil should be dilated and topical steroids used, although it may be advisable to use the latter only in moderate amounts because steroid therapy may delay absorption of the lens material (35). The IOP usually returns to normal after the lens material has been absorbed. When the IOP cannot be adequately controlled medically, the residual lens material should be surgically removed by irrigation if the material is loose or with vitrectomy instruments when it is adherent to ocular structures.

Phacoanaphylaxis

Terminology

In 1922, Verhoeff and Lemoine (49) reported that a few individuals were hypersensitive to lens protein and that rupture of the lens capsule in these cases led to an intraocular inflammation, which they called endophthalmitis phacoanaphylactica. Although such cases are apparently rare, evidence shows that a true phacoanaphylaxis does occur in response to lens protein antigen (50), with subsequent inflammation and occasional open-angle glaucoma.

Clinical Features

As in the case of lens particle glaucoma, a preceding disruption of the lens capsule by extracapsular cataract surgery or penetrating injury usually occurs (51). The distinguishing feature, however, is a latent period during which sensitization to lens protein occurs. A particularly likely setting for the development of phacoanaphylaxis is when lens material, especially the nucleus, is retained in the vitreous. The typical physical finding is a chronic, relentless, granulomatous-type inflammation that centers on lens material in the primarily involved eye or in the fellow eye after it has undergone extracapsular cataract surgery or phacoemulsification. Associated glaucoma is only rarely a feature of phacoanaphylaxis.

Theories of Mechanism

It has been demonstrated in rabbits that autologous lens protein is antigenic (50), and the lens capsule was assumed to isolate the lenticular antigens from the immune response, with sensitization occurring only when the capsule is violated. This concept was not supported by human studies, which failed to demonstrate lens antibodies after injury to the lens and showed an equal incidence of antibody in patients with cataracts and controls (52). The same study did show a higher prevalence of antibodies in a small group with hypermature cataracts and more frequent postoperative uveitis in patients with antibodies in preoperative blood specimens, although the latter observation was not statistically significant. In the rabbit study, considerable variation in the response to autologous lens antigen was observed, which may explain the infrequency with which phacoanaphylaxis is seen clinically (50). The cellular appearance of the immune response is characterized by polymorphonuclear leukocytes and lymphoid, epithelioid, and giant cells, usually around a nidus of lens material. The occasional glaucoma in phacoanaphylaxis may be related to the accumulation of these cells in the trabecular meshwork, although lens protein or particles may also be present and could account for the glaucoma.

Differential Diagnosis

Other chronic forms of uveitis, especially sympathetic ophthalmia, may occur in association with phacoanaphylaxis. Phacolytic and lens particle glaucomas must also be considered. Microscopic examination of the aqueous may be helpful, although variations in cytology have not been fully studied in this condition and the diagnosis may require histologic examination of the surgically removed lens material.

Management

Steroid therapy should be used to control the uveitis, with antiglaucoma medication administered as required. When medical measures are inadequate, the retained lens material should be surgically removed.

Intumescent Lens Phacomorphic Glaucoma

In some eyes with advanced cataract formation, the lens may become swollen or intumescent, with progressive reduction in the anterior chamber angle eventually leading to a form of angle-closure glaucoma (**Fig. 18.10**). This condition has been referred to as phacomorphic glaucoma (53). The angle closure may be caused by an enhanced pupillary block mechanism or by forward displacement of the lens–iris diaphragm. In either case, the condition is usually diagnosed by observing a mature, intumescent cataract associated with a central anterior chamber depth that is significantly shallower than that of the fellow eye. The treatment is initial medical reduction of the IOP with hyperosmotics, carbonic anhydrase inhibitors, and topical β-blockers or α2-agonists, followed by extraction of the cataract (54). However, in a small study of patients with phacomorphic glaucoma, the acute angle-closure glaucoma attack was relieved in all cases by laser iridotomy (55), which may help to bring the pressure under control before proceeding with cataract surgery. If the mechanism of glaucoma is felt to be partly related to chronic angle closure with formation of peripheral anterior synechiae, goniosynechialysis in conjunction with cataract extraction can be considered.

KEY POINTS

- The lens may be associated with glaucoma when it is dislocated, which may occur with trauma or certain inherited disorders, such as Marfan syndrome, homocystinuria, and Weill–Marchesani syndrome.
- Mechanisms by which a dislocated lens may be associated with glaucoma include pupillary block, degenerative changes of the lens, and concomitant damage of the anterior chamber angle.
- A cataractous lens may also lead to glaucoma by obstruction of the trabecular meshwork with lens protein and macrophages (i.e., phacolytic glaucoma), lens particles and debris (i.e., lens particle glaucoma), or inflammatory cells as part of an immune response (i.e., phacoanaphylaxis). An intumescent lens may lead to pupillary block and secondary angle-closure glaucoma.

REFERENCES

1. Chandler PA. Choice of treatment in dislocation of the lens. *Arch Ophthalmol.* 1964;71:765–786.
2. Jarrett WH. Dislocation of the lens: a study of 166 hospitalized cases. *Arch Ophthalmol.* 1967;78:289–296.
3. Nelson LB, Maumenee IH. Ectopia lentis. *Surv Ophthalmol.* 1982;27:143–160.
4. Goldberg MF. Clinical manifestations of ectopia lentis et pupillae in 16 patients. *Ophthalmology.* 1988;95:1080–1087.
5. Byles DB, Nischal KK, Cheng H. Ectopia lentis et pupillae: a hypothesis revisited. *Ophthalmology.* 1998;105:1331–1336.
6. Seefelder R. Anatomischer Befund in einem Falle von angeborener Ektopie der Pupille mit Linsenluxation. *Z Augenheilkd.* 1911;25:353–361.
7. Fuchs E. ber flchenhafte Wucherung des ziliaren Epithels, nebst Bemerkungen über Ektopie der Linse. *Klin Monatsbl Augenheilkd.* 1920;64:1.
8. Zeeman WPC. ber Ectopia pupillae et lentis congenita. *Klin Monatsbl Augenheilkd.* 1925;74:325–338.
9. Tsipouras P, Del Mastro R, Sarfarazi M, et al. Genetic linkage of the Marfan syndrome, ectopia lentis, and congenital contractural arachnodactyly to the fibrillin genes on chromosomes 15 and 5. *N Engl J Med.* 1992;326:905–909.
10. Maumenee IH. The eye in the Marfan syndrome. *Trans Am Ophthalmol Soc.* 1981;79:684–733.
11. Challa P, Hauser M, Luna C, et al. Juvenile bilateral lens dislocation and glaucoma associated with a novel mutation in fibrillin 1 gene. *Mol Vis.* 2006;12:1009–1015.
12. Izquierdo NJ, Traboulsi EI, Enger C, et al. Glaucoma in the Marfan syndrome. *Trans Am Ophthalmol Soc.* 1992;90:111–117.
13. Cross HE, Jensen AD. Ocular manifestations in the Marfan syndrome and homocystinuria. *Am J Ophthalmol.* 1973;75:405–420.

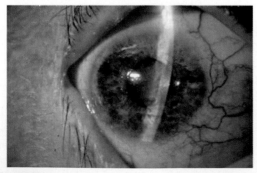

Figure 18.10 Phacomorphic glaucoma caused by an intumescent lens in an older adult. Note the extremely shallow anterior chamber centrally and peripherally. (From Mandelcorn E, Gupta N. Lens-related glaucomas. In: Tasman W, Jaeger EA, eds. *Duane's Clinical Ophthalmology.* Vol 3. Philadelphia, PA: Lippincott Williams & Wilkins, 2009:chap 54A.)

14. Burke JP, O'Keefe M, Bowell R, et al. Ocular complications in homocystinuria—early and late treated. *Br J Ophthalmol.* 1989;73:427–431.

15. Harrison DA, Mullaney PB, Mesfer SA, et al. Management of ophthalmic complications of homocystinuria. *Ophthalmology.* 1998;105:1886–1890.

16. Weill G. Ectopie des cristallins et malformations générales. *Ann Ocul (Paris).* 1932;169:21–44.

17. Marchesani O. Brachydaktylie und angeborene Kugellinse als Systemerkrankung. *Klin Monatsbl Augenheilkd.* 1939;103:392–406.

18. Jensen AD, Cross HE, Patton D. Ocular complications in the Weill–Marchesani syndrome. *Am J Ophthalmol.* 1974;77:261–269.

19. Dietlein TS, Jacobi PC, Krieglstein GK. Ciliary body is not hyperplastic in Weill–Marchesani syndrome. *Acta Ophthalmol Scand.* 1998; 76:623–624.

20. Fujiwara H, Takigawa Y, Ueno S, et al. Histology of the lens in the Weill–Marchesani syndrome. *Br J Ophthalmol.* 1990;74:631–634.

21. Wright KW, Chrousos GA. Weill–Marchesani syndrome with bilateral angle-closure glaucoma. *J Pediatr Ophthalmol Strabismus.* 1985;22: 129–132.

22. Ritch R, Solomon LD. Argon laser peripheral iridoplasty for angle-closure glaucoma in siblings with Weill–Marchesani syndrome. *J Glaucoma.* 1992;1:243–247.

23. Pavlin CJ, Buys YM, Pathmanatham T. Imaging zonular abnormalities using ultrasound biomicroscopy. *Arch Opthalmol.* 1998;116:854–857.

24. Pollard ZF. Phacolytic glaucoma secondary to ectopia lentis. *Ann Ophthalmol.* 1975;7:999–1001.

25. Friberg TR. Retinal perivasculitis in phacolytic glaucoma. *Am J Ophthalmol.* 1981;91:761–763.

26. Jay B. Glaucoma associated with spontaneous displacement of the lens. *Br J Ophthalmol.* 1972;56:258–262.

27. Ritch R, Wand M. Treatment of the Weill–Marchesani syndrome. *Ann Ophthalmol.* 1981;13:665–667.

28. Chandler PA. Completely dislocated hypermature cataract and glaucoma. *Trans Am Ophthalmol Soc.* 1959;57:242–253.

29. Gifford H. Danger of the spontaneous cure of senile cataracts. *Am J Ophthalmol.* 1900;17:289–293.

30. Zeeman WPC. Zwei Falle von Glaucoma phacogeneticum mit anatomischem Befund. *Ophthalmologica.* 1943;106:136–142.

31. Irvine SR, Irvine AR Jr. Lens-induced uveitis and glaucoma. Part III. "Phacogenetic glaucoma": lens-induced glaucoma; mature or hypermature cataract; open iridocorneal angle. *Am J Ophthalmol.* 1952;35:489–499.

32. Flocks M, Littwin CS, Zimmerman LE. Phacolytic glaucoma: a clinicopathologic study of one hundred thirty-eight cases of glaucoma associated with hypermature cataract. *Arch Ophthalmol.* 1955;54:37–45.

33. Epstein DL, Jedziniak JA, Grant WM. Obstruction of aqueous outflow by lens particles and by heavy-molecular-weight soluble lens proteins. *Invest Ophthalmol Vis Sci.* 1978;17:272–277.

34. Epstein DL, Jedziniak JA, Grant WM. Identification of heavy-molecular-weight soluble protein in aqueous humor in human phacolytic glaucoma. *Invest Ophthalmol Vis Sci.* 1978;17:398–402.

35. Epstein DL. Diagnosis and management of lens-induced glaucoma. *Ophthalmology.* 1982;89:227–230.

36. Bartholomew RS, Rebello PF. Calcium oxalate crystals in the aqueous. *Am J Ophthalmol.* 1979;88:1026–1028.

37. Brooks AMV, Grant G, Gillies WE. Comparison of specular microscopy and examination of aspirate in phacolytic glaucoma. *Ophthalmology.* 1990;97:85–89.

38. Brooks AMV, Drewe RH, Grant GB, et al. Crystalline nature of the iridescent particles in hypermature cataracts. *Br J Ophthalmol.* 1994; 78:581–582.

39. Thomas R, Braganza A, George T, et al. Vitreous opacities in phacolytic glaucoma. *Ophthalmic Surg Lasers.* 1996;27:839–843.

40. Goldberg MF. Cytological diagnosis of phacolytic glaucoma utilizing Millipore filtration of the aqueous. *Br J Ophthalmol.* 1967;51:847–853.

41. Tomita G, Watanabe K, Funahashi M, et al. Lens induced glaucoma—histopathological study of the filtrating angle. *Folia Ophthalmol Jpn.* 1984;35:1345.

42. Ueno H, Tamai A, Iyota K, et al. Electron microscopic observation of the cells floating in the anterior chamber in a case of phacolytic glaucoma. *Jpn J Ophthalmol.* 1989;33:103–113.

43. Yanoff M, Scheie HG. Cytology of human lens aspirate: its relationship to phacolytic glaucoma and phacoanaphylactic endophthalmitis. *Arch Ophthalmol.* 1968;80:166–170.

44. Jedziniak JA, Kinoshita JH, Yates EM, et al. On the presence and mechanism of formation of heavy molecular weight aggregates in human normal and cataractous lenses. *Exp Eye Res.* 1973;15:185–192.

45. Chandler PA. Problems in the diagnosis and treatment of lens-induced uveitis and glaucoma. *Arch Ophthalmol.* 1958;60:828–841.

46. Braganza A, Thomas R, George T, et al. Management of phacolytic glaucoma: experience of 135 cases. *Indian J Ophthalmol.* 1998;46:139–143.

47. Mandal AK, Gothwal VK. Intraocular pressure control and visual outcome in patients with phacolytic glaucoma managed by extracapsular cataract extraction with or without posterior chamber intraocular lens implantation. *Ophthalmic Surg Lasers.* 1998;29:880–889.

48. Muller H. Phacolytic glaucoma and phacogenic ophthalmia (lens-induced uveitis). *Trans Ophthalmol Soc U K.* 1963;83:689–704.

49. Verhoeff FH, Lemoine AN. Endophthalmitis phacoanaphylactica. In: *Transactions of the International Congress of Ophthalmologists.* Washington, DC: William F Fell; 1922:234.

50. Rahi AHS, Misra RN, Morgan G. Immunopathology of the lens. III. Humoral and cellular immune responses to autologous lens antigens and their roles in ocular inflammation. *Br J Ophthalmol.* 1977;61:371–379.

51. Perlman EM, Albert DM. Clinically unsuspected phacoanaphylaxis after ocular trauma. *Arch Ophthalmol.* 1977;95:244–246.

52. Nissen SH, Andersen P, Andersen HMK. Antibodies to lens antigens in cataract and after cataract surgery. *Br J Ophthalmol.* 1981;65:63–66.

53. Duke-Elder S. *System of Ophthalmology.* Vol II. London: Henry Kimpton; 1969:662.

54. Prajna NV, Ramakrishnan R, Krishnadas R, et al. Lens induced glaucomas—visual results and risk factors for final visual acuity. *Indian J Ophthalmol.* 1996;44:149–155.

55. Tomey KF, Al-Rajhi AA. Neodymium: YAG laser iridotomy in the initial management of phacomorphic glaucoma. *Ophthalmology.* 1992;99:660–665.

19

Glaucomas Associated with Disorders of the Retina, Vitreous, and Choroid

Several types of glaucoma are associated with diseases of the retina. The most common of these is neovascular glaucoma, which is usually associated with one of several retinal disorders, although some cases are associated with other ocular or extraocular conditions. Retinal detachments and a variety of less common disorders of the retina, vitreous, or choroid may cause or occur in association with various forms of glaucoma.

NEOVASCULAR GLAUCOMA

Terminology

In 1906, Coats (1) described new vessel formation on the iris in eyes with central retinal vein occlusion. This neovascularization of the iris is commonly known as rubeosis iridis and is now recognized as a complication of many diseases of the retina and other ocular and extraocular disorders. Rubeosis iridis is frequently associated with a severe form of glaucoma, which has been given different names on the basis of various clinical features: hemorrhagic glaucoma, referring to the hyphema that is present in some cases; congestive glaucoma, describing the frequently acute nature of the condition; and thrombotic glaucoma, implying an underlying vascular thrombotic cause. However, none of these terms accurately describes the glaucoma in all cases, and more nonspecific names are preferable, such as rubeotic glaucoma or neovascular glaucoma, which was proposed by Weiss and colleagues and is the term found most often in the current literature (2,3).

Factors Predisposing to Rubeosis Iridis

Most cases of rubeosis iridis are preceded by hypoxic disease of the retina. Diabetic retinopathy, central retinal vein occlusion, and carotid ischemic disease are the most common causes (4). However, many additional retinal diseases and certain other ocular or extraocular disorders have been recognized, resulting in a long list of conditions that may predispose to rubeosis iridis (**Table 19.1**).

Diabetic Retinopathy

Approximately one third of patients with rubeosis iridis have diabetic retinopathy. Tight metabolic control of blood glucose results in delayed onset of diabetic retinopathy and slows or prevents progression to nonproliferative and proliferative retinopathy (5). The frequency with which rubeosis iridis is associated with diabetic retinopathy is greatly influenced by surgical interventions. After pars plana vitrectomy for diabetic

retinopathy, the reported incidence of rubeosis iridis ranges from 25% to 42%, whereas that for neovascular glaucoma ranges from 10% to 23% (6–8), with most of these cases developing during the first 6 months after surgery (9). In these cases, rubeosis iridis and neovascular glaucoma occur more often in aphakic eyes (7,8,10). In one series, vitreous cavity lavage of hemorrhage after pars plana vitrectomy for diabetic retinopathy was associated with rubeosis iridis in 76% of aphakic eyes and 14% of phakic eyes (10). Postoperative neovascular glaucoma is also more common when rubeosis iridis is present before vitrectomy (11).

An unrepaired retinal detachment after vitrectomy for diabetic retinopathy is also a risk factor for postoperative rubeosis iridis. The acute onset or exacerbation of rubeosis iridis after diabetic vitrectomy can indicate the presence of a peripheral traction retinal detachment (12). Successful surgical reattachment of the retina during vitrectomy for diabetic retinopathy often leads to regression of preoperative rubeosis iridis, especially in phakic patients (13). A completely attached retina and aggressive anterior or peripheral photocoagulation therapy are the most important factors in controlling or preventing neovascular glaucoma after vitrectomy for proliferative diabetic retinopathy (12,14). Intraocular silicone oil also reduces the incidence of anterior segment neovascularization, possibly by acting as a diffusion or convection barrier to the posterior movement of oxygen from the anterior chamber or the anterior movement of an angiogenesis factor (15).

Nonproliferative and preproliferative diabetic retinopathy may progress after cataract surgery (4). Intracapsular cataract surgery alone in eyes with diabetic retinopathy has been associated with an increased incidence of postoperative rubeosis iridis and neovascular glaucoma. The incidence is similar with extracapsular extraction and a primary capsulotomy. Leaving the posterior capsule intact appears to reduce the likelihood of this complication, although a subsequent laser capsulotomy in patients with diabetes may lead to neovascular glaucoma.

Retinal Vascular Occlusive Disorders

Central retinal vein occlusion accounted for 28% of all cases of rubeosis iridis in one series (16). Elevated intraocular pressure (IOP), with or without glaucomatous damage, is thought by most (17–19) investigators to be a predisposing factor for retinal vein occlusion. Optic disc cupping was reported to be a significant risk factor for central and branch retinal vein occlusions in the Beaver Dam Eye Study (20). Other risk factors for central or branch retinal vein occlusion include systemic hypertension, diabetes, and male sex (19). Retinal vein occlusion may occur in a

Table 19.1	**Conditions Predisposing to Rubeosis Iridis and Neovascular Glaucoma**

RETINAL ISCHEMIC DISEASE

Diabetic retinopathy
Central retinal vein occlusion
Central retinal artery occlusion
Branch retinal vein occlusion
Branch retinal artery occlusion
Retinal detachment
Hemorrhagic retinal disorders
Coat exudative retinopathy
Eales disease
Leber congenital amaurosis
Retinopathy of prematurity
Persistent hyperplastic primary vitreous
Sickle-cell retinopathy
Syphilitic retinal vasculitis
Retinoschisis
Stickler syndrome (inherited vitreoretinal degeneration)
Optic nerve glioma with subsequent venous stasis retinopathy

IRRADIATION

Photoradiation
External beam
Charged particle: proton, helium ion radiation
Plaques

TUMORS

Choroidal melanoma
Ring melanoma of the ciliary body
Iris melanoma
Retinoblastoma
Large-cell lymphoma

INFLAMMATORY DISEASES

Uveitis: chronic iridocyclitis, Behçet disease
Vogt–Koyanagi–Harada syndrome
Sympathetic ophthalmia
Endophthalmitis
Crohn disease with retinal vasculitis

SURGICAL CAUSES

Carotid endarterectomy
Cataract extraction
Pars plana vitrectomy or lensectomy
Nd:YAG capsulotomy
Laser coreoplasty

EXTRAOCULAR VASCULAR DISORDERS

Carotid artery obstructive disease
Carotid–cavernous fistula
Internal carotid artery occlusion

Adapted from Sivak-Callcott JA, O'Day DM, Gass DM, et al. Evidence-based recommendations for the diagnosis and treatment of neovascular glaucoma. *Ophthalmology.* 2001;108:1767–1778.

wide range of ages (14 to 92 years in one large study, although 51% of these patients were 65 years or older) (21).

Rubeosis iridis and neovascular glaucoma are associated with central retinal artery occlusion, and they are less commonly associated with central vein occlusion. In two series of patients with central retinal artery occlusion, the incidence of rubeosis iridis was 16.67% and 18.2%, respectively (22,23). Patients who develop neovascular glaucoma in association with central retinal artery occlusion are usually elderly with severe carotid artery disease and atherosclerosis, which may be predisposing factors for retinal artery occlusion and, in some cases, ocular neovascularization (24,25). Branch retinal vein occlusion may rarely cause rubeosis iridis and neovascular glaucoma (16). Branch retinal artery occlusion has also been reported as a rare cause of rubeosis iridis (25,26), although the association with neovascular glaucoma is uncertain.

Other Retinal Disorders

Rubeosis iridis may be associated with a rhegmatogenous retinal detachment (27), especially when complicated by proliferative vitreoretinopathy (28). In some cases, the detachment may overlie a choroidal melanoma. A chronic retinal detachment with associated glaucoma should always raise the suspicion of melanoma. Neovascular glaucoma may also be associated with sickle-cell retinopathy and many other retinal disorders, which are listed in Table 19.1.

Other Ocular Disorders

Uveitis was present in 11% of rubeotic eyes in one series and in 1.5% of another study (16,29). An iris melanoma has also been associated with neovascular glaucoma, which resolved after the tumor was excised (30). End-stage glaucoma (open-angle or angle-closure) has been said to give rise to rubeosis iridis (16), which may be related to associated central retinal vein occlusion.

Extraocular Vascular Disorders

Carotid artery obstructive disease is probably the third most common cause of neovascular glaucoma, accounting for 13% of all cases in one series (29). These eyes may initially be normotensive or even hypotensive as a result of decreased perfusion of the ciliary body with reduced aqueous production, and fluorescein angiography may reveal an increased arm-to-retina time and leakage from the major retinal arterioles. A carotid–cavernous fistula may also cause rubeosis iridis and neovascular glaucoma as a result of decreased arterial flow and subsequent reduction in the ocular perfusion pressure, which may occur before or after treatment of the fistula (31,32). Internal carotid artery occlusion may create an ophthalmic artery steal phenomenon with associated rubeosis iridis (33).

Theories of Neovasculogenesis

The mechanisms by which the aforementioned clinical situations lead to rubeosis iridis are not fully understood, although the following theories have been proposed (4).

Retinal Hypoxia

Because most of the conditions associated with rubeosis iridis involve diminished perfusion of the retina, retinal hypoxia may be one factor in the formation of new vessels on the iris and anterior chamber angle and on the retina and optic nerve head. This concept is supported by the clinical observation that rubeosis iridis in association with proliferative diabetic retinopathy or central retinal vein occlusion is more likely to occur when significant capillary nonperfusion is present.

Angiogenesis Factors

The existence of an angiogenic substance regulating normal development of retinal blood vessels was hypothesized in 1948 (34). It has since been demonstrated that tumors possess a diffusible factor, tumor angiogenesis factor, that can elicit new vessel growth toward the tumor (35). Subsequent studies have suggested that human and animal retinas and other vascular ocular tissues have similar angiogenic activity related to a key angiogenic peptide, vascular endothelial growth factor (VEGF), which explains why ocular neovascularization can occur in areas remote from the site of retinal capillary nonperfusion. Several cell types in the retina synthesize VEGF, but under conditions of retinal ischemia, Müller cells appear to be the primary source. Four VEGF isoforms ($VEGF_{121}$, $VEGF_{165}$, $VEGF_{189}$, and $VEGF_{206}$) have been identified, which are generated by alternative mRNA splicing from the same gene (36). $VEGF_{165}$ is the most abundant form in the majority of tissues. VEGF is a potent angiogenic stimulator, promoting several steps of angiogenesis, including proliferation, migration, proteolytic activity, and capillary tube formation, thus playing a crucial role in both normal and pathologic angiogenesis. It is also known as a vascular permeability factor on the basis of its ability to induce vascular hyperpermeability and endothelial cell proliferation as well as migration.

Vasoinhibitory Factors

It has been postulated that ocular tissues may produce substances that inhibit neovascularization. The vitreous and lens are possible sources of these vasoinhibitory factors (37,38), which could explain why vitrectomy or lensectomy increases the risk for rubeosis iridis in eyes with diabetic retinopathy. Retinal pigment epithelial cells release an inhibitor of neovascularization (39).

Clinicopathologic Course

The clinical and histologic events that lead from a predisposing factor through rubeosis iridis to advanced neovascular glaucoma may be thought of in four stages (**Fig. 19.1**).

Prerubeosis Stage

In patients with a predisposing factor, such as diabetic retinopathy or central retinal vein occlusion, it is helpful to understand what the likelihood is for development of rubeosis iridis and what the chances are for progression to neovascular glaucoma. Additional circumstances, especially with the two mentioned predisposing factors, may increase the risk for neovascular glaucoma to the extent that treatment may be indicated even before rubeosis is detected.

Diabetic Retinopathy

The prevalence of rubeosis iridis among patients with diabetes mellitus ranges from 0.25% to 20% according to various reports (40). Diabetes usually exists for many years before rubeosis develops, and concomitant proliferative diabetic retinopathy is usually found. In populations of patients with proliferative diabetic retinopathy, rubeosis iridis is reported to occur in approximately one-half of the cases (40,41). Rubeosis iridis may rarely occur in an eye with nonproliferative retinopathy (40), although other predisposing factors, such as carotid artery disease, should be considered in these cases.

The risk for rubeosis iridis and neovascular glaucoma in patients with diabetic retinopathy is greatly increased when arteriolar or capillary nonperfusion is present or after vitrectomy or lensectomy. There is also a highly significant correlation between rubeosis iridis and optic disc neovascularization (42) as well as a rhegmatogenous retinal detachment (13,14). The demonstration of peripupillary leakage by iris fluorescein angiography correlates with the presence of abnormal iris vessels and the risk for rubeosis iridis after vitrectomy for diabetic retinopathy (**Fig. 19.2**). Slit-lamp biomicroscopy is less reliable than angiography in detecting the presence of diabetic iris lesions (43). It is important to pay close attention to the pupillary margin of the iris, where neovascularization is typically seen first (44), when looking for the earliest biomicroscopic evidence of anterior segment rubeosis. However, gonioscopy is also important, because angle neovascularization may occasionally precede that of the iris (45).

Central Retinal Vein Occlusion

During the early months after a central retinal vein occlusion, hypotony may develop (46). The explanation for this is unclear, although the possible influences of anterior segment ischemia or an angiogenic factor have been proposed.

As in diabetic retinopathy, the incidence of rubeosis iridis and neovascular glaucoma in eyes with central retinal vein occlusion is significantly correlated with the extent of retinal capillary nonperfusion. In one study, the incidence of rubeosis iridis after central retinal vein occlusion was 60% when retinal ischemia was demonstrated by fluorescein angiography, compared with 1% in eyes with good capillary perfusion (47).

Fluorescein angiography is the most direct method of evaluating capillary nonperfusion but is not always feasible because of obstruction of visualization by blood or other media opacities. The ophthalmoscopic findings may be helpful in determining the risk for neovascular glaucoma, which has been reported in 14% to 27% of eyes with hemorrhagic retinopathy (complete venous occlusion) but in no cases of venous stasis retinopathy (incomplete occlusion) (48,49). Several other techniques have predictive value. Fluorescein angiography of the iris reveals abnormal, leaking vessels in virtually all eyes with extensive retinal capillary closure after central retinal vein occlusion (50). Aqueous protein and cell concentrations, as indicated by a laser flare–cell meter, have been shown to correlate with fluorescein angiographic findings and the severity of retinal vein occlusion (51). A relative afferent

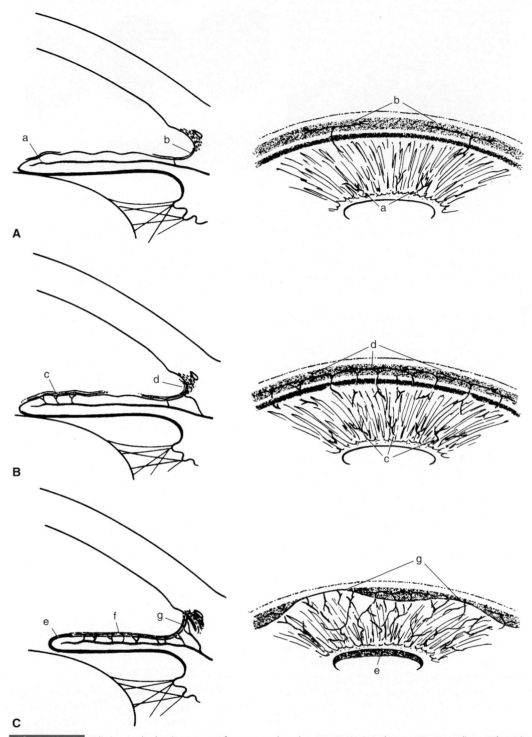

Figure 19.1 Clinicopathologic stages of neovascular glaucoma. **A:** Preglaucoma stage (i.e., rubeosis iridis), characterized by new vessels on the surface of the iris (*a*) and in the anterior chamber angle (*b*). **B:** Open-angle glaucoma stage, characterized by an increase in neovascularization and a fibrovascular membrane on the iris (*c*) and in the anterior chamber angle (*d*). **C:** Angle-closure glaucoma stage, characterized by contracture of the fibrovascular membrane, causing corectopia, ectropion uvea (*e*), flattening of the iris (*f*), and peripheral anterior synechiae (*g*).

pupillary defect also indicates an increased risk for rubeosis iridis after central retinal vein occlusion (52), and infrared pupillometry is an objective method of documenting this finding (53). Electroretinography also has useful predictive value (54). The most diagnostic findings include a B-wave implicit time delay and a reduced B-wave–A-wave amplitude ratio. Flicker electroretinography also has diagnostic value (55). Blood-flow velocities of the central retinal vein and artery can be measured with color Doppler imaging and provide a high degree of predictability regarding the risk for iris neovascularization (56).

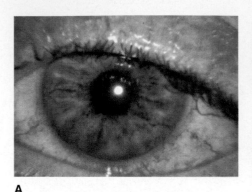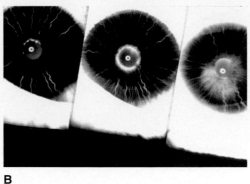

A   **B**

Figure 19.2   **A:** Slitlamp view of a diabetic patient with neovascular glaucoma. Neovascularization of the iris is seen through the edematous cornea that is secondary to uncontrolled IOP. **B:** Fluorescein angiographic view of another patient demonstrates fluorescein leakage along the superior papillary margin. In subsequent frames, the area of fluorescein leakage enlarges. (From Reiss GR, Sipperley JO. Glaucoma associated with retinal disorders and retinal surgery. In: Tasman W, Jaeger EA, eds. *Duane's Clinical Ophthalmology.* Vol. 3. Philadelphia, PA: Lippincott Williams & Wilkins:chap 54E.)

Despite evidence of good perfusion and a low risk for iris neovascularization by any of the noted techniques, all patients with central retinal vein occlusion should be followed for the possibility of rubeosis iridis and neovascular glaucoma. In some patients, perfused retinas will progress to nonperfusion. In one study, this was seen in 15% of cases (57). Time and age appear to influence this percentage. In one study, the cumulative probability of converting from nonischemic to ischemic central retinal vein occlusion in 6 and 18 months was 13.2% and 18.6%, respectively, in persons 65 years or older and 6.7% and 8.1%, respectively, in persons 45 to 64 years of age (21). The study also found that 83% of patients with indeterminate perfusion eventually developed nonperfusion or neovascularization of the iris or anterior chamber angle (58).

Preglaucoma Stage: Rubeosis Iridis

Clinical Features

The preglaucoma stage is characterized by a normal IOP, unless preexisting chronic open-angle glaucoma (COAG) is present. Slitlamp biomicroscopy early in the disease process typically reveals dilated tufts of preexisting capillaries and fine, randomly oriented vessels on the surface of the iris near the pupillary margin (**Fig. 19.3**). The new vessels are also characterized by leakage of fluorescein. Neovascularization in most cases is first seen on the peripupillary iris, although it may be first seen in the

anterior chamber angle in patients with diabetes and central retinal vein occlusion (45,59). Gonioscopy therefore may reveal a normal anterior chamber angle or may show a variable amount of angle neovascularization. The latter is characterized by single vascular trunks crossing the ciliary body band and scleral spur and arborizing on the trabecular meshwork.

Histopathologic Features

The rubeosis iridis begins intrastromally and then develops on the surface of the iris (37,60). Experimental retinal vein occlusion in monkey eyes indicates that the rubeosis iridis begins with dilatation of normal iris vessels and marked increase in metabolism of vascular endothelial cells followed by new vessel formation (61). Silicone-injection studies indicate that the new vessels on the iris arise from normal iris arteries and drain primarily into iris and ciliary body veins, whereas new vessels in the angle arise from arteries of the iris and ciliary body and connect with the peripheral neovascular network on the iris (62). Although the clinical appearance of rubeosis iridis is said to be the same in cases of diabetes and central retinal vein occlusion, the silicone injections show tighter and more evenly distributed neovascularization in the diabetic eye (62). The silicone-injection studies also show that new vessels in the angle run circumferentially in the trabecular meshwork, with branches coursing into the fibrosed Schlemm canal and occasionally into collector channels (62). The new vessels are characterized histologically as having thin fenestrated walls and are arranged in irregular patterns (60). The ultrastructure of iris neovascularization associated with sickle-cell retinopathy is said to be similar to that in diabetes and retinal occlusive disease with open interendothelial cell junctions, attenuated intraendothelial cytoplasm, and pericyte formation (63).

Open-Angle Glaucoma Stage

Clinical Features

Neovascular glaucoma does not invariably follow the development of rubeosis iridis (40,41,63,64), and the latter condition may rarely resolve spontaneously, especially that associated with diabetic retinopathy (40). The reported incidence of

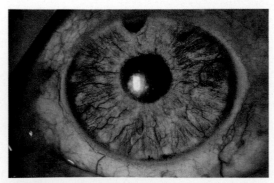

Figure 19.3   Slitlamp view of iris in a patient with rubeosis iridis shows tortuous vessels on the surface of the iris.

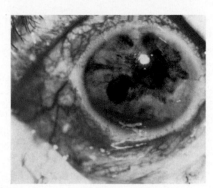

Figure 19.4 Slitlamp appearance of the iris in a patient with neovascular glaucoma shows marked rubeosis and hyphema.

neovascular glaucoma in diabetic patients with rubeosis iridis ranges from 13% to 41% (40,41,64), whereas that associated with central retinal vein occlusion is probably significantly higher. The latter condition typically occurs 8 to 15 weeks after the vascular occlusive event (63). It has been called 90-day glaucoma because the average time interval was thought to be 3 months. However, the glaucoma can develop during the first month or any time after a central retinal vein occlusion.

The rubeosis iridis is typically more florid in this stage, and biomicroscopic examination of the aqueous often reveals an inflammatory reaction and sometimes a hyphema (**Fig. 19.4**). By gonioscopy, the anterior chamber angle is still open, but the neovascularization may be intense (**Fig. 19.5**). The IOP is elevated and may rise suddenly, causing the patient to present with acute-onset glaucoma.

Histopathologic Features

The hallmark of the open-angle glaucoma stage is a fibrovascular membrane that covers the anterior chamber angle and anterior surface of the iris and may even extend onto the posterior iris (60,65). Chronic inflammatory changes are also typically seen on histologic examination (60,65). The glaucoma in this stage probably results from obstruction of the trabecular meshwork by the fibrovascular membrane, with variable contribution from the inflammation and hemorrhage. One histopathologic report of an eye with neovascular glaucoma and without a fibrovascular membrane covering the iridocorneal angle found that the spaces between the trabecular beams were lined by a single layer of vascular endothelium and were filled with red blood cells in this patient, suggesting that neovascular tissue found in the trabecular spaces might be one of the factors responsible for IOP elevation in eyes with neovascular glaucoma (66).

Angle-Closure Glaucoma Stage
Clinical Features

In the angle-closure glaucoma stage, the stroma of the iris has become flattened, with a smooth, glistening appearance. Ectropion uvea is frequently present, and the iris is often dilated and pulled anteriorly from the lens (**Fig. 19.6**). In the anterior chamber angle, the contracture leads to formation of peripheral anterior synechia, with eventual total synechial closure of the angle. The glaucoma in this stage is typically severe and usually requires surgical intervention.

Histopathologic Features

The clinically observed alterations of the iris and anterior chamber angle in this stage result from contracture of tissue overlying these structures. Histopathologic studies reveal peripheral anterior synechiae and flattening of the anterior iris surface by a confluent fibrovascular membrane (67,68). Overlying the new vessels is a clinically inapparent, superficial layer of myofibroblasts (i.e., fibroblastic cells with smooth-muscle differentiation), which may be responsible for the tissue contraction (67). A layer

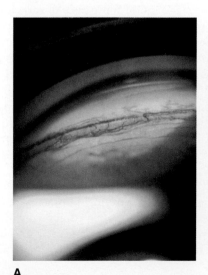

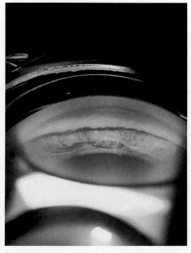

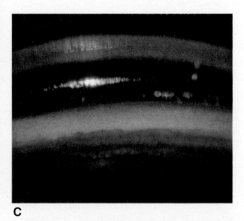

A   **B**   **C**

Figure 19.5 **A:** Angle neovascularization in a patient with a central retinal vein occlusion. Note vessels are superficial and found on the ciliary body band and trabecular meshwork. The angle is open although aqueous outflow is impaired. **B:** Neovascular glaucoma has progressed to angle closure in this patient. (A, B, courtesy of Joseph A. Halabis, OD.) **C:** A patient with open-angle neovascular glaucoma, with heavy neovascularization of the open angle. The angle, however, is beginning to close, as seen by the low synechia to the left of the view.

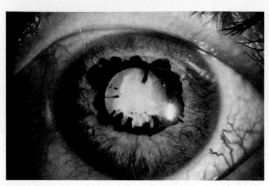

Figure 19.6 Slitlamp view of a patient with the angle-closure stage of neovascular glaucoma shows numerous new vessels on the iris, with pupillary dilatation and ectropion uvea due to contracture of the fibrovascular membrane.

of endothelium, continuous with the corneal endothelium at the pseudoangle, is also seen in some cases and has been observed to possess features of myoblastic differentiation (68,69), which may explain the origin of these cells.

Differential Diagnosis

In the open-angle stage, neovascular glaucoma must be distinguished from other glaucomas with acute onset, such as angle-closure glaucoma and glaucoma associated with anterior uveitis. This differentiation can usually be made on the basis of new vessels on the iris and in the anterior chamber angle with neovascular glaucoma, although eyes with uveitis often have dilatation of normal iris vessels that may be confused with neovascularization, especially with blue irides. Patients with Fuchs heterochromic iridocyclitis also typically have new vessels in the anterior chamber angle (see Chapter 22). In the angle-closure stage of neovascular glaucoma, the new vessels may be less apparent, and the differential diagnosis must include other causes of iris distortion and peripheral anterior synechiae, such as the iridocorneal endothelial syndrome (see Chapter 16) and old trauma (see Chapter 25).

Management

Panretinal Photocoagulation

Ablation of the peripheral retina with laser (usually argon) photocoagulation is the first line of therapy for most cases of neovascular glaucoma. This procedure has been shown to significantly reduce or eliminate anterior segment neovascularization in many cases and to reduce the chances of developing rubeosis iridis in eyes with diabetic retinopathy or central retinal vein occlusion (47,64,70–79). The mechanism by which panretinal photocoagulation influences neovascularization is uncertain, although it may be related to decreasing the retinal oxygen demand, which is consistent with the reported observation that the photoreceptor–retinal pigment epithelial complex accounts for two thirds of the total retinal oxygen consumption (80). This may reduce the stimulus for release of an angiogenesis factor or may reduce the hypoxia in the anterior ocular segment. However, in 27 eyes with ischemic central

retinal vein occlusion treated with panretinal photocoagulation, 5 developed posterior neovascularization, which had not been present preoperatively, suggesting that photocoagulation does not always eliminate retinal ischemia (81).

Prophylactic Therapy

Panretinal photocoagulation is most effective as prophylaxis against the development of neovascular glaucoma. It was once thought by some surgeons that photocoagulation should be performed during the prerubeosis stage in central retinal vein occlusion, if the risk for rubeosis iridis was sufficiently high. However, a multicenter, randomized clinical trial revealed that prophylactic photocoagulation does not totally prevent iris and angle neovascularization and that prompt regression of the rubeosis is more likely to occur in response to photocoagulation in eyes that have not been treated previously (82). With regard to central retinal vein occlusion, it is apparently better to follow patients closely and intervene promptly with panretinal photocoagulation at the early signs of rubeosis.

The risk for rubeosis iridis is more difficult to predict in eyes with diabetic retinopathy than in those with central retinal vein occlusion, but vitrectomy or lensectomy, especially in association with peripupillary fluorescein leakage, may be indications for prophylactic therapy. The latter is often performed as endophotocoagulation in conjunction with pars plana vitrectomy for diabetic retinopathy. By the time rubeosis iridis appears (preglaucoma stage), panretinal photocoagulation is indicated in all cases, including those resulting from central retinal artery occlusion and carotid artery insufficiency (83). Although neovascular glaucoma does not invariably follow rubeosis iridis, it does so with sufficient frequency that prophylactic laser therapy is justified in nearly all of these cases.

Treatment of Glaucoma

Panretinal photocoagulation may reverse IOP elevation in the open-angle glaucoma stage and in some cases of early angle-closure neovascular glaucoma, provided that the synechial closure has not exceeded 270 degrees (70,71,73,84). Even in the latter situation, panretinal photocoagulation may be useful in reducing anterior segment neovascularization before intraocular surgery (85). However, one study showed that panretinal photocoagulation before vitrectomy for diabetic retinopathy did not prevent postoperative rubeosis iridis (86). In these cases, intraocular panretinal photocoagulation at the time of vitrectomy may be the procedure of choice (87).

Panretinal Cryotherapy

When cloudy media preclude panretinal photocoagulation, transscleral panretinal cryotherapy, often combined with cyclocryotherapy, in eyes with neovascular glaucoma can control the IOP and reduce or abolish the neovascularization (88,89).

Anti-VEGF Agents

Many case reports have attempted to ascertain the value of intraocular anti-VEGF therapy with bevacizumab as an adjunctive treatment of iris neovascularization associated with glaucoma (36). These reports in patients with either diabetes or central retinal vein occlusion and associated neovascular glaucoma involved injecting 1.25-mg bevacizumab in the vitreous cavity or 1.0- to 1.25-mg bevacizumab in the anterior chamber before or concomitant with panretinal photocoagulation. Virtually all treated eyes had significant regression of anterior segment neovascularization within 48 hours, many with a concomitant reduction in IOP. The injected medication was reported to be safe and well tolerated. The effect of bevacizumab lasted for a number of weeks, and thereafter, new vessel formation was noted to resume in some eyes. Hence, it is important to proceed with panretinal photocoagulation as soon as practical to help prevent recurrent neovascularization. Intraocular injections of bevacizumab can be repeated, but how often eyes can be reinjected remains to be determined (90).

Medical Management of Glaucoma and Inflammation

When the IOP begins to rise, medical therapy is usually required and is frequently sufficient to control the pressure during the open-angle glaucoma stage. The mainstay of the therapy at this stage is drugs that reduce aqueous production, such as carbonic anhydrase inhibitors, topical β-blockers, and α$_2$-agonists. Prostaglandin analogues are rarely effective because access to the uveoscleral route is generally compromised from angle closure, and there is a theoretical concern regarding exacerbation of inflammation. Miotics are not helpful in the acute situation and should usually be avoided because they may increase the inflammation and discomfort. Topical corticosteroids may be useful in minimizing the inflammation and pain (91). Intravitreal triamcinolone has reduced retinal neovascularization in rabbit eyes (92), raising the question of a possible direct benefit of topical steroids on rubeotic vessels. In far-advanced or blind eyes, atropine is helpful for relief of pain. Hyperosmotic agents may also be required for temporary control of cases with marked IOP elevation.

Glaucoma Surgical Procedures

Cyclodestructive Procedures

If the disease follows its natural course to the angle-closure glaucoma stage, medical therapy usually becomes ineffective and surgical intervention is required. Even at this stage, panretinal photocoagulation may be beneficial by reducing the anterior segment neovascularization to allow filtration surgery. With active rubeosis, however, standard filtering surgery has a low chance of success, and a cyclodestructive procedure may be preferable.

Although good results have been reported by some surgeons with the use of cyclocryotherapy for neovascular glaucoma (93,94), other reports have been less encouraging (95–97). In one 2-year follow-up of 50 eyes, one third were uncontrolled and one third developed phthisis (95). Alternative cyclodestructive procedures include transscleral Nd:YAG cyclophotocoagulation and diode laser cyclophotocoagulation (98). Preliminary experience suggests that diode laser cyclophotocoagulation provides less postoperative inflammation and

better IOP control than Nd:YAG cyclophotocoagulation and has become the surgical procedure of choice for neovascular glaucoma when filtering surgery is not thought to be indicated (99,100).

Filtering Surgery

It has been a general belief that standard filtering procedures in eyes with neovascular glaucoma are rarely successful, primarily because of the high risk for intraoperative bleeding and postoperative progression of the fibrovascular membrane. However, a successful panretinal photocoagulation, combined with anti-VEGF treatment, can reduce neovascularization sufficiently to make it possible to perform a standard filtering operation, such as trabeculectomy. In one study, the adjunctive use of 5-fluorouracil provided success rates of 71% and 67% in the first and second postoperative years, respectively, although this fell to 41% and 28% by the fourth and fifth years, respectively (101). In another study, the use of mitomycin C during trabeculectomy yielded success rates of 62.6%, 58.2%, and 51.7% at 1, 2, and 5 years, respectively. Younger age and previous vitrectomy were prognostic factors for surgical failure (102). Other techniques for filtering surgery in neovascular glaucoma that may be helpful include a modified trabeculectomy with intraocular bipolar cautery of peripheral iris and ciliary processes and creation of a small iridectomy or avoidance of an iridectomy if the chamber is deep and pupillary block is absent (103,104).

Glaucoma Drainage-Device Surgery

Encouraging results have been reported with the implantation of drainage tubes or valves into the anterior chamber and through the pars plana (when combined with a vitrectomy) in eyes with neovascular glaucoma (105–107). Adjunctive bevacizumab may improve the success of glaucoma drainage-device surgery in these eyes (108). (Details regarding the techniques and reported results of these procedures are considered in Section III.)

Other Surgical Procedures

Several other techniques have been evaluated for the treatment of neovascular glaucoma. Endoscopic cyclophotocoagulation (see Chapter 41) may be helpful in lowering IOP, particularly in eyes that have reasonable visual potential and are not good candidates for aqueous drainage procedures. Silicone oil injection during revision of vitrectomy after unsuccessful diabetic vitreous surgery achieved stabilization or regression of anterior ocular neovascular changes in 83% of eyes in one study (109). Intravitreal injection of crystalline triamcinolone acetonide has also been demonstrated to decrease the degree of rubeosis iridis in neovascular glaucoma attributable to peripheral diabetic retinopathy or central retinal vein occlusion (110). Exposure to 100% oxygen under hyperbaric conditions significantly increases the partial pressure of oxygen in the aqueous humor of animal eyes, a mechanism that may have an application in treating hypoxic diseases of the anterior segment, including rubeosis iridis (111).

ALTERATIONS OF IOP ASSOCIATED WITH RETINAL DETACHMENT

Reduced IOP and Retinal Detachment

An eye with a rhegmatogenous retinal detachment typically has a reduced IOP. Experimental studies with retinal detachments in monkeys suggest that an early, transient pressure drop may result from inflammation and reduced aqueous production (112), whereas more prolonged hypotony may be caused by posterior flow of aqueous through the retinal hole (113). A study with kinetic vitreous fluorophotometry indicated a posterior flow, presumably through a break in the retinal pigment epithelium, in patients with vitreous and rhegmatogenous retinal detachments (114). Campbell (115) described a condition, the iris retraction syndrome, in which a patient presents with a rhegmatogenous retinal detachment, a secluded pupil, and angle closure with iris bombé. Pharmacologic suppression of aqueous production in these individuals leads to hypotony and a posterior retraction of the iris, presumably due to a shift in the predominant direction of aqueous flow toward the subretinal space.

Glaucomas Associated with Retinal Detachment

The coexistence of glaucoma and a retinal detachment in the same eye occurs under three circumstances: (a) glaucoma associated with retinal detachment, for which a cause-and-effect relationship is uncertain; (b) glaucoma directly related to retinal detachment; and (c) glaucoma after treatment of retinal detachment. (The first two situations are discussed in this chapter, and the third is considered in Chapter 26.)

Chronic Open-Angle Glaucoma and Retinal Detachment

Epidemiology

COAG is more common in eyes with a rhegmatogenous retinal detachment than in the general population. In one study of 817 cases of retinal detachment, COAG was present in 4%, and an additional 6.5% had elevated IOP without glaucomatous damage (116).

Theories of Mechanism

It is not known why COAG and rhegmatogenous retinal detachment occur in the same eye more frequently than would be anticipated on the basis of chance occurrence. Neither myopia nor the use of miotics has been found to be the common denominator (116). In 30 cases of spontaneous rhegmatogenous retinal detachment, 53% had a cup-to-disc ratio greater than 0.3, and 20% were high topical steroid responders (117). These values are significantly higher than those in the general population and resemble the findings in groups of patients with COAG, which led investigators to suggest that the two diseases might be related genetically by multifactorial inheritance.

Management

When COAG and retinal detachment coexist, one disorder may mask the presence of the other, necessitating careful attention to certain details during the management of either condition. When following a patient with COAG, the peripheral retina should be examined before initiating therapy and at least annually or whenever warning signs appear, such as floaters, flashing lights, loss of peripheral vision, or a sudden decrease in the IOP. Although the role of miotics in the pathogenesis of rhegmatogenous retinal detachment has not been clearly established, circumstantial evidence indicates that particular caution is warranted when these drugs are used (118).

In an eye with a rhegmatogenous retinal detachment, the reduced IOP may mask a preexisting glaucoma. Applanation tonometry should be performed before and after retinal detachment surgery, and the optic nerve head should be carefully inspected during the fundus examination to avoid missing coexisting glaucoma.

The success of retinal detachment surgery is not adversely affected by the presence of glaucoma, although the visual outcome may be worse because of the concomitant glaucomatous optic atrophy (116,119). After retinal detachment surgery, particularly in nondiabetic patients, regression of iris neovascularization may occur (120). After surgery, special caution should be given to the use of topical steroids because of the increased incidence of high topical steroid responders (117), and miotics should be used with caution in either eye.

Pigmentary Glaucoma and Retinal Detachment

Patients with the pigment dispersion syndrome, with or without glaucoma, may have an increased incidence of retinal detachment. Patients with retinal detachment are reported to have various degrees of pigment dispersion in the anterior chamber angle in a significant number of cases (121). As in the case of COAG, no definite cause-and-effect relationship has been established, but the same considerations as mentioned earlier must be employed in the management of coexisting pigmentary glaucoma and retinal detachment.

Schwartz Syndrome

A rhegmatogenous retinal detachment is typically associated with a slight reduction in the IOP. However, Schwartz described a rare condition in which the patient presents with unilateral pressure elevation, a retinal detachment, and an open anterior chamber angle with aqueous cells and flare (122). The condition is generally known as Schwartz syndrome.

Theories of Mechanism

Photoreceptor outer segments with few inflammatory cells have been demonstrated by Matsuo and colleagues in the aqueous of patients with Schwartz syndrome (123), and the injection of rod outer segments into human autopsy and living cat eyes has been shown to significantly reduce outflow facility by obstructing the trabecular meshwork (124). Other mechanisms that have been considered include ocular trauma with concomitant damage to the trabecular meshwork, anterior uveitis from the retinal detachment and obstruction of the trabecular meshwork by pigment from the retinal pigment epithelium, or glycosaminoglycans from the visual cells (122,125,126).

Management

Treatment of rhegmatogenous retinal detachment and the associated glaucoma is repair of the detachment, which typically results in resolution of the glaucoma within a few days (122). In the differential diagnosis, it is important to remember that an eye with a retinal detachment and glaucoma may harbor a malignant melanoma.

Glaucoma Associated with Other Forms of Retinal Detachment

In addition to rhegmatogenous retinal detachment, several other forms of retinal detachment may be associated with glaucoma. These include traction detachments, as with proliferative diabetic retinopathy and retinopathy of prematurity (discussed in this chapter); exudative retinal detachments (see Chapter 22); and detachments associated with neoplasia, such as melanomas and retinoblastoma (see Chapter 21). Each of these conditions may lead to neovascular or angle-closure glaucoma.

ANGLE-CLOSURE GLAUCOMAS ASSOCIATED WITH DISORDERS OF THE RETINA, VITREOUS, AND CHOROID

Central Retinal Vein Occlusion

Neovascular glaucoma occurring after retinal vascular occlusive disease was discussed earlier in this chapter. A few cases have been described in which shallowing of the anterior chamber after a central retinal vein occlusion led to transient angle-closure glaucoma (127–130).

Examination typically reveals a forward shift of the lens–iris diaphragm in the involved eye and a normal anterior chamber depth in the fellow eye. The mechanism of the angle closure is uncertain, although it has been postulated that transudation of fluid from the retinal vessels into the vitreous leads to forward displacement of the lens with a subsequent pupillary block (128). The differential diagnosis should include pupillary block glaucoma, which may lead to occlusion of the central retinal vein, and neovascular glaucoma, which can cause synechial closure of the anterior chamber angle. The former situation may be recognized by a potentially occludable angle in the fellow eye, and the latter can usually be identified by the presence of rubeosis iridis.

Treatment should usually be medical, because the angle returns to normal depth over several weeks. In general, aqueous suppressants, such as topical or oral carbonic anhydrase inhibitors, topical β-blockers, and α₂-agonists, in conjunction with topical cycloplegic agents are generally effective (129).

Hemorrhagic Retinal or Choroidal Detachment

Acute angle-closure glaucoma may follow a spontaneous massive hemorrhagic retinal or choroidal detachment (131). The hemorrhagic detachment is typically caused by a disciform macular lesion, and associated conditions include systemic hypertension, primary clotting disorders, and the systemic use of anticoagulants and thrombolytic agents (131,132). The mechanism of the angle closure is thought to be the abrupt, forward displacement of the lens–iris diaphragm by the massively detached retina and choroid (131). Visual prognosis is poor in these eyes, and the management is directed primarily at relief of pain through IOP control with antiglaucoma medications or cyclodestructive surgery.

Hemorrhagic choroidal detachment may also occur during or after intraocular surgery, especially filtering surgery, with associated IOP elevation and flattening of the anterior chamber. (This is discussed in Section III as a complication of trabeculectomy.)

Ciliochoroidal Effusion

In the following conditions, uveal effusion with ciliochoroidal detachment may lead to a forward rotation of the lens–iris diaphragm and angle-closure glaucoma.

Nanophthalmos

Nanophthalmos is a rare inherited disorder characterized by a small eye with a small cornea, shallow anterior chamber, narrow angle, and high lens-to-eye volume ratio (133–135). The eyes are highly hyperopic because of the short axial length (<20 mm by most definitions) and frequently develop angle-closure glaucoma in the fourth to sixth decades of life. Additional reported retinal disorders include pigmentary retinal dystrophy and a family with pigmentary retinal degeneration and cystic macular degeneration in an autosomal recessive syndrome (136,137). Uveal effusion and nonrhegmatogenous retinal detachment may follow intraocular surgery in these cases (133–135,138). There is also evidence in some patients that the uveal effusion and retinal detachment may precede the surgery and cause the angle-closure glaucoma by producing a forward shift of the lens–iris diaphragm, leading to a pupillary block mechanism (139).

Histopathologic studies reveal an unusually thick sclera with irregular, interlacing collagen bundles, fraying of collagen fibrils, reduced levels of glycosaminoglycans, and elevated levels of fibronectin (140–143). Altered metabolism of glycosaminoglycans and fibronectin may be related to the development of abnormal sclera in nanophthalmos (140,141,143). Tissue culture studies of sclerocytes from a patient with nanophthalmos revealed modified glycosaminoglycan metabolism, which may contribute to the abnormal packing of collagen bundles and thickening of the sclera (144). Uveal effusion may be caused by reduced scleral permeability to proteins by the thickened sclera or compression of venous drainage channels by the dense collagen around the vortex veins (145,146). However, no collagen abnormality was seen in three patients of one study, leading the investigators to suggest that nanophthalmos may result from several distinct defects (142).

This form of glaucoma responds poorly to conventional surgical therapy and has a high complication rate that is associated primarily with the uveal effusion (134,138). Medical therapy may be effective, although miotics may increase the pupillary block (134). Laser iridectomy and laser gonioplasty (i.e., retraction of the peripheral iris) have the highest success rates and are the procedures of choice (134,139), although these are not uniformly successful. One suggested approach to managing the uveal effusion is to decompress the vortex veins by making large scleral flaps over the veins and, in some cases, draining choroidal or subretinal fluid with air injection into the vitreous cavity (146). Lamellar sclerectomy, by dissecting areas of sclera to two-thirds thickness, is also reported to relieve the IOP elevation and the shallow anterior chamber (147).

Uveal Effusion Syndrome

The uveal effusion syndrome has similarities to nanophthalmos; the main exception is an eye of normal size. The uveal effusion syndrome occurs more frequently in male patients and is characterized by dilated episcleral vessels, thickened or detached choroid and ciliary body, and nonrhegmatogenous retinal detachment (145). As with nanophthalmos, the sclera may be thickened and impermeable, although one ultrastructural study revealed increased glycosaminoglycan-like deposits between the scleral fibers and dilated, rough endoplasmic reticulum and large intracellular glycogen-like granules in scleral cells (148). The IOP may be normal, unless angle-closure glaucoma is present, which reportedly responds to cycloplegic agents, aqueous suppressants, and corticosteroids (149). If surgical intervention is required, subscleral sclerectomy (i.e., sclerectomy under two scleral flaps located at the equator) may be helpful in inducing resolution of the subretinal fluid, especially in eyes that are smaller than the average size (<23 mm) (150).

Other Causes of Ciliochoroidal Effusion

Several additional causes of ciliochoroidal effusion are considered in subsequent chapters: arteriovenous malformation (see Chapter 20), tumors (see Chapter 21), inflammatory conditions (see Chapter 22), trauma (see Chapter 25), and surgery (see Chapter 26). Drugs, mostly sulfa-related compounds, rarely can produce uveal effusions. These include acetazolamide and topiramate (an anticonvulsant medication) (151).

Retinopathy of Prematurity

Contracture of the retrolental mass in retinopathy of prematurity (retrolental fibroplasia) can cause progressive shallowing of the anterior chamber with eventual angle-closure glaucoma. This complication coincides with the cicatricial phase of the disease, which usually has its onset at 3 to 6 months of age. However, the angle-closure glaucoma may occur later in childhood or even in young adulthood (152,153), and continued observation is needed. Although the typical mechanism of glaucoma is angle closure due to the retrolental mass, anterior chamber angle abnormalities, including hypopigmentation of the iris root, a translucent material in the angle, and a prominent Schwalbe line, suggest a developmental origin in some cases (154).

The glaucoma usually does not respond well to medical therapy, although some success has been reported with the use of cycloplegic agents and topical corticosteroids (155,156). Iridectomy or trabeculectomy may be effective in some cases (153). Lens aspiration, with anterior vitrectomy, has been successful in other patients in controlling the IOP, although the procedure is usually only to relieve pain and avoid enucleation

because useful vision is often lost by this stage (152). Vitrectomy techniques to reattach the retina have resulted in improved vision in some cases (157,158), although patients with concomitant glaucoma usually have a poor visual outcome despite reattachment of the retina (159). In one case, however, an infant regained vision after treatment of the glaucoma with antihypertensive medication (160).

Persistent Hyperplastic Primary Vitreous

Retention and hyperplasia of the primary vitreous is usually unilateral and is often associated with microphthalmia and elongated ciliary processes (161). Because of anastomotic vessels between the anterior and posterior tunica vasculosa lentis, the presence of small pupillary notches may be a helpful sign of persistent hyperplastic primary vitreous, especially when the diagnosis is obscured by an opaque lens (162). The appearance of persistent hyperplastic primary vitreous by computed tomography is sufficiently characteristic as to also make this a useful diagnostic modality (163).

Glaucoma is usually a late finding with persistent hyperplastic primary vitreous. Angle-closure mechanisms are most common, resulting from anterior displacement of the lens–iris diaphragm due to contracture of the fibrous retrolenticular mass or a swollen lens. Other cases of angle-closure glaucoma may have extensive peripheral anterior synechiae. Open-angle mechanisms may include chronic uveitis, intraocular hemorrhage, and abnormal development of the anterior chamber angle.

If left untreated, most of these eyes undergo progressive deterioration (164). The recommended treatment is aspiration of the lens and removal of the fibrovascular mass with scissors or vitrectomy instruments (164–166). Because the retina in these cases often extends as far anteriorly as the pars plicata, a pars plana incision is thought to be contraindicated (167), and success with a limbal incision has been reported (164). This treatment may prevent or eliminate the angle-closure glaucoma, although postoperative visual rehabilitation is difficult and treatment to avoid amblyopia is usually required (165,166).

Attention should also be given to the fellow eye in these cases, because two adult patients with uncomplicated unilateral persistent hyperplastic primary vitreous were found to have open-angle glaucoma in the contralateral eye, associated with anomalous blood vessels in the entire circumference of the anterior chamber angle, band keratopathy, and heterochromia iridis (167).

Retinal Dysplasia

This condition is usually bilateral and is associated with multiple congenital anomalies, especially in trisomy 13–15 (168). The dysplastic retina may be pulled up behind the lens, and glaucoma may result from angle closure or an associated dysgenesis of the anterior chamber angle.

Retinitis Pigmentosa

Retinitis pigmentosa has been described in association with glaucoma, which appears most often to be of the open-angle type (169). However, the association is infrequent, and a true cause-and-effect relationship has not been established.

KEY POINTS

■ Neovascular glaucoma is a relatively common and serious complication of several retinal disorders, especially diabetic retinopathy, central retinal vein occlusion, and ocular ischemia, as well as certain other ocular and extraocular conditions.

■ The pathophysiology of neovascular glaucoma involves abnormally high levels of VEGF within the eye and growth of a fibrovascular membrane on the iris surface and in the anterior chamber angle, which initially obstructs aqueous outflow in an open-angle glaucoma and then contracts to produce an angle-closure form of glaucoma.

■ The most effective long-term treatment of neovascularization of the iris or neovascular glaucoma is panretinal photocoagulation in the early stages of the disease to reduce the stimulus for anterior segment neovascularization. Intravitreal or intracameral injection of anti-VEGF agents cause regression of anterior segment neovascularization and can thus be a very useful short-term adjunct.

■ Retinal detachments are usually associated with a reduction in IOP, although some patients may have concomitant retinal detachment and glaucoma, which may or may not have a cause-and-effect relationship.

■ A group of conditions in which angle-closure glaucoma may be associated with a retinal, choroidal, or vitreous disorder include central retinal vein occlusion, nanophthalmos, retinopathy of prematurity, persistent hyperplastic primary vitreous, and retinal dysplasia.

REFERENCES

1. Coats G. Further cases of thrombosis of the central vein. *Roy Lond Ophthalmol Hosp Rep.* 1906;16:516.
2. Smith RJ. Rubeotic glaucoma. *Br J Ophthalmol.* 1981;65:606–609.
3. Weiss DI, Shaffer RN, Nehrenberg TR. Neovascular glaucoma complicating carotid-cavernous fistula. *Arch Ophthalmol.* 1963;69:304–307.
4. Sivak-Callcott JA, O'Day DM, Gass DM, et al. Evidence-based recommendations for the diagnosis and treatment of neovascular glaucoma. *Ophthalmology.* 2001;108:1767–1778.
5. Diabetes Control and Complications Trial (DCCT) Research Group. The effect of intensive treatment of diabetes on the development and progression of long-term complications in insulin-dependent diabetes mellitus. *N Engl J Med.* 1993;329:977–986.
6. Mandelcorn MS, Blankenship G, Machemer R. Pars plana vitrectomy for the management of severe diabetic retinopathy. *Am J Ophthalmol.* 1976;81:561–570.
7. Blankenship G, Cortez R, Machemer R. The lens and pars plana vitrectomy for diabetic retinopathy complications. *Arch Ophthalmol.* 1979;97:1263–1267.
8. Machemer R, Blankenship G. Vitrectomy for proliferative diabetic retinopathy associated with vitreous hemorrhage. *Ophthalmology.* 1981;88:643–646.
9. Blankenship GW, Machemer R. Long-term diabetic vitrectomy results: report of 10 year follow-up. *Ophthalmology.* 1985;92:503–506.
10. Blankenship GW. Management of vitreous cavity hemorrhage following pars plana vitrectomy for diabetic retinopathy. *Ophthalmology.* 1986;93:39–44.
11. Blankenship GW. Preoperative iris rubeosis and diabetic vitrectomy results. *Ophthalmology.* 1980;87:176–182.
12. Bopp S, Lucke K, Laqua H. Acute onset of rubeosis iridis after diabetic vitrectomy can indicate peripheral traction retinal detachment. *Ger J Ophthalmol.* 1992;1:375–381.
13. Scuderi JJ, Blumenkranz MS, Blankenship GW. Regression of diabetic rubeosis iridis following successful surgical reattachment of the retina by vitrectomy. *Retina.* 1982;2:193–196.
14. Wand M, Madigan JC, Gaudio AR, et al. Neovascular glaucoma following pars plana vitrectomy for complications of diabetic retinopathy. *Ophthalmic Surg.* 1990;21:113–118.
15. de Juan E Jr, Hardy M, Hatchell DL, et al. The effect of intraocular silicone oil on anterior chamber oxygen pressure in cats. *Arch Ophthalmol.* 1986;104:1063–1064.
16. Hoskins HD Jr. Neovascular glaucoma: current concepts. *Trans Am Acad Ophthalmol Otolaryngol.* 1974;78:330–333.
17. Gartner S, Henkind P. Neovascularization of the iris (rubeosis iridis). *Surg Ophthalmol.* 1978;22:291–312.
18. David R, Zangwill L, Badarna M, et al. Epidemiology of retinal vein occlusion and its association with glaucoma and increased intraocular pressure. *Ophthalmologica.* 1988;197:69–74.
19. Rath EZ, Frank RN, Shin DH, et al. Risk factors for retinal vein occlusions: a case-control study. *Ophthalmology.* 1992;99:509–514.
20. Klein B, Meuer S, Knudtson M, et al. The relationship of optic disk cupping to retinal vein occlusion: the Beaver Dam Eye Study. *Am J Ophthalmol.* 2006;141(5):859–862.
21. Hayreh SS, Zimmerman MB, Podhajsky P. Incidence of various types of retinal vein occlusion and their recurrence and demographic characteristics. *Am J Ophthalmol.* 1994;117:429–441.
22. Duker JS, Brown GC. Iris neovascularization associated with obstruction of the central retinal artery. *Ophthalmology.* 1988;95:1244–1250.
23. Duker JS, Sivalingam A, Brown GC, et al. A prospective study of acute central retinal artery obstruction: the incidence of secondary ocular neovascularization. *Arch Ophthalmol.* 1991;109:339–342.
24. Peternel P, Keber D, Videcnik V. Carotid arteries in central retinal vessel occlusion as assessed by Doppler ultrasound. *Br J Ophthalmol.* 1989;73:880–883.
25. Hayreh SS, Podhajsky P. Ocular neovascularization with retinal vascular occlusion. II. Occurrence in central and branch retinal artery occlusion. *Arch Ophthalmol.* 1982;100:1585–1596.
26. Bresnick GH, Gay AJ. Rubeosis iridis associated with branch retinal arteriolar occlusions. *Arch Ophthalmol.* 1967;77:176–180.
27. Tanaka S, Ideta H, Yonemoto J, et al. Neovascularization of the iris in rhegmatogenous retinal detachment. *Am J Ophthalmol.* 1991;112:632–634.
28. Comaratta MR, Chang S, Sparrow J. Iris neovascularization in proliferative vitreoretinopathy. *Ophthalmology.* 1992;99:898–905.
29. Brown GC, Magargal LE, Schachat A, et al. Neovascular glaucoma: etiologic considerations. *Ophthalmology.* 1984;91:315–320.
30. Shields MB, Proia AD. Neovascular glaucoma associated with an iris melanoma: a clinicopathologic report. *Arch Ophthalmol.* 1987;105:672–674.
31. Sugar HS. Neovascular glaucoma after carotid-cavernous fistula formation. *Ann Ophthalmol.* 1979;11:1667–1669.
32. Harris GJ, Rice PR. Angle closure in carotid-cavernous fistula. *Ophthalmology.* 1979;86:1521–1529.
33. Huckman MS, Haas J. Reversed flow through the ophthalmic artery as a cause of rubeosis iridis. *Am J Ophthalmol.* 1972;74:1094–1099.
34. Michaelson IC. The mode of development of the vascular system of the retina with some observations of its significance in certain retinal diseases. *Trans Ophthalmol Soc UK.* 1948;68:137–180.
35. Folkman J, Merler E, Abernathy C, et al. Isolation of a tumor factor responsible for angiogenesis. *J Exp Med.* 1971;133:275–288.
36. Ichhpujani P, Ramasubramanian A, Kaushik S, et al. Bevacizumab in glaucoma: a review. *Can J Ophthalmol.* 2007;42:812–815.
37. Henkind P. Ocular neovascularization. *Am J Ophthalmol.* 1978;85:287–301.
38. Williams GA, Eisenstein R, Schumacher B, et al. Inhibitor of vascular endothelial cell growth in the lens. *Am J Ophthalmol.* 1984;97:366–371.
39. Glaser BM, Campochiaro PA, Davis JL Jr, et al. Retinal pigment epithelial cells release inhibitors of neovascularization. *Ophthalmology.* 1987;94:780–784.
40. Ohrt V. The frequency of rubeosis iridis in diabetic patients. *Acta Ophthalmol.* 1971;49:301–307.
41. Madsen PH. Rubeosis of the iris and haemorrhagic glaucoma in patients with proliferative diabetic retinopathy. *Br J Ophthalmol.* 1971;55:368–371.
42. Bonnet M, Jourdain M, Francoz-Taillanter N. Clinical correlation between rubeosis iridis and optic disc neovascularization [in French]. *J Fr Ophthalmol.* 1981;4:405–410.
43. Bandello F, Brancato R, Lattanzio R, et al. Biomicroscopy versus fluorescein angiography of the iris in the detection of diabetic iridopathy. *Graefes Arch Clin Exp Ophthalmol.* 1993;231:444–448.
44. Browning DJ. Risk of missing angle neovascularization by omitting screening gonioscopy in patients with diabetes mellitus. *Am J Ophthalmol.* 1991;112:212.

45. Blinder KJ, Friedman SM, Mames RN. Diabetic iris neovascularization. *Am J Ophthalmol.* 1995;120:393–395.

46. Hayreh S, March W, Phelps CD. Ocular hypotony following retinal vein occlusion. *Arch Ophthalmol.* 1978;96:827–833.

47. Tasman W, Magargal LE, Augsburger JJ. Effects of argon laser photocoagulation on rubeosis iridis and angle neovascularization. *Ophthalmology.* 1980;87:400–402.

48. Priluck IA, Robertson DM, Hollenhorst RW. Long-term follow-up of occlusion of the central retinal vein in young adults. *Am J Ophthalmol.* 1980;90:190–202.

49. Zegarra H, Gutman FA, Conforto J. The natural course of central retinal vein occlusion. *Ophthalmology.* 1979;86:1931–1942.

50. Laatikainen L, Blach RK. Behavior of the iris vasculature in central retinal vein occlusion: a fluorescein angiographic study of the vascular response of the retina and the iris. *Br J Ophthalmol.* 1977;61:272–277.

51. Nguyen NX, Küchle M. Aqueous flare and cells in eyes with retinal vein occlusion—correlation with retinal fluorescein angiographic findings. *Br J Ophthalmol.* 1993;77:280–283.

52. Servais GE, Thompson HS, Hayreh SS. Relative afferent pupillary defect in central retinal vein occlusion. *Ophthalmology.* 1986;93:301–303.

53. Bloom PA, Papakostopoulos D, Gogolitsyn Y, et al. Clinical and infrared pupillometry in central retinal vein occlusion. *Br J Ophthalmol.* 1993; 77:75–80.

54. Sabates R, Hirose T, McMeel JW. Electroretinography in the prognosis and classification of central retinal vein occlusion. *Arch Ophthalmol.* 1983;101:232–235.

55. Severns ML, Johnson MA. Predicting outcome in central retinal vein occlusion using the flicker electroretinogram. *Arch Ophthalmol.* 1993; 111:1123–1130.

56. Williamson TH, Baxter GM. Central retinal vein occlusion, an investigation by color Doppler imaging: blood velocity characteristics and prediction of iris neovascularization. *Ophthalmology.* 1994;101: 1362–1372.

57. Chen JC, Klein ML, Watzke RC, et al. Natural course of perfused central retinal vein occlusion. *Can J Ophthalmol.* 1995;30:21–24.

58. Central Vein Occlusion Study Group. Baseline and early natural history report: the Central Vein Occlusion Study [comment]. *Arch Ophthalmol.* 1993;111:1087–1095.

59. Browning DJ, Scott AQ, Peterson CB, et al. The risk of missing angle neovascularization by omitting screening gonioscopy in acute central retinal vein occlusion. *Ophthalmology.* 1998;105:776–784.

60. Schulze RR. Rubeosis iridis. *Am J Ophthalmol.* 1967;63:487–495.

61. Nork TM, Tso MO, Duvall J, et al. Cellular mechanisms of iris neovascularization secondary to retinal vein occlusion. *Arch Ophthalmol.* 1989;107:581–586.

62. Jocson VL. Microvascular injection studies in rubeosis iridis and neovascular glaucoma. *Am J Ophthalmol.* 1977;83:508–517.

63. Goldberg MF, Tso MO. Rubeosis iridis and glaucoma associated with sickle cell retinopathy: a light and electron microscopic study. *Ophthalmology.* 1978;85:1028–1041.

64. Wand M, Dueker DK, Aiello LM, et al. Effects of panretinal photocoagulation on rubeosis iridis, angle neovascularization, and neovascular glaucoma. *Am J Ophthalmol.* 1978;86:332–339.

65. Anderson DM, Morin JD, Hunter WS. Rubeosis iridis. *Can J Ophthalmol.* 1971;6:183–188.

66. Kubota T, Tawara A, Hata Y, et al. Neovascular tissue in the intertrabecular spaces in eyes with neovascular glaucoma. *Br J Ophthalmol.* 1996;80:750–754.

67. John T, Sassani JW, Eagle RC Jr. The myofibroblastic component of rubeosis iridis. *Ophthalmology.* 1983;90:721–728.

68. Nomura T. Pathology of anterior chamber angle in diabetic neovascular glaucoma: extension of corneal endothelium onto iris surface. *Jpn J Ophthalmol.* 1983;27:193–200.

69. Harris M, Tso AY, Kaba FW, et al. Corneal endothelial overgrowth of angle and iris: evidence of myoblastic differentiation in three cases. *Ophthalmology.* 1984;91:1154–1160.

70. Little HL, Rosenthal AR, Dellaporta A, et al. The effect of pan-retinal photocoagulation on rubeosis iridis. *Am J Ophthalmol.* 1976;81: 804–809.

71. Laatikainen L. Preliminary report on effect of retinal panphotocoagulation on rubeosis iridis and neovascular glaucoma. *Br J Ophthalmol.* 1977;61:278–284.

72. Laatikainen L, Kohner EM, Khoury D, et al. Panretinal photocoagulation in central retinal vein occlusion: a randomised controlled clinical study. *Br J Ophthalmol.* 1977;61:741–753.

73. Jacobson DR, Murphy RP, Rosenthal AR. The treatment of angle neovascularization with panretinal photocoagulation. *Ophthalmology.* 1979;86:1270–1277.

74. Murphy RP, Egbert PR. Regression of iris neovascularization following panretinal photocoagulation. *Arch Ophthalmol.* 1979;97:700–702.

75. Pavan PR, Folk JC, Weingeist TA, et al. Diabetic rubeosis and panretinal photocoagulation: a prospective, controlled, masked trial using iris fluorescein angiography. *Arch Ophthalmol.* 1983;101:882–884.

76. Magargal LE, Brown GC, Augsburger JJ, et al. Neovascular glaucoma following central retinal vein obstruction. *Ophthalmology.* 1981;88: 1095–1101.

77. Magargal LE, Brown GC, Augsburger JJ, et al. Efficacy of panretinal photocoagulation in preventing neovascular glaucoma following ischemic central retinal vein obstruction. *Ophthalmology.* 1982;89:780–784.

78. Laatikainen L. A prospective follow-up study of panretinal photocoagulation in preventing neovascular glaucoma following ischaemic central retinal vein occlusion. *Graefes Arch Clin Exp Ophthalmol.* 1983;220: 236–239.

79. Kaufman SC, Ferris FL III, Swartz M, et al. Intraocular pressure following panretinal photocoagulation for diabetic retinopathy: diabetic retinopathy report no. 11. *Arch Ophthalmol.* 1987;105:807–809.

80. Weiter JJ, Zuckerman R. The influence of the photoreceptor-RPE complex on the inner retina: an explanation of the beneficial effects of photocoagulation. *Ophthalmology.* 1980;87:1133–1139.

81. Murdoch IE, Rosen PH, Shilling JS. Neovascular response in ischaemic central retinal vein occlusion after panretinal photocoagulation. *Br J Ophthalmol.* 1991;75:459–461.

82. The Central Vein Occlusion Study Group. A randomized clinical trial of early panretinal photocoagulation for ischemic central vein occlusion: the Central Vein Occlusion Study Group N Report [comment]. *Ophthalmology.* 1995;102:1434–1444.

83. Duker JS, Brown GC. The efficacy of panretinal photocoagulation for neovascularization of the iris after central retinal artery obstruction. *Ophthalmology.* 1989;96:92–95.

84. Teich SA, Walsh JB. A grading system for iris neovascularization: prognostic implications for treatment. *Ophthalmology.* 1981;88:1102–1106.

85. Flanagan DW, Blach RK. Place of panretinal photocoagulation and trabeculectomy in the management of neovascular glaucoma. *Br J Ophthalmol.* 1983;67:526–528.

86. Goodart R, Blankenship G. Panretinal photocoagulation influence on vitrectomy results for complications of diabetic retinopathy. *Ophthalmology.* 1980;87:183–188.

87. Miller JB, Smith MR, Boyer DS. Intraocular carbon dioxide laser photocautery: indications and contraindications at vitrectomy. *Ophthalmology.* 1980;87:1112–1120.

88. May DR, Bergstrom TJ, Parmet AJ, et al. Treatment of neovascular glaucoma with transscleral panretinal cryotherapy. *Ophthalmology.* 1980; 87:1106–1111.

89. Vernon SA, Cheng H. Panretinal cryotherapy in neovascular disease. *Br J Ophthalmol.* 1988;72:401–405.

90. Moraczewski AL, Lee RK, Palmberg PF, et al. Outcomes of treatment of neovascular glaucoma with intravitreal bevacizumab. *Br J Ophthalmol.* 2009;93(5):589–593.

91. Drews RC. Corticosteroid management of hemorrhagic glaucoma. *Trans Am Acad Ophthalmol Otolaryngol.* 1974;78:334–336.

92. Tano Y, Chandler D, Machemer R. Treatment of intraocular proliferation with intravitreal injection of triamcinolone acetonide. *Am J Ophthalmol.* 1980;90:810–816.

93. Feibel RM, Bigger JF. Rubeosis iridis and neovascular glaucoma: evaluation of cyclocryotherapy. *Am J Ophthalmol.* 1972;74:862–867.

94. Boniuk M. Cryotherapy in neovascular glaucoma. *Trans Am Acad Ophthalmol Otolaryngol.* 1974;78:337–343.

95. Krupin T, Mitchell KB, Becker B. Cyclocryotherapy in neovascular glaucoma. *Am J Ophthalmol.* 1978;86:24–26.

96. Faulborn J, Birnbaum F. Cyclocryotherapy of haemorrhagic glaucoma: clinical long time and histopathologic results [in German]. *Klin Monatsbl Augenheilkd.* 1977;170:651–656.

97. Faulborn J, Hoster K. Results of cyclocryotherapy in case of hemorrhagic glaucoma [in German]. *Klin Monatsbl Augenheilkd.* 1973;162:513–518.

98. Hampton C, Shields MB, Miller KN, et al. Evaluation of a protocol for transscleral Neodymium:YAG cyclophotocoagulation in one hundred patients. *Ophthalmology.* 1990;97:910–917.

99. Bloom PA, Tsai JC, Sharma K, et al. "Cyclodiode": trans-scleral diode laser cyclophotocoagulation in the treatment of advanced refractory glaucoma. *Ophthalmology.* 1997;104:1508–1519.

100. Oguri A, Takahashi E, Tomita G, et al. Transscleral cyclophotocoagulation with the diode laser for neovascular glaucoma. *Ophthalmic Surg Lasers.* 1998;29:722–727.

101. Tsai JC, Feuer WJ, Parrish RK II, et al. 5-Fluorouracil filtering surgery and neovascular glaucoma: long-term follow-up of the original pilot study. *Ophthalmology.* 1995;102:887–892.

102. Takihara Y, Inatani M, Fukushima M, et al. Trabeculectomy with mitomycin C for neovascular glaucoma: prognostic factors for surgical failure. *Am J Ophthalmol.* 2009;147(5):912–918, 918.e1.

103. Herschler J, Agness D. A modified filtering operation for neovascular glaucoma. *Arch Ophthalmol.* 1979;97:2339–2341.

104. Parrish R, Herschler J. Eyes with end-stage neovascular glaucoma: natural history following successful modified filtering operation. *Arch Ophthalmol.* 1983;101:745–746.

105. Sidoti PA, Dunphy TR, Baerveldt G, et al. Experience with the Baerveldt glaucoma implant in treating neovascular glaucoma. *Ophthalmology.* 1995;102:1107–1118.

106. Krupin R, Kaufman P, Mandell A, et al. Filtering valve implant surgery for eyes with neovascular glaucoma. *Am J Ophthalmol.* 1980;89:338–343.

107. Scott IU, Alexandrakis G, Flynn HW Jr, et al. Combined pars plana vitrectomy and glaucoma drainage implant placement for refractory glaucoma. *Am J Ophthalmol.* 2000;129:334–343.

108. Eid TM, Radwan A, el-Manawy W, et al. Intravitreal bevacizumab and aqueous shunting surgery for neovascular glaucoma: safety and efficacy. *Can J Ophthalmol.* 2009;44(4):451–456.

109. McCuen BW II, Rinkoff JS. Silicone oil for progressive anterior ocular neovascularization after failed diabetic vitrectomy [erratum]. *Arch Ophthalmol.* 1989;107:677–682.

110. Jonas JB, Hayler JK, Sofker A, et al. Regression of neovascular iris vessels by intravitreal injection of crystalline cortisone. *J Glaucoma.* 2001; 10:284–287.

111. Jampol LM, Orlin C, Cohen SB, et al. Hyperbaric and transcorneal delivery of oxygen to the rabbit and monkey anterior segment. *Arch Ophthalmol.* 1988;106:825–829.

112. Pederson JE, MacLellan HM. Experimental retinal detachment. I. Effect of subretinal fluid composition on reabsorption rate and intraocular pressure. *Arch Ophthalmol.* 1982;100:1150–1154.

113. Cantrill HL, Pederson JE. Experimental retinal detachment. III. Vitreous fluorophotometry. *Arch Ophthalmol.* 1982;100:1810–1813.

114. Tsuboi S, Taki-Noie J, Emi K, et al. Fluid dynamics in eyes with rhegmatogenous retinal detachments. *Am J Ophthalmol.* 1985;99:673–676.

115. Campbell DG. Iris retraction associated with rhegmatogenous retinal detachment syndrome and hypotony: a new explanation. *Arch Ophthalmol.* 1984;102:1457–1463.

116. Phelps CD, Burton TC. Glaucoma and retinal detachment. *Arch Ophthalmol.* 1977;95:418–422.

117. Shammas HF, Halasa AH, Faris BM. Intraocular pressure, cup-disc ratio, and steroid responsiveness in retinal detachment. *Arch Ophthalmol.* 1976;94:1108–1109.

118. Pape LG, Forbes M. Retinal detachment and miotic therapy. *Am J Ophthalmol.* 1978;85:558–566.

119. Burton TC, Lambert RW Jr. A predictive model for visual recovery following retinal detachment surgery. *Ophthalmology.* 1978;85:619–625.

120. Barile GR, Chang S, Horowitz JD, et al. Neovascular complications associated with rubeosis iridis and peripheral retinal detachment after retinal detachment surgery. *Am J Ophthalmol.* 1998;126:379–389.

121. Sebestyen JG, Schepens CL, Rosenthal ML. Retinal detachment and glaucoma. I. Tonometric and gonioscopic study of 160 cases. *Arch Ophthalmol.* 1962;67:736–745.

122. Schwartz A. Chronic open-angle glaucoma secondary to rhegmatogenous retinal detachment. *Am J Ophthalmol.* 1973;75:205–211.

123. Matsuo N, Takabatake M, Ueno H, et al. Photoreceptor outer segments in the aqueous humor in rhegmatogenous retinal detachment. *Am J Ophthalmol.* 1986;101:673–679.

124. Lambrou FH, Vela MA, Woods W. Obstruction of the trabecular meshwork by retinal rod outer segments. *Arch Ophthalmol.* 1989;107:742–745.

125. Davidorf FH. Retinal pigment epithelial glaucoma. *Ophthalmol Digest.* 1976;38:11.

126. Baba H. Probability of the presence of glycosaminoglycans in aqueous humor. *Graefes Arch Clin Exp Ophthalmol.* 1983;220:117–121.

127. Hyams SW, Neumann E. Transient angle-closure glaucoma after retinal vein occlusion: report of two cases. *Br J Ophthalmol.* 1972;56:353–355.

128. Grant WM. Shallowing of the anterior chamber following occlusion of the central retinal vein. *Am J Ophthalmol.* 1973;75:384–387.

129. Bloome MA. Transient angle-closure glaucoma in central retinal vein occlusion. *Ann Ophthalmol.* 1977;9:44–48.

130. Mendelsohn AD, Jampol LM, Shoch D. Secondary angle-closure glaucoma after central retinal vein occlusion. *Am J Ophthalmol.* 1985; 100:581–585.

131. Pesin SR, Katz LJ, Augsburger JJ, et al. Acute angle-closure glaucoma from spontaneous massive hemorrhagic retinal or choroidal detachment: an updated diagnostic and therapeutic approach. *Ophthalmology.* 1990;97:76–84.

132. Steinemann T, Goins K, Smith T, et al. Acute closed-angle glaucoma complicating hemorrhagic choroidal detachment associated with parenteral thrombolytic agents. *Am J Ophthalmol.* 1988;106:752–753.

133. Brockhurst RJ. Nanophthalmos with uveal effusion: a new clinical entity. *Arch Ophthalmol.* 1975;93:1989–1999.

134. Singh OS, Simmons RJ, Brockhurst RJ, et al. Nanophthalmos: a perspective on identification and therapy. *Ophthalmology.* 1982;89: 1006–1012.

135. Ryan EA, Zwann J, Chylack LT Jr. Nanophthalmos with uveal effusion: clinical and embryologic considerations. *Ophthalmology.* 1982;89: 1013–1017.

136. Ghose S, Sachdev MS, Kumar H. Bilateral nanophthalmos, pigmentary retinal dystrophy, and angle closure glaucoma—a new syndrome? *Br J Ophthalmol.* 1985;69:624–628.

137. MacKay CJ, Shek MS, Carr RE, et al. Retinal degeneration with nanophthalmos, cystic macular degeneration, and angle closure glaucoma: a new recessive syndrome. *Arch Ophthalmol.* 1987;105:366–371.

138. Calhoun FP Jr. The management of glaucoma in nanophthalmos. *Trans Am Ophthalmol Soc.* 1975;73:97–122.

139. Kimbrough RL, Trempe CS, Brockhurst RJ, et al. Angle-closure glaucoma in nanophthalmos. *Am J Ophthalmol.* 1979;88:572–579.

140. Trelstad RL, Silbermann NN, Brockhurst RJ. Nanophthalmic sclera: ultrastructural, histochemical, and biochemical observations. *Arch Ophthalmol.* 1982;100:1935–1938.

141. Yue BY, Duvall J, Goldberg MF, et al. Nanophthalmic sclera: morphologic and tissue culture studies. *Ophthalmology.* 1986;93:534–541.

142. Stewart DH III, Streeten BW, Brockhurst RJ, et al. Abnormal scleral collagen in nanophthalmos: an ultrastructural study. *Arch Ophthalmol.* 1991;109:1017–1025.

143. Yue BY, Kurosawa A, Duvall J, et al. Nanophthalmic sclera: fibronectin studies. *Ophthalmology.* 1988;95:56–60.

144. Shiono T, Shoji A, Mutoh T, et al. Abnormal sclerocytes in nanophthalmos. *Graefes Arch Clin Exp Ophthalmol.* 1992;230:348–351.

145. Gass JD. Uveal effusion syndrome: a new hypothesis concerning pathogenesis and technique of surgical treatment. *Retina.* 1983;3:159–163.

146. Brockhurst RJ. Vortex vein decompression for nanophthalmic uveal effusion. *Arch Ophthalmol.* 1980;98:1987–1990.

147. Wax MB, Kass MA, Kolker AE, et al. Anterior lamellar sclerectomy for nanophthalmos. *J Glaucoma.* 1992;1:222–227.

148. Ward RC, Gragoudas ES, Pon DM, et al. Abnormal scleral findings in uveal effusion syndrome. *Am J Ophthalmol.* 1988;106:139–146.

149. Fourman S. Angle-closure glaucoma complicating ciliochoroidal detachment. *Ophthalmology.* 1989;96:646–653.

150. Uyama M, Takahashi K, Kozaki J, et al. Uveal effusion syndrome: clinical features, surgical treatment, histologic examination of the sclera, and pathophysiology. *Ophthalmology.* 2000;107:441–449.

151. Sankar PS, Pasquale LR, Grosskreutz CL. Uveal effusion and secondary angle-closure glaucoma associated with topiramate use [comment]. *Arch Ophthalmol.* 2001;119:1210–1211.

152. Pollard ZF. Secondary angle-closure glaucoma in cicatricial retrolental fibroplasia. *Am J Ophthalmol.* 1980;89:651–653.

153. Michael AJ, Pesin SR, Katz LJ, et al. Management of late-onset angle-closure glaucoma associated with retinopathy of prematurity. *Ophthalmology.* 1991;98:1093–1098.

154. Hartnett ME, Gilbert MM, Richardson TM, et al. Anterior segment evaluation of infants with retinopathy of prematurity. *Ophthalmology.* 1990;97:122–130.

155. Kushner BJ. Ciliary block glaucoma in retinopathy of prematurity. *Arch Ophthalmol.* 1982;100:1078–1079.

156. Kushner BJ, Sondheimer S. Medical treatment of glaucoma associated with cicatricial retinopathy of prematurity. *Am J Ophthalmol.* 1982; 94:313–317.

157. Machemer R. Closed vitrectomy for severe retrolental fibroplasia in the infant. *Ophthalmology.* 1983;90:436–441.

158. Trese MT. Surgical results of stage V retrolental fibroplasia and timing of surgical repair. *Ophthalmology.* 1984;91:461–466.

159. Hartnett ME, Gilbert MM, Hirose T, et al. Glaucoma as a cause of poor vision in severe retinopathy of prematurity. *Graefes Arch Clin Exp Ophthalmol.* 1993;231:433–438.

160. Hartnett ME, Katsumi O, Hirose T, et al. Improved visual function in retinopathy of prematurity after lowering high intraocular pressure. *Am J Ophthalmol.* 1994;117:113–115.

161. Reese AB. Persistent hyperplastic primary vitreous. *Am J Ophthalmol.* 1955;40:317–331.

162. Meisels HI, Goldberg MF. Vascular anastomoses between the iris and persistent hyperplastic primary vitreous. *Am J Ophthalmol.* 1979;88:179–185.

163. Goldberg MF, Mafee M. Computed tomography for diagnosis of persistent hyperplastic primary vitreous (PHPV). *Ophthalmology.* 1983;90:442–451.

164. Stark WJ, Lindsey PS, Fagadau WR, et al. Persistent hyperplastic primary vitreous: surgical treatment. *Ophthalmology.* 1983;90:452–457.

165. Smith RE, Maumenee AE. Persistent hyperplastic primary vitreous: results of surgery. *Trans Am Acad Ophthalmol Otolaryngol.* 1974;78:911.

166. Nankin SJ, Scott WE. Persistent hyperplastic primary vitreous: roto-extraction and other surgical experience. *Arch Ophthalmol.* 1977;95:240–243.

167. Awan KJ, Humayun M. Changes in the contralateral eye in uncomplicated persistent hyperplastic primary vitreous in adults. *Am J Ophthalmol.* 1985;99:122–124.

168. Hoepner J, Yanoff M. Ocular anomalies in trisomy 13–15: an analysis of 13 eyes with two new findings. *Am J Ophthalmol.* 1972;74:729–737.

169. Kogbe OI, Follmann P. Investigations into the aqueous humour dynamics in primary pigmentary degeneration of the retina. *Ophthalmologica.* 1975;171:165–175.

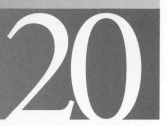

Glaucomas Associated with Elevated Episcleral Venous Pressure

EPISCLERAL VENOUS PRESSURE

The episcleral venous pressure is one factor that contributes to the intraocular pressure (IOP). The normal episcleral venous pressure is approximately 8 to 10 mm Hg (1–5), although recorded values vary according to the measurement technique used. (The instruments for measuring episcleral venous pressure are described in Chapter 2 (1,2,4,5).)

It is commonly thought that for every mm Hg increase in episcleral venous pressure, there is an equal rise in IOP, although the magnitude of IOP rise may be greater than the rise in venous pressure (6). Studies of chronic open-angle glaucoma have revealed no significant abnormality of episcleral venous pressure (2,5,7). In one study, however, the episcleral venous pressure was slightly higher in patients with primary open-angle glaucoma (12.1 mm Hg) or normal-tension glaucoma (11.6 mm Hg) than in control eyes (9.5 mm Hg) (8). There are, in fact, various conditions in which elevated episcleral venous pressure can produce characteristic forms of associated glaucoma. These conditions are the subject of this chapter.

GENERAL FEATURES OF ELEVATED EPISCLERAL VENOUS PRESSURE

The following findings are common to most eyes with abnormally elevated episcleral venous pressure.

External Examination

The most consistent feature is variable degrees of dilatation and tortuosity of the episcleral and bulbar conjunctival vessels. Additional findings may include chemosis, proptosis, orbital bruit, and pulsations over the orbit; however, these findings are inconsistent and depend on the underlying cause of the elevated episcleral venous pressure.

Intraocular Pressure

The rise in IOP is approximately equal to the rise in episcleral venous pressure. The resultant tension is typically in the mid-20s to mid-30s, and the ocular pulse amplitude is often increased (9).

Gonioscopy

The anterior chamber angle is typically open, and the only abnormality may be blood reflux into the Schlemm canal. However, the latter feature is of limited diagnostic value, because it is found inconsistently in eyes with elevated episcleral venous pressure and may be seen in healthy eyes.

Tonography

The facility of aqueous outflow is characteristically normal. A study with monkeys revealed that elevated venous pressure was associated with increased outflow (10), which may partly result from a widening of the Schlemm canal. However, prolonged elevation of episcleral venous pressure often leads to reduced outflow facility, which may persist after the venous pressure has normalized (9).

CLINICAL FORMS OF ELEVATED EPISCLERAL VENOUS PRESSURE

The various causes of elevated episcleral venous pressure may be considered to fall into three categories: obstruction to venous flow, arteriovenous fistulas, and idiopathic episcleral venous pressure elevation (5).

Venous Obstruction

Thyroid-Associated Ophthalmopathy

Thyroid-associated ophthalmopathy is also referred to as endocrine exophthalmos or Graves ophthalmopathy. The precise hormonal basis for the condition is uncertain, although the ocular pathology consists of orbital infiltration, including the extraocular muscles, with lymphocytes, mast cells, and plasma cell. This is the most common cause of unilateral and bilateral proptosis. In addition to glaucoma, other serious complications of thyroid-associated ophthalmopathy include corneal exposure due to proptosis or lid retraction and optic nerve compression from the orbital mass.

The glaucoma may occur by several mechanisms. The episcleral venous pressure may be elevated in severe cases of thyroid-associated ophthalmopathy with marked proptosis and orbital congestion due to obstruction of venous flow through the orbit (**Figs. 20.1** and **20.2**). This increases the IOP. A less common mechanism of glaucoma is anterior chamber inflammation, which may result from corneal exposure and ulceration.

Contracture of extraocular muscles, which occurs in the later, fibrotic phases of the infiltrative ophthalmopathy, may affect the IOP in different fields of gaze. Typically, fibrosis of the inferior rectus muscle causes resistance to upgaze, which is associated with a rise in the measured IOP when the patient looks up. In some cases, an artificial pressure elevation may be

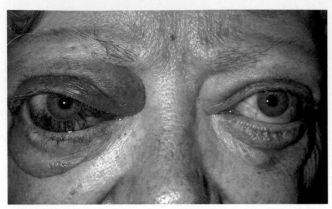

Figure 20.1 Asymmetrical exophthalmos, with congestive features greater in the right eye, in a patient with thyroid-associated ophthalmopathy. (Courtesy of Julie A. Woodward, MD.)

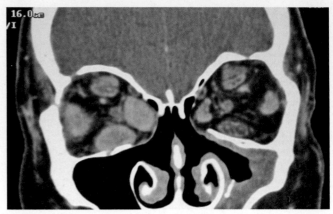

Figure 20.2 Orbital computed tomography scan of the patient in Figure 20.1 with thyroid-associated ophthalmopathy. Note the massively enlarged rectus muscles in the right orbit. (Courtesy of Julie A. Woodward, MD.)

recorded with gaze in the usual straight-ahead position, and the patient should be allowed to change the direction of gaze to their "resting" position (11). Ideally, the IOP should be measured in several fields of gaze to avoid this potential artifact of testing. Thyroid dysfunction may be associated with abnormal scleral rigidity; the IOP in patients with thyroid dysfunction should be measured by using applanation tonometry or another tonometer that affects scleral rigidity only minimally (as described in Chapter 2).

Superior Vena Cava Syndrome

Lesions of the upper thorax may obstruct venous return from the head, causing elevated episcleral venous pressure in association with exophthalmos, edema, and cyanosis of the face and neck, and dilated veins of the head, neck, chest, and upper extremities (12).

Orbital Amyloidosis

Rare cases of localized orbital amyloidosis with secondary glaucoma related to elevated episcleral venous pressure have been reported (13,14). Nelson and colleagues (14) postulate that perivascular infiltration of amyloid around extraocular vessels may contribute to raising the episcleral venous pressure. Other conditions that may occasionally obstruct orbital venous drainage include retrobulbar tumors and cavernous sinus thrombosis.

Arteriovenous Fistulas

Carotid–Cavernous Sinus Fistulas

Carotid–cavernous sinus fistulas can be subdivided into two categories. About three fourths of these fistulas are caused by trauma and are characterized by a direct vascular communication and high blood flow. The remaining cases occur spontaneously and typically have an indirect or dural communication with low flow (15).

Traumatic Fistulas

The typical trauma is severe head injury, which results in a large fistula between the internal carotid artery and the surrounding cavernous sinus venous plexus. This condition is characterized by pulsating exophthalmos, a bruit over the globe, conjunctival chemosis, engorgement of epibulbar veins, restriction of motility, and evidence of ocular ischemia (15–18). The shunting of blood through the internal carotid–cavernous sinus fistula increases blood flow and produces high venous pressure (15,19).

Spontaneous Fistulas

Spontaneous carotid–cavernous sinus fistula occurs most often in middle-aged or older women with no history of trauma. A small fistula in these cases is fed by a meningeal branch of the intracavernous internal carotid artery or external carotid artery, which empties directly into the cavernous sinus or an adjacent dural vein that connects with the cavernous sinus (19,20). The mixing of arterial and venous blood leads to a reduction in arterial pressure and an increase in orbital venous pressure, which increases the episcleral venous pressure. Patients with this condition have prominent episcleral and conjunctival veins—often their reason for seeking care—but they have minimal proptosis and no pulsations or bruit. The small fistula results in low-flow, low-pressure shunting (19). Most patients have elevated IOPs. The condition has been called red-eyed shunt syndrome (19) or dural shunt syndrome (20).

Orbital Varices

The condition of orbital varices is characterized by intermittent exophthalmos and elevated episcleral venous pressure, usually associated with stooping over or the Valsalva maneuver (6,21). Because venous pressure is typically normal between episodes, associated glaucoma is uncommon. However, glaucomatous damage has been reported to occur, and it has been suggested that management with antiglaucoma medications may be effective and should be tried before surgical intervention is considered (6).

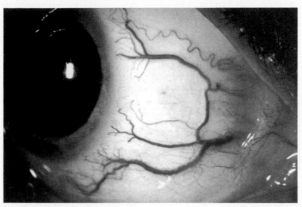

Figure 20.3 Temporal quadrant in a patient with idiopathic elevated episcleral venous pressure. Note how the episcleral veins begin as small, tapered vessels just behind the limbus and become larger as they coalesce and course posteriorly. This contrasts with anterior ciliary arteries, which are more tortuous than the episcleral veins in the normal state and end abruptly just behind the limbus. One such artery is seen in the upper portion of the image. Although arteries normally are more prominent than episcleral veins are, the opposite is true in eyes with elevated episcleral venous pressure.

Sturge–Weber Syndrome

One mechanism of IOP elevation in Sturge–Weber syndrome is believed to be elevated episcleral venous pressure due to the episcleral hemangiomas with arteriovenous fistulas (22,23). (The Sturge–Weber syndrome is discussed in more detail in Chapter 21.)

Idiopathic Episcleral Venous Pressure Elevation

Several reported cases have involved dilated episcleral veins (**Fig. 20.3**) and open-angle glaucoma without exophthalmos or any explanation for the venous congestion (24–30). The typical patient is elderly with no family history of the condition, although it may be seen in young adults and has been described in a mother and daughter (24). Most cases are unilateral, and those in which episcleral venous pressure has been measured have all had elevated venous pressures (24,27,30). The cause of the elevated episcleral venous pressure is unknown. In one series of five patients with unilateral elevation of episcleral venous pressure and open-angle glaucoma, venous outflow was determined to be normal by orbital venography, and the mechanism was presumed to be a localized venous obstruction in the region of the extraocular muscles (30). The associated glaucoma may be severe, with advanced glaucomatous damage.

MECHANISMS OF ASSOCIATED GLAUCOMA

Elevated episcleral venous pressure may lead to glaucoma by several mechanisms. Some are common to all forms of episcleral venous pressure elevation, whereas others are associated with specific conditions.

Direct Effect

Episcleral venous pressure is a component of the normal IOP, and a rise in episcleral venous pressure is associated with approximately the same amount of increase in IOP. Eyes with elevated episcleral venous pressure typically have a wide-open anterior chamber angle, often with blood in the Schlemm canal. This is the most common mechanism of glaucoma associated with elevated episcleral venous pressure.

Outflow Resistance

Although facility of outflow typically is normal, if not improved (10), when the episcleral venous pressure is elevated, prolonged elevation may lead to reduced outflow even after venous pressure is normalized (9). A trabeculectomy specimen from one idiopathic case revealed compression of the trabecular meshwork near the Schlemm canal, with extracellular deposits and hyalinization of the trabecular beams (29); whether this represents a primary or secondary alteration is unclear, however.

Acute Angle Closure

Angle-closure glaucoma has been associated with arteriovenous fistulas (31–33). The mechanism appears to be venous stasis in the vortex veins, leading to a serous choroidal detachment (31,32,34) or a suprachoroidal hemorrhage (33) and subsequent forward displacement of the lens–iris diaphragm. These conditions have been associated with the dural shunt syndrome (31–33) and an orbital arteriovenous fistula (32).

Neovascular Glaucoma

Reduced arterial flow in these cases may lead to ocular ischemia with neovascularization of the iris and angle (17,35,36). It has also been proposed, on the basis of experimental models and mathematic analysis, that the visual field loss in glaucoma associated with elevated venous pressure is caused by intraocular vein collapse and retardation of intraocular blood flow (37).

MANAGEMENT

Elevated Episcleral Venous Pressure

In many cases, the initial therapy should be directed toward eliminating the cause of the elevated episcleral venous pressure. This is particularly true in patients with thyroid-associated ophthalmopathy, superior vena cava syndrome, retrobulbar tumors, or cavernous sinus thrombosis. However, in cases of carotid–cavernous sinus fistula and orbital varices, the risk of surgical intervention may be such that other measures of glaucoma control should be considered first (6,17,18). Surgical intervention in the latter cases usually consists of intra-arterial balloon occlusion or embolization (15,38). Reported success rates range from 58% to 100% (15), but complications do occur, including anterior segment ischemia, ischemia of the optic nerve, and cerebral ischemia or stroke (17,18). A transvenous approach through the ipsilateral superior ophthalmic vein has been described as a safer way to pass a detachable balloon into the cavernous sinus (39) or to pass platinum coils for primary embolization (40). Attempted superior ophthalmic vein embolization in a patient with a dural carotid–cavernous sinus fistula caused uncontrolled proptosis, neovascular glaucoma, and severe vision loss (41). Because many fistulas close spontaneously, especially in patients with the dural shunt syndrome, conservative management is advisable in mild cases, with embolization reserved for those with visual disability or progressive signs (38).

Associated Glaucoma

When treatment of the associated glaucoma is required, drugs that reduce aqueous production, such as β-blockers, α_2-agonists, and carbonic anhydrase inhibitors, should be used, because agents that improve conventional outflow are rarely effective. Cases with acute angle closure associated with the dural shunt syndrome and uveal effusion may respond to these medications (32), whereas those with a suprachoroidal hemorrhage may require drainage of the blood (33). If surgical intervention becomes necessary, a filtering procedure should be used in most cases. However, the risk of uveal effusion and expulsive hemorrhage is increased when eyes with elevated episcleral venous pressure undergo filtering, especially in patients with the Sturge–Weber syndrome. It has been recommended that prophylactic sclerotomies for drainage of suprachoroidal fluid should be performed at the time of surgery (42). Nonpenetrating, deep sclerectomy followed by goniopuncture (i.e., a staged trabeculectomy) has been reported to reasonably control IOP over a 5-year period in a patient with idiopathic elevated episcleral venous pressure (43). Another option to consider in eyes deemed high risk for intraocular surgery or with poor visual potential is transscleral diode laser cyclophotocoagulation (described in Chapter 40).

KEY POINTS

- The episcleral venous pressure normally contributes 8 to 10 mm Hg to the IOP.
- Elevated episcleral venous pressure may be associated with several forms of glaucoma:
  - Obstruction to venous flow, as with thyroid-associated ophthalmopathy, superior vena cava syndrome, retrobulbar tumors, and cavernous sinus thrombosis
  - Arteriovenous fistulas, which include carotid–cavernous sinus fistula, orbital varices, and the Sturge–Weber syndrome
  - Idiopathic forms
- Mechanisms of associated glaucoma include
  - Direct effect of elevated episcleral venous pressure on IOP
  - Chronic outflow obstruction
  - Acute angle closure
  - Neovascular glaucoma
- Management is usually directed first at the cause of the venous pressure elevation, with medical, surgical, and laser glaucoma therapy as required.

REFERENCES

1. Brubaker RF. Determination of episcleral venous pressure in the eye. A comparison of three methods. *Arch Ophthalmol.* 1967;77:110–114.
2. Podos SM, Minas TF, Macri FJ. A new instrument to measure episcleral venous pressure. Comparison of normal eyes and eyes with primary open-angle glaucoma. *Arch Ophthalmol.* 1968;80:209–213.
3. Krakau CE, Widakowich J, Wilke K. Measurements of the episcleral venous pressure by means of an air jet. *Acta Ophthalmol (Copenh).* 1973;51:185–196.
4. Phelps CD, Armaly MF. Measurement of episcleral venous pressure. *Am J Ophthalmol.* 1978;85:35–42.
5. Talusan ED, Schwartz B. Episcleral venous pressure. Differences between normal, ocular hypertensive, and primary open angle glaucomas. *Arch Ophthalmol.* 1981;99:824–828.
6. Kollarits CR, Gaasterland D, Di Chiro G, et al. Management of a patient with orbital varices, visual loss, and ipsilateral glaucoma. *Ophthalmic Surg.* 1977;8:54–62.
7. Linner E. The outflow pressure in normal and glaucomatous eyes [in French]. *Acta Ophthalmol (Copenh).* 1955;33:101–116.
8. Selbach JM, Posielek K, Steuhl KP, et al. Episcleral venous pressure in untreated primary open-angle and normal-tension glaucoma. *Ophthalmologica.* 2005;219:357–361.
9. Chandler PA, Grant WM. *Glaucoma.* 2nd ed. Philadelphia, PA: Lea & Febiger; 1979:267.
10. Bárány EH. The influence of extraocular venous pressure on outflow facility in Cercopithecus ethiops and Macaca fascicularis. *Invest Ophthalmol Vis Sci.* 1978;17:711–717.
11. Buschmann W. Glaucoma in endocrine exophthalmus [in German]. *Klin Monatsbl Augenheilkd.* 1986;188:138–140.
12. Alfano JE, Alfano PA. Glaucoma and the superior vena caval obstruction syndrome. *Am J Ophthalmol.* 1956;42:685–696.
13. Bansal RK, Gupta A, Agarwal A. Primary orbital amyloidosis with secondary glaucoma: a case report. *Orbit.* 1991;10:105.
14. Nelson GA, Edward DP, Wilensky JT. Ocular amyloidosis and secondary glaucoma. *Ophthalmology.* 1999;106:1363–1366.
15. Keltner JL, Satterfield D, Dublin AB, et al. Dural and carotid cavernous sinus fistulas. Diagnosis, management, and complications. *Ophthalmology.* 1987;94:1585–1600.
16. Henderson JW, Schneider RC. The ocular findings in carotid-cavernous fistula in a series of 17 cases. *Am J Ophthalmol.* 1959;48:585–597.
17. Sanders MD, Hoyt WF. Hypoxic ocular sequelae of carotid-cavernous fistulae. Study of the causes of visual failure before and after neurosurgical treatment in a series of 25 cases. *Br J Ophthalmol.* 1969;53:82–97.
18. Palestine AG, Younge BR, Piepgras DG. Visual prognosis in carotid-cavernous fistula. *Arch Ophthalmol.* 1981;99:1600–1603.
19. Phelps CD, Thompson HS, Ossoinig KC. The diagnosis and prognosis of atypical carotid-cavernous fistula (red-eyed shunt syndrome). *Am J Ophthalmol.* 1982;93:423–436.
20. Grove AS Jr. The dural shunt syndrome. Pathophysiology and clinical course. *Ophthalmology.* 1984;91:31–44.
21. Wright JE. Orbital vascular anomalies. *Trans Am Acad Ophthalmol Otolaryngol.* 1974;78:OP606–OP616.
22. Weiss DI. Dual origin of glaucoma in encephalotrigeminal haemangiomatosis. *Trans Ophthalmol Soc UK.* 1973;93:477–493.
23. Phelps CD. The pathogenesis of glaucoma in Sturge–Weber syndrome. *Ophthalmology.* 1978;85:276–286.
24. Minas TF, Podos SM. Familial glaucoma associated with elevated episcleral venous pressure. *Arch Ophthalmol.* 1968;80:202–208.
25. Radius RL, Maumenee AE. Dilated episcleral vessels and open-angle glaucoma. *Am J Ophthalmol.* 1978;86:31–35.
26. Benedikt O, Roll P. Dilatation and tortuosity of episcleral vessels in open-angle glaucoma [in German]. *Klin Monatsbl Augenheilkd.* 1980;176:292–296.
27. Talusan ED, Fishbein SL, Schwartz B. Increased pressure of dilated episcleral veins with open-angle glaucoma without exophthalmos. *Ophthalmology.* 1983;90:257–265.
28. Ruprecht KW, Naumann GO. Unilateral secondary open-angle glaucoma with idiopathically dilated episcleral vessels [in German]. *Klin Monatsbl Augenheilkd.* 1984;184:23–27.
29. Roll P, Benedikt O. Dilatation and tortuosity of episcleral vessels in open-angle glaucoma. II. Electron microscopy study of the trabecular meshwork [in German]. *Klin Monatsbl Augenheilkd.* 1980;176:297–301.
30. Jørgensen JS, Guthoff R. Pathogenesis of unilateral dilated episcleral vessels and increase in intraocular pressure [in German]. *Klin Monatsbl Augenheilkd.* 1987;190:428–430.

31. Harris GJ, Rice PR. Angle closure in carotid-cavernous fistula. *Ophthalmology.* 1979;86:1521–1529.

32. Fourman S. Acute closed-angle glaucoma after arteriovenous fistulas. *Am J Ophthalmol.* 1989;107:156–159.

33. Buus DR, Tse DT, Parrish RK II. Spontaneous carotid cavernous fistula presenting with acute angle closure glaucoma. *Arch Ophthalmol.* 1989;107:596–597.

34. Jørgensen JS, Payer H. Increased episcleral venous pressure in uveal effusion [in German]. *Klin Monatsbl Augenheilkd.* 1989;195:14–16.

35. Spencer WH, Thompson HS, Hoyt WF. Ischaemic ocular necrosis from carotid-cavernous fistula. Pathology of stagnant anoxic "inflammation" in orbital and ocular tissues. *Br J Ophthalmol.* 1973;57:145–152.

36. Weiss DI, Shaffer RN, Nehrenberg TR. Neovascular glaucoma complicating carotid-cavernous fistula. *Arch Ophthalmol.* 1963;69:304–307.

37. Moses RA, Grodzki WJ Jr. Mechanism of glaucoma secondary to increased venous pressure. *Arch Ophthalmol.* 1985;103:1701–1703.

38. Kupersmith MJ, Berenstein A, Choi IS, et al. Management of nontraumatic vascular shunts involving the cavernous sinus. *Ophthalmology.* 1988;95:121–130.

39. Hanneken AM, Miller NR, Debrun GM, et al. Treatment of carotid-cavernous sinus fistulas using a detachable balloon catheter through the superior ophthalmic vein. *Arch Ophthalmol.* 1989;107:87–92.

40. Goldberg RA, Goldey SH, Duckwiler G, et al. Management of cavernous sinus-dural fistulas. Indications and techniques for primary embolization via the superior ophthalmic vein. *Arch Ophthalmol.* 1996;114:707–714.

41. Gupta N, Kikkawa DO, Levi L, et al. Severe vision loss and neovascular glaucoma complicating superior ophthalmic vein approach to carotid-cavernous sinus fistula. *Am J Ophthalmol.* 1997;124:853–855.

42. Bellows AR, Chylack LT Jr, Epstein DL, et al. Choroidal effusion during glaucoma surgery in patients with prominent episcleral vessels. *Arch Ophthalmol.* 1979;97:493–497.

43. Libre PE. Nonpenetrating filtering surgery and goniopuncture (staged trabeculectomy) for episcleral venous pressure glaucoma. *Am J Ophthalmol.* 2003;136:1172–1174.

Glaucomas Associated with Intraocular Tumors

A variety of intraocular tumors and tumor-like ocular disorders can give rise to glaucoma (**Table 21.1**) (1). In one survey of 2597 patients with intraocular tumors, 5% of the tumor-containing eyes had tumor-induced elevated intraocular pressure (IOP) at the time of the tumor diagnosis (2). In some cases, the mass lesions represent life-threatening malignancies, whereas other tumors are benign, creating critical problems with diagnosis and management.

Glaucoma secondary to intraocular tumors should be considered in all cases of unilateral or heavily asymmetric glaucoma, particularly when certain features such as iris heterochromia, lack of response to IOP-lowering treatment, or lack of response to steroids, which may indicate pseudouveitis, are present (1). B-scan ultrasonography and ultrasonographic biomicroscopy (UBM), as well as other diagnostic techniques (**Table 21.2**) (1), may be essential to demonstrate the presence of an intraocular tumor, particularly when it may be masked by a cataract, vitreous hemorrhage, retinal detachment, or other opacity in the ocular media. For patients with an intraocular malignant tumor, the emphasis shifts from the prevention of blindness to the preservation of life, but care must be taken in eyes with benign lesions to avoid loss of vision from unnecessary treatment. In this chapter, we consider the differential diagnosis and management of glaucomas associated with intraocular tumors.

PRIMARY UVEAL MELANOMAS

Melanomas of the uveal tract, the most common primary intraocular malignancy, are frequently associated with glaucoma by several mechanisms and with a variety of clinical presentations. In one large histopathologic study of eyes with malignant melanomas involving one or more portions of the uveal tract, the overall prevalence of glaucoma was 20% (3). Anterior uveal melanomas lead to IOP elevation more frequently than posterior melanomas, with reports of 41% and 45% of patients in two series, and choroidal melanomas were found to have associated glaucoma in 14% in one study (3,4). These figures are undoubtedly skewed, because one series represents histopathologic material and the other involves primarily patients referred to a glaucoma service (3,4). A clinical series from an oncology service may provide more meaningful statistics, in which 3% of 2111 eyes with uveal melanomas had associated IOP elevation, including 7% with iris melanomas, 17% with ciliary body melanomas, and 2% with choroidal melanomas (2). (Metastatic melanomas are rarely found in the eye but can cause glaucoma and are discussed later, under "Systemic Malignancies.")

Anterior Uveal Melanomas

Clinical Presentations and Mechanisms of Glaucoma

Melanomas of the anterior uveal tract most often arise from the ciliary body. These may be difficult to visualize directly because they often manifest as a smooth-domed elevation of the overlying iris. Wide dilatation may allow gonioscopic visualization of the lesion, which is typically seen as a dark brown mass between the iris and lens. In other cases, a primary melanoma of the ciliary body may extend through the peripheral iris and become visible as a nodular mass on the iris stroma and in the anterior chamber angle. Primary melanomas of the iris are usually easily seen by slitlamp biomicroscopy and gonioscopy, typically as slightly elevated, brown masses on the stroma (**Fig. 21.1**) with attendant hyperchromic heterochromia. Some melanomas of the iris, however, may be amelanotic and often have an associated, secondary vasculature and hypochromic heterochromia.

Melanomas of the anterior uvea may manifest as unilateral glaucoma. They may lead to glaucoma by open-angle or angle-closure mechanisms; the former mechanism is more common (**Fig. 21.2**). Aqueous humor outflow in the open anterior chamber angle can be obstructed by direct extension of the tumor or by trabecular meshwork seeding by tumor cells or melanin granules (1) (**Fig. 21.3**). In some eyes, the melanoma may arise from the iris, ciliary body, or iridociliary junction and spread circumferentially, creating a ring melanoma. A review of 14 patients with ring melanoma of the anterior chamber angle found that all patients presented with elevated IOP in the affected eye (5). In a rare presentation, a ring melanoma also masqueraded as pigmentary glaucoma (6). An anterior uveal melanoma may also extend posteriorly, causing a retinal detachment and giving the impression of a choroidal tumor. Others may extend into the anterior chamber, causing elevated IOP due to infiltration of the angle with occasional iris nodularity and heterochromia (7). Patients with ciliary body melanomas can present with chronic uveitis and refractory glaucoma (8). In melanomalytic glaucoma, macrophages containing melanin from a necrotic melanoma obstruct the trabecular meshwork (3,9). Ultrastructural studies reveal infiltration of the angle with melanin-laden macrophages, phagocytosis of melanin by trabecular endothelial cells, and tumor cells on the iris and in the meshwork (1).

Another variation of anterior uveal melanoma and glaucoma occurs with a tapioca iris melanoma. This rare melanoma of the iris creates a nodular appearance resembling tapioca

Table 21.1	Tumors and Tumor-Like Disorders Associated with Glaucoma		
Disorder	**Glaucoma, %**	**Glaucoma Mechanisms**	**Comments**
Anterior uveal malignant melanoma	41–45	Direct invasion of the angle Pigment dispersion	
Ring melanoma of the angle	100	Seeding of the meshwork with macrophages (melanomalytic) or pigment	
Ciliary body melanoma	—[a]	Anterior rotation of ciliary body Direct invasion of the angle Melanomalytic Uveitis Pigment dispersion	Can masquerade as a ciliary body cyst
Posterior uveal malignant melanoma	14	Neovascularization of the iris/angle (56%) Melanomalytic	
Uveal malignant melanoma, overall	3–20		
Melanocytoma	—[a]	Necrotic tumor cells (with or without macrophages) seeding meshwork Pigment dispersion	Iris, ciliary body, or choroidal lesions
Tapioca melanoma of the iris	33		
Metastasis to anterior segment	56–64	Infiltration of angle by tumor Seeding of meshwork by macrophages	Breast (40%) and lung (28%) are the most common primary sites
Metastasis to posterior segment	67	Angle closure from ciliary body or iris compression	
Metastasis to globe, overall	—[a]	Peripheral anterior synechiae Infiltration of Schlemm canal or collector channels Orbital infiltration, raising EVP	
Leukemia	—[a]	Hyphema (can be spontaneous) and migration of malignant cells into angle Hypopyon uveitis Neovascular Angle closure (anterior uveal infiltration, subretinal hemorrhage, or orbital infiltration) Elevated EVP (if orbital involvement)	Acute lymphocytic leukemia and acute myeloid leukemia most commonly associated with glaucoma Glaucoma can occur with childhood leukemias
Primary intraocular lymphoma with or without extraocular non-Hodgkin lymphoma	—[a,b]	Direct infiltration of iris and angle Inflammatory pseudouveitis Neovascular glaucoma	Often has retinal infiltrates and vitreous cells with cells with markedly elevated IOP
Histiocytosis X	—[a]	Involvement of anterior segment	Rare
Multiple myeloma	—[a]	Plasma cells obstructing TM Central vein occlusion (from increased plasma viscosity) with neovascular glaucoma Pars plana cysts with angle closure	Can masquerade as anterior uveitis
Myelodysplastic syndrome	—[a]	Acute angle closure caused by uveal effusion and nonrhegmatogenous retinal detachment and hemorrhage	

(continued)

Table 21.1	Tumors and Tumor-Like Disorders Associated with Glaucoma (*Continued*)		
Disorder	**Glaucoma, %**	**Glaucoma Mechanisms**	**Comments**
Retinoblastoma	17–23[c]	Neovascularization of the iris (70%) Angle closure from massive, exudative retinal detachment (27%) Obstruction of TM with tumor cells or inflammatory cells Elevated EVP if extrascleral/orbital involvement	
Juvenile xanthogranuloma	—[a]	Inflammatory cells Spontaneous hyphema	Histiocytic disorder that can masquerade as uveitis or tumor
Medulloepithelioma	46	Neovascularization of iris/angle Angle closure (ciliary body enlargement) Peripheral anterior synechiae	
Rhabdomyosarcoma	—[a]		Can rarely arise from iris or ciliary body
Benign anterior uveal tumors	—[a]		Nevi, melanocytosis, adenomas, and leiomyomas
Uveal melanocytoma	—[a]	Direct spread into the angle Dispersion of pigment from necrotic lesion	
Melanosis iridis	—[a]	Pigment dispersion	
Melanosis oculi	—[a]	Pigment dispersion	
Oculodermal melanocytosis	—[a]	Melanocytes in the meshwork	
Primary cysts of ciliary body or iris	—[a]	Angle closure (pseudoplateau iris) Pigment dispersion Mucus-producing epithelial cyst	
Sturge–Weber syndrome	71	Elevated EVP Developmental anomaly of the angle Neovascularization of the angle	Glaucoma associated with ipsilateral upper-eyelid cutaneous hemangioma
Von Recklinghausen neurofibromatosis	—[a]	Infiltration of the angle with tumor Angle closure due to thickening of ciliary body, fibrovascular membrane, resembling neovascular glaucoma failure of normal anterior chamber angle development	Glaucoma more likely if upper eyelid involved
Von Hippel–Lindau disease	—[a]	Rubeosis iridis or iridocyclitis	

[a]Unknown.
[b]Not common.
[c]Developed countries.
EVP, episcleral venous pressure; IOP, intraocular pressure; TM, trabecular meshwork.
Data from Radcliffe NM, Finger PT. Eye cancer related glaucoma: current concepts [review]. *Surv Ophthalmol.* 2009;54(1):47–73.

pudding and typically consists of low-grade spindle-type cells, although a case with epithelioid-type cells and metastases has been reported (10). Glaucoma is reported to occur in one third of the cases with tapioca melanoma (11).

An alternate mechanism of IOP elevation with an iris melanoma is neovascular glaucoma, which may resolve after excision of the tumor (12). Ciliary body melanomas may also cause an angle-closure form of glaucoma due to compression of the root of the iris into the anterior chamber angle or forward displacement of the lens–iris diaphragm (13) (**Fig. 21.4**).

Some eyes with a melanoma confined to the ciliary body may have a slightly lower IOP than that of the fellow eye (14). Any alteration in tension can be an indication of an anterior uveal melanoma.

Table 21.2	Diagnostic Techniques Helpful in Uncovering Intraocular Malignant Neoplasms
Technique	**Findings**
Gonioscopy	Mass in the angle, iris elevation, focal angle closure, neovascularization of anterior segment
Transillumination of globe (bright light placed on the eye)	Transillumination defect present in ciliary body/anterior uveal melanoma
UBM	Excellent tool for evaluating and following iris, angle, and ciliary body masses; ability to distinguish between solid tumors and nonmalignant cystic masses
Fine-needle aspiration biopsy	Helpful for atypical or metastatic tumors, particularly when diagnosis required for treatment
Vitrectomy-associated biopsy	Helpful in select situations (e.g., vitritis, intraocular lymphoma)
Finger iridectomy technique (clear cornea incision with 25-g aspiration cutter)	Helpful for obtaining tissue-sized specimens from iris masses
Anterior chamber aqueous aspiration (paracentesis)	Helpful if anterior segment cells or hypopyon is present
Fluorescein angiography of iris or choroid	Can be helpful in distinguishing melanomas from benign lesions
Diagnostic radiology (e.g., CT, MRI)	Orbital as well as CNS and systemic involvement as appropriate

CNS, central nervous system; CT, computed tomography; MRI, magnetic resonance imaging; UBM, ultrasonographic biomicroscopy.
Data from Radcliffe NM, Finger PT. Eye cancer related glaucoma: current concepts [review]. *Surv Ophthalmol.* 2009;54(1):47–73.

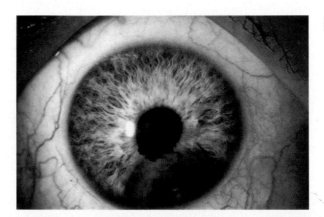

Figure 21.1 Slitlamp view of a malignant melanoma of the iris.

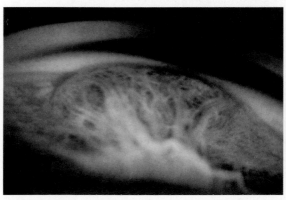

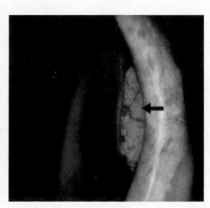

Figure 21.2 **A:** Gonioscopic view shows elevation of the peripheral iris in a patient with ciliary body melanoma. **B:** After wide dilation of the same eye, one can see a solid mass with irregular pigmentation between the iris and lens.

A

B

Light microscopic view of malignant melanoma cells seeding the anterior chamber angle causing glaucoma (**A**) and solid tumor involving the angle (**B**).

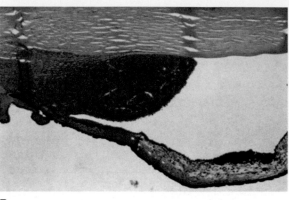

B

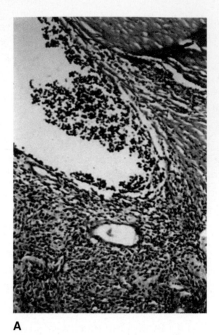

A

Differential Diagnosis

Several conditions can be confused with glaucoma and an anterior uveal melanoma. Associated changes may mask an underlying melanoma, whereas other mass lesions may simulate an anterior uveal melanoma. For example, iritis may appear to be present in some cases of glaucoma and melanoma, which usually represents tumor cells in the anterior chamber (4), whereas other eyes may have primary iritis with inflammatory nodules that may be confused with a malignancy (15). In one large series, a primary cyst of the iris was the most common lesion to be confused with a melanoma of the iris (16). However, anterior uveal melanomas can masquerade as cysts of the iris or ciliary body because of separation of the two epithelial layers by an eosinophilic exudate (4,13). Iris nevi may be especially

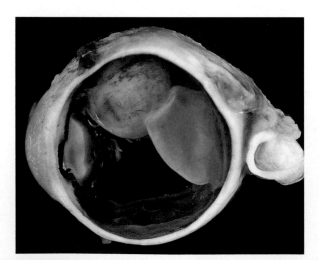

Gross appearance of a sectioned eye, showing a malignant melanoma of the ciliary body and anterior uvea adjacent to the lens, creating closure of the anterior chamber angle. (Courtesy of Prithvi Mruthyunjaya, MD.)

difficult to distinguish from iris melanomas clinically and histologically. (Other benign tumors and metastatic malignancies must be included in the differential diagnosis of uveal melanomas and are discussed later in this chapter.)

Choroidal Melanomas

Occasionally, a patient with a melanoma of the choroid may present with acute angle-closure glaucoma. This is usually caused by the forward displacement of the lens–iris diaphragm by a large posterior tumor, which is commonly associated with a total retinal detachment. The finding of a retinal detachment, especially if serous, and glaucoma in the same eye should alert the clinician to the possibility of an underlying malignant melanoma. Other reported mechanisms of IOP elevation in association with choroidal melanomas include neovascular glaucoma and pigment dispersion in the vitreous with melanomalytic glaucoma (3,17). In addition to retinal detachment, other conditions that may mask the presence of a choroidal melanoma include intraocular inflammation and hemorrhage, and a dislocated lens nucleus may mimic a choroidal melanoma, especially when inflammatory glaucoma is also present (18,19).

Diagnostic Adjuncts

The difficulty in detecting a uveal melanoma and distinguishing it from other intraocular tumors occasionally necessitates the use of special diagnostic measures.

Ultrasonography

UBM is a valuable tool to help determine the location, size, and extent of uveal melanomas (20–22). It can also help in differentiating retroiridal cysts from tumors (23), but it cannot distinguish between benign and malignant tumors. B-scan ultrasonography may be useful in demonstrating the presence

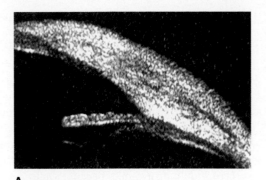
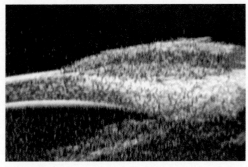

A   **B**

Figure 21.5 UBM features of malignant melanoma of the iris. **A:** Iridociliary melanoma replacing the peripheral iris and ciliary body and filling the anterior chamber angle. Mass is slightly sonolucent compared with normal iris stroma. **B:** Larger iridociliary melanoma. Iris appears to arise from the side of the mass. (From Corrêa ZM, Augsburger JJ. Ultrasound biomicroscopy of the anterior ocular segment. In: Tasman W, Jaeger EA, eds. *Duane's Foundations of Clinical Ophthalmology.* Vol 2. Philadelphia, PA: Lippincott Williams & Wilkins; 2008:chap 106.)

of a ciliary body melanoma (**Fig. 21.5**) or a choroidal melanoma when the latter is masked by a retinal detachment, vitreous hemorrhage, or other opacity in the ocular media. However, this technique does not always distinguish a neoplasm from other masses of the posterior ocular segment (24).

Fluorescein Angiography of the Iris

Fluorescein angiography of the iris has been useful in distinguishing melanomas from benign lesions of the iris, such as leiomyomas and benign melanocytic tumors (25–27). The angiographic characteristic of a melanoma of the iris is diffuse and eventually confluent fluorescence emanating from ill-defined vascular foci (27).

Cytopathologic Studies

An aqueous or vitreous aspirate may provide sufficient material for a histopathologic diagnosis of a primary or metastatic malignancy (28,29). This may be especially useful for suspected melanomas of the anterior uvea when cells can be seen in the aqueous by slitlamp biomicroscopy (**Fig. 21.6**). The technique involves aspiration of aqueous with a small-gauge needle

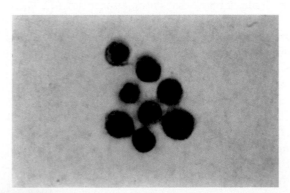

Figure 21.6 Light microscopic view of melanoma cells aspirated from the aqueous of an eye with anterior uveal melanoma (Papanicolaou, ×400). (From Ritch R, Shields MB, eds. *The Secondary Glaucomas.* St. Louis, MO: CV Mosby; 1982, with permission.)

through the limbus or peripheral cornea. For neoplastic cells, cytologic preservation is best with a Millipore filter (29).

A fine-needle aspiration biopsy may also be used to obtain material for cytopathologic study from a suspected anterior uveal or choroidal melanoma (30).

Frozen Section Diagnoses

A frozen section may be helpful in identifying a tumor of the iris and in determining the surgical resection margins of the lesion (31). In sending the iridectomy specimen to the pathologist, care must be taken to identify the orientation of the tissue and to avoid curling of the edges (31).

Prognosis

When a uveal melanoma is associated with glaucoma, the prognosis appears to be worse for metastasis and death, compared with that for a melanoma without glaucoma. In one study, three of four patients with a primary melanoma of the ciliary body and glaucoma died of metastatic disease within 2.5 years after enucleation (4), and another investigation of uveal melanomas in children and adolescents identified glaucoma as a predominant factor relating to a fatal outcome (32). Histopathologic studies of eyes with a ciliary body melanoma and glaucoma often reveal tumor cells in the aqueous outflow system, which is a potential route of extraocular metastasis (4). Patients with choroidal melanomas and glaucoma also have a more guarded prognosis, because the tumor is usually large by the time the glaucoma has developed.

Melanomas of the iris generally have a better prognosis than other uveal melanomas (33,34). The relatively benign nature may reflect the earlier detection and small size at the time of detection, allowed by the more obvious anterior location. However, metastases have been reported to occur. In one series of 1043 reported iris melanomas, 31 (3%) eventually metastasized (35). In another series of 169 microscopically proven iris melanomas, 5% developed distant metastasis over 10 years (36). In the latter series, metastases were significantly more likely to develop in older patients who demonstrated tumors of iris root or angle location with elevated IOP and extraocular extension. The cell type influences the rate of metastasis, with none among spindle A tumors in one series, 2.6% with spindle B tumors, 6.9% with epithelioid tumors, and 10.5% with mixed-cell tumors (35). The presence of glaucoma with an iris melanoma may also increase the risk for metastasis. Ring melanoma of the trabecular meshwork and angle structures, despite the relatively small tumor volume, has resulted in liver metastases in 25% of patients over a mean follow-up of 6 years (5).

Observed growth of iris lesions may be the best indicator of malignant potential. However, one study of 175 patients with melanocytic tumors of the iris, followed for 1 to 12 years, reported only a 4.6% incidence of tumor growth, and the growth was not always indicative of the presence of malignant cells (37). This low incidence may in part reflect the slow growth of iris melanomas in some patients. In one case report, an iris melanoma was followed over 41 years before producing glaucoma and resulting in enucleation (38). Continued close observation is essential in managing these patients.

Management

Considering the poor prognosis in cases of ciliary body or choroidal melanoma associated with glaucoma, the recommended management most often is enucleation, although fine-needle aspiration biopsy can be considered first to confirm the presence of malignancy if deemed appropriate. By the time glaucoma has developed, the melanoma is usually too large or diffuse for local treatment. However, there are exceptions, especially when the eye with the melanoma is the patient's only eye with useful vision. In such cases, local excision of an anterior uveal melanoma or radiotherapy of anterior or posterior tumors is occasionally attempted. In one series of 52 patients undergoing iridocyclectomy for lesions of the iris or ciliary body, one half of the excised lesions were benign and almost one third of the group eventually required enucleation (39). Radiotherapy, especially with anterior tumors, may be complicated by hemorrhage and further pressure elevation, as well as failure to eradicate the melanoma. Palladium-103 radiation therapy has been associated with fewer sight-limiting complications than iodine-125 and with excellent local tumor control (40).

Care must be taken to avoid artificial elevation of the IOP during diagnostic and surgical maneuvers for fear that this may accelerate extraocular dissemination of tumor cells (41–43). Enucleation techniques have been developed to minimize intraoperative pressure elevation, which include manometric pressure-regulating systems and the use of a wire snare to cut the optic nerve (42–44).

Iris melanoma and glaucoma are usually managed more conservatively because the tumors are typically small when first detected and can be observed for evidence of growth. However, iris melanomas may metastasize, and the degree to which associated glaucoma increases this risk is uncertain. In general, iris melanomas should be documented by photography (and UBM, when practical) and followed for evidence of growth. If slight growth is detected, continued close observation is still reasonable, whereas pronounced and progressive growth requires surgical intervention (45). This usually consists of complete excision by a sector iridectomy, although photocoagulation may be used to eradicate some iris melanomas (46). However, if the tumor has disseminated or diffusely extended in the anterior segment, which is often the case when associated glaucoma is present, enucleation is usually indicated.

The management of the associated glaucoma in eyes with a uveal melanoma is best limited to medical therapy. Filtering surgery should be avoided, because seeding of iris melanoma cells through a trabeculectomy site into the filtering bleb with extraocular dissemination and fatal metastases have been documented in such cases (37,47). When additional intervention for the glaucoma is required, especially in eyes with iris melanomas, an ab externo cyclodestructive procedure may be the procedure of choice.

SYSTEMIC MALIGNANCIES

Metastatic Carcinomas

Two large studies have been reported in which at least one eye from autopsy cases with known malignancies was examined for ocular metastases (48,49). The most common primary sites for metastasis to the eye were the lung and breast. The two studies reported similar results regarding the incidence of ocular metastases from the lung (6% and 6.7%), although the results differed for metastases from the breast (37% and 9.7%) and the overall incidence of metastasis from all primary carcinomas (12% and 4%) (39,48–50). Metastatic carcinoma of the eye is reported to be the most common form of intraocular malignancy (51).

The most common site of ocular metastasis is the posterior uvea, although glaucoma is more often associated with metastases to the anterior segment (1). In one study of 227 cases of carcinoma metastatic to the eye and orbit, glaucoma was detected in 7.5% of the total group and in 56% of the 26 cases with anterior ocular metastasis (52,53). In another series of 256 eyes with uveal metastases, associated IOP elevation was present in 5% of the total group but in 64% and 67% of eyes with iris and ciliary body metastases, respectively (2). The clinical appearance of metastatic carcinomas of the anterior uvea is a gelatinous or translucent mass, which may be a single lesion or multiple nodules on the iris, often associated with rubeosis iridis, iridocyclitis, or hyphema.

Mechanisms of glaucoma in eyes with anterior uveal metastatic carcinoma include obstructions of the trabecular meshwork by sheets of tumor cells or by infiltration with neoplastic tissue. Other mechanisms include angle closure due to compression of the iris from the tumor or by peripheral anterior synechiae. In some cases, ocular signs or symptoms may be the first manifestation of metastatic malignancies.

In the management of metastatic carcinoma to the anterior uvea, paracentesis with aqueous aspiration for cytopathologic examination is often helpful in establishing the diagnosis (Table 21.2). When the cytology is nondiagnostic, a serologic tumor marker (e.g., in the aqueous) has been used to make the diagnosis (54). Treatment of the metastatic carcinoma usually includes radiation therapy and occasional chemotherapy (1). Enucleation is usually reserved for blind, painful eyes. If the associated glaucoma persists, it should be controlled medically whenever possible.

Metastatic Melanomas

Although ocular melanomas usually are primary malignancies, metastatic melanomas of the eye occur and can occasionally cause glaucoma (28). A unique form has been called black hypopyon, in which a disseminated cutaneous malignant melanoma metastasized to the eye, where it became necrotic, possibly in response to immunotherapy or irradiation, resulting in a hypopyon of tumor cells and pigment-laden macrophages with associated glaucoma (55).

Leukemias

In an autopsy survey of 117 eyes of individuals who died of acute or chronic leukemia, the incidence of leukemic infiltrates in the ocular tissues was 28% (49). In a slitlamp study of 39 children with acute leukemia, the same percentage of cases was found to have flare or cells in the anterior chamber (56). In another series of childhood leukemias, the 5-year survival rate for patients with ocular manifestations was 21.4%, compared with 45.7% for those without ophthalmic involvement (57). Although this series began in 1972, when treatment was less effective than it is today (58), these findings emphasize that any child with leukemia and apparent iritis should be regarded as having a relapse, and anterior chamber aspiration and iris biopsy are essential procedures in establishing this diagnosis (58,59). In a series of 135 patients who had fatal leukemia, ocular leukemic infiltration was found in one third of the cases, most often in the choroid (60).

A leukemic infiltration of the anterior ocular segment leads to glaucoma in some cases, which may present in association with hyphema and hypopyon (Table 21.2). These patients more often have acute lymphocytic leukemia. In adults, acute and chronic leukemias may also have ocular involvement, with reported cases manifesting variously as bilateral hypopyon or a massive subretinal hemorrhage with acute angle-closure glaucoma. Aqueous aspirates may need to be studied to confirm that the patient is in relapse. In most cases, after the diagnosis has been established by cytologic examination of the aqueous aspirate, treatment usually includes irradiation and chemotherapy. In one reported case, the glaucoma cleared after washing necrotic tumor cells from the anterior chamber (61).

Other Neoplasias

Lymphomas

An autopsy review of 60 eyes from patients with lymphomas revealed ocular involvement in 4 (6.7%) (49). The anterior ocular segment may be involved, presenting as iridocyclitis, with occasional IOP elevation (62).

Histiocytosis X

This uncommon multisystem disorder, characterized by accumulation of histiocytes in various tissues, includes three clinical subsets: eosinophilic granuloma (i.e., lesions confined to bone), Hand–Schüller–Christian disease (i.e., bone and soft-tissue involvement), and Letterer–Siwe disease (i.e., predominantly soft-tissue involvement in infants). Histiocytosis X can involve the anterior chamber with associated glaucoma (63). This situation is apparently rare, because a study of 76 children with histiocytosis X revealed 18 with orbital involvement but none with intraocular involvement (64).

Multiple Myeloma

Apparent nongranulomatous anterior uveitis with associated glaucoma in a patient with multiple myeloma was found by cytologic examination to represent an infiltrate of neoplastic plasma cells (65). Mechanisms of glaucoma are summarized in Table 21.2.

Myelodysplastic Syndrome

In patients with the myelodysplastic syndrome, hematopoietic precursors of all three cell lines (i.e., erythroid, myeloid, and megakaryocytic lines) are abundant but morphologically abnormal, and 10% to 30% of cases are fatal because of acute blastic transformation of nonlymphocytic leukemia. Cases have been reported in which patients presented with acute angle-closure glaucoma associated with uveal effusion and nonrhegmatogenous retinal detachment and hemorrhage (66,67).

OCULAR TUMORS OF CHILDHOOD

In addition to leukemia and other systemic neoplasia in which the eye may be involved secondarily, there are certain childhood tumors in which the ocular involvement is a primary part of the disorder. These include retinoblastoma, medulloepithelioma, and rhabdomyosarcoma. Juvenile xanthogranuloma, a histiocytic lesion, is included in this category because it can mimic malignancy and also give rise to glaucoma.

Retinoblastoma

Incidence of Glaucoma

Although glaucoma is not commonly recognized clinically in children with retinoblastoma, histopathologic studies suggest that glaucoma is a frequent complication of this disease. One study of 149 eyes found histologic evidence of a glaucoma-inducing mechanism in 50% of the cases, although an elevated IOP had been clinically recorded in only 23% (68). In another series of 303 eyes with retinoblastoma, 17% had documented pressure elevation (2). Glaucoma was found in one study to be the presenting sign in 7% of eyes with retinoblastoma, with leukocoria (i.e., white pupillary reflex) and strabismus being the most common presentations, at 60% and 20%, respectively (69).

Mechanisms of Glaucoma

Neovascularization of the iris is a frequent histopathologic finding in eyes with retinoblastoma and is the most common cause of the associated glaucoma (1). Angiogenesis may be mediated by vascular endothelial growth factor (70). Rubeosis iridis and neovascular glaucoma are frequently overlooked clinically and should be considered in all cases of retinoblastoma. Two additional causes of glaucoma are angle closure due to massive exudative retinal detachment and obstruction of the anterior chamber angle by inflammatory cells or necrotic tumor tissue (2,68). In a review of 1500 patients with retinoblastoma, anterior chamber tumor involvement was seen in 30 cases and was found to indicate a poor prognosis (71). Specular microscopy has demonstrated clusters of retinoblastoma cells on the corneal endothelium as a bright, lacy network of reflections within a dark area (72).

Differential Diagnosis

Conditions that simulate retinoblastoma have been called pseudogliomas and include retinopathy of prematurity, persistent hyperplastic primary vitreous, retinal dysplasia, Coats disease, toxocariasis, and infantile retinal detachment (73,74). Each of these conditions also has a high incidence of rubeosis iridis so that this factor is not helpful in distinguishing retinoblastoma from the pseudogliomas (73,75).

Management

The presence of rubeosis iridis, with or without glaucoma, indicates a worse prognosis for patients with retinoblastoma (75). This is also true when glaucoma is present without iris neovascularization, because it usually indicates a large tumor with angle closure or dissemination of tumor cells into the anterior chamber (71). Although many treatments are available for retinoblastoma, including chemoreduction, laser photocoagulation, thermotherapy, cryotherapy, and plaque radiotherapy (76), enucleation is often indicated when glaucoma mechanisms are present.

Medulloepithelioma

Medulloepithelioma, or diktyoma, is a primary tumor of childhood that arises most often from nonpigmented ciliary epithelium. The clinical appearance is a whitish-gray mass or cyst of the iris or ciliary body. In a study of 56 cases, glaucoma was observed clinically in 26 eyes (77). Histopathologic evidence of glaucoma was seen in 18 cases, 11 of which had rubeosis iridis. Peripheral anterior synechiae and shallow anterior chambers were also commonly observed. In one report, glaucoma was associated with two white flocculi floating in the anterior chamber, delicate iris neovascularization, and a globular ciliary body mass (78). Some medulloepitheliomas are malignant, although the mortality rate is low. Although enucleation may be required for malignant cases, success has been reported with iridocyclectomy, and local excision has been recommended when the tumor is small and well circumscribed (77).

Rhabdomyosarcoma

Rhabdomyosarcoma is the most common malignant orbital tumor of childhood. It is rarely intraocular but has been reported to arise from the iris or ciliary body (79).

Juvenile Xanthogranuloma

Juvenile xanthogranuloma is a benign, self-limiting histiocytic disease of infants and young children, with rare cases occurring in young adults (80). It is characterized by discrete, yellow, papular cutaneous lesions primarily of the head and neck and by salmon-colored to lightly pigmented lesions of the iris. It is usually diagnosed by a biopsy of a skin lesion or an aqueous tap and iris biopsy, the histology of which reveals foamy histiocytes and Touton giant cells. The iris lesions are typically unilateral and may cause spontaneous hyphema. Glaucoma may occur from invasion of the anterior chamber angle with histiocytes or from the hyphema or a secondary uveitis. Treatment for eyes with juvenile xanthogranuloma and associated glaucoma includes topical and subconjunctival corticosteroids and occasional external-beam irradiation. Invasive surgery should be avoided if possible because prognosis is poor (81).

BENIGN TUMORS OF THE ANTERIOR UVEA

In the differential diagnosis of anterior uveal tumors, several benign lesions must be considered. These include nevi, cysts, melanocytoses, melanocytomas, adenomas, and leiomyomas. Glaucoma may be associated with several of these conditions, further complicating diagnosis and treatment. UBM may be a useful adjunct in distinguishing between some malignant and benign lesions.

Nevi of the Iris

One or more nevi on the stromal surface of the iris are a common clinical finding. They are usually recognized as small, discrete, flat, or slightly elevated lesions of variable pigmentation. Some, however, may be confused with melanomas, which has led to unnecessary surgical intervention. In a retrospective clinicopathologic study of 189 lesions of the anterior uvea that were originally diagnosed as melanomas, 80% were reclassified as nevi of several cell types (82). These investigators found no clinical features to distinguish benign from malignant tumors, including diffuse spread or the presence of glaucoma. In another study of melanocytic iris tumors, however, five clinical variables were associated with a higher risk for malignancy: diameter greater than 3 mm, pigment dispersion, prominent tumor vascularity, elevated IOP, and tumor-related ocular symptoms (83). Fluorescein angiography of the iris, aqueous aspiration for cytologic examination, or biopsy may aid in the important differentiation between melanomas and benign lesions of the iris. Diffuse, pigmented, and nonpigmented nevi of the iris can cause glaucoma by direct extension across the trabecular meshwork (82,84). This is rare in children, but the case of a 16-year-old girl has been reported in which an aggressive iris nevus caused glaucoma by invading the trabecular meshwork (85).

A specific form of iris nevus with associated glaucoma is the iris nevus syndrome. In these cases, diffuse nevi of the iris are associated with progressive synechial closure of the angle and subsequent IOP elevation (86). A subset of the iridocorneal endothelial syndrome, the Cogan–Reese syndrome, has a similar clinical appearance, but the pedunculated nodules on the surface of the iris are composed of tissue resembling iris stroma (87). The benign lesions of the iris in both of these conditions have been mistaken for malignant melanomas, which has led to enucleation in some patients. (These conditions are discussed further in Chapter 16.)

Cysts

Cysts of the iris are classified as primary and secondary, with the former arising from the epithelial layers of the iris and ciliary body or, less often, from the iris stroma (88). Most primary cysts are stationary lesions, rarely progressing or causing visual complications. However, families have been described in which multiple cysts of the iris and ciliary body, presumably of autosomal dominant inheritance, caused angle-closure glaucoma (89). Other reported mechanisms of IOP elevation associated with iris cysts include pigment dispersion (90) and a mucus-producing epithelial cyst of the iris stroma of unknown origin (91). Iris cysts have been successfully treated by laser cystotomy, although others may require surgical excision if uncontrolled IOP or other symptoms persist.

Secondary cysts of the iris may result from surgery, trauma, or neoplasia and are more likely than primary cysts to lead to inflammation and glaucoma (88,92). Ultrasonography has been a useful diagnostic adjunct for primary and secondary iris cysts.

Melanocytomas

These tumors are classified as benign nevi and are seen clinically as darkly pigmented lesions, usually on the optic nerve head and, less often, in the choroid, ciliary body, or iris. Tumors in the latter location can cause glaucoma by direct spread into the anterior chamber angle or by dispersion of pigment into the angle from a necrotic melanocytoma (93,94).

Melanoses

Melanosis iridis is characterized by verrucous-like elevations on the surface of a darkly pigmented, velvety iris. It is usually unilateral and sometimes sectorial, although bilateral involvement has been reported (95). Melanosis oculi has additional hyperpigmentation of the episclera, choroid, or both and has been reported in association with open-angle glaucoma in which the mechanism appears to be heavy pigmentation of the trabecular meshwork (96). A similar condition has been observed in oculodermal melanocytosis (nevus of Ota, which is considered later in this chapter).

Adenomas

Benign adenomas may arise from the epithelium of the anterior uvea, especially the ciliary body (Fuchs adenoma) (97). They occur predominantly in adults, although they have been observed in a child with associated hyperplastic primary vitreous (98). Although common among the elderly, adenomas are rarely observed clinically (99). Some can involve the iris primarily or secondarily and have caused glaucoma from pigment dispersion (100,101). Adenomas must be distinguished from anterior uveal cysts and melanomas (100). Adenocarcinomas may also arise from the ciliary body epithelium and may cause glaucoma (102).

Leiomyomas

These rare tumors may appear as a slow-growing grayish-white, vascularized nodule on the surface of the iris. Glaucoma is not a typical complication.

PHAKOMATOSES

In 1932, Van der Hoeve (103) coined the term phakomatosis, meaning "mother spot" or "birthmark," to denote a group of disorders that are characterized by hamartomas, which are congenital tumors arising from tissue that is normally found in the involved area. The hamartomas primarily involve the eye, skin, and nervous system, although other systems may be involved to a lesser degree, including pulmonary, cardiovascular, gastrointestinal, renal, and skeletal. In some cases, the anomalies are present at birth, whereas others become manifest later in life. The four conditions that traditionally comprise the phakomatoses are the von Hippel–Lindau syndrome, von Recklinghausen neurofibromatosis, tuberous sclerosis or Bourneville disease, and the Sturge–Weber syndrome. Several other disorders subsequently have been included by various investigators. The following discussion is limited to phakomatoses that frequently or occasionally are associated with glaucoma.

Sturge–Weber Syndrome

General Features

The hamartoma occurring in the Sturge–Weber syndrome (i.e., encephalotrigeminal angiomatosis) arises from vascular tissue and produces a characteristic port-wine hemangioma of the skin along the trigeminal distribution (**Fig. 21.7**) and an ipsilateral leptomeningeal angioma. The angiomata are present at birth and are usually unilateral, although bilateral cases also occur. In one review of 51 patients, the condition was recognized before 24 months of age in more than half the cases (104). The nervous system involvement frequently causes seizure disorders, hemispheric motor or sensory defects, and intellectual deficiency. A characteristic radiographic finding is cortical calcifications that develop after several years and appear as double densities or "railroad tracks." There is no race or sex predilection, and no hereditary pattern has been established.

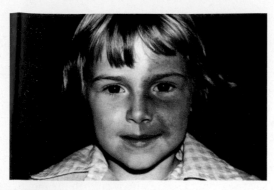

Figure 21.7 Child with the Sturge–Weber syndrome and unilateral glaucoma. Notice the typical port-wine hemangioma of the skin along the distribution of the left trigeminal nerve.

Ocular Features

Glaucoma occurs in approximately one half of the cases in which the port-wine stain involves the ophthalmic and maxillary divisions of the trigeminal nerve. Slitlamp examination typically reveals a dense episcleral vascular plexus and occasional ampulliform dilatations of conjunctival vessels. These findings are on the side of the cutaneous lesion. Some patients also have a choroidal hemangioma. In the study of 51 patients previously mentioned, 69% had conjunctival or episcleral hemangiomas, 55% had choroidal hemangiomas, and 71% had glaucoma (104).

Theories of Glaucoma Mechanism

The cause of glaucoma in the Sturge–Weber syndrome has been a controversial issue. Weiss (105) described two mechanisms, the more common of which occurs in infants, with a developmental anomaly of the anterior chamber angle similar to that of congenital glaucoma. One histopathologic report described a partial developmental anomaly of the anterior chamber angle (106), and another study revealed neovascularization in the trabecular meshwork (107). Cibis and associates (108) found aging changes, similar to those seen in chronic open-angle glaucoma in the trabecular meshwork of three eyes with the Sturge–Weber syndrome.

The other mechanism of glaucoma appears later in life and is associated with an open anterior chamber angle and small arteriovenous fistulas in the episcleral vessels. Phelps (109) observed episcleral hemangiomas in all cases and elevated episcleral venous pressure whenever this parameter could be studied but saw no abnormalities of the anterior chamber angle. He thought that elevated episcleral venous pressure was the most common glaucoma mechanism in all ages of patients with the Sturge–Weber syndrome.

Management

Medical therapy may suffice to control glaucoma that occurs in later life, whereas the infantile form usually requires surgical intervention (105). In most cases of glaucoma associated with elevated episcleral venous pressure, medical therapy has limited efficacy, and this appears to be true for prostaglandins (110). In one report, use of latanoprost was associated with development of an anterior uveal effusion (111). Success has been

reported with a trabeculectomy in children and adults (112,113). However, filtering surgery in these patients is associated with intraoperative choroidal effusion and occasionally with expulsive hemorrhage. In one study of 30 patients, goniotomy was not associated with these complications and was the investigator's first choice in most cases (113). Because whether the glaucoma is caused by an anterior chamber angle anomaly or elevated episcleral venous pressure is not certain, a combined trabeculotomy–trabeculectomy may improve the chances of success by treating both possible sources of elevated IOP (114,115), although it does not reduce the potential for serious complications.

Some surgeons prefer to perform one or more prophylactic posterior sclerotomies just before filtration surgery or any other intraocular procedure to reduce the risk for choroidal or retinal effusion and expulsive hemorrhage. Another surgical approach to reduce pressure in these patients, while minimizing intraocular complications, is implantation of a valved or nonvalved glaucoma drainage device. One case series reported good outcomes after two-staged implantation of Baerveldt glaucoma drainage devices (116). In this situation, the Baerveldt implant is placed in the appropriate location; the tube is reflected to an adjacent subconjunctival location and anchored to sclera. Six weeks later, the tube is dissected free and inserted into the anterior chamber. A final technique that may be considered is a cyclodestructive procedure that avoids incisional surgery.

Von Recklinghausen Neurofibromatosis

General Features

The principal systemic lesions in this condition involve the skin and include café-au-lait spots, which are flat, hyperpigmented lesions with well-circumscribed borders, and neurofibromas, which appear as soft, flesh-colored, pedunculated masses. The latter lesions arise from Schwann cells. Central nervous system involvement is uncommon, although neurofibromas may develop from cranial nerves, especially the acoustic nerve. Two subsets of neurofibromatosis have been distinguished: peripheral (von Recklinghausen neurofibromatosis), characterized by the skin lesions, and central, characterized by bilateral acoustic schwannomas (117). Both are inherited by an autosomal dominant mode with variable expressivity. Genetic analysis of a kindred with von Recklinghausen neurofibromatosis indicated that the responsible gene is located near the centromere on chromosome 17 (118).

Ocular Features

In the peripheral form, the eyelids, conjunctiva, iris, ciliary body, and choroid may be involved with the neurofibromas. The hamartomatous lesions of the iris are called Lisch nodules (119). They are usually bilateral and characterized by well-defined, clear to yellow or brown, dome-shaped, gelatinous elevations on the iris stroma (**Fig 21.8**). An ultrastructural study indicates that they are of melanocytic origin (120). Lisch nodules are a nearly constant feature of von Recklinghausen neurofibromatosis, occurring in 92% of one series of 77 patients (121). In another study of 64 patients, the nodules were seen

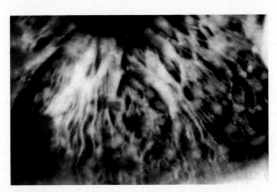

Figure 21.8 Slitlamp view of Lisch nodules on the iris of a patient with von Recklinghausen neurofibromatosis. (Courtesy of George Rosenwasser, MD.)

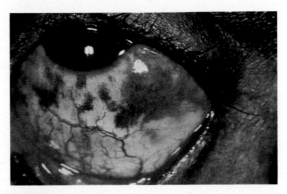

Figure 21.9 Abnormal pigmentation of the episclera in a patient with oculodermal melanocytosis (nevus of Ota).

in 95% and in all patients aged 16 years or older (122). Chorioretinal hamartomas and gliomas of the optic nerve are occasionally present. A fluorescein angiographic study of the choroidal lesions revealed avascular patches of hypofluorescence similar to multiple, small choroidal nevi (122). The central form of neurofibromatosis does not typically have ocular findings other than presenile posterior subcapsular or nuclear cataracts (117).

IOP elevation is more likely to occur in neurofibromatosis when the lids are involved with neurofibromas. Possible mechanisms of glaucoma include infiltration of the angle with neurofibromatous tissue, closure of the anterior chamber angle caused by nodular thickening of the ciliary body and choroid, fibrovascular membrane resembling neovascular glaucoma, and failure of normal anterior chamber angle development (123,124).

Management

In treating the glaucoma, medical measures should be attempted first, because surgical approaches are often not satisfactory. An infant with unilateral glaucoma underwent five unsuccessful operations before ocular neurofibromatosis was discovered 2 years later (125).

Von Hippel–Lindau Disease

This phakomatosis is characterized by angiomatosis of the retina and, in a small percentage of cases, the cerebellum. Most cases are not familial. Glaucoma may occur as a late sequela of rubeosis iridis or iridocyclitis.

Nevus of Ota

The nevus of Ota (i.e., oculodermal melanocytosis) is not included in all reported classifications of the phakomatoses, but it does fit the broader definition of the disease group.

General Features

The hamartoma in this condition represents an abnormally large accumulation of melanocytes in ocular tissues, especially the episclera (**Fig. 21.9**), the skin in the distribution of the trigeminal nerve, and occasionally the nasal or buccal mucosa.

In a study of 194 patients, 67 had only dermal involvement, 12 had only ocular involvement, and 115 had both (126). The condition is nearly always unilateral with a preponderance of females and a tendency toward races with darker pigmentation (127). Degeneration to malignant melanomas may occur in white patients but are rare in nonwhite patients (128).

Glaucoma

Evidence of chronic glaucoma has been observed in patients with the nevus of Ota (129). Elevated IOP, with or without glaucomatous damage, was seen in 10% of cases in one series (124). The involved eye typically has unusually heavy pigmentation of the trabecular meshwork, and histopathologic studies have revealed melanocytes in the meshwork (130,131).

Management

Medical management, as with other forms of open-angle glaucoma, should be tried first. If this fails, laser trabeculoplasty may be effective (96), although filtering surgery will most likely be required.

Phakomatosis Pigmentovascularis

Phakomatosis pigmentovascularis represents an overlap syndrome with combined oculodermal vascular malformation (nevus flammeus, similar to Klippel–Trenaunay–Weber syndrome and Sturge–Weber syndrome) and oculodermal melanocytosis (132). It has only been described in Asian patients.

Congenital glaucoma developed in all eyes that had 360-degree involvement of the episclera by the vascular malformation and melanocytosis. When one or both are present with only partial involvement, elevated IOP may develop later in life. Vascular malformation plays a more important role in the predisposition to glaucoma in these patients than does oculodermal melanocytosis.

KEY POINTS

- Glaucoma secondary to intraocular tumor should be considered in all cases of unilateral or heavily asymmetric glaucoma, particularly in the context of certain features: lack of response to IOP-lowering treatment, chronic pseudouveitis that is unresponsive to steroid treatment, iris heterochromia, unilateral pigment dispersion, serous retinal detachment with elevated IOP, dilated episcleral sentinel vessels, or media opacity precluding a good view of posterior segment.

- In general, management of glaucoma related to intraocular malignant tumors involves treatment of the underlying tumor and managing IOP with medical therapy, cyclophotocoagulation, or both. Incisional glaucoma procedures, such as trabeculectomy and glaucoma drainage-device surgery, are contraindicated in most cases of intraocular malignant tumors. In refractory cases, enucleation may be the preferred option.

- Primary malignant melanomas of the uvea may cause open-angle forms of glaucoma by direct extension or seeding of tumor cells, pigment granules, or macrophages into the anterior chamber angle. Less often, these tumors may cause angle-closure glaucoma by a mass effect behind the iris or lens or via iris neovascularization.

- Ultrasonography and cytology of aqueous aspirates are useful diagnostic adjuncts, and most confirmed cases are managed by enucleation. B-scan ultrasonography and UBM should be considered in all blind or painful eyes, particularly when a cloudy media prevents a clear view of the fundus and ciliary body region.

- Systemic malignancies, including metastatic carcinomas and melanomas, leukemias, and lymphomas, may occasionally cause glaucoma, usually by invasion of the anterior chamber angle.

- Ocular tumors of childhood that may cause glaucoma include retinoblastoma and medulloepithelioma.

- Some of the phakomatoses—most notably Sturge–Weber syndrome, von Recklinghausen neurofibromatosis, and nevus of Ota—may also have associated glaucoma.

REFERENCES

1. Radcliffe NM, Finger PT. Eye cancer related glaucoma: current concepts [review]. *Surv Ophthalmol.* 2009;54(1):47–73.
2. Shields CL, Shields JA, Shields MB, et al. Prevalence and mechanisms of secondary intraocular pressure elevation in eyes with intraocular tumors. *Ophthalmology.* 1987;94(7):839–846.
3. Yanoff M. Glaucoma mechanisms in ocular malignant melanomas. *Am J Ophthalmol.* 1970;70(6):898–904.
4. Shields MB, Klintworth GK. Anterior uveal melanomas and intraocular pressure. *Ophthalmology.* 1980;87(6):503–517.
5. Demirci H, Shields CL, Shields JA, et al. Ring melanoma of the anterior chamber angle: a report of fourteen cases. *Am J Ophthalmol.* 2001;132(3):336–342.
6. Chaudhry IM, Moster MR, Augsburger JJ. Iris ring melanoma masquerading as pigmentary glaucoma. *Arch Ophthalmol.* 1997;115(11):1480–1481.
7. Omulecki W, Pruszczynski M, Borowski J. Ring melanoma of the iris and ciliary body. *Br J Ophthalmol.* 1985;69(7):514–518.
8. Nguyen QD, Foster CS. Ciliary body melanoma masquerading as chronic uveitis. *Ocul Immunol Inflamm.* 1998;6(4):253–256.
9. Yanoff M, Scheie HG. Melanomalytic glaucoma. Report of a case. *Arch Ophthalmol.* 1970;84(4):471–473.
10. Zakka KA, Foos RY, Sulit H. Metastatic tapioca iris melanoma. *Br J Ophthalmol.* 1979;63(11):744–749.
11. Reese AB, Mund ML, Iwamoto T. Tapioca melanoma of the iris. 1. Clinical and light microscopy studies. *Am J Ophthalmol.* 1972;74(5):840–850.
12. Shields MB, Proia AD. Neovascular glaucoma associated with an iris melanoma. A clinicopathologic report. *Arch Ophthalmol.* 1987;105(5):672–674.
13. Hopkins RE, Carriker FR. Malignant melanoma of the ciliary body. *Am J Ophthalmol.* 1958;45(6):835–843.
14. Foos RY, Hull SN, Straatsma BR. Early diagnosis of ciliary body melanomas. *Arch Ophthalmol.* 1969;81(3):336–344.
15. Gupta K, Hoepner JA, Streeten BW. Pseudomelanoma of the iris in herpes simplex keratoiritis. *Ophthalmology.* 1986;93(12):1524–1527.
16. Shields JA, Sanborn GE, Augsburger JJ. The differential diagnosis of malignant melanoma of the iris. A clinical study of 200 patients. *Ophthalmology.* 1983;90(6):716–720.
17. el Baba F, Hagler WS, De la Cruz A, et al. Choroidal melanoma with pigment dispersion in vitreous and melanomalytic glaucoma. *Ophthalmology.* 1988;95(3):370–377.
18. Fraser DJ Jr, Font RL. Ocular inflammation and hemorrhage as initial manifestations of uveal malignant melanoma. Incidence and prognosis. *Arch Ophthalmol.* 1979;97(7):1311–1314.
19. Alward WL, Byrne SF, Hughes JR, et al. Dislocated lens nuclei simulating choroidal melanomas. *Arch Ophthalmol.* 1989;107(10):1463–1464.
20. Pavlin CJ, McWhae JA, McGowan HD, et al. Ultrasound biomicroscopy of anterior segment tumors. *Ophthalmology.* 1992;99(8):1220–1228.
21. Maberly DA, Pavlin CJ, McGowan HD, et al. Ultrasound biomicroscopic imaging of the anterior aspect of peripheral choroidal melanomas. *Am J Ophthalmol.* 1997;123(4):506–514.
22. Marigo FA, Finger PT, McCormick SA, et al. Iris and ciliary body melanomas: ultrasound biomicroscopy with histopathologic correlation. *Arch Ophthalmol.* 2000;118(11):1515–1521.
23. Marigo FA, Esaki K, Finger PT, et al. Differential diagnosis of anterior segment cysts by ultrasound biomicroscopy. *Ophthalmology.* 1999;106(11):2131–2135.
24. Gitter KA, Meyer D, Sarin LK. Ultrasound to evaluate eyes with opaque media. *Am J Ophthalmol.* 1967;64(1):100–113.
25. Christiansen JM, Wetzig PC, Thatcher DB, et al. Diagnosis and management of anterior uveal tumors. *Ophthalmic Surg.* 1979;10(1):81–88.
26. Brovkina AF, Chichua AG. Value of fluorescein iridography in diagnosis of tumours of the iridociliary zone. *Br J Ophthalmol.* 1979;63(3):157–160.
27. Jakobiec FA, Depot MJ, Henkind P, et al. Fluorescein angiographic patterns of iris melanocytic tumors. *Arch Ophthalmol.* 1982;100(8):1288–1299.
28. Char DH, Schwartz A, Miller TR, et al. Ocular metastases from systemic melanoma. *Am J Ophthalmol.* 1980;90(5):702–707.
29. Green WR. Diagnostic cytopathology of ocular fluid specimens. *Ophthalmology.* 1984;91(6):726–749.
30. Midena E, Segato T, Piermarocchi S, et al. Fine needle aspiration biopsy in ophthalmology. *Surv Ophthalmol.* 1985;29(6):410–422.
31. Karcioglu ZA, Caldwell DR. Frozen section diagnosis in ophthalmic surgery. *Surv Ophthalmol.* 1984;28(4):323–332.
32. Barr CC, McLean IW, Zimmerman LE. Uveal melanoma in children and adolescents. *Arch Ophthalmol.* 1981;99(12):2133–2136.
33. Rones B, Zimmerman LE. The prognosis of primary tumors of the iris treated by iridectomy. *Arch Ophthalmol.* 1958;60(2):193–205.
34. Dunphy EB, Dryja TP, Albert DM, et al. Melanocytic tumor of the anterior uvea. *Am J Ophthalmol.* 1978;86(5):680–683.
35. Geisse LJ, Robertson DM. Iris melanomas. *Am J Ophthalmol.* 1985;99(6):638–648.
36. Shields CL, Shields JA, Materin M, et al. Iris melanoma: risk factors for metastasis in 169 consecutive patients. *Ophthalmology.* 2001;108(1):172–178.
37. Territo C, Shields CL, Shields JA, et al. Natural course of melanocytic tumors of the iris. *Ophthalmology.* 1988;95(9):1251–1255.
38. Charteris DG. Progression of an iris melanoma over 41 years. *Br J Ophthalmol.* 1990;74(9):566–567.
39. Memmen JE, McLean IW. The long-term outcome of patients undergoing iridocyclectomy. *Ophthalmology.* 1990;97(4):429–432.
40. Finger PT. Plaque radiation therapy for malignant melanoma of the iris and ciliary body. *Am J Ophthalmol.* 2001;132(3):328–335.
41. Zimmerman LE, McLean IW, Foster WD. Statistical analysis of follow-up data concerning uveal melanomas, and the influence of enucleation. *Ophthalmology.* 1980;87(6):557–564.
42. Kramer KK, La Piana FG, Whitmore PV. Enucleation with stabilization of intraocular pressure in the treatment of uveal melanomas. *Ophthalmic Surg.* 1980;11(1):39–43.

43. Blair CJ, Guerry RK, Stratford TP. Normal intraocular pressure during enucleation for choroidal melanoma. *Arch Ophthalmol.* 1983;101(12): 1900–1902.

44. Migdal C. Effect of the method of enucleation on the prognosis of choroidal melanoma. *Br J Ophthalmol.* 1983;67(6):385–388.

45. McGalliard JN, Johnston PB. A study of iris melanoma in Northern Ireland. *Br J Ophthalmol.* 1989;73(8):591–595.

46. Cleasby GW, Van Westenbrugge JA. Treatment of iris melanoma by photocoagulation: a case report. *Ophthalmic Surg.* 1987;18(1):42–44.

47. Grossniklaus HE, Brown RH, Stulting RD, et al. Iris melanoma seeding through a trabeculectomy site. *Arch Ophthalmol.* 1990;108(9):1287–1290.

48. Bloch RS, Gartner S. The incidence of ocular metastatic carcinoma. *Arch Ophthalmol.* 1971;85(6):673–675.

49. Nelson CC, Hertzberg BS, Klintworth GK. A histopathologic study of 716 unselected eyes in patients with cancer at the time of death. *Am J Ophthalmol.* 1983;95(6):788–793.

50. Foulds WS, Lee WR. The significance of glaucoma in the management of melanomas of the anterior segment. *Trans Ophthalmol Soc UK.* 1983;103(pt 1):59–63.

51. Scholz R, Green WR, Baranano EC, et al. Metastatic carcinoma to the iris. Diagnosis by aqueous paracentesis and response to irradiation and chemotherapy. *Ophthalmology.* 1983;90(12):1524–1527.

52. Ferry AP, Font RL. Carcinoma metastatic to the eye and orbit. I. A clinicopathologic study of 227 cases. *Arch Ophthalmol.* 1974;92(4):276–286.

53. Ferry AP, Font RL. Carcinoma metastatic to the eye and orbit. II. A clinicopathological study of 26 patients with carcinoma metastatic to the anterior segment of the eye. *Arch Ophthalmol.* 1975;93(7):472–482.

54. Johnson BL. Bilateral glaucoma caused by nasal carcinoma obstructing schlemm's canal. *Am J Ophthalmol.* 1983;96(4):550–552.

55. Wormald RP, Harper JI. Bilateral black hypopyon in a patient with self-healing cutaneous malignant melanoma. *Br J Ophthalmol.* 1983;67(4):231–235.

56. Abramson A. Anterior chamber activity in children with acute leukemia. *Ann Ophthalmol.* 1980;12:553–556.

57. Ohkoshi K, Tsiaras WG. Prognostic importance of ophthalmic manifestations in childhood leukaemia. *Br J Ophthalmol.* 1992;76(11):651–655.

58. Rennie I. Ophthalmic manifestations of childhood leukaemia. *Br J Ophthalmol.* 1992;76(11):641.

59. Novakovic P, Kellie SJ, Taylor D. Childhood leukaemia: relapse in the anterior segment of the eye. *Br J Ophthalmol.* 1989;73(5):354–359.

60. Leonardy NJ, Rupani M, Dent G, et al. Analysis of 135 autopsy eyes for ocular involvement in leukemia. *Am J Ophthalmol.* 1990;109(4):436–444.

61. Kozlowski IM, Hirose T, Jalkh AE. Massive subretinal hemorrhage with acute angle-closure glaucoma in chronic myelocytic leukemia. *Am J Ophthalmol.* 1987;103(6):837–838.

62. Saga T, Ohno S, Matsuda H, et al. Ocular involvement by a peripheral T-cell lymphoma. *Arch Ophthalmol.* 1984;102(3):399–402.

63. Epstein DL, Grant WM. Secondary open-angle glaucoma in histiocytosis X. *Am J Ophthalmol.* 1977;84(3):332–336.

64. Moore AT, Pritchard J, Taylor DS. Histiocytosis X: an ophthalmological review. *Br J Ophthalmol.* 1985;69(1):7–14.

65. Shakin EP, Augsburger JJ, Eagle RC Jr, et al. Multiple myeloma involving the iris. *Arch Ophthalmol.* 1988;106(4):524–526.

66. Smith DL, Skuta GL, Trobe JD, et al. Angle-closure glaucoma as initial presentation of myelodysplastic syndrome. *Can J Ophthalmol.* 1990;25(6):306–308.

67. Wohlrab TM, Pleyer U, Rohrbach JM, et al. Sudden increase in intraocular pressure as an initial manifestation of myelodysplastic syndrome. *Am J Ophthalmol.* 1995;119(3):370–372.

68. Yoshizumi MO, Thomas JV, Smith TR. Glaucoma-inducing mechanisms in eyes with retinoblastoma. *Arch Ophthalmol.* 1978;96(1):105–110.

69. Ellsworth RM. The practical management of retinoblastoma. *Trans Am Ophthalmol Soc.* 1969;67:462–534.

70. Pe'er J, Neufeld M, Baras M, et al. Rubeosis iridis in retinoblastoma. Histologic findings and the possible role of vascular endothelial growth factor in its induction. *Ophthalmology.* 1997;104(8):1251–1258.

71. Haik BG, Dunleavy SA, Cooke C, et al. Retinoblastoma with anterior chamber extension. *Ophthalmology.* 1987;94(4):367–370.

72. Roberts CW, Iwamoto M, Haik BC. Ultrastructural correlation of specular microscopy in retinoblastoma. *Am J Ophthalmol.* 1986;102(2):182–187.

73. Moazed K, Albert D, Smith TR. Rubeosis iridis in "pseudogliomas". *Surv Ophthalmol.* 1980;25(2):85–90.

74. Shields JA. Ocular toxocariasis. A review. *Surv Ophthalmol.* 1984;28(5):361–381.

75. Spaulding G. Rubeosis iridis in retinoblastoma and pseudoglioma. *Trans Am Ophthalmol Soc.* 1978;76:584–609.

76. Shields CL, Shields JA, Cater J, et al. Plaque radiotherapy for retinoblastoma: long-term tumor control and treatment complications in 208 tumors. *Ophthalmology.* 2001;108(11):2116–2121.

77. Broughton WL, Zimmerman LE. A clinicopathologic study of 56 cases of intraocular medulloepitheliomas. *Am J Ophthalmol.* 1978;85(3):407–418.

78. Jakobiec FA, Howard GM, Ellsworth RM, et al. Electron microscopic diagnosis of medulloepithelioma. *Am J Ophthalmol.* 1975;79(2):321–329.

79. Wilson ME, McClatchey SK, Zimmerman LE. Rhabdomyosarcoma of the ciliary body. *Ophthalmology.* 1990;97(11):1484–1488.

80. Bruner WE, Stark WJ, Green WR. Presumed juvenile xanthogranuloma of the iris and ciliary body in an adult. *Arch Ophthalmol.* 1982;100(3):457–459.

81. Casteels I, Olver J, Malone M, et al. Early treatment of juvenile xanthogranuloma of the iris with subconjunctival steroids. *Br J Ophthalmol.* 1993;77(1):57–60.

82. Jakobiec FA, Silbert G. Are most iris "melanomas" really nevi? A clinicopathologic study of 189 lesions. *Arch Ophthalmol.* 1981;99(12):2117–2132.

83. Harbour JW, Augsburger JJ, Eagle RC Jr. Initial management and follow-up of melanocytic iris tumors. *Ophthalmology.* 1995;102(12):1987–1993.

84. Nik NA, Hidayat A, Zimmerman LE, et al. Diffuse iris nevus manifested by unilateral open angle glaucoma. *Arch Ophthalmol.* 1981;99(1):125–127.

85. Carlson DW, Alward WL, Folberg R. Aggressive nevus of the iris with secondary glaucoma in a child. *Am J Ophthalmol.* 1995;119(3):367–368.

86. Scheie HG, Yanoff M. Iris nevus (Cogan–Reese) syndrome. A cause of unilateral glaucoma. *Arch Ophthalmol.* 1975;93(10):963–970.

87. Cogan DG, Reese AB. A syndrome of iris nodules, ectopic Descemet's membrane, and unilateral glaucoma. *Doc Ophthalmol.* 1969;26:424–433.

88. Shields JA, Kline MW, Augsburger JJ. Primary iris cysts: a review of the literature and report of 62 cases. *Br J Ophthalmol.* 1984;68(3):152–166.

89. Vela A, Rieser JC, Campbell DG. The heredity and treatment of angle-closure glaucoma secondary to iris and ciliary body cysts. *Ophthalmology.* 1984;91(4):332–337.

90. Alward WL, Ossoinig KC. Pigment dispersion secondary to cysts of the iris pigment epithelium. *Arch Ophthalmol.* 1995;113(12):1574–1575.

91. Albert DL, Brownstein S, Kattleman BS. Mucogenic glaucoma caused by an epithelial cyst of the iris stroma. *Am J Ophthalmol.* 1992;114(2):222–224.

92. Finger PT, McCormick SA, Lombardo J, et al. Epithelial inclusion cyst of the iris. *Arch Ophthalmol.* 1995;113(6):777–780.

93. Nakazawa M, Tamai M. Iris melanocytoma with secondary glaucoma. *Am J Ophthalmol.* 1984;97(6):797–799.

94. Shields JA, Annesley WH Jr, Spaeth GL. Necrotic melanocytoma of iris with secondary glaucoma. *Am J Ophthalmol.* 1977;84(6):826–829.

95. Traboulsi EI, Maumenee IH. Bilateral melanosis of the iris. *Am J Ophthalmol.* 1987;103(1):115–116.

96. Goncalves V, Sandler T, O'Donnell FE Jr. Open angle glaucoma in melanosis oculi: response to laser trabeculoplasty. *Ann Ophthalmol.* 1985;17(1):33–36.

97. Lieb WE, Shields JA, Eagle RC Jr, et al. Cystic adenoma of the pigmented ciliary epithelium. Clinical, pathologic, and immunohistopathologic findings. *Ophthalmology.* 1990;97(11):1489–1493.

98. Doro S, Werblin TP, Haas B, et al. Fetal adenoma of the pigmented ciliary epithelium associated with persistent hyperplastic primary vitreous. *Ophthalmology.* 1986;93(10):1343–1350.

99. Zaidman GW, Johnson BL, Salamon SM, et al. Fuchs' adenoma affecting the peripheral iris. *Arch Ophthalmol.* 1983;101(5):771–773.

100. Shields CL, Shields JA, Cook GR, et al. Differentiation of adenoma of the iris pigment epithelium from iris cyst and melanoma. *Am J Ophthalmol.* 1985;100(5):678–681.

101. Shields JA, Augsburger JJ, Sanborn GE, et al. Adenoma of the iris-pigment epithelium. *Ophthalmology.* 1983;90(6):735–739.

102. Papale JJ, Akiwama K, Hirose T, et al. Adenocarcinoma of the ciliary body pigment epithelium in a child. *Arch Ophthalmol.* 1984;102(1):100–103.

103. Van der Hoeve J. Eye symptoms in phakomatoses. *Trans Ophthalmol Soc UK.* 1932;52:380–401.

104. Sullivan TJ, Clarke MP, Morin JD. The ocular manifestations of the Sturge–Weber syndrome. *J Pediatr Ophthalmol Strabismus.* 1992;29(6):349–356.

105. Weiss DI. Dual origin of glaucoma in encephalotrigeminal haemangiomatosis. *Trans Ophthalmol Soc U K.* 1973;93(0):477–493.

106. Christensen GR, Records RE. Glaucoma and expulsive hemorrhage mechanisms in the Sturge–Weber syndrome. *Ophthalmology.* 1979; 86(7):1360–1366.

107. Mwinula JH, Sagawa T, Tawara A, et al. Anterior chamber angle vascularization in Sturge–Weber syndrome. Report of a case. *Graefes Arch Clin Exp Ophthalmol.* 1994;232(7):387–391.

108. Cibis GW, Tripathi RC, Tripathi BJ. Glaucoma in Sturge–Weber syndrome. *Ophthalmology.* 1984;91(9):1061–1071.

109. Phelps CD. The pathogenesis of glaucoma in Sturge–Weber syndrome. *Ophthalmology.* 1978;85(3):276–286.

110. Altuna JC, Greenfield DS, Wand M, et al. Latanoprost in glaucoma associated with Sturge–Weber syndrome: benefits and side-effects. *J Glaucoma.* 1999;8(3):199–203.

111. Sakai H, Sakima N, Nakamura Y, et al. Ciliochoroidal effusion induced by topical latanoprost in a patient with Sturge–Weber syndrome. *Jpn J Ophthalmol.* 2002;46(5):553–555.

112. Ali MA, Fahmy IA, Spaeth GL. Trabeculectomy for glaucoma associated with Sturge–Weber syndrome. *Ophthalmic Surg.* 1990;21(5):352–355.

113. Iwach AG, Hoskins HD Jr, Hetherington J Jr, et al. Analysis of surgical and medical management of glaucoma in Sturge–Weber syndrome. *Ophthalmology.* 1990;97(7):904–909.

114. Board RJ, Shields MB. Combined trabeculotomy–trabeculectomy for the management of glaucoma associated wih Sturge–Weber syndrome. *Ophthalmic Surg.* 1981;12(11):813–817.

115. Agarwal HC, Sandramouli S, Sihota R, et al. Sturge–Weber syndrome: management of glaucoma with combined trabeculotomy-trabeculectomy. *Ophthalmic Surg.* 1993;24(6):399–402.

116. Budenz DL, Sakamoto D, Eliezer R, et al. Two-staged Baerveldt glaucoma implant for childhood glaucoma associated with Sturge–Weber syndrome. *Ophthalmology.* 2000;107(11):2105–2110.

117. Pearson-Webb MA, Kaiser-Kupfer MI, Eldridge R. Eye findings in bilateral acoustic (central) neurofibromatosis: association with presenile lens opacities and cataracts but absence of Lisch nodules. *N Engl J Med.* 1986;315(24):1553–1554.

118. Barker D, Wright E, Nguyen K, et al. Gene for von Recklinghausen neurofibromatosis is in the pericentromeric region of chromosome 17. *Science.* 1987;236(4805):1100–1102.

119. Lubs ML, Bauer MS, Formas ME, et al. Lisch nodules in neurofibromatosis type 1. *N Engl J Med.* 1991;324(18):1264–1266.

120. Perry HD, Font RL. Iris nodules in von Recklinghausen's Neurofibromatosis. Electron microscopic confirmation of their melanocytic origin. *Arch Ophthalmol.* 1982;100(10):1635–1640.

121. Lewis RA, Riccardi VM. Von Recklinghausen neurofibromatosis. Incidence of iris hamartomata. *Ophthalmology.* 1981;88(4):348–354.

122. Huson S, Jones D, Beck L. Ophthalmic manifestations of neurofibromatosis. *Br J Ophthalmol.* 1987;71(3):235–238.

123. Grant WM, Walton DS. Distinctive gonioscopic findings in glaucoma due to neurofibromatosis. *Arch Ophthalmol.* 1968;79(2):127–134.

124. Wolter JR, Bulter RG. Pigment spots of the iris and ectropion uveae. *Am J Ophthalmol.* 1963;56:964–973.

125. Brownstein S, Little JM. Ocular neurofibromatosis. *Ophthalmology.* 1983;90(12):1595–1599.

126. Teekhasaenee C, Ritch R, Rutnin U, et al. Ocular findings in oculodermal melanocytosis. *Arch Ophthalmol.* 1990;108(8):1114–1120.

127. Mishima Y, Mevorah B. Nevus Ota and nevus Ito in American Negroes. *J Invest Dermatol.* 1961;36:133–154.

128. Albert DM, Scheie HG. Nevus of Ota with malignant melanoma of the choroids: report of a case. *Arch Ophthalmol.* 1963;69(6):774–777.

129. Fishman GR, Anderson R. Nevus of Ota. Report of two cases, one with open-angle glaucoma. *Am J Ophthalmol.* 1962;54:453–457.

130. Sugar HS. Glaucoma with trabecular melanocytosis. *Ann Ophthalmol.* 1982;14(4):374–375.

131. Futa R, Shimizu T, Okura F, et al. A case of open-angle glaucoma associated with nevus Ota: electron microscopic study of the anterior chamber angle and iris. *Folia Ophthalmol Jpn.* 1984;35:501.

132. Teekhasaenee C, Ritch R. Glaucoma in phakomatosis pigmentovascularis. *Ophthalmology.* 1997;104(1):150–157.

Glaucomas Associated with Ocular Inflammation

22

Any portion of the eye can be affected by inflammatory processes, including the uveal tract (i.e., uveitis), cornea (i.e., keratitis), sclera (i.e., scleritis), and episclera (i.e., episcleritis). Uveitis is by far the most common of these diseases and can have an acute or chronic course. Most of the acute cases involve the anterior uvea (i.e., iritis or iridocyclitis), whereas the chronic forms, which have been defined as persisting for 3 months or longer, have been subclassified into four groups: anterior uveitis (i.e., iritis or iridocyclitis), intermediate uveitis (i.e., pars planitis), posterior uveitis (i.e., choroiditis or chorioretinitis), and anterior and posterior uveitis (i.e., panuveitis) (1). The relative frequencies of these four types of chronic uveitis, based on a survey of 400 consecutive patients from a uveitis service in Israel, were 45.8%, 15.3%, 14.5%, and 24.5%, respectively (1), similar to results of studies conducted in the United States and England (2–4).

The form of ocular inflammation that most frequently produces intraocular pressure (IOP) elevation is iridocyclitis (5). When glaucoma is associated with other types of ocular inflammation, there is usually secondary involvement of the anterior uveal tract. We therefore consider the clinical forms of iridocyclitis and the mechanisms and management of the associated glaucomas and then review the other forms of ocular inflammation that may be associated with glaucoma. The clinician should also keep in mind that the differential diagnosis of a patient who presents with "uveitis" and refractory glaucoma includes serious intraocular disease, such as infection (e.g., endophthalmitis), tumor (e.g., melanoma, lymphoma), acute angle-closure glaucoma, neovascular glaucoma, and secondary reaction to intraocular foreign body.

IRIDOCYCLITIS

Terminology

The general forms of iridocyclitis are classified primarily according to the clinical presentation and duration of active disease. A specific case of iridocyclitis, however, may manifest one or all of these clinical forms at different times during the course of the disease.

Acute Iridocyclitis

The characteristic history for this type of iridocyclitis is the sudden onset of mild to moderate ocular pain, photophobia, and blurred vision. Physical examination typically reveals ciliary flush, slight constriction of the pupil, and variable degrees of aqueous flare and cells (**Fig. 22.1**). In many cases, one will find inflammatory precipitates on the corneal endothelium (keratic precipitates). The IOP is often lower than in the fellow eye, although some patients present with a marked elevation of the pressure, which may be associated with severe pain and corneal edema.

Subacute Iridocyclitis

Some cases of ocular inflammation produce minimal or no symptoms. The diagnosis may be made during a routine eye examination or as part of a workup for a related systemic disease. This form of iridocyclitis can have serious consequences because complications such as associated glaucoma may go undetected until advanced damage has occurred.

Chronic Iridocyclitis

The clinical presentation in this form of iridocyclitis ranges from acute to subacute but is characterized by a protracted course of months to years, often with remissions and exacerbations. Complicating sequelae include the formation of posterior and peripheral anterior synechiae, cataracts, and band keratopathy. This form of iridocyclitis is particularly likely to cause glaucoma. In a study of 100 patients with uveitis, all of whom had anterior uveal involvement, glaucoma was present in 23 cases, of which 20 represented chronic uveitis and 3 acute uveitis (6).

Clinical Forms of Iridocyclitis and Glaucoma

Acute Anterior Uveitis

This is the most common form of ocular inflammation, with a lifetime cumulative incidence of approximately 0.2% in the general population (7). It represents a group of conditions characterized by acute iridocyclitis, although the pathogenesis of most cases is unknown except for the close association in many patients with the genetic marker HLA-B27. Patients with acute anterior uveitis are often classified as HLA-B27–positive and HLA-B27–negative populations. HLA-B27–positive acute anterior uveitis appears to represent a distinct clinical entity, accounting for approximately half of all cases in white patients (8). Compared with patients with HLA-B27–negative acute anterior uveitis, the HLA-B27–positive form occurs more in white individuals, has a younger age of onset (median age in the early 30s), has a slight preponderance of men, and is typically unilateral or unilateral alternating, although bilateral cases do occur (9–11). Ocular findings may be severe, such as fibrin in the anterior chamber, although mutton-fat keratic precipitates are not a typical finding (8). Ocular complications, including cataracts, posterior synechiae, elevated IOP, and cystoid macular edema, are also more common than in HLA-B27–negative cases (9–11), although the long-term visual

Figure 22.1 **A:** Slitlamp view of an eye with acute iritis shows the typical ciliary flush (*arrows*). (Courtesy of Gary N. Foulks, MD.) **B:** Slitlamp view of cell and flare in a patient with active uveitis. (Courtesy of Joseph A. Halabis, OD.)

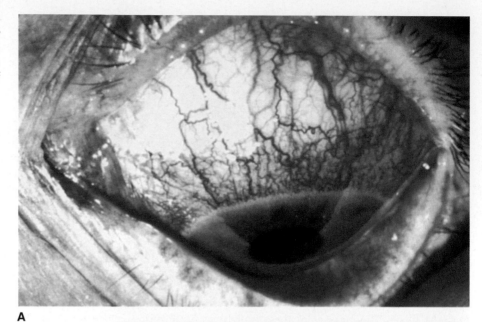

A

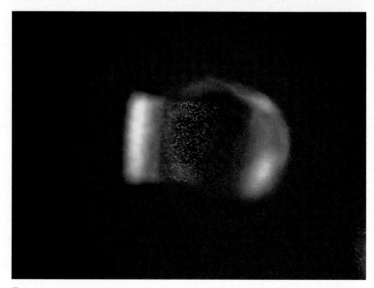

B

outcome is not significantly different (9,10). Anterior segment fluorophotometry suggests that HLA-B27–positive patients have more severe inflammation on the basis of blood–aqueous barrier disruption (12).

Rheumatologic complications, including ankylosing spondylitis, are seen in one half to two thirds of HLA-B27–positive patients, but they are uncommon in the HLA-B27–negative population (8–10). The former patients also have a higher-than-normal prevalence of first-degree relatives with HLA-B27–positive acute anterior uveitis and ankylosing spondylitis (11,13).

Some topical glaucoma medications have been associated with anterior uveitis. These include metipranolol and brimonidine (14,15). Whether latanoprost is also implicated remains a subject of controversy (16).

Patients with acute anterior uveitis usually respond to nonspecific anti-inflammatory therapy (as discussed later in this chapter), although it is important to rule out related ocular or systemic disease, which may require more specific therapy (17).

Sarcoidosis

This multisystem inflammatory disorder of uncertain origin has a predilection for young adults and blacks. The typical histopathologic finding is noncaseating granulomas, and systemic involvement commonly includes pulmonary hilar lymphadenopathy, peripheral lymphadenopathy, and cutaneous lesions. In a review of 532 cases of sarcoidosis, 202 (38%) had ocular involvement (18), but in another survey of 159 patients with systemic sarcoidosis, more than one half presented with ocular lesions as the initial manifestation (19). Ocular findings include chorioretinitis, retinal periphlebitis, and occasional involvement of the optic nerve, orbit, or lacrimal glands, although the most common ocular abnormality is anterior uveitis (18,19).

Iridocyclitis. Acute iridocyclitis with the previously described features of ciliary flush, aqueous flare and cells, and occasional fine or large (mutton-fat) keratic precipitates was noted in

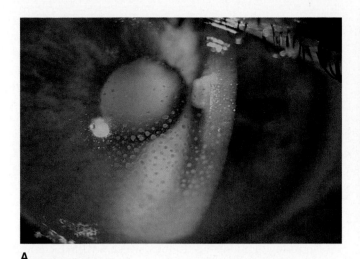

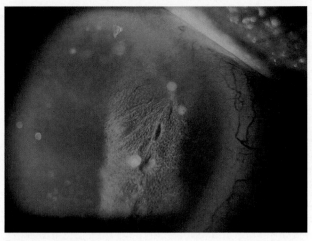

A   **B**

Figure 22.2   **A:** Slitlamp view of an eye with sarcoid uveitis shows the typical large ("mutton-fat") keratic precipitates. **B:** Busacca iris nodules in a patient with sarcoid uveitis. (Courtesy of Joseph A. Halabis, OD.)

approximately 15% of 202 patients with ocular sarcoid (18). In the acute phase, the inflammation was usually unilateral. The most common ocular manifestation of sarcoidosis is a chronic granulomatous uveitis, which was reported in more than one half of the 202 cases (18). It is more often bilateral, has a protracted course, and is typified by mutton-fat keratic precipitates, synechiae, and iris nodules (**Fig. 22.2**). The nodules, which were seen in 23 (11.4%) of the 202 cases of ocular sarcoid (18), may involve the pupillary border (Koeppe nodules) and stroma of the iris (Busacca nodules), as well as the anterior chamber angle and the ciliary body (19,20). In one series of 102 eyes of 52 patients with ocular sarcoidosis, 35% of eyes had iris nodules, 49% had nodules in the angle, and 42% had ciliary nodules (20). Gonioscopy may also reveal inflammatory precipitates on the trabecular meshwork and whitish spots on the ciliary body band, which hyperfluoresce during fluorescein gonioangiography and may represent granulomas of the ciliary body (21,22).

Chronic ocular sarcoidosis is associated with a worse visual prognosis than the acute form. In a series of 21 patients with sarcoid uveitis, 8 had a monophasic course and a favorable visual outcome, and 13 had a relapsing course with severe visual loss in five eyes (23). The course of the ocular disease does not always parallel that of the systemic manifestations. In one series of 33 patients with ocular and systemic sarcoidosis, all had chronic systemic manifestations, defined as a minimum duration of 5 years, whereas the anterior uveitis was chronic in only 18 patients (24). In another series of patients with chronic ocular sarcoidosis, approximately one half had no systemic manifestations (23). Sarcoidosis may also masquerade as many other conditions. In one report, five patients with clinical signs compatible with Fuchs heterochromic uveitis (discussed later) were found to have sarcoidosis on the basis of elevated serum angiotensin-converting enzyme levels or a positive Kveim test result (25).

Glaucoma. This complication of the iridocyclitis occurred in 22 of the 202 patients (10.9%) with ocular sarcoid (18). Chronic uveitis and associated glaucoma are poor prognostic

signs, with 8 of 11 such patients experiencing severe visual loss in one study (24). The most common mechanism of glaucoma associated with the iridocyclitis of sarcoidosis is obstruction of the trabecular meshwork by inflammatory debris or nodules (26). A more chronic form of glaucoma may be associated with inflammatory cell infiltration around the inner and outer walls of the Schlemm canal and with iris bombé or goniosynechiae (26,27), and a subacute form has been described with precipitates on the trabecular meshwork (21). Neovascularization of the iris and angle has also been reported as a mechanism of glaucoma in association with sarcoidosis (28).

Juvenile Rheumatoid Arthritis

Juvenile rheumatoid arthritis is a spectrum of arthritic disorders in children. One form is characterized by monarticular, or pauciarticular (involvement of four joints or less) onset, a predilection for girls, and minimal additional systemic manifestations. Other types of juvenile rheumatoid arthritis have polyarticular onset or additional acute systemic involvement.

Iridocyclitis. The prevalence of iridocyclitis in patients with the monarticular or pauciarticular form of juvenile rheumatoid arthritis has been variously reported at 16%, 19%, and 29% (20,29,31), whereas the other types of juvenile rheumatoid arthritis are rarely associated with this ocular finding (30–34). Juvenile rheumatoid arthritis is by far the most common systemic finding in children who have anterior uveitis associated with a specific systemic disease, accounting for 81% of one large series (35). The ocular inflammation may have an acute onset, with the typical features of acute iridocyclitis. However, many cases are asymptomatic, emphasizing the need for periodic ocular examinations of children with juvenile rheumatoid arthritis (30,31). The onset of the arthritis typically precedes that of the uveitis, although iridocyclitis may persist in adult life, whereas the arthritis usually disappears (32). Children with iridocyclitis rarely have a positive serology for rheumatoid factor, but they frequently have antinuclear antibody and HLA-B27 antigen, and some eventually are found to have typical ankylosing spondylitis (32,34).

Complications that may cause significant visual loss in children with iridocyclitis and juvenile rheumatoid arthritis include cataracts, band keratopathy, and glaucoma. These are more common when the uveitis is the initial manifestation. In one series, 67% of such patients had a poor visual outcome, compared with only 6% of those in whom the arthritis preceded the uveitis (36). The prevalence and severity of the complications and visual loss also correlate with the degree and duration of the ocular inflammation. In one report of 60 patients, an aggressive stepladder, steroid-sparing, therapeutic algorithm (topical and regional corticosteroids, systemic nonsteroidal anti-inflammatory drugs, systemic steroids, and systemic immunosuppressive chemotherapy) was thought to control the iridocyclitis while reducing the prevalence of cataract formation and retinal pathology (37). Those cases requiring cataract surgery responded well to phacoemulsification and anterior vitrectomy after at least 3 months of complete freedom from inflammation (37).

Glaucoma. The reported prevalence of glaucoma in children with juvenile rheumatoid arthritis and iridocyclitis ranges from 14% to 27% (32–34,36). Glaucoma is a particularly serious complication, with one of the eyes in one study having a vision of 20/200 or less (34). The glaucoma mechanism is usually a pupillary block, although it may also be related to alterations in the trabecular meshwork early in the course of the disease. Histopathologic studies of two advanced cases revealed peripheral anterior synechiae and occlusion of the pupil in one (38), and a dense inflammatory infiltrate composed primarily of plasma cells in the iris and ciliary body with angle closure in the other patient (39). Treatment is typically difficult, with many eyes responding only partially to corticosteroids. The addition of nonsteroidal anti-inflammatory agents may be helpful in these cases (33,34). Antiglaucoma drugs may be required to control IOP elevation, and glaucoma surgery is occasionally needed, although reported results in these cases are poor (32).

Ankylosing Spondylitis: Marie–Strumpell Disease

Ankylosing spondylitis is a form of arthritis that typically involves the cervical or lumbosacral spine and is associated with an intermittent acute iridocyclitis in 3.5% to 12.5% of reported cases (30). A high percentage of these patients have the HLA-B27 antigen (40). Recurrent uveitis may precede the arthritic symptoms, and there is evidence, based on HLA typing and sensitive bone scans, that the ocular inflammation may occur in the absence of overt symptoms or radiologic evidence of the spondylitis (41). There is an apparent overlap between this condition and HLA-B27–positive acute anterior uveitis and the iridocyclitis with juvenile rheumatoid arthritis (8–13,34). Glaucoma may result from trabecular damage or synechiae formation.

Pars Planitis

Pars planitis is a protracted ocular inflammatory disorder that has also been referred to as intermediate uveitis or chronic cyclitis (1,42). It primarily involves the ciliary body. Typical findings include a "snowbank" appearance of the vitreous base overlying the pars plana inferiorly, retinal phlebitis, and a cystoid maculopathy (43). In a series of 100 cases with a 4- to

20-year follow-up, the incidence of glaucoma was 8% (42), whereas another group of 58 eyes had glaucoma in 7% (43). A clinicopathologic study of seven cases of pars planitis revealed glaucoma in five, and possible mechanisms of pressure elevation included peripheral anterior synechiae, iris bombé, and rubeosis iridis (44). Topical corticosteroid and antiglaucoma therapy may be effective in some cases. Decreased visual acuity, which is usually caused by cystoid maculopathy, may require the long-term use of oral and periocular steroids, cryotherapy in the area of the snowbank, and systemic antimetabolites as the final step (43).

Glaucomatocyclitic Crisis: Posner–Schlossman Syndrome

In 1948, Posner and Schlossman (45) described a uniocular disease in young to middle-aged adults, which was characterized by recurrent attacks of mild anterior uveitis with marked elevations of IOP. Many patients have associated systemic disorders, including various allergic conditions and gastrointestinal diseases, most notably peptic ulcers (46). In one series of 22 patients, HLA-Bw54 was present in 41%, suggesting that immunogenetic factors play an important role in the pathogenesis of glaucomatocyclitic crisis (47). The possible role of herpes simplex virus was also suggested by a study that revealed DNA evidence of the virus in all aqueous specimens of 3 patients during acute attacks, but in none of 10 healthy controls (48).

Iridocyclitis. The typical symptoms are slight ocular discomfort, blurred vision, and halos, which last several hours up to a few weeks or, rarely, longer and tend to recur on a monthly or yearly basis (45). Physical findings are minimal, with occasional mild ciliary flush, slight pupillary constriction, and corneal epithelial edema. Hypochromia of the iris is not a consistent finding, but it has been reported in up to 40% of various series (49). Early segmental iris ischemia with late congestion and leakage on fluorescein angiography has also been described (50). Slit-lamp biomicroscopy reveals occasional faint flare and a few fine, nonpigmented keratic precipitates, and gonioscopy shows a normal, open angle with occasional debris and the characteristic absence of synechiae (45,49).

Glaucoma. The IOP is typically elevated in the range of 40 to 60 mm Hg and coincides with the duration of the uveitis. IOP and facility of aqueous outflow usually return to normal between attacks, although severe cases with optic nerve head and visual field damage have been reported (51,52). One study found that patients with 10 years or more of disease have a 2.8 times higher risk of developing glaucomatous disc and field damage, compared with patients with fewer than 10 years of disease (53). The glaucoma may be related to inflammatory changes in the trabecular meshwork. Histologic evaluation of a trabeculectomy specimen obtained during an acute attack revealed numerous mononuclear cells in the meshwork (54). Other theories of mechanism include increased aqueous production, possibly due to elevated levels of aqueous prostaglandins (55), and an association with chronic open-angle glaucoma (50,51). During attacks, most cases can be controlled with corticosteroids and antiglaucoma agents that reduce aqueous production (37,56). Apraclonidine has been reported to be

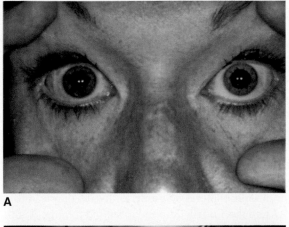

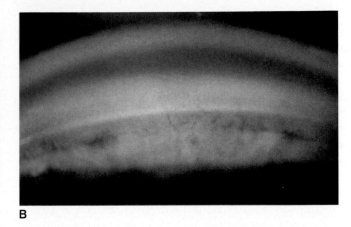

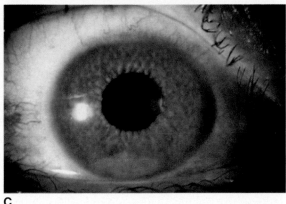

Figure 22.3 Some features of Fuchs heterochromic iridocyclitis. **A:** Heterochromia. **B:** The anterior chamber angle is open and characteristically free of synechiae, although fine vessels can be seen extending onto the trabecular meshwork. These vessels can be associated with an inflammatory membrane over the angle that may impede aqueous outflow. **C:** Iris nodules are seen in some patients with Fuchs heterochromic iridocyclitis.

especially effective during acute attacks (57). Rare, severe cases, however, may require filtering surgery (52,54).

Fuchs Heterochromic Cyclitis

In 1906, Fuchs (58) described a condition characterized by mild anterior uveitis, heterochromia, cataracts, and occasional glaucoma (**Fig. 22.3A**). The similarities and differences between this disease and glaucomatocyclitic crisis should be observed to avoid confusing the two. Fuchs heterochromic cyclitis (also referred to as uveitis or iridocyclitis) is usually unilateral, although bilateral involvement has been reported in up to 13% of the cases (59). The typical age of onset is in the third or fourth decade and there is an equal incidence between men and women (59,60). It is said to be the most commonly misdiagnosed form of uveitis (61), especially in black patients in whom the heterochromia may be less obvious (62).

Several etiologic theories have been considered; the most likely mechanism is true inflammation of immunologic origin, possibly related to depression of suppressor T-cell activity (61). Cellular immunity to corneal antigens has been found in most patients (63), with autoantibodies against corneal epithelium in almost 90% of cases (64). Immune deposits have been found in the vessel walls of iris biopsy specimens (65). The search for HLA-linked genetic factors is inconclusive, although preliminary evidence suggests a decrease in the frequency of HLA-CW3 (66). Fuchs heterochromic cyclitis has been reported in a father and son with associated retinitis pigmentosa (67), although the reported discordance in monozygotic twins suggests little or no genetic predisposition (68). A

few patients have associated congenital Horner syndrome, suggesting the possibility of a neurogenic mechanism in these cases (69). A clinical association between Fuchs heterochromic cyclitis and toxoplasmosis raised the possibility of a causal relationship (70,71), although a study of 88 patients with the former condition revealed no association with toxoplasmosis by indirect immunofluorescence antibody tests, enzyme-linked immunosorbent assay, or cellular immunity tests to toxoplasma antigen (72). Clinical similarities with sarcoidosis have also been reported (25).

Iridocyclitis. The uveitis in this disease is mild and tends to run a single, very protracted course, although it may be intermittent initially. The patient is usually unaware of any difficulty until visual disturbance, primarily from cataract formation, becomes apparent. Although hypochromia of the iris is more common than in glaucomatocyclitic crisis, it is not a constant feature, and tends to develop gradually during the course of the disease (59,60). In one series, it was seen in 92% of 54 white patients and 76% of 13 black patients (62).

Gross signs of ocular inflammation are typically absent, although slitlamp biomicroscopy may reveal minimal aqueous flare and cells. Characteristic fine, stellate keratic precipitates are usually seen on the lower half of the cornea but may also involve the upper half (73). The iris frequently has extensive stromal atrophy, and transillumination of the iris is reported to demonstrate a characteristic light, even translucence (74). One study revealed translucency not only of the iris but also of the surrounding ocular wall (75). Electron microscopic studies of the iris have revealed a scant number of deep stromal melanocytes with immature melanin granules, abundant plasma cells, an increase in mast cells, and a membranous degeneration of nerve fibers (76,77).

Patients may have neovascularization of the anterior chamber angle and iris, and nodules on the iris (66) (**Fig. 22.3B, C**). The nodules typically occur along the pupillary border, similar to the Koeppe nodules of sarcoidosis, although may appear across the whole surface of the iris (78). In one series, the nodules were seen in 20% of white patients and 30% of black patients (62). The finding of unilateral iris nodules may be especially helpful in making the diagnosis of Fuchs cyclitis in black individuals, in whom the heterochromia may be less apparent (78). Anterior segment fluorescein angiography has shown delayed filling, sector ischemia, leakage, and neovascularization, and fluorophotometry has revealed an abnormal permeability of the blood–aqueous barrier (79–81). A high percentage of patients may also have chorioretinal scars, which are often consistent with toxoplasmosis (70,71,82,83).

Cataract. Cataract formation is a typical feature of Fuchs heterochromic cyclitis. In approaching cataract surgery in these patients, intensive perioperative steroid therapy is advised, and synechialysis may be required during the procedure (84). Postoperative complications of marked anterior uveitis, hyphema, IOP elevation, and cystoid macular edema are more common than in routine cataract surgery (84). However, most reports describe good visual outcomes with cataract extraction and posterior chamber intraocular lens implantation (84–86).

Glaucoma. IOP elevation is not as common as with glaucomatocyclitic crisis but may occur as a late, serious complication. The reported incidence varies from 13% to 59% (73,87–89), with the higher figures seen in series with long-term follow-up. The glaucoma typically persists after the uveitis has subsided. The anterior chamber angle is open and characteristically free of synechiae, although fine vessels, which may hemorrhage, are often seen extending onto the trabecular meshwork (87). Histopathologic examination of the anterior chamber angle structures in one case revealed rubeosis, trabeculitis, and an inflammatory membrane over the angle (90), whereas another study showed extensive atrophy of the Schlemm canal and the trabecular endothelium (91). The glaucoma typically does not respond to steroid therapy but requires standard medical or surgical management (60,73,89). In one series of 30 patients, maximum medical therapy was unsuccessful in 73%, but surgical interventions (mostly trabeculectomy, one half with 5-fluorouracil [5-FU]) were successful in 72% of the cases (89).

Behçet Disease

Behçet disease is a multisystem disease that is caused by an occlusive vasculitis. It is characterized by uveitis, aphthous lesions of the mouth, and ulcerations of the genitalia (92,93). Additional systemic findings include erythema nodosum, arthropathy, thrombophlebitis, and a necrotizing vasculitis of the central nervous system, which may be fatal. The most common ocular disorder is iridocyclitis. Behçet disease is relatively common

in the Mediterranean basin and was found to be the most common associated condition with chronic uveitis in a uveitis service in Israel (1), although it is much less common in the United States and England (2–4). The iridocyclitis may be associated with a sterile hypopyon. In a study of 49 patients followed up for 10 years, 17 developed a hypopyon, which typically appears late in the course of the disease but was the initial finding in three patients (94). Posterior uveitis and necrotizing retinal vasculitis are also commonly found in this disorder (93,95). In the 10-year study, all patients developed anterior and posterior involvement within 2 years (94). The uveitis tends to occur late in the course of the disease and is eventually bilateral. The anterior uveitis may lead to glaucoma. All patients initially respond to steroid treatment, although the uveitis, in most cases, eventually requires cytotoxic–immunosuppressive agents such as chlorambucil (94). Even with this therapy, the prognosis is poor, with loss of useful visual acuity in 74% of eyes in the 10-year study (94).

Reiter Syndrome

Reiter syndrome is a multisystem disease that is characterized by conjunctivitis, urethritis, arthritis, and mucocutaneous lesions. It typically afflicts young men, with a high frequency of the HLA-B27 genotype (96). In a review of 113 patients, there were 98% with rheumatologic manifestations, 74% with genitourinary, 58% with ocular, and 42% with mucocutaneous findings (96). Conjunctivitis was seen in all patients with ocular manifestations and is characterized by a papillary reaction with a mucopurulent discharge. A nongranulomatous iridocyclitis without hypopyon was the second most common ocular manifestation, occurring in 12% of the total group, although glaucoma was only seen in 1 of the 113 patients.

Grant Syndrome: Glaucoma Associated with Precipitates on the Trabecular Meshwork

Chandler and Grant (97) described an uncommon form of open-angle glaucoma in which the only evidence of ocular inflammation was precipitates on the trabecular meshwork (**Fig. 22.4**). Because the condition is usually bilateral and the eyes are generally quiet, it may be mistaken for chronic open-angle glaucoma. However, careful goniosic examination reveals

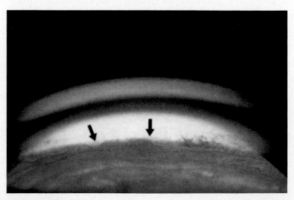

Figure 22.4 Keratitic precipitates on the trabecular meshwork (i.e., Grant syndrome).

gray or slightly yellow precipitates on the meshwork and irregular peripheral anterior synechiae, which often attach to the trabecular precipitates (21). The cause is unknown, although some patients eventually develop sarcoidosis, rheumatoid arthritis, ankylosing spondylitis, episcleritis, glaucomatocyclitic crisis, or chronic uveitis (21). The glaucoma, which is presumed to be caused by inflammatory changes in the trabecular meshwork, usually clears promptly with topical corticosteroid therapy, although antiglaucoma drugs that reduce aqueous production may be temporarily required for pressure control. The condition often recurs, and the patients must be followed closely. Untreated cases may progress to synechial closure of the angle.

Epidemic Dropsy

Epidemic dropsy is an acute toxic disease that results from the unintentional ingestion of sanguinarine in *Argemone mexicana* oil as an adulterant of cooking oils. It is characterized by the explosive onset of leg edema, with tenderness, erythema, and rash over the edematous parts; gastrointestinal symptoms; low-grade fever; and congestive heart failure that may be fatal (98,99). Ocular features include glaucoma and retinal vascular dilatation, tortuosity, and hemorrhage (98). The glaucoma is bilateral with open angles, normal outflow facility, and normal trabecular meshwork by histopathologic and histochemical testing (99). Although there are no signs of anterior segment inflammation, aqueous assays reveal elevated prostaglandin E_2 levels, histamine activity, and total protein levels, suggesting hypersecretion as the mechanism of IOP elevation (99).

Infectious Diseases

The following infectious processes may cause an iridocyclitis with the occasional association of glaucoma.

Congenital Rubella. This disorder predominantly affects the heart, auditory apparatus, and eyes (100), although virtually any organ may be involved. Ocular defects occur in 30% to 60% of the cases and include cataracts, microphthalmia, retinopathy, and glaucoma (101). Corneal edema may occur because of co-existent glaucoma or in the absence of elevated IOP (102). The associated glaucoma can occur in 2% to 15% of children with congenital rubella (103). Contrary to earlier reports, the cataracts and glaucoma occur together at a frequency that would be anticipated with each occurring independently (103). The glaucoma may be associated with hypoplasia of the iris stroma and hypoperfusion by iris angiography (104). The glaucoma is particularly severe, with blindness occurring in 8 of 15 children in one follow-up study (105). Mechanisms of the glaucoma include iridocyclitis, angle anomalies, and angle-closure glaucoma due to microphthalmia, an intumescent lens, or pupillary block after cataract extraction. Although the ocular abnormalities are most often observed in the neonatal period, the glaucoma may also occur later in childhood or in young adults, usually in association with microphthalmia and cataracts (106).

Syphilis. Congenital syphilis may cause iridocyclitis with glaucoma in the early or late stages of the disease. (Glaucoma associated with the interstitial keratitis of congenital syphilis is discussed later in this chapter.) Acquired syphilis in adults may also cause iridocyclitis and IOP elevation (107). Mass lesions of the iris and ciliary body have also been associated with this condition (108).

Hansen Disease. Uveitis is common in lepromatous leprosy and typically involves the iris and ciliary body (109–111). Four forms have been described: chronic iridocyclitis; acute plastic iridocyclitis; iris pearls or miliary lepromata, which is pathognomonic of the disease; and nodular lepromata, characterized by larger, less discrete masses on the iris (109). Complications of keratitis and iridocyclitis are the main causes of blindness in this disease (111). The chronic iridocyclitis may be associated with iris atrophy and small nonreacting pupils, which aggravate the visual impairment (112,113). In a study of 100 cases, 19 had acute or chronic iridocyclitis, and 12 had evidence of glaucoma, which was usually associated with chronic anterior uveitis (114). In another study of 193 patients, glaucoma was found in 10%, one half of whom had associated uveitis, although all had been previously treated with dapsone or clofazimine, or both (115).

Patients with Hansen disease more typically have lower-than-normal IOP and a significant postural change in IOP from the upright to the supine position. In some cases, this may be associated with chronic plastic iridocyclitis (113,116,117). However, these same IOP anomalies may be seen in patients without clinical evidence of anterior uveal inflammation and even in household contacts of patients with Hansen disease (118). These findings are thought to suggest early subclinical ciliary body autonomic neuropathy and may be useful in the early diagnosis of the disease. In cases with active anterior uveitis, however, the mechanism for the hypotension may be reduced aqueous production or increased uveoscleral outflow secondary to the inflammation (113,117).

Active iridocyclitis is reported to respond to treatment with dapsone, corticosteroids, and rifampin (109). There is evidence that effective antimicrobial and anti-inflammatory therapy may significantly minimize the ocular complications (119).

Disseminated Meningococcemia. These patients may have associated iridocyclitis or endophthalmitis with acute glaucoma (120,121), presumably due to obstruction of the anterior chamber by a blanket of cells.

Hemorrhagic Fever with Renal Syndrome (Nephropathia Epidemica). This disease is caused by the Puumala virus and is characterized by fever, chills, malaise, nausea, vomiting, and headache, which progresses to back and abdominal pain, uremia, hematuria, oliguria, and proteinuria. Three patients have been described with associated transient angle-closure glaucoma that was thought to be caused by swelling of the ciliary body (122). However, in a prospective study of 37 patients during the acute phase of the disease, the anterior chamber was shallower than after clinical recovery, but the IOP was below baseline and there were no cases of acute angle-closure attacks (123).

Acquired Immune Deficiency Syndrome (AIDS). This viral disorder has severe defects of immunoregulation, leading to life-threatening opportunistic infections, Kaposi sarcoma, or both. Bilateral acute angle-closure glaucoma has been reported in these patients, which appears to be due to choroidal effusion with anterior rotation of the ciliary body (124–126). B-scan echography is helpful in establishing the diagnosis by demonstrating diffuse choroidal thickening with ciliochoroidal effusion (126,127). These cases do not respond to miotics or iridotomy, although peripheral iridoplasty was successful in one case (125). Treatment with aqueous suppressants, cycloplegics, and topical steroids has been reported to achieve complete resolution of the angle closure (126).

Listeria Monocytogenes. Patients with *Listeria monocytogenes* endophthalmitis may present with a "dark hypopyon" and markedly elevated IOP. The dark appearance results from associated pigment dispersion, and the diagnosis can be established by culture and histopathologic examination of ocular fluid (128).

Theories of Mechanisms for Associated Glaucoma

The possible mechanisms by which iridocyclitis may lead to an elevated IOP already have been mentioned with regard to certain specific forms of iridocyclitis and are now summarized. In general, iridocyclitis affects both aqueous production and resistance to aqueous outflow, with the subsequent change in IOP representing a balance between these two factors.

Aqueous Production

Inflammation of the ciliary body usually leads to reduced aqueous production. If this outweighs a concomitant increased resistance to outflow, the IOP will be reduced, which is often the case with acute iridocyclitis. Experimental iridocyclitis in monkeys suggests that the hypotony may be due to reduced aqueous humor flow and increased uveoscleral outflow (129). However, prostaglandins, which have been demonstrated in the aqueous of eyes with uveitis, are known to cause elevated IOP without a reduction in outflow facility (130–133), suggesting that increased aqueous production may occur in some cases of uveitis, such as Posner–Schlossman syndrome.

Aqueous Outflow

When the aqueous outflow system is involved in an ocular inflammatory disease, increased resistance to outflow may result from a variety of acute and chronic mechanisms.

Acute Mechanisms of Obstruction

During the active phase of iridocyclitis, several mechanisms of obstruction to aqueous outflow may lead to a relatively sudden, but usually reversible, rise in IOP. In most cases, the anterior chamber angle is open, which is an important observation in ruling out pupillary block glaucoma. Obstruction of the trabecular meshwork may occur in several ways.

A disruption in the blood–aqueous barrier allows inflammatory cells and fibrin to enter the aqueous and accumulate in the trabecular meshwork. Normal serum components have been shown to reduce outflow when perfused in enucleated human eyes (134). Prostaglandins were demonstrated to increase aqueous protein content (132,133,135,136), and it has been suggested that an accumulation of cyclic adenosine

monophosphate (cAMP) due to prostaglandins or certain non-prostaglandin agents causes the barrier damage (137).

In other cases, swelling or dysfunction of the trabecular lamellae or endothelium may lead to aqueous outflow obstruction. Precipitates on the trabecular meshwork, as previously discussed, may also occur in eyes with ocular inflammation and elevated IOP (21,97). The use of corticosteroids in treating the inflammation may create yet another mechanism of IOP elevation (steroid-induced glaucoma, which is discussed in the next chapter).

Much less commonly, ocular inflammation may lead to acute closure of the anterior chamber angle by uveal effusion with forward rotation of the ciliary body. If a significant posterior uveitis is present, angle closure may result from displacement of the lens–iris diaphragm due to massive exudative retinal detachment.

Chronic Elevation of IOP

Several sequelae of inflammation may lead to chronic mechanisms of obstruction. Obstruction of aqueous outflow may result from scarring and obliteration of outflow channels, or from the overgrowth of an endothelial-cuticular or fibrovascular membrane in the open angle. The membranes may eventually contract, leading to synechial closure of the angle. In addition to the effect of membrane contraction, peripheral anterior synechiae may result from the protein and inflammatory cells in the angle, which pull the iris toward the cornea. Posterior synechiae may be sequelae of anterior uveitis and can cause iris bombé with closure of the anterior chamber angle.

Management

In treating an eye with iridocyclitis and glaucoma, control of the inflammatory component alone frequently leads to normalization of the IOP, and this is usually the first approach in the treatment plan. However, if the magnitude of the pressure elevation poses an immediate threat to vision or the IOP does not respond adequately to anti-inflammatory therapy, medical and even surgical management of the glaucoma may be indicated. The following basic principles of management apply to most cases of iridocyclitis, as well as other forms of ocular inflammation, with exceptions as noted in the discussions of the specific diseases. Differences between children and adults should be considered, including differences in the type of uveitis, higher risk of some ocular complications such as uveitic glaucoma, and the presence of other special complications, such as amblyopia (138).

Management of the Inflammation
Corticosteroids

This group of drugs constitutes the first-line defense in most cases of ocular inflammation. Topical administration is preferred for anterior segment disease and commonly used steroids include prednisolone, 1.0%, and dexamethasone, 0.1%. In a rabbit model of anterior uveitis, frequent topical administration of prednisolone acetate, 1.0%, caused a significant decrease in protein levels and leukocytes in the anterior chamber (139). Administration of the steroid every hour may be required initially, with gradual reduction in frequency as the inflammation subsides. In a rabbit model of keratitis, instillation every 15 minutes was even more effective than the hourly regimen, although five doses at 1-minute intervals each hour were equivalent to the effect achieved by administration every 15 minutes (140). When the response to topical administration is insufficient, periocular injections (e.g., dexamethasone phosphate, prednisolone succinate, triamcinolone acetate, or methylprednisolone acetate) or a systemic corticosteroid (e.g., prednisone) may be required. With any form of administration, the many side effects of corticosteroids must be considered, including steroid-induced glaucoma. Children with uveitis may have special dosing requirements and drug-associated risks, such as growth retardation with systemic corticosteroids (138).

Nonsteroidal Anti-inflammatory Agents

When the use of corticosteroids is contraindicated or inadequate, other anti-inflammatory drugs may be helpful. Prostaglandin synthetase inhibitors such as aspirin, imidazole, indoxyl, indomethacin, and dipyridamole have been effective in some cases of uveitis (141–144). With severe cases, immunosuppressive agents such as methotrexate, azathioprine, or chlorambucil may be indicated (145–147). In a study of 25 patients with severe chronic uveitis with poor response or unresponsiveness to corticosteroid therapy, all responded to long-term daily administration of prednisone (10 to 15 mg) combined with azathioprine (2.0 to 2.5 mg) or chlorambucil (6 to 8 mg) (148). These patients must be monitored closely for hematologic reactions.

Newer cyclooxygenase inhibitors such as flurbiprofen, ketorolac, suprofen, and diclofenac may provide useful anti-inflammatory effects without the risk of steroid-induced IOP elevation. Another class of anti-inflammatory agent is the 21-aminosteroids, which were developed as free radical scavengers and showed promise in rabbit models (149).

In conjunction with anti-inflammatory agents, a mydriatic–cycloplegic drug, such as atropine, 1%, homatropine, 1% to 5%, or cyclopentolate, 0.5% to 1%, is usually indicated to avoid posterior synechiae and to relieve the discomfort of ciliary muscle spasm.

Management of the Glaucoma
Medical Management

Because miotics and prostaglandins are generally contraindicated in the inflamed eye, a topical β-blocker, α_2-agonist, or carbonic anhydrase inhibitor is usually the first-line antiglaucoma drug in the treatment of glaucoma associated with ocular inflammation. An oral carbonic anhydrase inhibitor may also be needed, and a hyperosmotic agent is occasionally required as a short-term emergency measure.

In eyes with acute fibrinous anterior uveitis and impending pupillary block with or without peripheral anterior synechiae, it may be reasonable to consider use of intracameral tissue plasminogen activator (6.25 to 12.5 μg) (150).

Surgical Management

Intraocular surgery should be avoided whenever possible in eyes with active inflammation. However, when medical therapy is inadequate, surgery may be required. In these cases, it is best to do the least amount of surgery possible. A laser iridectomy is safer than an incisional iridectomy when an angle-closure mechanism is present, although fibrin may tend to close a small iridotomy in an inflamed eye. Laser trabeculoplasty is not effective in eyes with uveitis and open-angle glaucoma, and it may cause an additional, significant rise in IOP and is generally contraindicated in these cases. Filtering surgery with heavy steroid therapy is one approach in uveitis cases that are uncontrolled on maximum tolerable medical therapy. Adjuvant use of subconjunctival 5-FU may improve the success rate in these cases (148,149), and adjunctive use of mitomycin C is probably even more effective than 5-FU (151). Glaucoma drainage-device surgery can be an effective intervention in these cases, especially when significant postoperative inflammation is likely (152,153).

A technique called trabeculodialysis has also been described, in which a goniotomy knife is used to incise above the trabecular meshwork and then peel the meshwork downward (154). This was successful in a preliminary series of eyes with anterior uveitis and glaucoma (154), although a subsequent study of 30 eyes in 23 children and young adults achieved success in only 60%, with most of these requiring concomitant antiglaucoma medication (155). Goniotomy may be a safe and effective alternative in refractive glaucoma associated with chronic childhood uveitis, although patients may require use of glaucoma medication after the procedure (156). Cyclodestructive surgery, such as transscleral Nd:YAG cyclophotocoagulation, may be another reasonable surgical option, especially in aphakic and pseudophakic eyes with limited visual potential.

OTHER FORMS OF OCULAR INFLAMMATION

Choroiditis and Retinitis

In the following conditions, inflammation that is predominantly posterior may cause glaucoma by an associated anterior inflammatory component or by angle closure from a posterior mass effect.

Vogt–Koyanagi–Harada Syndrome

Vogt–Koyanagi–Harada disease is a chronic, granulomatous, systemic autoimmune disease with ophthalmic manifestations. The target of attack seems to be antigens associated with melanocytes. Patients are usually of Asian, Middle Eastern, Asian Indian, Native American, or Hispanic ethnicity, and they report neurologic symptoms, quickly followed by decreased vision (157). The systemic findings in this disorder include alopecia, poliosis, vitiligo, and central nervous system and auditory signs. Ocular manifestations consist of bilateral, diffuse granulomatous uveitis with exudative retinal detachment. In two reviews of 51 and 42 patients, glaucoma was found in 20% and 38%, respectively (158,159). In the first of these groups, a mild anterior uveitis was seen in all patients, posterior synechiae occurred in 36%, keratic precipitates occurred in 30%, and nodules occurred on the iris in 8.4% (158). Mechanisms of glaucoma may include an open angle in association with anterior uveitis or angle closure, which apparently results from swelling of the ciliary body caused by severe choroiditis (159–162). In the series of 42 patients, those with glaucoma had open angles in 56% and angle closure in 44% (159). These conditions may respond to corticosteroid therapy and antiglaucoma medication, although a high percentage requires surgical intervention (159,160). Complications that may limit visual acuity include cataract, glaucoma, choroidal neovascular membrane formation, and subretinal fibrosis.

Sympathetic Ophthalmia

This form of ocular inflammation typically occurs weeks or months after traumatic or surgical penetration of the fellow eye. The severity of the inflammation is related to the degree of ocular pigmentation, and the choroid is predominantly affected with frequent involvement of the overlying retina (163,164). The condition bears striking clinical and histopathologic similarities to the Vogt–Koyanagi–Harada syndrome and the two disorders may share a common immunopathologic inflammatory mechanism (164). In a study of 17 cases with an average follow-up of 10.6 years, 7 (43%) had glaucoma (163). The mechanism of the glaucoma is unknown, although in a histopathologic study of 105 cases, a high percentage had plasma cell infiltration of the iris and ciliary body (163), suggesting an immune reaction near the area of aqueous outflow. Whatever the cause, the glaucoma is typically difficult to treat, requiring frequent adjustments of corticosteroids and occasional surgical intervention (165).

Other Forms of Retinitis or Choroiditis

Cytomegalic inclusion retinitis was described in two adult patients who underwent renal transplantation, both of whom developed open-angle glaucoma presumably due to an associated anterior uveitis (166). The common ocular form of toxocariasis, characterized by retinitis and vitreitis, may also have anterior uveitis with posterior synechiae, iris bombé, and associated glaucoma (167).

Whipple disease can present as a posterior uveitis with or without gastrointestinal symptoms such as malabsorption (168). When suspected, the patient should be referred for possible jejunal biopsy to look for the presence of *Tropheryma whippelii*. Malaria (*Plasmodium vivax*–related) can be associated with acute bilateral panuveitis and secondary glaucoma (169). Clinical clues include a history of travel to an endemic area and multiple blotchy retinal hemorrhages.

Keratitis

Interstitial Keratitis

As a feature of congenital syphilis, interstitial keratitis typically appears late in the course of the disease, between 5 and 16 years of age, although it may appear as early as birth or as late as 30 years of age (170). The presenting symptoms of interstitial keratitis include marked ciliary flush, lacrimation, photophobia, and pain. The mechanisms of glaucoma associated with interstitial keratitis, in addition to the previously discussed concomitant iridocyclitis, include open-angle and angle-closure forms that usually appear later in life (171,172).

With the open-angle glaucomas, the eye may have irregular pigmentation of the anterior chamber angle, with occasional columnar peripheral anterior synechiae, and one histopathologic study revealed endothelium and a glassy membrane over the angle (171). This condition responds poorly to medical therapy but may be controlled by filtering surgery. Another mechanism of open-angle glaucoma in the adults is the recurrence of iridocyclitis in an eye that had interstitial keratitis in younger life (171). The residual ghost vessels in the cornea may help in making this diagnosis.

Eyes with interstitial keratitis in infancy often have small anterior segments and narrow angles, which can lead to angle-closure glaucoma later in life. This is usually subacute and responds well to peripheral iridotomy (171,173). In some cases, multiple cysts of the iris may lead to angle closure.

Interstitial keratitis may also be associated with vertigo, tinnitus, and deafness, which is referred to as Cogan syndrome. An atypical form may have noncorneal ocular inflammation (174), which may involve the anterior uvea with associated glaucoma.

Herpes Simplex Keratouveitis

This viral infection may cause recurrent conjunctivitis, keratitis, and uveitis. In one study of patients with herpes simplex keratouveitis, 28% had IOP elevation and 10% had glaucomatous damage (175). The keratitis in cases with associated IOP elevation is typically disciform or stromal, rather than a superficial ulcer, and may be associated with keratic precipitates (**Fig. 22.5**) (175). The pressure usually remains elevated for several weeks, and a rabbit model suggests a biphasic IOP response in which the uveitis during the first few days represents active infection, but subsequently is due to immune mechanisms (176). An analysis of aqueous from 33 patients with herpes revealed herpes simplex virus in 8 cases, all of whom had associated glaucoma (177). Histopathology of rabbit eyes with experimental herpetic keratouveitis showed mononuclear cells in the trabecular meshwork and peripheral anterior synechiae (178).

Management of this condition requires attention to the infection, inflammation, and glaucoma, and one suggested regimen includes topical trifluorothymidine, corticosteroids, and cycloplegics along with antiglaucoma agents that reduce aqueous production (177). One study indicated that the severity of the uveitis and IOP rise in experimental secondary herpes simplex uveitis was lessened with dexamethasone, 0.1%, administered twice daily, but not with use of aspirin or cyclophosphamide (179).

Herpes Zoster Keratouveitis

In addition to causing the characteristic cutaneous vesicular eruptions along the trigeminal distribution, this viral disease may produce a keratitis and uveitis. The anterior uveitis commonly leads to glaucoma. Sectoral iris atrophy can occur and there may be associated mutton-fat keratitic precipitates (**Fig. 22.6**). In one series of 86 patients with herpes zoster ophthalmicus, 37 had uveitis and 10 of these had associated glaucoma (180). In another study, 5 of 14 patients with keratouveitis had transient high IOPs (181). Intraocular inflammation and sectoral iris atrophy can also occur without a

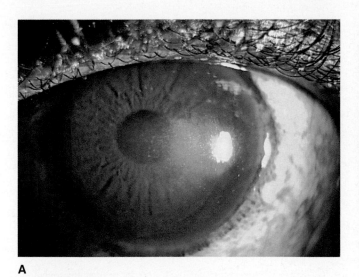

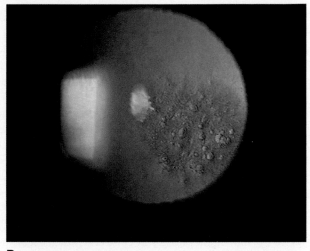

A   **B**

Figure 22.5   Slitlamp view of an eye with herpes simplex keratitis. **A:** Typical appearance of disciform keratitis in a patient with elevated IOP. **B:** In the same patient, retroillumination reveals fine keratic precipitates and overlying bullous corneal edema. (Courtesy of Joseph A. Halabis, OD.)

cutaneous component—that is, zoster sine herpete (182). Topical acyclovir has been shown to be superior to topical steroids in the treatment of herpes (183).

Adenovirus Type 10

Adenovirus type 10 has been reported to cause keratoconjunctivitis with a transient increase in IOP (184).

Scleritis

Scleritis is an extremely painful, potentially disastrous form of ocular inflammation, which may primarily involve the anterior or posterior segment of the eye (185). The anterior forms may present as diffuse or nodular anterior scleritis, characterized by episcleral congestion and scleral edema. These are painful and often recurrent, but relatively benign. Necrotizing scleritis is a more severe condition, with extensive granulomatous infiltration of the conjunctiva, episclera, and sclera and degradation of scleral collagen (186,187). It is typically painful and progressive, although a variation, scleromalacia perforans, which is

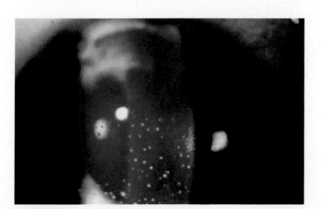

Figure 22.6   Slitlamp view of an eye with herpes zoster–related anterior uveitis. Notice the mutton-fat keratitic precipitates and sectoral iris atrophy.

seen primarily in patients with rheumatoid arthritis, has no pain or redness. Anterior segment fluorescein angiography helps to distinguish the more benign forms, which have vasodilatation and rapid flow, from the necrotizing cases, which have gross vascular abnormalities and delayed flow (188). Posterior scleritis, which is more difficult to diagnose, may present with pars planitis, exudative retinal detachment, optic nerve head edema, or proptosis.

In two large studies, the prevalence of glaucoma was 11.6% and 13% (185,189), and in another series elevated IOP was present in 18.7% with rheumatoid scleritis and 12% with non-rheumatoid scleritis (190). A histopathologic study of 92 enucleated eyes revealed evidence of increased IOP in 49% (191). In most cases, the glaucoma is associated with anterior scleritis, and mechanisms of pressure elevation in these patients include trabecular meshwork damage by iridocyclitis, overlying corneoscleral inflammation, and peripheral anterior synechiae (191). Other reported mechanisms include steroid-induced glaucoma, iris neovascularization (191), and elevated episcleral venous pressure in an eye with anterior diffuse scleritis in relapsing polychondritis (192). Bilateral glaucoma with marked IOP elevations, presumably of an open-angle mechanism, has been described in a 14-year-old boy with scleritis, a fibrinous anterior uveitis, and rheumatic fever (193). Glaucoma associated with posterior scleritis is much less common, but angle-closure mechanisms may result from a forward shift of the lens–iris diaphragm or an anterior rotation of the ciliary body in association with choroidal effusion (194,195).

Treatment of the scleritis generally consists of topical and systemic corticosteroids and nonsteroidal anti-inflammatory agents. A combination of oral prednisone and indomethacin proved to be more effective than either drug used alone and allowed lower doses of each (10 to 60 mg and 50 to 150 mg daily, respectively) (196). Antiglaucoma agents are used as needed, and surgical intervention for the glaucoma should be resorted to only when necessary.

Episcleritis

In contrast to scleritis, episcleritis produces only mild discomfort and does not typically lead to serious sequelae. The characteristic appearance is congestion of the episcleral vessels, which may be diffuse with chemosis and occasional lid edema (simple episcleritis), or localized with nodules in the episcleral tissue (nodular episcleritis) (185). Associated glaucoma is uncommon in this condition (185,190) but has been reported (189,197). In one series of 127 eyes of 94 patients, glaucoma was present in 4% (188). Presumed mechanisms of open-angle glaucoma include inflammation of the angle structures and steroid-induced glaucoma (185,197). Angle-closure glaucoma has also been observed in association with episcleritis (190,198), which was caused by ciliochoroidal effusion in one patient with immunoglobulin A nephropathy (198). In most cases, the episcleritis and the secondary glaucoma respond to topical corticosteroids, although iridotomy may be required for an angle-closure mechanism (198).

KEY POINTS

- The type of ocular inflammation most often associated with IOP elevation is iridocyclitis in a primary form or resulting from inflammation elsewhere in the eye.
- The anterior uveitis may be acute, subacute, or chronic; may occur as an isolated finding of uncertain origin (i.e., acute anterior uveitis, pars planitis, glaucomatocyclitic crises, and Fuchs heterochromic cyclitis); or may be associated with a systemic inflammatory disorder (i.e., sarcoidosis, some forms of rheumatoid arthritis, Behçet disease, and many infectious conditions).
- The mechanisms by which iridocyclitis leads to obstruction of aqueous outflow include acute, usually reversible forms (e.g., accumulation of inflammatory elements in the intertrabecular spaces, edema of the trabecular lamellae, or angle closure due to ciliary body swelling) and chronic forms (e.g., scar formation or membrane overgrowth in the anterior chamber angle). Uveitis may also cause increased aqueous production in some cases.
- The role of steroids should also be considered when thinking through the mechanism of the glaucoma in a patient with uveitis.
- Treatment of combined iridocyclitis and glaucoma involves steroidal and nonsteroidal anti-inflammatory agents and antiglaucoma drugs, with surgical intervention reserved for medical failures.
- Other forms of ocular inflammation that may be associated with glaucoma include choroiditis and retinitis, keratitis, scleritis, and episcleritis.

REFERENCES

1. Weiner A, Ben Ezra D. Clinical patterns and associated conditions in chronic uveitis. *Am J Ophthalmol.* 1991;112:151–158.
2. Darrel RW, Wagener HP, Kurland LT. Epidemiology of uveitis: incidence and prevalence in a small urban community. *Arch Ophthalmol.* 1962; 68:502–514.
3. Perkins ES, Folk J. Uveitis in London and Iowa. *Ophthalmologica.* 1984;189:36–40.
4. Henderly DE, Genstler AJ, Smith RE, et al. Changing patterns of uveitis. *Am J Ophthalmol.* 1987;103:131–136.
5. Merayo-Lloves J, Power WJ, Rodriguez A, et al. Secondary glaucoma in patients with uveitis. *Ophthalmologica.* 1999;213:300–304.
6. Panek WC, Holland GN, Lee DA, et al. Glaucoma in patients with uveitis. *Br J Ophthalmol.* 1990;74:223–227.
7. Linssen A, Rothova A, Valkenburg HA, et al. The lifetime cumulative incidence of acute anterior uveitis in a normal population and its relation to ankylosing spondylitis and histocompatibility antigen HLA-B27. *Invest Ophthalmol Vis Sci.* 1991;32:2568–2578.
8. Brewerton DA, Caffrey M, Nicholls A, et al. Acute anterior uveitis and HLA 27. *Lancet.* 1973;2:994–996.
9. Rothova A, van Veenedaal WG, Linssen A, et al. Clinical features of acute uveitis. *Am J Ophthalmol.* 1987;103:137–145.
10. Linssen A, Meenken C. Outcomes of HLA-B27-positive and HLA-B27-negative acute anterior uveitis. *Am J Ophthalmol.* 1995;120:351–361.
11. Tay-Kearney ML, Schwam BL, Lowder C, et al. Clinical features and associated systemic diseases of HLA-B27 uveitis. *Am J Ophthalmol.* 1996;121:47–56.
12. Fearnley IR, Spalton DJ, Smith SE. Anterior segment fluorophotometry I acute anterior uveitis. *Arch Ophthalmol.* 1987;105:1550–1555.
13. Derhaag PJ, Linssen A, Broekema N, et al. A familial study of the inheritance of HLA-B27-positive acute anterior uveitis. *Am J Ophthalmol.* 1988;105:603–606.
14. Patel NP, Patel KH, Moster MR, et al. Metipranolol-associated nongranulomatous anterior uveitis. *Am J Ophthalmol.* 1997;123:843–844.
15. Byles DB, Frith P, Salmon JF. Anterior uveitis as a side effect of topical brimonidine. *Am J Ophthalmol.* 2000;130:287–291.
16. Schumer RA, Camras CB, Mandahl AK. Putative side effects of prostaglandin analogs. *Surv Ophthalmol.* 2002;47(suppl 1):S219.
17. Moorthy RS, Mermoud A, Baerveldt G, et al. Glaucoma associated with uveitis. *Surv Ophthalmol.* 1997;41:361–394.
18. Obenauf CD, Shaw HE, Sydnor CF, et al. Sarcoidosis and its ophthalmic manifestations. *Am J Ophthalmol.* 1978;86:648–655.
19. Ohara K, Okubo A, Sasaki H, et al. Intraocular manifestations of systemic sarcoidosis. *Jpn J Ophthalmol.* 1992;36:452–457.
20. Mizuno K, Takahashi J. Sarcoid cyclitis. *Ophthalmology.* 1986;93:511–517.
21. Roth M, Simmons RJ. Glaucoma associated with precipitates on the trabecular meshwork. *Ophthalmology.* 1979;86:1613–1619.
22. Kimura R. Hyperfluorescent dots in the ciliary body band in patients with granulomatous uveitis. *Br J Ophthalmol.* 1982;66:322–325.
23. Karma A, Huhti E, Poukkula A. Course and outcome of ocular sarcoidosis. *Am J Ophthalmol.* 1988;106:467–472.
24. Jabs DA, Johns CJ. Ocular involvement in chronic sarcoidosis. *Am J Ophthalmol.* 1986;102:297–301.
25. Goble RR, Murray PI. Fuchs' heterochromic uveitis and sarcoidosis. *Br J Ophthalmol.* 1995;79:1021–1023.
26. Iwata K, Nanba K, Sobue K, et al. Ocular sarcoidosis: evaluation of intraocular findings. *Ann N Y Acad Sci.* 1976;278:445–454.
27. Hamanaka T, Takei A, Takemura T, et al. Pathological study of cases with secondary open-angle glaucoma due to sarcoidosis. *Am J Ophthalmol.* 2002;134:17–26.
28. Mayer J, Brouillette G, Corriveau LA. Sarcoidose et rubeosis iridis. *Can J Ophthalmol.* 1983;18:197–198.
29. Korner-Stiefbold U, Sauvain MJ, Gerber N, et al. Ophthalmological complications in patients with juvenile chronic arthritis (JCA) [in German]. *Klin Monatsbl Augenheilkd.* 1993;202:269–280.
30. Calabro JJ, Parrino GR, Atchoo PD, et al. Chronic iridocyclitis in juvenile rheumatoid arthritis. *Arthritis Rheum.* 1970;13:406–413.
31. Schaller J, Kupfer C, Wedgwood RJ. Iridocyclitis in juvenile rheumatoid arthritis. *Pediatrics.* 1969;44:92–100.
32. Key SN III, Kimura SJ. Iridocyclitis associated with juvenile rheumatoid arthritis. *Am J Ophthalmol.* 1975;80:425–429.
33. Chylack LT Jr, Bienfang DC, Bellows R, et al. Ocular manifestations of juvenile rheumatoid arthritis. *Am J Ophthalmol.* 1975;79:1026–1033.
34. Kanski JJ. Anterior uveitis in juvenile rheumatoid arthritis. *Arch Ophthalmol.* 1977;95:1794–1797.
35. Kanski JJ, Shun-Shin GA. Systemic uveitis syndromes in childhood: an analysis of 340 cases. *Ophthalmology.* 1984;91:1247–1252.
36. Wolf MD, Lichter PR, Ragsdale CG. Prognostic factors in the uveitis of juvenile rheumatoid arthritis. *Ophthalmology.* 1987;94:1242–1248.
37. Foster CS, Barrett F. Cataract development and cataract surgery in patients with juvenile rheumatoid arthritis-associated iridocyclitis. *Ophthalmology.* 1993;100:809–817.

38. Sabates R, Smith T, Apple D. Ocular histopathology in juvenile rheumatoid arthritis. *Ann Ophthalmol.* 1979;11:733–737.

39. Merriam JC, Chylack LT, Albert DM. Early-onset pauciarticular juvenile rheumatoid arthritis: a histopathologic study. *Arch Ophthalmol.* 1983;101:1085–1092.

40. Brewerton DA, Hart FD, Nicholls A, et al. Ankylosing spondylitis and HL-A 27. *Lancet.* 1973;1:904–907.

41. Russell AS, Lentle BC, Percy JS, et al. Scintigraphy of sacroiliac joints in acute anterior uveitis: a study of thirty patients. *Ann Intern Med.* 1976;85:606–608.

42. Smith RE, Godfrey WA, Kimura SJ. Complications of chronic cyclitis. *Am J Ophthalmol.* 1976;82:277–282.

43. Henderly DE, Genstler AJ, Rao NA, et al. Pars planitis. *Trans Ophthalmol Soc U K.* 1986;105:227–232.

44. Pederson JE, Kenyon KE, Green WR, et al. Pathology of pars planitis. *Am J Ophthalmol.* 1978;86:762–774.

45. Posner A, Schlossman A. Syndrome of unilateral recurrent attacks of glaucoma with cyclitic symptoms. *Arch Ophthalmol.* 1948;39:517–535.

46. Knox DL. Glaucomatocyclitic crises and systemic disease: peptic ulcer, other gastrointestinal disorders, allergy, and stress. *Trans Am Ophthalmol Soc.* 1988;86:473–495.

47. Hirose S, Ohno S, Matsuda H. HLA-Bw54 and glaucomatocyclitic crisis. *Arch Ophthalmol.* 1985;103:1837–1839.

48. Yamamoto S, Pavan-Langston D, Tada R, et al. Possible role of herpes simplex virus in the origin of Posner-Schlossman syndrome. *Am J Ophthalmol.* 1995;119:796–798.

49. Hollwich F. Clinical aspects and therapy of the Posner-Schlossman-syndrome [in German]. *Klin Monatsbl Augenheilkd.* 1978;172:736–744.

50. Raitta C, Vannas A. Glaucomatocyclitic crisis. *Arch Ophthalmol.* 1977;95:608–612.

51. Kass MA, Becker B, Kolker AE. Glaucomatocyclitic crisis and primary open-angle glaucoma. *Am J Ophthalmol.* 1973;75:668–673.

52. Hung PT, Chang JM. Treatment of glaucomatocyclitic crises. *Am J Ophthalmol.* 1974;77:169–172.

53. Jap A, Sivakumar M, Chee SP. Is Posner-Schlossman syndrome benign? *Ophthalmology.* 2001;108:913–918.

54. Harstad HK, Ringvold A. Glaucomatocyclitic crises (Posner-Schlossman syndrome): a case report. *Acta Ophthalmol.* 1986;64:146–151.

55. Nagataki S, Mishima S. Aqueous humor dynamics in glaucomato-cyclitic crisis. *Invest Ophthalmol.* 1976;15:365–370.

56. de Roetth A Jr. Glaucomatocyclitic crisis. *Am J Ophthalmol.* 1970;69:370–371.

57. Hong C, Yung Song KY. Effect of apraclonidine hydrochloride on the attack of Posner-Schlossman syndrome. *Korean J Ophthalmol.* 1993;7:28–33.

58. Fuchs E. Uber Komplikationen der Heterochromie. *Z Augenheilkd.* 1906;15:191–212.

59. Franceschetti A. Heterochromic cyclitis (Fuchs' syndrome). *Am J Ophthalmol.* 1955;39:50–58.

60. Kimura SJ, Hogan MJ, Thygeson P. Fuchs' syndrome of heterochromic cyclitis. *Arch Ophthalmol.* 1955;54:179–186.

61. O'Connor GR. Heterochromic iridocyclitis. *Trans Ophthalmol Soc UK.* 1985;104:219–231.

62. Tabbut BR, Tessler HH, Williams D. Fuchs' heterochromic iridocyclitis in blacks. *Arch Ophthalmol.* 1988;106:1688–1690.

63. van der Gaag R, Broersma L, Rothova A, et al. Immunity to a corneal antigen in Fuchs' heterochromic cyclitis patients. *Invest Ophthalmol Vis Sci.* 1989;30:443–448.

64. La Hey E, Baarsma GS, Rothova A, et al. High incidence of corneal epithelium antibodies in Fuchs' heterochromic cyclitis. *Br J Ophthalmol.* 1988;72:921–925.

65. La Hey E, Mooy CM, Baarsma GS, et al. Immune deposits in iris biopsy specimens from patients with Fuchs' heterochromic iridocyclitis. *Am J Ophthalmol.* 1992;113:75–80.

66. De Bruyere M, Dernouchamps JP, Sokal G. HLA antigens in Fuchs' heterochromic iridocyclitis. *Am J Ophthalmol.* 1986;102:392–393.

67. van den Born LI, van Schooneveld MJ, de Jong PT, et al. Fuchs' heterochromic uveitis associated with retinitis pigmentosa in a father and son. *Br J Ophthalmol.* 1994;78:504–505.

68. Jones NP, Read AP. Is there a genetic basis for Fuchs' heterochromic uveitis? Discordance in monozygotic twins. *Br J Ophthalmol.* 1992;76:22–24.

69. Regenbogen LS, Naveh-Floman N. Glaucoma in Fuchs' heterochromic cyclitis associated with congenital Horner's syndrome. *Br J Ophthalmol.* 1987;71:844–849.

70. Schwab IR. The epidemiologic association of Fuchs' heterochromic iridocyclitis and ocular toxoplasmosis. *Am J Ophthalmol.* 1991;111:356–362.

71. La Heiji E, Rothova A. Fuchs's heterochromic cyclitis in congenital ocular toxoplasmosis. *Br J Ophthalmol.* 1991;75:372–373.

72. La Hey E, Rothova A, Baarsma GS, et al. Fuchs' heterochromic iridocyclitis is not associated with ocular toxoplasmosis. *Arch Ophthalmol.* 1992;110:806–811.

73. Liesegang TJ. Clinical features and prognosis in Fuchs' uveitis syndrome. *Arch Ophthalmol.* 1982;100:1622–1626.

74. Saari M, Vuorre I, Nieminen H. Infra-red transillumination stereophotography of the iris in Fuchs's heterochromic cyclitis. *Br J Ophthalmol.* 1978;62:110–115.

75. La Hey E, Ijspeert JK, van den Berg TJ, et al. Quantitative analysis of iris translucency in Fuchs' heterochromic cyclitis. *Invest Ophthalmol Vis Sci.* 1993;34:2931–2942.

76. Melamed S, Lahav M, Sandbank U, et al. Fuchs' heterochromic iridocyclitis: an electron microscopic study of the iris. *Invest Ophthalmol Vis Sci.* 1978;17:1193–1199.

77. McCartney AC, Bull TB, Spalton DJ. Fuchs' heterochromic cyclitis: an electron microscopy study. *Trans Ophthalmol Soc UK.* 1986;105:324–329.

78. Rothova A, La Hey E, Baarsma GS, et al. Iris nodules in Fuchs' heterochromic uveitis. *Am J Ophthalmol.* 1994;18:338–342.

79. Saari M, Vuorre I, Nieminen H. Fuchs' heterochromic cyclitis: a simultaneous bilateral fluorescein angiographic study of the iris. *Br J Ophthalmol.* 1978;62:715–721.

80. Berger BB, Tessler HH, Kottow MH. Anterior segment ischemia in Fuchs' heterochromic cyclitis. *Arch Ophthalmol.* 1980;98:499–501.

81. Johnson D, Liesegang TJ, Brubaker RF. Aqueous humor dynamics in Fuchs' uveitis syndrome. *Am J Ophthalmol.* 1983;95:783–787.

82. Arffa RC, Schlaegel TF. Chorioretinal scars in Fuchs' heterochromic iridocyclitis. *Arch Ophthalmol.* 1984;102:1153–1155.

83. De Abreu MT, Belfort R Jr, Hirata PS. Fuchs' heterochromic cyclitis and ocular toxoplasmosis. *Am J Ophthalmol.* 1982;93:739–744.

84. Daus W, Schmidbauer J, Buschendorff P, et al. Results of extracapsular cataract extraction with intraocular lens implantation in eyes with uveitis and Fuchs' heterochromic iridocyclitis. *Ger J Ophthalmol.* 1992;1:399–402.

85. Baarsma GS, de Vries J, Hammudoglu CD. Extracapsular cataract extraction with posterior chamber lens implantation in Fuchs's heterochromic cyclitis. *Br J Ophthalmol.* 1991;75:306–308.

86. O'Neill D, Murray PI, Patel BC, et al. Extracapsular cataract surgery with and without intraocular lens implantation in Fuchs' heterochromic cyclitis. *Ophthalmology.* 1995;102:1362–1368.

87. Huber A. Das Glaukom bei komplizierter heterochromic Fuchs [in German]. *Ophthalmologica.* 1961;142:66–115.

88. Daus W, Kraus-Mackiw E. Fuchs' heterochromic cyclitis case reports of patients treated at Heidelberg University Eye Hospital since 1978. *Klin Monatsbl Augenheilkd.* 1984;185:410.

89. La Hey E, de Vries J, Langerhorst CT, et al. Treatment and prognosis of secondary glaucoma in Fuchs' heterochromic iridocyclitis. *Am J Ophthalmol.* 1993;116:327–340.

90. Perry HD, Yanoff M, Scheie HG. Rubeosis in Fuchs heterochromic iridocyclitis. *Arch Ophthalmol.* 1975;93:337–339.

91. Benedikt O, Roll P, Zirm M. The glaucoma in heterochromic cyclitis Fuchs: gonioscopic studies and electron microscopic investigations of the trabecular meshwork [in German]. *Klin Monatsbl Augenheilkd.* 1978;173:523–533.

92. Colvard DM, Robertson DM, O'Duffy JD. The ocular manifestations of Behçet's disease. *Arch Ophthalmol.* 1977;95:1813–1817.

93. Michelson JB, Chisari FV. Behçet's disease. *Surv Ophthalmol.* 1982;26:190–203.

94. Benezra D, Cohen E. Treatment and visual prognosis in Behçet's disease. *Br J Ophthalmol.* 1986;70:589–592.

95. James DG, Spiteri MA. Behçet's disease. *Ophthalmology.* 1982;89:1279–1284.

96. Lee DA, Barker SM, Su WP, et al. The clinical diagnosis of Reiter's syndrome: ophthalmic and nonophthalmic aspects. *Ophthalmology.* 1986;93:350–356.

97. Chandler PA, Grant WM. *Lectures on Glaucoma.* Philadelphia, PA: Lea & Febiger; 1954:257.

98. Rathore MK. Ophthalmological study of epidemic dropsy. *Br J Ophthalmol.* 1982;66:573–575.

99. Sachdev MS, Sood NN, Verma LK, et al. Pathogenesis of epidemic dropsy glaucoma. *Arch Ophthalmol.* 1988;106:1221–1223.

100. Cooper LZ, Ziring PR, Ockerse AB, et al. Rubella: clinical manifestations and management. *Am J Dis Child.* 1969;118:18–29.

101. Rudolph AJ, Desmond MM. Clinical manifestations of the congenital rubella syndrome. *Int Ophthalmol Clin.* 1972;12:3–19.

102. deLuise VP, Cobo LM, Chandler D. Persistent corneal edema in the congenital rubella syndrome. *Ophthalmology.* 1983;90:835–839.

103. Boniuk M. Glaucoma in the congenital rubella syndrome. *Int Ophthalmol Clin.* 1972;12:121–136.
104. Brooks AMV, Gillies WE. Glaucoma associated with congenital hypoplasia of the iris stroma in rubella. *Glaucoma.* 1989;11:36–41.
105. Wolff SM. The ocular manifestations of congenital rubella. *Trans Am Ophthalmol Soc.* 1972;70:577–614.
106. Boger WP III. Late ocular complications in congenital rubella syndrome. *Ophthalmology.* 1980;87:1244–1252.
107. Schwartz LK, O'Connor GR. Secondary syphilis with iris papules. *Am J Ophthalmol.* 1980;90:380–384.
108. Scully RE, Mark EJ, McNeely BU. Mass in the iris and a skin rash in a young man. *N Engl J Med.* 1984;310:972–981.
109. Michelson JB, Roth AM, Waring GO III. Lepromatous iridocyclitis diagnosed by anterior chamber paracentesis. *Am J Ophthalmol.* 1979;88: 674–679.
110. Malla OK, Brandt F, Anten JG. Ocular findings in leprosy patients in an institution in Nepal (Khokana). *Br J Ophthalmol.* 1981;65:226–230.
111. Joffrion VC, Brand ME. Leprosy of the eye—a general outline. *Lepr Rev.* 1984;55:105–114.
112. Ffytche TJ. Role of iris changes as a cause of blindness in lepromatous leprosy. *Br J Ophthalmol.* 1981;65:231–239.
113. Lewallen S, Courtright P, Lee HS. Ocular autonomic dysfunction and intraocular pressure in leprosy. *Br J Ophthalmol.* 1989;73:946–949.
114. Shields JA, Waring GO III, Monte LG. Ocular findings in leprosy. *Am J Ophthalmol.* 1974;77:880–890.
115. Walton RC, Ball SF, Joffrion VC. Glaucoma in Hansen's disease. *Br J Ophthalmol.* 1991;75:270–272.
116. Brandt F, Malla OK, Anten JG. Influence of untreated chronic plastic iridocyclitis on intraocular pressure in leprous patients. *Br J Ophthalmol.* 1981;65:240–242.
117. Hussein N, Courtright P, Ostler HB, et al. Low intraocular pressure and postural changes in intraocular pressure in patients with Hansen's Disease. *Am J Ophthalmol.* 1989;108:80–83.
118. Hussein N, Chiang T, Ehsan Q, et al. Intraocular pressure decrease in household contacts of patients with Hansen's disease and endemic control subjects. *Am J Ophthalmol.* 1992;114:479–483.
119. Spaide R, Nattis R, Lipka A, et al. Ocular findings in leprosy in the United States. *Am J Ophthalmol.* 1985;100:411–416.
120. deLuise VP, Stern JT, Paden P. Uveitic glaucoma caused by disseminated meningococcemia. *Am J Ophthalmol.* 1983;95:707–708.
121. Jensen AD, Naidoff MA. Bilateral meningococcal endophthalmitis. *Arch Ophthalmol.* 1973;90:396–398.
122. Saari KM. Acute glaucoma in hemorrhagic fever with renal syndrome (nephropathia epidemica). *Am J Ophthalmol.* 1976;81:455–461.
123. Kontkanen MI, Puustjarvi TJ, Lhdevirta JK. Intraocular pressure changes in nephropathia epidemica. *Ophthalmology.* 1995;102:1813–1817.
124. Ullman S, Wilson RP, Schwartz L. Bilateral angle-closure glaucoma in association with the acquired immune deficiency syndrome. *Am J Ophthalmol.* 1986;101:419–424.
125. Koster HR, Liebmann JM, Ritch R, et al. Acute angle-closure glaucoma in a patient with acquired immunodeficiency syndrome successfully treated with argon laser peripheral iridoplasty. *Ophthalmol Surg.* 1990;21:501–502.
126. Nash RW, Lindquist TD. Bilateral angle-closure glaucoma associated with uveal effusion: presenting sign of HIV infection. *Surv Ophthalmol.* 1992;36:255–258.
127. Joshi N, Constable PH, Margolis TP, et al. Bilateral angle closure glaucoma and accelerated cataract formation in a patient with AIDS. *Br J Ophthalmol.* 1994;78:656–657.
128. Eliott D, O'Brien TP, Green WR, et al. Elevated intraocular pressure, pigment dispersion and dark hypopyon in endogenous endophthalmitis from *Listeria* monocytogenes. *Surv Ophthalmol.* 1992;37:117–124.
129. Toris CB, Pederson JE. Aqueous humor dynamics in experimental iridocyclitis. *Invest Ophthalmol Vis Sci.* 1987;28:477–481.
130. Chiang TS, Thomas RP. Ocular hypertension following intravenous infusion of prostaglandin E$_1$. *Arch Ophthalmol.* 1972;88:418–420.
131. Chiang TS, Thomas RP. Consensual ocular hypertensive response to prostaglandin E$_2$. *Invest Ophthalmol.* 1972;11:845–849.
132. Kass MA, Podos SM, Moses RA, et al. Prostaglandin E$_1$ and aqueous humor dynamics. *Invest Ophthalmol.* 1972;11:1022–1027.
133. Podos SM, Becker B, Kass MA. Prostaglandin synthesis, inhibition, and intraocular pressure. *Invest Ophthalmol.* 1973;12:426–433.
134. Epstein DL, Hashimoto JM, Grant WM. Serum obstruction of aqueous outflow in enucleated eyes. *Am J Ophthalmol.* 1978;86:101–105.
135. Neufeld AH, Sears ML. The site of action of prostaglandin E$_2$ on the disruption of the blood-aqueous barrier in the rabbit eye. *Exp Eye Res.* 1973;7:445–448.
136. Kulkarni PS, Srinivasan BD. The effect of intravitreal and topical prostaglandins on intraocular inflammation. *Invest Ophthalmol Vis Sci.* 1982;23:383–392.
137. Bengtsson E. The effect of theophylline on the breakdown of the blood-aqueous barrier in the rabbit eye. *Invest Ophthalmol Vis Sci.* 1977;16: 636–640.
138. Holland GN, Stiehm ER. Special considerations in the evaluation and management of uveitis in children. *Am J Ophthalmol.* 2003;135:867–878.
139. Bolliger GA, Kupferman A, Leibowitz HM. Quantitation of anterior chamber inflammation and its response to therapy. *Arch Ophthalmol.* 1980;98:1110–1114.
140. Leibowitz HM, Kupferman A. Optimal frequency of topical prednisolone administration. *Arch Ophthalmol.* 1979;97:2154–2156.
141. Marsettio M, Siverio CE, Oh JO. Effects of aspirin and dexamethasone on intraocular pressure in primary uveitis produced by herpes simplex virus. *Am J Ophthalmol.* 1976;81:636–641.
142. Kass MA, Palmberg P, Becker B. The ocular anti-inflammatory action of imidazole. *Invest Ophthalmol Vis Sci.* 1977;16:66–69.
143. Spinelli HM, Krohn DL. Inhibition of prostaglandin-induced iritis: topical indoxole vs. indomethacin therapy. *Arch Ophthalmol.* 1980;98:1106–1109.
144. Podos SM. Effect of dipyridamole on prostaglandin-induced ocular hypertension in rabbits. *Invest Ophthalmol Vis Sci.* 1979;18:646–648.
145. Wong VG, Hersh EM. Methotrexate in the therapy of cyclitis. *Trans Am Acad Ophthalmol Otolaryngol.* 1965;69:279–293.
146. Andrasch RH, Pirofsky B, Burns RP. Immunosuppressive therapy for severe chronic uveitis. *Arch Ophthalmol.* 1978;96:247–251.
147. Fiscella R, Gagliano DA, Peachey NS, et al. Intravitreal U75412E: a new free radical scavenger. *Ophthalmol Surg.* 1991;22:740–744.
148. Jampel HD, Jabs DA, Quigley HA. Trabeculectomy with 5-fluorouracil for adult inflammatory glaucoma. *Am J Ophthalmol.* 1990;109:168–173.
149. Patitsas CJ, Rockwood EJ, Meisler DM, et al. Glaucoma filtering surgery with postoperative 5-fluorouracil in patients with intraocular inflammatory disease. *Ophthalmology.* 1992;99:594–599.
150. Skolnick CA, Fiscella RG, Tessler HH, et al. Tissue plasminogen activator to treat impending pupillary block glaucoma in patients with acute fibrinous HLA-B27 positive iridocyclitis. *Am J Ophthalmol.* 2000;129:363–366.
151. Prata JA, Neves RA, Minckler DS, et al. Trabeculectomy with mitomycin C in glaucoma associated with uveitis. *Ophthalmol Surg.* 1994;25:616–620.
152. Hill RA, Nguyen QH, Baerveldt G, et al. Trabeculectomy and Molteno implantation for glaucomas associated with uveitis. *Ophthalmology.* 1993;100:903–908.
153. Gil-Carrasco F, Salinas-VanOrman E, Recillas-Gispert C, et al. Ahmed valve implant for uncontrolled uveitic glaucoma. *Ocul Immunol Inflamm.* 1998;6:27–37.
154. Hoskins HD Jr, Hetherington J Jr, Shaffer RN. Surgical management of the inflammatory glaucomas. *Perspect Ophthalmol.* 1977;1:173–181.
155. Kanski JJ, McAllister JA. Trabeculodialysis for inflammatory glaucoma in children and young adults. *Ophthalmology.* 1985;92:927–930.
156. Freedman SF, Rodriguez-Rosa RE, Rojas MC, et al. Goniotomy for glaucoma secondary to chronic childhood uveitis. *Am J Ophthalmol.* 2002;133:617–621.
157. Read RW. Vogt-Koyanagi-Harada disease. *Ophthalmol Clin North Am.* 2002;15:333–341.
158. Ohno S, Char DH, Kimura SJ, et al. Vogt-Koyanagi-Harada syndrome. *Am J Ophthalmol.* 1977;83:735–740.
159. Forster DJ, Rao NA, Hill RA, et al. Incidence and management of glaucoma in Vogt-160. Koyanagi-Harada syndrome. *Ophthalmology.* 1993;100:613–618.
160. Shirato S, Hayashi K, Masuda K. Acute angle closure glaucoma as an initial sign of Harada's disease: report of two cases. *Jpn J Ophthalmol.* 1980;24:260–266.
161. Kimura R, Sakai M, Okabe H. Transient shallow anterior chamber as initial symptom in Harada's syndrome. *Arch Ophthalmol.* 1981;99:1604–1606.
162. Kimura R, Kasai M, Shoji K, et al. Swollen ciliary processes as an initial symptom in Vogt-Koyanagi-Harada syndrome. *Am J Ophthalmol.* 1983;95:402–403.
163. Lubin JR, Albert DM, Weinstein M. Sixty-five years of sympathetic ophthalmia: a clinicopathologic review of 105 cases (1913–1978). *Ophthalmology.* 1980;87:109–121.
164. Marak GE Jr. Recent advances in sympathetic ophthalmia. *Surv Ophthalmol.* 1979;24:141–156.
165. Makley TA Jr, Azar A. Sympathetic ophthalmia: a long-term follow-up. *Arch Ophthalmol.* 1978;96:257–262.
166. Merritt JC, Callender CO. Adult cytomegalic inclusion retinitis. *Ann Ophthalmol.* 1978;10:1059–1063.
167. Shields JA. Ocular toxocariasis: a review. *Surv Ophthalmol.* 1984;28: 361–381.

168. Nishimura JK, Cook BE Jr, Pach JM. Whipple disease presenting as posterior uveitis without prominent gastrointestinal symptoms. *Am J Ophthalmol.* 1998;126:130–132.

169. Biswas J, Fogla R, Srinivasan P, et al. Ocular malaria: a clinical and histopathologic study. *Ophthalmology.* 1996;103:1471–1475.

170. Tavs LE. Syphilis. *Major Probl Clin Pediatr.* 1978;19:222–256.

171. Grant WM. Late glaucoma after interstitial keratitis. *Am J Ophthalmol.* 1975;79:87–91.

172. Tsukahara S. Secondary glaucoma due to inactive congenital syphilitic interstitial keratitis. *Ophthalmologica.* 1977;174:188–194.

173. Sugar HS. Late glaucoma associated with inactive syphilitic interstitial keratitis. *Am J Ophthalmol.* 1962;53:602–605.

174. Cobo LM, Haynes BF. Early corneal findings in Cogan's syndrome. *Ophthalmology.* 1984;91:903–907.

175. Falcon MG, Williams HP. Herpes simplex kerato-uveitis and glaucoma. *Trans Ophthalmol Soc U K.* 1978;98:101–104.

176. Oh JO. Effect of cyclophosphamide on primary herpes simplex uveitis in rabbits. *Invest Ophthalmol Vis Sci.* 1978;17:769–773.

177. Sundmacher R, Neumann-Haefelin D. Herpes simplex virus isolations from the aqueous of patients suffering from focal iritis, endotheliitis, and prolonged disciform keratitis with glaucoma [in German]. *Klin Monatsbl Augenheilkd.* 1979;175:488–501.

178. Townsend WM, Kaufman HE. Pathogenesis of glaucoma and endothelial changes in herpetic kerato-uveitis in rabbits. *Am J Ophthalmol.* 1971;71:904–910.

179. Dennis RF, Oh JO. Aspirin, cyclophosphamide, and dexamethasone effects on experimental secondary herpes simplex uveitis. *Arch Ophthalmol.* 1979;97:2170–2174.

180. Womack LW, Liesegang TJ. Complications of herpes zoster ophthalmicus. *Arch Ophthalmol.* 1983;101:42–45.

181. Reijo A, Antti V, Jukka M. Endothelial cell loss in herpes zoster keratouveitis. *Br J Ophthalmol.* 1983;67:751–754.

182. Nakamura M, Tanabe M, Yamada Y, et al. Zoster sine herpete with bilateral ocular involvement. *Am J Ophthalmol.* 2000;129:809–810.

183. McGill J, Chapman C. A comparison of topical acyclovir with steroids in the treatment of herpes zoster keratouveitis. *Br J Ophthalmol.* 1983;67:746–750.

184. Hara J, Ishibashi T, Fujimoto F, et al. Adenovirus type 10 keratoconjunctivitis with increased intraocular pressure. *Am J Ophthalmol.* 1980;90:481–484.

185. Watson PG, Hayreh SS. Scleritis and episcleritis. *Br J Ophthalmol.* 1976;60:163–191.

186. Young RD, Watson PG. Microscopical studies of necrotising scleritis. I. Cellular aspects. *Br J Ophthalmol.* 1984;68:770–780.

187. Young RD, Watson PG. Microscopical studies of necrotising scleritis. II. Collagen degradation in the scleral stroma. *Br J Ophthalmol.* 1984;68:781–789.

188. Watson PG, Bovey E. Anterior segment fluorescein angiography in the diagnosis of scleral inflammation. *Ophthalmology.* 1985;92:1–11.

189. de La Maza MS, Jabbur NS, Foster CS. Severity of scleritis and episcleritis. *Ophthalmology.* 1994;101:389–396.

190. McGavin DD, Williamson J, Forrester JV, et al. Episcleritis and scleritis: a study of their clinical manifestations and association with rheumatoid arthritis. *Br J Ophthalmol.* 1976;60:192–226.

191. Wilhelmus KR, Grierson I, Watson PG. Histopathologic and clinical associations of scleritis and glaucoma. *Am J Ophthalmol.* 1981;91:697–705.

192. Chen CJ, Harisdangkul V, Parker L. Transient glaucoma associated with anterior diffuse scleritis in relapsing polychondritis. *Glaucoma.* 1982;4:109–111.

193. Ortiz JM, Kamerling JM, Fischer D, et al. Scleritis, uveitis, and glaucoma in a patient with rheumatic fever. *Am J Ophthalmol.* 1995;120:538–539.

194. Quinlan MP, Hitchings RA. Angle-closure glaucoma secondary to posterior scleritis. *Br J Ophthalmol.* 1978;62:330–335.

195. Mangouritsas G, Ulbig M. Secondary angle closure glaucoma in posterior scleritis [in German]. *Klin Monatsbl Augenheilkd.* 1991;199:40–44.

196. Mondino BJ, Phinney RB. Treatment of scleritis with combined oral prednisone and indomethacin therapy. *Am J Ophthalmol.* 1988;106:473–479.

197. Harbin TS Jr, Pollack IP. Glaucoma in episcleritis. *Arch Ophthalmol.* 1975;93:948–950.

198. Pavlin CJ, Easterbrook M, Harasiewicz K, et al. An ultrasound biomicroscopic analysis of angle-closure glaucoma secondary to ciliochoroidal effusion in IgA nephropathy. *Am J Ophthalmol.* 1993;116:341–345.

23

Steroid-Induced Glaucoma

A certain percentage of the general population responds to repeated instillation of systemic or ocular corticosteroids with a variable increase in the intraocular pressure (IOP) (see Chapter 11). This appears to have been reported first by McLean in 1950, after administration of corticotropin (ACTH) and cortisone systemically (1), and then by François (2), after local administration of cortisone. It occurs more commonly in individuals who have chronic open-angle glaucoma (COAG) or a family history of the disease. There are many unknown facets regarding the pressure response to steroids, such as the precise distribution of steroid responders in the general population, the reproducibility of these responses, and hereditary influences. Nevertheless, the critical fact is that certain people do manifest this response to long-term steroid therapy, whether given by the topical, systemic, periocular, or intraocular route, and the IOP elevation can lead to glaucomatous optic atrophy and loss of vision. Such a condition is referred to as steroid-induced glaucoma.

CLINICAL FEATURES

The typical clinical presentation of steroid-induced glaucoma is associated with topical, periocular, intraocular, or oral steroid therapy, although it can occur with any type of steroid administration. IOP elevation usually develops within a few weeks with potent topical or intraocular corticosteroids or in months with the weaker steroids (3,4). The clinical picture resembles that of COAG, with an open, normal-appearing anterior chamber angle and absence of symptoms. Much less often, the condition may have an acute presentation, and pressure rises have been observed within hours after steroid administration in eyes with open angles (3,5). This reaction has been seen with intensive systemic steroid therapy, with the topical use of potent corticosteroids, and with the use of intravitreal triamcinolone in patients with pseudophakia.

Although children appear to have a lower incidence of positive steroid responses than adults do (6), IOP elevation has been reported with treatment of external diseases in infants with corticosteroids, with nasal and inhalational steroids, and with corticosteroid eyedrops after strabismus surgery in children younger than 10 years (7–9). After strabismus surgery and the use of topical dexamethasone, IOP increased in a dose- and age-dependent manner in Chinese children; children younger than 6 years were especially at high risk (10). However, long-term, low-dose oral prednisone therapy in children was not associated with higher-than-normal IOPs in one study (11).

IOP elevation may occur in the first few weeks after a trabeculectomy despite a good filtering bleb, possibly because of the influence of topical steroid therapy (12). Steroid-induced glaucoma may also mimic low-tension glaucoma when the steroid-induced pressure elevation has damaged the optic nerve head and visual field in the past, but the IOP has subsequently returned to normal with cessation of steroid use (13).

Since the early 1990s, with the advent of laser refractive surgery and concomitant use of postoperative steroids, cases of severe IOP elevation and serious optic nerve damage have been reported (14,15). One explanation for this may be a failure to recognize the elevated IOP because of refractive surgery–induced errors in the accuracy of applanation tonometry (16). Reasons for a falsely low IOP reading after refractive surgery that can mask steroid-induced glaucoma include central corneal thinning, ocular rigidity changes, corneal edema, or fluid accumulation beneath a laser in situ keratomileusis (LASIK) flap (17,18).

IOP elevation secondary to steroid use has also been reported as a mechanism for glaucoma after Descemet-stripping endothelial keratoplasty (19).

THEORIES OF MECHANISM

It is generally agreed that the IOP elevation due to steroid administration results from reduction in facility of aqueous outflow. (Detailed references in this regard can be found in review articles by Jones and Rhee (4) and Kersey and Broadway (20).) The precise mechanism responsible for the obstruction to outflow is unknown, but the following observations and theories have been reported.

Nuclear Transport of Glucocorticoid Receptor

Glucocorticoids have been shown to alter trabecular meshwork cell morphology by causing an increase in nuclear size and DNA content (21). Experiments on cultured human trabecular meshwork cells exposed to dexamethasone have demonstrated that the FK506-binding immunophilin FKBP51 mediates nuclear transport of the human glucocorticoid receptor GRbeta (22), suggesting that this plays a role in increased glucocorticoid responsiveness.

Influence on Extracellular Matrix

François (23–25) postulated that glycosaminoglycans in the polymerized form become hydrated, producing a "biologic edema" that may increase resistance to aqueous outflow.

Hyaluronidase in lysosomes depolymerizes hyaluronate, and corticosteroids stabilize the lysosomal membrane, which may lead to an accumulation of polymerized glycosaminoglycans in the trabecular meshwork.

Animal and tissue culture and organ perfusion experiments have demonstrated outflow obstruction in response to corticosteroids. Topical dexamethasone–induced IOP elevation in rabbits was associated with an increase in chondroitin sulfate in the aqueous outflow pathway but a decrease in hyaluronic acid (26). Dexamethasone can decrease the synthesis of collagen in normal human trabecular meshwork explants and decrease the extracellular activity of tissue plasminogen activator (27,28). In cultured human trabecular meshwork cells, glucocorticoids increased the expression of the extracellular matrix protein fibronectin, glycosaminoglycans, and elastin, increased depositions of which are also seen in the outflow pathways of patients with COAG (29,30).

Influence on Phagocytosis

Endothelial cells lining the trabecular meshwork have phagocytic properties, which may help to clean the aqueous of debris before it reaches the inner wall of the Schlemm canal. Corticosteroids are known to suppress phagocytic activity, and suppressed phagocytosis of the trabecular endothelium may allow debris in the aqueous to accumulate in the meshwork and act as a barrier to outflow (31). In support of this are experiments that demonstrate the formation of cross-linked actin networks in the trabecular meshwork cytoskeleton with exposure to dexamethasone (32). This theory of reduced phagocytic activity is also consistent with ultrastructural studies showing marked depositions of amorphous and fibrous or linear material in the juxtacanalicular meshwork of eyes with steroid-induced glaucoma (33,34).

Genetic Influences

With the discovery that mutations in several genes are associated with familial COAG and with the knowledge that patients with COAG and their relatives are at increased risk for steroid-induced IOP elevation, there has been interest in searching for the involvement of these genes in humans and in animal models of steroid-induced glaucoma. Studies have shown no evidence for a link between myocilin or optineurin mutations and steroid-induced ocular hypertension (35). Microarrays and macroarrays have been used to study differential gene expression between cultured human trabecular meshwork cells, with and without exposure to dexamethasone. These experiments, which require confirmation, have revealed multiple genes that may be involved in protective and damaging mechanisms with IOP elevation that are upregulated with dexamethasone (in addition to myocilin): α_1-antichymotrypsin, pigment epithelium–derived factor, cornea-derived transcript 6, prostaglandin D_2 synthase, growth arrest specific 1, decorin, insulin-like growth factor binding protein 2, ferritin light chain, and fibulin-1C (36–38). Much more work needs to be done to determine which of these genes are upregulated in vivo and which

of these and other genes play a role in increasing outflow resistance in response to steroid application.

Outflow Obstruction by Steroid Particles

In a case series by Singh and colleagues, three patients experienced a rapid rise in IOP after receiving intravitreal triamcinolone injections for diabetic macular edema (39). All three patients had pseudophakia and required surgical intervention to control their IOP. A peculiar finding was the presence of white crystals in the angle of one patient, suggesting direct physical obstruction of the trabecular meshwork with crystalline steroid particles. Another study that monitored the elevation of IOP after administration of a single dose of intravitreal triamcinolone noted that four of six eyes requiring topical administration of IOP-lowering agents after the injection had postinjection abnormalities in the inferior angle—characterized by pigmented particulate matter—that had not been present at the baseline examination (40).

Animal Models

Animal models of steroid-induced glaucoma have been reported in monkeys, beagles, and sheep, although the pathogenic mechanisms are unclear (41–43).

PREVENTION

To avoid loss of vision from steroid-induced glaucoma, physicians must know how to prevent or minimize the chances of its occurrence. This requires close attention to the patient's history and to the selection and use of steroids.

Patient Selection

Individuals with COAG or a family history of the disease are more likely than other persons to respond to long-term steroid therapy with a significant rise in IOP. The same is true for young children and older adults, and persons with highly myopic eyes, diabetes mellitus, or connective tissue disease (especially rheumatoid arthritis) (**Table 23.1**) (44–49). All such persons who undergo long-term steroid treatment are therefore at increased risk for steroid-induced glaucoma. However, because it is impossible to predict which individuals will have a pressure rise, all patients should be observed closely. Physicians should avoid steroid use when a safer drug will suffice. If a steroidal agent must be used, the patient should receive the lowest possible amount of drug over the shortest duration needed. In addition, it is wise to establish a baseline IOP before initiation of corticosteroid therapy, and the tension should be monitored closely for the duration of the therapy.

Drug Selection

When corticosteroid therapy is required for any disorder, the optimum drug is the one that can achieve the desired therapeutic response by the safest route of administration in the

Table 23.1	Factors Associated with an Increased Risk for Steroid Response

COAG
First-degree relative with COAG
Very young age or older adult
High myopia
Previous steroid response
Type 1 diabetes mellitus
Connective tissue disease (e.g., rheumatoid arthritis)
Penetrating keratoplasty, particularly in eyes with Fuchs endothelial dystrophy or keratoconus

COAG, chronic open-angle glaucoma.

lowest concentration and with the fewest potential adverse reactions. With regard to the IOP response, the following observations should be considered.

Routes of Administration

Topical Therapy

IOP rise after corticosteroid therapy occurs more often with topical administration than with systemic administration. The IOP rise may occur with drops or ointment applied directly to the eye and with steroid preparations used in treating the skin of the eyelids (50).

Periocular Therapy

Periocular injection of a long-acting corticosteroid is the most dangerous route of administration from the standpoint of steroid-induced glaucoma. IOP elevation may occur in response to subconjunctival, sub-Tenon, or retrobulbar injection of steroids (51). Patients' response to earlier topical steroid therapy does not always predict their response to periocular corticosteroid use (52). Use of repository steroids is particularly dangerous because of the prolonged duration of action, and it may occasionally be necessary to surgically excise the remaining drug before the pressure can be brought under control (52,53). Histopathologic study of excised specimens has revealed granular or foamy eosinophilic material in the subepithelial connective tissue (54). If repository steroids must be used, they should be injected in an inferior quadrant and an anterior location to avoid compromising the superior sites for possible future filtering surgery and to enable easy excision, should this be required.

Intravitreal Therapy

Intravitreal steroid use can also cause a rise in IOP. Injection of triamcinolone acetonide to treat intraocular neovascular or inflammatory diseases increases the IOP by several mm Hg in about half of the patients treated, within 2 to 4 weeks after the start of treatment; in some cases (e.g., in eyes that have pseudophakia or have undergone vitrectomy), pressure may rise even more rapidly (4,55,56). Placement of a depot steroid implant in the vitreous has also been reported to produce serious

elevation of IOP in a large percentage of patients. This was observed in patients with fluocinolone acetonide implants for posterior uveitis. Seventy-five percent of the eyes required some form of IOP-lowering treatment over time (57).

Systemic Therapy

Systemic administration of corticosteroids is least likely to induce glaucoma, although cases have been described (58). If pressure does rise, it is reported that this response does not correlate with the dosage or duration of treatment but is associated with the degree of pressure response to topical steroid use (58,59). IOP elevation has been associated with the use of inhalational and nasal corticosteroids (60), and amounts of corticosteroids sufficient to affect the IOP can be absorbed from skin application in areas remote from the eyes (61).

Relative Pressure-Inducing Effects of Topical Steroids

Although topical corticosteroid use is more likely than systemic steroid use to cause elevated IOP, the topical route of administration is still generally preferred for ocular conditions to avoid the additional dangers associated with systemic corticosteroid therapy. Although no topical steroid is totally free of a pressure-inducing effect, the following observations have been reported about the relative tendencies of these drugs to increase the IOP.

Corticosteroids

In general, the pressure-inducing effect of a topical steroid is proportional to its anti-inflammatory potency. Betamethasone, dexamethasone, and prednisolone are commonly used potent corticosteroids with a significant tendency to produce steroid-induced glaucoma. However, the pressure-inducing potency is related to the dosage of the drug used. In a study of high topical steroid responders, betamethasone, 0.01%, caused significantly less pressure elevation than the 0.1% concentration did (62). The formulation may cause some dissociation of anti-inflammatory and pressure-inducing effects. In a rabbit study, dexamethasone acetate, 0.1%, had a better anti-inflammatory effect than dexamethasone alcohol, 0.1%, or dexamethasone sodium phosphate, 0.1%, did, and use of the acetate and sodium phosphate preparations had the same effect on IOP elevation in humans (63).

Flurandrenolide, a less commonly used corticosteroid, has also been reported to cause steroid-induced glaucoma (64). Another corticosteroid with high topical activity, clobetasone butyrate, 0.1%, has been evaluated in comparison with prednisolone phosphate, 0.5%, and betamethasone phosphate, 0.1% (65). Although the results vary somewhat by study, clobetasone butyrate had similar or slightly weaker anti-inflammatory effects but also was less likely to increase the IOP.

Nonadrenal Steroids

A group of drugs closely related to progesterone has been shown to have useful anti-inflammatory properties with significantly less pressure-inducing effects than most corticosteroids. Medrysone is primarily of value in the treatment of extraocular disorders because it has limited corneal penetration, although one study found it to be effective in treating iritis (66). Most reports describe little or no associated IOP elevation, although a slight pressure response in some patients has been observed (62). The steroid antagonist mifepristone has been shown to reduce the hypertensive effect of medrysone in rabbits (67). Fluorometholone, 0.1%, is more efficacious than medrysone in treating inflammation of the anterior ocular segment. Although the pressure-inducing effect of fluorometholone is substantially less than that of the potent corticosteroids (65,68, 69), significant pressure rises have been observed with the use of this drug (69). Fluorometholone, 0.25%, is also less likely to increase IOP in corticosteroid responders than dexamethasone, 0.1%, is (70), although the increased concentration does not appear to significantly enhance the drug's anti-inflammatory effect (65). Formulation of fluorometholone as an acetate derivative, however, does appear to increase its effectiveness, rendering it as effective as prednisolone acetate, 1.0%, in one study (65). Despite the greater margin of safety with regard to IOP elevation, the same precautions must be taken with nonadrenal steroid use as with corticosteroid use.

Nonsteroidal Anti-Inflammatory Drugs

Topical nonsteroidal anti-inflammatory drugs (NSAIDs), which act primarily as cyclooxygenase inhibitors, may be effective in treating anterior ocular segment inflammation, apparently by reducing the breakdown of the blood–aqueous barrier. Preliminary experience with topical oxyphenbutazone, flurbiprofen, and diclofenac indicates that these NSAID agents do not cause an elevation of IOP (71–73). Other commercially available drugs in this class include suprofen and ketorolac. It has also been shown that flurbiprofen does not block corticosteroid-induced pressure elevation (72).

MANAGEMENT

Discontinuation of Steroid Use

Discontinuation of the use of the steroid is the first line of defense and is often all that is required. The chronic form is said to normalize in 1 to 4 weeks, whereas the acute form typically resolves within days of stopping the steroid use (5). In rare cases, the glaucoma may persist despite stopping all steroid use. The latter situation occurred in 6 of 210 patients (2.8%) in one series, and all of these patients had a family history of glaucoma (3). The duration of steroid therapy also appears to influence the reversibility of the IOP elevation. In a study of 22 patients with steroid-induced glaucoma, the pressures normalized in all cases in which the drug was used for less than 2 months, whereas the tension remained chronically elevated in all patients who used the steroid for more than 4 years (74). If continued corticosteroid therapy is essential, it may be possible to control the IOP with the additional use of antiglaucoma medications or by changing to a steroid with less pressure-inducing potential.

Excision of Depot Steroid

In all cases where depot steroid appears to be responsible for the rise in IOP, the optimal treatment, if medical management fails, is to excise the depot steroid (52–54). This can often be done as a minor procedure and can dramatically lower IOP within a few days. If the depot steroid cannot be removed because it is deemed essential or because of its location, filtering surgery may be required. In cases of intravitreal triamcinolone injection, vitrectomy has also been helpful in reducing the IOP (4).

Glaucoma Therapy

The medical management of these cases is essentially the same as for COAG. Laser trabeculoplasty (selective or argon) can help reduce the IOP temporarily, particularly in eyes treated with intravitreal triamcinolone (75,76). Another approach is anterior sub-Tenon injection of anecortave acetate, which has also been reported to be effective in these patients (77). Trabeculectomy or glaucoma-drainage device implantation is indicated when the glaucoma is uncontrolled on maximum tolerable medication. Trabeculotomy has also been reported to be successful in one paper (78).

KEY POINTS

- It takes approximately 2 weeks for the IOP to increase after administration of steroids. The degree of IOP elevation is related to the potency of the steroid and the route of administration. Risk factors for steroid-induced glaucoma include a personal or family history of COAG, type 1 diabetes mellitus, myopia, and rheumatoid arthritis.
- The mechanism of steroid-induced glaucoma is related to increased resistance to outflow, possibly through an influence on the extracellular matrix or endothelial cells of the trabecular meshwork. Genetic influences are also being disclosed.
- After refractive surgery, the IOP reading may be falsely reduced, making detection of a steroid-induced IOP elevation difficult. Ultrasonographic biomicroscopy can be helpful in detecting intrastromal fluid after LASIK, which can yield an artifactually low IOP measurement.
- Prevention of a steroid-induced rise in IOP should be attempted by judicious use of anti-inflammatory agents.
- When steroid-induced glaucoma occurs, the steroid therapy should be stopped, or the steroid excised, as appropriate, and persistent pressure elevation should be managed with medication or surgery as required.

REFERENCES

1. McLean JM. Use of ACTH and cortisone. *Trans Am Ophthalmol Soc.* 1950;48:293–296.
2. François J. Cortisone et tension oculaire [in French]. *Ann D'Oculist.* 1954;187:805–816.

3. François J. Corticosteroid glaucoma. *Ann Ophthalmol.* 1977;9(9):1075–1080.

4. Jones R III, Rhee DJ. Corticosteroid-induced ocular hypertension and glaucoma: a brief review and update of the literature. *Curr Opin Ophthalmol.* 2006;17(2):163–167.

5. Weinreb RN, Polansky JR, Kramer SG, et al. Acute effects of dexamethasone on intraocular pressure in glaucoma. *Invest Ophthalmol Vis Sci.* 1985;26(2):170–175.

6. Biedner BZ, David R, Grudsky A, et al. Intraocular pressure response to corticosteroids in children. *Br J Ophthalmol.* 1980;64(6):430–431.

7. Gnad HD, Martenet AC. Kongenitales Glaukom und Cortison [in German]. *Klin Monatsbl Augenheilkd.* 1973;162(1):86–90.

8. Desnoeck M, Casteels I, Casteels K. Intraocular pressure elevation in a child due to the use of inhalation steroids—a case report. *Bull Soc Belge Ophtalmol.* 2001;280:97–100.

9. Ohji M, Kinoshita S, Ohmi E, et al. Marked intraocular pressure response to instillation of corticosteroids in children. *Am J Ophthalmol.* 1991;112(4):450–454.

10. Lam DS, Fan DS, Ng JS, et al. Ocular hypertensive and anti-inflammatory responses to different dosages of topical dexamethasone in children: a randomized trial. *Clin Experiment Ophthalmol.* 2005;33(3):252–258.

11. Kaye LD, Kalenak JW, Price RL, et al. Ocular implications of long-term prednisone therapy in children. *J Pediatr Ophthalmol Strabismus.* 1993;30(3):142–144.

12. Wilensky JT, Snyder D, Gieser D. Steroid-induced ocular hypertension in patients with filtering blebs. *Ophthalmology.* 1980;87(3):240–244.

13. Sugar HS. Low tension glaucoma: a practical approach. *Ann Ophthalmol.* 1979;11(8):1155–1171.

14. Morales J, Good D. Permanent glaucomatous visual loss after photorefractive keratectomy. *J Cataract Refract Surg.* 1998;24(5):715–718.

15. Shaikh NM, Shaikh S, Singh K, et al. Progression to end-stage glaucoma after laser in situ keratomileusis. *J Cataract Refract Surg.* 2002;28(2):356–359.

16. Damji KF, Muni RH, Munger RM. Influence of corneal variables on accuracy of intraocular pressure measurement. *J Glaucoma.* 2003;12(1):69–80.

17. Hamilton DR, Manche EE, Rich LF, et al. Steroid-induced glaucoma after laser in situ keratomileusis associated with interface fluid. *Ophthalmology.* 2002;109(4):659–665.

18. Najman-Vainer J, Smith RJ, Maloney RK. Interface fluid after LASIK: misleading tonometry can lead to end-stage glaucoma. *J Cataract Refract Surg.* 2000;26(4):471–472.

19. Lee WB, Jacobs DS, Musch DC, et al. Descemet's stripping endothelial keratoplasty: safety and outcomes: a report by the American Academy of Ophthalmology. *Ophthalmology.* 2009;116(9):1818–1830.

20. Kersey JP, Broadway DC. Corticosteroid-induced glaucoma: a review of the literature. *Eye.* 2006;20(4):407–416.

21. Wordinger RJ, Clark AF. Effects of glucocorticoids on the trabecular meshwork: towards a better understanding of glaucoma. *Prog Retin Eye Res.* 1999;18(5):629–667.

22. Zhang X, Clark AF, Yorio T. FK506-binding protein 51 regulates nuclear transport of the glucocorticoid receptor beta and glucocorticoid responsiveness. *Invest Ophthalmol Vis Sci.* 2008;49:1037–1047.

23. François J. Tissue culture of ocular fibroblasts. *Ann Ophthalmol.* 1975;7(12):1551–1554.

24. François J. The importance of the mucopolysaccharides in intraocular pressure regulation. *Invest Ophthalmol.* 1975;14(3):173–176.

25. François J, Victoria-Troncoso V. Mucopolysaccharides and pathogenesis of cortisone glaucoma [in German]. *Klin Monatsbl Augenheilkd.* 1974;165(1):5–10.

26. Knepper PA, Collins JA, Frederick R. Effects of dexamethasone, progesterone, and testosterone on IOP and GAGs in the rabbit eye. *Invest Ophthalmol Vis Sci.* 1985;26(8):1093–1100.

27. Hernandez MR, Weinstein BI, Dunn MW, et al. The effect of dexamethasone on the synthesis of collagen in normal human trabecular meshwork explants. *Invest Ophthalmol Vis Sci.* 1985;26(12):1784–1788.

28. Seftor RE, Stamer WD, Seftor EA, et al. Dexamethasone decreases tissue plasminogen activator activity in trabecular meshwork organ and cell cultures. *J Glaucoma.* 1994;3(4):323–328.

29. Johnson DH, Bradley JM, Acott TS. The effect of dexamethasone on glycosaminoglycans of human trabecular meshwork in perfusion organ culture. *Invest Ophthalmol Vis Sci.* 1990;31(12):2568–2571.

30. Steely HT, Browder SL, Julian MB, et al. The effects of dexamethasone on fibronectin expression in cultured human trabecular meshwork cells. *Invest Ophthalmol Vis Sci.* 1992;33(7):2242–2250.

31. Bill A. The drainage of aqueous humor [editorial]. *Invest Ophthalmol.* 1975;14(1):1–3.

32. Clark AF, Wilson K, McCartney MD, et al. Glucocorticoid-induced formation of cross-linked actin networks in cultured human trabecular meshwork cells. *Invest Ophthalmol Vis Sci.* 1994;35(1):281–294.

33. Rohen JW, Linner E, Witmer R. Electron microscopic studies on the trabecular meshwork in two cases of corticosteroid-glaucoma. *Exp Eye Res.* 1973;17(1):19–31.

34. Roll P, Benedikt O. Electron microscopic studies of the trabecular meshwork in corticosteroid glaucoma [in German]. *Klin Monatsbl Augenheilkd.* 1979;174(3):421–428.

35. Fingert JH, Clark AF, Craig JE, et al. Evaluation of the myocilin (MYOC) glaucoma gene in monkey and human steroid-induced ocular hypertension. *Invest Ophthalmol Vis Sci.* 2001;42(1):145–152.

36. Fan BJ, Wang DY, Tham CC, et al. Gene expression profiles of human trabecular meshwork cells induced by triamcinolone and dexamethasone. *Invest Ophthalmol Vis Sci.* 2008;49(5):1886–1897.

37. Lo WR, Rowlette LL, Caballero M, et al. Tissue differential microarray analysis of dexamethasone induction reveals potential mechanisms of steroid glaucoma. *Invest Ophthalmol Vis Sci.* 2003;44(2):473–485.

38. Ishibashi T, Takagi Y, Mori K, et al. cDNA microarray analysis of gene expression changes induced by dexamethasone in cultured human trabecular meshwork cells. *Invest Ophthalmol Vis Sci.* 2002;43(12):3691–3697.

39. Singh IP, Ahmad SI, Yeh D, et al. Early rapid rise in intraocular pressure after intravitreal triamcinolone acetonide injection. *Am J Ophthalmol.* 2004;138(2):286–287.

40. Im L, Allingham RR, Singh I, et al. A prospective study of early intraocular pressure changes after a single intravitreal triamcinolone injection. *J Glaucoma.* 2008;17(2):128–132.

41. Clark AF, Steely HT, Dickerson JE, Jr., et al. Glucocorticoid induction of the glaucoma gene MYOC in human and monkey trabecular meshwork cells and tissues. *Invest Ophthalmol Vis Sci.* 2001;42(8):1769–780.

42. Gelatt KN, Mackay EO. The ocular hypertensive effects of topical 0.1% dexamethasone in beagles with inherited glaucoma. *J Ocul Pharmacol Ther.* 1998;14(1):57–66.

43. Gerometta R, Podos SM, Danias J, et al. Steroid-induced ocular hypertension in normal sheep. *Invest Ophthalmol Vis Sci.* 2009;50(2):669–673.

44. Podos SM, Becker B, Morton WR. High myopia and primary open-angle glaucoma. *Am J Ophthalmol.* 1966;62(6):1038–1043.

45. Becker B. Diabetes mellitus and primary open-angle glaucoma. *Am J Ophthalmol.* 1971;1(1 pt 1):1–16.

46. Armaly MF. Effect of corticosteroids on intraocular pressure and fluid dynamics. I. The effect of dexamethasone in the normal eye. *Arch Ophthalmol.* 1963;70:482–491.

47. Armaly MF. Effect of corticosteroids on intraocular pressure and fluid dynamics. II. The effect of dexamethasone in the glaucomatous eye. *Arch Ophthalmol.* 1963;70:492–499.

48. Gaston H, Absolon MJ, Thurtle OA, et al. Steroid responsiveness in connective tissue diseases. *Br J Ophthalmol.* 1983;67(7):487–490.

49. Erdurmus M, Cohen EJ, Yildiz EH, et al. Steroid-induced intraocular pressure elevation or glaucoma after penetrating keratoplasty in patients with keratoconus or Fuchs dystrophy. *Cornea.* 2009;28(7):759–764.

50. Zugerman C, Saunders D, Levit F. Glaucoma from topically applied steroids. *Arch Dermatol.* 1976;112(9):1326.

51. Nozik RA. Periocular injection of steroids. *Trans Am Acad Ophthalmol Otolaryngol.* 1972;76(3):695–705.

52. Herschler J. Increased intraocular pressure induced by repository corticosteroids. *Am J Ophthalmol.* 1976;82(1):90–93.

53. Herschler J. Intractable intraocular hypertension induced by repository triamcinolone acetonide. *Am J Ophthalmol.* 1972;74(3):501–504.

54. Ferry AP, Harris WP, Nelson MH. Histopathologic features of subconjunctivally injected corticosteroids. *Am J Ophthalmol.* 1987;103(5):716–718.

55. Vedantham V. Intraocular pressure rise after intravitreal triamcinolone. *Am J Ophthalmol.* 2005;139(3):575.

56. Breusegem C, Vandewalle E, Van Calster J, et al. Predictive value of a topical dexamethasone provocative test before intravitreal triamcinolone acetonide injection. *Invest Ophthalmol Vis Sci.* 2009;50(2):573–576.

57. Bollinger KE, Smith SD. Prevalence and management of elevated intraocular pressure after placement of an intravitreal sustained-release steroid implant. *Curr Opin Ophthalmol.* 2009;20(2):99–103.

58. Godel V, Feiler-Ofry V, Stein R. Systemic steroids and ocular fluid dynamics. I. Analysis of the sample as a whole: influence of dosage and duration of therapy. *Acta Ophthalmol (Copenh).* 1972;50(5):655–663.

59. Godel V, Feiler-Ofry V, Stein R. Systemic steroids and ocular fluid dynamics. II. Systemic versus topical steroids. *Acta Ophthalmol (Copenh)*. 1972;50(5):664–676.

60. Opatowsky I, Feldman RM, Gross R, et al. Intraocular pressure elevation associated with inhalation and nasal corticosteroids. *Ophthalmology*. 1995;102(2):177–179.

61. Schwartzenberg GW, Buys YM. Glaucoma secondary to topical use of steroid cream. *Can J Ophthalmol*. 1999;34(4):222–225.

62. Kitazawa Y. Increased intraocular pressure induced by corticosteroids. *Am J Ophthalmol*. 1976;82(3):492–495.

63. Leibowitz HM, Kupferman A, Stewart RH, et al. Evaluation of dexamethasone acetate as a topical ophthalmic formulation. *Am J Ophthalmol*. 1978;86(3):418–423.

64. Brubaker RF, Halpin JA. Open-angle glaucoma associated with topical administraion of flurandrenolide to the eye. *Mayo Clin Proc*. 1975;50(6):322–326.

65. Leibowitz HM, Ryan WJ Jr, Kupferman A. Comparative anti-inflammatory efficacy of topical corticosteroids with low glaucoma-inducing potential. *Arch Ophthalmol*. 1992;110(1):118–120.

66. Bedrossian RH, Eriksen SP. The treatment of ocular inflammation with medrysone. *Arch Ophthalmol*. 1969;81(2):184–191.

67. Green K, Cheeks L, Slagle T, et al. Interaction between progesterone and mifepristone on intraocular pressure in rabbits. *Curr Eye Res*. 1989;8(3):317–320.

68. Mindel JS, Tavitian HO, Smith H Jr, et al. Comparative ocular pressure elevation by medrysone, fluorometholone, and dexamethasone phosphate. *Arch Ophthalmol*. 1980;98(9):1577–1578.

69. Morrison E, Archer DB. Effect of fluorometholone (FML) on the intraocular pressure of corticosteroid responders. *Br J Ophthalmol*. 1984;68(8):581–584.

70. Kass M, Cheetham J, Duzman E, et al. The ocular hypertensive effect of 0.25% fluorometholone in corticosteroid responders. *Am J Ophthalmol*. 1986;102(2):159–163.

71. Wilhelmi E. Experimental and clinical investigation of a non-hormonal anti-inflammatory eye ointment. *Ophthalmic Res*. 1973;5(5):253–289.

72. Gieser DK, Hodapp E, Goldberg I, et al. Flurbiprofen and intraocular pressure. *Ann Ophthalmol*. 1981;13(7):831–833.

73. Strelow SA, Sherwood MB, Broncato LJ, et al. The effect of diclofenac sodium ophthalmic solution on intraocular pressure following cataract extraction. *Ophthalmic Surg*. 1992;23(3):170–175.

74. Espildora J, Vicuna P, Diaz E. Cortisone-induced glaucoma: a report on 44 affected eyes [in French]. *J Fr Ophthalmol*. 1981;4(6–7):503–508.

75. Ricci F, Missiroli F, Parravano M. Argon laser trabeculoplasty in triamcinolone acetonide induced ocular hypertension refractory to maximal medical treatment. *Eur J Ophthalmol*. 2006;16(5):756–757.

76. Rubin B, Taglienti A, Rothman RF, et al. The effect of selective laser trabeculoplasty on intraocular pressure in patients with intravitreal steroid-induced elevated intraocular pressure. *J Glaucoma*. 2008;17(4):287–292.

77. Robin AL, Suan EP, Sjaarda RN, et al. Reduction of intraocular pressure with anecortave acetate in eyes with ocular steroid injection-related glaucoma. *Arch Ophthalmol*. 2009;127(2):173–178.

78. Honjo M, Tanihara H, Inatani M, et al. External trabeculotomy for the treatment of steroid-induced glaucoma. *J Glaucoma*. 2000;9(6):483–485.

24

Glaucomas Associated with Intraocular Hemorrhage

Intraocular hemorrhage is most commonly caused by trauma or surgery. Hyphemas may occur spontaneously in association with several ocular disorders, most of which are discussed in other chapters. Whatever the initial cause, intraocular hemorrhage frequently leads to intraocular pressure (IOP) elevation when the aqueous outflow channels become obstructed by blood in various forms. In this chapter, we consider the mechanisms and management of the blood-induced glaucomas and some specific causes of intraocular hemorrhage that are not covered in other chapters.

GLAUCOMAS ASSOCIATED WITH HYPHEMA

Blunt Trauma

A common source of hyphema, or blood in the anterior chamber, is blunt trauma. This usually results from a tear in the iris or ciliary body, causing bleeding from the small branches of the major arterial circle.

General Features

Young age and male sex appear to be risk factors for blunt ocular trauma. In one large series, 77% of the patients with traumatic hyphemas were younger than 30 years of age (1). In another large study, the annual incidence of traumatic hyphema was significantly increased among men, and sports-related injuries were identified as a cause for a recent rise in the incidence rate (2).

The initial clinical finding may be a microscopic hyphema, which is characterized by red blood cells circulating in the aqueous. In other cases, the quantity of blood may be sufficient to create a layered hyphema. These range in size from a small layer of blood in the inferior quadrant of the anterior chamber, which is the more common situation, to a total hyphema, in which the entire anterior chamber is filled with blood (**Fig. 24.1**). In most cases, the blood clears within a few days, primarily through the trabecular meshwork, and the prognosis is good unless the associated trauma has caused other ocular injuries. However, complications may occur during the postinjury course that can have devastating results.

Complications

Recurrent Hemorrhage

The reported frequency with which eyes rebleed after traumatic hyphema ranges from 4% to 35%, with a rate of fewer than 10% in most reported series (2–28). Rebleeding usually occurs during the first week after the initial injury, which is probably related to the normal lysis and retraction of the clot. Studies vary considerably on risk factors for recurrent bleeding. Some investigators have found no identifiable factors (22,23); others have observed that an increased frequency is associated with the size of the initial hyphema, the degree of reduced visual acuity, and delayed medical attention (24). Use of aspirin can increase the frequency of rebleeding (9,14,29). Elevated IOP is a risk factor for recurrent hemorrhage, but hypotony may also increase the risk for rebleeding (3,5,24). Studies have also suggested that black race is another risk factor for recurrent hemorrhage (21,30).

Although studies may differ regarding the frequency of rebleeding and the risk factors by which this complication can be predicted, nearly all reported series agree that recurrent hemorrhage, as compared with the initial hyphema, is associated with significantly more complications and a more-frequent need for surgical intervention.

Associated Glaucoma

Although IOP elevation may occur after the initial bleed, it is more common after a recurrent hemorrhage and constitutes the most serious complication of a traumatic hyphema. The incidence of glaucoma associated with a traumatic hyphema is partially related to the size of the hemorrhage. In one study of 235 cases, glaucoma occurred in 13.5% of the eyes in which the hyphema filled less than one half of the anterior chamber, in 27% of those with a bleed involving more than one half of the chamber, and in 52% of the eyes with a total hyphema (17). In another study, in addition to hyphema, factors that predicted

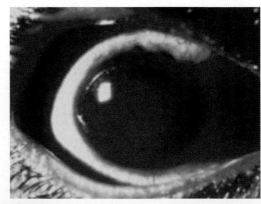

Figure 24.1 A total hyphema in an 11-year-old boy. Although initially normal, the IOP increased to 40 mm Hg within 24 hours. (From Crouch ER Jr, Crouch ER. Trauma: ruptures and bleeding. In: Tasman W, Jaeger EA, eds. *Duane's Clinical Ophthalmology.* Vol. 4. Lippincott Williams & Wilkins; 2009:chap 61.)

chronically elevated IOP after blunt trauma included increased angle pigmentation, a higher baseline IOP, angle recession, and lens displacement and cataract (31). It is important to distinguish between a total hyphema with bright red blood and an "eight-ball" hyphema, characterized by dark red-black blood, because the latter carries a worse prognosis relative to associated glaucoma (4). In one series of 113 cases, IOP was elevated in one third of those with a rebleed but in all cases with "eight-ball" hyphemas (4).

The mechanism of pressure elevation is related to obstruction of the trabecular meshwork in most cases of traumatic hyphema. Although fresh red blood cells are known to pass through the conventional aqueous outflow system with relative ease, it appears to be the overwhelming numbers of cells, combined with plasma, fibrin, and debris, that may lead to a transient obstruction of aqueous outflow (**Fig. 24.2**) (32). On the basis of the effect of melanin on traumatic hyphema in rabbits, one study suggested that in darker-pigmented individuals, release of melanin into the anterior chamber with trauma may prolong the course of hyphema and affect the rate of rebleeding (33). In cases of eight-ball hyphema, it is presumably the formation of a clot, occasionally with degenerated red blood cells from an associated vitreous hemorrhage, that further impedes the outflow.

Sickle cell hemoglobinopathies, including sickle cell trait, increase the incidence of IOP elevation in association with hyphema (34–36). Erythrocytes in these disorders have an increased tendency to sickle in the aqueous humor (34,35,37), and the elongated, rigid cells pass more slowly through the trabecular meshwork (38), leading to IOP elevation even with small amounts of intracameral blood (34,35). Even moderately elevated pressure may affect the optic nerve head more deleteriously in patients with sickle cell anemia than in other patients, possibly because of reduced vascular perfusion (34,35). Given that IOPs that would normally be considered safe to simply watch carefully (e.g., in the range of 20– to 30–mm Hg) can result in severe vision loss, such patients need to be observed

diligently and treated more aggressively to keep IOP in the normal range. Another mechanism of glaucoma associated with sickle cell hemoglobinopathies is obstruction to aqueous outflow due to sickled erythrocytes in the Schlemm canal, which has been observed after blunt trauma and in one case with no antecedent trauma (36).

Diabetes mellitus may be associated with delayed clearing of blood from the anterior chamber. Erythrocytes from patients with diabetes have decreased deformability and increased adherence, resulting in delayed clearance time from the rabbit anterior chamber, compared with red blood cells from healthy human participants (39).

Corneal Bloodstaining

Corneal bloodstaining typically results from a prolonged total hyphema that is usually but not always associated with elevated IOP (40). This complication occurred in 6 of 289 patients (2%) with traumatic hyphema, all of whom had a recurrent total hyphema (38). The earliest pathologic event may be corneal endothelial decompensation associated with the passage of hemoglobin and hemoglobin products into the stroma (41). The cornea may initially have a red discoloration, which in rabbit studies is associated with extracellular hemoglobin particles and oxyhemoglobin (41). The hemoglobin is apparently phagocytized by keratocytes and degraded to hemosiderin (41,42). The cornea takes on a brownish discoloration at this stage, which is associated with methemoglobin in the stroma (41). Clearing of the corneal bloodstaining begins in the peripheral and posterior stroma, apparently because of diffusion of hemoglobin breakdown products out of the cornea, and may take up to 3 years to clear completely (42,43).

Management
Conservative Management of Hyphema

There is general agreement that the uncomplicated hyphema should be managed nonsurgically with the aims of accelerating resorption of the hyphema and minimizing rebleeding. Historically, bed rest and patching were advised for patients with hyphemas. However, little evidence supports these adjuncts to treatment. In most cases, all that is needed is limiting the patient's ambulation, avoiding use of aspirin and nonsteroidal anti-inflammatory agents, and using a shield simply to protect the injured eye. Hospitalization is rarely necessary unless the hyphema is large, there is associated ocular trauma, sickle cell disease or trait is present, or the patient cannot be relied on to maintain limited activity or to return for recommended follow-up visits.

Acceleration of Hyphema Clearance

Various drugs have been used by some physicians to accelerate resorption of the hyphema, but no agent has proven to be efficacious for safely accelerating hyphema resorption. Rabbit studies have not supported the efficacy of atropine, pilocarpine, or acetazolamide use for this purpose (44–46), although the use of hyperosmotic agents may accelerate resorption of a clotted hyphema (47). Intracameral tissue plasminogen activator,

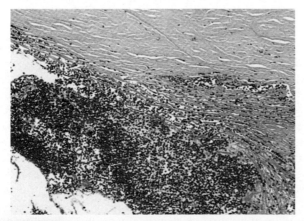

Figure 24.2 Red blood cells and their products of degeneration obstruct the trabecular meshwork in hyphema (hematoxylin–eosin, ×40). (From Callahan CE, Sassani JW. Pathology of glaucoma. In: Tasman W, Jaeger EA, eds. *Duane's Foundations of Clinical Ophthalmology.* Vol. 3. Lippincott Williams & Wilkins; 2008: chap 19.)

a clot-specific fibrinolytic agent, has been shown to accelerate the clearance of experimental hyphema in rabbits, although it may also increase the risk of rebleeding (47–49).

Prevention of Rebleeding

Numerous drugs have also been evaluated regarding their ability to prevent rebleeding, with reported results that have been conflicting. Some investigators found that use of oral prednisone significantly reduced the rebleeding rate (8), whereas others found neither steroids nor estrogen to be of value in this regard (4,15). Antifibrinolytic agents (including tranexamic acid and aminocaproic acid (11–13,21,26–28)) have been used in an effort to minimize rebleeding by delaying the natural lysis of the clot. Most reports indicate that the use of either drug is associated with a significant reduction in rebleeds (11,13,26,28). Tranexamic acid has been evaluated in several series of traumatic hyphemas in children (28,50,51). In a study of hospitalized children, the rebleeding rate was 3% with use of tranexamic acid (25 mg/kg every 8 hours for 5 days), compared with 8% without use of antifibrinolytic therapy (28). One group of children with small hyphemas treated with systemic tranexamic acid therapy and limited activity at home had no recurrent hemorrhage (51). A randomized, placebo-controlled trial of 238 patients found tranexamic acid to be more effective than oral prednisolone or no treatment in preventing rebleeding (rebleed rates, 10%, 18%, and 26%, respectively) (52).

Some studies have found no significant difference between tranexamic or aminocaproic acid and placebo therapy (12,53). Aminocaproic acid is typically given as 100 mg/kg every 4 hours, up to a maximum of 30 g daily for 5 days, which is associated with frequent side effects, including lightheadedness, nausea, vomiting, and systemic hypotension. A half dose of 50 mg/kg reduced the incidence of dizziness and hypotension without adversely affecting the reduced rate of recurrent hemorrhage, but it did not lower the incidence of nausea and vomiting (54). In a randomized comparison of aminocaproic acid (50 mg/kg every 4 hours for 5 days) with oral prednisone (40 mg daily), the rebleed rate was 7.1% in each group (27). Another reported complication is elevated IOP associated with the accelerated clot dissolution (55). Use of topical aminocaproic acid has been found to be a safe and effective alternative to systemic administration to prevent secondary hemorrhage. The use of the topical formulation (30% aminocaproic acid in 2% carboxypolymethylene gel) was associated with no systemic side effects (56).

The influence of hydrostatic pressure on the damaged vessels has also been studied, and one report described fewer rebleeds with medical reduction of systemic blood pressure and elevation of the head of the bed (57). The use of aspirin may increase the chances of recurrent hemorrhage (9,14), and therefore, any drug that may increase the risk of bleeding should be avoided for the first week after the trauma or until the hyphema has cleared completely.

Management of Associated IOP Elevation

Medical treatment of elevated IOP is occasionally needed to protect the optic nerve head and enhance the resorption of the hyphema. IOP reduction is best accomplished with use of an aqueous suppressant, such as a topical β-blocker or carbonic anhydrase inhibitor. However, caution should be exercised with the use of carbonic anhydrase inhibitors in patients with sickle cell hemoglobinopathies, because use of these agents increases the concentration of ascorbic acid in the aqueous humor, leading to more sickling in the anterior chamber (58). In the management of patients with sickle cell trait, control of the IOP during the first 24 hours was associated with a good prognosis, and lack of control in that period was associated with continued difficulty in managing the pressure (59). Hyperbaric oxygen therapy can significantly reduce the percentage of sickled cells injected intracamerally in rabbits by raising the aqueous PO_2, which may be of value in patients with sickle cell hyphema (60). In one study, using transcorneal oxygen therapy (humidified oxygen 1 to 3 L/min) dramatically reduced the IOP in patients with glaucoma due to sickle cell hyphema (61).

Surgical intervention becomes necessary when a sustained IOP elevation cannot be controlled medically and threatens to damage the optic nerve or is associated with corneal blood-staining. The critical pressure level depends on the status of the optic nerve head (if this is known): Healthy discs usually tolerate pressures of 40 to 50 mm Hg for 5 or 6 days, but an optic nerve head with preexisting glaucomatous optic atrophy may experience further damage at pressures less than 30 mm Hg within 24 to 48 hours. A total hyphema for more than 4 days is an additional indication for surgical intervention. Special attention must be given to patients with sickle cell anemia or trait because their optic nerve heads are especially vulnerable to damage at minimal to moderate elevations in IOP. A pressure in the mid-20s (mm Hg) for more than 1 day may be an indication to surgically intervene in these patients (59).

The surgical approach most often used is evacuation of the hyphema, which usually includes clotted blood, from the anterior chamber. It is also possible to remove the liquefied portion of the hyphema by gently irrigating the anterior chamber through a paracentesis wound and allowing the residual clot to resorb (62). This technique is of particular value when a sudden increase in pressure requires emergency measures to avoid irreversible loss of vision, as may occur with sickle cell disease (63). A corneal transfixing needle has been developed for simultaneously irrigating the anterior chamber and evacuating a fluid hyphema (64).

Many surgeons prefer to also remove the clot, and fibrinolytic agents such as urokinase and fibrinolysin have been used to facilitate clot lysis and irrigation (65,66). Other reported surgical techniques to remove the clot include cryoextraction, ultrasonic emulsification and extraction, and removal with vitrectomy instruments (67–70). Viscoelastic agents, such as sodium hyaluronate, have also been used to mechanically dissect a clot from the iris and express it through a corneoscleral incision (71,72). The fourth day after injury is said to be the optimum time for removal of the clot because it has usually retracted from the adjacent structures by then (73,74).

Other surgeons have advocated a trabeculectomy and iridectomy combined with gentle irrigation of the anterior chamber (75,76). During any surgical attempt to evacuate the hyphema, the iris may prolapse into the incision because of a pupillary block, necessitating an iridectomy (77). Complete resorption of the hyphema may follow iridectomy alone (78). When recurrent bleeding occurs during clot extraction, raising the IOP to 50 mm Hg for 5 minutes has been used to stop the bleeding (70).

Penetrating Injuries

Intraocular hemorrhage is also frequently associated with penetrating injuries, although associated glaucoma is less common than with blunt trauma in the early postinjury period because of the open wound. However, IOP elevation may follow closure of the wound, especially if meticulous care is not given to reconstruction of the anterior chamber and treatment of the associated inflammation in the early postoperative period (79).

Hyphemas Associated with Intraocular Surgery

Bleeding in the eye can be a serious complication of any intraocular procedure and may occur during the operation or in the early or even late postoperative period.

During Surgery

As an intraoperative complication, bleeding is usually associated with damage to the ciliary body, as can occur when a filtering procedure or iridectomy is performed. Intraoperative bleeding can usually be controlled by placing a large air bubble or viscoelastic agent in the anterior chamber for a few minutes, which raises the IOP and acts as a tamponade. Applying direct, gentle pressure with the tip of a sponge or Gel-Foam, or applying epinephrine (1:1000), to the ciliary body for 1 to 2 minutes can also help stop ciliary body bleeding. Cautery is generally avoided in these cases, although use of an intraocular, bipolar unit may be effective.

After Surgery

Bleeding in the early postoperative period is usually not associated with serious sequelae and should be managed conservatively with limited activity and elevation of the head. Small hyphemas after intraocular surgery normally clear rapidly, although the time may be considerably longer in eyes with preexisting glaucoma because of delayed passage of red blood cells through the trabecular meshwork. When a postoperative hyphema is associated with elevated IOP or excessive fibrin, conservative medical management should be instituted as required, by using drugs that lower aqueous production or hyperosmotics if necessary. Frequent topical steroid use can assist in clearing fibrin, and if this is unsuccessful, then intracameral use of tissue plasminogen activator (6.25 μg or 12.5 μg) can be helpful (80). Surgical intervention is reserved for critical cases, although the indications may be somewhat more liberal than with a traumatic hyphema if there is danger of rupturing a corneoscleral wound or causing further atrophy to an optic nerve that has previously been damaged by glaucoma.

Hemorrhage in the late postoperative period may result from the reopening of a uveal wound or from disruption of new vessels growing across a corneoscleral incision (81). In a study of 58 eyes 5 to 10 years after cataract extraction, 12% had vessels in the inner aspects of the incision site and nearly one half of these had evidence of mild intraocular hemorrhage (82). Direct argon laser therapy may be used to treat such vessels when they can be visualized gonioscopically (81), and use of transscleral Nd:YAG laser or diode photocoagulation may be effective if direct argon laser therapy is unsuccessful (83). Fortunately, postoperative hyphema is far less common because of the introduction of small incision and clear cornea cataract surgery.

Spontaneous Hyphemas

Hyphemas may also develop spontaneously in various conditions, most of which are considered in other chapters. In some cases, the hyphema may cause or contribute to an increase in the IOP.

Intraocular Tumors

A spontaneous hyphema may occur in a child with juvenile xanthogranuloma or retinoblastoma, and intraocular hemorrhage may be a manifestation of an ocular malignant melanoma or other intraocular neoplasm (see Chapter 21).

Neovascularization

New blood vessels in the anterior ocular segment, which may lead to a spontaneous hyphema, are seen in neovascular glaucoma (discussed in Chapter 19), Fuchs heterochromic cyclitis (Chapter 22), and other chronic uveitides.

Vascular Tufts at the Pupillary Margin

Vascular tufts at the pupillary margin, also called neovascular tufts or iris microhemangiomas, represent yet another source of spontaneous hyphema. Slitlamp biomicroscopy may reveal multiple vascular tufts along the pupillary margin, and fluorescein angiography of the iris has revealed small areas of staining and leakage from the lesions (84). One histopathologic study revealed thin-walled new vessels at the pupillary margin of the iris with a mild inflammatory cell infiltration (85), and another report described the vascular abnormality as a hamartoma of the capillary hemangioma type (86). Although more common in older adults, this condition occurs in adults of all ages. Most patients have no systemic disease, although associations with diabetes mellitus and myotonic dystrophy have been reported (84,87,88). Spontaneous hyphemas occur in a few of these cases, occasionally causing transient IOP elevation (89,90). Laser photocoagulation has been reported to successfully eradicate bleeding vascular tufts (85,91). However, because having recurrent hyphemas or permanent damage related to the transiently elevated IOP is rare, it is best to withhold treatment until one or more recurrences of bleeding are documented.

Dilatation and Posterior Synechiae

Spontaneous hyphemas may result in individuals with posterior synechiae in whom dilation drops are used. As the iris pulls away from the synechiae, hemorrhage may occur (**Fig. 24.3**).

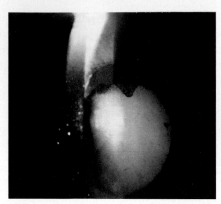

Figure 24.3 Spontaneous hyphema in a patient with posterior synechiae whose eye has been dilated. Note the hemorrhage at the 12-o'clock position of the pupil.

GLAUCOMAS ASSOCIATED WITH DEGENERATED OCULAR BLOOD

Ghost Cell Glaucoma

In 1976, Campbell and coworkers (92) described a form of glaucoma in which degenerated red blood cells (ghost cells) develop in the vitreous cavity and subsequently enter the anterior chamber, where they temporarily obstruct aqueous outflow.

Theories of Mechanism

Having entered the vitreous cavity by one of several mechanisms (trauma, surgery, or retinal disease), fresh erythrocytes are transformed from their typical biconcave, pliable nature to tan- or khaki-colored, spherical, less-pliable structures, referred to as ghost cells (92). Histologically, these cells have thin walls and appear hollow except for clumps of denatured hemoglobin, called Heinz bodies. Unlike fresh red blood cells, ghost cells do not pass readily through a 5-μm Millipore filter or human trabecular meshwork. The ghost cells develop within 7 to 10 days and may remain in the vitreous cavity for many months, until a disruption of the anterior hyaloid allows them to enter the anterior chamber. Once in the anterior chamber, the abnormal cells accumulate in the trabecular meshwork, where they may cause a temporary, but occasionally marked, elevation of IOP.

Specific Causes

Several situations can lead to ghost cell glaucoma.

Cataract Extraction

Cataract extraction may be associated with glaucoma due to ghost cells in one of three ways (93). First, a large hyphema with vitreous hemorrhage occurs in the early postoperative period. As the hyphema clears, ghost cells, which developed in the vitreous, come forward and obstruct aqueous outflow. Second, a vitreous hemorrhage is present before cataract surgery, and disruption of the anterior hyaloid due to the operation allows the ghost cells to enter the anterior chamber. Third, a vitreous hemorrhage develops at some point after cataract extraction because of retinal disease, and the ghost cells develop and come

forward through previously made defects in the anterior hyaloid. Ghost cell glaucoma has also been associated with intraocular lens implantation, especially when anterior chamber or iris-fixation lenses were used (94).

Vitrectomy

Vitrectomy may lead to ghost cell glaucoma in eyes with preexisting vitreous hemorrhage if the anterior hyaloid is disrupted and the vitreous and cells are not completely removed (95).

Vitreous Hemorrhage without Surgery

Vitreous hemorrhage without surgery may also lead to ghost cell glaucoma. The vitreous hemorrhage may be caused by trauma or associated with a retinal disorder, such as diabetic retinopathy (96,97). Bilateral vitreous hemorrhage and ghost cell glaucoma may occur after poisonous snakebites, especially those from crotalids, because proteolytic enzymes can disrupt vascular integrity and act as hemorrhagic factors (98). The traumatic cases may have associated hyphema, which may clear before the ghost cell glaucoma develops or may persist and mask the actual mechanism of the glaucoma. The route of ghost cells to the anterior chamber in these phakic eyes is presumed to be a defect in the anterior hyaloid face (96,97).

Clinical Features

Depending on the number of ghost cells in the anterior chamber, the IOP ranges from normal to marked elevation with pain and corneal edema (92). Slitlamp biomicroscopy reveals characteristic khaki-colored cells in the aqueous and on the corneal endothelium (**Fig. 24.4A,B**). If present in large quantities, the ghost cells may layer out inferiorly, creating a pseudohypopyon, which is occasionally associated with a layer of fresher red blood cells (known as a "candy-stripe sign") (**Fig. 24.4C,D**). On gonioscopy, the anterior chamber angle is typically open and may appear normal, or may be covered by scant to heavy amounts of khaki-colored cells.

Differential Diagnosis

Glaucoma due to ghost cells may be confused with the less common hemolytic and hemosiderotic glaucomas. Neovascular glaucoma and glaucoma due to inflammation must be ruled out. Although the diagnosis is usually made easily on the basis of history and clinical features, it may be confirmed by examination of an aqueous aspirate, which reveals the typical ghost cells. This examination may be performed with phase contrast microscopy or by routine light microscopy of a paraffin-embedded specimen stained with hematoxylin and eosin (92,99).

Management

Glaucoma due to ghost cells is not a permanent condition, but it may last for months before the abnormal cells eventually clear from the anterior chamber angle. In the interim, the IOP can often be controlled with the use of standard antiglaucoma medications. Some cases, however, require surgical intervention, which usually involves removal of the ghost cells from the anterior chamber by irrigation or removal of all ocular ghost cells by vitrectomy (92,100). After ghost cells are surgically removed,

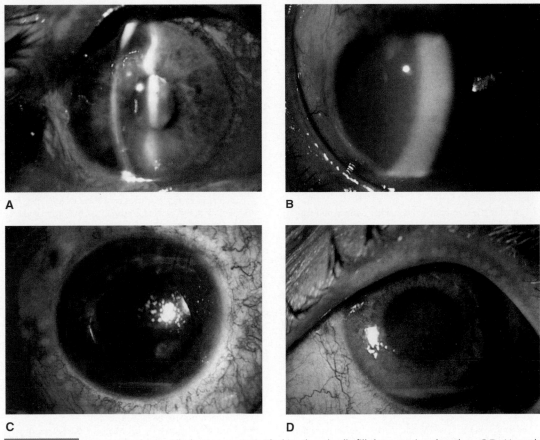

Figure 24.4 Eyes with ghost cell glaucoma. **A,B:** Khaki-colored cells fill the anterior chamber. **C,D:** Note the layering of ghost cells inferiorly, creating a pseudohypopyon. The eye in D shows a classic "candy-stripe sign."

the IOP promptly returns to normal in most cases in the absence of preexisting glaucoma.

Hemolytic Glaucoma

Fenton and Zimmerman (101) described a form of glaucoma associated with intraocular hemorrhage in which macrophages ingest contents of the red blood cells and then accumulate in the trabecular meshwork, where they temporarily obstruct aqueous outflow. Clinically, numerous red-tinted cells are seen floating in the aqueous, and the anterior chamber angle is typically open, with reddish-brown pigment covering the trabecular meshwork (102). Cytologic examination of the aqueous reveals macrophages containing golden-brown pigment (102). An ultrastructural study of seven eyes revealed red blood cells and macrophages with phagocytized blood and pigment in the trabecular spaces; the endothelial cells of the trabecular meshwork were degenerated and had phagocytized blood (103). The condition is self-limiting and should be managed medically, if possible. When surgical intervention is required, anterior chamber lavage has been recommended (102).

Hemosiderotic Glaucoma

Hemoglobin from lysed red blood cells in the anterior chamber is phagocytized by endothelial cells of the trabecular meshwork in this rare condition. Iron in the hemoglobin subsequently causes siderosis, which is believed to produce tissue alterations in the trabecular meshwork, eventually resulting in obstruction to aqueous outflow (104). However, an association between iron staining of the trabecular meshwork and impairment of aqueous outflow has yet to be clearly established.

KEY POINTS

- Red blood cells in a fresh or degenerated form in the anterior chamber may lead to elevated IOP by obstructing aqueous outflow through the trabecular meshwork.
- The most common cause of a new hyphema is blunt trauma. Glaucoma may result from the initial hemorrhage, but more often from a rebleed, and initial therapy is directed toward accelerating resorption of the hyphema and minimizing rebleeding.
- When glaucoma occurs, medical management may control the IOP until the hyphema clears, although some cases require surgical intervention, which includes removal of the blood. Hyphema in the setting of sickle cell hemoglobinopathies requires aggressive management, as even moderately elevated IOP can produce rapid damage to the optic nerve.
- Other causes of new hyphemas include spontaneous bleeding from tumors; neovascularization; or, rarely, vascular tufts at the pupillary margin.

- The most common form of glaucoma associated with degenerated ocular blood is ghost cell glaucoma, in which degenerating erythrocytes obstruct aqueous outflow. This may follow cataract extraction, vitrectomy, or trauma.
- Other situations in which degenerated blood may lead to glaucoma include hemolytic glaucoma and hemosiderotic glaucoma.

REFERENCES

1. Pilger IS. Medical treatment of traumatic hyphema. *Surv Ophthalmol.* 1975;20:28–34.
2. Kennedy RH, Brubaker RF. Traumatic hyphema in a defined population. *Am J Ophthalmol.* 1988;106:123–130.
3. Howard GM, Hutchinson BT, Frederick AR Jr. Hyphema resulting from blunt trauma: gonioscopic, tonographic, and ophthalmoscopic observations following resolution of the hemorrhage. *Trans Am Acad Ophthalmol Otolaryngol.* 1965;69:294–305.
4. Spaeth GL, Levy PM. Traumatic hyphema: its clinical characteristics and failure of estrogens to alter its course—a double-blind study. *Am J Ophthalmol.* 1966;62:1098–1106.
5. Milstein BA. Traumatic hyphema: a study of 83 consecutive cases. *South Med J.* 1971;64:1081–1085.
6. Giles CL, Bromley WG. Traumatic hyphema: a retrospective analysis from the University of Michigan Teaching Hospitals. *J Pediatr Ophthalmol.* 1972;9:90.
7. Edwards WC, Layden WE. Traumatic hyphema: a report of 184 consecutive cases. *Am J Ophthalmol.* 1973;75:110–116.
8. Yasuna E. Management of traumatic hyphema. *Arch Ophthalmol.* 1974;91:190–191.
9. Crawford JS, Lewandowski RL, Chan W. The effect of aspirin on rebleeding in traumatic hyphema. *Am J Ophthalmol.* 1975;80:543–545.
10. Fritch CD. Traumatic hyphema. *Ann Ophthalmol.* 1976;8:1223–1225.
11. Crouch ER Jr, Frenkel M. Aminocaproic acid in the treatment of traumatic hyphema. *Am J Ophthalmol.* 1976;81:355–360.
12. Mortensen KK, Sjølie AK. Secondary hemorrhage following traumatic hyphaema: a comparative study of conservative and tranexamic acid treatment. *Acta Ophthalmol.* 1978;56:763–768.
13. Bramsen T. Fibrinolysis and traumatic hyphaema. *Acta Ophthalmol.* 1979;57:447–454.
14. Gorn RA. The detrimental effect of aspirin on hyphema rebleed. *Ann Ophthalmol.* 1979;11:351–355.
15. Spoor TC, Hammer M, Belloso H. Traumatic hyphema: failure of steroids to alter its course—a double-blind prospective study. *Arch Ophthalmol.* 1980;98:116–119.
16. Rakusin W. Traumatic hyphema. *Am J Ophthalmol.* 1972;74:284–292.
17. Coles WH. Traumatic hyphema: an analysis of 235 cases. *South Med J.* 1968;61:813–816.
18. Cassel GH, Jeffers JB, Jaeger EA. Wills Eye Hospital traumatic hyphema study. *Ophthalmic Surg.* 1985;16:441–443.
19. Thomas MA, Parrish RK II, Feuer WJ. Rebleeding after traumatic hyphema. *Arch Ophthalmol.* 1986;104:206–210.
20. Agapitos PJ, Noel LP, Clarke WN. Traumatic hyphema in children. *Ophthalmology.* 1987;94:1238–1241.
21. Spoor TC, Kwitko GM, O'Grady JM, et al. Traumatic hyphema in an urban population. *Am J Ophthalmol.* 1990;109:23–27.
22. Kearns P. Traumatic hyphaema: a retrospective study of 314 cases. *Br J Ophthalmol.* 1991;75:137–141.
23. Ng CS, Strong NP, Sparrow JM, et al. Factors related to the incidence of secondary haemorrhage in 462 patients with traumatic hyphema. *Eye (Lond).* 1992;6(pt 3):308–312.
24. Fong LP. Secondary hemorrhage in traumatic hyphema. *Ophthalmology.* 1994;101:1583–1588.
25. Volpe NJ, Larrison WI, Hersh PS, et al. Secondary hemorrhage in traumatic hyphema. *Am J Ophthalmol.* 1991;112:507–513.
26. Wilson TW, Jeffers JB, Nelson LB. Aminocaproic acid prophylaxis in traumatic hyphema. *Ophthalmic Surg.* 1990;21:807–809.
27. Farber MD, Fiscella R, Goldberg MF. Aminocaproic acid versus prednisone for the treatment of traumatic hyphema: a randomized clinical trial. *Ophthalmology.* 1991;98:279–286.
28. Deans R, Noël LP, Clarke WN. Oral administration of tranexamic acid in the management of traumatic hyphema in children. *Can J Ophthalmol.* 1992;27:181–183.
29. Ganley JP, Geiger JM, Clement JR, et al. Aspirin and recurrent hyphema after blunt ocular trauma. *Am J Ophthalmol.* 1983;96:797–801.
30. Lai JC, Fekrat S, Barron Y, et al. Traumatic hyphema in children: risk factors for complications. *Arch Ophthalmol.* 2001;119:64–70.
31. Sihota R, Kumar S, Gupta V, et al. Early predictors of traumatic glaucoma after closed globe injury trabecular pigmentation, widened angle recess, and higher baseline intraocular pressure. *Arch Ophthalmol.* 2008;126:921–926.
32. Sternberg P Jr, Tripathi RC, Tripathi BJ, et al. Changes in outflow facility in experimental hyphema. *Invest Ophthalmol Vis Sci.* 1980;19:1388–1390.
33. Lai WW, Bhavnani VD, Tessler HH, et al. Effect of melanin on traumatic hyphema in rabbits. *Arch Ophthalmol.* 1999;117:789–793.
34. Goldberg MF. The diagnosis and treatment of secondary glaucoma after hyphema in sickle cell patients. *Am J Ophthalmol.* 1979;87:43–49.
35. Goldberg MF. Sickled erythrocytes, hyphema, and secondary glaucoma. I. The diagnosis and treatment of sickled erythrocytes in human hyphemas. *Ophthalmic Surg.* 1979;10:17–31.
36. Friedman AH, Halpern BL, Friedberg DN, et al. Transient open-angle glaucoma associated with sickle cell trait: report of 4 cases. *Br J Ophthalmol.* 1979;63:832–836.
37. Goldberg MF. Sickled erythrocytes, hyphema, and secondary glaucoma. IV. The rate and percentage of sickling of erythrocytes in rabbit aqueous humor, in vitro and in vivo. *Ophthalmic Surg.* 1979;10:62–69.
38. Goldberg MF, Tso MO. Sickled erythrocytes, hyphema, and secondary glaucoma. VII. The passage of sickled erythrocytes out of the anterior chamber of the human and monkey eye: light and electron microscopic studies. *Ophthalmic Surg.* 1979;10:89–123.
39. Williams GA, Hatchell DL, Collier BD, et al. Clearance from the anterior chamber of RBCs from human diabetics. *Arch Ophthalmol.* 1984;102:930–931.
40. Beyer TL, Hirst LW. Corneal blood staining at low pressures. *Arch Ophthalmol.* 1985;103:654–655.
41. Gottsch JD, Messmer EP, McNair DS, et al. Corneal blood staining: an animal model. *Ophthalmology.* 1986;93:797–802.
42. McDonnell PJ, Green WR, Stevens RE, et al. Blood staining of the cornea: light microscopic and ultrastructural features. *Ophthalmology.* 1985;92:1668–1674.
43. Brodrick JD. Corneal blood staining after hyphaema. *Br J Ophthalmol.* 1972;56:589–593.
44. Rose SW, Coupal JJ, Simmons G, et al. Experimental hyphema clearance in rabbits: drug trials with 1% atropine and 2% and 4% pilocarpine. *Arch Ophthalmol.* 1977;95:1442–1444.
45. Masket S, Best M. Therapy in experimental hyphema. II. Acetazolamide. *Arch Ophthalmol.* 1972;87:222–224.
46. Masket S, Best M, Fisher LV, et al. Therapy in experimental hyphema. *Arch Ophthalmol.* 1971;85:329–333.
47. Lambrou FH, Snyder RW, Williams GA. Use of tissue plasminogen activator in experimental hyphema. *Arch Ophthalmol.* 1987;105:995–997.
48. Howard GR, Vukich J, Fiscella RG, et al. Intraocular tissue plasminogen activator in a rabbit model of traumatic hyphema. *Arch Ophthalmol.* 1991;109:272–274.
49. Williams DF, Han DP, Abrams GW. Rebleeding in experimental traumatic hyphema treated with intraocular tissue plasminogen activator. *Arch Ophthalmol.* 1990;108:264–266.
50. Uusitalo RJ, Ranta-Kemppainen L, Tarkkanen A. Management of traumatic hyphema in children: an analysis of 340 cases. *Arch Ophthalmol.* 1988;106:1207–1209.
51. Clarke WN, Noël LP. Outpatient treatment of microscopic and rim hyphemas in children with tranexamic acid. *Can J Ophthalmol.* 1993;28:325–327.
52. Rahmani B, Jahadi HR. Comparison of tranexamic acid and prednisolone in the treatment of traumatic hyphema. *Ophthalmology.* 1999;106:375–379.
53. Kraft SP, Christianson MD, Crawford JS, et al. Traumatic hyphema in children: treatment with epsilon-aminocaproic acid. *Ophthalmology.* 1987;94:1232–1237.
54. Palmer DJ, Goldberg MF, Frenkel M, et al. A comparison of two dose regimens of epsilon aminocaproic acid in the prevention and management of secondary traumatic hyphemas. *Ophthalmology.* 1986;93:102–108.
55. Dieste MC, Hersh PS, Kylstra JA, et al. Intraocular pressure increase associated with epsilon-aminocaproic acid therapy for traumatic hyphema. *Am J Ophthalmol.* 1988;106:383–390.

56. Crouch ER Jr, Williams PB, Gray MK, et al. Topical aminocaproic acid in the treatment of traumatic hyphema. *Arch Ophthalmol.* 1997;115: 1106–1112.

57. Macdougald TJ. The treatment of traumatic hyphaema. *Trans Ophthalmol Soc U K.* 1972;92:815–817.

58. Goldberg MF. Sickled erythrocytes, hyphema, and secondary glaucoma. V. The effect of vitamin C on erythrocyte sickling in aqueous humor. *Ophthalmic Surg.* 1979;10:70–77.

59. Deutsch TA, Weinreb RN, Goldberg MF. Indications for surgical management of hyphema in patients with sickle cell trait. *Arch Ophthalmol.* 1984;102:566–569.

60. Wallyn CR, Jampol LM, Goldberg MF, et al. The use of hyperbaric oxygen therapy in the treatment of sickle cell hyphema. *Invest Ophthalmol Vis Sci.* 1985;26:1155–1158.

61. Benner JD. Transcorneal oxygen therapy for glaucoma associated with sickle cell hyphema. *Am J Ophthalmol.* 2000;130:514–515.

62. Belcher CD III, Brown SV, Simmons RJ. Anterior chamber washout for traumatic hyphema. *Ophthalmic Surg.* 1985;16:475–479.

63. Wax MB, Ridley ME, Magargal LE. Reversal of retinal and optic disc ischemia in a patient with sickle cell trait and glaucoma secondary to traumatic hyphema. *Ophthalmology.* 1982;89:845–851.

64. Tripathi RC. A corneal transfixing irrigation/perfusion device: a new method for evacuation of hyphema. *Ophthalmic Surg.* 1980;11:569–571.

65. Rakusin W. The role of urokinase in the management of traumatic hyphaema. *Ophthalmologica.* 1973;167:373–382.

66. Oosterhuis JA. Fibrinolysin irrigation in traumatic secondary hyphema. *Ophthalmologica.* 1968;155:357–378.

67. Hill K. Cryoextraction of total hyphema. *Arch Ophthalmol.* 1968;80: 368–370.

68. Kelman CD, Brooks DL. Ultrasonic emulsification and aspiration of traumatic hyphema: a preliminary report. *Am J Ophthalmol.* 1971;71: 1289–1291.

69. McCuen BW, Fung WE. The role of vitrectomy instrumentation in the treatment of severe traumatic hyphema. *Am J Ophthalmol.* 1979;88:930–934.

70. Stern WH, Mondal KM. Vitrectomy instrumentation for surgical evacuation of total anterior chamber hyphema and control of recurrent anterior chamber hemorrhage. *Ophthalmic Surg.* 1979;10:34–37.

71. Sholiton DB, Solomon OD. Surgical management of black ball hyphema with sodium hyaluronate. *Ophthalmic Surg.* 1981;12:820–822.

72. Bartholomew RS. Viscoelastic evacuation of traumatic hyphaema. *Br J Ophthalmol.* 1987;71:27–28.

73. Sears ML. Surgical management of black ball hyphema. *Trans Am Acad Ophthalmol Otolaryngol.* 1970;74:820–825.

74. Wolter JR, Henderson JW, Talley TW. Histopathology of a black ball blood clot removed four days after total traumatic hyphema. *J Pediatr Ophthalmol.* 1971;8:15.

75. Weiss JS, Parrish RK, Anderson DR. Surgical therapy of traumatic hyphema. *Ophthalmic Surg.* 1983;14:343–345.

76. Graul TA, Ruttum MS, Lloyd MA, et al. Trabeculectomy for traumatic hyphema with increased intraocular pressure. *Am J Ophthalmol.* 1994;117:155–159.

77. Heinze J. The surgical management of total hyphaema. *Aust J Ophthalmol.* 1975;3:20.

78. Parrish R, Bernardino V Jr. Iridectomy in the surgical management of eight-ball hyphema. *Arch Ophthalmol.* 1982;100:435–437.

79. Richardson K. Acute glaucoma after trauma. In: Freeman H, Mac K, eds. *Ocular Trauma.* New York, NY: Appleton-Century-Croft; 1979:161–166.

80. Damji KF, O'Connor M, Hill V. Tissue plasminogen activator for treatment of fibrin in endophthalmitis. *Can J Ophthalmol.* 2001;36:269–271.

81. Bene C, Hutchins R, Kranias G. Cataract wound neovascularization: an often overlooked cause of vitreous hemorrhage. *Ophthalmology.* 1989; 96:50–53.

82. Watzke RC. Intraocular hemorrhage from vascularization of the cataract incision. *Ophthalmology.* 1980;87:19–23.

83. Kramer TR, Brown RH, Lynch MG, et al. Transscleral Nd:YAG photocoagulation for cataract incision vascularization associated with recurrent hyphema. *Am J Ophthalmol.* 1989;107:681–682.

84. Cobb B. Vascular tufts at the pupillary margin: a preliminary report on 44 patients. *Trans Ophthalmol Soc U K.* 1968;88:211–221.

85. Coleman SL, Green WR, Patz A. Vascular tufts of pupillary margin of iris. *Am J Ophthalmol.* 1977;83:881–883.

86. Meades KV, Francis IC, Kappagoda MB, et al. Light microscopic and electron microscopic histopathology of an iris microhaemangioma. *Br J Ophthalmol.* 1986;70:290–294.

87. Mason GI. Iris neovascular tufts: relationship to rubeosis, insulin, and hypotony. *Arch Ophthalmol.* 1979;97:2346–2352.

88. Cobb B, Shilling JS, Chisholm IH. Vascular tufts at the pupillary margin in myotonic dystrophy. *Am J Ophthalmol.* 1970;69:573–582.

89. Perry HD, Mallen FJ, Sussman W. Microhaemangiomas of the iris with spontaneous hyphaema and acute glaucoma. *Br J Ophthalmol.* 1977; 61:114–116.

90. Mason GI, Ferry AP. Bilateral spontaneous hyphema arising from iridic microhemangiomas. *Ann Ophthalmol.* 1979;11:87–91.

91. Hagen AP, Williams GA. Argon laser treatment of a bleeding iris vascular tuft. *Am J Ophthalmol.* 1986;101:379–380.

92. Campbell DG, Simmons RJ, Grant WM. Ghost cells as a cause of glaucoma. *Am J Ophthalmol.* 1976;81:441–450.

93. Campbell DG, Essigmann EM. Hemolytic ghost cell glaucoma: further studies. *Arch Ophthalmol.* 1979;97:2141–2146.

94. Summers CG, Lindstrom RL. Ghost cell glaucoma following lens implantation. *J Am Intraocul Implant Soc.* 1983;9:429–433.

95. Campbell DG, Simmons RJ, Tolentino FI, et al. Glaucoma occurring after closed vitrectomy. *Am J Ophthalmol.* 1977;83:63–69.

96. Brooks AM, Gillies WE. Haemolytic glaucoma occurring in phakic eyes. *Br J Ophthalmol.* 1986;70:603–606.

97. Mansour AM, Chess J, Starita R. Nontraumatic ghost cell glaucoma—a case report. *Ophthalmic Surg.* 1986;17:34–36.

98. Rojas L, Ortiz G, Gutierrez M, et al. Ghost cell glaucoma related to snake poisoning. *Arch Ophthalmol.* 2001;119:1212–1213.

99. Cameron JD, Havener VR. Histologic confirmation of ghost cell glaucoma by routine light microscopy. *Am J Ophthalmol.* 1983;96:251–252.

100. Singh H, Grand MG. Treatment of blood-induced glaucoma by trans pars plana vitrectomy. *Retina.* 1981;1:255–257.

101. Fenton RH, Zimmerman LE. Hemolytic glaucoma: an unusual cause of acute open-angle secondary glaucoma. *Arch Ophthalmol.* 1963;70: 236–239.

102. Phelps CD, Watzke RC. Hemolytic glaucoma. *Am J Ophthalmol.* 1975;80: 690–695.

103. Grierson I, Lee WR. Further observations on the process of haemophagocytosis in the human outflow system. *Albrecht Von Graefes Arch Klin Exp Ophthalmol.* 1978;208:49–64.

104. Vannas S. Hemosiderosis in eyes with secondary glaucoma after delayed intraocular hemorrhages. *Acta Ophthalmol.* 1960;38:254–267.

CONTUSION INJURIES

General Features

Blunt injuries involving the eye are not uncommon; fortunately, many can be prevented with the use of appropriate protective eyewear. A survey of data derived from hospital discharge abstracts in the United States between 1984 and 1987 revealed a rate of 13.2 cases per 100,000 for any ocular trauma as a principal diagnosis, of which approximately 40% were coded as contusion of the eyeball or adnexa or orbital blowout fracture (1). Young men appear to be most prone to such trauma. In a series of 205 patients with ocular contusion injuries, 85% were males and 75% were younger than 30 years (2). Sporting and domestic accidents accounted for almost two thirds of these injuries, with the remaining known causes divided between unintentional industrial injuries and malicious acts. Among 32 patients hospitalized for sport-related ocular contusion, ball games were the most common cause (3). Boxing is an especially high-risk sport for ocular trauma; in one series of 74 asymptomatic boxers, 66% of the men evaluated had one or more ocular injury (4). An increasingly common source of severe ocular trauma is air bag inflation in a motor vehicle accident (5).

Data from the U.S. Eye Injury Registry on 6021 patients with blunt ocular contusion suggest that the 6-month incidence of posttraumatic glaucoma is 3.4% (6). The same study identified several independently predictive factors associated with the development of posttraumatic glaucoma, including poor initial visual acuity, advancing age, lens injury, angle recession, and hyphema. Another study compared 40 consecutive eyes with closed globe injury and a chronically elevated intraocular pressure (IOP) for a minimum of 3 months with 52 eyes that had closed globe injury and no evidence of glaucoma. Increased pigmentation at the angle, elevated baseline IOP, hyphema, lens displacement, and angle recession of more than 180 degrees were associated with the occurrence of chronic glaucoma after closed globe injury (7).

Clinical Findings

The anterior segment is the portion of the eye most frequently damaged by blunt trauma, and hyphema is the most common mode of clinical presentation (**Fig. 25.1**), occurring in 81% of the 212 eyes in one series (2). A late sign that is almost pathognomonic of hyphema is pigment clumps on the trabecular meshwork (**Fig. 25.2**). (The management of traumatic hyphema is discussed in Chapter 24.) As the blood clears, ruptures in various structures of the anterior segment may be found (**Fig. 25.3**). The most common of these is angle recession (**Fig. 25.4A–C**), which is seen by gonioscopy as an irregular widening of the ciliary body band. Histologically, this represents a tear between the longitudinal and circular muscles of the ciliary body. The reported prevalence of angle recession in eyes with traumatic hyphemas ranges from 60% to 94% (8–12). Angle abnormalities occurred in more than one half of the 32 patients with sports-related ocular contusions and in 19% of the 74 boxers (3,4). When gonioscopic examination was included in a population-based glaucoma survey, some degree of

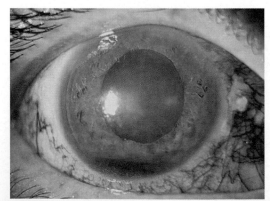

Figure 25.1 An eye with a traumatic hyphema. Slitlamp view reveals layered blood in the anterior chamber. (Courtesy of Joseph A. Halabis, OD.)

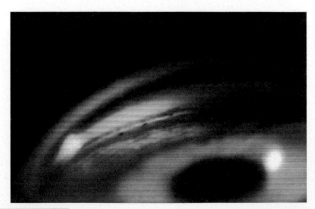

Figure 25.2 Gonioscopic view of an angle demonstrates pigment balls or clumps on the trabecular meshwork. These are virtually pathognomonic of previous traumatic hyphema.

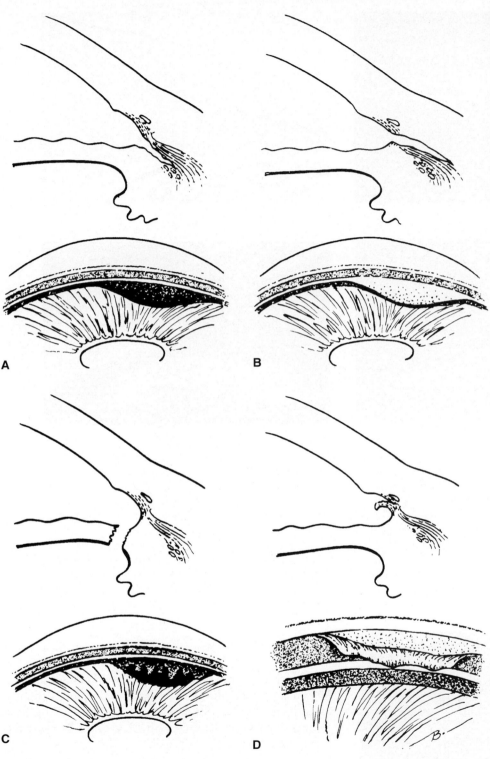

Figure 25.3 Forms of anterior chamber angle injury associated with blunt trauma, showing cross-sectional and corresponding gonioscopic appearances. **A:** Angle recession (i.e., tear between the longitudinal and circular muscles of the ciliary body). **B:** Cyclodialysis (i.e., separation of the ciliary body from the scleral spur, with widening of the suprachoroidal space). **C:** Iridodialysis (i.e., tear in the root of the iris). **D:** Trabecular damage (i.e., tear in the anterior portion of the meshwork, creating a flap that is hinged at the scleral spur).

angle recession was found in 14.8% of the people studied, 5.5% of whom had glaucoma (13). Other associated injuries include iridodialysis, a tear in the root of the iris (**Fig. 25.5**), and cyclodialysis, which is a separation of the ciliary body from the scleral spur (**Fig. 25.4D**). Another finding associated with recurrent trauma, angle recession, and glaucoma is iridoschisis, or separation of layers of iris stroma, which is different from that seen in older adults, because it is more patchy and involves the superior and inferior quadrants (14). Patients with blunt ocular

trauma may also present with iritis, cataracts, dislocation of the lens, or chorioretinal trauma.

Severe blunt ocular injuries can occur with air bag deployment in adults and children (5). In one report of seven children who sustained air bag injuries, serious injuries included corneal edema in one patient and traumatic hyphema with secondary glaucoma and cataract in another. Fortunately, there were no permanent visual sequelae among these children (15). The investigator, however, recommended that infants and children

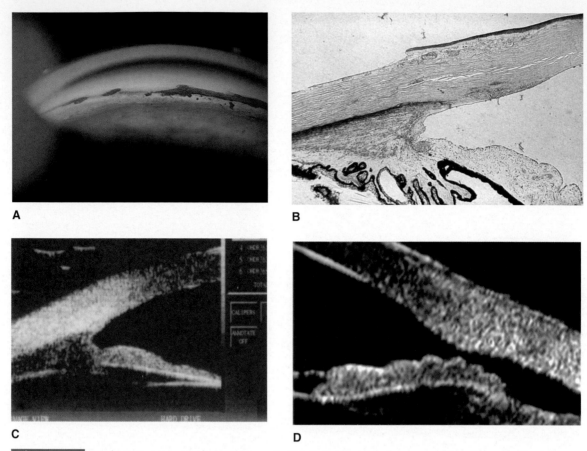

A

B

C

D

Figure 25.4 Ocular trauma to angle structures. **A:** Gonioscopic view of an eye with angle recession, characterized by the irregular widening of the ciliary body band and pigment clumps. (Courtesy of Joseph A. Halabis, OD.) **B:** Histologic section through the anterior chamber angle of an eye with angle recession shows the deep tear into the face of the ciliary body. The trabecular meshwork, which is considerably anterior to the recessed ciliary body, is partly hyalinized and is covered on its inner aspect by an abnormal proliferation of Descemet membrane, another mechanism of glaucoma associated with trauma. (Courtesy of Ramesh C. Tripathi, MD, PhD.) **C:** Ultrasonographic biomicroscopy shows angle recession. **D:** Ultrasonographic biomicroscopy reveals a cyclodialysis cleft. (From Corrêa ZM, Augsburger JJ. Ultrasound biomicroscopy of the anterior ocular segment. In: Tasman W, Jaeger EA, eds. *Duane's Foundations of Clinical Ophthalmology.* Vol. 2. Philadelphia, PA: Lippincott Williams & Wilkins; 2008: chap 31.)

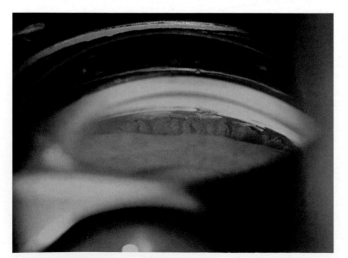

Figure 25.5 Gonioscopic view of an eye with iridodialysis. The ciliary processes are easily viewed through the opening in the iris. (Courtesy of Joseph A. Halabis, OD.)

travel in the rear seat of automobiles to minimize their risk of injury.

Ultrasonographic biomicroscopy should be kept in mind for evaluating mechanisms of trauma (see Chapter 3). In some cases, there may be a traumatic cyclodialysis cleft or weak zonules that can be detected with relative ease by using this technology (16).

Mechanisms of Glaucoma

Early Postinjury Period

A patient with a recent blunt ocular injury may present with a slightly reduced IOP. This may result from a reduction in aqueous production due to the associated iritis or possibly a temporary increase in outflow facility because of the disruption of structures in the anterior chamber angle.

Other patients may have an elevated IOP during the early postcontusion period. In some cases, this may be a transient elevation, which lasts up to several weeks and occurs in the absence of any other obvious damage to the eye. However, there is usually an associated traumatic iritis, hyphema, or dislocation of the lens, the mechanisms of which are discussed elsewhere in this textbook (in Chapters 22, 24, and 18, respectively). Other reported mechanisms of elevated IOP associated with blunt trauma to the eye include shallowing of the anterior chamber due to uveal effusion, vitreous filling a deep anterior chamber, and Schwartz–Matsuo syndrome, which may include fluctuations in IOP in association with retinal detachment accompanied by tears of the nonpigmented epithelium of the ciliary body (17–20).

Late Postinjury Period

Although elevated IOP after blunt ocular trauma is transient in most cases, it is important to follow up these patients indefinitely, because 4% to 9% of those with angle recession greater than 180 degrees eventually—often many years later—develop glaucoma (9,11,21,22). This condition has been called angle-recession glaucoma, although the term is somewhat of a misnomer, because the angle recession is not the actual cause of the obstruction to aqueous outflow. The clinicopathologic correlation between blunt injury to the eye and the delayed development of glaucoma was reported by Wolff and Zimmerman (23), who suggested that the angle recession provided evidence of past injury but was not the actual cause of the glaucoma. They suggested that initial trauma to the trabecular meshwork stimulated proliferative or degenerative changes in the trabecular tissue, which led to obstruction of aqueous outflow. Herschler (24) supported this concept by observations of clinical cases and animal studies, which revealed tears in the trabecular meshwork just posterior to the Schwalbe line during the early posttraumatic period. This produced a flap of trabecular tissue, which was hinged at the scleral spur (Fig. 25.3). With time, scarring ensued, causing the initial trabecular injury to be less apparent, but leading to chronic obstruction in portions of the aqueous outflow system.

In addition to alterations in the trabecular meshwork, another mechanism of delayed IOP elevation is the extension of an endothelial layer with a Descemet-like membrane from the cornea over the anterior chamber angle (23,25,26). Additional factors may influence which eyes with a history of blunt trauma will develop chronic glaucoma. For example, most eyes that eventually develop glaucoma after blunt injury appear to have an underlying predisposition to reduced aqueous outflow, as evidenced by frequent alterations of IOP in the fellow eye (12,24,27). Among 13 patients who developed angle-recession glaucoma an average of 34 years after trauma, 7 had definite or suspicious glaucomatous visual field loss in the fellow eye (27). Older adults also are more susceptible to late-postcontusion pressure elevation (22).

Management of Glaucoma

If possible, elevated IOP in the early postinjury period is best controlled medically, primarily with the use of drugs that reduce aqueous production, such as β-blockers, carbonic anhydrase inhibitors, and α_2-agonists. Concomitant disorders, such as inflammation, hyphema, and subluxation of the lens, must also be managed, as discussed in other chapters. Eyes with a shallow anterior chamber and uveal effusion may respond to corticosteroids and mydriatic cycloplegics (17).

Chronic IOP elevation due to trabecular damage does not respond well to miotic therapy. In one reported case with associated angle recession, use of pilocarpine caused a paradoxic pressure rise, and use of cycloplegics lowered the tension (28). The investigators theorized that the reduction in conventional outflow combined with a tear in the ciliary body might have shifted the eye to a predominantly uveoscleral mechanism of aqueous outflow, which is known to be impaired by miotics. Prostaglandin agents may be helpful in some cases of trauma but are generally used after acute signs of inflammation have subsided and a trial of aqueous suppressants has failed to adequately reduce the IOP. Drugs that reduce aqueous production are known to be efficacious in eyes with scarring of the trabecular meshwork.

Laser trabeculoplasty does not have a high success rate in this form of glaucoma, although it can be tried after medical therapy has failed but before filtering surgery is attempted. An alternative laser procedure, Nd:YAG laser trabeculopuncture, in which an energy of 1.0 to 2.5 mJ is applied to the meshwork in a manner similar to argon laser trabeculoplasty, has been reported to offer significant advantages over trabeculoplasty in the treatment of angle-recession glaucoma (29).

When medical and laser therapies have failed, an incisional outflow operation is usually indicated. In a study comparing three procedures (i.e., trabeculectomy without antimetabolite, trabeculectomy with adjunctive 5-fluorouracil or mitomycin C, or a Molteno single-plate implantation), trabeculectomy with antimetabolite therapy was the most effective, although late bleb infection is a significant risk (30). In another study examining long-term outcomes in 38 patients who underwent implantation of a Molteno drainage device for traumatic glaucoma, IOP was controlled in 76% of cases (with adjunctive use of medications) at a mean follow-up of 10.9 years (31). An alternative to outflow surgery, especially in eyes with limited visual potential, is transscleral cyclophotocoagulation or one of the other cyclodestructive procedures. In cases of traumatic aniridia, in which the ciliary process tips can be visualized by gonioscopy, transpupillary argon cyclophotocoagulation offers another option (32).

PENETRATING INJURIES

General Features

Penetrating injuries of the eye may result from blunt force, sharp lacerations, or missiles. In a study of 453 patients, the relative frequencies of these three sources of trauma were 22%, 37%, and 41%, respectively (33). As with the nonpenetrating injuries, young men are most vulnerable to these types of injuries, and many of these injuries could be prevented with the use of appropriate protective eyewear. Of the patients in the study, 86% were male, and the mean age of the entire group was 26 years (33).

The IOP immediately after a penetrating injury is frequently reduced because of the open wound or the associated iridocyclitis. After closure of the corneal or scleral wound, however, glaucoma may develop because of intraocular tissue changes induced by the penetrating injury. Among 3627 patients in the U.S. Eye Injury Registry who experienced penetrating ocular injuries, the 6-month incidence of glaucoma was 2.67%. Factors associated with the development of posttraumatic glaucoma included advancing age, lens injury, poor visual acuity, and intraocular inflammation (34).

Mechanisms of Glaucoma

Tissue Disruption

During the early postinjury period, the IOP may be elevated due to inflammation, hyphema, or angle closure from a swollen, disrupted lens. As these conditions subside, chronic mechanisms of glaucoma may follow. In some cases, a cyclitic membrane may develop because of inflammatory material. This arises from the nonpigmented ciliary epithelium and organizes on a scaffold of lens, iris, anterior hyaloid, or whatever tissue may remain after the injury (35). The membrane may lead to closure of the anterior chamber angle by forward displacement of the lens–iris diaphragm or by seclusion of the pupil with subsequent iris bombé. Failure to reform a flat anterior chamber or adequately treat the inflammation may lead to chronic pressure elevation due to peripheral anterior synechiae. Additional, rare causes of delayed IOP elevation include sympathetic ophthalmia and epithelial ingrowth.

Retained Intraocular Foreign Bodies

Retained intraocular foreign bodies may be associated with the same tissue disruption and associated glaucoma as noted earlier. Prolonged intraocular retention of certain metallic foreign bodies may lead to delayed tissue alterations. Siderosis results from the intraocular retention of ferrous metal (iron), but it may also be caused by intraocular hemorrhage (the ionized form of iron is indistinguishable from hemosiderin). This material can cause structural alterations in tissues throughout the eye. Glaucoma may be a complication of advanced cases, although there is no proof that trabecular outflow is impaired by iron staining of the trabecular structures. Copper is also oxidized in the eye and can lead to chalcosis, with tissue damage that is nearly as severe as that encountered with ferrous foreign bodies. Glaucoma appears to be less common in these patients, although retinal changes can lead to visual field defects that may be confused with those of glaucoma (36).

Management of Glaucoma

The best way to avoid loss of vision from glaucoma after penetrating ocular injuries is to minimize the development of chronic aqueous outflow obstruction by properly treating the initial injury. This may include removal of portions of incarcerated uveal tissue; aspiration of the lens, if disrupted or swollen; anterior vitrectomy; removal of foreign bodies; meticulous closure of the wound; and reformation of the anterior chamber. In some cases, it is necessary to close the wound initially and perform the intraocular surgery with vitreous instruments later. In a series of 112 such patients, the final visual result was best when the vitrectomy was done within 72 hours of the injury (35). Corticosteroid therapy to avoid cyclitic membranes and scarring in the anterior chamber angle is also important in the early postinjury period, and antibiotic therapy is needed as prophylaxis against endophthalmitis.

Antiglaucoma medication may be needed for control of transient pressure elevations during the early postinjury period and during subsequent chronic glaucoma, and use of drugs that reduce aqueous production is preferable in both situations. When medical therapy is insufficient, especially in the chronic cases, surgical intervention is indicated. Laser trabeculoplasty is usually not possible because of peripheral anterior synechia, in which case filtering surgery should be recommended. In siderosis bulbi, removal of the intraocular foreign body by using vitrectomy techniques may be beneficial in some cases (37).

CHEMICAL AND THERMAL BURNS

Alkali Burns

Alkali burns of the eye may produce a rapid initial rise in the IOP. This is often followed by a return to normal or subnormal pressure and then a slower, sustained elevation of the ocular tension (38). Possible mechanisms of the early pressure rise include shrinkage of the cornea and sclera and an increase in uveal blood flow (38,39). The altered blood-flow dynamics may be mediated by using prostaglandins (39), which may also be associated with the later IOP elevation (38). A hypopyon may also develop and contribute to the pressure rise.

In managing the glaucoma associated with an alkali burn of the cornea, use of topical corticosteroids may be helpful if a significant inflammatory component is present. It has been shown in rabbits that topical steroids can be used for the first week without increasing the risk for corneal melting, but not thereafter (40). The presence of prostaglandins during the delayed pressure rise suggests that the early use of drugs such as indomethacin and imidazole, which inhibit prostaglandin synthesis, may be beneficial. Use of antiglaucoma agents, especially those that reduce aqueous production, is also frequently needed in these circumstances. Miotics and prostaglandins should usually be avoided.

Acid Burns

Acid burns of the cornea have been shown to cause an IOP response in rabbits similar to that seen with alkali burns (41). A rapid tension increase, lasting up to 3 hours, probably results from shrinkage of the outer ocular coats, and a subsequent sustained rise is considered to be mediated by prostaglandin release (41). Treatment of the associated glaucoma in these patients is similar to that for alkali burns.

Thermal Burns

Thermal burns of the face often involve the eyelids, although the globes tend to be spared except for occasional corneal injury. However, in severely burned patients, in whom the administration of large quantities of intravenous fluids to maintain blood pressure is the key therapeutic measure, orbital congestion and massive periorbital swelling may lead to marked IOP elevations (42). In three reported cases, lateral canthotomies resulted in a significant relief of the potentially damaging high pressures (42).

RADIATION DAMAGE

Radiation therapy to structures near the eyes may increase the IOP (43). The mechanism of the pressure rise is not well understood, although in some eyes the cause may be neovascular glaucoma or intraocular hemorrhage due to retinal radiation damage. Medical therapy should be used when possible, although surgical intervention, such as filtering surgery or a cyclodestructive procedure, is often needed. The prognosis is generally poor.

KEY POINTS

- The most common form of ocular trauma that may lead to IOP elevation is blunt or contusion injuries. These injuries may cause an early pressure rise due to iritis, hyphema, or lens dislocation, or they may cause delayed development of glaucoma from scarring of the damaged trabecular meshwork.
- Penetrating injuries may also cause an elevation of tension due to tissue disruption in the anterior chamber angle or in association with the retention of intraocular foreign bodies, such as iron and copper.
- Chemical burns by alkali or acid may cause a pressure rise, the mechanisms of which may include collagen shrinkage and prostaglandin release.
- Thermal burns and radiation damage are other, rare causes of elevated IOP.
- Eye protection in sports and occupations involving potential damage to the eye is critical to prevent sharp or blunt trauma.

REFERENCES

1. Klopfer J, Tielsch JM, Vitale S, et al. Ocular trauma in the United States: eye injuries resulting in hospitalization, 1984 through 1987. *Arch Ophthalmol.* 1992;110:838–842.
2. Canavan YM, Archer DB. Anterior segment consequences of blunt ocular injury. *Br J Opthalmol.* 1982;66:549–555.
3. Gracner B, Kurelac Z. Gonioscopic changes in ocular contusions sustained in sports [in German]. *Klin Monatsbl Augenheilkd.* 1985;186:128–130.
4. Giovinazzo VJ, Yannuzzi LA, Sorenson JA, et al. The ocular complications of boxing. *Ophthalmology.* 1987;94:587–596.
5. Lesher MP, Durrie DS, Stiles MC. Corneal edema, hyphema, and angle recession after air bag inflation. *Arch Ophthalmol.* 1993;111:1320–1322.
6. Girkin CA, McGwin G Jr, Long C, et al. Glaucoma after ocular contusion: a cohort study of the United States Eye Injury Registry. *J Glaucoma.* 2005;14(6):470–473.
7. Kumar SR, Gupta S, Dada V, et al. Early predictors of traumatic glaucoma after closed globe injury: trabecular pigmentation, widened angle recess, and higher baseline intraocular pressure. *Arch Opthalmol.* 2008;126(7):921–926.
8. Howard GM, Hutchinson BT, Frederick AR. Hyphema resulting from blunt trauma: gonioscopic, tonographic, and ophthalmoscopic observations following resolution of the hemorrhage. *Trans Am Acad Ophthalmol Otolaryngol.* 1965;69:294.
9. Blanton FM. Anterior chamber angle recession and secondary glaucoma: a study of the after effects of traumatic hyphemas. *Arch Ophthalmol.* 1964;72:39.
10. Tonjum AM. Gonioscopy in traumatic hyphema. *Acta Opthalmol.* 1966;44:650–664.
11. Mooney D. Angle recession and secondary glaucoma. *Br J Ophthalmol.* 1973;57:608–612.
12. Spaeth GL. Traumatic hyphema, angle recession, dexamethasone hypertension, and glaucoma. *Arch Opthalmol.* 1967;78:714–721.
13. Salmon JF, Mermoud A, Ivey A, et al. The detection of post-traumatic angle recession by gonioscopy in a population-based glaucoma survey. *Ophthalmology.* 1994;101:1844–1850.
14. Salmon JF. The association of iridoschisis and angle-recession glaucoma. *Am J Ophthalmol.* 1992;114:766–767.
15. Lueder GT. Air bag-associated ocular trauma in children. *Ophthalmology.* 2000;107:1472–1475.
16. Ozdal MP, Mansour M, Deschenes J. Ultrasound biomicroscopic evaluation of the traumatized eyes. *Eye (Lond).* 2003;17(4):467–472.
17. Dotan S, Oliver M. Shallow anterior chamber and uveal effusion after nonperforating trauma to the eye. *Am J Ophthalmol.* 1982;94:782–784.
18. Kutner BN. Acute angle closure glaucoma in nonperforating blunt trauma. *Arch Ophthalmol.* 1988;106:19–20.
19. Samples JR, Van Buskirk EM. Open-angle glaucoma associated with vitreous humor filling the anterior chamber. *Am J Ophthalmol.* 1986;102:759–761.
20. Matsuo T, Muraoka N, Shiraga F, et al. Schwartz-Matsuo syndrome in retinal detachment with tears of the nonpigmented epithelium of the ciliary body. *Acta Ophthalmol Scand.* 1998;76:481–485.
21. Kaufman JH, Tolpin DW. Glaucoma after traumatic angle recession: a ten-year prospective study. *Am J Ophthalmol.* 1974;79:648–654.
22. Thiel HJ, Aden G, Pulhorn G. Changes in the chamber angle following ocular contusions. *Klin Monatsbl Augenheilkd.* 1980;177:165–173.
23. Wolff SM, Zimmerman LE. Chronic secondary glaucoma: associated with retrodisplacement of iris root and deepening of the anterior chamber angle secondary to contusion. *Am J Ophthalmol.* 1962;54:547–563.
24. Herschler J. Trabecular damage due to blunt anterior segment injury and its relationship to traumatic glaucoma. *Trans Sect Ophthalmol Am Acad Ophthalmol Otolaryngol.* 1977;83:239–248.
25. Lauring L. Anterior chamber glass membranes. *Am J Ophthalmol.* 1969;68:308–312.
26. Iwamoto T, Witmer R, Landolt E. Light and electron microscopy in absolute glaucoma with pigment dispersion phenomena and contusion angle deformity. *Am J Ophthalmol.* 1971;72:420–434.
27. Tesluk GC, Spaeth GL. The occurrence of primary open-angle glaucoma in the fellow eye of patients with unilateral angle-cleavage glaucoma. *Ophthalmology.* 1985;92(7):904–911.
28. Bleiman BS, Schwartz AL. Paradoxical intraocular pressure response to pilocarpine: a proposed mechanism and treatment. *Arch Ophthalmol.* 1979;97:1305–1306.
29. Fukuchi T, Iwata K, Sawaguchi S, et al. Nd:YAG laser trabeculopuncture (YLT) for glaucoma with traumatic angle recession. *Graefes Arch Clin Exp Ophthalmol.* 1993;231:571–576.
30. Mermoud A, Salmon JF, Barron A, et al. Surgical management of post-traumatic angle recession glaucoma. *Ophthalmology.* 1993;100:634–642.

31. Fuller JR, Bevin TH, Molteno AC. Long-term follow-up of traumatic glaucoma treated with Molteno implants. *Ophthalmology.* 2001;108:1796–1800.

32. Kim DD, Moster MR. Transpupillary argon laser cyclophotocoagulation in the treatment of traumatic glaucoma. *J Glaucoma.* 1999;8:340–341.

33. deJuan E Jr, Sternberg P Jr, Michels RG. Penetrating ocular injuries: types of injuries and visual results. *Ophthalmology.* 1983;90:1318–1322.

34. Girkin CA, McGwin G Jr, Morris R, et al. Glaucoma following penetrating ocular trauma: a cohort study of the United States Eye Injury Registry. *Am J Opthalmol.* 2005;139(1):100–105.

35. Coleman DJ. Early vitrectomy in the management of the severely traumatized eye. *Am J Ophthalmol.* 1982;93:543–551.

36. Rosenthal AR, Marmor MF, Leuenberger P, et al. Chalcosis: a study of natural history. *Ophthalmology.* 1979;86:1956–1972.

37. Sneed SR, Weingeist TA. Management of siderosis bulbi due to a retained iron-containing intraocular foreign body. *Ophthalmology.* 1990;97: 375–379.

38. Paterson CA, Pfister RR. Intraocular pressure changes after alkali burns. *Arch Ophthalmol.* 1974;91:211–218.

39. Green K, Paterson CA, Siddiqui A. Ocular blood flow after experimental alkali burns and prostaglandin administration. *Arch Ophthalmol.* 1985;103:569–571.

40. Donshik PC, Berman MB, Dohlman CH, et al. Effect of topical corticosteroids on ulceration in alkali-burned corneas. *Arch Ophthalmol.* 1978;96:2117–2120.

41. Paterson CA, Eakins KE, Paterson E, et al. The ocular hypertensive response following experimental acid burns in the rabbit eye. *Invest Ophthalmol Vis Sci.* 1979;18:67–74.

42. Evans LS. Increased intraocular pressure in severely burned patients. *Am J Ophthalmol.* 1991;111:56–58.

43. Barron A, McDonald JE, Hughes WF. Long-term complications of beta radiation therapy in ophthalmology. *Trans Am Ophthalmol Soc.* 1970;68:113–128.

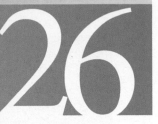

Glaucomas after Ocular Surgery

Many diverse forms of glaucomas occur as complications of various ocular surgical procedures, including glaucoma surgery, cataract extraction and related procedures, corneal transplantation, and vitreoretinal surgery.

MALIGNANT (CILIARY BLOCK) GLAUCOMA

Terminology

In 1869, von Graefe (1) described a rare complication of certain ocular procedures that was characterized by shallowing or flattening of the anterior chamber and an elevation of the intraocular pressure (IOP). He called the condition malignant glaucoma because of the poor response to conventional therapy. The concept of malignant glaucoma has been expanded to include various clinical situations, which have these common denominators: shallowing or flattening of the central and peripheral anterior chambers, elevation of the IOP, and unresponsiveness to or aggravation by use of miotics but frequent relief with cycloplegic–mydriatic therapy (2,3).

Studies of the mechanism of malignant glaucoma (considered later in this chapter) led some investigators to recommend new terms for this group of diseases. On the basis of the theory that obstruction of normal aqueous flow is caused by apposition of the ciliary processes against the equator of the lens or the anterior hyaloid, the name ciliary block glaucoma was proposed (4,5). The term aqueous misdirection is also commonly used to denote the concept of posterior diversion of the aqueous due to the ciliary block. To describe the concept that a forward shift of the lens pushes peripheral iris into the anterior chamber angle, the term direct lens block angle closure has been suggested (6). There is no universal agreement on the terminology for this group of conditions; the traditional term, malignant glaucoma, is retained for purposes of discussion in this text. When discussing this term with patients, however, the physician should be aware that the term malignant may have unintended and undesirable connotations, and it is therefore advisable to provide appropriate context when using this term or to use an alternative term.

Clinical Forms

Whether all the clinical conditions called malignant glaucoma should actually be included in a single disease category is not yet established. Nevertheless, the following disorders have been described under that name.

Classic Malignant Glaucoma

Classic malignant glaucoma is the prototype and most common form of the disease group. It typically follows incisional surgical intervention for angle-closure glaucoma and is reported to complicate 0.6% to 4% of these cases (2,3,7). Neither the type of surgery nor the IOP immediately before surgical intervention appears to be related to the postoperative development of malignant glaucoma (3). However, partial or total closure of the anterior chamber angle at the time of surgery is associated with an increased incidence of this complication (3). An acute angle-closure attack may be a predisposing factor, because when malignant glaucoma occurs, it frequently does so in an eye with previous angle closure, although the angle may have been open preoperatively (7). Conversely, the condition rarely follows a prophylactic iridectomy when the angle is open at the time of surgery (7).

The classic presentation is a unilateral disorder in the early postoperative period after incisional surgery. However, cases have been reported after laser iridotomy, and bilateral cases have been reported with both incisional and laser procedures that, although the actual mechanisms may differ, do clinically resemble classic forms of the disease (8–10). Some cases may not have an elevated IOP (11); others may occur months to years later, after the cessation of cycloplegic therapy or the institution of miotic drops (2,3,10).

Malignant Glaucoma in Aphakia

Although classic malignant glaucoma typically occurs in phakic eyes, it may persist after lens removal for treatment of the disease or develop after cataract extraction in eyes without preexisting glaucoma (3). It is important to differentiate malignant glaucoma in aphakia and in its other forms from pupillary block glaucoma and delayed suprachoroidal hemorrhage (discussed later in this chapter).

Malignant Glaucoma in Pseudophakia

Malignant glaucoma may be associated with an intraocular lens implant in the anterior chamber, presumably by the same mechanism as malignant glaucoma in aphakia (12). It has also been observed in eyes with posterior chamber implants, with or without an associated glaucoma filtering procedure (**Fig. 26.1**) (13). Malignant glaucoma has also occurred after implantation of an intraocular lens in the posterior chamber of a phakic eye (i.e., malignant glaucoma induced by a phakic intraocular lens in the posterior chamber of a patient with myopia) (14).

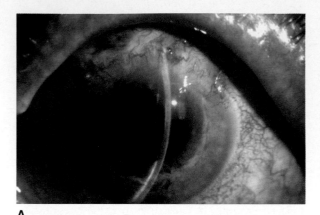
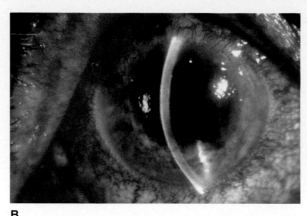

A B

Figure 26.1 Ciliary block after cataract extraction and posterior chamber lens implantation. **A:** The central chamber is shallow; the peripheral chamber is flat. The intraocular lens is pushed forward, and the haptic posterior to the iris is indenting the iris surface. **B:** After disruption of the posterior capsule and anterior hyaloid face with Nd:YAG laser, the chamber immediately deepens; the intraocular lens is no longer pressed against the iris. (Courtesy of E. Hodapp, MD. From Werner MA, Grajewski AL. Glaucoma in aphakia and pseudophakia. In: Tasman W, Jaeger EA, eds. *Duane's Clinical Ophthalmology*. Vol 3. Philadelphia, PA:Lippincott Williams & Wilkins; 2008:chap 54G.)

Miotic-Induced Malignant Glaucoma

The onset of classic malignant glaucoma may correspond to the institution of miotic therapy, suggesting a causal relationship (15). Although the precise mechanism behind this relationship is unknown, the action of miotics may produce malignant glaucoma through contraction of the ciliary body or associated forward shift of the lens with shallowing of the anterior chamber. Similar clinical pictures have been described in unoperated eyes receiving miotic therapy and in an eye treated with miotics after a filtering procedure for open-angle glaucoma (16,17).

Malignant Glaucoma Associated with Bleb Needling

A case of malignant glaucoma after needling of a trabeculectomy bleb has been reported (18). It is possible that bleb needling results in a shallowing of the anterior chamber that predisposes to malignant glaucoma.

Malignant Glaucoma Associated with Inflammation and Infection

Inflammation and trauma are also precipitating factors of malignant glaucoma (6). A form of malignant glaucoma is associated with endophthalmitis caused by fungal keratomycosis and the atypical bacterium *Nocardia asteroides* (19).

Malignant Glaucoma Associated with Other Ocular Disorders

Retinal detachment surgery caused the malignant glaucoma syndrome in a patient who developed choroidal detachments after a buckling procedure (20). However, the anterior chamber shallowing in this situation may be secondary to an anterior uveal effusion with forward rotation of the lens or iris diaphragm, producing a secondary angle-closure glaucoma that resembles malignant glaucoma. Several cases of malignant

glaucoma–like syndrome have been reported after pars plana vitrectomy (21,22), and one case reported after diode laser cyclophotocoagulation (23). The condition has also been noted in children with retinopathy of prematurity and in a patient with corneal hydrops in keratoconus (24,25).

Spontaneous Malignant Glaucoma

Malignant glaucoma may rarely develop spontaneously in an eye without previous surgery, miotic therapy, or other apparent cause (26).

Theories of Mechanism

There is a lack of general agreement regarding the sequence of events responsible for the development of malignant glaucoma, although the following are the more popular theories.

Posterior Pooling of Aqueous

Shaffer (27) hypothesized that an accumulation of aqueous behind a posterior vitreous detachment causes the forward displacement of the iris–lens or iris–vitreous diaphragm. The concept was subsequently expanded to include the pooling of aqueous in vitreous pockets. This theory is supported by an ultrasonographic study of eyes with malignant glaucoma in aphakia demonstrating echo-free zones in the vitreous from which aqueous was reportedly aspirated (28). The mechanisms leading to the posterior diversion of aqueous are uncertain, although strong evidence supports the following possibilities.

Ciliolenticular (Ciliovitreal) Block

In cases of malignant glaucoma, the tips of the ciliary processes rotate forward and press against the lens equator in the phakic eye or against the anterior hyaloid in aphakia, which may create the obstruction to forward flow of aqueous (4,29) (**Figs. 26.2** and **26.3**, respectively). Studies involving ultrasonographic

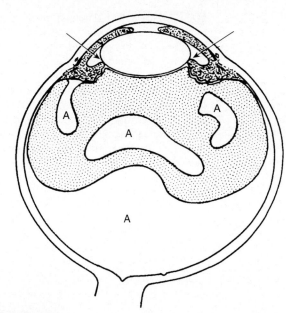

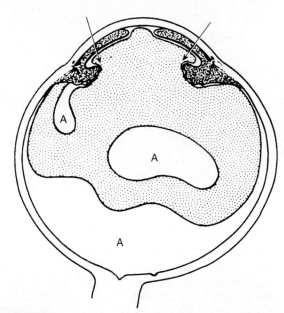

Figure 26.2 Concept of ciliolenticular block as the mechanism of malignant glaucoma. Apposition of the ciliary processes to the lens equator *(arrows)* causes a posterior diversion of aqueous *(A)*, which pools in and behind the vitreous with a forward shift of the lens–iris diaphragm.

Figure 26.3 Concept of ciliovitreal block as the mechanism of malignant glaucoma in aphakia. Apposition of ciliary processes against the anterior hyaloid *(arrows)* leads to posterior diversion of aqueous *(A)*, which causes a forward shift of the vitreous and iris.

biomicroscopy have confirmed the anterior rotation of the ciliary processes (30,31); two studies also showed a shallow collection of supraciliary fluid (31,32). This concept led to the proposed term ciliary block glaucoma as a substitute for malignant glaucoma (4).

Anterior Hyaloid Obstruction

The anterior hyaloid may contribute to ciliolenticular block, and breaks in the hyaloid near the vitreous base possibly allow the posterior diversion of aqueous (5) (**Fig. 26.4**). The hyaloid breaks, however, have a one-way valve effect, because fluid coming anteriorly closes the vitreous face against the ciliary body, preventing forward flow (5). Some investigators have observed the ciliolenticular contact but noticed that the spaces between the ciliary processes were open, with vitreous visible behind them, suggesting that the obstruction to anterior aqueous flow is the anterior vitreous face, which is compressed forward

against the ciliary processes in phakic and aphakic forms of malignant glaucoma (3).

In perfusion studies with animal and human eyes, resistance to flow of a fluid through vitreous increases significantly with an elevation of pressure in the eye (33–35). The increased resistance might be caused by compression of the vitreous and its displacement against the ciliary body, lens, and iris, thereby reducing the available area of anterior hyaloid through which fluid could flow (34,35). These clinical and laboratory observations support the concept that an intact anterior hyaloid may be important in preventing the forward movement of aqueous as it travels anteriorly.

Slackness of Lens Zonules

Chandler and Grant (36) postulated that the forward movement of the lens–iris diaphragm in malignant glaucoma might be caused by abnormal slackness or weakness of the zonules of

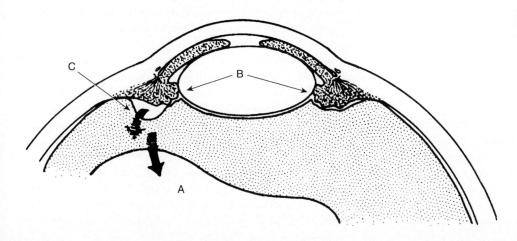

Figure 26.4 The anterior hyaloid may contribute to the ciliolenticular block *(B)*, and breaks in the hyaloid near the vitreous base *(C)* may allow the aqueous *(A)* to be diverted posteriorly *(arrows)*.

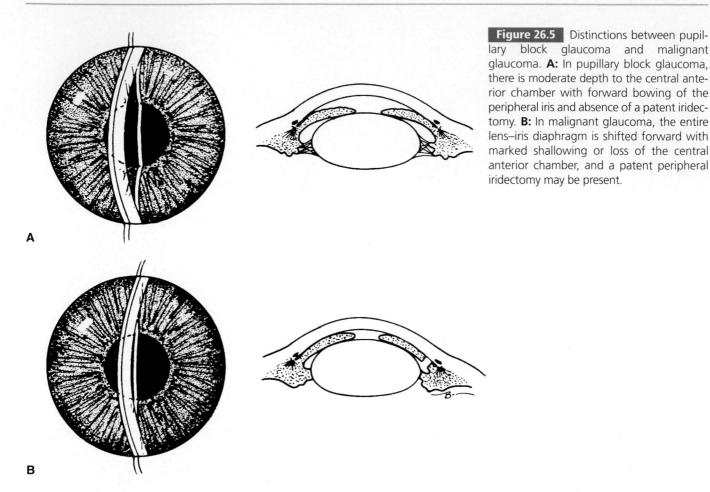

Figure 26.5 Distinctions between pupillary block glaucoma and malignant glaucoma. **A:** In pupillary block glaucoma, there is moderate depth to the central anterior chamber with forward bowing of the peripheral iris and absence of a patent iridectomy. **B:** In malignant glaucoma, the entire lens–iris diaphragm is shifted forward with marked shallowing or loss of the central anterior chamber, and a patent peripheral iridectomy may be present.

A

B

the lens as well as pressure from the vitreous. Others have also advocated this theory and suggested that the laxity of the zonules might be the result of severe, prolonged angle closure (7), or ciliary muscle spasm induced by surgery, miotics, inflammation, trauma, or other unknown factors (6). The concept that the lens subsequently pushes the peripheral iris into the anterior chamber angle led to the proposed term of direct lens block angle closure (6).

It seems likely that malignant glaucoma is a multifactorial disorder, in which one or more elements of the aforementioned mechanisms may be involved, depending on the clinical context.

Differential Diagnosis

The diagnosis of malignant glaucoma requires the exclusion of the following conditions (3,5).

Pupillary Block Glaucoma

Pupillary block is the most difficult entity to distinguish from malignant glaucoma but must be ruled out before the latter diagnosis can be made. During slitlamp biomicroscopy, attention should be focused on two questions. First, is the central anterior chamber moderately deep with bowing of the peripheral iris into the chamber angle, as typically noted in pupillary block, or is the entire iris–lens diaphragm shifted forward with

marked shallowing or loss of the central anterior chamber, more consistent with malignant glaucoma (**Fig. 26.5**)? Second, and probably of more diagnostic value, is a patent iridectomy present? If the iridectomy is clearly patent, a pupillary block mechanism is unlikely. However, if patency cannot be confirmed, the diagnosis of pupillary block cannot be ruled out, and one should proceed with a definitive laser iridotomy.

Choroidal Detachments

Choroidal separation with serous fluid is common after glaucoma filtering procedures and might be confused with malignant glaucoma because of the shallow or flat anterior chamber. These eyes typically are hypotonus. However, when the anterior chamber is flat, IOP measurements by Goldmann applanation tonometry, pneumotonometry, or a Tono-Pen are often highly inaccurate, tending to overestimate the IOP, and therefore cannot be relied on to distinguish between excessive filtration and malignant glaucoma (37). A more helpful diagnostic finding is the presence of a choroidal detachment, which is easily seen if there is adequate visibility of the posterior segment—or alternatively, the presence of choroidal fluid observed by ultrasonography.

Most serous choroidal detachments will resolve spontaneously as IOP rises. However, those that are persistent or massive with central touch can be approached surgically by making scleral incisions in the inferior quadrants. If a characteristic straw-colored fluid is obtained from the suprachoroidal space, the diagnosis of serous choroidal detachment is confirmed, and the procedure is completed by draining as much suprachoroidal fluid as possible and reforming the anterior chamber with air or saline, or both.

A case series has been reported of patients with occult annular ciliary body detachment giving rise to angle-closure glaucoma that is clinically indistinguishable from malignant glaucoma (38). Ultrasonographic biomicroscopy facilitated the diagnosis and guided subsequent management.

Suprachoroidal Hemorrhage

Suprachoroidal hemorrhage may occur hours or days after ocular surgery and create shallowing or loss of the anterior chamber, which is typically associated with pain and elevated IOP. It is often preceded by ocular hypotony. The eye is usually more inflamed than with serous choroidal detachment, and the choroidal elevation is frequently dark reddish–brown. The surgical approach is the same as that for serous choroidal detachments, with drainage of the blood from the suprachoroidal space though the sclerotomies and reformation of the anterior chamber.

Management of Malignant Glaucoma

Medical Management

Chandler and Grant (36) reported in 1962 that mydriatic–cycloplegic treatment was effective for malignant glaucoma, and the next year Weiss and colleagues (39) recommended the use of hyperosmotics to combat this condition. Cycloplegics, by virtue of stimulating contraction of the ciliary body, help pull the lens back by tightening the zonules, helping to break the ciliary block, whereas the presumed benefit of a hyperosmotic agent is to reduce the pressure exerted by the vitreous (5,36,39). These two measures, along with the use of aqueous suppressants, help reduce the flow of aqueous that perpetuates shallowing of the anterior chamber and resultant malignant glaucoma. A standard medical regimen includes the use of topical atropine two to three times daily, intravenous mannitol, topical β-blocker or α$_2$-agonist (or both), and oral or topical carbonic anhydrase inhibitors. After the attack is broken, the patient should be maintained indefinitely on atropine therapy to prevent recurrences.

Surgical Management

Medical treatment of malignant glaucoma is effective in approximately one half of cases within 5 days (2,3). If the condition persists beyond this time, surgical intervention is usually indicated.

Laser Techniques

Argon laser photocoagulation of the ciliary processes that can be visualized through an iridectomy or transscleral diode laser cyclophotocoagulation has been reported to relieve malignant glaucoma, presumably by breaking the ciliolenticular block (40,41). Nd:YAG laser can also be effective in treating aphakic and pseudophakic malignant glaucoma by disrupting the anterior hyaloid face or the posterior lens capsule and hyaloid face (42).

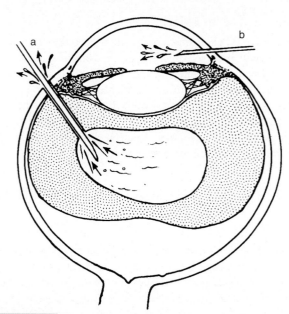

Figure 26.6   Posterior sclerotomy and air injection in the management of malignant glaucoma. Fluid is drained or aspirated from the vitreous by means of a pars plana incision *(a)* and the anterior chamber is deepened with air *(b)*.

Slitlamp Needle Revision

When the anterior hyaloid face is accessible in the anterior segment and an Nd:YAG laser is not accessible, performing transcorneal needling to disrupt the anterior vitreous face and reform the anterior chamber may be possible (43).

Posterior Sclerotomy and Air Injection

A pars plana incision with aspiration of liquid vitreous with reformation of the anterior chamber with an air bubble (**Fig. 26.6**) is felt by some to be the incisional surgical procedure of choice for classic malignant glaucoma (2,3,5). It has been suggested that the sclerotomy should be placed 3 mm posterior to the limbus to break the anterior hyaloid, thereby reducing its contribution to the blockade (5). Postoperatively, patients are generally maintained on atropine to avoid recurrence.

Anterior Pars Plana Vitrectomy

Other surgeons prefer a careful removal of the anterior vitreous including the anterior hyaloid with vitrectomy instruments (44–46). Failure to include the anterior hyaloid may result in recurrence of malignant glaucoma. Results with posterior sclerotomy and anterior vitrectomy techniques are favorable, but both have the potential for serious complications. The preferred method of treatment depends on the surgeon's experience and preference.

Lens Extraction

This is favored by some surgeons as the incisional surgical procedure of choice, whereas others use this approach if the posterior sclerotomy and air injection or anterior vitrectomy fails (47). To be effective, lens extraction should be combined with an incision of the anterior hyaloid and possibly with deep incisions into fluid pockets in the vitreous (2,3).

Management of the Fellow Eye

When malignant glaucoma has already occurred in one eye, the fellow eye will also probably develop the condition if it undergoes intraocular surgery. For this reason, it is best to do a prophylactic laser iridotomy, if indicated. However, if angle-closure glaucoma is present, every effort should be made to break the attack before surgery and, if the attack cannot be broken, mydriatic–cycloplegic therapy should be used vigorously after iridotomy and continued indefinitely.

GLAUCOMAS IN APHAKIA OR PSEUDOPHAKIA

Terminology

The term aphakic or pseudophakic glaucoma is occasionally seen in the literature. It is mentioned in this text only to discourage its use because it implies that a single form of glaucoma is associated with aphakia or pseudophakia. There are many mechanisms by which cataract extraction, with or without intraocular lens implantation, can lead to glaucoma, and it is best to refer to these glaucomas in aphakia or pseudophakia by terms that describe the particular events leading to the IOP elevation.

Incidence

The IOP may be elevated transiently in the early postoperative period or may become chronically elevated at any time after cataract surgery.

Aphakia

In the days before intraocular lens implantation, a rise in IOP during the first several days after cataract extraction was not uncommon, although the frequency of this complication varied according to the surgical technique used for wound closure (48). Chronic glaucoma in aphakia was much less common than the early, transient pressure rise. In one series of 203 uncomplicated cataract extractions, persistent glaucoma occurred in 3% of the eyes (49). However, these chronic cases posed a much greater threat to vision and a much more difficult therapeutic challenge than the eyes with transient pressure elevation did.

Pseudophakia

The advent of extracapsular cataract extraction and posterior chamber intraocular lens implantation was generally associated with a reduced incidence of long-term IOP elevation (50). In one series of 373 eyes undergoing cataract surgery, those receiving intracapsular extraction and anterior chamber (133 eyes) or iris fixation (31 eyes) lenses had a late mean IOP rise of 0.8 mm Hg, whereas those undergoing extracapsular surgery with posterior chamber implants (209 eyes) had a mean IOP fall of 0.6 mm Hg (51). Eyes undergoing phacoemulsification cataract extraction also had IOP lowering of 1.1 to 2.5 mm Hg for at least 6 months postoperatively (52). However, extracapsular and phacoemulsification cataract surgeries are associated with pressure complications in the early and late postoperative periods. In eyes without preexisting glaucoma, more than one

half in one series had an IOP of 25 mm Hg or more 2 to 3 hours postoperatively (53), and the IOP exceeded 23 mm Hg on the first postoperative day in 29% of eyes in another study (54). Chronic glaucoma was seen in 4% of eyes after standard extracapsular extraction in one series and in 2.1% of another large series (54,55). Postoperative glaucoma also occurred in 11.3% of eyes receiving secondary anterior chamber implants (56).

With any cataract procedure, early and late postoperative IOP elevations can occur by a wide variety of mechanisms.

Mechanism of Intraocular Pressure Elevation

Influence of Viscoelastic Substances

To protect the corneal endothelium and maintain anterior chamber depth during certain stages of cataract extraction and intraocular lens implantation, filling the anterior chamber with a viscous aqueous substitute has become common practice. The viscoelastic substance that has received the most extensive evaluation for this purpose is sodium hyaluronate (Healon). Although some surgeons have found no significant postoperative pressure rises associated with the use of sodium hyaluronate (57), others have documented high pressures in the first few days after surgery (58). Sodium hyaluronate injected into the anterior chamber of rabbit and monkey eyes caused marked pressure rises (59), and perfusion in enucleated human eyes decreased the outflow facility by 65% (60). This was not reversed by vigorous anterior chamber irrigation, but facility was restored to baseline by irrigation with hyaluronidase. The most likely mechanism of IOP elevation is temporary obstruction of the trabecular meshwork by the viscoelastic.

Alternative viscoelastic substances have also been evaluated. Chondroitin sulfate caused minimal pressure elevation when used during lens implantation in various animal eyes or when injected as a 10% concentration into the anterior chamber of rabbit and monkey eyes (59,61). A formulation of chondroitin sulfate and sodium hyaluronate (Viscoat) was compared with sodium hyaluronate and was less advantageous during cataract surgery in one study and caused IOP rises in the immediate postoperative period in many patients (62). In another study, the duration of IOP elevation was found to be shorter with formulation including chondroitin sulfate (63). A modified sodium hyaluronate viscoelastic (Healon GV), which has a higher molecular weight, viscosity, and sodium hyaluronate concentration than Healon, was associated with a similar postoperative IOP course to that of the latter agent (64). Patients receiving a newer viscoelastic, Healon 5, with special rheologic properties had a lower IOP in the postoperative period, compared with patients receiving Viscoat (65); however, in other studies, postoperative IOP spike did not differ between patients receiving Healon 5 and those receiving other viscoelastics (66,67). Use of ethylcellulose (1% to 2%) did not cause a significant postoperative pressure rise in animal or human eyes and appeared to provide good protection of the corneal endothelium (60,68). In comparative trials, hydroxypropyl methylcellulose, 2%, was found to have the same effect on corneal thickness as balanced salt solution with no rise in IOP and the same early, mild IOP elevation as with sodium hyaluronate 1% (69,70).

Inflammation and Hemorrhage

Transient postoperative inflammation occurs to some degree after every cataract extraction. When excessive, obstruction of the trabecular meshwork by inflammatory cells and fibrin may lead to IOP elevations. The inflammatory response and associated glaucoma may be particularly prominent when lens fragments are retained in the vitreous after extracapsular cataract extraction (71).

Intraocular lens implants increase the risk of serious postoperative uveitis, especially with anterior chamber lenses and, historically, with iris-supported lenses (72). This may be associated with hyphema and glaucoma, which has been referred to as the uveitis, glaucoma, and hemorrhage (UGH) syndrome (73). Uveitis was particularly common with the iris-supported lenses, apparently because of the movement of the lens against the iris and the subsequent cellular reaction (74,75). The inflammation and hemorrhage with anterior chamber lenses is thought to be caused by the contact of the rough posterior surface of the lens with the iris. This has been borne out on ultrasonographic biomicroscopy, which can help detect malpositioned haptics (especially with posterior chamber lenses) and be used to plan subsequent surgical intervention (76). The degree to which lens–iris contact liberates pigment may be related to the design and quality of the specific lens (73,77). Posterior chamber lenses are least likely to induce uveitis. Fluorophotometric studies have shown that pseudophakic eyes with a posterior chamber lens and an intact posterior lens capsule have minimal alteration in the blood–aqueous barrier (78).

In addition to hyphema associated with uveitis, bleeding in the aqueous or vitreous compartments may be seen immediately after cataract surgery or as a late or recurring complication. One source of the late hemorrhage is new vessels in the corneoscleral wound (79). Intraocular lens implantation may also be complicated by late or recurrent hemorrhage, which has been reported with anterior chamber, iris fixation, and posterior chamber implants (80–82). Posterior chamber implants usually have sulcus fixation, and the mechanism in all cases is presumably erosion into the adjacent tissue. Postoperative bleeding from any source may lead to IOP elevation by the mechanisms discussed in Chapter 24, including ghost cell glaucoma from a vitreous hemorrhage (83).

Pigment Dispersion

Variable amounts of pigment granules, primarily from the iris pigment epithelium, are dispersed into the anterior chamber with all cataract operations. Excessive pigment dispersion can lead to transiently elevated IOP in aphakic or pseudophakic eyes, with the latter occasionally leading to a chronic form of glaucoma.

Pseudophakic pigmentary glaucoma is most often associated with posterior chamber lenses (84,85). Pigment dispersion is produced by rubbing of the iris pigment epithelium against the optic and loops of the intraocular lens. This leads to the dispersion of pigment granules, which cause obstruction of the trabecular meshwork—a process similar to phakic pigmentary glaucoma. Acute pigmentary glaucoma has been

reported with one-piece lenses in which one of the haptics has dislocated into the sulcus. Pigment granules on the central corneal endothelium (i.e., Krukenberg spindle) are occasionally noted. Pigment granules may be visualized circulating in the aqueous humor in the anterior chamber, especially after pupillary dilatation. The most useful diagnostic finding is iris transillumination defects at the site of contact with the lens implant. Gonioscopy typically reveals heavy pigmentation of the trabecular meshwork.

Unilateral IOP elevation and bilateral pigmentary dispersion syndrome have been reported after implantation of phakic refractive intraocular lenses (86). Acquired pigmentary glaucoma should be considered for patients with phakic intraocular lenses. These patients should be monitored for this condition.

Vitreous Filling the Anterior Chamber

Grant (87) described a mechanism of acute open-angle glaucoma in which vitreous humor fills the anterior chamber after cataract surgery; this could be cured in some cases by mydriasis to minimize pupillary block, but other eyes required miosis to draw the vitreous from the angle. Simmons (88) observed that many cases resolve spontaneously in several months. When surgical intervention is required, an iridotomy may be curative, but other eyes will require an anterior vitrectomy (89).

Pupillary Block

In Aphakia

This is a relatively rare complication of intracapsular cataract extraction (90). It is more likely to occur weeks after a transient flat anterior chamber secondary to a wound leak. The condition may also be more common after surgery for congenital cataracts. A combination of sector and peripheral iridectomies may minimize this complication (91). Modern approaches to congenital cataract surgery render these measures unnecessary, although a peripheral iridectomy is still advisable.

The pathogenesis of pupillary block in aphakia can be caused by adherence between the iris and anterior vitreous face, which increases the resistance of aqueous humor flow into the anterior chamber through the pupil or iridectomy. In these cases, the aqueous humor accumulates behind the iris, causing a forward shift of the iris and narrowing of the anterior chamber angle (**Fig. 26.7**). The mechanism may be dependent on an intact anterior hyaloid, because fluorescein studies have shown that aqueous will flow preferentially through spontaneous openings in the vitreous face (92). This condition may be distinguished from the much less common malignant glaucoma in aphakia by the deeper central anterior chamber and forward bowing of the peripheral iris in the eyes with aphakic pupillary block glaucoma (93) (**Fig. 26.8**).

In Pseudophakia

Pupillary block glaucoma in pseudophakia was once seen most often with anterior chamber and iris-supported lenses, although there are numerous reports of this complication occurring with posterior chamber lenses (94,95). It usually appears early after surgery but may rarely be delayed months or years.

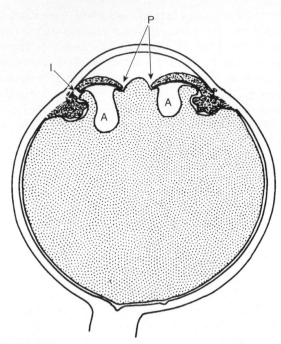

Figure 26.7 Pupillary block in aphakia. An adherence between the iris and anterior vitreous face blocks the flow of aqueous into the anterior chamber at the pupil *(P)* and iridectomy site *(I)*. The posterior accumulation of aqueous *(A)* causes forward bowing of the peripheral iris with closure of the anterior chamber angle.

Many cases are asymptomatic and are discovered on routine postoperative examination. Some may even have a normal IOP, although peripheral anterior synechiae and chronic pressure elevation usually follow if the peripheral anterior chamber depth is not promptly restored. With anterior chamber lenses, the iris bulges forward on either side of the lens (**Fig. 26.9**), whereas the mechanism with posterior chamber lenses appears to be excessive inflammation with posterior synechiae to the intraocular lens or the anterior lens capsule (96).

With modern cataract techniques and intraocular lens implantation in the posterior chamber, the incidence of pupillary

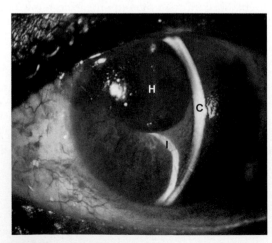

Figure 26.8 Slitlamp view of an eye with pupillary block in a patient with aphakia shows the hyaloid face *(H)* well back from the cornea *(C)* centrally but peripheral anterior bowing of the iris *(I)* with closure of anterior chamber angle.

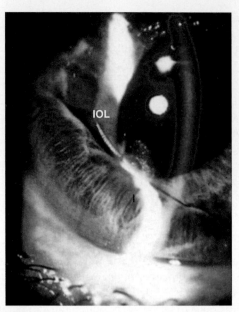

Figure 26.9 Slitlamp view of pupillary block in a pseudophakic eye shows forward bulging of the iris *(I)* peripheral to the margin of the anterior chamber intraocular lens *(IOL)*.

block glaucoma in pseudophakia is sufficiently low that a peripheral iridectomy is no longer a routine part of cataract surgery. However, when excessive postoperative inflammation is anticipated or when combined with a filtering procedure, an iridectomy is still advisable in most cases.

Peripheral Anterior Synechiae or Trabecular Damage

In most cases of chronic glaucoma in aphakia or pseudophakia, peripheral anterior synechiae are present, presumably because of a flat anterior chamber or the presence of inflammation or debris in the early postoperative period. Flat anterior chambers after cataract surgery may be caused by a wound leak with subsequent hypotony and choroidal detachments. To avoid the complication of peripheral anterior synechiae and chronic glaucoma, a flat anterior chamber should be corrected promptly. In one series of 203 uncomplicated cataract extractions, 47% had some degree of peripheral anterior synechiae, and all of those with associated glaucoma had peripheral anterior synechiae present in more than one quarter of the filtering angle (49).

In other cases of glaucoma in aphakia or pseudophakia, the angle may be open in all quadrants and appear essentially normal. The mechanism of aqueous outflow obstruction in cases of chronic open-angle glaucoma (COAG) in aphakia or pseudophakia is uncertain, but it most likely is related to alterations in the trabecular meshwork due to the surgery and possibly a preexisting reduction in outflow facility. In many of these patients, COAG may have been present but undiagnosed preoperatively.

Distortion of the Anterior Chamber Angle

Kirsch and colleagues (97) described the gonioscopic appearance of an internal white ridge resembling an inverted snowbank along the inner margins of the corneoscleral incision after routine cataract extraction. For approximately the first 2 weeks, the ridge typically obscures visualization of the trabecular meshwork and then gradually recedes over the next few months. There is some controversy regarding the pathogenesis of the internal ridge. Campbell and Grant (98) provided evidence that distortion of the anterior chamber angle is induced by tight corneoscleral sutures, whereas Kirsch and colleagues suggested that edema of the deep corneal stroma is the mechanism (97). Whatever the initiating factors may be, the ridge is known to be associated with the formation of peripheral anterior synechiae, vitreous adhesions, and hyphema. In some cases, it is likely that the white ridge contributes to the early, transient pressure elevation after cataract surgery. In one study of 95 cataract extractions, early IOP rise occurred in 23% of the eyes with limbal incisions but in none with corneal incisions, suggesting that distortion produced by the corneoscleral wound temporarily affects the adjacent trabecular meshwork and aqueous outflow (99).

Glaucoma after Congenital Cataract Surgery

Children tend to have a higher incidence of glaucoma after cataract extraction than adults do. In the United Kingdom, the overall annual incidence of postoperative glaucoma was approximately 5% and the median time to development of glaucoma was 1.3 years (range, 0.4 months to 6.7 years) (100). Younger age at detection of cataract was independently associated with the development of glaucoma. In other studies, the reported prevalence of glaucoma after congenital cataract surgery ranged from 6.1% to 24% (101–103). Although most of the reported cases have involved an open-angle mechanism, a pupillary block mechanism is not uncommon in children with aphakic or pseudophakia. This may be another situation in which an iridectomy is indicated as a part of the cataract surgery. The use of a vitrectomy instrument to aspirate the cataract, with wide excision of the posterior capsule, may reduce the incidence of postoperative glaucoma in children (101). However, even with automated lensectomy and vitrectomy in children, some studies reveal glaucoma rates of 12.5% to 24% (102,103). One study found an increased risk for glaucoma in eyes that underwent postoperative secondary membranectomy for visual axis occlusion, especially when secondary membranectomy was performed within 1 year of primary surgery (104).

Influence of α-Chymotrypsin

Glaucoma via this mechanism is rarely seen today but was common in the era of intracapsular surgery. In 1958, Barraquer (105) demonstrated the value of the enzymatic zonulolysis with α-chymotrypsin in facilitating intracapsular cataract extraction, and the enzyme was commonly used for that purpose. In 1964, Kirsch (106) reported a transient pressure rise in 75% of the eyes in which 2 to 4 mL of a 1:5000 dilution of the enzyme was used, compared with a 24% incidence of high pressures in a group without enzyme. The complication was somewhat more common in patients with preexisting COAG (107).

Nd:YAG Laser Posterior Capsulotomy

Another cause of IOP elevation after extracapsular cataract extraction or phacoemulsification is the use of Nd:YAG laser to perform a discission in the posterior lens capsule when that structure becomes significantly opacified after the initial surgery. In numerous studies, the procedure was associated with significant pressure elevation. The pressure rise may be detected in the first few hours, and the IOP usually returns to its baseline level within 1 week; in some eyes, however, the IOP elevation may last for several weeks, and several large series have revealed persistent or late-onset pressure elevations in 0.8% to 6% of the cases (108,109). Cases have been reported in which the laser-induced pressure elevation caused progressive glaucomatous visual field loss or transient loss of light perception, requiring emergency paracentesis (110,111). Other causes of visual loss after Nd:YAG capsulotomy include cystoid macular edema and retinal detachment (112). Risk factors for significant IOP elevations after Nd:YAG capsulotomy differ among studies, but they include preexisting glaucoma or a preoperative IOP greater than 20 mm Hg, large capsulotomies, a sulcus rather than capsular fixed posterior chamber lens, the absence of a posterior chamber lens, myopia, vitreoretinal disease, vitreous prolapse into the anterior chamber, and the total amount of laser energy used (113–115).

The mechanism of IOP elevation after Nd:YAG capsulotomy is not fully understood, although tonographic studies have shown that it is related to reduced aqueous outflow (115,116). Most cases have an open-angle mechanism, and the obstruction of the trabecular meshwork may be with fibrin and inflammatory cells due to a breakdown in the blood–aqueous barrier or debris from the capsule or cortical remnants (117). Other reported mechanisms of IOP elevation include pupillary block due to forward movement of the vitreous and herniated vitreous occluding a preexisting glaucoma surgical fistula (118,119). Pretreatment with topical apraclonidine, timolol, brimonidine, or topical carbonic anhydrase inhibitors is done to minimize the early postoperative rise in IOP (120).

Management

Preoperative Considerations

In preparing for a cataract operation, certain considerations may help to minimize the risk of postoperative complications related to glaucoma, particularly in eyes with preexisting glaucoma.

Pressure Reduction

Many surgeons elect to reduce the vitreous volume and IOP by applying external pressure to the globe before surgery to maintain a deep anterior chamber and to minimize the potential complications of vitreous loss and expulsive hemorrhage. The external force may be accomplished by digital pressure, a rubber ball with an elastic band around the head, or a pneumatic rubber balloon (i.e., a Honan IOP reducer). Each technique has the potential risk of optic atrophy or arterial occlusion from the excessive or prolonged application of pressure, and the Honan device may be the safest in this regard by allowing monitoring of the pressure in the balloon. Although the IOP does not correlate directly or linearly with the pressure in the Honan balloon, studies suggest that it is safe in normotensive eyes, especially when the instrument is set at 30 mm Hg for 5 minutes (121). However, the induced IOP rise is a function of the initial ocular tension, and marked pressure elevations may occur in eyes with initial levels above 30 mm Hg, indicating the need for extreme caution in these cases. Use of these approaches may be unnecessary if topical or subconjunctival anesthesia is used.

Selection of Intraocular Lens

Intraocular lens implantation in the posterior chamber in association with extracapsular cataract extraction and phacoemulsification, although not devoid of potential glaucoma-related complications, is generally associated with a slight reduction in postoperative IOP and is well tolerated even in eyes with advanced preexisting glaucoma where IOP is satisfactorily controlled. Anterior chamber lenses, however, are more problematic, and preoperative glaucoma or anterior chamber angle abnormalities are relative contraindications to their use. In one study of 18 normotensive eyes with angle-supported lenses, synechiae developed around the haptics in 12 cases (94), which can lead to aqueous outflow obstruction, especially in eyes with preexisting glaucoma. In another study, anterior chamber lens implantation in eyes with preoperative peripheral anterior synechiae was associated with corneal endothelial cell loss, fibrous endothelial metaplasia, and angle cicatrization (122).

Intraoperative Considerations

Attention to gentle handling of tissues, hemostasis, and minimal intraocular manipulation may reduce the risk of postoperative IOP rise associated with hemorrhage or excessive inflammation or pigment dispersion. One study found that the technique of wound closure (specifically, a sutureless sclerocorneal tunnel incision) and the surgeon's experience were more important than prophylactic medications in preventing IOP elevation after phacoemulsification (123). Judicious use of intraocular agents such as viscoelastic substances and thorough irrigation to remove the material at the end of the case, especially in eyes with preexisting glaucoma, may help to minimize the risk of postoperative glaucoma complications.

The miotic agents, acetylcholine and carbachol, are often injected into the eye during cataract surgery to constrict the pupil, especially after implantation of a posterior chamber intraocular lens. Use of acetylcholine, compared with balanced salt solution, was associated with lower IOPs at 3 and 6 hours postoperatively but was not statistically significantly different at 24 hours (124). Use of the combination of preoperative acetazolamide and intraoperative acetylcholine was more effective than either drug alone in controlling postoperative IOP elevation (125). Carbachol was associated with lower postoperative pressures, compared with acetylcholine or balanced salt solution, at 24 hours, 2 days, and 3 days postoperatively (126). The intracameral use of carbachol therefore may be helpful in avoiding early IOP rises, especially in eyes with preexisting glaucoma.

Early Postoperative Period

The IOP can rise a few hours after routine cataract extraction but generally returns to normal within 1 to 3 days. A modest pressure rise (e.g., <30 mm Hg) in a nonglaucomatous eye with a deep anterior chamber is usually of no consequence and requires no antiglaucoma therapy. However, high pressures may cause pain and occasional disruption of the corneoscleral wound. Eyes with preexisting glaucoma and advanced glaucomatous optic atrophy may have further nerve damage with even short episodes of pressure elevation. Anterior ischemic optic neuropathy has occurred during these periods of elevated pressure in eyes with vulnerable optic nerve head circulation (127). If there is pain or a threat to the optic nerve head, cornea, or cataract incision, temporary medical measures should be used.

Several drugs have been evaluated for their efficacy in controlling the early IOP rise in eyes with open anterior chamber angles. Although the results from various studies are somewhat conflicting, a randomized trial showed that topical brinzolamide, brimonidine, 0.2%, timolol, 0.5%, intracameral acetylcholine, and acetazolamide, 250 mg, administered immediately after cataract surgery were more effective than use of no ocular hypotensive medication at reducing the IOP at 6 hours and 20 to 24 hours after surgery (128). Another randomized trial comparing various antiglaucoma drops found that use of a combination of timolol, 0.5%, and dorzolamide, 2%, produced the greatest IOP reduction in the first 24 hours after phacoemulsification cataract surgery (129). Steroids were ineffective in one study (130), but they may help control the pressure when inflammation is excessive. Indomethacin and aspirin have also reduced the postoperative pressure rise (131), presumably by inhibiting prostaglandin synthesis. When uveitis and glaucoma are associated with retained lens fragments in the vitreous, pars plana vitrectomy is reported to yield good results (71).

Uveitis, glaucoma, and hyphema may be managed by using mydriatic agents to minimize iris movement against the lens in mild cases. In more severe cases, steroids should be used for the iritis, and a carbonic anhydrase inhibitor or topical β-blocker or α₂-agonist for the glaucoma. Argon laser photocoagulation may be effective in controlling the hemorrhage in the rare cases in which the bleeding site is visible (132). Recurrent hyphema and glaucoma is usually an indication to remove the lens implant, although this is often difficult and can lead to serious intraoperative complications. When glaucoma and hyphema are associated with vitreous hemorrhage, pars plana vitrectomy has been recommended (133). Pigment dispersion in pseudophakia can usually be controlled medically and gradually becomes easier to manage in most cases; removal of the lens implant is rarely required.

Pupillary block in aphakia may initially be treated with mydriasis to break the block, although an iridotomy is usually required. To be effective, the iridotomy must be placed over a pocket of aqueous behind the iris, rather than an area in which the vitreous is in broad apposition to the posterior surface of the iris. The laser is particularly useful in these cases, because more than one iridotomy can be made until an aqueous pocket is found as evidenced by a deepening of the peripheral anterior chamber. Suggested alternative surgical approaches include separating the iris from the vitreous adhesions with laser iridoplasty, an iris repositor, or pars plana vitrectomy.

Pupillary block in pseudophakia may be broken with mydriatic therapy by enlarging the pupil beyond the edges of an anterior chamber lens or by lysing posterior synechiae from a posterior chamber lens. Use of one or more of the following agents may also be required as an emergency measure: carbonic anhydrase inhibitor, hyperosmotic agent, β-blocker, α₂-agonist. The definitive treatment is an iridotomy, which is best achieved with a laser as soon as possible. The laser may also be used to break the block by dilating the pupil (134). Closed vitrectomy has also been used to relieve pseudophakic pupillary block (135).

Late Postoperative Period

Most patients with chronic glaucoma in aphakia or pseudophakia can and should be managed medically. This is usually done with the use of drugs that reduce aqueous production, such as carbonic anhydrase inhibitors, β-blockers, and α₂-agonists, although miotic therapy can also be effective. Surgical intervention is reserved for cases that are uncontrolled on maximum tolerable medical therapy. Laser trabeculoplasty may be effective in cases that do not have extensive peripheral anterior synechiae and is the initial surgical procedure of choice (136). When strict IOP and visual acuity criteria were used to define success in one study, no surgical procedure was highly effective for chronic glaucoma in aphakia or pseudophakia (137). In one series of trabeculectomies in 82 aphakic eyes, fewer than half were successful (138). Other surgeons, however, have had somewhat better results and feel that trabeculectomy with antimetabolite is the procedure of choice if trabeculoplasty fails or is not possible (136). When conjunctival scarring does not allow performance of a trabeculectomy in a superior quadrant, implantation of a glaucoma drainage device is usually indicated. Transscleral cyclophotocoagulation can also be attempted (see Chapter 41), although it should usually be reserved for patients with poor visual potential or in whom incisional surgery is not possible or thought to have a poor chance of success.

When Nd:YAG capsulotomy is required in the late postoperative period, apraclonidine (1.0% or 0.5%), timolol, or acetazolamide given 1 hour before or immediately after the procedure, or both, effectively minimizes the postlaser pressure rise.

GLAUCOMAS ASSOCIATED WITH EPITHELIAL INGROWTH AND OTHER CELLULAR PROLIFERATIONS

A group of rare but potentially devastating conditions may complicate cataract surgery, incisional glaucoma procedures, or any other incisional operation, and some forms of trauma. These conditions have as their common denominator a proliferation of cells into the anterior chamber.

Epithelial Ingrowth

Clinical Features

With this condition, also referred to as epithelial downgrowth, an epithelial membrane grows into the eye through a penetrating wound. It extends over the posterior surface of the cornea, causing corneal edema, and grows down across the anterior chamber angle and onto the iris, which may lead to a refractory form of glaucoma. It occurs in 0.09% to 0.12% of eyes after cataract surgery (139–142). The incidence appears to be declining with newer cataract techniques, although a case has been reported with a sutureless scleral tunnel incision (142). It may also occur after penetrating trauma, penetrating keratoplasty, and glaucoma surgery (143–145).

Early in the disease process, a wound leak may be present. By slitlamp biomicroscopy, the epithelial ingrowth on the cornea is seen as a thin gray translucent or transparent membrane with a scalloped, thickened leading edge (**Fig. 26.10A**). Specular microscopy may reveal a characteristic pattern of cell borders, which may have some diagnostic value (142). Fluorophotometry has also been reported to have diagnostic value by showing a delayed disappearance of the topically applied fluorescein in the area overlying the membrane (142). The membrane on the iris is more difficult to see, but it typically causes a flattening of the stroma and can be delineated by the characteristic white burns that result from diagnostic application of argon laser photocoagulation (Fig. 26.10B) (146). In one case with a

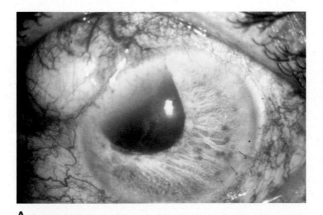

A

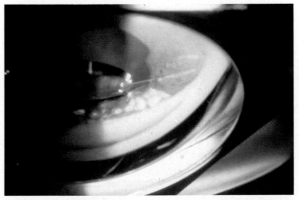

B

Figure 26.10 Epithelial downgrowth. **A:** Clinical appearance of epithelial downgrowth. Note advancing epithelial line located on the corneal endothelium. **B:** Gonioscopic image of white, coagulated areas of epithelium on the iris surface after confirmatory surface treatment with argon laser. (Courtesy of E. Hodapp, MD. From Werner MA, Grajewski AL. Glaucoma in aphakia and pseudophakia. In: Tasman W, Jaeger EA, eds. *Duane's Clinical Ophthalmology*. Vol 3. Philadelphia, PA:Lippincott Williams & Wilkins; 2008:chap 54G.)

penetrating foreign body, the membrane had a gelatinous appearance, which by histology revealed goblet cells and mucinous material (143). Gonioscopy often reveals peripheral anterior synechiae. Cytologic evaluation of an aqueous aspirate has been described as a diagnostic aid (147), although the clinical features are usually sufficient to establish the diagnosis.

Mechanisms of Ingrowth and Glaucoma

A wound leak is generally felt to be the initial factor leading to epithelial ingrowth and is frequently seen at the time of diagnosis (146). Ultrastructural studies show well-developed epithelium, resembling that of the bulbar conjunctiva, growing over posterior cornea, anterior chamber angle, and the iris (148,149). Mechanisms that have been proposed for the glaucoma associated with epithelial ingrowth include the growth of epithelium over the trabecular meshwork, areas of necrosis in the trabecular meshwork, peripheral anterior synechiae, pupillary block, and desquamated epithelium or mucinous material in the aqueous outflow system (139,143,150).

Management

When epithelial ingrowth is present, radical surgical intervention is usually required. Maumenee (146) described a technique of excising the fistula and involved iris and destroying the epithelium on the posterior cornea with cryotherapy. Subsequent modifications have included en bloc excision of the involved chamber angle tissues, excision of all involved tissue followed by keratoplasty, and the use of vitrectomy instruments to remove involved iris and vitreous (151–153). In an eye treated with filtering surgery and adjunctive subconjunctival 5-fluorouracil (5-FU), the epithelial membrane grew rapidly to involve the entire posterior cornea when the injections were stopped (154). A case report described intracameral application of 5-FU resulting in complete clearance of the epithelial membrane (155). Implantation of a Molteno drainage device has provided effective palliative treatment for the associated glaucoma in these cases (156), and a double-plate Molteno shunt combined with penetrating keratoplasty provided IOP control and restoration of vision in two cases (157).

Fibrous Proliferation

Two forms of this condition have been described: fibrous ingrowth and retrocorneal membranes. Fibrous ingrowth is the result of inadequate wound closure after intraocular surgery or penetrating trauma. It has been reported to occur in approximately one third of eyes enucleated after cataract extraction (158). The hallmark of this form of fibrous proliferation is a break in the corneal endothelium and Descemet membrane, which allows fibroblasts to enter the anterior chamber from subepithelial connective tissue or from corneal or limbal stroma (159–161). The fibrous tissue, which is often vascularized, may grow over the corneal endothelium, the anterior chamber angle, and the iris, and into the vitreous cavity. Peripheral anterior synechiae are frequently seen in these cases (161). Clinically, the condition may be difficult to distinguish from epithelial ingrowth, although it is usually less progressive

and less destructive. When glaucoma is present, it may be the result of damage from the surgery or trauma or from the direct effect of the fibrous tissue in the anterior chamber angle. Treatment is generally confined to controlling the IOP, preferably with use of medications, although surgery, such as a cyclodestructive procedure, may be necessary.

Retrocorneal membranes may result from various inflammatory or traumatic insults to the cornea. Descemet membrane is typically intact and the fibrous tissue is believed to represent metaplastic endothelial cells (162). Glaucoma is not commonly associated but may result from the initial insult.

Melanocyte Proliferation

A proliferation of melanocytes from the iris across the trabecular meshwork and posterior surface of the cornea has also been described as a mechanism of glaucoma after cataract extraction (163).

GLAUCOMAS ASSOCIATED WITH CORNEAL PROCEDURES

Penetrating Keratoplasty

Incidence

Penetrating keratoplasty, by using modern techniques of tight wound closure, is complicated by a significant incidence of IOP elevation in both the early and late postoperative periods, although reported incidences vary considerably. One study revealed a 31% incidence of early increases in IOP and a 29% incidence of late (>3 months) increases (164); another large survey had a 9% incidence of immediate postoperative glaucoma and an 18% incidence of chronic postkeratoplasty glaucoma (165). Late, chronic glaucoma is more likely to occur in eyes that had early postoperative pressure rise (166). Factors associated with glaucoma after penetrating keratoplasty include recipient age older than 60 years, aphakia, preexisting glaucoma, preoperative diagnosis of adherent leukoma, bullous keratopathy, herpetic keratitis, trauma or keratoconus, associated vitrectomy, and anterior segment reconstruction (164–170). In one series, the average maximum pressure in the first week was 24 mm Hg in phakic eyes, 40 mm Hg in aphakic eyes, and 50 mm Hg in eyes that had combined cataract extraction and keratoplasty (171). When keratoplasty was combined with cataract extraction, the incidence of glaucoma was higher with intracapsular extraction than with extracapsular surgery (172). The incidence of postkeratoplasty glaucoma is also increased after repeated penetrating keratoplasty (173). Glaucoma after corneal grafting is dangerous not only from the standpoint of glaucomatous optic atrophy but also from the high incidence of associated graft failures (174).

Clinical Findings and Glaucoma Mechanisms

Early Postoperative Period

In some cases, the postoperative glaucoma after penetrating keratoplasty has the same pressure-elevating mechanisms associated with other intraocular procedures, including uveitis, hemorrhage, pupillary block, and steroid-induced glaucoma (175). However, additional mechanisms of early postoperative glaucoma are unique to eyes that have undergone penetrating keratoplasty, especially when aphakia is also present. Two such mechanisms have been postulated.

Collapse of the Trabecular Meshwork. Collapse of the trabecular meshwork may result from the loss of anterior support due to the incision in the Descemet membrane, which may be compounded in the aphakic eye by a reduction in posterior support from the loss of zonular tension (176,177). This hypothesis is supported by the observation that through-and-through suturing in one study was associated with better facility of outflow in autopsy eyes and lower early postoperative IOP, compared with conventional suturing (176,177). Some surgeons, however, report less postoperative pressure rise with use of superficial sutures, which they believe prevents angle distortion (178).

Compression of the Anterior Chamber Angle. Compression of the anterior chamber angle may be caused by the conventional techniques of penetrating keratoplasty, causing an early postoperative IOP rise and subsequent chronic glaucoma due to peripheral anterior synechiae (178,179). (Modified techniques that may help to avoid this complication are discussed under "Management.")

Late Postoperative Period

Gradual flattening of the anterior chamber several months after aphakic keratoplasty has been described (180). This phenomenon appears to be related to an intact anterior vitreous face, and prophylactic vitrectomy has been suggested to avoid this complication. IOP elevation may also occur in association with graft rejection, which may require long-term steroid and antiglaucoma therapy (181). The pigment dispersion syndrome may also be seen with pseudophakic eyes that have undergone corneal transplantation; in these patients, the syndrome has the unique feature of an inferior linear pigmented endothelial line, and it should not be confused with an allograft reaction (182). Another late-developing glaucoma occurs after keratoplasty for congenitally opaque corneas (183). It is not associated with peripheral anterior synechiae, and the mechanism is unknown. Other forms of late-onset glaucoma may result from peripheral anterior synechiae, the long-term use of steroids, or epithelial ingrowth (144,175,184).

Management

Preventive Measures

On the basis of a mathematical model, angle compression may be minimized and trabecular support improved by the following factors: a donor graft that is larger than the recipient trephine; looser or shorter suture bites to minimize tissue compression; smaller trephine size; a thinner peripheral host cornea; and a larger host corneal diameter (179,185). Reports conflict regarding whether an oversized corneal donor graft improves outflow and reduces postkeratoplasty glaucoma. A perfusion study with autopsy eyes revealed no improvement in outflow, and the use of 0.5-mm oversized grafts in a clinical series afforded no protection against postoperative glaucoma (186,187). However, other clinical studies indicate that the use of oversized grafts is associated with deeper anterior chamber depths, a lower incidence of progressive angle closure, and significantly lower postoperative pressures, compared with use of same-sized grafts (188–191). Oversized grafts, however, are contraindicated in treating keratoconus because they cause a significant increase in myopia (192). Another technique to prevent postkeratoplasty angle-closure glaucoma is the placement of sutures near the pupillary portion of a flaccid iris to create a taut iris (193). In addition, glaucoma after keratoplasty can be minimized by using meticulous wound closure and extensive postoperative steroids (194) (with caution for steroid-responsive patients).

Treatment of Glaucoma

Medical Therapy. Medical therapy should be tried first, unless a specific, treatable condition, such as pupillary block, is apparent. However, attempts to alter the early postoperative pressure rise are frequently unsuccessful. Carbonic anhydrase inhibitors were not found to be significantly efficacious in this situation (195), although they may be useful in treating the chronic glaucoma. Reported results with timolol have been conflicting (195), although the drug does appear to have some value, especially in controlling chronic glaucoma after keratoplasty (175). Miotics may occasionally be of value.

Surgical Therapy. Surgical therapy is indicated when the optic nerve head or the graft is threatened by a persistently elevated IOP. No glaucoma operation has been found to be entirely suitable for controlling IOP and preserving graft clarity. One investigation found a 30% incidence of graft failure after any intraocular procedure (196). When penetrating keratoplasty was performed after trabeculectomy in one series, the 5-year probability of successfully maintaining IOP control and a clear graft was only 27%, which increased to 50% in another series of combined trabeculectomy and penetrating keratoplasty (197). Implantation of a Molteno drainage device achieved IOP control of 21 mm Hg or less with one or more procedures in a series of 17 eyes, although seven had allograft rejections (198). In another series, involving 26 eyes with glaucoma drainage devices, final IOP was less than 18 mm Hg in 96% of the eyes but graft failure occurred in 42% (199). Cyclocryotherapy was once the most commonly used surgical procedure for glaucoma after penetrating keratoplasty (200), although the high incidence of serious complications limits its usefulness. Transscleral cyclophotocoagulation has largely replaced cyclocryotherapy as the cyclodestructive procedure of choice. However, in one series of 39 patients, 77% had a final IOP between 7 and 21 mm Hg, but 44% of those with clear grafts before cyclophotocoagulation had graft decompensation (201).

Descemet-Stripping Endothelial Keratoplasty

Glaucoma after Descemet-stripping endothelial keratoplasty has been reported to occur in 0% to 15% of cases by two mechanisms: pupillary block related to the air bubble in the immediate postoperative period and obstruction of the trabecular meshwork resulting from long-term steroid use (202). Management involves use of IOP-lowering medication and release of air from a paracentesis as deemed appropriate.

GLAUCOMA ASSOCIATED WITH KERATOPROSTHESIS

A keratoprosthesis, such as the Boston keratoprosthesis or the osteo-odonto-keratoprosthesis, can be used to provide an optically clear pathway in cases of severe corneal opacification and vascularization—for example, after chemical burns or with autoimmune disorders, such as Stevens–Johnson syndrome. Preexisting glaucoma appears to be a significant risk factor for elevated IOP and visual loss postoperatively (203,204), and as a result, implantation of a glaucoma drainage device at the time of the keratoprosthesis surgery has been suggested (**Fig. 26.11**). Close monitoring of patients for development or exacerbation of glaucoma is warranted in the postoperative period, and if medical management does not sufficiently control the IOP, transscleral diode laser cyclophotocoagulation may be a useful adjunctive measure (205). Measuring IOP in these patients remains problematic.

GLAUCOMAS ASSOCIATED WITH VITREOUS AND RETINAL PROCEDURES

Glaucomas after Pars Plana Vitrectomy

Incidence

IOP elevation is the most common major complication after pars plana vitreous surgery. The reported incidence of postoperative glaucoma ranges from 20% to 26% (206–208). In one prospective study of 222 cases, an IOP rise of 5 to 22 mm Hg during the first 48 hours occurred in 61% of eyes, and an increase of 30 mm Hg occurred in 35% (209).

Clinical Findings and Glaucoma Mechanisms

Many of the factors that lead to IOP elevation after pars plana vitrectomy and the management of these conditions are considered in other chapters. These various mechanisms are reviewed here according to the time frame in which they occur after vitreous surgery.

First Day

Air or long-acting gases such as sulfur hexafluoride and perfluorocarbons (perfluoropropane and perfluoroethane) are occasionally injected into the vitreous cavity to tamponade the retina. The expansion of these gases during the early postoperative period can lead to significant IOP elevation (206–208). Perfluorocarbons are capable of greater expansion and longevity than sulfur hexafluoride (210). In one study of 10 patients receiving 0.3 mL of perfluoropropane, all eyes had an immediate increase in IOP, which was sufficient in four eyes to collapse the central retinal artery (211). However, the pressure fell to baseline level in 30 to 60 minutes and did not rise again for the subsequent 5 days.

Monitoring IOP in the early postoperative period is important when using any long-acting gas, and attention must be given to the tonometer used. Pneumatic tonometry underestimated IOP in gas-filled human autopsy eyes, whereas Perkins applanation tonometry gave the most accurate readings when using a mercury manometer as a reference standard (212). In a clinical study of 84 gas-filled eyes, the Tono-Pen gave pressure readings similar to those obtained by Goldmann applanation tonometry, but pneumatic tonometry again underestimated the IOP (212).

Occasionally, it is necessary to remove a portion of the gas to relieve extremely high IOPs (206). Patients with a gas-filled eye should be cautioned regarding air travel, although expansion of a 0.6-mL bubble during ascent is usually compensated for by accelerated aqueous outflow without a significant IOP rise (213,214). On descent, the eye may become hypotonus, and drugs that reduce aqueous production should be avoided, because they may prolong the hypotony, leading to uveal effusion (214).

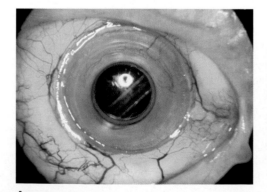

A

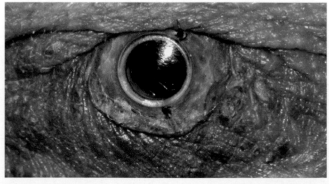

B

Figure 26.11 Slitlamp photographs of patients with keratoprostheses. Glaucoma is a challenging accompaniment in many patients with these devices. **A:** Type I keratoprosthesis used in a patient with intact conjunctiva and adequate tear function. This patient required placement of a glaucoma drainage device for uncontrolled glaucoma. Note the silicone tube in the pupillary space. **B:** Type II keratoprosthesis used for patients with inadequate tear function or conjunctiva. The keratoprosthesis extends through the closed eyelid. (Courtesy of Natalie Afshari, MD.)

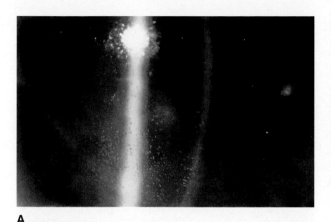
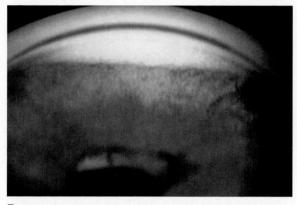

A   B

Figure 26.12 Pupillary block by silicone oil. **A:** IOP is elevated by minute silicone oil bubbles in the anterior chamber angle, seen here to the left of the corneal reflex and on either side of the line of iris illumination. **B:** Gonioscopic view of the superior quadrant, where an accumulated bank of silicone bubbles has created an "inverse pseudohypopyon."

Another class of agents, heavier-than-water perfluorocarbon liquids, can be used to hydrokinetically manipulate the retina, to remove dislocated intraocular lenses and lens fragments, and as short-term tamponade. One of these, perfluoroperhydrophenanthrene (Vitreon), was associated with chronically elevated IOP in 11% of cases (215). The mechanism of the associated glaucoma appears to be angle closure (216).

Severe choroidal and ciliary body hemorrhage, the equivalent of an expulsive hemorrhage in open-eye surgery, can also cause angle-closure glaucoma in the immediate postoperative period (207).

First Week

IOP elevation during this period is most likely caused by hyphema, ghost cells, or hemolytic glaucoma (see Chapter 24); retained lens material with phacolytic glaucoma (see Chapter 18); uveitis (see Chapter 22); or preexisting glaucoma. Another cause of IOP elevation in the early postvitrectomy period is overfill of the anterior chamber (with an open angle) or fibrin pupillary block (217). The latter has been successfully treated with the use of argon laser to make holes in the fibrin pupillary membrane and by the intracameral injection of recombinant tissue plasminogen activator to dissolve the fibrin clot (218,219).

Two to Four Weeks After Surgery

Between 2 and 4 weeks postoperatively, the cause of newly developed glaucoma is most often neovascular glaucoma (discussed in Chapter 19).

Silicone oil is occasionally used as a retinal tamponade in unusually difficult vitreoretinal procedures. The reported frequencies with which this technique is associated with postoperative IOP elevation vary widely, ranging from 5% to 50% (217), and one series showed no influence of silicone on ocular tension (220). This discrepancy may be related to the numerous variables produced by the intraocular silicone and to the underlying disease of the eye, which may reduce aqueous outflow and inflow, with the resulting IOP representing a balance of the two. Most studies, however, suggest that a high percentage of patients do have a transient postoperative pressure rise, with a small proportion retaining chronic glaucoma.

Mechanisms of IOP elevation that are directly attributable to the silicone include pupillary block and silicone oil in the anterior chamber (**Fig. 26.12**). Histologic studies have shown obstruction of the trabecular meshwork by minute silicone bubbles, pigmented cells, and silicone-laden macrophages (221). However, these findings are not always associated with glaucoma. In one study, new glaucoma developed in 10% of eyes with emulsified silicone oil in the anterior chamber (222). The absence of glaucoma in other cases may result from the pressure-lowering effect of ciliary-body detachment by cyclitic membranes or total retinal detachments (223,224). Fibrous tissue has been shown to form around silicone vesicles, the retraction of which may lead to these detachments (224).

An iridectomy may relieve the pupillary-block mechanism and some cases of COAG by allowing the silicone to fall back into the vitreous cavity. Because the silicone oil rises to the top of the eye, the iridectomy should be placed inferiorly, and this should be a standard part of all vitreoretinal procedures that include use of silicone oil. It has been suggested, however, that the iridectomy should be placed peripherally and should be no larger than 2 mm, because a larger, more centrally located inferior iridectomy may allow silicone oil to enter the anterior chamber, creating a form of reverse pupillary block with a deep anterior chamber (225). When the iridectomy does not relieve the chronic IOP elevation, antiglaucoma medications may be adequate, but other patients may require surgical intervention, including removal of the silicone oil, implantation of a glaucoma drainage device, or a cyclodestructive procedure (226).

GLAUCOMAS AFTER SCLERAL BUCKLING PROCEDURES

Scleral buckling procedures are reported to cause a transient shallowing of the anterior chamber with elevation of the IOP in 4% to 7% of cases (227). However, this is frequently asymptomatic and may go undetected unless slitlamp biomicroscopy

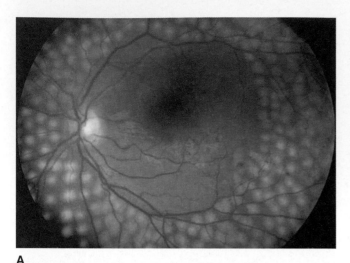

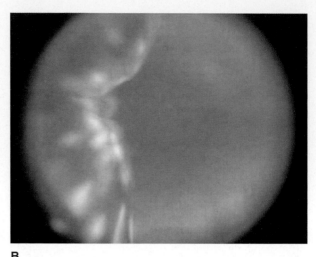

A

B

Figure 26.13 Panretinal photocoagulation with elevated IOP. **A:** The IOP increased in the first few hours after scatter laser photocoagulation of proliferative diabetic retinopathy. **B:** The patient had blurred vision 4 days later and was found to have peripheral choroidal detachments, a closed peripheral angle, and an IOP of 35 mm Hg. Use of cycloplegics, topical corticosteroids, timolol maleate, and acetazolamide rapidly reduced the pressure. The choroidal detachments resolved in 10 days. (From Reiss GR, Sipperley JO. Glaucoma associated with retinal disorders and retinal surgery. In: Tasman W, Jaeger EA, eds. *Duane's Clinical Ophthalmology*. Vol 3. Philadelphia, PA:Lippincott Williams & Wilkins; chap 54E.)

and tonometry are performed in the early postoperative period. Findings of an experimental study with monkeys suggest that occlusion of the vortex veins by an encircling band or sectoral scleral indentation causes congestion and forward rotation of the ciliary body with subsequent shallowing of the anterior segment (228). The same study showed that occlusion of the vortex veins also caused the ciliary processes to produce a protein-rich aqueous, which might further reduce outflow. These changes in the early postoperative period rarely lead to serious sequelae. Many eyes have reduced IOP months after retinal detachment surgery, which is caused by a decrease in aqueous production (229). However, peripheral anterior synechiae may develop with subsequent chronic glaucoma. The physician must be alert for this because reduced scleral rigidity in these patients may give falsely low IOP readings, especially with indentation tonometry (230).

Treatment of angle closure after scleral buckling includes use of atropine to relieve ciliary muscle spasm and use of corticosteroids to reduce the inflammation and prevent synechia formation. Carbonic anhydrase inhibitors, β-blockers, and α₂-agonists may be used when necessary for temporary pressure control. When surgical intervention is required, drainage of suprachoroidal fluid is usually the procedure of choice. A peripheral iridectomy is rarely of value in these cases.

Scleral buckling surgery also causes marked intraoperative IOP elevations. One study, using a pars plana infusion cannula attached to an electronic pressure transducer, documented pressures as high as 210 mm Hg during scleral depression and cryopexy, although the long-term consequences of these pressure elevations are unknown (231). Scleral buckling also may reduce ocular blood flow because of decreased ophthalmic perfusion pressure (232).

GLAUCOMAS AFTER RETINAL PHOTOCOAGULATION

An elevated IOP may follow extensive laser photocoagulation of the retina (**Fig. 26.13**) (233,234). In many cases, the anterior chamber angle remains open, and the mechanism of pressure elevation in these eyes is unknown. Other patients have a closed angle initially or later in the course of the pressure elevation. The mechanism of angle closure is thought to be swelling of the ciliary body or an outpouring of fluid from the choroid to the vitreous with subsequent forward displacement of the lens–iris diaphragm (233). The condition is temporary, with normal or slightly reduced pressures recorded after 1 month (235), although an analysis of data from the Diabetic Retinopathy Study did not support the belief that panretinal photocoagulation could reduce IOP (236). Pretreatment with apraclonidine reduced the incidence of IOP elevations greater than 6 mm Hg during the first 3 hours after laser surgery, compared with placebo drops (25% vs. 32%, respectively), although the difference was not statistically significant (237). The pressure rise should be managed medically in the same manner described for early pressure rise and shallow anterior chamber after scleral buckling.

KEY POINTS

- Malignant or ciliary block glaucoma:
  - Malignant or ciliary block glaucoma occurs most often as a complication of anterior segment incisional surgery in patients with angle-closure glaucoma or shallow anterior chambers.

- The mechanism appears to be increased aqueous flow resistance into the anterior chamber, producing accumulation of aqueous humor in the posterior segment, which leads to a collapse of the anterior chamber from forward vitreous displacement.
- Atropine is the mainstay of medical therapy for malignant glaucoma, although about half of the patients require laser or incisional surgery.

■ Elevated IOP after cataract extraction:
- Causes of increased pressure during the early postoperative period include inflammation, hemorrhage, pigment dispersion, anterior chamber angle distortion, angle closure, vitreous in the anterior chamber, and the use of viscoelastic.
- Chronic glaucoma after cataract surgery may result from peripheral anterior synechiae or trabecular meshwork damage. The implantation of an intraocular lens may induce some additional mechanisms of glaucoma associated with pupillary block, inflammation, hemorrhage, or pigment dispersion.
- YAG laser capsulotomy can also lead to IOP elevation in association with cataract surgery.

■ Epithelial ingrowth and other cellular proliferations in the anterior chamber may be the mechanism of glaucoma after incisional procedures involving the anterior segment and some forms of trauma.

■ Penetrating keratoplasty may be complicated by associated glaucoma, with the common glaucoma mechanism being angle closure.

■ Newer corneal procedures, such as Descemet-stripping endothelial keratoplasty, can also be associated with glaucoma. Vitreoretinal procedures, including vitrectomy, the intravitreal injection of gas or silicone oil, scleral buckling, and retinal photocoagulation, may also be associated with postoperative IOP elevation.

REFERENCES

1. von Graefe A. Beitrage zur pathologie und therapie des glaucoms. *Arch Fur Ophthalmol.* 1869;15:108.
2. Chandler PA, Simmons RJ, Grant WM. Malignant glaucoma: medical and surgical treatment. *Am J Ophthalmol.* 1968;66:495–502.
3. Simmons RJ. Malignant glaucoma. *Br J Ophthalmol.* 1972;56:263–272.
4. Weiss DI, Shaffer RN. Ciliary block (malignant) glaucoma. *Trans Am Acad Ophthalmol Otolaryngol.* 1972;76:450–461.
5. Shaffer RN, Hoskins HD Jr. Ciliary block (malignant) glaucoma. *Ophthalmology.* 1978;85:215–221.
6. Levene R. A new concept of malignant glaucoma. *Arch Ophthalmol.* 1972;87:497.
7. Lowe RF. Malignant glaucoma related to primary angle closure glaucoma. *Aust J Ophthalmol.* 1979;7:11.
8. Cashwell LF, Martin TJ. Malignant glaucoma after laser iridotomy. *Ophthalmology.* 1992;99:651–658.
9. Aminlari A, Sassani JW. Simultaneous bilateral malignant glaucoma following laser iridotomy. *Graefes Arch Clin Exp Ophthalmol.* 1993;231:12–14.
10. Saunders PPR, Douglas GR, Feldman F, et al. Bilateral malignant glaucoma. *Can J Ophthalmol.* 1992;27:19.
11. Burgansky-Eliash Z, Ishikawa H, Schuman JS. Hypotonous malignant glaucoma: aqueous misdirection with low intraocular pressure. *Ophthalmic Surg Lasers Imaging.* 2008;39(2):155–159.
12. Hanish SJ, Lamberg RL, Gordon JM. Malignant glaucoma following cataract extraction and intraocular lens implant. *Ophthalmic Surg.* 1982;13:713–714.
13. Tomey KF, Senft SH, Antonios SR, et al. Aqueous misdirection and flat chamber after posterior chamber implants with and without trabeculectomy. *Arch Ophthalmol.* 1987;105:770–773.
14. Kodjikian L, Gain P, Donate D, et al. Malignant glaucoma induced by a phakic posterior chamber intraocular lens for myopia. *J Cataract Refract Surg.* 2002;28:2217–2221.
15. Pecora JL. Malignant glaucoma worsened by miotics in a postoperative angle-closure glaucoma patient. *Ann Ophthalmol.* 1979;11:1412–1414.
16. Rieser JC, Schwartz B. Miotic-induced malignant glaucoma. *Arch Ophthalmol.* 1972;87:706–712.
17. Merritt JC. Malignant glaucoma induced by miotics postoperatively in open-angle glaucoma. *Arch Ophthalmol.* 1977;95:1988–1989.
18. Mathur R, Gazzard G, Oen F. Malignant glaucoma following needling of a trabeculectomy bleb. *Eye.* 2002;16:667–668.
19. Lass JH, Thoft RA, Bellows AR, et al. Exogenous nocardia asteroides endophthalmitis associated with malignant glaucoma. *Ann Ophthalmol.* 1981;13:317–321.
20. Weiss IS, Deiter PD. Malignant glaucoma syndrome following retinal detachment surgery. *Ann Ophthalmol.* 1974;6:1099–1104.
21. Massicotte EC, Schuman JS. A malignant glaucoma-like syndrome following pars plana vitrectomy [Comment in: *Ophthalmology.* 2000;107:1220–1222]. *Ophthalmology.* 1999;106:1375–1379.
22. Francis BA, Babel D. Malignant glaucoma (aqueous misdirection) after pars plana vitrectomy [Comment in: *Ophthalmology.* 1999;106:1375–1379]. *Ophthalmology.* 2000;107:1220–1222.
23. Azuara-Blanco A, Dua HS. Malignant glaucoma after diode laser cyclophotocoagulation. *Am J Ophthalmol.* 1999;127:467–469.
24. Kushner BJ. Ciliary block glaucoma in retinopathy of prematurity. *Arch Ophthalmol.* 1982;100:1078–1079.
25. Jacoby B, Reed JW, Cashwell LF. Malignant glaucoma in a patient with Down's syndrome and corneal hydrops. *Am J Ophthalmol.* 1990;110:434–435.
26. Schwartz AL, Anderson DR. "Malignant glaucoma" in an eye with no antecedent operation or miotics. *Arch Ophthalmol.* 1975;93:379–381.
27. Shaffer RN. The role of vitreous detachment in aphakic and malignant glaucoma. *Trans Am Acad Ophthalmol Otolaryngol.* 1954;58:217–231.
28. Buschmann W, Linnert D. Echography of the vitreous body in case of aphakia and malignant aphakic glaucoma [in German]. *Klin Monatsbl Augenheilkd.* 1976;168:453–461.
29. Lippas J. Mechanics and treatment of malignant glaucoma and the problem of a flat anterior chamber. *Am J Ophthalmol.* 1964;57:620–627.
30. Tello C, Chi T, Shepps G, et al. Ultrasound biomicroscopy in pseudophakic malignant glaucoma. *Ophthalmology.* 1993;100:1330–1334.
31. Trope GE, Pavlin CJ, Bau A, et al. Malignant glaucoma: clinical and ultrasound biomicroscopic features. *Ophthalmology.* 1994;101:1030–1035.
32. Liu L, Wang T, Li Z. Studies of mechanism of malignant glaucoma using ultrasound biomicroscope [in Chinese]. *Zhonghua Yan Ke Za Zhi.* 1998;34:178.
33. Fatt I. Hydraulic flow conductivity of the vitreous gel. *Invest Ophthalmol Vis Sci.* 1977;16:555–558.
34. Epstein DL, Hashimoto JM, Anderson PJ, et al. Experimental perfusions through the anterior and vitreous chambers with possible relationships to malignant glaucoma. *Am J Ophthalmol.* 1979;88:1078–1086.
35. Quigley HA. Malignant glaucoma and fluid flow rate. *Am J Ophthalmol.* 1980;89:879–880.
36. Chandler PA, Grant WM. Mydriatic-cycloplegic treatment in malignant glaucoma. *Arch Ophthalmol.* 1962;68:353–359.
37. Wright MM, Grajewski AL. Measurement of intraocular pressure with a flat anterior chamber. *Ophthalmology.* 1991;98:1854–1857.
38. Liebmann JM, Weinreb RN, Ritch R. Angle-closure glaucoma associated with occult annular ciliary body detachment. *Arch Ophthalmol.* 1998;116:731–735.
39. Weiss DI, Shaffer RN, Harrington DO. Treatment of malignant glaucoma with intravenous mannitol infusion: medical reformation of the anterior chamber by means of an osmotic agent—a preliminary report. *Arch Ophthalmol.* 1963;69:154–158.
40. Herschler J. Laser shrinkage of the ciliary processes: a treatment for malignant (ciliary block) glaucoma. *Ophthalmology.* 1980;87:1155–1159.
41. Stumpf TH, Austin M, Bloom PA, et al. Transscleral cyclodiode laser photocoagulation in the treatment of aqueous misdirection syndrome. *Ophthalmology.* 2008;115(11):2058–2061.

42. Epstein DL, Steinert RF, Puliafito CA. Neodymium-YAG laser therapy to the anterior hyaloid in aphakic malignant (ciliovitreal block) glaucoma. *Am J Ophthalmol.* 1984;98:137–143.

43. Francis BA, Wong RM, Minckler DS. Slit-lamp needle revision for aqueous misdirection after trabeculectomy. *J Glaucoma.* 2002;11:183–188; author reply 184–185.

44. Sugar HS. Bilateral aphakic malignant glaucoma. *Arch Ophthalmol.* 1972;87:347–351.

45. Koerner FH. Anterior pars plana vitrectomy in ciliary and iris block glaucoma. *Graefes Arch Clin Exp Ophthalmol.* 1980;214:119–127.

46. Byrnes GA, Leen MM, Wong TP, et al. Vitrectomy for ciliary block (malignant) glaucoma. *Ophthalmology.* 1995;102:1308–1311.

47. Bastian A, Kohler U. Therapy and functional results in malignant glaucoma. *Klin Monatsbl Augenheilkd.* 1972;161:316–321.

48. Tuberville A, Tomoda T, Nissenkorn I, et al. Postsurgical intraocular pressure elevation. *J Am Intraocul Implant Soc.* 1983;9:309–312.

49. Racz P, Szilvassy I, Pinter E. Findings in the anterior chamber angle after cataract extraction without complication. *Klin Monatsbl Augenheilkd.* 1974;164:218–220.

50. Hansen TE, Naeser K, Nilsen NE. Intraocular pressure $2\frac{1}{2}$ years after extracapsular cataract extraction and sulcus implantation of posterior chamber intraocular lens. *Acta Ophthalmol.* 1991;69:225–228.

51. Radius RL, Schultz K, Sobocinski K, et al. Pseudophakia and intraocular pressure. *Am J Ophthalmol.* 1984;97:738–742.

52. Tong JT, Miller KM. Intraocular pressure change after sutureless phacoemulsification and foldable posterior chamber lens implantation. *J Cataract Refract Surg.* 1998;24:256–262.

53. Gross JG, Meyer DR, Robin AL, et al. Increased intraocular pressure in the immediate postoperative period after extracapsular cataract extraction. *Am J Ophthalmol.* 1988;105:466–469.

54. Kooner KS, Dulaney DD, Zimmerman TJ. Intraocular pressure following extracapsular cataract extraction and posterior chamber intraocular lens implantation. *Ophthalmic Surg.* 1988;19:471–474.

55. David R, Tessler Z, Yagev R, et al. Persistently raised intraocular pressure following extracapsular cataract extraction. *Br J Ophthalmol.* 1990;74:272–274.

56. Kooner KS, Dulaney DD, Zimmerman TJ. Intraocular pressure following secondary anterior chamber lens implantation. *Ophthalmic Surg.* 1988;19:274–276.

57. Holmberg ÅS, Philipson BT. Sodium hyaluronate in cataract surgery. II. Report on the use of Healon in extracapsular cataract surgery using phacoemulsification. *Ophthalmology.* 1984;91:53–59.

58. Ruusuvaara P, Pajari S, Setala K. Effect of sodium hyaluronate on immediate postoperative intraocular pressure after extracapsular cataract extraction and IOL implantation. *Acta Ophthalmol.* 1990;68:721–727.

59. Mac Rae SM, Edelhauser HF, Hyndiuk RA, et al. The effects of sodium hyaluronate, chondroitin sulfate, and methylcellulose on the corneal endothelium and intraocular pressure. *Am J Ophthalmol.* 1983;95:332–341.

60. Berson FG, Patterson MM, Epstein DL. Obstruction of aqueous outflow by sodium hyaluronate in enucleated human eyes. *Am J Ophthalmol.* 1983;95:668–672.

61. Harrison SE, Soll DB, Shayegan M, et al. Chondroitin sulfate: a new and effective protective agent for intraocular lens insertion. *Ophthalmology.* 1982;89:1254–1260.

62. Alpar JJ, Alpar AJ, Baca J, et al. Comparison of Healon and Viscoat in cataract extraction and intraocular lens implantation. *Ophthalmic Surg.* 1988;19:636–642.

63. Burke S, Sugar J, Farber MD. Comparison of the effects of two viscoelastic agents, Healon and Viscoat, on postoperative intraocular pressure after penetrating keratoplasty. *Ophthalmic Surg.* 1990;21:821–826.

64. Caporossi A, Baiocchi S, Sforzi C, et al. Healon GV versus Healon in demanding cataract surgery. *J Cataract Refract Surg.* 1995;21:710–713.

65. Schwenn O, Dick HB, Krummenauer F, et al. Healon5 versus Viscoat during cataract surgery: intraocular pressure, laser flare and corneal changes. *Graefes Arch Clin Exp Ophthalmol.* 2000;238:861–867.

66. Arshinoff SA, Albiani DA, Taylor-Laporte J. Intraocular pressure after bilateral cataract surgery using Healon, Healon5, and Healon GV. *J Cataract Refract Surg.* 2002;28:617–625.

67. Holzer MP, Tetz MR, Auffarth GU, et al. Effect of Healon5 and 4 other viscoelastic substances on intraocular pressure and endothelium after cataract surgery. *J Cataract Refract Surg.* 2001;27:213–218.

68. Aron-Rosa D, Cohn HC, Aron J-J, et al. Methylcellulose instead of Healon in extracapsular surgery with intraocular lens implantation. *Ophthalmology.* 1983;90:1235–1238.

69. Bigar F, Gloor B, Schimmelpfennig B, et al. Tolerance and safety of intraocular use of 2% hydroxypropylmethylcellulose [in German]. *Klin Monatsbl Augenheilkd.* 1988;193:21–24.

70. Storr-Paulsen A. Analysis of the short-term effect of two viscoelastic agents on the intraocular pressure after extracapsular cataract extraction: sodium hyaluronate 1% vs hydroxypropyl methylcellulose 2%. *Acta Ophthalmol.* 1993;71:173–176.

71. Hutton WL, Snyder WB, Vaiser A. Management of surgically dislocated intravitreal lens fragments by pars plana vitrectomy. *Ophthalmology.* 1978;85:176–189.

72. Layden WE. Pseudophakia and glaucoma. *Ophthalmology.* 1982;89:875–879.

73. Ellingson FT. The uveitis-glaucoma-hyphema syndrome associated with the Mark-VII Choyce anterior chamber lens implant. *J Am Intraocul Implant Soc.* 1978;4:50–53.

74. Miller D, Doane MG. High-speed photographic evaluation of intraocular lens movements. *Am J Ophthalmol.* 1984;97:752–759.

75. Sievers H, von Domarus D. Foreign-body reaction against intraocular lenses. *Am J Ophthalmol.* 1984;97:743–751.

76. Piette S, Canlas OA, Tran HV, et al. Ultrasound biomicroscopy in uveitis-glaucoma-hyphema syndrome. *Am J Ophthalmol.* 2002;133:839–841.

77. Keates RH, Ehrlich DR. "Lenses of chance" complications of anterior chamber implants. *Ophthalmology.* 1978;85:408–414.

78. Sawa M, Sakanishi Y, Shimizu H. Fluorophotometric study of anterior segment barrier functions after extracapsular cataract extraction and posterior chamber intraocular lens implantation. *Am J Ophthalmol.* 1984;97:197–204.

79. Bene C, Hutchins R, Kranias G. Cataract wound neovascularization: an often overlooked cause of vitreous hemorrhage. *Ophthalmology.* 1989;96:50–53.

80. Wiley RG, Neville RG, Martin WG. Late postoperative hemorrhage following intracapsular cataract extraction with the IOLAB 91Z anterior chamber lens. *J Am Intraocul Implant Soc.* 1983;9:466–469.

81. Magargal LE, Goldberg RE, Uram M, et al. Recurrent microhyphema in the pseudophakic eye. *Ophthalmology.* 1983;90:1231–1234.

82. Johnson SH, Kratz RP, Olson PF. Iris transillumination defect and microhyphema syndrome. *J Am Intraocul Implant Soc.* 1984;10:425–428.

83. Summers CG, Lindstrom RL. Ghost cell glaucoma following lens implantation. *J Am Intraocul Implant Soc.* 1983;9:429–433.

84. Woodhams JT, Lester JC. Pigmentary dispersion glaucoma secondary to posterior chamber intraocular lenses. *Ann Ophthalmol.* 1984;16:852–855.

85. Huber C. The gray iris syndrome: an iatrogenic form of pigmentary glaucoma. *Arch Ophthalmol.* 1984;102:397–398.

86. Brandt JD, Mockovak ME, Chayet A. Pigmentary dispersion syndrome induced by a posterior chamber phakic refractive lens. *Am J Ophthalmol.* 2001;131:260–263.

87. Grant WM. Open-angle glaucoma associated with vitreous filling the anterior chamber. *Trans Am Ophthalmol Soc.* 1963;61:196–218.

88. Simmons RJ. The vitreous in glaucoma. *Trans Ophthalmol Soc UK.* 1975;95:422–428.

89. Samples JR, Van Buskirk EM. Open-angle glaucoma associated with vitreous humor filling the anterior chamber. *Am J Ophthalmol.* 1986;102:759–761.

90. Chandler PA. Glaucoma in aphakia. *Trans Am Acad Ophthalmol Otolaryngol.* 1963;67:483–487.

91. Chandler PA. Surgery of congenital cataract. *Trans Am Acad Ophthalmol Otolaryngol.* 1968;72:341–354.

92. Zauberman H, Yassur Y, Sachs U. Fluorescein pupillary flow in aphakics with intact and spontaneous openings of the vitreous face. *Br J Ophthalmol.* 1977;61:450–453.

93. Boke W, Teichmann KD. Differential diagnosis of postoperative glaucoma following iridectomy and filtering procedures [in German]. *Klin Monatsbl Augenheilkd.* 1980;177:545–550.

94. Van Buskirk EM. Pupillary block after intraocular lens implantation. *Am J Ophthalmol.* 1983;95:55–59.

95. Werner D, Kaback M. Pseudophakic pupillary-block glaucoma. *Br J Ophthalmol.* 1977;61:329–333.

96. Naveh N, Wysenbeek Y, Solomon A, et al. Anterior capsule adherence to iris leading to pseudophakic pupillary block. *Ophthalmic Surg.* 1991;22:350–352.

97. Kirsch RE, Levine O, Singer JA. Further studies on the ridge at the internal edge of the cataract incision. *Trans Am Acad Ophthalmol Otolaryngol.* 1977;83:224–231.

98. Campbell DG, Grant WM. Trabecular deformation and reduction of outflow facility due to cataract and penetrating keratoplasty sutures. *Invest Ophthalmol Vis Sci.* 1977;16(suppl):126.

99. Rothkoff L, Biedner B, Blumental M. The effect of corneal section on early increased intraocular pressure after cataract extraction. *Am J Ophthalmol.* 1978;85:337–338.

100. Chak M, Rahi JS. Incidence of and factors associated with glaucoma after surgery for congenital cataract: findings from the British Congenital Cataract Study. *Ophthalmology.* 2008;115(6):1013–1018.

101. Chrousos GA, Parks MM, O'Neill JF. Incidence of chronic glaucoma, retinal detachment and secondary membrane surgery in pediatric aphakic patients. *Ophthalmology.* 1984;91:1238–1241.

102. Egbert JE, Wright MM, Dahlhauser KF, et al. A prospective study of ocular hypertension and glaucoma after pediatric cataract surgery. *Ophthalmology.* 1995;102:1098–1101.

103. Simon JW, Mehta N, Simmons ST, et al. Glaucoma after pediatric lensectomy/vitrectomy. *Ophthalmology.* 1991;98:670–674.

104. Lee AF, Lee SM, Chou JC, et al. Glaucoma following congenital cataract surgery. *Zhonghua Yi Xue Za Zhi (Taipei).* 1998;61:65–70.

105. Barraquer J. Zonulolisis enzymatica. *Ann Med Chir.* 1958;34:148.

106. Kirsch RE. Glaucoma following cataract extraction associated with use of alpha-chymotrypsin. *Arch Ophthalmol.* 1964;72:612–620.

107. Lantz JM, Quigley JH. Intraocular pressure after cataract extraction: effects of alpha-chymotrypsin. *Can J Ophthalmol.* 1973;8:339–343.

108. Keates RH, Steinert RF, Puliafito CA, et al. Long-term follow-up of Nd:YAG laser posterior capsulotomy. *J Am Intraocul Implant Soc.* 1984;10:164–168.

109. Fourman S, Apisson J. Late-onset elevation in intraocular pressure after Neodymium-YAG laser posterior capsulotomy. *Arch Ophthalmol.* 1991;109:511–513.

110. Kurata F, Krupin T, Sinclair S, et al. Progressive glaucomatous visual field loss after neodymium-YAG laser capsulotomy. *Am J Ophthalmol.* 1984;98:632–634.

111. Vine AK. Ocular hypertension following Nd:YAG laser capsulotomy: a potentially blinding complication. *Ophthalmic Surg.* 1984;15:283–284.

112. Steinert RF, Puliafito CA, Kumar SR, et al. Cystoid macular edema, retinal detachment, and glaucoma after Nd:YAG laser posterior capsulotomy. *Am J Ophthalmol.* 1991;112:373–380.

113. Gimbel HV, Van Westenbrugge JA, Sanders DR, et al. Effect of sulcus vs. capsular fixation on YAG-induced pressure rises following posterior capsulotomy. *Arch Ophthalmol.* 1990;108:1126–1129.

114. Schubert HD. Vitreoretinal changes associated with rise in intraocular pressure after Nd:YAG capsulotomy. *Ophthalmic Surg.* 1987;18:19–22.

115. Wetzel W. Ocular aqueous humor dynamics after photodisruptive laser surgery procedures. *Ophthalmic Surg.* 1994;25:298–302.

116. Richter CU, Arzeno G, Pappas HR, et al. Intraocular pressure elevation following Nd:YAG laser posterior capsulotomy. *Ophthalmology.* 1985; 92:636–640.

117. Mitchell PG, Blair NP, Deutsch TA, et al. The effect of neodymium:YAG laser shocks on the blood-aqueous barrier. *Ophthalmology.* 1987;94:488–490.

118. Ruderman JM, Mitchell PG, Kraff M. Pupillary block following Nd:YAG laser capsulotomy. *Ophthalmic Surg.* 1983;14:418–419.

119. Shrader CE, Belcher CD III, Thomas JV, et al. Acute glaucoma following Nd:YAG laser membranotomy. *Ophthalmic Surg.* 1983;14:1015.

120. Pollack IP, Brown RH, Crandall AS, et al. Prevention of the rise in intraocular pressure following neodymium-YAG posterior capsulotomy using topical 1% apraclonidine. *Arch Ophthalmol.* 1988;106:754–757.

121. McDonnell PJ, Quigley HA, Maumenee AE, et al. The Honan intraocular pressure reducer: an experimental study. *Arch Ophthalmol.* 1985;103: 422–425.

122. Rowsey JJ, Gaylor JR. Intraocular lens disasters: peripheral anterior synechia. *Ophthalmology.* 1980;87:646–664.

123. Bömer TG, Lagréze W-DA, Funk J. Intraocular pressure rise after phacoemulsification with posterior chamber lens implantation: effect of prophylactic medication, wound closure, and surgeon's experience. *Br J Ophthalmol.* 1995;79:809–813.

124. Hollands RH, Drance SM, Schulzer M. The effect of acetylcholine on early postoperative intraocular pressure. *Am J Ophthalmol.* 1987;103:749–753.

125. West J, Burke J, Cunliffe I, et al. Prevention of acute postoperative pressure rises in glaucoma patients undergoing cataract extraction with posterior chamber lens implant. *Br J Ophthalmol.* 1992;76:534–537.

126. Ruiz RS, Rhem MN, Prager TC. Effects of carbachol and acetylcholine on intraocular pressure after cataract extraction. *Am J Ophthalmol.* 1989;107:7–10.

127. Hayreh SS. Anterior ischemic optic neuropathy. IV. Occurrence after cataract extraction. *Arch Ophthalmol.* 1980;98:1410–1416.

128. Borazan M, Karalezli A, Akman A, et al. Effect of antiglaucoma agents on postoperative intraocular pressure after cataract surgery with Viscoat. *J Cataract Refract Surg.* 2007;33(11):1941–1945.

129. Schwenn O, Xia N, Krummenauer F, et al. Prevention of early postoperative increase in intraocular pressure after phacoemulsification: comparison of different antiglaucoma drugs [in German]. *Ophthalmology.* 2001;98:934–943.

130. Bloomfield S. Failure to prevent enzyme glaucoma: a negative report. *Am J Ophthalmol.* 1968;64:405–406.

131. Rich WJCC. Prevention of postoperative ocular hypertension by prostaglandin inhibitors. *Trans Ophthalmol Soc UK.* 1977;97:268–271.

132. Pazandak B, Johnson S, Kratz R, et al. Recurrent intraocular hemorrhage associated with posterior chamber lens implantation. *J Am Intraocul Implant Soc.* 1983;9:327–329.

133. Brucker AJ, Michels RG, Green WR. Pars plana vitrectomy in the management of blood-induced glaucoma with vitreous hemorrhage. *Ann Ophthalmol.* 1978;10:1427–1437.

134. Obstbaum SA, Galin MA, Barasch KR, et al. Laser photomydriasis in pseudophakic pupillary block. *J Am Intraocul Implant Soc.* 1981;7:28–30.

135. Mackool RJ. Closed vitrectomy and the intraocular implant. *Ophthalmology.* 1981;88:414–424.

136. Bellows AR, Johnstone MA. Surgical management of chronic glaucoma in aphakia. *Ophthalmology.* 1983;90:807–813.

137. Gross RL, Feldman RM, Spaeth GL, et al. Surgical therapy of chronic glaucoma in aphakia and pseudophakia. *Ophthalmology.* 1988;95:1195–1201.

138. Heuer DK, Gressel MG, Parrish RD II, et al. Trabeculectomy in aphakic eyes. *Ophthalmology.* 1984;91:1045.

139. Bernardino VB, Kim JC, Smith TR. Epithelialization of the anterior chamber after cataract extraction. *Arch Ophthalmol.* 1969;82:742–750.

140. Theobald GD, Haas JS. Epithelial invasion of the anterior chamber following cataract extraction. *Trans Am Acad Ophthalmol Otolaryngol.* 1948;52:470–485.

141. Weiner MJ, Trentacoste J, Pon DM, et al. Epithelial downgrowth: a 30-year clinicopathological review. *Br J Ophthalmol.* 1989;73:6–11.

142. Holliday JN, Buller CR, Bourne WM. Specular microscopy and fluorophotometry in the diagnosis of epithelial downgrowth after a sutureless cataract operation. *Am J Ophthalmol.* 1993;116:238–240.

143. Küchle M, Naumann GOH. Mucogenic secondary open-angle glaucoma in diffuse epithelial ingrowth treated by block-excision. *Am J Ophthalmol.* 1991;111:230–234.

144. Sugar A, Meyer RF, Hood CI. Epithelial downgrowth following penetrating keratoplasty in the aphake. *Arch Ophthalmol.* 1977;95:464–467.

145. Smith RE, Parrett C. Specular microscopy of epithelial downgrowth. *Arch Ophthalmol.* 1978;96:1222–1224.

146. Maumenee AE. Treatment of epithelial downgrowth and intraocular fistula following cataract extraction. *Trans Am Ophthalmol Soc.* 1964;62:153–166.

147. Calhoun FP Jr. An aid to the clinical diagnosis of epithelial downgrowth into the anterior chamber following cataract extraction. *Am J Ophthalmol.* 1966;61:1055–1059.

148. Iwamoto T, Srinivasan BD, DeVoe AG. Electron microscopy of epithelial downgrowth. *Ann Ophthalmol.* 1977;9:1095–1110.

149. Zavala EY, Binder PS. The pathologic findings of epithelial ingrowth. *Arch Ophthalmol.* 1980;98:2007–2014.

150. Jensen P, Minckler DS, Chandler JW. Epithelial ingrowth. *Arch Ophthalmol.* 1977;95:837–842.

151. Naumann GOH, Rummelt V. Block excision of cystic and diffuse epithelial ingrowth of the anterior chamber: report on 32 consecutive patients. *Arch Ophthalmol.* 1992;110:223–227.

152. Friedman AH. Radical anterior segment surgery for epithelial invasion of the anterior chamber: report of three cases. *Trans Am Acad Ophthalmol Otolaryngol.* 1977;83:216–223.

153. Stark WJ, Michels RG, Maumenee AE, et al. Surgical management of epithelial ingrowth. *Am J Ophthalmol.* 1978;85:772–780.

154. Loane ME, Weinreb RN. Glaucoma secondary to epithelial downgrowth and 5-fluorouracil. *Ophthalmic Surg.* 1990;21:704–706.

155. Shaikh AA, Damji KF, Mintsioulis G, et al. Bilateral epithelial downgrowth managed in one eye with intraocular 5-fluorouracil. *Arch Ophthalmol.* 2002;120:1396–1398.

156. Fish LA, Heuer DK, Baerveldt G, et al. Molteno implantation for secondary glaucomas associated with advanced epithelial ingrowth. *Ophthalmology.* 1990;97:557–561.

157. Costa VP, Katz LJ, Cohen EJ, et al. Glaucoma associated with epithelial downgrowth controlled with Molteno tube shunts. *Ophthalmic Surg.* 1992;23:797–800.

158. Allen JC. Epithelial and stromal ingrowths. *Am J Ophthalmol.* 1968; 65:179–182.

159. Swan KC. Fibroblastic ingrowth following cataract extraction. *Arch Ophthalmol.* 1973;89:445–449.

160. Sherrard ES, Rycroft PV. Retrocorneal membranes. II. Factors influencing their growth. *Br J Ophthalmol.* 1967;51:387–393.

161. Friedman AH, Henkind P. Corneal stromal overgrowth after cataract extraction. *Br J Ophthalmol.* 1970;54:528–534.

162. Michels RG, Kenyon KR, Maumenee AE. Retrocorneal fibrous membrane. *Invest Ophthalmol.* 1972;11:822.

163. Ueno H, Green WR, Kenyon KR, et al. Trabecular and retrocorneal proliferation of melanocytes and secondary glaucoma. *Am J Ophthalmol.* 1979;88:592–597.

164. Karesh JW, Nirankari VS. Factors associated with glaucoma after penetrating keratoplasty. *Am J Ophthalmol.* 1983;96:160–164.

165. Foulks GN. Glaucoma associated with penetrating keratoplasty. *Ophthalmology.* 1987;94:871–874.

166. Olson RF, Kaufman HE. Prognostic factors of intraocular pressure after aphakic keratoplasty. *Am J Ophthalmol.* 1978;86:510.

167. Goldberg DB, Schanzlin DJ, Brown SI. Incidence of increased intraocular pressure after keratoplasty. *Am J Ophthalmol.* 1981;92:372–377.

168. Sihota R, Sharma N, Panda A, et al. Post-penetrating keratoplasty glaucoma: risk factors, management and visual outcome. *Aust N Z J Ophthalmol.* 1998;26:305–309.

169. Allouch C, Borderie V, Touzeau O, et al. Incidence and factors influencing glaucoma after penetrating keratoplasty [in French]. *J Fr Ophthalmol.* 2003;26:553–561.

170. Franca ET, Arcieri ES, Arcieri RS, et al. A study of glaucoma after penetrating keratoplasty. *Cornea.* 2003;22:91; author reply 91. *Cornea.* 2002;21:284–288.

171. Irvine AR, Kaufman HE. Intraocular pressure following penetrating keratoplasty. *Am J Ophthalmol.* 1969;68:835–844.

172. Brightbill FS, Stainer GA, Hunkeler JD. A comparison of intracapsular and extracapsular lens extraction combined with keratoplasty. *Ophthalmology.* 1983;90:34–37.

173. Robinson CH Jr. Indications, complications and prognosis for repeat penetrating keratoplasty. *Ophthalmic Surg.* 1979;10:27–34.

174. Heydenreich A. Corneal regeneration and intraocular tension. *Klin Monatsbl Augenheilkd.* 1966;148:500.

175. Lass JH, Pavan-Langston D. Timolol therapy in secondary angle-closure glaucoma post penetrating keratoplasty. *Ophthalmology.* 1979;86:51–59.

176. Zimmerman TJ, Krupin T, Grodzki W, et al. The effect of suture depth on outflow facility in penetrating keratoplasty. *Arch Ophthalmol.* 1978;96:505–506.

177. Zimmerman TJ, Waltman SR, Sachs U, et al. Intraocular pressure after aphakic penetrating keratoplasty "through-and-through" suturing. *Ophthalmic Surg.* 1979;10:49–52.

178. Nissenkorn I, Wood TO. Intraocular pressure following aphakic transplants. *Ann Ophthalmol.* 1983;15:1168–1171.

179. Olson RJ, Kaufman HE. A mathematical description of causative factors and prevention of elevated intraocular pressure after keratoplasty. *Invest Ophthalmol Vis Sci.* 1977;16:1085–1092.

180. Gnad HD. Athalamia as a late complication after keratoplasty on aphakic eyes. *Br J Ophthalmol.* 1980;64:528–530.

181. Polack FM. Graft rejection and glaucoma. *Am J Ophthalmol.* 1986;101:294–297.

182. Insler MS, McShrerry Zatzkis S. Pigment dispersion syndrome in pseudophakic corneal transplants. *Am J Ophthalmol.* 1986;102:762–765.

183. Schanzlin DJ, Goldberg DB, Brown SI. Transplantation of congenitally opaque corneas. *Ophthalmology.* 1980;87:1253–1264.

184. Yamaguchi T, Polack FM, Valenti J. Electron microscopic study of epithelial downgrowth after penetrating keratoplasty. *Br J Ophthalmol.* 1981;65:374–382.

185. Olson RJ. Aphakic keratoplasty: determining donor tissue size to avoid elevated intraocular pressure. *Arch Ophthalmol.* 1978;96:2274–2276.

186. Zimmerman TJ, Krupin T, Grodzki W, et al. Size of donor corneal button and outflow facility in aphakic eyes. *Ann Ophthalmol.* 1979;11:809–811.

187. Perl T, Charlton KH, Binder PS. Disparate diameter grafting: astigmatism, intraocular pressure, and visual acuity. *Ophthalmology.* 1981;88:774–781.

188. Heidemann DG, Sugar A, Meyer RF, et al. Oversized donor grafts in penetrating keratoplasty: a randomized trial. *Arch Ophthalmol.* 1985;103:1807–1811.

189. Foulks GN, Perry HD, Dohlman CH. Oversize corneal donor grafts in penetrating keratoplasty. *Ophthalmology.* 1979;86:490–494.

190. Zimmerman T, Olson R, Waltman S, et al. Transplant size and elevated intraocular pressure: postkeratoplasty. *Arch Ophthalmol.* 1978;96:2231–2233.

191. Bourne WM, Davison JA, O'Fallon WM. The effects of oversize donor buttons on postoperative intraocular pressure and corneal curvature in aphakic penetrating keratoplasty. *Ophthalmology.* 1982;89:242–246.

192. Perry HD, Foulks GN. Oversize donor buttons in corneal transplantation surgery for keratoconus. *Ophthalmic Surg.* 1987;18:751–752.

193. Cohen EJ, Kenyon KR, Dohlman CH. Iridoplasty for prevention of post-keratoplasty angle closure and glaucoma. *Ophthalmic Surg.* 1982;13:994–996.

194. Thoft RA, Gordon JM, Dohlman CH. Glaucoma following keratoplasty. *Trans Am Acad Ophthalmol Otolaryngol.* 1974;78:352–364.

195. Olson RJ, Kaufman HE, Zimmerman TJ. Effects of timolol and Daranide on elevated intraocular pressure after aphakic keratoplasty. *Ann Ophthalmol.* 1979;11:1833–1836.

196. Lemp MA, Pfister RR, Dohlman CG. The effect of intraocular surgery on clear corneal grafts. *Am J Ophthalmol.* 1970;70:719–721.

197. Kirkness CM, Steele AD, Ficker LA, et al. Coexistent corneal disease and glaucoma managed by either drainage surgery and subsequent keratoplasty or combined drainage surgery and penetrating keratoplasty. *Br J Ophthalmol.* 1992;76:146–152.

198. McDonnell PJ, Robin JB, Schanzlin DJ, et al. Molteno implant for control of glaucoma in eyes after penetrating keratoplasty. *Ophthalmology.* 1988;95:364–369.

199. Sherwood MB, Smith MF, Driebe WT Jr, et al. Drainage tube implants in the treatment of glaucoma following penetrating keratoplasty. *Ophthalmic Surg.* 1993;24:185–189.

200. Binder PS, Abel R Jr, Kaufman HE. Cyclocryotherapy for glaucoma after penetrating keratoplasty. *Am J Ophthalmol.* 1975;79:489–492.

201. Threlkeld AB, Shields MB. Noncontact transscleral Nd:YAG cyclophotocoagulation for glaucoma after penetrating keratoplasty. *Am J Ophthalmol.* 1995;120:569–576.

202. Lee WB, Jacobs DS, Musch DC, et al. Descemet's stripping endothelial keratoplasty: safety and outcomes: a report by the American Academy of Ophthalmology. *Ophthalmology.* 2009;116(9):1818–1830.

203. Sayegh RR, Ang LP, Foster CS, et al. The Boston keratoprosthesis in Stevens–Johnson syndrome. *Am J Ophthalmol.* 2008;145(3):438–444.

204. Kumar RS, Tan DT, Por YM, et al. Glaucoma management in patients with osteo-odonto-keratoprosthesis (OOKP): the Singapore OOKP Study. *J Glaucoma.* 2009;18(5):354–360.

205. Rivier D, Paula JS, Kim E, et al. Glaucoma and keratoprosthesis surgery: role of adjunctive cyclophotocoagulation. *J Glaucoma.* 2009;18(4):321–324.

206. Faulborn J, Conway BP, Machemer R. Surgical complications of pars plana vitreous surgery. *Ophthalmology.* 1978;85:116–125.

207. Aaberg TM, Van Horn DL. Late complications of pars plana vitreous surgery. *Ophthalmology.* 1978;85:126–140.

208. Ghartey KN, Tolentino FI, Freeman HM, et al. Closed vitreous surgery. XVII. Results and complications of pars plana vitrectomy. *Arch Ophthalmol.* 1980;98:1248–1252.

209. Han DP, Lewis H, Lambrou FH Jr, et al. Mechanisms of intraocular pressure elevation after pars plana vitrectomy. *Ophthalmology.* 1989;96:1357–1362.

210. Crittenden JJ, deJuan E Jr, Tiedeman J. Expansion of long-acting gas bubbles for intraocular use: principles and practice. *Arch Ophthalmol.* 1985;103:831–834.

211. Coden DJ, Freeman WR, Weinreb RN. Intraocular pressure response after pneumatic retinopexy. *Ophthalmic Surg.* 1988;19:667–669.

212. Hines MW, Jost BF, Fogelman KL. Oculab Tono-Pen, Goldmann applanation tonometry, and pneumatic tonometry for intraocular pressure assessment in gas-filled eyes. *Am J Ophthalmol.* 1988;106:174–179.

213. Lincoff H, Weinberger D, Reppucci V, et al. Air travel with intraocular gas. I. The mechanisms for compensation. *Arch Ophthalmol.* 1989;107:902–906.

214. Lincoff H, Weinberger D, Stergiu P. Air travel with intraocular gas. II. Clinical considerations. *Arch Ophthalmol.* 1989;107:907–910.

215. Adile SL, Peyman GA, Greve MDJ, et al. Postoperative chronic pressure abnormalities in the Vitreon study. *Ophthalmic Surg.* 1994;25:584–589.

216. Foster RE, Smiddy WS, Alfonso EC, et al. Secondary glaucoma associated with retained perfluorophenanthrene. *Am J Ophthalmol.* 1994;118:253–255.

217. Ichhpujani P, Jindal A, Jay Katz L. Silicone oil induced glaucoma: a review. *Graefes Arch Clin Exp Ophthalmol.* 2009;247(12):1585–1593.

218. Lewis H, Han D, Williams GA. Management of fibrin pupillary-block glaucoma after pars plana vitrectomy with intravitreal gas injection. *Am J Ophthalmol.* 1987;103:180–182.

219. Jaffe GJ, Lewis H, Han DP, et al. Treatment of postvitrectomy fibrin pupillary block with tissue plasminogen activator. *Am J Ophthalmol.* 1989;108:170–175.

220. Watzke RC. Silicone retinopiesis for retinal detachment: a long-term clinical evaluation. *Arch Ophthalmol.* 1967;77:185–196.

221. Ni C, Wang W-J, Albert DM, et al. Intravitreous silicone injection: histopathologic findings in a human eye after 12 years. *Arch Ophthalmol.* 1983;101:1399–1401.

222. Valone J Jr, McCarthy M. Emulsified anterior chamber silicone oil and glaucoma. *Ophthalmology.* 1994;101:1908–1912.

223. Sugar HS, Okamura ID. Ocular findings six years after intravitreal silicone injection. *Arch Ophthalmol.* 1976;94:612–615.

224. Laroche L, Pavlakis C, Saraux H, et al. Ocular findings following intravitreal silicone injection. *Arch Ophthalmol.* 1983;101:1422–1425.

225. Bartov E, Huna R, Ashkenazi I, et al. Identification, prevention, and treatment of silicone oil pupillary block after an inferior iridectomy. *Am J Ophthalmol.* 1991;111:501–504.

226. Nguyen QH, Lloyd MA, Heuer DK, et al. Incidence and management of glaucoma after intravitreal silicone oil injection for complicated retinal detachments. *Ophthalmology.* 1992;99:1520–1526.

227. Sebestyen JG, Schepens CL, Rosenthal ML. Retinal detachment and glaucoma. I. Tonometric and gonioscopic study of 160 cases. *Arch Ophthalmol.* 1962;67:736.

228. Hayreh SS, Baines JAB. Occlusion of the vortex veins: an experimental study. *Br J Ophthalmol.* 1973;57:217–238.

229. Araie M, Sugiura Y, Minota K, et al. Effects of the encircling procedure on the aqueous flow rate in retinal detachment eyes: a fluorometric study. *Br J Ophthalmol.* 1987;71:510–515.

230. Johnson MW, Han DP, Hoffman KE. The effect of scleral buckling on ocular rigidity. *Ophthalmology.* 1990;97:190–195.

231. Gardner TW, Quillen DA, Blankenship GW, et al. Intraocular pressure fluctuations during scleral buckling surgery. *Ophthalmology.* 1993; 100:1050–1054.

232. Yoshida A, Hirokawa H, Ishiko S, et al. Ocular circulatory changes following scleral buckling procedures. *Br J Ophthalmol.* 1992;76:529–531.

233. Mensher JH. Anterior chamber depth alteration after retinal photocoagulation. *Arch Ophthalmol.* 1977;95:113–116.

234. Blondeau P, Pavan PR, Phelps CD. Acute pressure elevation following panretinal photocoagulation. *Arch Ophthalmol.* 1981;99:1239–1241.

235. Schidte SN. Changes in eye tension after panretinal xenon arc and argon laser photocoagulation in normotensive diabetic eyes. *Acta Ophthalmol.* 1982;60:692–700.

236. Kaufman SC, Ferris FL III, Swartz M, et al. Intraocular pressure following panretinal photocoagulation for diabetic retinopathy: diabetic retinopathy report no. 11. *Arch Ophthalmol.* 1987;105:807–809.

237. Tsai JC, Lee MB, WuDunn D, et al. Incidence of acute intraocular pressure elevation after panretinal photocoagulation. *J Glaucoma.* 1995;4:45–48.

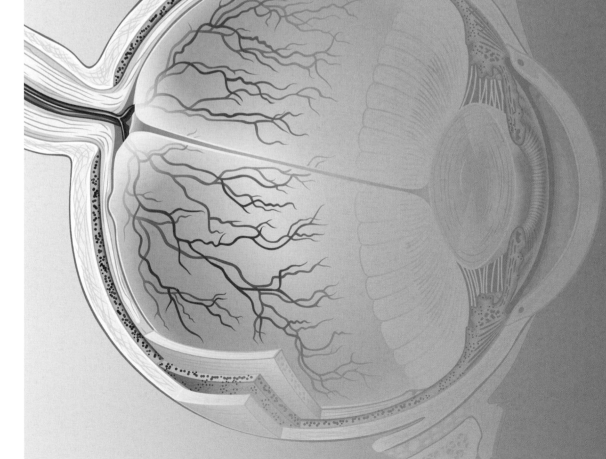

Management of Glaucoma

Principles of Medical Therapy and Management

This chapter covers the management of the patient with glaucoma using an evidence-based approach. The following factors will be considered: (a) making an accurate clinical diagnosis; (b) assessing the stage of disease; (c) assessing the risk factors for disease progression; (d) understanding the patient's access to health care and related factors; (e) considering the patient's lifestyle, health status, and life expectancy; and (f) implementing a treatment strategy on the basis of these factors and other considerations. All of these factors influence how aggressive the physician should be to achieve the target intraocular pressure (IOP) range to minimize the progression of glaucomatous optic neuropathy. In addition, given the current resources for information and technology through the Internet, literature, glaucoma support groups, and other sources, patients are better informed today (although sometimes misinformed) about their glaucomatous conditions. It is essential to make the patient a part of the team in his or her care, which includes discussion of treatment options from medical to laser or surgical interventions.

GATHERING EVIDENCE TO EVALUATE THE PATIENT

After gathering the data on the patient and making the clinical diagnosis (as described in the preceding chapters), the physician must understand the evidence from the results of major epidemiology studies (see Chapter 9) and glaucoma clinical trials to develop a management plan for the individual patient. Four major prospective National Institutes of Health–sponsored glaucoma clinical trials have shown that lowering IOP is important for "protecting" the susceptible optic nerve in patients with glaucoma (see Chapters 10 and 11, and the National Eye Institute's Web site: www.nei.nih.gov/neitrials/topics.asp#glaucoma). In addition, another glaucoma clinical trial reported on the benefit of reducing IOP in patients with normal-tension glaucoma (1). These large-scale randomized clinical trials were designed to study outcomes in a cohort of patients with different forms and stages of chronic open-angle glaucoma (COAG) or suspected glaucoma. Results of these studies can be used as we recommend management and treatment for the individual patient. The results are summarized below.

Ocular Hypertension Treatment Study

The Ocular Hypertension Treatment Study (OHTS) evaluated the safety and efficacy of topical ocular hypotensive medication in delaying or preventing the onset of COAG in participants with no initial glaucomatous damage and an IOP between 24 and 32 mm Hg (2,3). An important aspect of the design of this study was to evaluate the risk for glaucoma in patients of both European ancestry and black African descent. The 1636 participants were randomly assigned to observation or treatment with a target IOP reduction of 20%. The investigators found that topical ocular hypotensive medications can delay the onset of COAG in patients with elevated IOP, although not all patients with ocular hypertension require treatment. In the multivariate analysis, race was not a significant risk factor, which can be explained by the fact that African Americans in OHTS had overall thinner central corneas and larger optic discs. The clinical risk factors that increased the risk for glaucoma included older age, large cup-to-disc ratio, early visual field loss, thin central cornea, and elevated IOP.

Early Manifest Glaucoma Trial

The Early Manifest Glaucoma Trial (EMGT) assessed treatment versus observation without treatment in patients with early glaucoma and found that progression was less frequent and occurred later in treated patients (4,5). The EMGT demonstrated that the following factors were predictors of glaucoma progression: elevated IOP, older age, bilaterality, exfoliation, disc hemorrhages, and relatively thin central cornea. In addition, lower systolic perfusion pressure, lower systolic blood pressure, and cardiovascular disease history emerged as new predictors, suggesting a vascular role in glaucoma progression (6).

Collaborative Initial Glaucoma Treatment Study

The Collaborative Initial Glaucoma Treatment Study (CIGTS) evaluated the efficacy and safety of surgery versus medical treatment in patients with newly diagnosed, early glaucoma and found similar outcomes with the two treatment approaches (7). Investigators also found that when patients receive a glaucoma diagnosis, they may have symptoms that are not elicited by routine clinical testing, requiring discussion with the patient to reduce worries and unnecessary concerns about blindness and improving their quality of life (8).

Advanced Glaucoma Intervention Study

The Advanced Glaucoma Intervention Study (AGIS) investigated two surgical sequences in patients with advanced glaucoma. One sequence began with argon laser trabeculoplasty followed by trabeculectomy, if necessary; the other began with trabeculectomy and was followed by argon laser trabeculoplasty if the trabeculectomy failed. The study provided a weak suggestion that an initial argon laser trabeculoplasty delays the progression of glaucoma more effectively in black patients than in white patients (9). Retrospective evaluation of the study data suggest that consistent, low IOPs with minimal IOP variation is associated with reduced progression of visual field in patients with advanced glaucoma (10).

APPROACH TO THE PATIENT WITH GLAUCOMA

These clinical trials and other evidence from epidemiology studies have led to a better understanding of the management of patients with ocular hypertension and with early and advanced glaucoma (11,12). Given these evidence-based risk factors, it is important to consider that an individual patient may not be comparable with the study participants, who had to meet specific inclusion and exclusion criteria to be enrolled in the clinical trials. Thus, the recommendations to treat patients with various forms and disease stages of glaucoma should be guided by the results of these important clinical trials, while keeping in mind potential differences between the individual patient and the average clinical trial participant (13). Overall, when treating the individual patient, physicians should remember that IOP is a surrogate clinical endpoint and that the long-term goal is to preserve vision and the best quality of life for the patient. In the perspective of glaucoma and the vision spectrum (**Fig. 27.1**), our approach must change along the vision continuum to accommodate the knowledge gained from epidemiology studies, clinical trials, and long-term clinical experience.

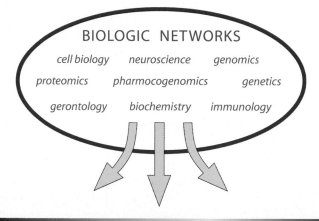

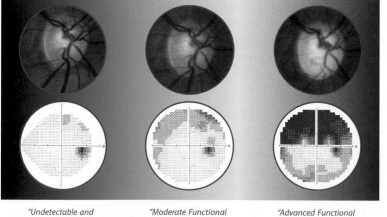

Figure 27.1 There is a broad spectrum of glaucoma, ranging from asymptomatic to advanced disease with optic nerve damage and visual field loss. This case demonstrates progression of glaucoma based on right optic disc photos and right visual fields over 18 years despite medical and surgical treatments with IOP reduction and fluctuation between 7 and 13 mm Hg. For such a patient, we need further advances beyond the risk factors identified in well-designed clinical trials. Such advances will develop from the research areas represented in the "biologic networks" and "environment." (Modified from Moroi SE, Richards JE. Glaucoma and genomic medicine. *Glaucoma Today.* 2008;1: 16–24.)

The New Patient

A new patient may or may not know whether he or she has glaucoma or know the type of glaucoma. If the patient has not been seen by an ophthalmologist previously, a full eye examination is indicated. This entails addressing the chief complaint; obtaining an ocular and medical history; testing visual acuity and refraction; performing tonometry and pachymetry; conducting an external examination with evaluation of the pupillary reaction, slitlamp biomicroscopy, and gonioscopy; assessing the retina and optic nerve head with photographic documentation; and testing the visual field.

When making a new diagnosis of glaucoma, physicians should explain the basics of glaucoma to the patient and help him or her understand that glaucoma can lead to irreversible blindness, but that this can be prevented with early diagnosis and proper care. It is also important to explain the type of glaucoma and to show the patient photographs of the optic disc or a computerized topographic analysis report and copies of the visual fields. It is worth explaining to patients that, unless the glaucoma is diagnosed in the very advanced stage, the prognosis for retaining their vision is excellent, especially with a good understanding of their disease combined with adherence to recommended treatment and frequent follow-up visits. In one study, white patients with glaucoma had an approximately 25% chance of monocular blindness and a 9% chance of bilateral blindness in 20 years, even if the glaucoma remained uncontrolled (14).

The Established Patient

For the established patient, the critical components of continuity of care are to evaluate adherence to glaucoma medical treatment, evaluate tolerance to the treatment, and assess stability of the optic nerve head and visual function. If the patient has had a surgical intervention, the surgical site should be examined carefully for signs of tissue breakdown or infection. Many patients are more interested in their IOP levels, often remembering the numbers from the previous visit. Although sharing this information with the patient is helpful, a discussion of the complete clinical picture allows the patient to be better educated, which may result in better adherence to the treatment plan.

THE TREATMENT PLAN

In general, the overall goal to managing all patients with glaucoma is to preserve visual function while maintaining the best possible quality of life. This goal can be achieved by preventing or slowing the progression of glaucomatous damage by lowering IOP to a level at which further damage is minimal. Although not universally accepted, guidelines for glaucoma treatment are available from various professional societies (e.g., American Academy of Ophthalmology, at http://one.aao.org/CE/PracticeGuidelines/PPP.aspx; International Council of Ophthalmology, at www.icoph.org; European Glaucoma Society, at www.eugs.org; and South East Asia Glaucoma Interest Group, at http://seagig.org), with approaches for managing the various clinical forms of glaucoma or ocular hypertension. In the medical management of a patient with glaucoma, physicians should consider when to initiate treatment, how to start, how to follow the patient, when to change the treatment, and when to move on to surgical intervention.

When to Treat

To avoid unnecessary treatment, physicians must decide whether treatment is really indicated. When elevated IOP is present without glaucomatous damage (i.e., ocular hypertension), the physician must evaluate the risk factors for progression to glaucoma before deciding whether to treat. Most patients who have ocular hypertension appear to do well without treatment (2). When the patient presents with established glaucomatous damage or dangerously high IOP, the indication to initiate treatment is usually clear.

How to Start

Initiating treatment involves establishing the target IOP or IOP range, selecting the appropriate medication, educating and instructing the patient, and establishing the efficacy and safety of the treatment at follow-up evaluations.

Establishing the Target Pressure

Elevated IOP is the most important causative risk factor for glaucoma development and progression, and it is the only one for which we have proven treatment. However, no single pressure value is appropriate for all patients. Rather, the physician must establish a target pressure or target IOP range that can prevent further glaucomatous damage. The IOP target is based on the status of the optic nerve head and other risk factors for progression. In most cases, reducing the IOP by 20% to 30% from baseline is recommended, which should result in a target IOP in the middle to high teens (mm Hg) for eyes with minimal damage (e.g., early neural rim thinning without visual field loss), the low to middle teens for eyes with moderate damage (e.g., cupping to the disc margin in one quadrant with early field loss), and the high single digits to low teens for eyes with advanced damage (e.g., extensive cupping and field loss).

Other risk factors that should be considered in establishing the target pressure include the central corneal thickness, with thin corneas having been identified as a major risk factor for patients with ocular hypertension (3,15). Older age, family history of glaucoma, African heritage, and myopia are also indicators of an increased risk for the presence and progression of COAG (11), whereas Asian heritage and hyperopia suggest an increased risk for angle-closure glaucoma (16). Growing evidence suggests that vascular factors, such as ocular ischemia and vasospastic disease, may contribute to the pathogenesis and increased risk for glaucoma (6,17,18), especially in normal-tension glaucoma (19). (Risk factors for specific forms of glaucoma are considered in more detail in Chapter 9.)

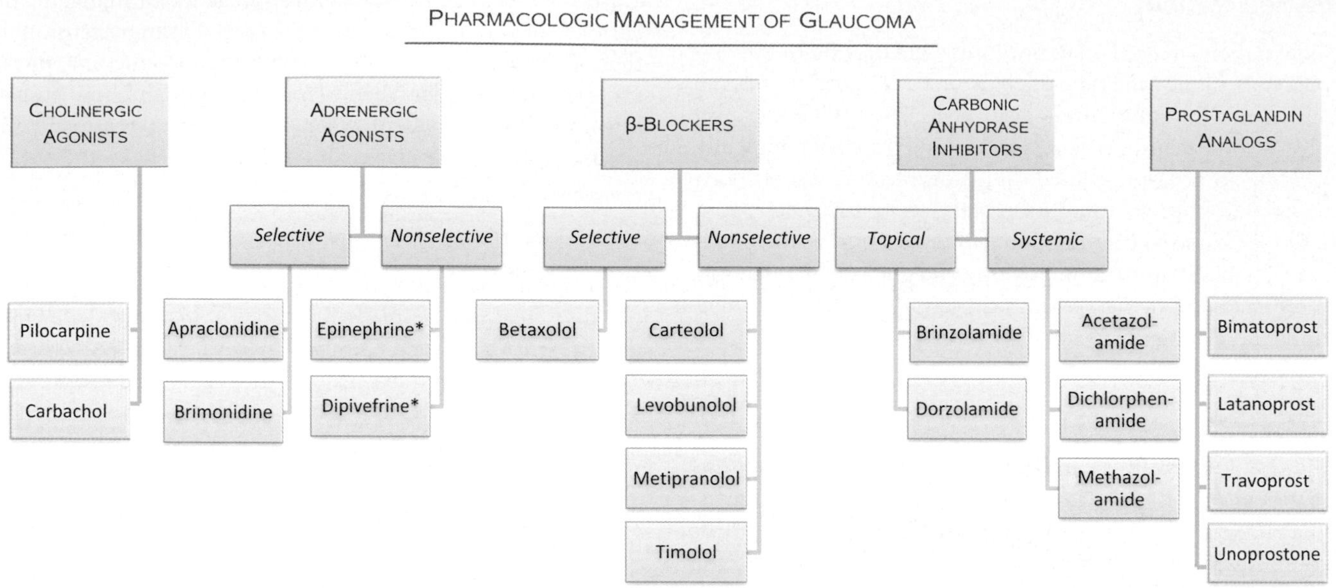

PHARMACOLOGIC MANAGEMENT OF GLAUCOMA

Figure 27.2 Medical therapy options for glaucoma treatment. Agents with an asterisk are no longer commercially available.

Selecting Initial Medication

In the United States, initial medical therapy remains the standard for most patients with newly diagnosed glaucoma. The treatment of most forms of open- and closed-angle glaucoma includes the use of topical and occasionally orally administered agents that lower IOP by enhancing aqueous outflow, reducing aqueous production, or both. Currently, five different classes of glaucoma medications are available for the long-term treatment of glaucoma: prostaglandin-related agents, or hypotensive lipids; β-adrenergic receptor antagonists, or β-blockers; adrenergic receptor agonists; carbonic anhydrase inhibitors; and cholinergics, or miotic agents. An overview of currently available glaucoma drugs is provided in **Figure 27.2** and their basic mechanism of action on aqueous humor dynamics is shown in **Figure 27.3**.

Exceptions to initiating glaucoma therapy with medications include patients with very high IOPs, which pose an immediate threat to vision; a history of medical treatment without success or with intolerable side effects; and problems with adherence to therapy. Acute angle-closure glaucomas and many forms of childhood glaucoma are managed with initial or early surgery.

One may initiate therapy using a uniocular trial; however, some investigators have recently questioned this approach (20). If the fellow untreated eye is used as a control, then physicians must keep in mind that some antiglaucoma eyedrops may produce a small consensual reduction in IOP in the untreated eye (21). Once-daily dosing has the benefits of increased adherence and possibly decreased side effects. However, if once-daily medication is not achieving the target IOP, then reassessment of treatment may be the next step. In general, the therapeutic goal is to use the least amount of medication that will accomplish the desired therapeutic effect with the fewest adverse reactions and that is affordable for the patient.

Pharmacokinetics of Topical Drugs

In using topical glaucoma medications, one should consider the basic pharmacokinetics, which deals with the absorption, distribution, metabolism, and elimination of an administered drug (22). The availability of these topically applied pharmacologic agents at the receptor site is influenced by (a) drug kinetics in the conjunctival cul-de-sac, (b) corneal and transconjunctival–scleral penetration, and (c) the distribution and rate of drug elimination within the eye (22).

Drug Kinetics in the Conjunctival Cul-de-Sac

Following topical instillation, a medication first mixes with the tears in the cul-de-sac, which normally contains 7 to 9 μL of fluid and has a maximum capacity of about 30 μL. The precorneal tear film is a dynamic trilaminar fluid layer conceptually described as an outer lipid layer, a middle aqueous layer, and an inner mucin layer (23,24). The drop size of commercial glaucoma medications ranges from 25.1 to 56.4 μL, with an average of 39 μL (25). Therefore, as much as one half of the medication may spill out from the lids at the time of instillation.

A large percentage of that which remains in the cul-de-sac enters the lacrimal drainage system as a result of the pumping action created by blinking of the eylids. The rate of loss of the drug in the tears is rapid, with the peak time occurring within the first few minutes after instillation. This drug loss not only reduces the amount of drug available for the pharmacologic effect within the eye but also increases the

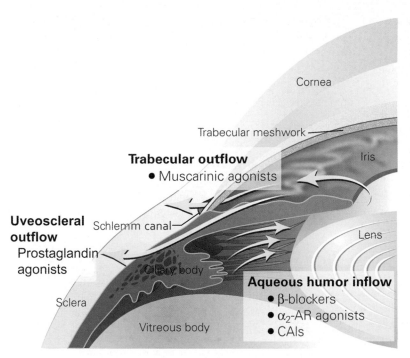

Cornea

Trabecular meshwork

Trabecular outflow
• Muscarinic agonists

Iris

Uveoscleral outflow
Prostaglandin agonists

Schlemm canal

Lens

Ciliary body

Sclera

Vitreous body

Aqueous humor inflow
• β-blockers
• α₂-AR agonists
• CAIs

Figure 27.3 Schematic of anterior portion of the human eye highlighting anatomy relevant to current glaucoma therapeutics. The aqueous humor is produced by the ciliary body and secreted by the ciliary body epithelial bilayer into the posterior chamber (*three small arrows* indicate the aqueous humor inflow pathway). The aqueous humor bathes and nourishes the crystalline lens and then circulates into the anterior chamber through the pupil (indicated by the *single arrow* going across the iris). The aqueous humor leaves the eye through the trabecular meshwork and into the Schlemm canal (trabecular outflow) and through the peripheral base of the iris, into the ciliary body, and through the sclera (uveoscleral outflow). Current glaucoma medical therapy modulates intraocular pressure by decreasing aqueous humor inflow (β-blockers, α₂-adrenergic receptor [*AR*] agonists, and carbonic anhydrase inhibitors [*CAIs*]), by enhancing trabecular outflow (muscarinic agonists), or by enhancing uveoscleral outflow (prostaglandin agonists). (Modified from McLaren NC, Moroi SE. Clinical implications of pharmacogenetics for glaucoma therapeutics. *Pharmacogenomics J.* 2003; 3:197–201.)

potential for systemic side effects by absorption into the systemic circulation via the nasopharyngeal mucosa. The degree to which this occurs can be influenced by nasolacrimal occlusion, which is discussed later in this chapter. Thus, the bioavailability of the drug for corneal and conjunctival–scleral penetration is significantly influenced by the degree to which a drug saturates the tear film and by the retention time in the cul-de-sac.

Corneal and Transconjunctival–Scleral Penetration

In order for the drug to reach the intraocular targets, the drug must penetrate the cornea and anterior conjunctival and scleral tissues (26). The cornea may be conceptualized as a "lipid–water–lipid" sandwich in that the lipid content of the epithelium and endothelium is approximately 100 times greater than that of the stroma (27). Consequently, the epithelium and endothelium are readily traversed by lipid-soluble substances (i.e., compounds in a nonionized or nonelectrolyte form) but are impermeable to water-soluble agents (i.e., ionized compounds or electrolytes). These permeability characteristics create a selective barrier, in that only drugs that can exist in both a water-soluble and lipid-soluble state are able to penetrate the intact cornea. This has been referred to as the differential solubility concept. On the basis of these biologic properties of the cornea, drugs tend to concentrate in various layers of the cornea. Some of the drug may be degraded at this level while another portion is temporarily stored in the cornea. The cornea therefore acts as a depot and a limiting factor for transfer of the drug to the aqueous humor (28). Another consideration for drug design and delivery takes advantage of the endogenous enzymes in the corneal epithelium that activate some glaucoma prodrugs into their active form, such as bimatoprost and presumably the other prostaglandin-like agents (29).

Intraocular Factors Influencing Drug Bioavailability

After penetrating the cornea, conjunctiva, and sclera, the drug must distribute to the appropriate structures in the anterior segment of the eye. The bioavailability of the drug is affected by local tissue binding (30,31), by local tissue metabolism, and by diffusion into the vascular system via the aqueous outflow system. In vitro studies with synthetic melanin revealed a binding rate up to 85% for β-blockers, compared with 40% for pilocarpine, 50% for epinephrine, and almost none for prostaglandins (32). These findings corresponded to results of in vivo studies, in which timolol and pilocarpine had a greater IOP-lowering effect in albino than pigmented rabbits, whereas prostaglandins had the same effect in both groups of animals (32). Another effect of tissue–drug binding is a potential drug depot effect whereby β-adrenergic inhibitors can be released very slowly from the pigmented uveal tissues, accounting for the longer duration of effect in pigmented eyes (33). Other drugs, including pilocarpine, are metabolized in the ocular tissues (34). Thus, the small portion of the instilled drop that escapes extraocular or intraocular elimination, tissue binding, or inactivation may finally reach the appropriate target where it exerts its pharmacologic effect.

Formulation of Topical Drugs

The pharmacokinetics of a particular drug can be greatly influenced by the manner in which it is formulated. This includes the vehicle, pH, concentration, and additives of the formulation. The vehicle in which a drug is delivered affects the amount of medication available for ocular penetration by influencing the rate of drug loss in the tears, the precorneal tear film saturation, and the length of time that the drug remains in contact with the cornea (35). Commonly used vehicles are soluble polymers, including methylcellulose and polyvinyl alcohol. They reduce the initial rapid drainage and prolong the drug–cornea contact time presumably by increasing tear viscosity, providing solution homogeneity (uniform suspension of drug particles in solution), and reducing surface tension.

Ointments significantly increase drug bioavailability by reducing loss in the tears, inhibiting dilution by the tears, providing a higher effective concentration of the drug, and increasing tissue contact time (36). They are limited, however, by interference with vision and aesthetic considerations. Soluble gels, emulsions, and suspensions have also been examined. Although no longer available, pilocarpine gel was formulated as a high-viscosity acrylic soluble gel that delivered a 24-hour pilocarpine dose following a single, nighttime application in the cul-de-sac (37).

Liposomes may be designed as small, homogenous unilamellar structures composed of phospholipids and water, which can be suitable for incorporating topical medications (35), but none is currently in clinical use. Various solid materials have been evaluated for their ability to release a drug at a sustained rate from a location on the cornea or in the conjunctival cul-de-sac. Although no longer available, a diffusional system released pilocarpine from between two polymeric membranes (38), which delivered the drug with zero-order kinetics because the amount of drug delivered per unit time was independent of the amount left undelivered.

As discussed earlier, the lipid–water solubility ratio (or partition coefficient) of a compound influences corneal penetration. Design of topically applied drugs must take into account both the ionized (i.e., more water-soluble) and nonionized (i.e., more lipid-soluble) forms. The two forms of the drug exist in equilibrium, with one form penetrating a particular layer of the cornea and then replenishing the other form to maintain the equilibrium. The pH at which a drug is formulated influences this ratio, with weak bases (which include most glaucoma medications) being absorbed through the cornea at a higher pH, whereas weak acids are absorbed better at a lower pH. Solution pH also affects drug stability and patient comfort on instillation. Fortunately, most weak bases at physiologic pH of 7.4 exist predominantly in the nonionized form (39).

Compounds with a molecular weight greater than 500 g/mol have poor corneal absorption. However, this is not a major factor because most ophthalmic drugs have a lower molecular weight. There is an optimal drug concentration to increase bioavailability of the drug at the target site, but this is balanced by the concern that at higher drug concentrations, a greater amount of drug is lost in the lacrimal drainage system, which increases the potential for systemic side effects.

The topic of additives used in glaucoma medications has received much attention relative to concerns of ocular surface irritation, dry eye, and long-term safety to the ocular tissues (40–43). The main additive is benzalkonium chloride, which not only serves as a "preservative" by providing bacteriostatic activity but also influences corneal penetration by decreasing the surface tension of nonpolar drugs, allowing them to mix more with the tear film, leading to enhanced corneal absorption. (More specific information on modifications in the additives is discussed in the individual chapters discussing specific glaucoma medications.) Additives do not, however, prevent bacterial contamination, and physicians must educate patients on the proper handling of eyedrop dispensers.

Glaucoma Medications

Prostaglandins (Hypotensive Lipids)

The prostaglandin-like compounds, or "hypotensive lipids," are the most recent class of drugs to be introduced for the long-term management of glaucoma. Although high concentrations of prostaglandins are associated with ocular inflammation and elevated IOP, very low concentrations effectively reduce the pressure by increasing uveoscleral outflow (44). In the United States, the first of these drugs to be released was latanoprost, followed by unoprostone, travoprost, and bimatoprost. (For further details regarding mechanism of action, side effects, and cost issues, see Chapter 28.)

β-Blocking Drugs

Of all the glaucoma drug classes, we have the most experience with topical β-blockers, the first of which was timolol maleate, which was approved for use by the U.S. Food and Drug Administration in 1978. These drugs, which lower IOP by reducing aqueous production, are available as nonselective (i.e., blocking β_1 and β_2 receptors) or selective (i.e., primarily blocking β_1 receptors) agents. Concentrations of β-blockers used in treating glaucoma range from 0.25% to 1.0% and are usually instilled once or twice per day. The β_1-selective β-blocker betaxolol causes fewer pulmonary and cardiovascular side effects, but it is less effective in lowering IOP than the nonselective β-blockers. (For further details regarding mechanism of action, side effects, and cost issues, see Chapter 29.)

α-Selective Adrenergic Drugs

The α_2-adrenergic agonists lower IOP primarily by reducing aqueous production. Apraclonidine in a 1% concentration was first used to prevent IOP spikes after anterior segment laser procedures but was later approved for treatment of chronic glaucoma. Apraclonidine in a 0.5% concentration can also be used short term in patients with glaucoma receiving maximally tolerated medical therapy who require additional reduction in IOP; however, its long-term use is limited by frequent allergic reactions.

Brimonidine is more selective than apraclonidine and appears to elicit a lower incidence of ocular allergic reactions. Like apraclonidine, brimonidine can be used to prevent IOP spikes after argon laser trabeculoplasty. It has been reported to cause clinically significant pulmonary depression in children (45–48). (For further details on mechanism of action, side effects, and cost issues, see Chapter 30.) Epinephrine compounds are no longer available to treat glaucoma, given the availability of newer drugs that are more effective and have fewer side effects.

Carbonic Anhydrase Inhibitors

This is the only class of systemic medications that can be used both topically and systemically for the treatment of glaucoma. These agents lower the IOP by reducing aqueous production through inhibition of the carbonic anhydrase enzyme. Acetazolamide is the prototype carbonic anhydrase inhibitor and may be administered orally or intravenously. Methazolamide is the other oral carbonic anhydrase inhibitor. The topical carbonic anhydrase inhibitors dorzolamide, 2%, and brinzolamide, 1%, are available for the long-term treatment of glaucoma. (For further details regarding mechanism of action, side effects, and cost issues, see Chapter 31.)

Miotic Agents

Pilocarpine is the oldest known therapy for glaucoma, which was introduced in the 1870s. It is a cholinergic agent most commonly used in the treatment of open-angle glaucoma. It is occasionally used in solution with concentrations ranging from 0.5% to 6%, typically administered four times daily. (For further details regarding mechanism of action, side effects, and cost issues, see Chapter 32.)

Educating and Instructing the Patient

The physician is ultimately responsible for educating the patient; the physician or another member of the health care team must discuss the basic aspects of the disease, prognosis, and treatment. This effort is an important investment for the physician–patient relationship. In addition to the physician, office personnel and educational resources should also be used. The most important ancillary individual is the office nurse or technician, who should be able to restate and expand on what the physician has said, instruct the patient on the instillation of eyedrops, work out the therapeutic regimen, and provide the necessary reinforcement of these matters at each follow-up visit. That individual should also be able to answer questions about use of the medications or possible side effects. Other important resource materials are available from several reliable health-related organizations. In some centers, classes or meetings are provided for patients to broaden their understanding of their condition. These are usually conducted by nurses, technicians, or social workers and may incorporate lectures, videos, question-and-answer sessions, or group discussions.

About the Disease

It is essential for patients to be made aware of their disease and its potential seriousness without creating undue apprehension. Patients should be told that they have glaucoma, what glaucoma is, and that it can lead to total and irreversible blindness but that the blindness can be prevented with proper treatment. It is not uncommon for patients to have been taking glaucoma medication for years but be unaware that they have glaucoma or relate it to blindness, whereas others may live in daily fear that they will inevitably go blind. The time taken to correct these misconceptions is one of the most important measures in preventing blindness and improving the general well-being of patients.

Why the Medications

Patients must understand that the purpose of taking their medications is to lower the IOP, which is the main treatable risk factor for slowing loss of vision from glaucomatous optic neuropathy. It should be made clear that this treatment will not improve their visual acuity and that any medication has potential side effects. Many patients stop using their eyedrops because "they did not seem to be helping."

Poor adherence to recommended medical therapy is a major problem in the prevention of blindness from glaucoma. Most forms of glaucoma represent chronic diseases in which symptoms are mild or absent, treatment is prophylactic, and the consequences of stopping therapy are delayed, all of which are associated with poor adherence to medical therapy. In an older study of 184 patients in which adherence to pilocarpine treatment was monitored electronically in the medication bottle, participants administered 76.0 ± 24.3% of the prescribed pilocarpine doses, but they reported taking 97.1 ± 5.9% of the prescribed pilocarpine doses (49). Another important observation was that the rate of adherence was significantly higher in the 24-hour period preceding the return appointment than in the entire observation period. In a similar study involving 110 patients, patients administered 82.7 ± 19.0% of the prescribed timolol doses (range, 20% to 100%) (50).

What can be done to improve patient adherence to treatment? This question has received serious attention recently, and practical patient-centered communication skills using open-ended questions will best engage the patient to adopt adherent self-management behaviors (51). Once poor adherence is recognized, the cause is usually found to be related to (a) patient factors, (b) medication regimen, (c) provider factors, or (d) situational or environmental factors (52). Learning from the experience in health behavior and hypertension, we should strive to simplify the glaucoma medication regimen, be cost conscious, and educate the patient about the pathophysiology of glaucoma and the importance of various treatments for glaucoma (53).

The Therapeutic Regimen

When told to use eyedrops more than once daily, some patients may not appropriately space the doses unless properly instructed. It is important to work out a daily schedule, especially if patients are using multiple medications. If they are taking more than one drop at the same time of day, they may be instilling them so close together that they are diluting or washing each other from the cul-de-sac. Thus, the physician should instruct the patient to wait at least 5 minutes between instillation of the eyedrops. The physician and patient should work out a schedule that fits the patient's daily activities and links the use of the eyedrops with specific daily functions, such as meals. It is advisable to record this schedule on a form that is large enough for the patient to see and can be kept in a convenient location (**Fig. 27.4**). It may also be helpful to make sure that the patient can distinguish between drugs by associating a drug with the color of the bottle top, although this is more difficult today because of a lack of standardized colors for different drug classes.

Figure 27.4 Example of a drug schedule that can be used to instruct the patient in the use of glaucoma medications and serve as a reminder for the patient.

DAILY DRUG REMINDER

PATIENT NAME: Johnston, M.   DATE: Oct. 1, 2010

DRUG	EYE R = Right L = Left B = Both	BREAKFAST	LUNCH	SUPPER	BEDTIME
Xalatan	L				✓
Cosopt	B	✓		✓	

Administration of Eyedrops

It should not be assumed that a patient knows how to instill eyedrops properly. Improper instillation has been identified as a major factor in failure of medical therapy. It is a good practice to observe the patient's technique and instruct her or him in the proper technique. **Figure 27.5** shows one effective method in which the patient can be instructed. Nasolacrimal occlusion for 5 minutes after instillation of a drop has been shown to significantly reduce drug loss through the tear ducts, with a marked reduction in systemic drug absorption and an increase

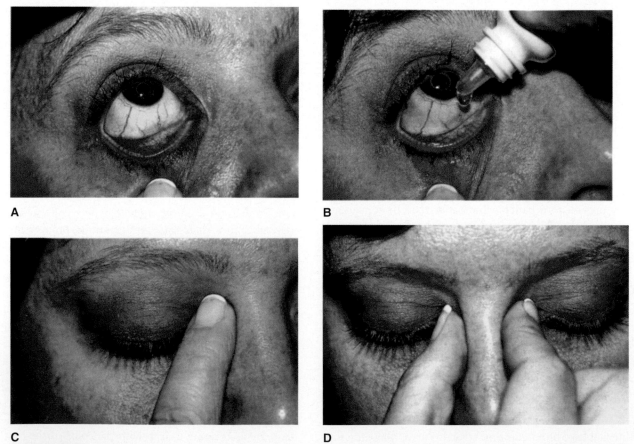

A

B

C

D

Figure 27.5 A technique for instilling eyedrops. **A:** Pinch the lower lid and pull it down to create a pocket. **B:** Place one drop in the pocket. **C:** Look down while bringing the lower lid up to touch the eye. **D:** Close the eye and apply gentle pressure over the lacrimal sac.

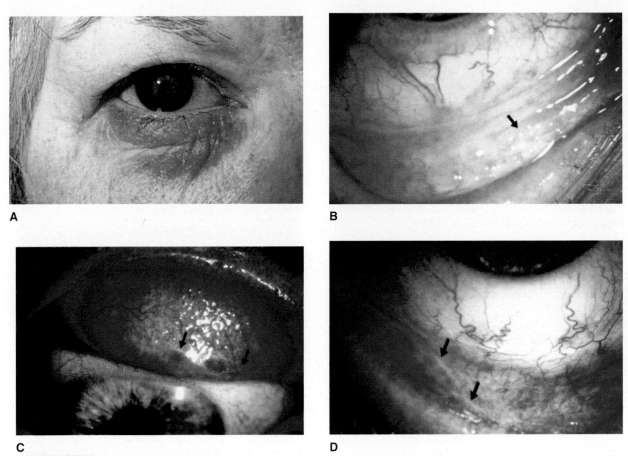

Figure 27.6 Reactions to long-term use of topical agents. **A:** Typical appearance of contact dermatitis of the lids, which can occur with any glaucoma drug. In many cases, the reaction is related to a preservative in the formulation; preservative-free preparations (e.g., with timolol and pilocarpine) are available. **B:** Slitlamp view of follicular conjunctivitis. Palpebral follicles are present (*arrow*). **C,D:** In most cases of cicatricial pemphigoid, the patient is using multiple glaucoma medications; virtually all glaucoma drugs have been implicated in this adverse reaction. In C, the patient has linear scars of the superior conjunctiva (*arrows*); D shows the foreshortening of the inferior conjunctival fornix, with linear scars (*arrows*).

in anterior chamber concentrations (54). Gentle eyelid closure for 5 minutes, which minimizes lacrimal drainage by eliminating the blink movements, appears to have a similar result (55).

Follow-up

Evaluation of Efficacy

Having started the patient on a new eyedrop, the physician should see the patient again to confirm IOP efficacy and evaluate adherence and side effects (**Fig. 27.6**). Unless the IOP is dangerously high, in which case the patient should be seen again within days of the first visit, it may be better to wait a month or two to get a better sense of the long-term benefit of the drug and how the patient is coping with it. A monocular trial of a medication to compare side effects in the treated eye versus the fellow untreated eye has some advantages; however, the role and value of the monocular trial in predicting the efficacy of the drug has been questioned (20).

After a stable and acceptable IOP reduction has been achieved, the patient is usually reevaluated every 3 to 6 months, depending on his or her individual situation. Over the years of

follow-up, one may consider temporarily discontinuing a drug in one eye to determine whether it is still contributing to the reduced IOP.

Diurnal Curve

In establishing the efficacy of a new drug, physicians must remember that IOP fluctuates considerably throughout a 24-hour cycle and that the pattern of this fluctuation differs among individual patients. Studies have suggested that healthy individuals and patients with glaucoma may experience their highest IOPs at night (56,57). Their blood pressure values may also be lowest at night, reducing blood flow to the optic nerve head below critical levels and increasing the risk for progressive glaucomatous damage (58,59). Although current tonometric technology and insurance limitations do not provide for user-friendly and accessible 24-hour IOP monitoring, checking the pressure at various times during office hours is advisable to determine whether a daytime spike occurs. Prescribing glaucoma medications that can maximally reduce IOP over 24 hours and minimally influence blood pressure have practical and theoretical advantages for the patient with glaucoma.

Patient Reinforcement

At every visit, patients should be asked about adherence and any problems they may be having with their medications. Asking about their general welfare is equally important, because patients often do not relate changes in their life, such as fatigue, with a drop that they are putting in their eye.

Contact with the Family Physician

It may be of value to maintain contact with the patient's family physician or other physicians who are caring for the patient to ensure that the medical history is accurate and to avoid potential drug interactions with the patient's glaucoma drugs and medications for other conditions.

WHEN AND HOW TO CHANGE OR COMBINE MEDICATIONS

When the target IOP is no longer being maintained with a particular medical regimen, the question is whether to replace or to add to the current drugs or to move on to surgery. A reverse uniocular trial, by temporarily discontinuing an eyedrop in one eye, may help to indicate whether the rising pressure is caused by loss of drug efficacy or worsening of the glaucoma. If this trial indicates the former, replacing the drug with one from another class may be appropriate, whereas the latter may suggest adding another drug to the existing therapy.

When evaluating the efficacy of adjunctive medical therapy, the first medication is likely to have a more significant IOP-lowering effect, compared with the effect of adding a second and possibly third medication. Having patients with glaucoma on more than three topical medications is uncommon and of questionable value, although there are exceptions. Important considerations when using several medications are whether each drug is making a significant IOP-lowering contribution, and the impact of multiple medications on the quality of life, adherence to a complex medication regimen, and the cost of the medications. These issues are the rationale for combining glaucoma medications into a single formulation, such as the fixed combination of dorzolamide, 2%, and timolol maleate, 0.5% (60), and that of brimonidine, 0.2%, and timolol, 0.5% (61), and thereby improving adherence. The fixed combination of prostaglandin agents and timolol is not yet available in the United States.

When to Quit and Move on to Surgery

Possibly the biggest mistake in treating patients with glaucoma is continuing to try various combinations of drugs when the target IOP is not being reached instead of moving on to laser or incisional surgical intervention. The indications for quitting medical therapy include an inability to maintain target IOP, progressive glaucomatous damage on maximum medical therapy, and the patient's inability to tolerate or adhere to the medical regimen.

PHARMACOGENETICS

The variations in the drug-mediated IOP response are due to a combination of factors, including adherence, biologic mechanisms related to aqueous humor dynamics (see Chapter 1), ocular and systemic conditions, and possibly environmental factors and genetics (**Fig. 27.7**). At present, certain environmental factors have been shown to contribute to variation in

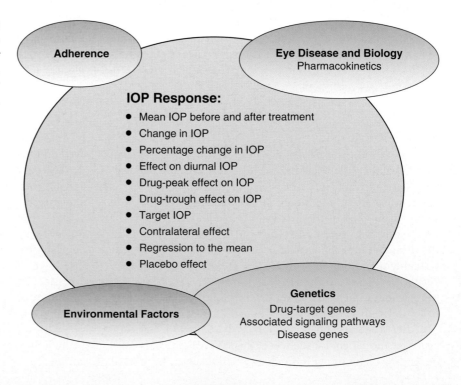

Figure 27.7 Overview of factors (*small ovals*) to consider for assessing the efficacy of a glaucoma drug on "IOP response" (*large center oval*). (Modified from McLaren NC, Moroi SE. Clinical implications of pharmacogenetics for glaucoma therapeutics. *Pharmacogenomics J.* 2003;3:197–201.)

IOP response to medications. Specifically, the concurrent use of some systemic medications, such as systemic β-blockers and calcium-channel blockers, may decrease the efficacy of topically applied β-blockers (21,62). The study of the impact of genetics on drug response is known as pharmacogenetics (63).

Pharmacogenetics attempts to determine whether differences in drug response, which may be related to either efficacy or toxicity, are attributable to the diversity in genes that are transmissible from one generation to the next. Most drug-response variations are of the Gaussian type, which tend to be viewed as environmentally determined but usually have some definable hereditary elements (64,65). The tails of the Gaussian distribution curves are of clinical interest: Those at the lower limits are typically identified as "nonresponders" and those with values at the upper limits are classified as "super responders." In the OHTS, patients who were randomly assigned to medical treatment showed a Gaussian-type distribution of IOP response following treatment with topical β-blockers (21). Recently, a medical record, population-based study found that among the four candidate genes of the $β_1$-, $β_2$-, and $β_3$-adrenergic receptor genes and the *CYP2D6* gene, one gene variation in the $β_2$-adrenergic receptor gene was associated with a 20% or greater IOP decrease with use of topical timolol (66). This has not yet been repeated, but because this gene is not a primary open-angle glaucoma locus (67), this genetic marker needs to be validated as a potential research tool for predicting drug response to topical β-blockers.

Informed expectations of glaucoma drug efficacy may be determined from clinical pharmacology trials. There is no clear definition of a "clinical responder" in the context of glaucoma medical treatment, but the selection of 15% reduction from baseline IOP at peak drug effect appears to have been first used in evaluating the efficacy of latanoprost (68). In another study, "nonresponders" to drug treatment were defined as patients whose IOP did not decrease by 10% (69). Prior to 1996, most glaucoma pharmacology trials defined efficacy on the basis of the mean IOP, and the variation in the IOP response had to be inferred from the standard errors of the mean and standard deviations. Since that time, the IOP response to a drug has been reported in numerous formats, which include the following: mean pretreatment IOP, mean posttreatment IOP, change in IOP, target change in IOP, percentage change in IOP, effect on diurnal IOP, "clinical success," and percentage of patients achieving a specified target IOP. Much of this shift in data reporting may be attributed to the defined treatment goals in the glaucoma clinical trials (discussed at the beginning of this chapter).

The challenge of genomics is to determine whether we can predict disease risk, disease progression, and treatment outcome despite the intricate biologic and physiologic interactions among expression of drug target genes, drug-metabolizing enzymes, and disease genes. Identification of genetic markers of "poor IOP responders" has the potential to target those patients with disease to more appropriate treatment, such as surgery, to lower IOP more effectively, thus minimizing progressive optic nerve damage and visual field loss. We imagine that a "genetic panel" will be developed with robust markers for common diseases, such as diabetes mellitus, hypertension, some cancers, macular degeneration, glaucoma, and commonly prescribed medications. Such genetic markers will need to be tested in stratified patient populations for predictive value and then validated in separate cohorts. A cost–benefit analysis with economic modeling will also need to demonstrate the health benefits and long-term cost savings to improve treatment outcomes and thereby decrease disease morbidity. The coverage of genetic testing will be determined through the process of technology assessment by national insurance and private payors. The future application of such a genetic profile could lead to fewer return office visits for follow-up for changed medical therapy, thus improving treatment outcomes.

KEY POINTS

- At the present time, we have solid evidence to inform patients with newly diagnosed glaucoma about the condition, its treatment, expected outcomes, and impact of this chronic disease and various treatments on their quality of life.
- Patient-centered communication is essential to modify health behaviors to assess the impact of treatment on the physical and social functioning and other quality-of-life parameters (51,70), including the cost of treating the disease.
- Relative elevation of IOP is the major causative risk factor for the development and progression of glaucoma. A target IOP should be established with minimal fluctuation over a 24-hour period under glaucoma treatment. This initial target IOP may need to be reassessed if there is glaucoma progression.
- Preventing progressive glaucomatous damage with the fewest medications in the lowest concentration needed to achieve the target IOP and considering the patient's quality of life should be the goals of therapy.
- Initiation or change of therapy with a uniocular trial can be helpful to assess side effects and efficacy.
- Patient-centered communication on the disease, treatment, simplified medical regimen, possible drug side effects, and proper eyedrop administration are essential for proper adherence to treatment.
- When medical treatment is ineffective, initially substitute (rather than add) medications. Stopping treatment periodically may help to assess its continuing efficacy.
- When the glaucoma is not controlled medically, the physician should not hesitate to move on to surgical intervention.

REFERENCES

1. Drance SM. Some clinical implications of the collaborative normal tension glaucoma study. *Klin Oczna.* 2004;106(4–5):588–592.
2. Kass MA, Heuer DK, Higginbotham EJ, et al. The Ocular Hypertension Treatment Study: a randomized trial determines that topical ocular hypotensive medication delays or prevents the onset of primary open-angle glaucoma. *Arch Ophthalmol.* 2002;120(6):701–713; discussion 829–830.

3. Gordon MO, Beiser JA, Brandt JD, et al. The Ocular Hypertension Treatment Study: baseline factors that predict the onset of primary open-angle glaucoma. *Arch Ophthalmol.* 2002;120(6):714–720; discussion 829–830.

4. Leske MC, Heijl A, Hussein M, et al. Factors for glaucoma progression and the effect of treatment: the Early Manifest Glaucoma Trial. *Arch Ophthalmol.* 2003;121(1):48–56.

5. Leske MC, Heijl A, Hyman L, et al. Early Manifest Glaucoma Trial: design and baseline data. *Ophthalmology.* 1999;106(11):2144–2153.

6. Leske MC, Heijl A, Hyman L, et al. Predictors of long-term progression in the early manifest glaucoma trial. *Ophthalmology.* 2007;114(11): 1965–1972.

7. Lichter PR, Musch DC, Gillespie BW, et al. Interim clinical outcomes in the Collaborative Initial Glaucoma Treatment Study comparing initial treatment randomized to medications or surgery. *Ophthalmology.* 2001;108(11):1943–1953.

8. Jampel HD, Frick KD, Janz NK, et al. Depression and mood indicators in newly diagnosed glaucoma patients. *Am J Ophthalmol.* 2007;144(2): 238–244.

9. AGIS I. The Advanced Glaucoma Intervention Study (AGIS): 9. Comparison of glaucoma outcomes in black and white patients within treatment groups. *Am J Ophthalmol.* 2001;132(3):311–320.

10. AGIS Investigators. The Advanced Glaucoma Intervention Study (AGIS): 7. The relationship between control of intraocular pressure and visual field deterioration. *Am J Ophthalmol.* 2000;130(4):429–440.

11. Coleman AL, Miglior S. Risk factors for glaucoma onset and progression. *Surv Ophthalmol.* 2008;53(suppl 1):S3–S10.

12. Thomas R, Kumar RS, Chandrasekhar G, et al. Applying the recent clinical trials on primary open angle glaucoma: the developing world perspective. *J Glaucoma.* 2005;14(4):324–327.

13. Singh K. The randomized clinical trial: beware of limitations. *J Glaucoma.* 2004;13(2):87–89.

14. Hattenhauer MG, Johnson DH, Ing HH, et al. The probability of blindness from open-angle glaucoma. *Ophthalmology.* 1998;105(11): 2099–2104.

15. Herndon LW, Weizer JS, Stinnett SS. Central corneal thickness as a risk factor for advanced glaucoma damage. *Arch Ophthalmol.* 2004;122(1):17–21.

16. Congdon N. Reducing the visual burden of glaucoma in Asia: what we know and what we need to know. *J Glaucoma.* 2009;18(1):88–92.

17. Miglior S, Torri V, Zeyen T, et al. Intercurrent factors associated with the development of open-angle glaucoma in the European glaucoma prevention study. *Am J Ophthalmol.* 2007;144(2):266–275.

18. Leske MC, Wu SY, Hennis A, et al. Risk factors for incident open-angle glaucoma: the Barbados Eye Studies. *Ophthalmology.* 2008;115(1):85–93.

19. Flammer J, Orgul S, Costa VP, et al. The impact of ocular blood flow in glaucoma. *Prog Retin Eye Res.* 2002;21(4):359–393.

20. Realini TD. A prospective, randomized, investigator-masked evaluation of the monocular trial in ocular hypertension or open-angle glaucoma. *Ophthalmology.* 2009;116(7):1237–1242.

21. Piltz J, Gross R, Shin DH, et al. Contralateral effect of topical beta-adrenergic antagonists in initial one-eyed trials in the ocular hypertension treatment study. *Am J Ophthalmol.* 2000;130(4):441–453.

22. Mishima S. Clinical pharmacokinetics of the eye. Proctor lecture. *Invest Ophthalmol Vis Sci.* 1981;21(4):504–541.

23. Tiffany JM. The normal tear film. *Dev Ophthalmol.* 2008;41:1–20.

24. Ohashi Y, Dogru M, Tsubota K. Laboratory findings in tear fluid analysis. *Clin Chim Acta.* 2006;369(1):17–28.

25. Lederer CM Jr, Harold RE. Drop size of commercial glaucoma medications. *Am J Ophthalmol.* 1986;101(6):691–694.

26. Schoenwald RD, Deshpande GS, Rethwisch DG, et al. Penetration into the anterior chamber via the conjunctival/scleral pathway. *J Ocul Pharmacol Ther.* 1997;13(1):41–59.

27. Benson H. Permeability of the cornea to topically applied drugs. *Arch Ophthalmol.* 1974;91(4):313–327.

28. Mindel JS, Smith H, Jacobs M, et al. Drug reservoirs in topical therapy. *Invest Ophthalmol Vis Sci.* 1984;25(3):346–350.

29. Maxey KM, Johnson JL, LaBrecque J. The hydrolysis of bimatoprost in corneal tissue generates a potent prostanoid FP receptor agonist. *Surv Ophthalmol.* 2002;47(4 suppl 1):S34–S40.

30. Salazar M, Shimada K, Patil PN. Iris pigmentation and atropine mydriasis. *J Pharmacol Exp Ther.* 1976;197(1):79–88.

31. Patil PM, Jacobowitz D. Unequal accumulation of adrenergic drugs by pigmented and nonpigmented iris. *Am J Ophthalmol.* 1974;78:470–477.

32. Nagata A, Mishima HK, Kiuchi Y, et al. Binding of antiglaucomatous drugs to synthetic melanin and their hypotensive effects on pigmented and nonpigmented rabbit eyes. *Jpn J Ophthalmol.* 1993;37(1):32–38.

33. Salminen L, Imre G, Huupponen R. The effect of ocular pigmentation on intraocular pressure response to timolol. *Acta Ophthalmol Suppl.* 1985;173:15–18.

34. Lee VH, Hui HW, Robinson JR. Corneal metabolism of pilocarpine in pigmented rabbits. *Invest Ophthalmol Vis Sci.* 1980;19(2):210–213.

35. Shell JW. Ophthalmic drug delivery systems. *Surv Ophthalmol.* 1984;29(2):117–128.

36. Trueblood JH, Rossomondo RM, Wilson LA, et al. Corneal contact times of ophthalmic vehicles. Evaluation by microscintigraphy. *Arch Ophthalmol.* 1975;93(2):127–130.

37. March WF, Stewart RM, Mandell AI, et al. Duration of effect of pilocarpine gel. *Arch Ophthalmol.* 1982;100(8):1270–1271.

38. Dohlman CH, Pavan-Langston D, Rose J. A new ocular insert device for continuous constant-rate delivery of medication to the eye. *Ann Ophthalmol.* 1972;4(10):823–832.

39. Akers MJ. Ocular bioavailability of topically applied ophthalmic drugs. *Am Pharm.* 1983;NS23(1):33–36.

40. Leung EW, Medeiros FA, Weinreb RN. Prevalence of ocular surface disease in glaucoma patients. *J Glaucoma.* 2008;17(5):350–355.

41. Ciancaglini M, Carpineto P, Agnifili L, et al. An in vivo confocal microscopy and impression cytology analysis of preserved and unpreserved levobunolol-induced conjunctival changes. *Eur J Ophthalmol.* 2008; 18(3):400–407.

42. Guenoun JM, Baudouin C, Rat P, et al. In vitro study of inflammatory potential and toxicity profile of latanoprost, travoprost, and bimatoprost in conjunctiva-derived epithelial cells. *Invest Ophthalmol Vis Sci.* 2005;46(7):2444–2450.

43. Manni G, Centofanti M, Oddone F, et al. Interleukin-1 beta tear concentration in glaucomatous and ocular hypertensive patients treated with preservative-free nonselective beta-blockers. *Am J Ophthalmol.* 2005; 139(1):72–77.

44. Toris CB, Camras CB, Yablonski ME, et al. Effects of exogenous prostaglandins on aqueous humor dynamics and blood-aqueous barrier function. *Surv Ophthalmol.* 1997;41(suppl 2):S69–S75.

45. Lai Becker M, Huntington N, Woolf AD. Brimonidine tartrate poisoning in children: frequency, trends, and use of naloxone as an antidote. *Pediatrics.* 2009;123(2):e305–e311.

46. Vanhaesebrouck S, Cossey V, Cosaert K, et al. Cardiorespiratory depression and hyperglycemia after unintentional ingestion of brimonidine in a neonate. *Eur J Ophthalmol.* 2009;19(4):694–695.

47. Fernandez MA, Rojas MD. Pediatric systemic poisoning resulting from brimonidine ophthalmic drops. *Pediatr Emerg Care.* 2009;25(1):59.

48. Enyedi LB, Freedman SF. Safety and efficacy of brimonidine in children with glaucoma. *J AAPOS.* 2001;5(5):281–284.

49. Kass MA, Meltzer DW, Gordon M, et al. Compliance with topical pilocarpine treatment. *Am J Ophthalmol.* 1986;101(5):515–523.

50. Kass MA, Gordon M, Morley RE Jr, et al. Compliance with topical timolol treatment. *Am J Ophthalmol.* 1987;103(2):188–193.

51. Hahn SR. Patient-centered communication to assess and enhance patient adherence to glaucoma medication. *Ophthalmology.* 2009;116(11 suppl):S37–S42.

52. Tsai JC. A comprehensive perspective on patient adherence to topical glaucoma therapy. *Ophthalmology.* 2009;116(11 suppl):S30–S36.

53. Budenz DL. A clinician's guide to the assessment and management of nonadherence in glaucoma. *Ophthalmology.* 2009;116(11 suppl):S43–S47.

54. Ellis PP, Wu PY, Pfoff DS, et al. Effect of nasolacrimal occlusion on timolol concentrations in the aqueous humor of the human eye. *J Pharm Sci.* 1992;81(3):219–220.

55. Zimmerman TJ, Kooner KS, Kandarakis AS, et al. Improving the therapeutic index of topically applied ocular drugs. *Arch Ophthalmol.* 1984;102(4):551–553.

56. Larsson LI. Intraocular pressure over 24 hours after repeated administration of latanoprost 0.005% or timolol gel-forming solution 0.5% in patients with ocular hypertension. *Ophthalmology.* 2001;108(8): 1439–1444.

57. Bagga H, Liu JH, Weinreb RN. Intraocular pressure measurements throughout the 24 h. *Curr Opin Ophthalmol.* 2009;20(2):79–83.

58. Hayreh SS, Zimmerman MB, Podhajsky P, et al. Nocturnal arterial hypotension and its role in optic nerve head and ocular ischemic disorders. *Am J Ophthalmol.* 1994;117(5):603–624.

59. Graham SL, Drance SM. Nocturnal hypotension: role in glaucoma progression. *Surv Ophthalmol.* 1999;43(suppl 1):S10–S16.

60. Choudhri S, Wand M, Shields MB. A comparison of dorzolamide-timolol combination versus the concomitant drugs. *Am J Ophthalmol.* 2000; 130(6):832–833.

61. Craven ER, Walters TR, Williams R, et al. Brimonidine and timolol fixed-combination therapy versus monotherapy: a 3-month randomized trial in patients with glaucoma or ocular hypertension. *J Ocul Pharmacol Ther.* 2005;21(4):337–338.

62. Schuman JS. Effects of systemic beta-blocker therapy on the efficacy and safety of topical brimonidine and timolol. Brimonidine Study Groups 1 and 2. *Ophthalmology.* 2000;107(6):1171–1177.

63. Moroi SE, Raoof DA, Reed DM, et al. Progress toward personalized medicine for glaucoma. *Expert Rev Ophthalmol.* 2009;4(2):146–161.

64. Kalow W. Pharmacogenetics in biological perspective [review]. *Pharmacol Rev.* 1997;49(4):369–379.

65. Vessell ES. Pharmacogenetic perspectives gained from twin and family studies. In: Kalow W, ed. *Pharmacogenetics of Drug Metabolism (International Encyclopedia of Pharmacology and Therapeutics Series).* Vol 137. New York, NY: Permagon Press; 1992:843–863.

66. McCarty CA, Burmester JK, Mukesh BN, et al. Intraocular pressure response to topical beta-blockers associated with an ADRB2 single-nucleotide polymorphism. *Arch Ophthalmol.* 2008;126(7):959–963.

67. McLaren N, Reed DM, Musch DC, et al. Evaluation of the beta2-adrenergic receptor gene as a candidate glaucoma gene in 2 ancestral populations. *Arch Ophthalmol.* 2007;125(1):105–111.

68. Alm A, Widengard I, Kjellgren D, et al. Latanoprost administered once daily caused a maintained reduction of intraocular pressure in glaucoma patients treated concomitantly with timolol [see comments]. *Br J Ophthalmol.* 1995;79(1):12–16.

69. Hedman K, Alm A. A pooled-data analysis of three randomized, double-masked, six-month clinical studies comparing the intraocular pressure reducing effect of latanoprost and timolol. *Eur J Ophthalmol.* 2000; 10(2):95–104.

70. Aspinall PA, Johnson ZK, Azuara-Blanco A, et al. Evaluation of quality of life and priorities of patients with glaucoma. *Invest Ophthalmol Vis Sci.* 2008;49(5):1907–1915.

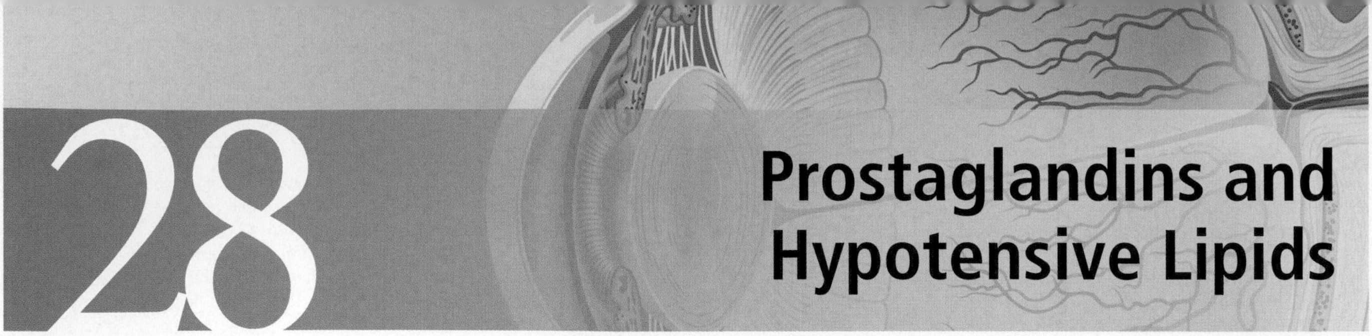

The prostaglandins, thromboxanes, and leukotrienes are eicosanoids, which are metabolic products of 20-carbon arachidonic acid (**Fig. 28.1**). After the prostaglandins are synthesized, they are released and transported out of cells by transporters (1). The prostaglandins that reach the systemic circulation are inactivated in the lung and liver (2). The earliest physiologic effect observed for prostaglandins was contraction of the human uterus after exposure to seminal fluid (3). The initial ocular observation of miosis in the cat was noted after exposure to iris extracts (4). In rabbits, the topical application of 25 to 200 μg of prostaglandins caused an initial rise in intraocular pressure (IOP), followed by pressure reduction for 15 to 20 hours, whereas a 5-μg dose produced ocular hypotension without an initial pressure rise (5). Early studies on relatively large doses of topical prostaglandins revealed inflammation with conjunctival hyperemia and breakdown of the blood–aqueous barrier (6). Subsequent studies indicated that smaller amounts of prostaglandins lowered IOP, which led to the development of this drug class for the medical management of glaucoma.

Several important chemical modifications were made to improve the bioavailability and to make it a more selective FP-receptor agonist (**Fig. 28.2**) (7). The addition of a phenyl ring to the omega chain (i.e., latanoprost, travoprost, and bimatoprost) improved the selectivity for the FP receptor. To improve solubility, the C-1 carboxyl group was modified with an ethyl amide in the case of bimatoprost or an isopropyl ester for latanoprost, travoprost, and unoprostone. This modification at the C-1 carboxyl group creates a lipophilic prodrug, which is hydrolyzed by the cornea into the free acid drug form (8).

MECHANISMS OF ACTION

The prostaglandins have a mixed pharmacologic response because of the diversity of the receptors. The prostaglandin or prostanoid receptors include four subtypes (EP, FP, IP, and TP) of receptors for the endogenous prostaglandins, PGD_2, PGE_2, $PGF_{2\alpha}$, and PGI_2 or TXA_2, respectively (9). The prostanoid receptors are in the family of the G protein–coupled receptors (10). The prostanoid FP receptor exists in two forms: type A for the full-length receptor and type B for the splice variant, which is truncated or shortened compared with the full-length form (11). Both FP receptor forms couple to phospholipase C,

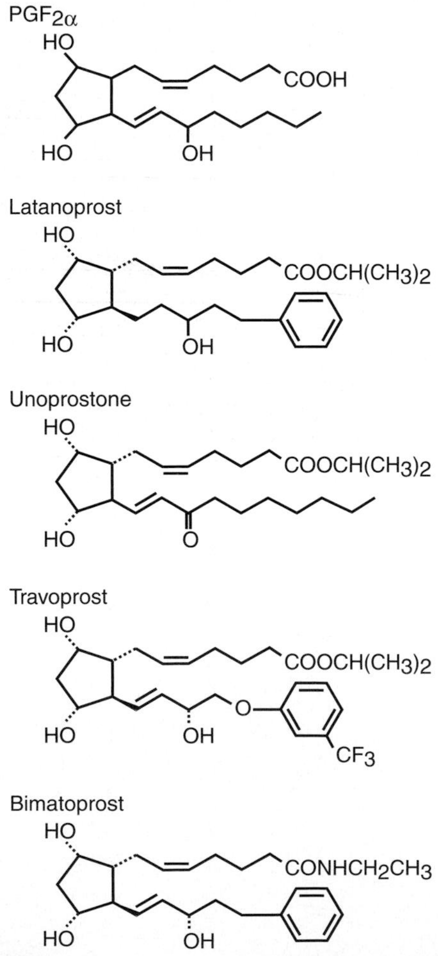

PGF$_{2\alpha}$

Latanoprost

Unoprostone

Travoprost

Bimatoprost

Figure 28.2 Representative structures for prostaglandin-related agents. For the prostaglandin (PG) nomenclature, the last letter refers to the ring structure chemical modifications, the subscripted number is the number of double bonds, and the Greek-letter subscript refers to the orientation of the hydroxyl group.

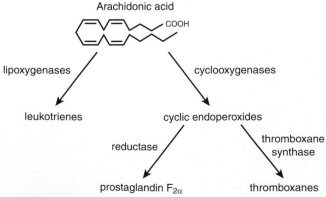

Figure 28.1 Overview of the products derived from arachidonic acid metabolism.

which triggers the release of the second messenger inositol phosphate production and subsequently activates a molecular transduction cascade that leads to IOP reduction.

The prostanoid receptors are distributed widely in ocular tissues, which accounts for the diverse biologic effects of prostaglandins on the eye (12). The expression and distribution of the prostanoid receptors in the human eye have been determined with radioligand receptor binding studies and a variety of molecular methods (13–15). In most animal and human studies, the ocular hypotensive effect of prostaglandins, or hypotensive lipids, was not explained by reducing aqueous production, reducing episcleral venous pressure, or increasing conventional aqueous outflow (16–19). After binding and activating the FP receptors in the ciliary smooth muscle, the precise mechanism by which prostaglandins improve uveoscleral outflow (see Chapter 2) is not fully understood. Two possible mechanisms that have been studied are relaxation of the ciliary muscle and remodeling the extracellular matrix of the ciliary muscle.

In monkey studies, pilocarpine, which causes contraction of the ciliary muscle (see Chapter 32) and is known to reduce uveoscleral outflow, antagonized the $PGF_{2\alpha}$-induced ocular hypotension (20). The in vitro studies of ciliary muscle response to $PGF_{2\alpha}$ have been conflicting. Prostaglandin $F_{2\alpha}$ consistently relaxed carbachol-precontracted fresh ciliary muscle strips from monkey eyes (21). Similarly, trabecular and ciliary muscle contraction induced by endothelin was blocked by unoprostone, a docosanoid, which is a metabolite of docosahexaenoic acid (22). Studies in monkeys suggest a dual action of $PGF_{2\alpha}$ on the ciliary muscle, involving a short-onset, long-lasting relaxation and narrowing of the muscle fiber bundles and a slowly developing, shorter-duration dissolution of the intermuscular connective tissue (23). It is apparent from these and other studies that the effects depend on the species studied and the effect of aging (24). The clinical use of pilocarpine and latanoprost is discussed in the section "Drug Interaction."

There is greater evidence to support the mechanism of remodeling the extracellular matrix of the ciliary muscle. In cultured smooth muscle cells, $PGF_{2\alpha}$ activates the FP receptors and initiates a signal transduction cascade that leads to the induction of the nuclear transcription factor and c-FOS (25). The c-FOS transcription factor binds to a special AP-1 transcription regulatory element in the promoter of certain genes, which leads to transcription of those particular genes (26). One gene class that is regulated by the AP-1 transcription regulatory element is the matrix metalloproteinase family (27). Specific molecules of the matrix metalloproteinase family degrade extracellular matrix substrates, such as certain collagens, fibronectin, or laminin. In ciliary muscle cultures, certain prostaglandin-like agents increase matrix metalloproteinases (28,29). Collagen types I, III, and IV, laminin, fibronectin, and hyalurons were reduced in cultured human ciliary muscle treated by the free acid of latanoprost and $PGF_{2\alpha}$ (30). This prostaglandin-mediated increase in certain matrix metalloproteinases and change in extracellular matrix molecules seen in vitro in the cultured cells were observed in vivo.

In monkeys, immunohistochemical methods have identified increased expression of certain matrix metalloproteinases in ciliary muscle, iris root, and sclera (31). Both collagen type IV and myocilin (*MYOC*), formerly known as trabecular meshwork–inducible glucocorticoid response gene (TIGR) (see Chapter 8), appear to be colocalized in ciliary muscle, and topical $PGF_{2\alpha}$-isopropyl ester treatment decreases *MYOC* expression in monkey eyes (32). Prostaglandin-mediated changes in extracellular matrix metalloproteinases have been identified in ciliary muscle (33), which correlates with the reduction in collagen molecules within the uveoscleral outflow pathways (34). The collective evidence of data supports that the prostaglandins enhance uveoscleral outflow by remodeling the extracellular matrix in the uveoscleral outflow pathway, with possible contributions from some relaxation of the ciliary muscle and change in cell shape by cytoskeletal alteration.

Other possible effects of this class of drugs have also been studied. The evidence on the potential effect of the prostaglandin agents on ocular blood flow in the various vascular beds of the anterior segment, retinal, choroidal, and retrobulbar hemodynamics is not well understood (35). The interaction between prostaglandin agents and adrenergic pathways has been suggested based on the observation that adrenergic antagonists blocked the PGE_2-induced increase in total outflow facility (36). It appears that the PGE class of prostaglandins has an additive effect in combination with latanoprost in lowering IOP in glaucomatous monkey eyes by enhancing trabecular outflow (37,38).

SPECIFIC AGENTS

Latanoprost

Approved for use in 1996, latanoprost was the first clinically practical prostaglandin for the treatment of glaucoma. Latanoprost, 0.005%, given once daily, has been compared with timolol, 0.5%, used twice daily in 6-month trials enrolling ocular hypertensive and glaucoma patients. Three studies included a total of 829 volunteers. In one of these trials, the diurnal IOP reduction at 6 months was 27% with timolol, 31% with latanoprost applied in the morning, and 35% with latanoprost used in the evening (39). In the other two comparative trials, latanoprost was given in the evening, with one study reporting 6-month diurnal IOP reductions of 32.7% and 33.7% for timolol and latanoprost, respectively, and the other reporting 6-month IOP reductions of 4.9 ± 2.9 mm Hg and 6.7 ± 3.4 mm Hg for timolol and latanoprost, respectively (40,41). Unlike timolol, latanoprost lowers the IOP at night and during the day, providing uniform, around-the-clock IOP reduction when administered once daily, alone or in combination with timolol (42).

The effect of latanoprost after 2 years of treatment was evaluated in 532 patients (496 and 113 were treated for 6 and 24 months, respectively) (43), who continued latanoprost monotherapy treatment as part of an open-label trial from the initial 6-month phase III study in Scandinavia and the United Kingdom (39). Over all, there was a similar mean IOP reduction at 2 years, with a decrease of 8.9 mm Hg (34%), compared with 6 months, with a decrease of 8.2 mm Hg (32%). Of the 532 total patients, 20% were withdrawn from treatment because of adverse events based on increased iris color, ocular adverse events, nonocular adverse events, high risk for increased iris color, or IOP treatment failure. For the patients with IOP treatment failure, insufficient IOP control was more common in persons with open-angle glaucoma than in those with ocular hypertension. Patients who initially started with higher baseline IOPs had a higher risk of IOP treatment failure with latanoprost monotherapy.

In addition to its effectiveness to treat ocular hypertension and open-angle glaucoma, latanoprost has also been examined in pediatric glaucoma. In general, latanoprost appears to be safe but tends to be less effective in lowering IOP in children, who have diverse forms of glaucoma treated with concomitant medical antiglaucoma therapies, compared with adults (44). Among the various forms of glaucoma in the pediatric population, it appeared that the older children and those with juvenile-onset open-angle glaucoma showed a better response to this drug (45).

Several prospective studies have examined the efficacy of latanoprost in lowering IOP in patients with chronic angle-closure glaucoma. A meta-analysis was conducted to evaluate the efficacy of prostaglandin analogs in 1090 patients from nine randomized clinical trials with chronic angle-closure glaucoma treated with latanoprost, bimatoprost, or travoprost monotherapy (46). The difference in absolute IOP reduction between the prostaglandin analogs and timolol varied from 0.4 to 1.6 mm Hg during the diurnal curve, 0.9 to 2.3 mm Hg at peak, and 1.3 to 2.4 mm Hg at trough. For latanoprost, the relative IOP reduction was 31% during the diurnal curve, 34% at peak effect, and 31% at trough effect. For timolol, the relative IOP reduction was 23% during the diurnal curve, 24% at peak, and 21% at trough. Based on this meta-analysis, latanoprost is at least as effective as timolol at reducing the IOP efficacy in eyes with chronic angle-closure glaucoma.

Another prospective observational case series of 137 Asian patients with chronic angle-closure glaucoma, which was defined as trabecular meshwork not visible for at least 180 degrees on gonioscopy, were treated with latanoprost (47). After 12 weeks of treatment, latanoprost reduced IOP from 25.0 ± 5.5 to 17.5 ± 5.0 mm Hg. The percentage change in IOP was not affected by the degree of angle narrowing or extent of synechial angle closure.

Three smaller studies also reported on the IOP-lowering effect of latanoprost in patients with chronic angle-closure glaucoma. In a study of 14 Korean patients with 360 degrees of peripheral anterior synechiae on gonioscopy, latanoprost, 0.005%, once daily reduced the IOP from 30.3 ± 4.5 mm Hg at baseline to 21.5 ± 5.9 mm Hg after 3 months of treatment (48). In a study of 36 Japanese patients with chronic angle-closure glaucoma treated by laser iridotomy, the effects of latanoprost alone versus the unfixed combination therapy of timolol maleate, 0.5%, and dorzolamide hydrochloride, 1%, were compared (49). After 12 weeks of treatment, latanoprost reduced the IOP by 33%, from 22.2 ± 2.0 to 14.8 ± 1.9 mm Hg. Timolol maleate and dorzolamide hydrochloride reduced IOP by 24%, from 22.5 ± 2.2 to 17.1 ± 2.7 mm Hg. Finally, in 32 patients who had previous peripheral iridectomy and inadequate IOP, half of the group was randomly assigned to latanoprost and the other half to timolol (50). Latanoprost lowered the IOP by 8.8 mm Hg (34% reduction from a baseline of 25.7 mm Hg), compared with 5.7 mm Hg for timolol (23% reduction from a baseline of 25.2 mm Hg). Thus, when IOP elevation persists after peripheral iridectomy in patients with primary angle-closure glaucoma, latanoprost is effective in lowering the IOP.

Unoprostone

Unlike the 20-carbon molecular skeleton of arachidonic acid, unoprostone, also known as UF-021, may be considered a docosanoid, which is a 22-carbon molecule (Fig. 28.2). Unoprostone has been in clinical use in Japan since 1994 in a 0.12% formulation. Unoprostone, 0.15%, became available for clinical use in the United States in 2000. Studies in Japan have shown that unoprostone, 0.12%, administered two times daily lowered IOP by 11% to 23% from baseline (51–53).

Comparison studies between unoprostone and timolol have shown that unoprostone is not as effective as timolol at decreasing the IOP (54,55). The effectiveness of unoprostone has also been compared with latanoprost. In a comparative parallel-group study in a total of 108 patients, there was a mean IOP reduction of 6.7 mm Hg in the group treated with latanoprost, compared with 3.3 mm Hg lowering in the unoprostone-treated group (56). Similar results showing better efficacy of latanoprost compared with unoprostone were shown in a smaller study of patients with ocular hypertension (57).

A recent study demonstrated that unoprostone increased activity of certain tissue inhibitors of matrix metalloproteinase in cultured human ciliary body smooth muscle cells, compared with bimatoprost and latanoprost (58). It is proposed that this differential effect of the prostaglandin agents may explain the lower clinical efficacy of unoprostone compared with the other agents.

Travoprost

Travoprost, also known as AL-6221, was approved for clinical use in the United States in 2001 (59). The effectiveness of travoprost has been compared with that of timolol and latanoprost.

In a 9-month clinical trial with 573 patients, travoprost showed a 30% to 33% decrease in IOP from baseline compared with a 25% to 29% decrease in IOP in patients using timolol, 0.5%, twice daily (60). In a 6-month comparative study of travoprost and timolol involving 605 patients, the IOP decrease from baseline ranged from −6.5 to −8.0 mm Hg for travoprost, 0.004%, and −5.2 to −7.0 mm Hg for timolol (61). In a 12-month comparative clinical trial of travoprost, latanoprost, and timolol involving 801 patients, the IOP-lowering effect of travoprost was greater than the timolol and similar to that of latanoprost (62). In another clinical trial of 426 patients with uncontrolled IOP on timolol alone, travoprost led to further, significant IOP reduction after 6 months of treatment (63).

Travoprost has also been shown to be effective in lowering IOP in patients with chronic angle-closure glaucoma (46,64).

Travoprost was observed to be more effective in lowering IOP compared with latanoprost in blacks compared with nonblack patients (62,65). However, subsequent studies have not reproduced this observation. In a small, randomized, investigator-masked multicenter study, 83 patients with open-angle glaucoma were self-identified as white or other (i.e., African, East Indian, Asian, or Hispanic) and were randomly assigned to receive one of three prostaglandin–prostamide drugs (66). After 24 weeks of treatment, there was a significant decrease in IOP compared with baseline. In this study, there were no differences in treatment effect between the three drugs or between the two ethnic groups, and there was no interaction between race and drug. The results from this smaller study confirmed the observation in the larger Ocular Hypertension Treatment Study (67). The IOP response to prostaglandin analogs was slightly greater in self-declared African American participants compared with whites, but this difference was not statistically significant. The greater IOP reduction was associated with a higher baseline IOP and a thinner central corneal measurement.

Bimatoprost

Bimatoprost, which was also known as AGN 192024, was approved for clinical use in the United States in 2001. Its chemical structure differs from $PGF_{2\alpha}$ and the other prostaglandin analogs (Fig. 28.2) with an amide ethyl group at the C-1 position. There is growing evidence to support the designation of this agent as a prostamide, given the identification of the cyclooxygenase-2 (COX-2)–derived oxidation products of the endocannabinoids and the recent discovery and development of prostamide antagonists (68–70).

Bimatoprost is hydrolyzed by the cornea to a lesser extent than with latanoprost, unoprostone, and travoprost into the active free acid form of the drug (8). The IOP lowering of bimatoprost (30.4% lowering with once-daily dosing) is greater than that of timolol (26.2% lowering with twice-daily dosing) (71). Similar treatment results have been shown in other clinical studies comparing bimatoprost and timolol (72,73). Bimatoprost has been compared with latanoprost and showed a similar IOP-lowering effect (74–76). In a community-based "switch study" involving 1283 patients who were changed from latanoprost to bimatoprost treatment, there was a mean IOP reduction of 3.4 mm Hg after 2 months of bimatoprost treatment (77). In such a "switch" study, however, the observed IOP reduction may simply reflect a regression to the mean with repeated IOP measurements over time (78).

Bimatoprost has also been shown to lower IOP in patients with chronic angle-closure glaucoma. In a meta-analysis of nine randomized clinical trials enrolling a total of 1090 patients, bimatoprost lowered the diurnal IOP curve by 26%, the peak IOP by 28%, and the trough IOP by 27% (46). Timolol lowered the diurnal IOP curve by 23%, the peak IOP by 24%, and the trough IOP by 21%. Other studies also showed that bimatoprost was effective compared with latanoprost in lowering IOP in chronic angle-closure glaucoma (79,80).

There is some evidence to support that bimatoprost has both FP-receptor agonist activity and possibly another mechanism of action related to trabecular outflow and an alternative signaling pathway based on an assay in feline iris (70,81,82).

ADMINISTRATION

Latanoprost, 0.005%, travoprost, 0.004%, and bimatoprost, 0.03%, are administered similarly as one drop daily to the eye. More frequent dosing of these particular agents resulted in reduced efficacy of the drug (71,83). In contrast, unoprostone, 0.15%, is administered as one drop two times daily to the eye.

The dosing regimen for this drug class is unusual given that the pharmacokinetic data indicate a very short plasma elimination half-life ($t_{1/2}$ life of 9.2 minutes after intravenous administration and 2.3 minutes after topical administration for latanoprost; $t_{1/2}$ life of 45 minutes after intravenous administration for bimatoprost) (84–86). This molecule is dosed at what appears to be homeopathic levels, but at this dose, it has profound clinical effects on IOP reduction in most patients. The explanation for this dosing regimen and the efficacy is not fully understood on the basis of our present knowledge of the pharmacology and mechanism of action of this drug class (as discussed in the earlier section).

The issue of the effect of storage temperature has been raised with these agents because one study reported that latanoprost exhibits thermal and ultraviolet instability (87). This raises issues related to chemical stability of the molecule and to the role of the composition of the dispensing system on bioavailability of the drug. A comparative study with the other agents in this drug class has not been reported. It has been suggested that unopened bottles of latanoprost be stored under refrigeration. Once opened, latanoprost may be stored at room temperature (as high as 25°C, or 77°F) for up to 6 weeks. The other agents are recommended to be stored at room temperature (15°C to 25°C, or 59°F to 77°F, for bimatoprost; 2°C to 25°C, or 36°F to 77°F, for travoprost and unoprostone).

DRUG INTERACTION

Given the additional 13% to 37% IOP lowering by combining a uveoscleral outflow drug together with the aqueous humor inflow suppressant timolol (88,89), fixed combinations of the prostaglandin agents with timolol have been studied. In other countries, the fixed combination of latanoprost, 0.005%, and timolol, 0.5%, was approved for clinical use in Europe during the summer of 2001 and has been shown to be effective and comparable with each component given separately (90–92). The fixed combination of travoprost, 0.004%, and timolol, 0.5%, and bimatoprost and timolol, 0.5%, are also available in other countries (93–97). At present, none of these agents are approved for use in the United States.

The combination of the prostaglandin agents in addition to oral and topical carbonic anhydrase inhibitors (CAIs) have been examined. In 24 patients with glaucoma, a mean IOP of 19.5 mm Hg was achieved while on treatment with acetazolamide (250 mg twice daily), which decreased to 16.8 mm Hg, which was a 15% IOP reduction, after 15 days of combination treatment with latanoprost (0.005% once daily) and acetazolamide (250 mg twice daily) (98). Topical CAIs were also shown to have additional IOP-lowering effect in combination with latanoprost (99). A similar effect was observed with travoprost (100,101).

The combination of the prostaglandin agent bimatoprost and the α_2-adrenergic agonist brimonidine has been compared with the combination of timolol and latanoprost in 28 patients (102). The mean IOP at baseline was 24.8 mm Hg. There was a decrease of 8.5 to 9.0 mm Hg after treatment with bimatoprost combined with brimonidine, and 7.5 to 7.7 mm Hg after treatment with latanoprost combined with timolol. Another study compared combination therapy of brimonidine and latanoprost to the fixed combination of timolol and dorzolamide in patients with glaucoma or ocular hypertension (103). The brimonidine and latanoprost combination was associated with a mean IOP reduction of 9.2 mm Hg. This IOP decrease with use of the combination of the prostaglandin-related drugs and brimonidine is greater than the decrease of 6.7 mm Hg with use of the timolol–dorzolamide fixed combination.

Initially, the interaction of latanoprost with miotic agents, such as pilocarpine, was not clear based on the early observation that pilocarpine antagonized $PGF_{2\alpha}$-induced ocular hypotension in monkeys (20). This observation was not surprising because pilocarpine contracts the ciliary muscle, which can both decrease uveoscleral outflow and increase trabecular outflow facility by pulling on the scleral spur (see Chapter 32). In contrast, latanoprost lowers IOP by improving uveoscleral outflow, possibly through relaxation of the ciliary muscle, but primarily through remodeling the extracellular matrix (see "Mechanisms of Action"). This is consistent with an ultrasound biomicroscopy study of 36 healthy young Japanese persons showing that pilocarpine, 2%, increased the ciliary body thickness by 8.3% and latanoprost, 0.005%, decreased the thickness by 3.3% (104).

However, in clinical trials, it became apparent that pilocarpine did not impair the IOP-lowering effect of latanoprost (105), and it was demonstrated that these drugs were additive by fluorophotometric, pneumotonometric, and venomanometric methods (106). In a study of 20 patients with ocular hypertension who were initially treated with pilocarpine, 2%, three times daily or latanoprost, 0.005%, twice daily, the IOP reduction at the end of 1 week was 14.3% on pilocarpine alone and 23.4% on latanoprost alone (107). When pilocarpine was then added to the latanoprost, the additional IOP reduction was 7.4%, compared with 14.2% when latanoprost was added to pilocarpine. In patients who were on maximal medical therapy that included miotics, latanoprost had an additive effect, with additional IOP lowering (108,109). Although the use of miotic therapies has declined with the availability of other drug classes with fewer ocular side effects and less frequent dosing, the miotic agents are expected to have an additive effect in combination with the prostaglandin-related drugs.

In general, there are few studies to support switching within the class of the prostaglandin agents. It has been suggested that unoprostone may have additive IOP lowering to latanoprost on the basis of a study of 41 patients (110). This additive effect was not supported in another study of 52 patients in which half the patients were initially treated with latanoprost for 6 weeks followed by adding unoprostone, and the other half of patients were treated initially with unoprostone and later adding latanoprost (111). The combination of unoprostone with latanoprost did not result in further IOP lowering compared with latanoprost alone. It appears that unoprostone is not likely very useful as an adjunctive prostaglandin agent in patients who are already on another prostaglandin agent.

There is awareness that a small number of patients are nonresponders to latanoprost (112,113), which would also be expected for the other prostaglandin-related agents. In 15 patients who were classified as nonresponders to latanoprost, which was defined as less than 10% IOP lowering after 6 to 8 weeks of latanoprost, 0.005%, administered once daily, bimatoprost (18.2 mm Hg on bimatoprost treatment) was more effective than latanoprost (24.1 mm Hg on latanoprost treatment) (114). The mechanism to explain the variation in IOP response to latanoprost versus bimatoprost in the same group of patients is not understood.

SIDE EFFECTS

Several side effects have been reported for the prostaglandin class of glaucoma medications that appear unique to this drug class compared with the other types of glaucoma medications. Most of these side effects are associated with use of latanoprost, because clinical experience has been longer with this agent than with unoprostone, bimatoprost, or travoprost. In general, these side effects are not common and a causal relationship has not been established. Although some of these side effects were not apparent in the well-designed glaucoma pharmacology clinical trial, it should be appreciated that new side effects or unanticipated effects are observed in the postmarketing use of a drug in individual patients who do not reflect the average participant in the clinical trials.

In general, based on the various clinical trials, the prostaglandin-related agents were associated with greater conjunctival hyperemia compared with timolol-treated eyes (39–41,60,71). The hyperemia frequency rates in the product labeling are 5% to 15% for latanoprost, 0.005%; 15% to 45% for bimatoprost, 0.03%; 35% to 50% for travoprost, 0.004%; and 10% to 25% for unoprostone, 0.15%. The tremendous variation in the frequency of this side effect among the clinical trials depended on the particular dosing regimen used and the method used to ascertain this clinical finding, which may be elicited by patient report, by discontinuation rate for hyperemia, by grading based on clinical photographs, or by investigators' severity scoring (115). Several studies have compared the prostaglandin-related drugs to each other, and in general,

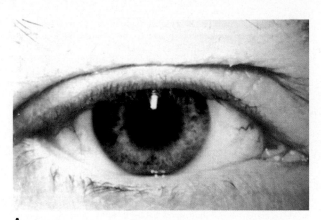
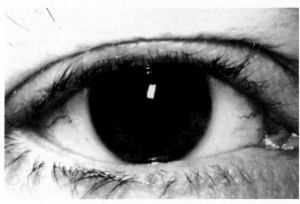

A   **B**

Figure 28.3 Increased pigmentation of the iris in a patient taking prostaglandin therapy for glaucoma for 10 months. This side effect occurs primarily in patients with green-brown or blue–gray-brown iris color. (From Watson P, Stjernschantz J. A six-month, randomized, double-masked study comparing latanoprost with timolol in open-angle glaucoma and ocular hypertension. The Latanoprost Study Group. *Ophthalmology.* 1996;103(1):126–137, with permission.)

all the prostaglandin-related agents were associated with some degree of conjunctival hyperemia (57,62,75,116).

The effect of latanoprost on conjunctival fibroblasts and conjunctiva has been examined. In rabbits treated with topical latanoprost, there was upregulation of matrix metalloproteinase type 3 compared with control and timolol-treated eyes (117). Latanoprost increased the number of fibroblasts that stained for proliferating cell nuclear antigen, a marker for proliferating cells, compared with control treated rabbit eyes (118). With 6 months of latanoprost treatment in patients, the drug appeared to have transient effects on goblet cell density and was associated with a decrease in conjunctival epithelial cell size based on impression cytology staining comparing the status before and after treatment (119). A control patient population was not examined in that study. The effect of these agents on conjunctival biology and function is not fully understood regarding the impact of glaucoma drugs on the tissues and outcome of filtration surgery.

The main concern for corneal toxicity associated with prostaglandin treatment is an eye with a history of herpes simplex keratitis. There are case reports of reactivation of herpes simplex keratitis in patients treated with latanoprost or bimatoprost (120,121). In a rabbit model, topical latanoprost increased the severity and recurrence or herpetic keratitis (122), and unoprostone did not (123). In a patient with a history of herpetic keratitis, an alternative drug class would be prudent for initial drug treatment for glaucoma. Superficial epithelial lesions of the cornea have been reported after latanoprost treatment (40,124). In a 1-year clinical trial comparing latanoprost, fixed-combination latanoprost–timolol, and timolol, all three treatments had similar long-term corneal effects with little change in corneal endothelial cell density and corneal thickness (125).

The intraocular inflammatory effects of aqueous cell and flare and miosis, which result from the administration of large doses of prostaglandins, were not seen in animal or human eyes in the doses associated with the ocular hypotensive response (126–128). The absorptive transport systems of the ciliary

processes appear to prevent topically applied prostaglandins and other eicosanoids from causing retinal toxicity (129). Although, in general, this class of drug is well tolerated in a large number of patients, a few patients developed anterior uveitis while on latanoprost or cystoid macular edema after treatment with latanoprost (130–134). Similarly, there are reported cases of cystoid macular edema associated with use of unoprostone, travoprost, and bimatoprost (135). Cautious use of this class of drugs is advised in eyes with risk factors for cystoid macular edema (135,136).

The most visible side effect of the prostaglandin drug class is increased pigmentation in the periocular skin and iris and alterations in the eyelid cilia. Increased periocular skin pigmentation has been reported with the use of the prostaglandin agents (137). Instructing patients to wipe off any excess drops on the periocular skin area is important to minimize exposure of this area to this effect, which is reversible upon cessation of the drug exposure. Darkening of the iris was seen in 10% of the patients in one study (39), and also with the other prostaglandin agents (138). This was reported to occur more commonly in eyes with mixed green-brown or blue–gray-brown iris color (**Fig. 28.3**) but has also been reported in a brown iris (39,139). The mechanism appears to be similar in the iris and epidermal melanocytes with upregulation of tyrosinase activity in melanocytes (140,141). In the pigmented rabbit model of lighter colored iris from sympathetic denervation, treatment of this eye with latanoprost darkened the iris in the denervated eye (142). Both light and electron microscopy studies indicate that the melanin content is increased in iris stromal melanocytes without proliferation of cells (143–145). Because the alteration in iris color relates to iris stromal melanocytes, this is not expected to be related to open-angle glaucoma related to pigment dispersion (see Chapter 17), which in general is related to release of intraocular pigment by disruption of the pigmented epithelium on the posterior surface of the iris.

Reports of prostaglandin-associated alterations in eyelid cilia include hypertrichosis and increased pigmentation (146).

Their effect on eyelash prominence is further highlighted by the recent U.S. Food and Drug Administration approval of bimatoprost, 0.03%, for treatment of hypotrichosis of eyelashes. For some patients, this side effect is beneficial and desirable, especially in the setting of chemotherapy-induced hair loss (147). The mechanism responsible for this side effect involves stimulating the growth phase of the hair cycle in the dermal papilla (148).

Other reactions reported to be associated with latanoprost include allergic contact dermatitis, iris cyst associated with latanoprost, and herpes simplex dermatitis (149–151).

With regard to systemic side effects, the amount of prostaglandin entering the circulation from the low doses of its ester that is required to lower the IOP is a small fraction of the amount of endogenous prostaglandins that are normally released from virtually all tissues of the body (129). No significant systemic reactions were reported with latanoprost in any of the clinical trials (39,40,152). In a crossover study comparing the effect of 6-day treatment with latanoprost and placebo, 24 patients with asthma had no alteration in respiratory function and asthmatic symptoms (153). Another study of 141 patients with newly diagnosed glaucoma included cardiovascular and respiratory examinations at baseline and after 3 months of treatment with betaxolol, brimonidine, latanoprost, or timolol (154). There were no statistically significant changes in the cardiovascular and spirometry measurements in the treated patients with the exception of timolol, which was associated with a decrease in peak flow. It appears that the prostaglandin agents have little clinical effect on cardiac and respiratory systems.

KEY POINTS

- The prostaglandin agents are effective in lowering IOP and are practically used as first-line treatment agents.
- At high levels, these ubiquitous local hormones produce ocular inflammation and ocular hypertension, but in smaller amounts, they reduce IOP. The prostaglandin agents are well tolerated and have virtually no systemic side effects.
- The main mechanism of action for reducing IOP is primarily by improving uveoscleral outflow with a proposed biochemical effect of altering the extracellular matrix.
- Caution should be used in considering alternative medical treatment to the prostaglandins if a patient has a history of uveitis or herpes simplex keratitis.

REFERENCES

1. Itoh S, Lu R, Bao Y, et al. Structural determinants of substrates for the prostaglandin transporter PGT. *Mol Pharmacol.* 1996;50(4):738–742.
2. Ferreira S, Vane JR. Prostaglandins: their disappearance and release into the circulation. *Nature.* 1967;216:868–873.
3. Kurzrok R, Lieb CC. Biochemical studies of human semen: II. The action of semen on the human uterus. *Proc Soc Exp Biol Med.* 1930;28:1056–1057.
4. Ambache N. Irin, a smooth-muscle contracting substance present in rabbit iris. *J Physiol.* 1955;129(3):65–66.
5. Camras C, Bito LZ, Eakins KE. Reduction of intraocular pressure by prostaglandins applied topically to the eyes of conscious rabbits. *Invest Ophthalmol Vis Sci.* 1977;16:1125–1134.
6. Giuffre G. The effects of prostaglandin F2 alpha in the human eye. *Graefes Arch Clin Exp Ophthalmol.* 1985;222(3):139–141.
7. Resul B, Stjernschantz J, Selen G, et al. Structure–activity relationships and receptor profiles of some ocular hypotensive prostanoids. *Surv Ophthalmol.* 1997;41(suppl 2):S47–S52.
8. Maxey KM, Johnson JL, LaBrecque J. The hydrolysis of bimatoprost in corneal tissue generates a potent prostanoid FP receptor agonist. *Surv Ophthalmol.* 2002;47(4 suppl 1):S34–S40.
9. Coleman RA, Smith WL, Narumiya S. International Union of Pharmacology classification of prostanoid receptors: properties, distribution, and structure of the receptors and their subtypes. *Pharmacol Rev.* 1994;46(2):205–229.
10. Pierce KL, Gil DW, Woodward DF, et al. Cloning of human prostanoid receptors. *Trends Pharmacol Sci.* 1995;16(8):253–256.
11. Pierce KL, Bailey TJ, Hoyer PB, et al. Cloning of a carboxyl-terminal isoform of the prostanoid FP receptor. *J Biol Chem.* 1997;272:883–887.
12. Bito LZ, Stjernschantz J, eds. *The Ocular Effects of Prostaglandins and Other Eicosanoids.* New York, NY: Alan R. Liss; 1989.
13. Matsuo T, Cynader MS. Localisation of prostaglandin F2 alpha and E2 binding sites in the human eye. *Br J Ophthalmol.* 1992;76(4):210–213.
14. Anthony TL, Pierce KL, Stamer WD, et al. Prostaglandin F2 alpha receptors in the human trabecular meshwork. *Invest Ophthalmol Vis Sci.* 1998;39(2):315–321.
15. Kamphuis W, Schneemann A, van Beek LM, et al. Prostanoid receptor gene expression profile in human trabecular meshwork: a quantitative real-time PCR approach. *Invest Ophthalmol Vis Sci.* 2001;42(13):3209–3215.
16. Lee PY, Podos SM, Severin C. Effect of prostaglandin F2 alpha on aqueous humor dynamics of rabbit, cat, and monkey. *Invest Ophthalmol Vis Sci.* 1984;25(9):1087–1093.
17. Crawford K, Kaufman PL, Gabelt BT. Effects of topical PGF2 alpha on aqueous humor dynamics in cynomolgus monkeys. *Curr Eye Res.* 1987;6(8):1035–1044.
18. Toris CB, Camras CB, Yablonski ME. Effects of PhXA41, a new prostaglandin F2 alpha analog, on aqueous humor dynamics in human eyes. *Ophthalmology.* 1993;100(9):1297–1304.
19. Serle JB, Podos SM, Kitazawa Y, et al. A comparative study of latanoprost (Xalatan) and isopropyl unoprostone (Rescula) in normal and glaucomatous monkey eyes. *Jpn J Ophthalmol.* 1998;42(2):95–100.
20. Crawford K, Kaufman PL. Pilocarpine antagonizes prostaglandin F2 alpha-induced ocular hypotension in monkeys. Evidence for enhancement of uveoscleral outflow by prostaglandin F2 alpha. *Arch Ophthalmol.* 1987;105(8):1112–1116.
21. Poyer JF, Millar C, Kaufman PL. Prostaglandin F2 alpha effects on isolated rhesus monkey ciliary muscle. *Invest Ophthalmol Vis Sci.* 1995;36(12):2461–2465.
22. Thieme H, Stumpff F, Ottlecz A, et al. Mechanisms of action of unoprostone on trabecular meshwork contractility. *Invest Ophthalmol Vis Sci.* 2001;42(13):3193–3201.
23. Crawford KS, Kaufman PL. Dose-related effects of prostaglandin F2 alpha isopropylester on intraocular pressure, refraction, and pupil diameter in monkeys. *Invest Ophthalmol Vis Sci.* 1991;32(3):510–519.
24. Gabelt BT, Gottanka J, Lutjen-Drecoll E, et al. Aqueous humor dynamics and trabecular meshwork and anterior ciliary muscle morphologic changes with age in rhesus monkeys. *Invest Ophthalmol Vis Sci.* 2003;44(5):2118–2125.
25. Lindsey JD, To HD, Weinreb RN. Induction of c-fos by prostaglandin F2 alpha in human ciliary smooth muscle cells. *Invest Ophthalmol Vis Sci.* 1994;35(1):242–250.
26. Karin M, Liu Z, Zandi E. AP-1 function and regulation. *Curr Opin Cell Biol.* 1997;9(2):240–246.
27. Woessner JF Jr. Matrix metalloproteinases and their inhibitors in connective tissue remodeling. *FASEB J.* 1991;5(8):2145–2154.
28. Weinreb RN, Kashiwagi K, Kashiwagi F, et al. Prostaglandins increase matrix metalloproteinase release from human ciliary smooth muscle cells. *Invest Ophthalmol Vis Sci.* 1997;38(13):2772–2780.
29. Kashiwagi K, Jin M, Suzuki M, et al. Isopropyl unoprostone increases the activities of matrix metalloproteinases in cultured monkey ciliary muscle cells. *J Glaucoma.* 2001;10(4):271–276.
30. Ocklind A. Effect of latanoprost on the extracellular matrix of the ciliary muscle. A study on cultured cells and tissue sections. *Exp Eye Res.* 1998;67(2):179–191.
31. Gaton DD, Sagara T, Lindsey JD, et al. Increased matrix metalloproteinases 1, 2, and 3 in the monkey uveoscleral outflow pathway after

topical prostaglandin F(2 alpha)-isopropyl ester treatment. *Arch Ophthalmol.* 2001;119(8):1165–1170.

32. Lindsey JD, Gaton DD, Sagara T, et al. Reduced TIGR/myocilin protein in the monkey ciliary muscle after topical prostaglandin F(2alpha) treatment. *Invest Ophthalmol Vis Sci.* 2001;42(8):1781–1786.

33. Weinreb RN, Lindsey JD. Metalloproteinase gene transcription in human ciliary muscle cells with latanoprost. *Invest Ophthalmol Vis Sci.* 2002;43(3):716–722.

34. Sagara T, Gaton DD, Lindsey JD, et al. Topical prostaglandin F2alpha treatment reduces collagen types I, III, and IV in the monkey uveoscleral outflow pathway. *Arch Ophthalmol.* 1999;117(6):794–801.

35. Costa VP, Harris A, Stefansson E, et al. The effects of antiglaucoma and systemic medications on ocular blood flow. *Prog Retin Eye Res.* 2003;22(6):769–805.

36. Green K, Kim K. Interaction of adrenergic antagonists with prostaglandin E2 and tetrahydrocannabinol in the eye. *Invest Ophthalmol.* 1976;15(2):102–111.

37. Wang RF, Podos SM, Serle JB, et al. Effect of latanoprost or 8-iso prostaglandin E2 alone and in combination on intraocular pressure in glaucomatous monkey eyes. *Arch Ophthalmol.* 2000;118(1):74–77.

38. Dijkstra BG, Schneemann A, Hoyng PF. Flow after prostaglandin E1 is mediated by receptor-coupled adenylyl cyclase in human anterior segments. *Invest Ophthalmol Vis Sci.* 1999;40(11):2622–2626.

39. Alm A, Stjernschantz J. Effects on intraocular pressure and side effects of 0.005% latanoprost applied once daily, evening or morning. A comparison with timolol. Scandinavian Latanoprost Study Group. *Ophthalmology.* 1995;102(12):1743–1752.

40. Watson P, Stjernschantz J. A six-month, randomized, double-masked study comparing latanoprost with timolol in open-angle glaucoma and ocular hypertension. The Latanoprost Study Group. *Ophthalmology.* 1996;103(1):126–137.

41. Camras CB. Comparison of latanoprost and timolol in patients with ocular hypertension and glaucoma: a six-month masked, multicenter trial in the United States. The United States Latanoprost Study Group. *Ophthalmology.* 1996;103(1):138–147.

42. Racz P, Ruzsonyi MR, Nagy ZT, et al. Around-the-clock intraocular pressure reduction with once-daily application of latanoprost by itself or in combination with timolol. *Arch Ophthalmol.* 1996;114(3):268–273.

43. Hedman K, Watson PG, Alm A. The effect of latanoprost on intraocular pressure during 2 years of treatment. *Surv Ophthalmol.* 2002;47(suppl 1):S65–S76.

44. Coppens G, Stalmans I, Zeyen T, et al. The safety and efficacy of glaucoma medication in the pediatric population. *J Pediatr Ophthalmol Strabismus.* 2009;46(1):12–18.

45. Enyedi LB, Freedman SF. Latanoprost for the treatment of pediatric glaucoma. *Surv Ophthalmol.* 2002;47(suppl 1):S129–S132.

46. Cheng JW, Cai JP, Li Y, et al. A meta-analysis of topical prostaglandin analogs in the treatment of chronic angle-closure glaucoma. *J Glaucoma.* 2009;18(9):652–657.

47. Aung T, Chan YH, Chew PT. Degree of angle closure and the intraocular pressure-lowering effect of latanoprost in subjects with chronic angle-closure glaucoma. *Ophthalmology.* 2005;112(2):267–271.

48. Kook MS, Cho HS, Yang SJ, et al. Efficacy of latanoprost in patients with chronic angle-closure glaucoma and no visible ciliary-body face: a preliminary study. *J Ocul Pharmacol Ther.* 2005;21(1):75–84.

49. Sakai H, Shinjyo S, Nakamura Y, et al. Comparison of latanoprost monotherapy and combined therapy of 0.5% timolol and 1% dorzolamide in chronic primary angle-closure glaucoma (CACG) in Japanese patients. *J Ocul Pharmacol Ther.* 2005;21(6):483–489.

50. Chew PT, Hung PT, Aung T. Efficacy of latanoprost in reducing intraocular pressure in patients with primary angle-closure glaucoma. *Surv Ophthalmol.* 2002;47(suppl 1):S125–S128.

51. Yamamoto T, Kitazawa Y, Azuma I, et al. Clinical evaluation of UF-021 (Rescula; isopropyl unoprostone). *Surv Ophthalmol.* 1997;41(suppl 2):S99–S103.

52. Azuma I, Masuda K, Kitazawa Y, et al. Double-masked comparative study of UF-021 and timolol ophthalmic solutions in patients with primary open-angle glaucoma or ocular hypertension. *Jpn J Ophthalmol.* 1993;37(4):514–525.

53. Takase M, Murao M, Koyano S, et al. Ocular effects of topical instillation of UF-021 ophthalmic solution in healthy volunteers [in Japanese]. *Nippon Ganka Gakkai Zasshi.* 1992;96(10):1261–1267.

54. Nordmann JP, Mertz B, Yannoulis NC, et al. A double-masked randomized comparison of the efficacy and safety of unoprostone with timolol and betaxolol in patients with primary open-angle glaucoma including exfoliation glaucoma or ocular hypertension. 6 month data. *Am J Ophthalmol.* 2002;133(1):1–10.

55. Stewart WC, Stewart JA, Kapik BM. The effects of unoprostone isopropyl 0.12% and timolol maleate 0.5% on diurnal intraocular pressure. *J Glaucoma.* 1998;7(6):388–394.

56. Susanna RJ, Giampani JJ, Borges AS, et al. A double-masked, randomized clinical trial comparing latanoprost with unoprostone in patients with open-angle glaucoma or ocular hypertension. *Ophthalmology.* 2001;108(2):259–263.

57. Kobayashi H, Kobayashi K, Okinami S. A comparison of intraocular pressure-lowering effect of prostaglandin F2-alpha analogues, latanoprost, and unoprostone isopropyl. *J Glaucoma.* 2001;10(6):487–492.

58. Ooi YH, Oh DJ, Rhee DJ. Effect of bimatoprost, latanoprost, and unoprostone on matrix metalloproteinases and their inhibitors in human ciliary body smooth muscle cells. *Invest Ophthalmol Vis Sci.* 2009;50(11):5259–5265.

59. Hellberg MR, McLaughlin MA, Sharif NA, et al. Identification and characterization of the ocular hypotensive efficacy of travoprost, a potent and selective FP prostaglandin receptor agonist, and AL-6598, a DP prostaglandin receptor agonist. *Surv Ophthalmol.* 2002;47(suppl 1):S13–S33.

60. Goldberg I, Cunha-Vaz J, Jakobsen JE, et al. Comparison of topical travoprost eye drops given once daily and timolol 0.5% given twice daily in patients with open-angle glaucoma or ocular hypertension. *J Glaucoma.* 2001;10(5):414–422.

61. Fellman RL, Sullivan EK, Ratliff M, et al. Comparison of travoprost 0.0015% and 0.004% with timolol 0.5% in patients with elevated intraocular pressure: a 6-month, masked, multicenter trial. *Ophthalmology.* 2002;109(5):998–1008.

62. Netland PA, Landry T, Sullivan EK, et al. Travoprost compared with latanoprost and timolol in patients with open-angle glaucoma or ocular hypertension. *Am J Ophthalmol.* 2001;132(4):472–484.

63. Orengo-Nania S, Landry T, Von Tress M, et al. Evaluation of travoprost as adjunctive therapy in patients with uncontrolled intraocular pressure while using timolol 0.5%. *Am J Ophthalmol.* 2001;132(6):860–868.

64. Chen MJ, Chen YC, Chou CK, et al. Comparison of the effects of latanoprost and travoprost on intraocular pressure in chronic angle-closure glaucoma. *J Ocul Pharmacol Ther.* 2006;22(6):449–454.

65. Netland PA, Robertson SM, Sullivan EK, et al. Response to travoprost in black and nonblack patients with open-angle glaucoma or ocular hypertension. *Adv Ther.* 2003;20(3):149–163.

66. Birt CM, Buys YM, Ahmed II, et al. Prostaglandin efficacy and safety study undertaken by race (The PRESSURE Study). *J Glaucoma* 2009;Dec 30 [Epub ahead of print]

67. Mansberger SL, Hughes BA, Gordon MO, et al. Comparison of initial intraocular pressure response with topical beta-adrenergic antagonists and prostaglandin analogues in African American and white individuals in the Ocular Hypertension Treatment Study. *Arch Ophthalmol.* 2007;125(4):454–459.

68. Porter AC, Felder CC. The endocannabinoid nervous system: unique opportunities for therapeutic intervention. *Pharmacol Ther.* 2001;90(1):45–60.

69. Yu M, Ives D, Ramesha CS. Synthesis of prostaglandin E2 ethanolamide from anandamide by cyclooxygenase-2. *J Biol Chem.* 1997;272(34):21181–21186.

70. Woodward DF, Liang Y, Krauss AH. Prostamides (prostaglandin-ethanolamides) and their pharmacology. *Br J Pharmacol.* 2008;153(3):410–419.

71. Brandt JD, VanDenburgh AM, Chen K, et al. Comparison of once- or twice-daily bimatoprost with twice-daily timolol in patients with elevated IOP: a 3-month clinical trial. *Ophthalmology.* 2001;108(6):1023–1031.

72. Higginbotham EJ, Schuman JS, Goldberg I, et al. One-year, randomized study comparing bimatoprost and timolol in glaucoma and ocular hypertension. *Arch Ophthalmol.* 2002;120(10):1286–1293.

73. Laibovitz RA, VanDenburgh AM, Felix C, et al. Comparison of the ocular hypotensive lipid AGN 192024 with timolol: dosing, efficacy, and safety evaluation of a novel compound for glaucoma management. *Arch Ophthalmol.* 2001;119(7):994–1000.

74. DuBiner H, Cooke D, Dirks M, et al. Efficacy and safety of bimatoprost in patients with elevated intraocular pressure: a 30-day comparison with latanoprost. *Surv Ophthalmol.* 2001;45(suppl 4):S353–S360.

75. Gandolfi S, Simmons ST, Sturm R, et al. Bimatoprost Study Group. Three-month comparison of bimatoprost and latanoprost in patients with glaucoma and ocular hypertension. *Adv Ther.* 2001;18(3):110–121.

76. Noecker RS, Dirks MS, Choplin NT, et al. A six-month randomized clinical trial comparing the intraocular pressure-lowering efficacy of

bimatoprost and latanoprost in patients with ocular hypertension or glaucoma. *Am J Ophthalmol.* 2003;135(1):55–63.

77. Bournias TE, Lee D, Gross R, et al. Ocular hypotensive efficacy of bimatoprost when used as a replacement for latanoprost in the treatment of glaucoma and ocular hypertension. *J Ocul Pharmacol Ther.* 2003; 19(3):193–203.

78. Bhorade AM, Gordon MO, Wilson B, et al. Variability of intraocular pressure measurements in observation participants in the Ocular Hypertension Treatment Study. *Ophthalmology.* 2009;116(4):717–724.

79. How AC, Kumar RS, Chen YM, et al. A randomised crossover study comparing bimatoprost and latanoprost in subjects with primary angle closure glaucoma. *Br J Ophthalmol.* 2009;93(6):782–786.

80. Chen MJ, Chen YC, Chou CK, et al. Comparison of the effects of latanoprost and bimatoprost on intraocular pressure in chronic angle-closure glaucoma. *J Ocul Pharmacol Ther.* 2007;23(6):559–566.

81. Wan Z, Woodward DF, Cornell CL, et al. Bimatoprost, prostamide activity, and conventional drainage. *Invest Ophthalmol Vis Sci.* 2007; 48(9):4107–4115.

82. Brubaker RF, Schoff EO, Nau CB, et al. Effects of AGN 192024, a new ocular hypotensive agent, on aqueous dynamics. *Am J Ophthalmol.* 2001;131(1):19–24.

83. Nagasubramanian S, Sheth GP, Hitchings RA, et al. Intraocular pressure-reducing effect of PhXA41 in ocular hypertension. Comparison of dose regimens. *Ophthalmology.* 1993;100(9):1305–1311.

84. Stjernschantz J, Selen G, Sjoquist B, et al. Preclinical pharmacology of latanoprost, a phenyl-substituted PGF2 alpha analogue. *Adv Prostaglandin Thromboxane Leukot Res.* 1995;23:513–518.

85. Woodward DF, Krauss AH, Chen J, et al. The pharmacology of bimatoprost (Lumigan). *Surv Ophthalmol.* 2001;45(suppl 4):S337–S345.

86. Sjoquist B, Stjernschantz J. Ocular and systemic pharmacokinetics of latanoprost in humans. *Surv Ophthalmol.* 2002;47(suppl 1):S6–S12.

87. Morgan PV, Proniuk S, Blanchard J, et al. Effect of temperature and light on the stability of latanoprost and its clinical relevance. *J Glaucoma.* 2001;10(5):401–405.

88. Villumsen J, Alm A. The effect of adding prostaglandin F2 alpha-isopropylester to timolol in patients with open angle glaucoma. *Arch Ophthalmol.* 1990;108(8):1102–1105.

89. Higginbotham EJ, Diestelhorst M, Pfeiffer N, et al. The efficacy and safety of unfixed and fixed combinations of latanoprost and other antiglaucoma medications. *Surv Ophthalmol.* 2002;47(suppl 1):S133–S140.

90. Polo V, Larrosa JM, Ferreras A, et al. Effect on diurnal intraocular pressure of the fixed combination of latanoprost 0.005% and timolol 0.5% administered in the evening in glaucoma. *Ann Ophthalmol (Skokie).* 2008;40(3–4):157–162.

91. Centofanti M, Oddone F, Vetrugno M, et al. Efficacy of the fixed combinations of bimatoprost or latanoprost plus timolol in patients uncontrolled with prostaglandin monotherapy: a multicenter, randomized, investigator-masked, clinical study. *Eur J Ophthalmol.* 2009;19(1): 66–71.

92. Calissendorff B, Sjoquist B, Hogberg G, et al. Bioavailability in the human eye of a fixed combination of latanoprost and timolol compared to monotherapy. *J Ocul Pharmacol Ther.* 2002;18(2):127–131.

93. Rossi GC, Pasinetti GM, Bracchino M, et al. Switching from concomitant latanoprost 0.005% and timolol 0.5% to a fixed combination of travoprost 0.004%/timolol 0.5% in patients with primary open-angle glaucoma and ocular hypertension: a 6-month, multicenter, cohort study. *Expert Opin Pharmacother.* 2009;10(11):1705–1711.

94. Konstas AG, Mikropoulos D, Haidich AB, et al. Twenty-four-hour intraocular pressure control with the travoprost/timolol maleate fixed combination compared with travoprost when both are dosed in the evening in primary open-angle glaucoma. *Br J Ophthalmol.* 2009;93(4): 481–485.

95. Gross RL, Sullivan EK, Wells DT, et al. Pooled results of two randomized clinical trials comparing the efficacy and safety of travoprost 0.004%/timolol 0.5% in fixed combination versus concomitant travoprost 0.004% and timolol 0.5%. *Clin Ophthalmol.* 2007;1(3):317–322.

96. Martinez A, Sanchez M. Efficacy and safety of bimatoprost/timolol fixed combination in the treatment of glaucoma or ocular hypertension. *Expert Opin Pharmacother.* 2008;9(1):137–143.

97. Brandt JD, Cantor LB, Katz LJ, et al. Bimatoprost/timolol fixed combination: a 3-month double-masked, randomized parallel comparison to its individual components in patients with glaucoma or ocular hypertension. *J Glaucoma.* 2008;17(3):211–216.

98. Rulo AH, Greve EL, Hoyng PF. Additive ocular hypotensive effect of latanoprost and acetazolamide. A short-term study in patients with elevated intraocular pressure. *Ophthalmology.* 1997;104(9):1503–1507.

99. Kimal Arici M, Topalkara A, Guler C. Additive effect of latanoprost and dorzolamide in patients with elevated intraocular pressure. *Int Ophthalmol.* 1998;22(1):37–42.

100. Boyer S, Gay D. Additive effect of dorzolamide hydrochloride to patients taking travoprost: a retrospective study. *Optometry.* 2008;79(9):501–504.

101. Reis R, Queiroz CF, Santos LC, et al. A randomized, investigator-masked, 4-week study comparing timolol maleate 0.5%, brinzolamide 1%, and brimonidine tartrate 0.2% as adjunctive therapies to travoprost 0.004% in adults with primary open-angle glaucoma or ocular hypertension. *Clin Ther.* 2006;28(4):552–559.

102. Netland PA, Michael M, Rosner SA, et al. Brimonidine Purite and bimatoprost compared with timolol and latanoprost in patients with glaucoma and ocular hypertension. *Adv Ther.* 2003;20(1):20–30.

103. Zabriskie N, Netland PA. Comparison of brimonidine/latanoprost and timolol/dorzolamide: two randomized, double-masked, parallel clinical trials. *Adv Ther.* 2003;20(2):92–100.

104. Mishima HK, Shoge K, Takamatsu M, et al. Ultrasound biomicroscopic study of ciliary body thickness after topical application of pharmacologic agents. *Am J Ophthalmol.* 1996;121(3):319–321.

105. Toris CB, Alm A, Camras CB. Latanoprost and cholinergic agonists in combination. *Surv Ophthalmol.* 2002;47(suppl 1):S141–S147.

106. Toris CB, Zhan GL, Zhao J, et al. Potential mechanism for the additivity of pilocarpine and latanoprost. *Am J Ophthalmol.* 2001;131(6):722–728.

107. Fristrom B, Nilsson SE. Interaction of PhXA41, a new prostaglandin analogue, with pilocarpine. A study on patients with elevated intraocular pressure. *Arch Ophthalmol.* 1993;111(5):662–665.

108. Patelska B, Greenfield DS, Liebmann JM, et al. Latanoprost for uncontrolled glaucoma in a compassionate case protocol. *Am J Ophthalmol.* 1997;124(3):279–286.

109. Shin DH, McCracken MS, Bendel RE, et al. The additive effect of latanoprost to maximum-tolerated medications with low-dose, high-dose, or no pilocarpine therapy. *Ophthalmology.* 1999;106(2):386–390.

110. Stewart WC, Sharpe ED, Stewart JA, et al. Additive efficacy of unoprostone isopropyl 0.12% (Rescula) to latanoprost 0.005%. *Am J Ophthalmol.* 2001;131(3):339–344.

111. Saito M, Takano R, Shirato S. Effects of latanoprost and unoprostone when used alone or in combination for open-angle glaucoma. *Am J Ophthalmol.* 2001;132(4):485–489.

112. Camras CB, Hedman K. Rate of response to latanoprost or timolol in patients with ocular hypertension or glaucoma. *J Glaucoma.* 2003;12(6):466–469.

113. Scherer WJ. A retrospective review of non-responders to latanoprost. *J Ocul Pharmacol Ther.* 2002;18(3):287–291.

114. Gandolfi SA, Cimino L. Effect of bimatoprost on patients with primary open-angle glaucoma or ocular hypertension who are nonresponders to latanoprost. *Ophthalmology.* 2003;110(3):609–614.

115. Feldman RM. Conjunctival hyperemia and the use of topical prostaglandins in glaucoma and ocular hypertension. *J Ocul Pharmacol Ther.* 2003;19(1):23–35.

116. Parrish RK, Palmberg P, Sheu WP. A comparison of latanoprost, bimatoprost, and travoprost in patients with elevated intraocular pressure: a 12-week, randomized, masked-evaluator multicenter study. *Am J Ophthalmol.* 2003;135(5):688–703.

117. Mietz H, Schlotzer-Schrehardt U, Strassfeld C, et al. Effect of latanoprost and timolol on the histopathology of the rabbit conjunctiva. *Invest Ophthalmol Vis Sci.* 2001;42(3):679–687.

118. Lark KK, Pasha AS, Yan X, et al. The effect of latanoprost and brimonidine on rabbit subconjunctival fibroblasts. *J Glaucoma.* 1999;8(1):72–76.

119. Moreno M, Villena A, Cabarga C, et al. Impression cytology of the conjunctival epithelium after antiglaucomatous treatment with latanoprost. *Eur J Ophthalmol.* 2003;13(6):553–559.

120. Wand M, Gilbert CM, Liesegang TJ. Latanoprost and herpes simplex keratitis. *Am J Ophthalmol.* 1999;127(5):602–604.

121. Kroll DM, Schuman JS. Reactivation of herpes simplex virus keratitis after initiating bimatoprost treatment for glaucoma. *Am J Ophthalmol.* 2002;133(3):401–403.

122. Kaufman HE, Varnell ED, Thompson HW. Latanoprost increases the severity and recurrence of herpetic keratitis in the rabbit. *Am J Ophthalmol.* 1999;127(5):531–536.

123. Kaufman HE, Varnell ED, Toshida H, et al. Effects of topical unoprostone and latanoprost on acute and recurrent herpetic keratitis in the rabbit. *Am J Ophthalmol.* 2001;131(5):643–646.

124. Sudesh S, Cohen EJ, Rapuano CJ, et al. Corneal toxicity associated with latanoprost. *Arch Ophthalmol.* 1999;117(4):539–540.

125. Lass JH, Eriksson GL, Osterling L, et al. Comparison of the corneal effects of latanoprost, fixed combination latanoprost-timolol, and timolol:

a double-masked, randomized, one-year study. *Ophthalmology.* 2001; 108(2):264–271.

126. Bito LZ, Draga A, Blanco J, et al. Long-term maintenance of reduced intraocular pressure by daily or twice daily topical application of prostaglandins to cat or rhesus monkey eyes. *Invest Ophthalmol Vis Sci.* 1983;24(3):312–319.

127. Camras CB, Friedman AH, Rodrigues MM, et al. Multiple dosing of prostaglandin F2 alpha or epinephrine on cynomolgus monkey eyes. III. Histopathology. *Invest Ophthalmol Vis Sci.* 1988;29(9):1428–1436.

128. Villumsen J, Alm A, Soderstrom M. Prostaglandin F2 alpha-isopropyl-lester eye drops: effect on intraocular pressure in open-angle glaucoma. *Br J Ophthalmol.* 1989;73(12):975–979.

129. Bito LZ. Prostaglandins and other eicosanoids: their ocular transport, pharmacokinetics, and therapeutic effects [review]. *Trans Ophthalmol Soc U K.* 1986;105(pt 2):162–170.

130. Fechtner RD, Khouri AS, Zimmerman TJ, et al. Anterior uveitis associated with latanoprost. *Am J Ophthalmol.* 1998;126(1):37–41.

131. Warwar RE, Bullock JD, Ballal D. Cystoid macular edema and anterior uveitis associated with latanoprost use. Experience and incidence in a retrospective review of 94 patients. *Ophthalmology.* 1998;105(2):263–268.

132. Ayyala RS, Cruz DA, Margo CE, et al. Cystoid macular edema associated with latanoprost in aphakic and pseudophakic eyes. *Am J Ophthalmol.* 1998;126(4):602–604.

133. Miyake K, Ota I, Maekubo K, et al. Latanoprost accelerates disruption of the blood-aqueous barrier and the incidence of angiographic cystoid macular edema in early postoperative pseudophakias. *Arch Ophthalmol.* 1999;117(1):34–40.

134. Moroi SE, Gottfredsdottir MS, Schteingart MT, et al. Cystoid macular edema associated with latanoprost therapy in a case series of patients with glaucoma and ocular hypertension. *Ophthalmology.* 1999;106(5): 1024–1029.

135. Wand M, Shields BM. Cystoid macular edema in the era of ocular hypotensive lipids. *Am J Ophthalmol.* 2002;133(3):393–397.

136. Miyake K, Ibaraki N. Prostaglandins and cystoid macular edema. *Surv Ophthalmol.* 2002;47(suppl 1):S203–S218.

137. Kook MS, Lee K. Increased eyelid pigmentation associated with use of latanoprost. *Am J Ophthalmol.* 2000;129(6):804–806.

138. Yamamoto T, Kitazawa Y. Iris-color change developed after topical isopropyl unoprostone treatment. *J Glaucoma.* 1997;6(6):430–432.

139. Chiba T, Kashiwagi K, Kogure S, et al. Iridial pigmentation induced by latanoprost ophthalmic solution in Japanese glaucoma patients. *J Glaucoma.* 2001;10(5):406–410.

140. Lindsey JD, Jones HL, Hewitt EG, et al. Induction of tyrosinase gene transcription in human iris organ cultures exposed to latanoprost. *Arch Ophthalmol.* 2001;119(6):853–860.

141. Kashiwagi K, Tsukamoto K, Suzuki M, et al. Effects of isopropyl unoprostone and latanoprost on melanogenesis in mouse epidermal melanocytes. *J Glaucoma.* 2002;11(1):57–64.

142. Zhan GL, Toris CB, Camras CB, et al. Prostaglandin-induced iris color darkening. An experimental model. *Arch Ophthalmol.* 1998;116(8): 1065–1068.

143. Tsai JC, Sivak-Callcott JA, Haik BG, et al. Latanoprost-induced iris heterochromia and open-angle glaucoma: a clinicopathologic report. *J Glaucoma.* 2001;10(5):411–413.

144. Grierson I, Lee WR, Albert DM. The fine structure of an iridectomy specimen from a patient with latanoprost-induced eye color change. *Arch Ophthalmol.* 1999;117(3):394–396.

145. Pfeiffer N, Grierson I, Goldsmith H, et al. Histological effects in the iris after 3 months of latanoprost therapy: the Mainz 1 study. *Arch Ophthalmol.* 2001;119(2):191–196.

146. Johnstone MA, Albert DM. Prostaglandin-induced hair growth. *Surv Ophthalmol.* 2002;47(suppl 1):S185–S202.

147. Moroi SE. Eyelash preservation during chemotherapy and topical prostaglandin therapy. *Arch Int Med.* 2010. In press.

148. Malkinson FD, Geng L, Hanson WR. Prostaglandins protect against murine hair injury produced by ionizing radiation or doxorubicin. *J Invest Dermatol.* 1993;101(1 suppl):135S–137S.

149. Jerstad KM, Warshaw E. Allergic contact dermatitis to latanoprost. *Am J Contact Dermat.* 2002;13(1):39–41.

150. Krohn J, Hove VK. Iris cyst associated with topical administration of latanoprost. *Am J Ophthalmol.* 1999;127(1):91–93.

151. Morales J, Shihab ZM, Brown SM, et al. Herpes simplex virus dermatitis in patients using latanoprost. *Am J Ophthalmol.* 2001;132(1):114–116.

152. Camras CB, Alm A, Watson P, et al. Latanoprost, a prostaglandin analog, for glaucoma therapy. Efficacy and safety after 1 year of treatment in 198 patients. Latanoprost Study Groups. *Ophthalmology.* 1996;103(11): 1916–1924.

153. Hedner J, Everts B, Moller CS. Latanoprost and respiratory function in asthmatic patients: randomized, double-masked, placebo-controlled crossover evaluation. *Arch Ophthalmol.* 1999;117(10):1305–1309.

154. Waldock A, Snape J, Graham CM. Effects of glaucoma medications on the cardiorespiratory and intraocular pressure status of newly diagnosed glaucoma patients. *Br J Ophthalmol.* 2000;84(7):710–713.

29

β-Adrenergic Receptor Antagonists

The adrenergic receptors are an important physiologic target, and within the eye these receptors have a major role in regulating aqueous humor dynamics (see Chapter 1). After the development of systemic β-adrenergic receptor antagonists, commonly called β-blockers, for cardiovascular applications, topical formulations of β-blockers were later developed for lowering intraocular pressure (IOP) in the treatment of glaucoma. The first commercially available β-blocker was propranolol, which was introduced in 1967 for the treatment of cardiac arrhythmias, angina pectoris, and systemic hypertension. This drug was found to reduce IOP when given orally, topically, or intravenously (1–3). Many of these compounds, however, caused adverse reactions, such as corneal anesthesia due to membrane-stabilizing activity, dry eye–related problems, subconjunctival fibrosis, corneal ulcers, and rash (2,4). With further development and research, several compounds in the β-blocker class of drugs were identified without these adverse reactions and were introduced into clinical use. α-Adrenergic receptor antagonists have also been developed, but this class of drugs appears to have minimal effects on aqueous humor dynamics and is not used in the long-term treatment of glaucoma.

β-ADRENERGIC RECEPTOR ANTAGONISTS

Mechanisms of Action

Aqueous humor flow is the main mechanism by which the β-blockers lower the IOP. Timolol has been shown to have its main IOP-lowering effect by reducing aqueous humor production based on studies using tonographic and fluorophotometric methods (5). The β-adrenergic receptors, predominantly of the β_2 subtype, have been identified in ciliary processes (6–9). The influence of timolol on aqueous humor formation may be related to inhibition of catecholamine-stimulated synthesis of cyclic adenosine monophosphate (AMP), which has been demonstrated in rabbit studies (10,11).

The mechanism by which an adrenergic antagonist reduces aqueous production relates to the physiology of the sympathetic system in the ciliary processes and on aqueous humor dynamics (see Chapter 1). In patients with sympathetic denervation from postganglionic Horner syndrome, neither aqueous humor flow nor IOP is affected (12). The possibility that tone could arise from circulating catecholamines was not supported by the observation that patients with bilateral adrenalectomies do not influence the circadian rhythm of aqueous flow nor the daytime effect of timolol on the flow (13). Another interesting observation is that timolol does not appear to be effective in sleeping human participants during which time the aqueous flow is normally less than half the daytime flow rate (14). However, timolol does lower aqueous flow at night in humans receiving systemic epinephrine (15). Based on these clinical observations in certain diseases known to affect the sympathetic nervous system and normal physiologic conditions, the precise mechanisms by which the sympathetic system regulates aqueous humor dynamics is complex and not fully understood (see Chapter 1).

Overall, the outflow facility does not appear to be influenced by timolol (16,17). However, topical timolol was associated with a small myopic shift in one human study, suggesting that sympathetic innervation is involved in the resting tone of the ciliary muscle (18). Furthermore, the β-adrenergic receptors, primarily of the β_2 subtype, have been demonstrated in human trabecular meshwork (19,20). A histologic study of the outflow apparatus in human eyes treated with timolol before enucleation for malignant melanoma revealed no morphologic changes suggestive of a pressure-lowering action by the drug (21). However, the trabecular meshwork in primates after long-term timolol therapy revealed degeneration of the trabecular cells, partial destruction of the beams, rarefaction of the meshwork, and disconnection of the trabecular lamellae from the ciliary muscle fibers (22).

The possible effect of β-blockers on ocular blood flow is complex and involves consideration of the various vascular beds, including the ciliary, retinal, choroidal, and retrobulbar vessels located within their respective tissues (23). There are conflicting effects of the topical β-blockers on ciliary systolic perfusion pressure (24). Carteolol and levobunolol were shown to increase ocular pulsatile blood flow (25,26). Another study showed that carteolol, compared with a placebo, had no significant effect on human retinal circulation with regard to changes in vessel diameter, maximum erythrocyte velocity, and volumetric blood flow rate (27). In a study of patients with normal-tension glaucoma, color Doppler imaging of orbital vessels showed an increase in end-diastolic velocity and a decrease in resistance index with betaxolol, but not with timolol (28). However, when the two drugs were evaluated in rabbits with an intraluminal microvascular corrosion casting technique, neither produced an observable vasomotor effect (29). With regard to ocular blood flow, levobunolol, betaxolol, and carteolol did not influence perimacular hemodynamics as determined by blue field entoptic simulation in normal volunteers, which the investigators thought suggested normal autoregulation (30). Whether β-blockers clinically influence ocular blood flow and whether there is a significant difference between nonselective and cardioselective agents is unclear.

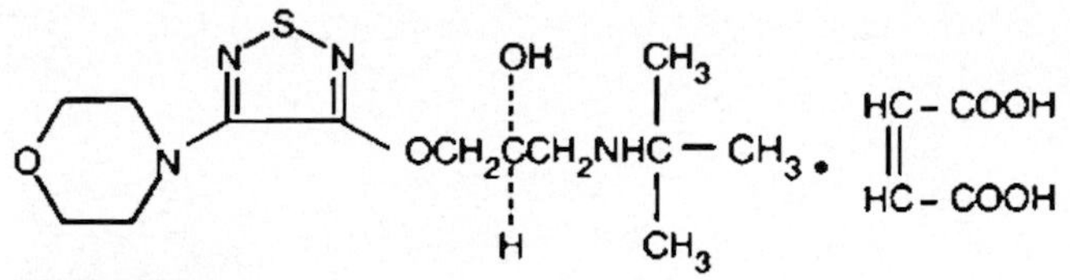

Figure 29.1 Chemical structure of timolol.

Other possible mechanisms for the effect of timolol on lowering IOP have been examined. It does not appear that timolol significantly influences the blood–aqueous barrier. Simultaneous bilateral fluorescein angiography of the iris revealed no effect of timolol on dye leakage (31). It also appears that the timolol mechanism is not prostaglandin mediated, because it is not altered by concurrent therapy with indomethacin or flurbiprofen (32,33). In a study with rabbit eyes, there was a suggestion that timolol might act as a dopaminergic antagonist to lower blood flow to the ciliary body (34). However, metoclopramide, a dopamine-2 antagonist, did not affect the ocular hypotensive action of timolol in healthy volunteers (35).

Specific Agents

The first topical β-blocker available as a topical agent for the treatment of glaucoma was timolol (**Fig. 29.1**). (The commercially available β-blockers are discussed in the following text and summarized in **Table 29.1**.) Other β-blockers were subsequently developed, and in general, although comparable with timolol, they vary according to relative β-blocking potency, selectivity for specific β-receptor, and other characteristics (**Table 29.2**) (36).

Timolol

Timolol is a nonselective, β_1- and β_2-adrenergic antagonist, which is produced by using various formulations. Timolol was found to lack the adverse effects related to corneal anesthesia and subconjunctival fibrosis compared with the earlier β-blockers (37). Rabbit studies revealed an IOP-lowering effect in both the treated and the fellow untreated eye (38,39). Primate studies have demonstrated a topical timolol effect on aqueous flow in the fellow, untreated eye, the degree of which is dose related (40). The contralateral effect of β-blockers has also been shown in patients with open-angle glaucoma and patients with ocular hypertension (41,42). The observation of the contralateral IOP lowering in the fellow untreated eye suggests that the drug is absorbed and exerts its effect through the systemic circulation (see "Side Effects").

Single doses of timolol in normotensive individuals and in patients with chronic open-angle glaucoma (COAG) lowered the IOP (42,43). Short-term, multiple-dose trials with patients with open-angle glaucoma demonstrated a sustained reduction in the IOP (44–47).

Comparative studies have shown the IOP-lowering efficacy of timolol to be greater than that of epinephrine (45,48) and equal to or slightly weaker than various concentrations of combined epinephrine and guanethidine (49). Compared with pilocarpine, timolol had an equivalent or slightly greater IOP-

Table 29.1	Commercially Available Topical β-Blockers	
Generic Preparation and Brand Names	**Concentrations, %**
Timolol maleate[a]	
Timoptic	0.25, 0.5
Timoptic XE	0.25, 0.5
Timolol GFS	0.5
Istalol	0.5
Timolol hemihydrate[a]	
Betimol	0.25, 0.5
Betaxolol HCl	
Betoptic S[b]	0.25
Levobunolol HCl[a]	
Betagan	0.25, 0.5
AkBeta	0.25, 0.5
Carteolol HCl[a]	
Ocupress	1.0
Metipranolol HCl[a]	
OptiPranolol	0.3
Timolol	0.5
With dorzolamide	
Cosopt[b]	0.2
With brimonidine tartrate	
Combigan[c]	0.2

[a]Other generic products may be available for timolol and levobunolol.
[b]Suspension.
[c]Fixed combination.

lowering effect (50–53). In a comparative study of timolol twice daily compared with pilocarpine four times daily, more patients receiving pilocarpine discontinued the study because of inadequate IOP control, and patients receiving pilocarpine had significantly greater visual field deterioration (54). In another comparative study, echothiophate iodide was more effective than timolol in the treatment of glaucoma in eyes with aphakia (55).

With the availability of timolol in the gel-forming solution, several clinical studies have shown equivalence in IOP lowering for timolol gel dosed once daily and timolol solution dosed twice daily (56,57). Similar studies comparing once-daily dosing of timolol gel and timolol solution have not been reported. This issue of designing clinical studies to compare the efficacy of β-blockers is clinically relevant, because once-daily instillation of levobunolol provided similar IOP control to twice-daily use of the same drug (58,59), which is discussed later.

Betaxolol

Unlike timolol and the other β-blockers, betaxolol hydrochloride is a cardioselective, β_1-adrenergic antagonist. It is currently available as a 0.25% suspension formulation. Although this drug is more selective on the β_1-receptors, receptor occupancy studies of human aqueous from betaxolol-treated eyes suggest a role of β_2-receptor blockade (60). The mechanism of ocular

Table 29.2	Pharmacologic Properties of Ocular β-Blockers				
Drug	**Relative β-Blocking Potency**	**Partial Agonist Activity (ISA)**	**β₁-Selectivity**	**Local Serum Anesthetic Effect**	**Half-Life, hr**
Timolol	510	0	0	±	35
Betaxolol	110	0	+	0	1220
Levobunolol	50	0	0	0	6
Metipranolol	1.8	0	0	±	2
Carteolol	1	+	0	0	37

ISA, intrinsic sympathomimetic activity; +, activity present; ±, weak effect; 0, no effect.
Data from Lee PS, Chruscicki DA. Pharmacology of ocular β-adrenoreceptor antagonists. In: Tasman W, Jaeger EA, eds. *Duane's Foundations of Clinical Ophthalmology*. Vol 3. Philadelphia, PA: Lippincott Williams & Wilkins; 2008:chap 32.

hypotension appears to be the same as that for timolol, with reduction of aqueous humor production and no effect on outflow resistance or pupillary diameter (61).

When compared with timolol at 0.25% and 0.5% doses, the magnitude of IOP reduction in most studies is slightly less with betaxolol, and there may be a greater need for adjunctive therapy than with timolol (62,63). In one study of 153 glaucoma patients whose IOPs were controlled on timolol, the 50% of patients who were switched to betaxolol in a masked and random fashion had a significant increase in IOP (64). However, when betaxolol, 0.5%, and timolol, 0.5%, both given twice daily, were compared in long-term, parallel trials of 18 to 30 months in patients with open-angle glaucoma, the timolol group had better IOP levels, but the betaxolol group had a more favorable course regarding retinal sensitivity as measured by static automated perimetry (65,66). (The possible explanation for this is discussed later.)

Several clinical studies have also compared the IOP-lowering efficacy of betaxolol and α-adrenergic agonists. In a 3-month comparative trial of betaxolol, 0.5%, and dipivefrin, 0.1%, IOP reductions were similar, with mean decreases of 4.1 and 3.5 mm Hg, respectively (67). In a 4-month masked, randomized trial comparing twice-daily treatment with betaxolol, 0.25%, or brimonidine, 0.2%, in 188 patients with glaucoma or ocular hypertension, IOP reductions measured near the peak effect of these drugs showed mean decreases of 5.9 mm Hg for brimonidine and 3.8 mm Hg for betaxolol (68).

Levobunolol

Levobunolol (1-bunolol), an analog of propranolol, is another nonselective β₁- and β₂-adrenergic antagonist. In short-term studies, the onset of an ocular hypotensive effect occurred within the first hour after instillation, peaked at 3 hours, and lasted up to 24 hours (69). In commercial bottles, a drop of the original levobunolol is significantly larger than that of timolol, which results from the dispensing system and the increased viscosity of levobunolol (70). However, the drop size does not appear to influence the efficacy or safety of the drug (71). Levobunolol is effective with once-daily administration in a high percentage of patients (72), with once-daily instillation of the 0.5% concentration providing similar IOP control to

twice-daily use of the same drug and the 0.25% concentration given once daily providing adequate control in many cases (58).

In comparative short-term and long-term clinical studies, levobunolol in various concentrations was equivalent to timolol with regard to ocular hypotensive efficacy and side effects when the two drugs were administered twice daily (73,74). It was also shown to be equivalent to the nonselective β-blocker metipranolol (75) but had significantly greater pressure-lowering efficacy than betaxolol in a 3-month study (76). It has also been shown to provide additional IOP reduction when added to dipivefrin, with efficacy and safety comparable with concomitant timolol and dipivefrin therapy (77).

Carteolol

Carteolol is a nonselective β-adrenergic antagonist with intrinsic sympathomimetic activity. The latter feature produces an early, transient adrenergic agonist response that is not found in the other topical β-blockers. Studies with systemic β-blockers indicate that intrinsic sympathomimetic activity does not interfere with the therapeutic benefits of β-blockers (78). In most studies comparing carteolol and timolol, there was no significant difference in the effects on pulse or blood pressure (79,80). Although the intrinsic sympathomimetic activity of carteolol does not appear to protect against cardiovascular effects such as reduced pulse and blood pressure, there is evidence that it may decrease the cardiovascular risks associated with cholesterol abnormalities. A comparative trial of carteolol, 1%, and timolol, 0.5%, in 58 healthy, normolipidemic adult men confirmed the earlier findings with regard to timolol and showed significantly less effect of carteolol on high-density lipoprotein (HDL) cholesterol (81). Carteolol therapy was associated with a 3.3% decrease in HDL level and a 4% increase in total cholesterol–HDL ratio, compared with 8% and 10%, respectively, with timolol. Although the implications of these findings are not clear for glaucoma populations, it underscores the importance of recommending nasolacrimal occlusion to minimize systemic absorption of topical β-blockers.

In a vehicle-controlled trial, carteolol, 1%, and carteolol, 2%, produced mean IOP reductions of 23% and 26%, respectively (82). When compared with timolol, the ocular hypotensive efficacy and duration of action were comparable in most studies (79,80). Carteolol has been shown, however, to cause less ocular irritation than timolol in the first few minutes after instillation (79). Carteolol has also been studied as a fixed combination with pilocarpine. Various combinations of carteolol, 1% and 2%, with pilocarpine, 2% and 4%, and of timolol, 0.5%, with pilocarpine, 2% and 4%, gave mean IOP reductions of 24% to 40% (82,83). However, carteolol or timolol in combination with pilocarpine was slightly less effective than when the two drugs were given separately (83).

Metipranolol

Metipranolol is a nonselective β-blocker that has been shown in a placebo-controlled trial to significantly lower the IOP by reducing the rate of aqueous flow with no effect on outflow (84). Comparative studies have shown that it is comparable with timolol and levobunolol with regard to efficacy and safety. Metipranolol is commercially available in a 0.3% concentration (85) (Table 29.1).

D-Timolol

Previous reference to timolol in this chapter has been to L-timolol, or the (S)-enantiomer, which is the stereoisomer form of the drug currently used in the treatment of glaucoma. The D-timolol, the (R)-enantiomer, is a significantly less potent β-adrenergic antagonist with regard to both IOP reduction and systemic effects (86,87).

Atenolol

Atenolol is a selective β_1-adrenergic antagonist with no intrinsic sympathomimetic or membrane-stabilizing properties (88). Oral atenolol, 25 to 100 mg, provided significant IOP reduction when compared with a placebo (89). Topical administration of atenolol, 2%, was similar to pilocarpine, 2% (90), and atenolol, 4%, was more effective than epinephrine, 1% (91). However, a long-term study showed that the initial pressure control gradually wore off in some patients (92).

Metoprolol

Metoprolol is a cardioselective β_1-adrenergic antagonist that, like betaxolol, has reduced IOP without the adverse respiratory side effects of the nonselective β-blockers (93). Prolonged ocular hypotensive action has been demonstrated with both oral administration of 100-mg tablets or topical instillation of metoprolol, 1% to 5% (93,94). Metoprolol, 3%, was similar to pilocarpine, 2% to 4%, in lowering IOP in one study and had roughly the equivalent ocular hypotensive effect to that of timolol in another evaluation (95,96).

Pindolol

Pindolol is a potent β-adrenergic antagonist with an intrinsic sympathomimetic effect and is reported to provide a good ocular hypotensive effect (97). Pindolol, 0.5% to 1%, has been shown to provide prolonged IOP reduction without significant ocular or systemic side effects (98), although reports are conflicting regarding the influence of pindolol on corneal anesthesia (97).

Nadolol

Oral administration of nadolol, a nonselective β-blocker, 10 to 80 mg daily, has been shown to cause a significant, dose-related reduction in IOP (99). Topical preparations also produce a significant dose-dependent IOP reduction, which lasts more than 9 hours with the higher concentrations of 1% to 2%, but this effect was not maintained with continued use (100). To overcome the issue of poor corneal penetration, the prodrug analog of nadolol, diacetyl nadolol, was developed and found to be as effective as timolol in lowering the IOP up to 8 hours with less efficacy thereafter (101). However, diacetyl nadolol, 2%, had a lower incidence of tolerance than did timolol, 0.5%, in a 3-month study (102).

Befunolol

Befunolol, 0.25% and 0.5%, provided good IOP reduction in a 3-month study (103), with no significant diminution of effect during 1-year follow-up (104). In a preliminary study, changing from timolol, 0.5%, to befunolol, 0.5%, was associated with a significant additional decrease in IOP (105).

Administration

Concentrations

Commercially available β-blockers are formulated in various concentrations (Table 29.1). Early experience with patients with COAG indicated that the maximum IOP-lowering effect of timolol maleate is achieved with the 0.5% concentration (37,43). In other studies, however, the 0.25% concentration was equally or more efficacious than the 0.5%, although the latter provided a somewhat longer duration of action (106,107). Dose–response studies of aqueous humor formation in primates showed that a dose of timolol as small as 2.5 μg can suppress aqueous flow by a 20%, suggesting that standard clinical doses may be greater than necessary (108). Nevertheless, individuals with darker irides appear to require higher concentrations of timolol (109). In one study, timolol had a significant ocular hypotensive effect 1 hour after instillation in patients with blue irides but no effect in brown-eyed patients, which probably relates to nonspecific binding of the drug to pigment (110).

Frequency

Good corneal penetration of timolol has been demonstrated in rabbit and human eyes, with peak aqueous humor concentrations in human eyes occurring within 1 to 2 hours (111,112). The IOP-lowering effect peaks approximately 2 hours after administration and lasts for at least 24 hours (37,43,113). The optimum frequency of administration in most cases is twice daily, although once-a-day treatment has been shown to be adequate in many cases (114,115). One study found no significant difference whether timolol, 0.5%, was given in the morning or evening (116). Timolol in a gel vehicle was found to elicit a 1 to 2 mm Hg greater efficacy than the solution during 24 hours after instillation (117). When timolol use is discontinued after long-term therapy, aqueous humor flow does not increase significantly until the fourth day, and the IOP effect may still be seen 14 days later (118). This may reflect the concentration of the drug in melanotic tissues and the slow release. In rabbits receiving topical timolol for 42 days, the drug was still present in pigmented ocular tissues 42 days after withdrawal of the drug (119).

Long-Term Efficacy

Numerous long-term studies have confirmed the continued efficacy of long-term timolol therapy for many patients (120–126). In a significant number of cases, however, the pressure responsiveness to timolol will decrease with continued administration. This occurs in two phases, which Boger (127) called short-term escape and long-term drift.

Short-Term Escape

Many patients will experience a dramatic reduction in IOP with the initiation of timolol therapy. However, the pressure usually rises during the next few days and plateaus at a maintenance level (50,128–130). The 1-hour IOP response to timolol does not predict which patients will have a significant loss of responsiveness 3 to 4 weeks later (130). It has been demonstrated that the number of β-receptors in ocular tissues increases during the first few days of timolol therapy (131), which may explain this escape phenomenon. In any case, it is good clinical practice to wait approximately 1 month after initiating timolol to determine the efficacy of therapy.

Long-Term Drift

When the IOP levels off after the initiation of timolol therapy, control can be maintained in most cases. Some patients, however, have a slow decline in pressure response to timolol, usually beginning 3 months to 1 year after starting treatment (120–126,132,133). Fluorophotometric studies indicate that aqueous humor flow is higher in most patients after 1 year of timolol therapy compared with the value 1 week after initiating treatment (134). Some patients regain responsiveness to timolol after a washout period. In one study of 39 eyes showing a long-term drift with timolol, 0.5%, 23 eyes received dipivefrin (a prodrug of epinephrine) during a 30- or 60-day timolol holiday, and the remainder received artificial tears in place of the timolol (135). When the timolol was reinstituted, the dipivefrin-treated group had a mean IOP decrease of 8.2 mm Hg, compared with 3.9 in the non–dipivefrin-treated group, and the response to timolol was more prolonged in eyes treated for 60 days with dipivefrin. Based on this observation, a treatment strategy of pulsatile therapy, in which timolol, 0.5%, is given for 6 months and then alternates with dipivefrin for 2 months, was studied and shown to minimize long-term drift, compared with continuous use of timolol (136).

Drug Interactions and Multiple-Agent Formulations

Numerous clinical studies have been conducted to examine the effect of combining topical β-blockers, primarily with timolol, 0.5%, with other antiglaucoma therapy. However, when instituting fixed-combination versus multiple-drug therapy, the possibility of changes in ocular and systemic drug absorption, adherence, and cost of the therapy must be considered (137,138).

There are two commercially available forms of fixed combination drugs formulated with timolol, 0.5% (138). The combination of brimonidine tartrate, 0.2%, with timolol, 0.5% (Combigan), was developed because of the efficacy of IOP lowering with the individual components of the α₂-adrenergic agonist brimonidine and timolol, 0.5% (139) (see Chapter 30). The other fixed combination is dorzolamide, 2.0%, with timolol, 0.5% (Cosopt; also available in generic formulation) (140). However, in general, there is greater efficacy in IOP lowering when combining timolol with the oral carbonic anhydrase inhibitors (CAIs) (141–143), compared with topical CAIs (see Chapter 31). (The interaction between timolol and the prostaglandin agents is discussed in Chapter 28.)

For timolol, the combined effect of timolol and a miotic is, for most patients, significantly greater than the effect of either medication alone (141,144–146). Although no longer available in the United States, a combined formulation of timolol, 0.5%, and pilocarpine, 2% to 4% (TP2 and TP4), administered twice daily, provides IOP reduction similar to timolol and pilocarpine when given separately (147).

Another important clinical question is the efficacy and safety of combined topical β-blockers and oral β-blockers. The oral β-blockers are commonly used for the treatment of various cardiovascular disorders and have improved the outcome of patients with congestive heart failure (148,149). These systemic β-blockers may also affect the IOP, and the concurrent use of a systemic and topical β-blocker may reduce the IOP-lowering efficacy of the topical β-blocker (150–152). In general, topical timolol can produce additional IOP reduction without altering pulse or blood pressure in patients pretreated with oral timolol, propranolol, alprenolol, or metoprolol (150,151,153).

Side Effects

Ocular Toxicity

Adverse ocular reactions are usually low with topical β-blocker therapy. This drug class does not affect the pupillary size or accommodation (154). The tear film may be altered in patients who have low baseline tear flow (155–157). Long-term therapy with timolol has been shown to affect the mucus layer of the tear film (158).

There have been, however, reports of allergic and toxic reactions. Burning and conjunctival hyperemia may occasionally occur and are frequently associated with superficial punctate keratopathy and corneal anesthesia (159–163). A serious ocular reaction is related to ocular cicatricial pemphigoid, which has been reported to occur in patients receiving topical timolol (164,165). In most of these cases, the patients were also receiving additional glaucoma medications, although a few were receiving timolol alone when the pemphigoid was diagnosed. Tissue culture studies with human Tenon fibroblasts suggest that β-blockers do not stimulate cell proliferation directly but may do so by chronic inflammation from the irritating effects of the antiglaucoma medications or preservatives (166). Exposure of the conjunctiva to these antiglaucoma medications or their preservatives has also been shown to change the appearance of the tissue and to increase the presence of inflammatory cells (167). This may have implications regarding the success of glaucoma filtering surgery.

Most human and animal investigations have revealed no toxicity of topical timolol therapy to the corneal endothelium (168–171). A small subgroup of patients treated with timolol may have markedly diminished corneal sensitivity (162,163). Corneal epithelial erosions were reported in two patients wearing gas permeable contact lenses soon after starting topical timolol therapy, and the combination of timolol and a contact lens in rabbits caused marked alterations in corneal epithelium and endothelium (172). Eight patients were described in which the combination of epithelial defects and topical steroid and β-blocker therapy led to a precipitation of calcium phosphate deposits in the superficial stroma (173).

A potentially serious ocular effect that has been the focus of considerable investigation is the influence of β-blockers on ocular blood flow (174). If the drug reduces vascular perfusion of the optic nerve head, this may cancel the benefit of reduced IOP. A rabbit study using injected microspheres indicated that both nonselective and cardioselective β-blockers decrease ocular blood flow (175). However, high-resolution Doppler ultrasonography suggested that timolol improves the flow velocity of the central retinal artery in healthy and diabetic individuals (176,177), but other studies suggest that timolol has no significant effect on the choroidal vasculature in healthy persons or retinal hemodynamics in patients with normal-tension glaucoma (178,179).

The most troublesome ocular reaction reported with metipranolol is a granulomatous anterior uveitis, characterized by mutton-fat keratic precipitates, flare and cells, and IOP elevation. In the United Kingdom, 15 cases were described in one report, with reference to 51 more cases from other parts of the country (180). Seven patients, rechallenged with metipranolol, all developed an adverse reaction within 14 days (181), and the drug was withdrawn from clinical use in the United Kingdom. A retrospective study of 1306 patients treated with metipranolol in Germany revealed a low risk of uveitis associated with the medication, and it was assumed that the problem was related to the unique formulation used in the United Kingdom (182). However, three cases have been reported in the United States (183,184), one of which recurred when inadvertently rechallenged treatment (184).

For betaxolol, one case was reported in which aphakic cystoid macular edema was associated with therapy (185), and three cases have been described of periocular cutaneous pigmentary changes, which returned to normal after discontinuation of topical betaxolol treatment (186).

Systemic Toxicity

After widespread and long-term use of the topical β-blockers in the treatment of glaucoma, it became apparent that topical use of this drug class can cause adverse systemic side effects (187). Systemic toxicity has been reported more often than ocular reactions and potentially constitutes the more significant adverse effect of topical β-blocker therapy (188). With the initial availability of timolol, there are notably more cases reporting the adverse systemic effects of this particular agent, but the other topical β-blocker agents are also associated with similar side effects.

Systemic Absorption

Measurable plasma levels of timolol are present within 8 minutes or less of topical application (189). In comparing plasma levels of timolol from systemic absorption of once-daily gel-forming solution compared with twice-daily solution in a crossover designed study, there appears to be slightly lower plasma levels detected when six healthy male participants were given the once-daily gel-forming solution instead of the twice-daily solution (190). The cardiovascular effects of these dosing regimens in 43 patients showed a comparable decrease in mean 24-hour heart rate, compared with placebo (191). Given the concerns for systemic absorption of both the gel-forming and solution formulations of timolol, the role of punctal occlusion after instillation of the drug (see Chapter 27) is important because there is evidence that this action significantly reduces plasma timolol levels (192), which may help to minimize the systemic side effects. In one study, drug instillation at 12 PM was shown to optimize the ratio of ocular to systemic absorption, possibly relating to drug absorption into the eye and bloodstream (193).

There is a reported difference in plasma concentrations comparing topical betaxolol, 0.5%, or timolol, 0.25%, which were given before cataract surgery. The plasma concentrations of betaxolol were lower than those of timolol, whereas the aqueous levels were twice as high for betaxolol as for timolol (194). In a related study, these same investigators determined that the higher plasma levels of the absorbed timolol compared with betaxolol could functionally bind with the β_1- and β_2-adrenergic receptors based on radioligand binding methods (60). In another study, timolol and carteolol (also a nonselective β-blocker) blocked both the β_1 and β_2 effects of isoproterenol, but betaxolol had minimal influence on either receptor effect (195). The latter investigators suggest that the low rate of systemic diffusion with betaxolol may relate to the high lipophilic and protein-binding properties, which favor a high level of local diffusion and a fixation to lacrimal proteins before the drug reaches the general circulation, where it binds to plasma proteins, leaving only a small amount to circulate freely (195).

Cardiovascular Effects

Blockade of β_1-adrenergic receptors slows the pulse rate and weakens myocardial contractility. In most healthy patients, these effects are of no consequence, but healthy individuals may be at risk under certain circumstances, such as the stress of surgery or heavy exercise (196–198). Topical timolol therapy has been associated with severe bradycardia, arrhythmias, heart failure, and syncope (159,199). The induced bradycardia may be more pronounced when timolol is used concomitantly with other drugs, such as quinidine or the calcium antagonist, verapamil (200,201). Topical betaxolol has also been associated with similar cardiovascular side effects, including arrhythmia, bradycardia, sinus arrest, and decompensation of congestive heart failure (202–204). Selecting another glaucoma drug class is prudent because of the potential for serious complications in patients with preexisting cardiac conditions such as sinus bradycardia, greater than first-degree heart block, and congestive heart failure. Oral β-blockers have a role in the management of patients with congestive heart failure (148,149,205). Obtaining an accurate medical history and assessing pulse rate and rhythm before initiating a topical β-blocker should identify most patients with potential cardiovascular contraindications (188). Communication with the patient's primary care physician about potential systemic side effects from topical antiglaucoma medical therapy should also be considered.

Respiratory Effects

Blockade of β_2-adrenergic receptors produces contraction of bronchial smooth muscle, which may cause bronchospasm and airway obstruction, especially in asthmatics or any patient with bronchospasm requiring xanthines or inhaled steroids (159,206,207). Thirteen cases of death in status asthmaticus after initiation of timolol therapy had been reported to the National Registry of Drug-Induced Ocular Side Effects by 1984 (208). Dyspnea and apneic spells may be more common in young children, and caution must be taken by nursing mothers, because high levels of timolol were found in the milk of a mother receiving topical timolol (209).

Central Nervous System Effects

Central nervous system effects can occur with timolol therapy and include depression, anxiety, confusion, dysarthria, hallucinations, lightheadedness, drowsiness, weakness, fatigue, tranquilization, dissociative behavior, disorientation, and emotional lability (159,210). Similar side effects have also been reported in association with betaxolol therapy (211).

Effect on Cholesterol Levels

Oral β-blockers are known to adversely alter plasma lipid profiles, and topical timolol, 0.5%, twice daily for 2 months, without nasolacrimal occlusion, has been shown to decrease plasma HDL cholesterol levels, which increases the risk of coronary artery disease (212). Another study found no significant adverse effects of topical timolol on serum lipoprotein levels (213), although the sample size was small in a heterogenous patient population with no controls. The issue of β-blockers on cholesterol is considered further in this chapter under the discussion of carteolol.

Other Systemic Reactions

Other systemic reactions that have been reported in association with timolol therapy include gastrointestinal distress (nausea, diarrhea, and cramping), dermatologic disorders (maculopapular rash, alopecia, and hives), and sexual impotence

(159,162,214,215). Because these observations were made in a predominantly elderly population, it is difficult to confirm a cause-and-effect relationship in all cases. Of greater concern with timolol therapy, however, is the exacerbation of myasthenia gravis and the altered response to hypoglycemic episodes in diabetic patients, which may mask symptoms of the attack (216,217).

α-ADRENERGIC RECEPTOR ANTAGONISTS

Mechanisms of Action

As mentioned in the introduction, α-adrenergic receptor antagonists are available. These receptors mediate the action of the neurotransmitter norepinephrine in the end-organ targets for the sympathetic nervous system. In the iris, the stimulation of the dilator muscle with α-adrenergic receptor agonists causes mydriasis or dilation of the pupil. Although α-adrenergic receptors have been detected by pharmacology receptor binding studies in the ciliary body of various species (218,219), their functional role in aqueous humor dynamics is not known. The clinical use of these agents is limited.

Specific Agents

Thymoxamine

Thymoxamine hydrochloride competes with norepinephrine for α-adrenergic receptors. As a result, it produces miosis by inhibiting the dilator muscle of the iris without influencing the ciliary muscle-induced facility of aqueous outflow (220). Thus, it has no effect on open-angle glaucoma (221). It does not affect the rate of aqueous humor formation, IOP, or anterior chamber volume (222). Because this agent does not cause shallowing of the anterior chamber or ciliary spasm, it provides safe, rapid reversal of the effects of an adrenergic mydriatic drug. Thymoxamine, 0.1%, is used to reverse mydriasis from phenylephrine (223).

Thymoxamine has a role in the management of angle-closure glaucoma because it causes miosis despite the presence of pressure-induced ischemia of the iris sphincter. Furthermore, it does not increase the posterior vector force of the iris, and thus does not potentially aggravate the pupillary block. In a study of patients with acute angle-closure glaucoma, thymoxamine, 0.5%, administered every minute for five times and then every 15 minutes for 2 to 3 hours broke the attack in all cases, except those with peripheral anterior synechiae or prolonged angle closure (224).

One theory for the mechanism of pigment dispersion in pigmentary glaucoma, as discussed in Section II, is contact between the iris pigment epithelium and packets of lens zonules. It has been suggested that miosis without cyclotropia, as produced by thymoxamine, provides an effective means of minimizing this effect (225).

Thymoxamine, 0.5%, causes a substantial narrowing of the palpebral fissure in many patients with eyelid retraction, especially cases occurring secondary to thyroid disease, and it has been suggested that this may have value in the diagnosis of thyroid eye disease and possibly in the medical treatment of eyelid retraction (226).

Dapiprazole

This α-adrenergic antagonist is similar in action to thymoxamine and is commercially available for the reversal of mydriasis after an ocular examination. It was evaluated in human volunteers and found to produce miosis and IOP reduction (227).

Other α₁-Adrenergic Receptor Antagonists

Other agents in this class have been examined but were not further developed for commercial use. Bunazosin lowers IOP in healthy persons in single doses of 0.025% to 0.2% and was effective for 1 week in a concentration of 0.1% (228). The mechanism of IOP reduction is presumed to be increased uveoscleral outflow, because it does not influence aqueous production, conventional outflow, or episcleral venous pressure (228). Prazosin is used as an oral medication to lower blood pressure and produce peripheral vasodilatation. Rabbit studies have shown that topical administration of prazosin, 0.001% to 0.1%, causes a dose-related lowering of IOP by reducing aqueous humor formation (229).

Corynanthine is a selective α₁-adrenergic antagonist produced IOP reduction in animals without altering conventional outflow facility or the rate of aqueous humor flow (230). Thus, it was postulated that the mechanism of pressure reduction might be an increase in uveoscleral outflow. In a clinical trial, 2% and 5% concentrations of corynanthine did lower the IOP, although a 3-week study with the 2% concentration did not reveal a sustained pressure reduction (231).

Labetalol is a combined α- and β-adrenergic blocking agent that has been shown to produce a significant, dose-related IOP reduction in rabbits (232,233), although it has a poor ocular hypotensive effect in human eyes (233,234).

KEY POINTS

- Topical β-blockers significantly lower IOP by reducing aqueous humor flow.
- Given the availability of generic formulations, this drug class is an inexpensive and effective antiglaucoma medication.
- Careful monitoring of potentially serious β-blocker–associated pulmonary and cardiac side effects is warranted to minimize prolonged exposure with this drug class.
- α-Adrenergic antagonists produce miosis by inhibiting the dilator muscle of the iris but have no clinically significant effect on aqueous humor dynamics.

REFERENCES

1. Pandolfi M, Ohrstrom A. Treatment of ocular hypertension with oral beta-adrenergic blocking agents. *Acta Ophthalmol (Copehn)*. 1974; 52(4):464–467.
2. Musini A, Fabbri B, Bergamaschi M, et al. Comparison of the effect of propranolol, lignocaine, and other drugs on normal and raised intraocular pressure in man. *Am J Ophthalmol*. 1971;72(4):773–781.
3. Takats I, Szilvassy I, Kerek A. Intraocular pressure and circulation of aqueous humour in rabbit eyes following intravenous administration of propranolol (Inderal) [German]. *Albrecht Von Graefes Arch Klin Exp Ophthalmol*. 1972;185(4):331–342.
4. Rahi AH, Chapman CM, Garner A, et al. Pathology of practolol-induced ocular toxicity. *Br J Ophthalmol*. 1976;60(5):312–323.
5. Coakes RL, Brubaker RF. The mechanism of timolol in lowering intraocular pressure in the normal eye. *Arch Ophthalmol*. 1978;96(11): 2045–2048.
6. Nathanson JA. Human ciliary process adrenergic receptor: pharmacological characterization. *Invest Ophthalmol Vis Sci*. 1981;21(6):798–804.
7. Trope GE, Clark B. Beta adrenergic receptors in pigmented ciliary processes. *Br J Ophthalmol*. 1982;66(12):788–792.
8. Wax MB, Molinoff PB. Distribution and properties of beta-adrenergic receptors in human iris-ciliary body. *Invest Ophthalmol Vis Sci*. 1987;28(3):420–430.
9. Bromberg BB, Gregory DS, Sears ML. Beta-adrenergic receptors in ciliary processes of the rabbit. *Invest Ophthalmol Vis Sci*. 1980;19(2):203–207.
10. Bartels SP, Roth HO, Jumblatt MM, et al. Pharmacological effects of topical timolol in the rabbit eye. *Invest Ophthalmol Vis Sci*. 1980;19(10): 1189–1197.
11. Nathanson JA. Adrenergic regulation of intraocular pressure: identification of beta 2-adrenergic-stimulated adenylate cyclase in ciliary process epithelium. *Proc Natl Acad Sci U S A*. 1980;77(12):7420–7424.
12. Wentworth WO, Brubaker RF. Aqueous humor dynamics in a series of patients with third neuron Horner's syndrome. *Am J Ophthalmol*. 1981;92(3):407–415.
13. Maus TL, Young WFJ, Brubaker RF. Aqueous flow in humans after adrenalectomy. *Invest Ophthalmol Vis Sci*. 1994;35(8):3325–3331.
14. Topper JE, Brubaker RF. Effects of timolol, epinephrine, and acetazolamide on aqueous flow during sleep. *Invest Ophthalmol Vis Sci*. 1985;26(10):1315–1319.
15. Rettig ES, Larsson LI, Brubaker RF. The effect of topical timolol on epinephrine-stimulated aqueous humor flow in sleeping humans. *Invest Ophthalmol Vis Sci*. 1994 ;35(2):554–559.
16. Zimmerman TJ, Harbin R, Pett M, Kaufman HE. Timolol and facility of outflow. *Invest Ophthalmol Vis Sci*. 1977;16(7):623–624.
17. Sonntag JR, Brindley GO, Shields MB. Effect of timolol therapy on outflow facility. *Invest Ophthalmol Vis Sci*. 1978;17(3):293–296.
18. Gilmartin B, Hogan RE, Thompson SM. The effect of Timolol Maleate on tonic accommodation, tonic vergence, and pupil diameter. *Invest Ophthalmol Vis Sci*. 1984;25(6):763–770.
19. Wax MB, Molinoff PB, Alvarado J, et al. Characterization of beta-adrenergic receptors in cultured human trabecular cells and in human trabecular meshwork. *Invest Ophthalmol Vis Sci*. 1989;30(1):51–57.
20. Jampel HD, Lynch MG, Brown RH, et al. Beta-adrenergic receptors in human trabecular meshwork. Identification and autoradiographic localization. *Invest Ophthalmol Vis Sci*. 1987;28(5):772–779.
21. McMenamin PG, Lee WR, Grierson I, et al. Giant vacuoles in the lining endothelium of the human Schlemm's canal after topical timolol maleate. *Invest Ophthalmol Vis Sci*. 1983;24(3):339–342.
22. Lutjen-Drecoll E, Kaufman, PL. Morphological changes in primate aqueous humor formation and drainage tissues after long-term treatment with antiglaucomatous drugs. *J Glaucoma*. 1993;2:316.
23. Costa VP, Harris A, Stefansson E, et al. The effects of antiglaucoma and systemic medications on ocular blood flow. *Prog Retin Eye Res*. 2003; 22(6):769–805.
24. Pillunat L, Stodtmeister R. Effect of different antiglaucomatous drugs on ocular perfusion pressures. *J Ocul Pharmacol*. 1988;4(3):231–242.
25. Yamazaki S, Baba H, Tokoro T. Effects of timolol and carteolol on ocular pulsatile blood flow. *Nippon Ganka Gakkai Zasshi*. 1992;96(8):973–977.
26. Bosem ME, Lusky M, Weinreb RN. Short-term effects of levobunolol on ocular pulsatile flow. *Am J Ophthalmol*. 1992;114(3):280–286.
27. Grunwald JE, Delehanty J. Effect of topical carteolol on the normal human retinal circulation. *Invest Ophthalmol Vis Sci*. 1992;33(6):1853–1856.
28. Harris A, Spaeth GL, Sergott RC, et al. Retrobulbar arterial hemodynamic effects of betaxolol and timolol in normal-tension glaucoma. *Am J Ophthalmol*. 1995;120(2):168–175.
29. Orgul S, Mansberger S, Bacon DR, et al. Optic nerve vasomotor effects of topical beta-adrenergic antagonists in rabbits. *Am J Ophthalmol*. 1995;120(4):441–447.
30. Harris A, Shoemaker JA, Burgoyne J, et al. Acute effect of topical beta-adrenergic antagonists on normal perimacular hemodynamics. *J Glaucoma*. 1995;4:36.

31. Airaksinen PJ, Alanko HI. Vascular effects of timolol and pilocarpine in the iris. A simultaneous bilateral fluorescein angiographic study. *Acta Ophthalmol (Copenh)*. 1983;61(2):195–205.

32. Goldberg HS, Feldman F, Cohen MM, et al. Effect of topical indomethacin and timolol maleate on intraocular pressure in normal subjects. *Am J Ophthalmol*. 1985;99(5):576–578.

33. Sulewski ME, Robin AL, Cummings HL, et al. Effects of topical flurbiprofen on the intraocular pressure lowering effects of apraclonidine and timolol. *Arch Ophthalmol*. 1991;109(6):807–809.

34. Watanabe K, Chiou GC. Action mechanism of timolol to lower the intraocular pressure in rabbits. *Ophthalmic Res*. 1983;15(3):160–167.

35. Mekki QA, Turner P. Dopamine-2 receptor blockade does not affect the ocular hypotensive action of timolol. *Br J Ophthalmol*. 1988;72(8):598–600.

36. Lee PS, Chruscicki DA. Pharmacology of ocular β-adrenoreceptor antagonists. In: Tasman W, Jaeger EA, eds. *Duane's Foundations of Clinical Ophthalmology*. Vol 3. Philadelphia, PA: Lippincott Williams & Wilkins; 2008:chap 32.

37. Katz IM, Hubbard WA, Getson AJ, et al. Intraocular pressure decrease in normal volunteers following timolol ophthalmic solution. *Invest Ophthalmol*. 1976;15(6):489–492.

38. Vareilles P, Silverstone D, Plazonnet B, et al. Comparison of the effects of timolol and other adrenergic agents on intraocular pressure in the rabbit. *Invest Ophthalmol Vis Sci*. 1977;16(11):987–996.

39. Radius RL, Diamond GR, Pollack IP, et al. Timolol. A new drug for management of chronic simple glaucoma. *Arch Ophthalmol*. 1978;96(6):1003–1008.

40. Bartels SP. Aqueous humor flow measured with fluorophotometry in timolol-treated primates. *Invest Ophthalmol Vis Sci*. 1988;29(10):1498–1504.

41. Spinelli D, Montanari P, Vigasio F, et al. Effects of timolol maleate on untreated contralateral eyes [author's transl]. *J Fr Ophtalmol*. 1982;5(3):153–158.

42. Piltz J, Gross R, Shin DH, et al. Contralateral effect of topical beta-adrenergic antagonists in initial one-eyed trials in the ocular hypertension treatment study. *Am J Ophthalmol*. 2000;130(4):441–453.

43. Zimmerman TJ, Kaufman HE. Timolol. A beta-adrenergic blocking agent for the treatment of glaucoma. *Arch Ophthalmol*. 1977;95(4):601–604.

44. Ritch R, Hargett N, Podos S, et al. Retail cost of antiglaucoma drugs in two cities. *Am J Ophthalmol*. 1978;86(1):1–7.

45. Moss AP, Ritch R, Hargett NA, et al. A comparison of the effects of timolol and epinephrine on intraocular pressure. *Am J Ophthalmol*. 1978;86(4):489–495.

46. Zimmerman TJ, Kass MA, Yablonski ME, et al. Timolol maleate: efficacy and safety. *Arch Ophthalmol*. 1979;97(4):656–658.

47. LeBlanc RP, Krip G. Timolol. Canadian multicenter study. *Ophthalmology*. 1981;88(3):224–228.

48. Sonntag JR, Brindley GO, Shields MB, et al. Timolol and epinephrine. Comparison of efficacy and side effects. *Arch Ophthalmol*. 1979;97(2):273–277.

49. Hoyng PF, Verbey NL. Timolol v guanethidine-epinephrine formulations in the treatment of glaucoma. An open clinical trial. *Arch Ophthalmol*. 1984;102(12):1788–1793.

50. Boger WP III, Steinert RF, Puliafito CA, et al. Clinical trial comparing timolol ophthalmic solution to pilocarpine in open-angle glaucoma. *Am J Ophthalmol*. 1978;86(1):8–18.

51. Hass I, Drance SM. Comparison between pilocarpine and timolol on diurnal pressures in open-angle glaucoma. *Arch Ophthalmol*. 1980;98(3):480–481.

52. Merte HJ, Merkle W. Experiences in a double-blind study with different concentrations of timolol and pilocarpine [author's transl]. *Klin Monatsbl Augenheilkd*. 1980;177(4):443–450.

53. Calissendorff B, Maren N, Wettrell K, et al. Timolol versus pilocarpine separately or combined with acetazolamide-effects on intraocular pressure. *Acta Ophthalmol (Copenh)*. 1980;58(4):624–631.

54. Vogel R, Crick RP, Mills KB, et al. Effect of timolol versus pilocarpine on visual field progression in patients with primary open-angle glaucoma. *Ophthalmology*. 1992;99(10):1505–1511.

55. Christakis C, Mangouritsas N. Comparative studies of the pressure-lowering effect of timolol and phospholine iodide [author's transl]. *Klin Monatsbl Augenheilkd*. 1981;179(3):197–200.

56. Schenker H, Maloney S, Liss C, et al. Patient preference, efficacy, and compliance with timolol maleate ophthalmic gel-forming solution versus timolol maleate ophthalmic solution in patients with ocular hypertension or open-angle glaucoma. *Clin Ther*. 1999;21(1):138–147.

57. Konstas AG, Mantziris DA, Maltezos A, et al. Comparison of 24 hour control with Timoptic 0.5% and Timoptic-XE 0.5% in exfoliation and primary open-angle glaucoma. *Acta Ophthalmol Scand*. 1999;77(5):541–543.

58. Derick RJ, Robin AL, Tielsch J, et al. Once-daily versus twice-daily levobunolol (0.5%) therapy. A crossover study. *Ophthalmology*. 1992;99(3):424–429.

59. Wandel T, Fishman D, Novack GD, et al. Ocular hypotensive efficacy of 0.25% levobunolol instilled once daily. *Ophthalmology*. 1988;95(2):252–255.

60. Vuori ML, Ali-Melkkila T, Kaila T, et al. Beta 1- and beta 2-antagonist activity of topically applied betaxolol and timolol in the systemic circulation. *Acta Ophthalmol (Copenh)*. 1993;71(5):682–685.

61. Reiss GR, Brubaker RF. The mechanism of betaxolol, a new ocular hypotensive agent. *Ophthalmology*. 1983;90(11):1369–1372.

62. Berry DP Jr, Van Buskirk EM, Shields MB. Betaxolol and timolol. A comparison of efficacy and side effects. *Arch Ophthalmol*. 1984;102(1):42–45.

63. Allen RC, Hertzmark E, Walker AM, et al. A double-masked comparison of betaxolol vs timolol in the treatment of open-angle glaucoma. *Am J Ophthalmol*. 1986;101(5):535–541.

64. Vogel R, Tipping R, Kulaga SF, et al. Changing therapy from timolol to betaxolol. Effect on intraocular pressure in selected patients with glaucoma. Timolol-Betaxolol Study Group. *Arch Ophthalmol*. 1989;107(9):1303–1307.

65. Messmer C, Flammer J, Stumpfig D. Influence of betaxolol and timolol on the visual fields of patients with glaucoma. *Am J Ophthalmol*. 1991;111(6):678–681.

66. Collignon-Brach J. Long-term effect of ophthalmic beta-adrenoceptor antagonists on intraocular pressure and retinal sensitivity in primary open-angle glaucoma. *Curr Eye Res*. 1992;11(1):1–3.

67. Albracht DC, LeBlanc RP, Cruz AM, et al. A double-masked comparison of betaxolol and dipivefrin for the treatment of increased intraocular pressure. *Am J Ophthalmol*. 1993;116(3):307–313.

68. Javitt J, Goldberg I. Comparison of the clinical success rates and quality of life effects of brimonidine tartrate 0.2% and betaxolol 0.25% suspension in patients with open-angle glaucoma and ocular hypertension. Brimonidine Outcomes Study Group II. *J Glaucoma*. 2000;9(5):398–408.

69. Duzman E, Ober M, Scharrer A, et al. A clinical evaluation of the effects of topically applied levobunolol and timolol on increased intraocular pressure. *Am J Ophthalmol*. 1982;94(3):318–327.

70. Schwartz JS, Christensen RE, Lee DA. Comparison of timolol maleate and levobunolol: doses and volume per bottle. *Arch Ophthalmol*. 1989;107(1):17.

71. Charap AD, Shin DH, Petursson G, et al. Effect of varying drop size on the efficacy and safety of a topical beta blocker. *Ann Ophthalmol*. 1989;21(9):351–357.

72. Rakofsky SI, Melamed S, Cohen JS, et al. A comparison of the ocular hypotensive efficacy of once-daily and twice-daily levobunolol treatment. *Ophthalmology*. 1989;96(1):8–11.

73. Long D, Zimmerman T, Spaeth G, et al. Minimum concentration of levobunolol required to control intraocular pressure in patients with primary open-angle glaucoma or ocular hypertension. *Am J Ophthalmol*. 1985;99(1):18–22.

74. Group TLS. Levobunolol. A four-year study of efficacy and safety in glaucoma treatment. *Ophthalmology*. 1989;96:642.

75. Krieglstein GK, Novack GD, Voepel E, et al. Levobunolol and metipranolol: comparative ocular hypotensive efficacy, safety, and comfort. *Br J Ophthalmol*. 1987;71(4):250–253.

76. Long DA, Johns GE, Mullen RS, et al. Levobunolol and betaxolol. A double-masked controlled comparison of efficacy and safety in patients with elevated intraocular pressure. *Ophthalmology*. 1988;95(6):735–741.

77. Allen RC, Robin AL, Long D, et al. A combination of levobunolol and dipivefrin for the treatment of glaucoma. *Arch Ophthalmol*. 1988;106(7):904–907.

78. Frishman W, Kostis, J. The significance of intrinsic sympathomimetic activity in beta-adrenoceptor blocking drugs. *Cardiovasc Rev Rep*. 1982;3:503.

79. Negishi C, Kanai A, Nakajima A, et al. Ocular effects of β-blocking agent carteolol on healthy volunteers and glaucoma patients. *Jpn J Ophthalmol*. 1981;25:464.

80. Scoville B, Mueller B, White BG, et al. A double-masked comparison of carteolol and timolol in ocular hypertension. *Am J Ophthalmol*. 198815;105(2):150–154.

81. Freedman SF, Freedman NJ, Shields MB, et al. Effects of ocular carteolol and timolol on plasma high-density lipoprotein cholesterol level. *Am J Ophthalmol*. 1993;116(5):600–611.

82. Keates E, Friedland BR, Steward RH, et al. Carteolol hydrochloride: controlled evaluations of its ocular hypotensive efficacy relative to its vehicle, and in combination with pilocarpine, relative to timolol. *J Glaucoma*. 1994;3:315.

83. Demailly P, Allaire C, Bron V, et al. Effectiveness and tolerance of beta-blocker/pilocarpine combination eye drops in primary open-angle glaucoma and high intraocular pressure. *J Glaucoma.* 1995;4(4):235–241.

84. Serle JB, Lustgarten JS, Podos SM. A clinical trial of metipranolol, a non-cardioselective beta-adrenergic antagonist, in ocular hypertension. *Am J Ophthalmol.* 1991;112(3):302–307.

85. Kruse W. Metipranolol—a new beta-blocker. *Klin Monatsbl Augenheilkd.* 1983;182(6):582–584.

86. Liu JH, Bartels SP, Neufeld AH. Effects of L- and D-timolol on cyclic AMP synthesis and intraocular pressure in water-loaded, albino and pigmented rabbits. *Invest Ophthalmol Vis Sci.* 1983;24(9):1276–1282.

87. Keates EU, Stone R. The effect of D-timolol on intraocular pressure in patients with ocular hypertension. *Am J Ophthalmol.* 1984;98(1):73–78.

88. Elliot MJ, Cullen PM, Phillips CI. Ocular hypotensive effect of atenolol (Tenormin, I.C.I.). A new beta-adrenergic blocker. *Br J Ophthalmol.* 1975;59(6):296–300.

89. Tutton MK, Smith RJ. Comparison of ocular hypotensive effects of 3 dosages of oral atenolol. *Br J Ophthalmol.* 1983;67(10):664–667.

90. Wettrell K, Wilke K, Pandolfi M. Topical atenolol versus pilocarpine: a double-blind study of the effect on ocular tension. *Br J Ophthalmol.* 1978;62(5):292–295.

91. Phillips CI, Gore SM, Gunn PM. Atenolol versus adrenaline eye drops and an evaluation of these two combined. *Br J Ophthalmol.* 1978; 62(5):296–301.

92. Brenkman RF. Long-term hypotensive effect of atenolol 4% eyedrops. *Br J Ophthalmol.* 1978;62(5):287–291.

93. Alm A, Wickstrom CP. Effects of systemic and topical administration of metoprolol on intraocular pressure in healthy subjects. *Acta Ophthalmol (Copenh).* 1980;58(5):740–747.

94. Krieglstein G. The long-term ocular systemic effects of topically applied metoprolol tartrate in glaucoma and ocular hypertension. *Acta Ophthalmol (Copenh).* 1981;59:15.

95. Nielsen PG, Ahrendt N, Buhl H, et al. Metoprolol eyedrops 3%, a short-term comparison with pilocarpine and a five-month follow-up study (multicenter). *Acta Ophthalmol (Copenh).* 1982;60(3):347–352.

96. Collignon-Brach J, Weekers R. Comparative clinical study of metoprolol and timolol [author's transl]. *J Fr Ophtalmol.* 1981;4(4):275–278.

97. Bonomi I, Steindler P. Effect of pindolol on intraocular pressure. *Br J Ophthalmol.* 1975;59(6):301–303.

98. Smith RJ, Blamires T, Nagasubramanian S, et al. Addition of pindolol to routine medical therapy: a clinical trial. *Br J Ophthalmol.* 1982; 66(2):102–108.

99. Williamson J, Atta HR, Kennedy PA, et al. Effect of orally administered nadolol on the intraocular pressure in normal volunteers. *Br J Ophthalmol.* 1985;69(1):38–40.

100. Krieglstein GK, Mohamed J. The comparative multiple-dose intraocular pressure responses of nadolol and timolol in glaucoma and ocular hypertension. *Acta Ophthalmol (Copenh).* 1982;60(2):284–292.

101. Duzman E, Chen CC, Anderson J, et al. Diacetyl derivative of nadolol. I. Ocular pharmacology and short-term ocular hypotensive effect in glaucomatous eyes. *Arch Ophthalmol.* 1982;100(12):1916–1919.

102. Duzman E, Rosen N, Lazar M. Diacetyl nadolol: 3-month ocular hypotensive effect in glaucomatous eyes. *Br J Ophthalmol.* 1983; 67(10):668–673.

103. Merte HJ, Stryz JR. Initial experience with the beta-blocker befunolol in the treatment of open-angle glaucoma in Europe. *Klin Monatsbl Augenheilkd.* 1984;184(1):55–58.

104. Merte HJ, Stryz JR. Additional experience with the beta blocker befunolol (Glaukonex) in open-angle glaucoma over a period of 1 year. *Klin Monatsbl Augenheilkd.* 1984;184(4):316–317.

105. Tanaka K, Nakaya H, Yamada Y, et al. Therapeutic results obtained in patients with glaucoma with alteration from 0.05% timolol eye solution to 0.5% befunolol eye solution. *Folia Ophthalmol Jpn.* 1985;36:741.

106. Collignon-Brach J, Weekers R. Timolol [author's transl]. *J Fr Ophtalmol.* 1979;2(11):603–607.

107. Mills KB. Blind randomised non-crossover long-term trial comparing topical timolol 0.25% with timolol 0.5% in the treatment of simple chronic glaucoma. *Br J Ophthalmol.* 1983;67(4):216–219.

108. Robinson J, Kaufman, PL. Dose-dependent suppression of aqueous humor formation by timolol in the cynomolgus monkey. *J Glaucoma.* 1993;2:251.

109. Katz IM, Berger ET. Effects of iris pigmentation on response of ocular pressure to timolol. *Surv Ophthalmol.* 1979;23(6):395–398.

110. Salminen L, Imre G, Huupponen R. The effect of ocular pigmentation on intraocular pressure response to timolol. *Acta Ophthalmol Suppl.* 1985;173:15–18.

111. Schmitt CJ, Lotti VJ, LeDouarec JC. Penetration of timolol into the rabbit eye. Measurements after ocular instillation and intravenous injection. *Arch Ophthalmol.* 1980;98(3):547–551.

112. Phillips CI, Bartholomew RS, Kazi G, et al. Penetration of timolol eye drops into human aqueous humour. *Br J Ophthalmol.* 1981;65(9): 593–595.

113. Zimmerman TJ, Kaufman HE. Timolol, dose response and duration of action. *Arch Ophthalmol.* 1977;95(4):605–607.

114. Soll DB. Evaluation of timolol in chronic open-angle glaucoma. Once a day vs twice a day. *Arch Ophthalmol.* 1980;98(12):2178–2181.

115. Yalon M, Urinowsky E, Rothkoff L, et al. Frequency of timolol administration. *Am J Ophthalmol.* 1981;92(4):526–529.

116. Letchinger SL, Frohlichstein D, Glieser DK, et al. Can the concentration of timolol or the frequency of its administration be reduced? *Ophthalmology.* 1993;100(8):1259–1262.

117. Laurence J, Holder D, Vogel R, et al. A double-masked, placebo-controlled evaluation of timolol in a gel vehicle. *J Glaucoma.* 1993;2:177.

118. Schlecht LP, Brubaker RF. The effects of withdrawal of timolol in chronically treated glaucoma patients. *Ophthalmology.* 1988;95(9):1212–1216.

119. Trope GE, Menon IA, Liu GS, et al. Ocular timolol levels after drug withdrawal: an experimental model. *Can J Ophthalmol.* 1994;29(5):217–219.

120. Krieglstein GK. A follow-up study on the intraocular pressure response of timolol eye drops [author's transl]. *Klin Monatsbl Augenheilkd.* 1979;175(5):627–633.

121. Merte HJ, Merkle W. Results of long-term treatment of glaucoma with timolol ophthalmic solution [author's transl]. *Klin Monatsbl Augenheilkd.* 1980;177(5):562–571.

122. Steinert RF, Thomas JV, Boger WP III. Long-term drift and continued efficacy after multiyear timolol therapy. *Arch Ophthalmol.* 1981; 99(1):100–103.

123. Airaksinen PJ, Valle O, Takki KK, et al. Timolol treatment of chronic open-angle glaucoma and ocular hypertension. A 2.5-year multicenter study. *Graefes Arch Clin Exp Ophthalmol.* 1982;219(2):68–71.

124. Blika S, Saunte E. Timolol maleate in the treatment of glaucoma simplex and glaucoma capsulare. A three-year follow up study. *Acta Ophthalmol (Copenh).* 1982;60(6):967–976.

125. Maclure GM. Chronic open angle glaucoma treated with Timolol. A four year study. *Trans Ophthalmol Soc U K.* 1983;103(pt 1):78–83.

126. LeBlanc RP, Saheb NE, Krip G. Timolol: long-term Canadian multicentre study. *Can J Ophthalmol.* 1985;20(4):128–130.

127. Boger WP III. Short term "escape" and long term "drift." The dissipation effects of the beta adrenergic blocking agents. *Surv Ophthalmol.* 1983;28(suppl):235–242.

128. Boger WP III, Puliafito CA, Steinert RF, et al. Long-term experience with timolol ophthalmic solution in patients with open-angle glaucoma. *Ophthalmology.* 1978;85(3):259–267.

129. Oksala A, Salminen L. Tachyphylaxis in timolol therapy for chronic glaucoma [author's transl]. *Klin Monatsbl Augenheilkd.* 1980;177(4):451–454.

130. Krupin T, Singer PR, Perlmutter J, et al. One-hour intraocular pressure response to timolol. Lack of correlation with long-term response. *Arch Ophthalmol.* 1981;99(5):840–841.

131. Neufeld AH, Zawistowski KA, Page ED, et al. Influences on the density of beta-adrenergic receptors in the cornea and iris—ciliary body of the rabbit. *Invest Ophthalmol Vis Sci.* 1978;17(11):1069–1075.

132. Lin LL, Galin MA, Obstbaum SA, et al. Longterm timolol therapy. *Surv Ophthalmol.* 1979;23(6):377–380.

133. Plane C, Boulmier A. Long-term treatment of chronic glaucoma with timolol drops: results after four years [author's transl]. *J Fr Ophtalmol.* 1981;4(11):751–756.

134. Brubaker RF, Nagataki S, Bourne WM. Effect of chronically administered timolol on aqueous humor flow in patients with glaucoma. *Ophthalmology.* 1982;89(3):280–283.

135. Gandolfi SA. Restoring sensitivity to timolol after long-term drift in primary open-angle glaucoma. *Invest Ophthalmol Vis Sci.* 1990;31(2):354–358.

136. Gandolfi SA, Vecchi M. Serial administration of adrenergic antagonist and agonist ("pulsatile therapy") reduces the incidence of long-term drift to timolol in humans. *Invest Ophthalmol Vis Sci.* 1996;37(4):684–688.

137. Hommer A, Thygesen J, Ferreras A, et al. A European perspective on costs and cost effectiveness of ophthalmic combinations in the treatment of open-angle glaucoma. *Eur J Ophthalmol.* 2008;18(5):778–786.

138. Woodward DF, Chen J. Fixed-combination and emerging glaucoma therapies. *Expert Opin Emerg Drugs.* 2007;12(2):313–327.

139. Sherwood MB, Craven ER, Chou C, et al. Twice-daily 0.2% brimonidine-0.5% timolol fixed-combination therapy vs monotherapy with timolol or brimonidine in patients with glaucoma or ocular hypertension: a 12-month randomized trial. *Arch Ophthalmol.* 2006;124(9):1230–1238.

140. Boyle JE, Ghosh K, Gieser DK, et al. A randomized trial comparing the dorzolamide-timolol combination given twice daily to monotherapy with timolol and dorzolamide. Dorzolamide-Timolol Study Group. *Ophthalmology.* 1998;105(10):1945–1951.

141. Keates EU. Evaluation of timolol maleate combination therapy in chronic open-angle glaucoma. *Am J Ophthalmol.* 1979;88(3 pt 2):565–571.

142. Berson FG, Epstein DL. Separate and combined effects of timolol maleate and acetazolamide in open-angle glaucoma. *Am J Ophthalmol.* 1981;92(6):788–791.

143. Kass MA, Korey M, Gordon M, et al. Timolol and acetazolamide. A study of concurrent administration. *Arch Ophthalmol.* 1982;100(6):941–942.

144. Smith RJ, Nagasubramanian S, Watkins R, et al. Addition of timolol maleate to routine medical therapy: a clinical trial. *Br J Ophthalmol.* 1980;64(10):779–781.

145. Nielsen NV, Eriksen JS. Timolol in maintenance treatment of ocular hypertension and glaucoma. *Acta Ophthalmol (Copenh).* 1979;57(6):1070–1077.

146. Kass MA. Efficacy of combining timolol with other antiglaucoma medications. *Surv Ophthalmol.* 1983;28(suppl):274–279.

147. Soderstrom MB, Wallin O, Granstrom PA, et al. Timolol-pilocarpine combined vs timolol and pilocarpine given separately [see comments]. *Am J Ophthalmol.* 1989;107(5):465–470.

148. Krum H, Roecker EB, Mohacsi P, et al. Effects of initiating carvedilol in patients with severe chronic heart failure: results from the COPERNICUS Study. *JAMA.* 2003;289(6):712–718.

149. Post SR, Hammond HK, Insel PA. Beta-adrenergic receptors and receptor signaling in heart failure [review] [107 refs]. *Annu Rev Pharmacol Toxicol.* 1999;39:343–360.

150. Blondeau P, Cote M, Tetrault L. Effect of timolol eye drops in subjects receiving systemic propranolol therapy. *Can J Ophthalmol.* 1983;18(1):18–21.

151. Gross F, Schuman JS. Reduced ocular hypotensive effect of topical beta-blockers in glaucoma patients receiving oral beta-blockers. *J Glaucoma.* 1992;1:174.

152. Schuman JS. Effects of systemic beta-blocker therapy on the efficacy and safety of topical brimonidine and timolol. Brimonidine Study Groups 1 and 2 [see comments]. *Ophthalmology.* 2000;107(6):1171–1177.

153. Batchelor ED, O'Day DM, Shand DG, et al. Interaction of topical and oral timolol in glaucoma. *Ophthalmology.* 1979;86(1):60–65.

154. Johnson SH, Brubaker RF, Trautman JC. Absence of an effect of timolol on the pupil. *Invest Ophthalmol Vis Sci.* 1978;17(9):924–926.

155. Nielsen NV, Eriksen JS. Timolol transitory manifestations of dry eyes in long term treatment. *Acta Ophthalmol (Copenh).* 1979;57(3):418–424.

156. Coakes RL, Mackie IA, Seal DV. Effects of long-term treatment with timolol on lacrimal gland function. *Br J Ophthalmol.* 1981;65(9):603–605.

157. Kuppens EV, Stolwijk TR, de Keizer RJ, et al. Basal tear turnover and topical timolol in glaucoma patients and healthy controls by fluorophotometry. *Invest Ophthalmol Vis Sci.* 1992;33(12):3442–3448.

158. Herreras JM, Pastor JC, Calonge M, et al. Ocular surface alteration after long-term treatment with an antiglaucomatous drug. *Ophthalmology.* 1992;99(7):1082–1088.

159. McMahon CD, Shaffer RN, Hoskins HD Jr, et al. Adverse effects experienced by patients taking timolol. *Am J Ophthalmol.* 1979;88(4):736–738.

160. Wilson RP, Spaeth GL, Poryzees E. The place of timolol in the practice of ophthalmology. *Ophthalmology.* 1980;87(5):451–454.

161. Van Buskirk EM. Adverse reactions from timolol administration. *Ophthalmology.* 1980;87(5):447–450.

162. Van Buskirk EM. Corneal anesthesia after timolol maleate therapy. *Am J Ophthalmol.* 1979;88(4):739–743.

163. Weissman SS, Asbell PA. Effects of topical timolol (0.5%) and betaxolol (0.5%) on corneal sensitivity. *Br J Ophthalmol.* 1990;74(7):409–412.

164. Tauber J, Melamed S, Foster CS. Glaucoma in patients with ocular cicatricial pemphigoid. *Ophthalmology.* 1989;96(1):33–37.

165. Fiore PM, Jacobs IH, Goldberg DB. Drug-induced pemphigoid. A spectrum of diseases [review] [13 refs]. *Arch Ophthalmol.* 1987;105(12):1660–1663.

166. Williams DE, Nguyen KD, Shapourifar-Tehrani S, et al. Effects of timolol, betaxolol, and levobunolol on human tenon's fibroblasts in tissue culture. *Invest Ophthalmol Vis Sci.* 1992;33(7):2233–2241.

167. Broadway DC, Grierson I, Sturmer J, et al. Reversal of topical antiglaucoma medication effects on the conjunctiva. *Arch Ophthalmol.* 1996;114(3):262–267.

168. Brubaker RF, Coakes RL, Bourne WM. Effect of timolol on the permeability of corneal endothelium. *Ophthalmology.* 1979;86(1):108–111.

169. Staatz WD, Radius RL, Van Horn DL, et al. Effects of timolol on bovine corneal endothelial cultures. *Arch Ophthalmol.* 1981;99(4):660–663.

170. Alanko HI, Airaksinen PJ. Effects of topical timolol on corneal endothelial cell morphology in vivo. *Am J Ophthalmol.* 1983;96(5):615–621.

171. Lass JH, Eriksson GL, Osterling L, et al.; Latanoprost Corneal Effects Study G. Comparison of the corneal effects of latanoprost, fixed combination latanoprost-timolol, and timolol: a double-masked, randomized, one-year study [comment]. *Ophthalmology.* 2001;108(2):264–271.

172. Arthur BW, Hay GJ, Wasan SM, et al. Ultrastructural effects of topical timolol on the rabbit cornea. Outcome alone and in conjunction with a gas permeable contact lens. *Arch Ophthalmol.* 1983;101(10):1607–1610.

173. Huige WM, Beekhuis WH, Rijneveld WJ, et al. Unusual deposits in the superficial corneal stroma following combined use of topical corticosteroid and beta-blocking medication. *Doc Ophthalmol.* 1991;78(3–4):169–175.

174. Harris A, Jonescu-Cuypers CP. The impact of glaucoma medication on parameters of ocular perfusion. *Curr Opin Ophthalmol.* 2001;12(2):131–137.

175. Chiou GC, Chen YJ. Effects of antiglaucoma drugs on ocular blood flow in ocular hypertensive rabbits. *J Ocul Pharmacol.* 1993;9(1):13–24.

176. Steigerwalt RD Jr, Belcaro G, Cesarone MR, et al. Doppler ultrasonography of the central retinal artery in normals treated with topical timolol. *Eye.* 1993;7(pt 3):403–406.

177. Steigerwalt RD Jr, Belcaro G, Cesarone MR, et al. Doppler ultrasonography of the central retinal artery in patients with diabetes and vascular disease treated with topical timolol. *Eye.* 1995;9(pt 4):495–501.

178. Grajewski AL, Ferrari-Dileo G, Feuer WJ, et al. Beta-adrenergic responsiveness of choroidal vasculature. *Ophthalmology.* 1991;98(6):989–995.

179. Truckenbrodt C, Klein S, Vilser W. Does timolol modify retinal hemodynamics in patients with normal pressure glaucoma? *Ophthalmologe.* 1992;89(6):452–454.

180. Akingbehin T, Villada JR. Metipranolol-associated granulomatous anterior uveitis. *Br J Ophthalmol.* 1991;75(9):519–523.

181. Akingbehin T, Villada JR, Walley T. Metipranolol-induced adverse reactions: I. The rechallenge study. *Eye.* 1992;6(pt 3):277–279.

182. Kessler C, Christ, T. Incidence of uveitis in glaucoma patients using metipranolol. *J Glaucoma.* 1993;2:166.

183. Schultz JS, Hoenig JA, Charles H. Possible bilateral anterior uveitis secondary to metipranolol (optipranolol) therapy. *Arch Ophthalmol.* 1993;111(12):1606–1607.

184. Melles RB, Wong IG. Metipranolol-associated granulomatous iritis. *Am J Ophthalmol.* 1994;118(6):712–715.

185. Hesse RJ, Swan JL II. Aphakic cystoid macular edema secondary to betaxolol therapy. *Ophthalmic Surg.* 1988;19(8):562–564.

186. Arnoult L, Bowman, ZL, Kimbrough, RL, et al. Periocular cutaneous pigmentary changes associated with topical betaxolol. *J Glaucoma.* 1995;4:263.

187. Vogel R, Strahlman E, Rittenhouse KD. Adverse events associated with commonly used glaucoma drugs [review] [82 refs]. *Int Ophthalmol Clin.* 1999;39(2):107–124.

188. Lama PJ. Systemic adverse effects of beta-adrenergic blockers: an evidence-based assessment. *Am J Ophthalmol.* 2002;134(5):749–760.

189. Kaila T, Salminen L, Huupponen R. Systemic absorption of topically applied ocular timolol. *J Ocul Pharmacol.* 1985;1(1):79–83.

190. Shedden AH, Laurence J, Barrish A, et al. Plasma timolol concentrations of timolol maleate: timolol gel-forming solution (TIMOPTIC-XE) once daily versus timolol maleate ophthalmic solution twice daily. *Doc Ophthalmol.* 2001;103(1):73–79.

191. Dickstein K, Hapnes R, Aarsland T. Comparison of aqueous and gellan ophthalmic timolol with placebo on the 24-hour heart rate response in patients on treatment for glaucoma. *Am J Ophthalmol.* 2001;132(5):626–632.

192. Passo MS, Palmer EA, Van Buskirk EM. Plasma timolol in glaucoma patients. *Ophthalmology.* 1984;91(11):1361–1363.

193. Ohdo S, Grass GM, Lee VH. Improving the ocular to systemic ratio of topical timolol by varying the dosing time. *Invest Ophthalmol Vis Sci.* 1991;32(10):2790–2798.

194. Vuori ML, Ali-Melkkila T, Kaila T, et al. Plasma and aqueous humour concentrations and systemic effects of topical betaxolol and timolol in man. *Acta Ophthalmol (Copenh).* 1993;71(2):201–206.

195. Le Jeunne C, Munera Y, Hugues FC. Systemic effects of three beta-blocker eyedrops: comparison in healthy volunteers of beta 1- and beta 2-adrenoreceptor inhibition. *Clin Pharmacol Ther.* 1990;47(5):578–583.

196. Caprioli J, Sears ML. Caution on the preoperative use of topical timolol. *Am J Ophthalmol.* 1983;95(4):561–562.

197. Doyle WJ, Weber PA, Meeks RH. Effect of topical timolol maleate on exercise performance. *Arch Ophthalmol.* 1984;102(10):1517–1518.

198. Leier CV, Baker ND, Weber PA. Cardiovascular effects of ophthalmic timolol. *Ann Intern Med.* 1986;104(2):197–199.

199. Nelson WL, Fraunfelder FT, Sills JM, et al. Adverse respiratory and cardiovascular events attributed to timolol ophthalmic solution, 1978–1985. *Am J Ophthalmol.* 1986;102(5):606–611.

200. Dinai Y, Sharir M, Naveh N, et al. Bradycardia induced by interaction between quinidine and ophthalmic timolol. *Ann Intern Med.* 1985;103(6 pt 1):890–891.

201. Pringle SD, MacEwen CJ. Severe bradycardia due to interaction of timolol eye drops and verapamil. *Br Med J (Clin Res Ed).* 1987;294(6565):155–156.

202. Nelson WL, Kuritsky JN. Early postmarketing surveillance of betaxolol hydrochloride, September 1985-September 1986. *Am J Ophthalmol.* 1987;103(4):592.

203. Zabel RW, MacDonald IM. Sinus arrest associated with betaxolol ophthalmic drops. *Am J Ophthalmol.* 1987;104(4):431.

204. Ball S. Congestive heart failure from betaxolol. Case report. *Arch Ophthalmol.* 1987;105(3):320.

205. Pinski SL. Continuing progress in the treatment of severe congestive heart failure. *JAMA.* 2003;289(6):754–756.

206. Jones FL Jr, Ekberg NL. Exacerbation of asthma by timolol. *N Engl J Med.* 1979;301(5):270.

207. Avorn J, Glynn RJ, Gurwitz JH, et al. Adverse pulmonary effects of topical beta blockers used in the treatment of glaucoma. *J Glaucoma.* 1993;2:158.

208. Van Buskirk EM, Fraunfelder FT. Ocular beta-blockers and systemic effects. *Am J Ophthalmol.* 1984;98(5):623–624.

209. Lustgarten JS, Podos SM. Topical timolol and the nursing mother. *Arch Ophthalmol.* 1983;101(9):1381–1382.

210. Coyle J. Timoptic and depression. *J Ocul Ther Surg.* 1983;2(6):311.

211. Orlando RG. Clinical depression associated with betaxolol. *Am J Ophthalmol.* 1986;102(2):275.

212. Coleman AL, Diehl DL, Jampel HD, et al. Topical timolol decreases plasma high-density lipoprotein cholesterol level. *Arch Ophthalmol.* 1990;108(9):1260–1263.

213. West J, Longstaff S. Topical timolol and serum lipoproteins. *Br J Ophthalmol.* 1990;74(11):663–664.

214. Fraunfelder FT. Interim report: National Registry of Possible Drug-induced Ocular Side Effects. *Ophthalmology.* 1980;87(2):87–90.

215. Fraunfelder FT, Meyer SM, Menacker SJ. Alopecia possibly secondary to topical ophthalmic beta-blockers. *JAMA.* 1990;263(11):1493–1494.

216. Shaivitz SA. Timolol and myasthenia gravis. *JAMA.* 1979;242(15):1611–1612.

217. Velde TM, Kaiser FE. Ophthalmic timolol treatment causing altered hypoglycemic response in a diabetic patient. *Arch Intern Med.* 1983;143(8):1627.

218. Wikberg-Matsson A, Uhlen S, Wikberg JE. Characterization of alpha(1)-adrenoceptor subtypes in the eye. *Exp Eye Res.* 2000;70(1):51–60.

219. Moroi SE, Hao Y, Inoue-Matsuhisa E, et al. Cell signaling in bovine ciliary epithelial organ culture. *J Ocul Pharmacol Ther.* 2000;16(1):65–74.

220. Wand M, Grant WM. Thymoxamine hydrochloride: an alpha-adrenergic blocker. *Surv Ophthalmol.* 1980;25(2):75–84.

221. Wand M, Grant WM. Thymoxamine hydrochloride: effects on the facility of outflow and intraocular pressure. *Invest Ophthalmol.* 1976;15(5):400–403.

222. Lee DA, Brubaker RF, Nagataki S. Effect of thymoxamine on aqueous humor formation in the normal human eye as measured by fluorophotometry. *Invest Ophthalmol Vis Sci.* 1981;21(6):805–811.

223. Relf SJ, Gharagozloo NZ, Skuta GL, et al. Thymoxamine reverses phenylephrine-induced mydriasis. *Am J Ophthalmol.* 1988;106(3):251–255.

224. Halasa AH, Rutkowski PC. Thymoxamine therapy for angle-closure glaucoma. *Arch Ophthalmol.* 1973;90(3):177–179.

225. Campbell DG. Pigmentary dispersion and glaucoma. A new theory. *Arch Ophthalmol.* 1979;97(9):1667–1672.

226. Dixon RS, Anderson RL, Hatt MU. The use of thymoxamine in eyelid retraction. *Arch Ophthalmol.* 1979;97(11):2147–2150.

227. Iuglio N. Ocular effects of topical application of dapiprazole in man. *Glaucoma.* 1984;6:110.

228. Oshika T, Araie M, Sugiyama T, et al. Effect of bunazosin hydrochloride on intraocular pressure and aqueous humor dynamics in normotensive human eyes. *Arch Ophthalmol.* 1991;109(11):1569–1574.

229. Krupin T, Feitl M, Becker B. Effect of prazosin on aqueous humor dynamics in rabbits. *Arch Ophthalmol.* 1980;98(9):1639–1642.

230. Serle JB, Stein AJ, Podos SM, et al. Corynanthine and aqueous humor dynamics in rabbits and monkeys. *Arch Ophthalmol.* 1984;102(9):1385–1388.

231. Serle JB, Podos SM, Lustgarten JS, et al. The effect of corynanthine on intraocular pressure in clinical trials. *Ophthalmology.* 1985;92(7):977–980.

232. Leopold IH, Murray DL. Ocular hypotensive action of labetalol. *Am J Ophthalmol.* 1979;88(3 pt 1):427–431.

233. Bonomi L, Perfetti S, Bellucci R, et al. Ocular hypotensive action of labetalol in rabbit and human eyes. *Albrecht Von Graefes Arch Klin Exp Ophthalmol.* 1981;217(3):175–181.

234. Krieglstein GK, Kontic D. Nadolol and labetalol: comparative efficacy of two beta-blocking agents in glaucoma. *Albrecht Von Graefes Arch Klin Exp Ophthalmol.* 1981;216(4):313–317.

30

Adrenergic Stimulators

Like the β-adrenergic receptors, the α-adrenergic receptors are part of the sympathetic nervous system that play a major role to regulate in part aqueous humor dynamics (see Chapter 1). Development of this class of glaucoma medications was based on the observation that a topical formulation of the antihypertensive agent clonidine lowered intraocular pressure (IOP) (1). The clinical value of clonidine as an ocular hypotensive agent was limited by the fact that it penetrates the blood–brain barrier, occasionally causing significant systemic hypotensive episodes, even with topical administration. Further research led to the approval of several α$_2$-adrenergic agonists for use in managing glaucoma. The nonselective α- and β-adrenergic receptor agonists epinephrine and the prodrug dipivefrin are no longer available but are summarized in this chapter for historical reasons.

MECHANISMS OF ACTION

The mechanism of action by which apraclonidine, clonidine, and brimonidine tartrate lower IOP is through reducing aqueous production (2). These agents have little, if any, effect on blood–aqueous barrier permeability (3). In one clinical trial, there was also a suggestion that apraclonidine may increase outflow facility and reduce episcleral venous pressure (4). Given the presence of α$_{2A}$-adrenergic receptors in cultured human trabecular meshwork cells (5), these agents may exert some effect on outflow facility. In contrast, brimonidine does not appear to have an effect on conventional aqueous humor outflow or episcleral venous pressure, but it increases uveoscleral outflow (6).

Another possible mechanism may involve an increase in prostaglandin levels. However, in studies involving healthy volunteers and patients with either ocular hypertension or glaucoma, pretreatment with flurbiprofen had no influenc on the IOP-lowering effect of apraclonidine (7,8).

Epinephrine, a neurohumoral transmitter, and norepinephrine, a neurotransmitter, stimulate adrenergic receptors and mediate the physiologic sympathetic actions on aqueous humor dynamics. Early studies of epinephrine and the prodrug dipivefrin showed multiple effects on aqueous humor dynamics. The effects of epinephrine have been described in three phases. In the early phase, within minutes after instillation of epinephrine, aqueous inflow is reduced, presumably due to the α-adrenergic effect of vasoconstriction, which reduces the ultrafiltration of plasma into the stroma of the ciliary processes (9). This α-adrenergic effect on aqueous production, however, is transient and not of sufficient magnitude to significantly influence IOP. The middle phase overlaps with the first phase and

is believed to be an early, moderate-sized α-adrenergic effect on true outflow facility. Fluorophotometric and tonographic studies in healthy (10,11) and ocular hypertensive human eyes suggest that IOP reduction for at least the first several hours after topical instillation of epinephrine is associated with improved facility of outflow (12). The late phase is believed to occur weeks to months after continued administration of epinephrine. The mechanism is thought to be related to metabolism of glycosaminoglycans in the trabecular meshwork (13).

SPECIFIC AGENTS

Apraclonidine

Apraclonidine is a para-amino derivative of clonidine, an α$_2$-adrenergic agonist that is used clinically as a potent systemic antihypertensive agent. Topical apraclonidine hydrochloride is available in a 1% concentration for the treatment of short-term IOP elevation, especially after anterior segment laser procedures, and in a 0.5% preparation for the long-term management of glaucoma. In a 90-day study comparing apraclonidine, 0.25% or 0.5%, three times a day and timolol, 0.5%, twice a day, the apraclonidine, 0.5%, reduced IOP more than apraclonidine, 0.25%, but no significant difference was observed between apraclonidine, 0.5%, and timolol, 0.5% (14).

Brimonidine

Brimonidine tartrate, 0.2%, has been similar to timolol, 0.5%, and greater than betaxolol, 0.25%, in IOP-lowering efficacy (15). As with apraclonidine, brimonidine is useful in controlling the IOP rise after anterior segment laser surgery. In two vehicle-controlled, multicenter trials involving 480 patients undergoing 360% argon laser trabeculoplasty, brimonidine, 0.5%, provided effective postoperative pressure control, whether it was given before, after, or before and after the procedure (16). Brimonidine, 0.2%, is as effective as apraclonidine, 0.5%, in preventing postoperative IOP elevation after anterior segment laser procedures (17).

In addition to lowering the IOP, brimonidine may prevent optic nerve damage through a neuroprotective mechanism. Brimonidine reduces loss of retinal ganglion cells in an optic nerve crush injury model in rats and mice (18). These findings have been supported by later studies examining the effect of brimonidine on retinal ganglion cell death in retinal ischemia models and laser-induced glaucoma models (19). However, these models of optic nerve injury are not directly comparable to glaucoma occurring in humans. Whether brimonidine provides neuroprotection in humans with glaucoma remains unknown.

Dipivefrin and Epinephrine

Dipivefrin, a prodrug of epinephrine, is a direct-acting sympathomimetic that stimulates both α- and β-adrenergic receptors. Neither dipivefrin nor epinephrine is currently available. Dipivefrin, or dipivalyl epinephrine, was a modification of epinephrine in which two pivalic acid groups were added to the parent drug. It was significantly more lipophilic than epinephrine, which increases the corneal penetration 17-fold (20). Dipivefrin was hydrolyzed to epinephrine after absorption into the eye, with most of the hydrolysis occurring in the cornea (21). Clinical trials indicate that the pressure-lowering effect of dipivefrin, 0.1%, is similar to that of betaxolol, 0.5% (22).

ADMINISTRATION

Topical 1% apraclonidine is indicated for short-term use generally to prevent and to manage postlaser IOP elevation. In a double-masked, randomized, 90-day trial involving patients with chronic open-angle glaucoma (COAG), apraclonidine, 0.25% and 0.5%, given three times daily, reduced the IOP an average of 3.6 and 5.4 mm Hg, respectively, compared with 5.0 mm Hg with timolol, 0.5%, administered twice daily (14). Apraclonidine also had a similar effect to β-adrenergic antagonists on daytime aqueous flow, with an average reduction of 30% (23). Unlike timolol, however, which does not affect aqueous flow during sleep, apraclonidine caused a 27% reduction of the spontaneous nocturnal rate (23).

Brimonidine is an effective agent for long-term management of glaucoma. For optimal IOP-lowering effect, it is recommended that brimonidine, 0.2%, be administered three times daily. Its effect is similar to that of timolol maleate, 0.5%, and superior to betaxolol, 0.25%, when administered twice daily (24). Given the additive effects of brimonidine and timolol, 0.5%, the fixed combination of these two medications was developed and shown to be slightly more effective compared with monotherapy alone (25). In another study, brimonidine, 0.2%, had an IOP effect similar to dorzolamide, 2%, when administered three times daily (26). Compared with latanoprost administered once daily, twice-daily brimonidine had a similar IOP-lowering effect at peak but did not lower IOP as effectively at trough (27).

Dipivefrin is available as a 0.1% solution. Like its predecessor epinephrine, dipivefrin is administered twice daily for maximal effect.

DRUG INTERACTIONS

A 4-month study ($n = 120$) was designed to compare the efficacy of brimonidine, dorzolamide, and brinzolamide in reducing IOP when used as adjunctive therapy to a once-daily prostaglandin analog of bimatoprost, latanoprost, or travoprost (28). Study eyes were randomly assigned to adjunctive treatment of three times daily brimonidine tartrate, 0.15% ($n = 41$); dorzolamide hydrochloride, 2% ($n = 40$); or brinzolamide, 1% ($n = 39$). At 4 months of adjunctive therapy, the mean IOP was lower and the mean change from baseline IOP was greater in the brimonidine group than in either the dorzolamide group or the brinzolamide group at 10 AM and 4 PM. The mean IOP reduction from baseline at 10 AM and 4 PM was 4.8 mm Hg (21%) and 3.8 mm Hg (19%) with brimonidine, 3.4 mm Hg (16%) and 2.8 mm Hg (14%) with dorzolamide, and 3.4 mm Hg (16%) and 2.6 mm Hg (13%) with brinzolamide. The addition of brimonidine to a prostaglandin agent provided greater IOP lowering than the addition of either dorzolamide or brinzolamide.

A pooled data analysis ($n = 180$) compared the IOP-lowering efficacy and ocular tolerability of the fixed-combination drugs brimonidine, 0.2%, with timolol, 0.5%, and dorzolamide, 2%, with timolol, 0.5%. Patients with glaucoma or ocular hypertension had been assigned to one of the two fixed-combination drugs, used as monotherapy or as an adjunctive to prostaglandin therapy. At 3 months, the mean ($\pm$SD) IOP reduction from baseline with fixed-combination monotherapy was 7.7 $\pm$ 4.2 mm Hg (32.3%) for brimonidine–timolol versus 6.7 $\pm$ 5.0 mm Hg (26.1%) for dorzolamide–timolol. The mean IOP reduction from prostaglandin-treated baseline with fixed-combination adjunctive therapy was 6.9 $\pm$ 4.8 mm Hg (29.3%) for brimonidine–timolol and 5.2 $\pm$ 3.7 mm Hg (23.5%) for dorzolamide–timolol ($P = 0.2$). At 3 months, the fixed-combination brimonidine–timolol provided the same or greater IOP lowering compared with fixed-combination dorzolamide–timolol (29).

Brimonidine is generally additive to other glaucoma agents, with the exception of apraclonidine, which is chemically and functionally similar. Brimonidine further reduced IOP by 17% to 19% when administered to healthy participants taking timolol maleate, 0.5% (30). As mentioned earlier, this additive effect leads to the development and release of the fixed combination of brimonidine, 0.2%, with timolol, 0.5%.

The interaction between epinephrine and dipivefrin with β-adrenergic blockers is less clear because epinephrine stimulates and β-blockers inhibit β-adrenergic receptors. When epinephrine therapy was added to eyes already receiving timolol, an additional reduction in IOP is usually small or absent (31). Continued therapy with dipivefrin in combination with timolol historically provided only a 1– to 3–mm Hg additional IOP reduction in most patients over that achieved with timolol alone (32).

SIDE EFFECTS

Ocular Toxicity

The most significant ocular side effect with apraclonidine is a follicular conjunctivitis with or without contact dermatitis. Of 64 patients on long-term therapy with the 1% concentration, 48% developed an allergic reaction (33). Similar ocular side effects have been reported for brimonidine. The rate of ocular allergies is substantially less than that encountered with the use of apraclonidine. In one study, 15% of patients developed ocular allergies, compared with a reported 36% or more of those taking apraclonidine (33). In a study of patients with known ocular allergy to apraclonidine, 10.5% developed allergic symptoms to brimonidine during 18-month follow-up (34).

Other ocular side effects that have been reported with apraclonidine include eyelid retraction, mydriasis, and conjunctival blanching (35), which are due to cross-reactivity with α_1-adrenergic receptors in Müller muscle, iris sphincter muscle, and arterial smooth muscle, respectively.

The ocular side effects of dipivefrin can include those described earlier, but in addition there are some side effects that are unique to this epinephrine prodrug. After an initial vasoconstrictive effect, reactive hyperemia occurs with epinephrine, and to a lesser extent with dipivefrin. Oxidation and polymerization of epinephrine convert the drug to adrenochrome, a pigment of the melanin family, which historically appears as dark deposits in several ocular structures. Another well-recognized side effect is epinephrine-associated cystoid macular edema, which was observed in some aphakic eyes receiving topical epinephrine.

Systemic Toxicity

Systemic side effects are similar between topical apraclonidine and brimonidine because they both act at the same receptors. Systemic effects of topically applied brimonidine include oral dryness, sedation, drowsiness, headache, and fatigue (36). These effects may be more common in the elderly and in the very young. Because of risks of pronounced central nervous system depression, brimonidine should be used with great caution or not at all in children younger than 5 years (37).

Since dipivefrin was a prodrug of epinephrine, there were less sympathetic adverse reactions, which included elevated blood pressure, tachycardia, arrhythmias, headaches, tremor, nervousness, and anxiety. Since dipivefrin is not converted to active epinephrine until it enters the eye, there were fewer systemic effects than the standard forms of epinephrine.

INDICATIONS

Among the adrenergic stimulators, apraclonidine and brimonidine are α_2-adrenergic agonists that are useful in controlling short-term pressure elevations, especially in association with certain laser procedures, as well as the long-term management of glaucoma. Since brimonidine is now available in several generic formulations, it is affordable. The main value of apraclonidine is to minimize short-term IOP elevations after laser procedures and after phacoemulsification and intraocular lens implantation (38). Apraclonidine, 0.5%, can be used in the long-term management of glaucoma, but the benefit is limited by the high incidence of allergic reactions (33). Brimonidine is an effective choice as a second-line drug for glaucoma management in adults but should be used cautiously, if at all, in young children. Epinephrine and dipivefrin, a prodrug of epinephrine, are no longer available.

KEY POINTS

- The α_2-adrenergic agonists include apraclonidine and brimonidine. They are useful to lower acute pressure elevations following laser procedures.
- These agents are considered second-line drugs for long-term management of COAG in adults.
- Given the ability of these drugs to cross the blood–brain barrier in young children and infants, they should not be used in this patient population due to reports of apnea and systemic hypotension.

REFERENCES

1. Krieglstein GK, Langham ME, Leydhecker W. The peripheral and central neural actions of clonidine in normal and glaucomatous eyes. *Invest Ophthalmol Vis Sci.* 1978;17(2):149–158.
2. Lee DA, Topper JE, Brubaker RF. Effect of clonidine on aqueous humor flow in normal human eyes. *Exp Eye Res.* 1984;38(3):239–246.
3. Gharagozloo NZ, Relf SJ, Brubaker RF. Aqueous flow is reduced by the alpha-adrenergic agonist, apraclonidine hydrochloride (ALO 2145). *Ophthalmology.* 1988;95(9):1217–1220.
4. Toris CB, Tafoya ME, Camras CB, et al. Effects of apraclonidine on aqueous humor dynamics in human eyes. *Ophthalmology.* 1995;102(3):456–461.
5. Stamer WD, Huang Y, Seftor RE, et al. Cultured human trabecular meshwork cells express functional alpha 2A adrenergic receptors. *Invest Ophthalmol Vis Sci.* 1996;37(12):2426–2433.
6. Toris CB, Gleason ML, Camras CB, et al. Effects of brimonidine on aqueous humor dynamics in human eyes. *Arch Ophthalmol.* 1995;113(12):1514–1517.
7. Sulewski ME, Robin AL, Cummings HL, et al. Effects of topical flurbiprofen on the intraocular pressure lowering effects of apraclonidine and timolol. *Arch Ophthalmol.* 1991;109(6):807–809.
8. McCannel C, Koskela T, Brubaker RF. Topical flurbiprofen pretreatment does not block apraclonidine's effect on aqueous flow in humans. *Arch Ophthalmol.* 1991;109(6):810–811.
9. Van Buskirk EM. The ciliary vasculature and its perturbation with drugs and surgery. *Trans Am Ophthalmol Soc.* 1988;86:794.
10. Townsend DJ, Brubaker RF. Immediate effect of epinephrine on aqueous formation in the normal human eye as measured by fluorophotometry. *Invest Ophthalmol Vis Sci.* 1980;19(3):256–266.
11. Nagataki S, Brubaker RF. Early effect of epinephrine on aqueous formation in the normal human eye. *Ophthalmology.* 1981;88(3):278–282.
12. Schenker HI, Yablonski ME, Podos SM, et al. Fluorophotometric study of epinephrine and timolol in human subjects. *Arch Ophthalmol.* 1981;99(7):1212–1216.
13. Sears ML. The mechanism of action of adrenergic drugs in glaucoma. *Invest Ophthalmol.* 1966;5:115.
14. Stewart WC, Laibovitz R, Horwitz B, et al. A 90-day study of the efficacy and side effects of 0.25% and 0.5% apraclonidine vs 0.5% timolol. Apraclonidine Primary Therapy Study Group. *Arch Ophthalmol.* 1996;114(8):938–942.
15. Javitt J, Goldberg I. Comparison of the clinical success rates and quality of life effects of brimonidine tartrate 0.2% and betaxolol 0.25% suspension in patients with open-angle glaucoma and ocular hypertension. Brimonidine Outcomes Study Group II. *J Glaucoma.* 2000;9(5):398–408.
16. Barnebey HS, Robin AL, Zimmerman TJ, et al. The efficacy of brimonidine in decreasing elevations in intraocular pressure after laser trabeculoplasty. *Ophthalmology.* 1993;100(7):1083–1088.
17. Chen TC, Ang RT, Grosskreutz CL, et al. Brimonidine 0.2% versus apraclonidine 0.5% for prevention of intraocular pressure elevations after anterior segment laser surgery. *Ophthalmology.* 2001;108(6):1033–1038.
18. Yoles E, Wheeler LA, Schwartz M. Alpha2-adrenoreceptor agonists are neuroprotective in a rat model of optic nerve degeneration. *Invest Ophthalmol Vis Sci.* 1999;40(1):65–73.
19. Wheeler L, WoldeMussie E, Lai R. Role of alpha-2 agonists in neuroprotection. *Surv Ophthalmol.* 2003;48(suppl 1):S47–S51.

20. Goldberg I, Kolker AE, Kass MA, et al. Dipivefrin: current concepts. *Aust J Ophthalmol.* 1980;8(2):147–150.
21. Mindel JS, Cohen G, Barker LA, et al. Enzymatic and nonenzymatic hydrolysis of D,L-dipivefrin. *Arch Ophthalmol.* 1984;102(3):457–460.
22. Albracht DC, LeBlanc RP, Cruz AM, et al. A double-masked comparison of betaxolol and dipivefrin for the treatment of increased intraocular pressure. *Am J Ophthalmol.* 1993;116(3):307–313.
23. Koskela T, Brubaker RF. Apraclonidine and timolol. Combined effects in previously untreated normal subjects. *Arch Ophthalmol.* 1991;109(6):804–806.
24. David R. Brimonidine (Alphagan): a clinical profile four years after launch. *Eur J Ophthalmol.* 2001;11(suppl 2):S72–S77.
25. Sherwood MB, Craven ER, Chou C, et al. Twice-daily 0.2% brimonidine-0.5% timolol fixed-combination therapy vs monotherapy with timolol or brimonidine in patients with glaucoma or ocular hypertension: a 12-month randomized trial. *Arch Ophthalmol.* 2006;124(9):1230–1238.
26. Stewart WC, Sharpe ED, Harbin TSJ, et al. Brimonidine 0.2% versus dorzolamide 2% each given three times daily to reduce intraocular pressure. *Am J Ophthalmol.* 2000;129(6):723–727.
27. Simmons ST, Earl ML, Alphagan/Xalatan Study G. Three-month comparison of brimonidine and latanoprost as adjunctive therapy in glaucoma and ocular hypertension patients uncontrolled on beta-blockers: tolerance and peak intraocular pressure lowering. *Ophthalmology.* 2002;109(2):307–314.
28. Bournias TE, Lai J. Brimonidine tartrate 0.15%, dorzolamide hydrochloride 2%, and brinzolamide 1% compared as adjunctive therapy to prostaglandin analogs. *Ophthalmology.* 2009;116(9):1719–1724.
29. Nixon DR, Yan DB, Chartrand JP, et al. Three-month, randomized, parallel-group comparison of brimonidine-timolol versus dorzolamide-timolol fixed-combination therapy. *Curr Med Res Opin.* 2009;25(7):1645–1653.
30. Maus TL, Nau C, Brubaker RF. Comparison of the early effects of brimonidine and apraclonidine as topical ocular hypotensive agents. *Arch Ophthalmol.* 1999;117(5):586–591.
31. Ohrstrom A, Pandolfi M. Regulation of intraocular pressure and pupil size by beta-blockers and epinephrine. *Arch Ophthalmol.* 1980;98(12):2182–2184.
32. Tsoy EA, Meekins BB, Shields MB. Comparison of two treatment schedules for combined timolol and dipivefrin therapy. *Am J Ophthalmol.* 1986;102(3):320–324.
33. Butler P, Mannschreck M, Lin S, et al. Clinical experience with the long-term use of 1% apraclonidine. Incidence of allergic reactions. *Arch Ophthalmol.* 1995;113(3):293–296.
34. Shin DH, Glover BK, Cha SC, et al. Long-term brimonidine therapy in glaucoma patients with apraclonidine allergy. *Am J Ophthalmol.* 1999;127(5):511–515.
35. Jampel HD, Robin AL, Quigley HA, et al. Apraclonidine. A one-week dose-response study. *Arch Ophthalmol.* 1988;106(8):1069–1073.
36. Novack GD, O'Donnell MJ, Molloy DW. New glaucoma medications in the geriatric population: efficacy and safety. *J Am Geriatr Soc.* 2002;50(5):956–962.
37. Enyedi LB, Freedman SF. Safety and efficacy of brimonidine in children with glaucoma. *J AAPOS.* 2001;5(5):281–284.
38. Brown RH, Stewart RH, Lynch MG, et al. ALO 2145 reduces the intraocular pressure elevation after anterior segment laser surgery. *Ophthalmology.* 1988;95(3):378–384.

31

Carbonic Anhydrase Inhibitors

Carbonic anhydrase inhibitors (CAIs) are the only class of drugs that are used as systemically administered agents in chronic glaucoma therapy. The CAIs belong to the sulfonamide class of drugs. In 1954, acetazolamide was introduced as an ocular hypotensive drug, and most of the information in this chapter is based on experience with this drug. Methazolamide is another commercially available systemic CAI, but dichlorphenamide (available in Europe and Australia) and ethoxyzolamide are no longer available in the United States. After overcoming the challenges for topical drug delivery due to limited ocular absorption and bioavailability, both topical CAI drugs, dorzolamide and brinzolamide, have assumed a role in the management of glaucoma. The CAIs all share the same basic mechanism of action of lowering intraocular pressure (IOP) by decreasing aqueous humor flow through inhibition of carbonic anhydrase (CA) in ciliary epithelium. Side effects of the oral compounds essentially differ only in degree and are much less with the use of topical drugs.

MECHANISMS OF ACTION

CA is responsible for the catalytic hydration of CO_2 and dehydration of H_2CO_3:

$$CO_2 + H_2O \overset{CA}{\rightleftarrows} H_2CO_3 \rightleftarrows HCO_3^- + H^+$$

The physiologic effects of CAIs are related to ion transport, metabolic acidosis, blood flow, and fluid transport that are described in the following text. There are 14 gene forms of CA encoding for CA isoenzymes that have various cellular and tissue distributions and physiologic effects (1,2). In the eye, four CA isoenzymes, CA I through CA IV, have been identified (3). The main therapeutic target of CAIs in the ciliary processes is the cytosolic CA II isoform (formerly called type C). In patients who have CA II deficiency, acetazolamide fails to decrease IOP, suggesting that this isozyme is inhibited by the drug (4).

Based on the catalytic reaction described earlier, the two effects of ion transport and acidosis are closely related. Changes in ion transport associated with aqueous humor secretion are expected to be altered by CAIs, which is the main mechanism of action of the CAIs to decrease aqueous humor formation. Acetazolamide decreases aqueous humor formation in the human eye about 30% compared with only 18% for topical dorzolamide (5). When added to timolol, which alone reduced daytime flow by 33%, the combination of the two aqueous suppressants reduced the flow rate by 44% (6).

When dorzolamide is added to timolol, there is an additive effect to suppress aqueous humor flow (7).

Acetazolamide creates a local acidic environment (8) that inhibits net chloride flux across the ciliary epithelium, but the principal ions affected by CAIs have not been established in human eyes. Metabolic acidosis is known to reduce IOP and may be another mechanism of action for oral CAIs (9). However, the ocular hypotensive effect of these drugs does not depend on alterations of pH in the blood or aqueous humor (10).

Ocular blood flow is complex and involves consideration of the various vascular beds, including the retinal, choroidal, and retrobulbar vessels located within their respective tissues (11). Acetazolamide increases blood flow and blood-flow velocity within the middle cerebral artery of the brain but not in the ophthalmic and central retinal arteries (12). In a recent review of 35 specific studies, the meta-analysis provided the evidence that topical CAIs increase ocular blood-flow velocities in the retinal circulation, central retinal, and short posterior ciliary arteries but not in the ophthalmic artery (13).

The other clinical effect of CA relates to the fluid movement from the retina toward the choroid (14). Acetazolamide has been shown to increase the rate of subretinal fluid absorption in experimental retinal detachment (15) and to increase the adhesion between retina and pigment epithelium (16). It may also be effective in the treatment of macular edema in patients with retinal pigment epithelial cell disease and uveitis (17,18). However, CAIs do not reduce macular edema associated with primary retinal vascular diseases (17).

ADMINISTRATION

Oral Carbonic Anhydrase Inhibitors

To achieve the therapeutic effect of reducing aqueous humor production, more than 90% of the CA activity needs to be inhibited (19). For this reason, the drug must be used in adequate doses (20). Because the free amount of drug determines the pharmacologic effect, understanding the protein binding of the drug (i.e., how much drug is taken up by serum proteins and blood cells) is important. Acetazolamide is highly bound compared with methazolamide, which explains why larger doses are required for acetazolamide to achieve its therapeutic effect compared with methazolamide. The drugs are not extensively metabolized and are primarily excreted in the urine (**Table 31.1**).

The traditional oral dose for long-term acetazolamide therapy in adults is 250-mg tablets every 6 hours or 500-mg sustained-release capsules twice each day (22). For children, the

Table 1.5	Commercial Carbonic Anhydrase Inhibitors					
Generic Preparation	**Brand Name**	**Strengths**	**Protein Binding, %**	**Metabolism, %**	**Renal Excretion, %**
ORAL					
Acetazolamide	Diamox, tablets	125 mg, 250 mg	95	—[a]	100
	Diamox Sequels	250 mg,[b] 500 mg	95	—[a]	100
	Diamox, parenteral	500 mg/vial	95	—[a]	100
Methazolamide	Neptazane	25 mg, 50 mg	55	75[c]	25
	GlaucTabs	25 mg, 50 mg	55	75[c]	25
	MZM	25 mg, 50 mg	55	75[c]	25
TOPICAL					
Dorzolamide	Trusopt	0.5%,[d] 1%,[d] 2%	33	25–40	60–75
Brinzolamide	Azopt	1%	60	Yes[e]	32

[a]Minimal.
[b]Diamox Sustets, 250 mg, are available in Europe.
[c]Presumed.
[d]Trusopt is available in the United States as 2%, but it is also available as 0.5% and 1% formulations in Japan.
[e]The percentage of drug metabolized is not published (21).

recommended dose of acetazolamide is 5 to 10 mg/kg of body weight every 4 to 6 hours (23). In tablet form, the ocular hypotensive effect peaks in 2 hours and lasts up to 6 hours, whereas that of the capsule peaks in 8 hours and persists beyond 12 hours. For more rapid action, acetazolamide may be given intravenously, which provides a peak effect in 15 minutes and lasts up to 4 hours. A useful routine for emergencies, such as acute angle-closure glaucoma, is to give 250 mg of acetazolamide intravenously if the patient is unable to tolerate oral administration of two 250-mg tablets.

An alternative oral regimen with methazolamide is to begin with 25 mg of methazolamide given twice daily, advancing to 50 mg twice daily and up to 100 mg taken three times daily (23). The advantage is that the drug can be used in smaller dosages, which cause fewer side effects, because the drug has a longer plasma half-life than acetazolamide and a lower rate of protein binding, allowing the free drug to distribute into tissues and be more active on a weight basis in reducing aqueous production (24). A 500-mg sustained-release capsule of acetazolamide had a greater ocular hypotensive effect and was better tolerated than methazolamide (25,26). Generic acetazolamide tablets and sequels are commercially available, providing significant cost savings.

Topical Carbonic Anhydrase Inhibitors

Dorzolamide

Approved in the United States in 1998, dorzolamide (**Fig. 31.1**) lowers the IOP by reducing aqueous humor flow by inhibiting the CA II isoenzyme in the ciliary body (27). At 2 hours after dosing, dorzolamide causes 14.7% to 27% reduction in IOP, and at 8 hours after dosing, 12.9% to 17.5% reduction in IOP (28,29). A 2% solution is the only strength available in the United States,

but 0.5% and 1% formulations are available in Japan. The recommended administration is three times daily because there is greater IOP lowering compared with two times daily. It is most frequently administered twice daily for adherence.

In a 1-year trial comparing timolol, 0.5%, and betaxolol, 0.5%, both given twice daily, the mean percentage IOP reduction with dorzolamide was 23%, compared with 25% and 21% with timolol and betaxolol, respectively (30). Adjunctive therapy studies have shown that twice-daily dorzolamide provides additional IOP lowering in patients being treated with timolol, 0.5%, twice daily (31). When compared with pilocarpine four times daily as a second drug in patients whose IOP was uncontrolled with timolol, 0.5%, dorzolamide three times daily gave similar additional IOP reduction and was preferred by patients because of reduced side effects (32). When dorzolamide, 2% three times daily, was added to once-daily latanoprost, IOP was reduced by an additional 15% (33).

Several studies have reported on the use of dorzolamide in the pediatric population. In a randomized study comparing dorzolamide, 2%, three times daily with timolol gel once daily combined with placebo two times daily in children with glaucoma or elevated IOP younger than 6 years, dorzolamide lowered IOP by as much as 23.3% and was well tolerated,

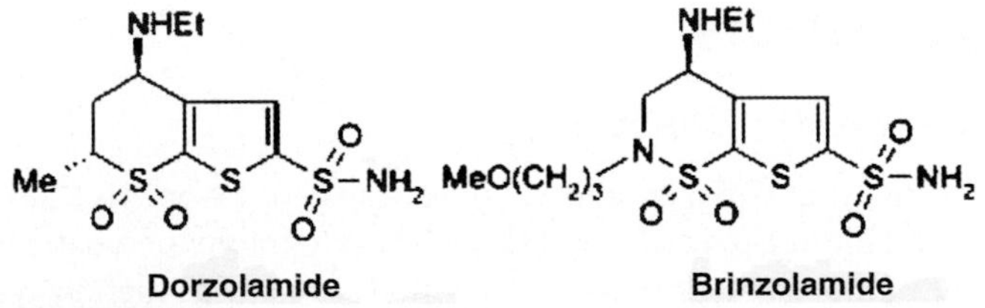

Figure 31.1 Chemical structure of dorzolamide (Trusopt) and brinzolamide (Azopt), topical CAIs.

compared with timolol (34). In a review of published studies reported on childhood glaucoma, additive therapy of twice-daily dorzolamide to once-daily timolol appeared to be the most effective and best tolerated compared with α_2-agonists and prostaglandin analogues (35).

The IOP-lowering effect of the fixed combination of dorzolamide, 2%, and timolol, 0.5%, (Cosopt) is similar to that of the same drugs dosed separately (36). In a randomized study comparing the 24-hour efficacy and tolerability of a fixed combination of dorzolamide, 2%, and timolol, 0.5%, versus timolol, 0.5%, the dorzolamide–timolol combination exhibited greater IOP lowering than timolol during the daytime but not at night (37). It is now available in generic form, providing considerable cost savings.

Brinzolamide

Approved in the United States in 1998, brinzolamide (Fig. 31.1) lowers IOP by inhibiting the CA II isoenzyme in the ciliary body (21). The Brinzolamide Dose-Response Study Group reported that brinzolamide caused a dose-related IOP reduction when dosed two times daily, with the 1% formulation being at the top of the dose-response curve (38). The IOP reduction at the peak effect 2 hours after dosing ranged from −3.3 to −5.3 mm Hg. At the trough effect 12 hours after dosing, the IOP was lower by −2.8 to −4.9 mm Hg.

When brinzolamide, 1%, was compared with dorzolamide, 2%, the absolute IOP lowering and percentage IOP lowering were similar, with up to 19.1% lowering with brinzolamide dosed three times daily and 20.1% lowering with dorzolamide dosed similarly (39). In adjunctive studies, brinzolamide, 1%, dosed three times daily was added in patients with open-angle glaucoma or ocular hypertension already treated with timolol, 0.5%, used twice daily and caused an additional IOP lowering up to 4.1 mm Hg, which was greater than with placebo (40). When comparing the additivity of twice-daily dorzolamide or brinzolamide with topical timolol, 0.5%, equivalence in IOP lowering was demonstrated for both dosing regimens (41). In a randomized trial comparing the additivity of twice-daily brinzolamide, 1%, with twice-daily brimonidine, 0.15%, in patients already receiving travoprost, the adjunctive brinzolamide therapy was marginally more effective than the adjunctive brimonidine therapy was at lowering the IOP (42). The fixed combination of brinzolamide, 1%, and timolol, 0.5%, is currently in phase III clinical trials (43,44).

SIDE EFFECTS

Ocular Side Effects

For the oral CAIs, an idiosyncratic, transient myopia is a sulfonamide-related reaction (45). Ultrasonography of a patient with induced myopia associated with sulfonamide therapy revealed shallowing of the anterior chamber without thickening of the lens, suggesting that ciliary body edema might cause forward movement of the lens–iris diaphragm (46), which can also account for a mechanism of angle closure due to the forward shift of the lens–iris diaphragm.

The most frequently experienced ocular adverse reactions with topical CAI use are irritation immediately after instillation, transient blurred vision, and occasional hypersensitivity reactions (47). It has been proposed that the lower pH of dorzolamide compared with brinzolamide possibly contributes to ocular discomfort (21). Periorbital dermatitis has been reported with topical CAI use, but benzalkonium chloride sensitivity is also an important consideration (48). In patients with open-angle glaucoma or ocular hypertension, mean corneal thickness increased after dorzolamide treatment, but this was not clinically significant (28,49). Potentially serious effects on the cornea are theoretically possible because CA isoenzymes I and II are expressed in corneal endothelium and are involved in maintaining corneal transparency (50). In healthy eyes, CA inhibition of the cornea may not be clinically significant (51). However, in susceptible individuals, clinically significant corneal edema has been associated with use of topical dorzolamide (52).

Systemic Side Effects

Systemic side effects are common with oral CAI therapy, frequently necessitating altering medical therapy (53). Paresthesia of the fingers and toes and around the mouth is a common side effect. Increased urinary frequency from the diuretic action is experienced by nearly all patients initially, but this diuretic effect is not a factor in reducing the IOP (54).

Serum electrolyte imbalances may create more debilitating problems. Metabolic acidosis, associated with bicarbonate depletion, occurs with the higher dosages of CAIs and should be avoided in patients with hepatic insufficiency, renal failure, adrenocortical insufficiency, hyperchloremic acidosis, depressed sodium or potassium levels, or severe pulmonary obstruction (55). The risk in patients with liver disease was re-emphasized in a case report of a patient with cirrhosis who developed hepatic encephalopathy due to ammonia intoxication within days after starting acetazolamide therapy (56). A symptom complex of malaise, fatigue, weight loss, anorexia, depression, and decreased libido is common in patients receiving oral CAI therapy and has been correlated with the degree of metabolic acidosis (57,58). High-dose aspirin combined with a CAI may cause serious acid–base imbalance and salicylate intoxication (59). Potassium depletion may occur during the initial phase of CAI therapy because of increased urinary excretion, especially if diuresis is brisk, and is the apparent explanation for the frequent paresthesias. However, this is normally transient and does not lead to significant hypokalemia unless it is given concomitantly with chlorothiazide diuretics, digitalis, corticosteroids, or adrenocorticotropic hormone, or in patients with hepatic cirrhosis (60). Potassium supplement is indicated only when significant hypokalemia is documented (61).

Also common are gastrointestinal symptoms, including vague abdominal discomfort, a peculiar metallic taste experienced particularly with ingestion of carbonated beverages, nausea, and diarrhea. These symptoms appear to be unrelated to any serum chemical change, and the cause is unknown. Taking the medication with meals may help to reduce the symptoms (57). A less common but debilitating side effect is renal calculi formation, which reportedly is increased in patients receiving acetazolamide and methazolamide (62,63).

The following sulfonamide-related reactions are typical with this drug class and constitute the most serious adverse reactions related to CAI therapy. Blood dyscrasias are rare, but thrombocytopenia, agranulocytosis, aplastic anemia, and neutropenia have been reported with acetazolamide or methazolamide therapy (64). The mechanism of this rare but serious reaction is suggested to be related to the development of immune-mediated mechanisms. These blood dyscrasias cannot be predicted by monitoring blood cell counts, and with the exception of aplastic anemia, the other blood dyscrasias are reversible on cessation of use of the drug. In contrast, aplastic anemia typically has a delayed, insidious onset and is frequently fatal. Most cases occur within less than 6 months of initiating therapy, and some patients have recovered after stopping use of the drug. Because monitoring blood cell counts is not a cost-effective way to monitor for these rare CAI-associated blood dyscrasias, an interval patient history should be obtained in order to be vigilant of potentially relevant hematologic symptoms that may rarely develop after starting CAI therapy.

Other sulfonamide-related side effects include maculopapular and urticarial types of skin eruptions (65), as well as Stevens–Johnson syndrome (66). Teratogenic effects have been observed in rats and in one human case, although the patient's mother was also receiving the anticholinergic agent dicyclomine during weeks 8 to 12 of pregnancy (67,68). Glaucoma treatment during pregnancy should be coordinated with the patient's obstetrician.

The main advantage of the topical CAIs, dorzolamide and brinzolamide, is the marked reduction in systemic side effects, compared with the oral agents. The minor, transient side effect of bitter taste has been reported after topical brinzolamide and dorzolamide administration (39). However, serious systemic reactions may occur in some patients, and thrombocytopenia and erythema multiforme have been reported with topical dorzolamide therapy (69,70).

KEY POINTS

- CAIs lower IOP by reducing aqueous humor production through an alteration in ion transport associated with aqueous humor secretion.
- The oral CAIs, although effective and inexpensive, have numerous side effects that limit their use in most cases to short-term therapy.
- The topical CAIs, although less potent than the systemic forms, have the advantage of causing fewer systemic side effects and are useful for the long-term management of glaucoma.

REFERENCES

1. Hewett-Emmett D. Evolution and distribution of the carbonic anhydrase gene families. *EXS.* 2000;90:29–76.
2. Supuran CT. Carbonic anhydrases—an overview. *Curr Pharm Des.* 2008;14(7):603–614.
3. Wistrand PJ. Carbonic anhydrase inhibition in ophthalmology: carbonic anhydrases in cornea, lens, retina and lacrimal gland. *EXS.* 2000;90:413–424.
4. Krupin T, Sly WS, Whyte MP, et al. Failure of acetazolamide to decrease intraocular pressure in patients with carbonic anhydrase II deficiency. *Am J Ophthalmol.* 1985;99(4):396–399.
5. Maus TL, Larsson LI, McLaren JW, et al. Comparison of dorzolamide and acetazolamide as suppressors of aqueous humor flow in humans. *Arch Ophthalmol.* 1997;115(1):45–49.
6. Dailey RA, Brubaker RF, Bourne WM. The effects of timolol maleate and acetazolamide on the rate of aqueous formation in normal human subjects. *Am J Opthalmol.* 1982;93(2):232–237.
7. Wayman LL, Larsson LI, Maus TL, et al. Additive effect of dorzolamide on aqueous humor flow in patients receiving long-term treatment with timolol. *Arch Ophthalmol.* 1998;116(11):1438–1440.
8. To CH, Do CW, Zamudio AC, et al. Model of ionic transport for bovine ciliary epithelium: effects of acetazolamide and HCO. *Am J Physiol Cell Physiol.* 2001;280(6):C1521–C1530.
9. Bietti G, Virno M, Pecori-Giraldi J, et al. Acetazolamide, metabolic acidosis, and intraocular pressure. *Am J Ophthalmol.* 1975;80(3 pt 1):360–369.
10. Mehra KS. Relationship of pH of aqueous and blood with acetazolamide. *Ann Ophthalmol.* 1979;11:63.
11. Costa VP, Harris A, Stefansson E, et al. The effects of antiglaucoma and systemic medications on ocular blood flow. *Prog Retin Eye Res.* 2003;22(6):769–805.
12. Harris A, Tippke S, Sievers C, et al. Acetazolamide and CO_2: acute effects on cerebral and retrobulbar hemodynamics. *J Glaucoma.* 1996;5(1):39–45.
13. Siesky B, Harris A, Brizendine E, et al. Literature review and meta-analysis of topical carbonic anhydrase inhibitors and ocular blood flow. *Surv Ophthalmol.* 2009;54(1):33–46.
14. Moldow B, Sander B, Larsen M, et al. Effects of acetazolamide on passive and active transport of fluorescein across the normal BRB. *Invest Ophthalmol Vis Sci.* 1999;40(8):1770–1775.
15. Marmor MF, Negi A. Pharmacologic modification of subretinal fluid absorption in the rabbit eye. *Arch Ophthalmol.* 1986;104(11):1674–1677.
16. Marmor MF, Maack T. Enhancement of retinal adhesion and subretinal fluid resorption by acetazolamide. *Invest Ophthalmol Vis Sci.* 1982;23(1):121–124.
17. Cox SN, Hay E, Bird AC. Treatment of chronic macular edema with acetazolamide. *Arch Ophthalmol.* 1988;106(9):1190–1195.
18. Farber MD, Lam S, Tessler HH, et al. Reduction of macular oedema by acetazolamide in patients with chronic iridocyclitis: a randomised prospective crossover study [comment]. *Br J Ophthalmol.* 1994;78(1):4–7.
19. Friedenwald JS. Current studies on acetazolamide (Diamox) and aqueous humor flow. *Am J Ophthalmol.* 1955;40:139.
20. Becker B. Misuse of acetazolamide. *Am J Ophthalmol.* 1957;43:799.
21. DeSantis L. Preclinical overview of brinzolamide. *Surv Ophthalmol.* 2000;44(suppl 2):S119–S129.
22. Joyce PW, Mills KB, Richardson T, et al. Equivalence of conventional and sustained release oral dosage formulations of acetazolamide in primary open angle glaucoma. *Br J Clin Pharmacol.* 1989;27(5):597–606.
23. Havener WH. *Ocular Pharmacology.* 5th ed. St. Louis, MO: CV Mosby; 1983.
24. Maren TH, Haywood JR, Chapman SK, et al. The pharmacology of methazolamide in relation to the treatment of glaucoma. *Invest Ophthalmol Vis Sci.* 1977;16(8):730–742.
25. Dahlen K, Epstein DL, Grant WM, et al. A repeated dose-response study of methazolamide in glaucoma. *Arch Ophthalmol.* 1978;96(12):2214–2218.
26. Lichter PR, Newman LP, Wheeler NC, et al. Patient tolerance to carbonic anhydrase inhibitors. *Am J Ophthalmol.* 1978;85(4):495–502.
27. Wang R-F, Serle JB, Podos SM, et al. MK-507 (L-671,152), a topically active carbonic anhydrase inhibitor, reduces aqueous humor production in monkeys. *Arch Ophthalmol.* 109(9):1297–1299.

28. Wilkerson M, Cyrlin M, Lippa EA, et al. Four-week safety and efficacy study of dorzolamide, a novel, active topical carbonic anhydrase inhibitor. *Arch Ophthalmol.* 1993;111(10):1343–1350.

29. Strahlman E, Tipping R, Vogel R. A six-week dose-response study of the ocular hypotensive effect of dorzolamide with a one-year extension: Dorzolamide Dose-Response Study Group. [Erratum appears in *Am J Ophthalmol.* 1996;122:928.] *Am J Ophthalmol.* 1996;122:183–194.

30. Strahlman E, Tipping R, Vogel R, et al. A double-masked, randomized 1-year study comparing dorzolamide (Trusopt), timolol, and betaxolol. *Arch Ophthalmol.* 1995;113:1009.

31. Petounis A, Mylopoulos N, Kandarakis A, et al. Comparison of the additive intraocular pressure-lowering effect of latanoprost and dorzolamide when added to timolol in patients with open-angle glaucoma or ocular hypertension: a randomized, open-label, multicenter study in Greece. *J Glaucoma.* 2001;10(4):316–324.

32. Laibovitz R, Strahlman ER, Barber BL, et al. Comparison of quality of life and patient preference of dorzolamide and pilocarpine as adjunctive therapy to timolol in the treatment of glaucoma. *J Glaucoma.* 1995;4(5):306–313.

33. Kimal Arici M, Topalkara A, Guler C. Additive effect of latanoprost and dorzolamide in patients with elevated intraocular pressure. *Int Ophthalmol.* 1998;22(1):37–42.

34. Ott EZ, Mills MD, Arango S, et al. A randomized trial assessing dorzolamide in patients with glaucoma who are younger than 6 years. *Arch Ophthalmol.* 2005;123(9):1177–1186.

35. Coppens G, Stalmans I, Zeyen T, et al. The safety and efficacy of glaucoma medication in the pediatric population. *J Pediatr Ophthalmol Strabismus.* 2009;46(1):12–18.

36. Hutzelmann J, Owens S, Shedden A, et al. Comparison of the safety and efficacy of the fixed combination of dorzolamide/timolol and the concomitant administration of dorzolamide and timolol: a clinical equivalence study. International Clinical Equivalence Study Group. *Br J Ophthalmol.* 1998;82(11):1249–1253.

37. Feldman RM, Stewart RH, Stewart WC, et al. 24-hour control of intraocular pressure with 2% dorzolamide/0.5% timolol fixed-combination ophthalmic solution in open-angle glaucoma. *Curr Med Res Opin.* 2008;24(8):2403–2412.

38. Silver LH. Dose-response evaluation of the ocular hypotensive effect of brinzolamide ophthalmic suspension (Azopt): Brinzolamide Dose-Response Study Group. *Surv Ophthalmol.* 2000;44(suppl 2):S147–S153.

39. Sall K. The efficacy and safety of brinzolamide 1% ophthalmic suspension (Azopt) as a primary therapy in patients with open-angle glaucoma or ocular hypertension: Brinzolamide Primary Therapy Study Group. *Surv Ophthalmol.* 2000;44(suppl 2):S155–S162.

40. Shin D. Adjunctive therapy with brinzolamide 1% ophthalmic suspension (Azopt) in patients with open angle glaucoma or ocular hypertension maintained on timolol therapy. *Surv Ophthalmol.* 2000;44(suppl 2):S163–S168.

41. Michaud JE, Friren B. Comparison of topical brinzolamide 1% and dorzolamide 2% eye drops given twice daily in addition to timolol 0.5% in patients with primary open-angle glaucoma or ocular hypertension. *Am J Ophthalmol.* 2001;132(2):235–243.

42. Feldman RM, Tanna AP, Gross RL, et al. Comparison of the ocular hypotensive efficacy of adjunctive brimonidine 0.15% or brinzolamide 1% in combination with travoprost 0.004%. *Ophthalmology.* 2007;114(7):1248–1254.

43. Hollo G, Bozkurt B, Irkec M. Brinzolamide/timolol fixed combination: a new ocular suspension for the treatment of open-angle glaucoma and ocular hypertension. *Expert Opin Pharmacother.* 2009;10(12):2015–2024.

44. Manni G, Denis P, Chew P, et al. The safety and efficacy of brinzolamide 1%/timolol 0.5% fixed combination versus dorzolamide 2%/timolol 0.5% in patients with open-angle glaucoma or ocular hypertension. *J Glaucoma.* 2009;18(4):293–300.

45. Grant W, Leopold I, eds. *Symposium on Ocular Therapy.* Vol 6. St. Louis, MO: Mosby; 1972:19.

46. Bovino JA, Marcus DF. The mechanism of transient myopia induced by sulfonamide therapy. *Am J Ophthalmol.* 1982;94(1):99–102.

47. Barnebey H, Kwok SY. Patients' acceptance of a switch from dorzolamide to brinzolamide for the treatment of glaucoma in a clinical practice setting. *Clin Ther.* 2000;22(10):1204–1212.

48. Delaney YM, Salmon JF, Mossa F, et al. Periorbital dermatitis as a side effect of topical dorzolamide. *Br J Ophthalmol.* 2002;86(4):378–380.

49. Inoue K, Okugawa K, Oshika T, et al. Influence of dorzolamide on corneal endothelium. *Jpn J Ophthalmol.* 2003;47(2):129–133.

50. Srinivas SP, Ong A, Zhai CB, et al. Inhibition of carbonic anhydrase activity in cultured bovine corneal endothelial cells by dorzolamide. *Invest Ophthalmol Vis Sci.* 2002;43(10):3273–3278.

51. Egan CA, Hodge DO, McLaren JW, et al. Effect of dorzolamide on corneal endothelial function in normal human eyes. *Invest Ophthalmol Vis Sci.* 1998;39(1):23–29.

52. Konowal A, Morrison JC, Brown SV, et al. Irreversible corneal decompensation in patients treated with topical dorzolamide. *Am J Ophthalmol.* 1999;127(4):403–406.

53. Lichter PR. Reducing side effects of carbonic anhydrase inhibitors. *Ophthalmology.* 1981;88(3):266–269.

54. Becker B. The mechanism of the fall in intraocular pressure induced by the carbonic anhydrase inhibitor, Diamox. *Am J Ophthalmol.* 1955;39(2 pt 2):177–184.

55. Block ER, Rostand RA. Carbonic anhydrase inhibition in glaucoma: hazard or benefit for the chronic lunger? *Surv Ophthalmol.* 1978;23(3):169–172.

56. Margo CE. Acetazolamide and advanced liver disease. *Am J Ophthalmol.* 1986;101(5):611–612.

57. Epstein DL, Grant WM. Carbonic anhydrase inhibitor side effects: serum chemical analysis. *Arch Ophthalmol.* 1977;95(8):1378–1382.

58. Wallace TR, Fraunfelder FT, Petursson GJ, et al. Decreased libido: a side effect of carbonic anhydrase inhibitor. *Ann Ophthalmol.* 1979;11(10):1563–1566.

59. Anderson CJ, Kaufman PL, Sturm RJ. Toxicity of combined therapy with carbonic anhydrase inhibitors and aspirin. *Am J Ophthalmol.* 1978;86(4):516–519.

60. Spaeth GL. Potassium, acetazolamide, and intraocular pressure. *Arch Ophthalmol.* 1967;78(5):578–582.

61. Critchlow AS, Freeborn S, Roddie RA. Potassium supplements during treatment of glaucoma with acetazolamide. *Br Med J.* 1984;289:21.

62. Kass MA, Kolker AE, Gordon M, et al. Acetazolamide and urolithiasis. *Ophthalmology.* 1981;88(3):261–265.

63. Ellis PP. Urinary calculi with methazolamide therapy. *Doc Ophthalmol.* 1973;34(1):137–142.

64. Fraundfelder FT, Meyer SM, Bagby GC Jr, et al. Hematologic reactions to carbonic anhydrase inhibitors. *Am J Ophthalmol.* 1985;100(1):79–81.

65. Gandham SB, Spaeth GL, Di Leonardo M, et al. Methazolamide-induced skin eruptions. *Arch Ophthalmol.* 1993;111(3):370–372.

66. Flach AJ, Smith RE, Fraunfelder FT. Stevens-Johnson syndrome associated with methazolamide treatment reported in two Japanese-American women. *Ophthalmology.* 1995;102(11):1677–1680.

67. Maren TH. Teratology and carbonic anhydrase inhibition. *Arch Ophthalmol.* 1971;85(1):1–2.

68. Worsham F, Beckman EN, Mitchell EH. Sacrococcygeal teratoma in a neonate. *JAMA.* 1978;240(3):251–252.

69. Martin XD, Danese M. Dorzolamide-induced immune thrombocytopenia: a case report and literature review. *J Glaucoma.* 2001;10(2):133–135.

70. Munshi V, Ahluwalia H. Erythema multiforme after use of topical dorzolamide. *J Ocul Pharmacol Ther.* 2008;24(1):91–93.

Cholinergic Stimulators and Hyperosmotic Agents

32

With the introduction of newer medications that have improved efficacy and few side effects, the cholinergic stimulators and hyperosmotic agents have a limited role in glaucoma management. Introduced in the 1870s, pharmacologic agents that mimic the cholinergic effects of acetylcholine are referred to as cholinergic agonists, parasympathomimetics stimulators, or miotics because of their effect on the pupil (**Fig. 32.1**). Among the acetylcholinesterase inhibitors, which have limited availability, only echothiophate iodide is discussed. The hyperosmotic agents are another class of compounds administered systemically (orally or intravenously) in short-term, emergency situations, such as with acute angle-closure glaucoma or other glaucomas involving dangerously high intraocular pressures (IOPs). Although many consider these drugs of historical interest, the cholinergic stimulators and hyperosmotic agents remain useful in specific clinical situations.

MECHANISMS OF ACTION

Cholinergic Stimulators

The cholinergic agents (**Table 32.1**) (1) are indicated for use in all forms of open-angle glaucoma where the aqueous outflow system is functionally intact. They share a common mechanism of action by stimulating muscarinic cholinergic receptors. Among the five receptor subtypes (2), the m3 muscarinic receptor is the predominant subtype expressed in human ciliary muscle cells and iris sphincter (3). They lower IOP by increasing facility of aqueous outflow (see the modified Goldmann equation in Chapter 2) by ciliary muscle contraction, which causes traction on the scleral spur and alters the configuration of the trabecular meshwork and Schlemm canal (**Fig. 32.2**). This mechanism is supported by primate and human studies. Disinserting the ciliary muscle from the scleral spur in monkeys eliminates the effect of pilocarpine on IOP and facility of outflow (4). Histologic studies of human eyes treated with pilocarpine before enucleation for malignant melanoma demonstrate a posterior, internal pull on the scleral spur, with trabecular space widening, endothelial meshwork distention, an increase in giant vacuoles, and larger, more frequent pores in the inner endothelium of the Schlemm canal (5). Primate studies suggest that the increase in giant vacuoles is a result of enhanced aqueous flow through the outflow system rather than a direct action of pilocarpine on the endothelium of the Schlemm canal (6).

Other aqueous humor dynamic effects have been investigated. Fluorophotometric studies in humans show minimal stimulation of aqueous humor formation with pilocarpine (7). Pilocarpine decreases uveoscleral outflow (8), which may have clinical significance in eyes with markedly reduced conventional or trabecular outflow. As these eyes become increasingly dependent on unconventional or uveoscleral drainage, pilocarpine may cause a paradoxical rise in IOP (9). Episcleral venous pressure does not appear to be altered by pilocarpine (10).

The miotic effect, caused by pilocarpine and related compounds, is produced by stimulating muscarinic receptors of the iris sphincter muscle. This effect "tightens" the iris and helps open the anterior chamber island, making pilocarpine a useful adjunct in the short-term management of angle closure resulting from relative pupillary block (see Chapter 12).

Hyperosmotic Agents

The most widely accepted mechanism of action for the hyperosmotic agents is reduction of vitreous volume due to a change in osmotic gradient between the blood and ocular tissues, which lowers IOP. This concept is supported by rabbit studies that demonstrate a reduction in vitreous body weight of approximately 3% to 4% after administration of mannitol (11). With time, a variable amount of the hyperosmotic agent may enter the eye, depending on the permeability of the blood–ocular barriers to the drug and the size of the drug molecules. As the compound is cleared from the systemic circulation, there may be a reversal of the osmotic gradient in some cases, resulting in a transient rise in IOP.

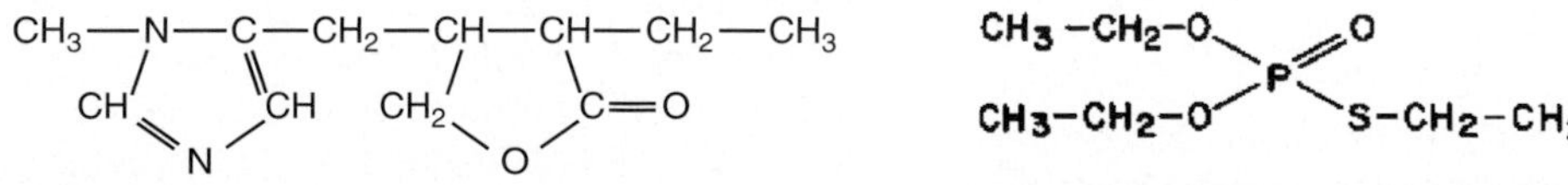

A

PILOCARPINE

B

ECHOTHIOPHATE (PHOSPHOLINE)

Figure 32.1 Chemical structures of the direct acting muscarinic agent, pilocarpine (**A**), and the indirect acting muscarinic agent, echothiophate (**B**).

Table 32.1	Commercial Miotic Preparations	
Preparations	**Brand Names**	**Concentrations**
PILOCARPINE SOLUTIONS		
Hydrochlorides	Isopto Carpine	0.25%, 1%, 2%, 4%
	Generic	0.5%, 1%, 2%, 3%, 4%, 6%
Gel	Pilopine HS gel	4%
Carbachol	Isopto Carbachol	1.5%, 3.0%
INTRACAMERAL INJECTIONS		
Acetylcholine	Miochol	20-mg powder in a vial with 2 mL diluent
Carbachol	Miostat	0.01 in a vial

Data from *Physicians' Desk Reference for Ophthalmic Medicines.* 36th ed. Montvale, NJ: Thomson; 2008.

ADMINISTRATION

Cholinergic Stimulators

Pilocarpine solution is applied topically and is largely degraded in the cornea (12), with less than 3% entering the anterior chamber (13). The IOP-lowering effect is dose related up to pilocarpine, 4% (14,15). In darkly pigmented eyes, pilocarpine, 6%, may produce additional IOP reduction (16). Based on pharmacokinetic studies in animals and pharmacodynamic studies in humans (13,14,17), pilocarpine is given four times daily. However, one study reported that pilocarpine, 2%, administered twice daily, followed by nasolacrimal occlusion gave maximal IOP response (18).

Although not commonly prescribed, another formulation of 4% pilocarpine hydrochloride is a high-viscosity acrylic vehicle (Pilopine), which is applied at bedtime and produces a significant IOP reduction for 24 hours (19). It was comparable to pilocarpine hydrochloride drops, four times daily (20,21), with less induced myopia and impaired visual acuity.

Although not commonly prescribed, carbachol is a dual-action parasympathomimetic that produces direct muscarinic receptor stimulation and an indirect parasympathomimetic effect by inhibiting acetylcholinesterase. Carbachol has poor corneal penetration and requires an adjuvant, such as benzalkonium chloride, to achieve therapeutic levels (22). The usual dosage is three times daily. A carbachol, 1.5%, three times daily—the usual dosage—was as potent and effective as pilocarpine, 2%, four times a day (23). There appears to be no significant difference in the effectiveness of pilocarpine compared with carbachol.

Even less commonly used are the acetylcholinesterase inhibitors, and only echothiophate iodide (phospholine iodide), 0.125%, is currently available in the United States. Echothiophate had the advantage of a prolonged duration of action, with the maximum effect occurring in 4 to 6 hours and a substantial residual present after 24 hours, allowing it to be used on a twice-daily regimen.

Another route of administration is intracameral injection of either carbachol or acetylcholine to achieve miosis during surgery. After cataract surgery, intracameral carbachol has been shown to provide better IOP control in the early postoperative period, compared with intracameral acetylcholine or placebo using balanced salt solution (24,25).

Hyperosmotic Agents

The systemic administration of a hyperosmotic agent is occasionally used as an emergency method of lowering the IOP or preoperatively to minimize the "posterior pressure" effect of the vitreous in a supine position. Although not widely used, glycerin (Osmoglyn) is administered orally in a dose of 1 to 1.5 g/kg (or 2 to 3 cc/kg) of body weight of a 50% solution (26,27). The ocular hypotensive effect occurs within 10 minutes of administration, peaks in 30 minutes, and lasts for approximately 5 hours (26,27).

Mannitol is administered intravenously with a filter administration set over 30 minutes in a dose of 1 to 2 g/kg of body weight of a 25% solution (27). If crystals are present in this 25% solution, then the vial should be warmed up to 60°C to 80°C to dissolve the crystals, and the solution should cool to body temperature before injection. However, lower doses are equally effective. In a study of patients awaiting cataract surgery, 100 mL of 20% mannitol, which is 20 g, given over 20 minutes had the same magnitude of IOP reduction and

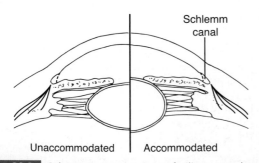

Figure 32.2 Schematic mechanism of ciliary muscle contraction on anterior segment anatomy. After applying a topical cholinergic medication, the ciliary muscle fibers contract, leading to traction on the scleral spur and altering aqueous outflow through the trabecular meshwork and Schlemm canal. An accommodative effect is also mediated by a decrease in concentric diameter of the ciliary body with "rounding" of the lens and a slight decrease in the anterior chamber depth.

deepening of the anterior chamber as 200 mL did, although the latter had a more rapid and sustained ocular hypotensive effect (27). The onset of action is in 20 to 60 minutes, and the duration varies from 2 to 6 hours (27,28). Mannitol may be indicated when glycerin is thought to be insufficient or when it is not tolerated. The drug is distributed in the extracellular fluid compartments and has poor ocular penetration (27).

DRUG INTERACTIONS

Cholinergic Stimulators and Other Glaucoma Medications

Since the miotic agents share a similar mechanism of action, they do not show an additive IOP-lowering effect within this drug class (29). In general with other drug classes' having a different mechanism of action, there is an additive effect using the combination of pilocarpine and the α_2-agonists apraclonidine and brimonidine (see Chapter 30). For the adrenergic receptor agonists, the fixed combinations of epinephrine and pilocarpine are no longer available. For adrenergic antagonists, two fixed combinations of timolol and pilocarpine (Timpilo and Fotil) are available in some parts of the world (30). Aqueous humor levels of pilocarpine, 2%, and timolol, 0.5%, in rabbits were not different whether the drugs were given alone or in fixed combination (31). Although pilocarpine reduces and prostaglandins increase uveoscleral outflow, the prostaglandin agents have an additive IOP-lowering effect when used with pilocarpine (Chapter 28). Pilocarpine may also be used effectively in combination with carbonic anhydrase inhibitors (see Chapter 31).

Hyperosmotic Agents and Other Glaucoma Medications

This drug class is not used for long-term medical management of glaucoma.

SIDE EFFECTS

Cholinergic Stimulators

The systemic effects of topically applied pilocarpine are uncommon but are similar to those of muscarine, with stimulation of glands, contraction of smooth muscle, and cardiac and central cognitive effects (32). Symptoms include diaphoresis, salivation, tearing, and bronchial secretion. Smooth muscle contraction may cause nausea, vomiting, diarrhea, bronchospasm, abdominal pain, and genitourinary effects. Third-degree atrioventricular block and cognitive dysfunction in patients with Alzheimer disease have been reported after administration of topical pilocarpine (33). The antidote for systemic pilocarpine toxicity is atropine.

Ocular side effects are common with pilocarpine and can interfere with quality of life and adherence (34). Ciliary muscle spasm leads to a brow ache, which usually subsides with continued therapy. Transient myopia is caused by an axial thickening and forward shift of the lens (Fig. 32.2), which begins

approximately 15 minutes after dosing, peaks in 45 to 60 minutes, and lasts for 1.5 to 2 hours (35). Miosis may dim vision and may alter visual fields (36), as discussed in Chapter 5, especially if cataracts are present.

Retinal detachment with use of miotics has been suspected, although a definite cause-and-effect relationship has not been established (37,38). The detachments are typically rhegmatogenous, and it is presumed that ciliary body contraction exerts vitreoretinal traction, which causes retinal tears. The degree of risk appears to be related to preexisting retinal pathology (37,38). A vitreous hemorrhage without a detectable retinal hole or detachment has also been reported in a patient 1 day after initiating pilocarpine therapy (39). When starting treatment with any miotic, it is good practice to review the patient's history for increased risk of retinal detachment and to perform a peripheral fundus examination. Macular holes have also been reported to develop within weeks after starting therapy with pilocarpine, 2% (40,41).

A cataractogenic effect of pilocarpine has been suggested from observing patients on long-term uniocular miotic therapy (42).

Various corneal effects have been reported. A subtle, diffuse, superficial corneal haze was observed in 20% to 28% of patients after prolonged use of Pilopine (43), which caused no symptoms or long-term consequences. Pilocarpine therapy was thought to be associated with corneal graft rejection in three patients, which the authors suggested might be related to intraocular inflammation (44). Intracameral carbachol has been associated with transient corneal swelling in rabbits (45), but a 1-year follow-up of cataract patients revealed no short-term or long-term adverse effects (46). Increased blood–aqueous barrier permeability to plasma proteins has been demonstrated clinically with a laser flare-cell meter and fluorophotometry after instillation of pilocarpine (47). In most patients, this may not be clinically significant, although it may increase postoperative inflammation, and constitutes a relative contraindication in uveitis or in the presence of anterior segment neovascularization.

Cicatricial pemphigoid has been reported in patients undergoing long-term topical glaucoma therapy (48,49), but the cause-and-effect relationship of this association is uncertain. Among 111 patients with cicatricial pemphigoid, 29 (26%) had glaucoma treated with multiple glaucoma drops, including pilocarpine (48). One study of 179 glaucoma patients and 420 controls suggested that long-term glaucoma therapy for 3 years or longer is associated with significant foreshortening of the inferior conjunctival fornix (50).

Hypersensitivity and toxic reactions may also result from the use of pilocarpine or the preservative. Allergic reactions typically involve the eyelids and conjunctiva, often with a giant papillary reaction of the superior tarsal conjunctiva, whereas toxic reactions cause a follicular response in the conjunctiva (51).

Hyperosmotic Agents

Side effects from hyperosmotics are common and can be serious or even fatal but are worse with intravenous mannitol (17). These effects include diuresis, headache, acidemia, anaphylactic reaction, backache, cardiovascular overload resulting from transient rise in blood volume, chills and fever, confusion and disorientation, diarrhea, headache, intracranial hemorrhage, pulmonary edema, and renal insufficiency (27,52). Death has been reported in a patient who developed pulmonary edema, acidemia, and anuria following mannitol therapy, and special caution is advised in patients with compromised cardiovascular or renal function (52). If diuresis becomes an issue during surgery, then it may be necessary to use an indwelling catheter. Mannitol has been shown to increase aqueous flare in humans (53), which may have implications regarding increased postoperative inflammation.

Nausea and vomiting are common, especially with the oral glycerin, presumably because of the heavy sweet taste. This is transient and usually of no consequence, but it can be a problem if the vomiting occurs during surgery or leads to loss of the medication or aspiration. The nausea can be minimized by serving the medication with ice and a tart flavoring. Glycerin is metabolized, which causes less diuresis and is safer than mannitol based on the side effects described earlier; however, the caloric content, 4.32 kcal/g (26), and dehydration can cause problems with repeated administration in patients with diabetes mellitus (54).

KEY POINTS

- Although not commonly used now, pilocarpine is useful because it is inexpensive and lowers IOP in patients with open-angle glaucoma by increasing aqueous outflow and in patients with angle-closure glaucoma by relieving pupillary block.
- Pilocarpine may be practically considered as medical treatment for open-angle glaucoma because it is inexpensive.
- The miotics share common ocular side effects, which include brow ache and induced myopia from ciliary muscle spasm, dimness of vision from the miosis in the presence of cataract, and an increased risk of retinal detachment.
- The hyperosmotic agents have a limited but specific role for the management of acute, short-term IOP reduction in emergency situations.
- The hyperosmotic agents are used to reduce the vitreous volume, which decreases "posterior pressure," before some intraocular surgical procedures, such as cataract surgery in "high-risk" eyes with nanophthalmos or a corneal transplant.

REFERENCES

1. *Physicians' Desk Reference for Ophthalmic Medicines.* 36th ed. Montvale, NJ: Thomson; 2008.
2. Eglen RM, Choppin A, Watson N. Therapeutic opportunities from muscarinic receptor research [review]. *Trends Pharmacol Sci.* 2001;22(8):409–414.
3. Nietgen GW, Schmidt J, Hesse L, et al. Muscarinic receptor functioning and distribution in the eye: molecular basis and implications for clinical diagnosis and therapy [review]. *Eye.* 1999;13(3a):285–300.
4. Kaufman PL, Barany EH. Loss of acute pilocarpine effect on outflow facility following surgical disinsertion and retrodisplacement of the ciliary muscle from the scleral spur in the cynomolgus monkey. *Invest Ophthalmol.* 1976;15(10):793–807.
5. Grierson I, Lee WR, Abraham S. Effects of pilocarpine on the morphology of the human outflow apparatus. *Br J Ophthalmol.* 1978;62(5):302–313.
6. Grierson I, Lee WR, Abraham S. The effects of topical pilocarpine on the morphology of the outflow apparatus of the baboon (*Papio cynocephalus*). *Invest Ophthalmol Vis Sci.* 1979;18(4):346–355.
7. Nagataki S, Brubaker RF. Effect of pilocarpine on aqueous humor formation in human beings. *Arch Ophthalmol.* 1982;100(5):818–821.
8. Bill A, Phillips CI. Uveoscleral drainage of aqueous humour in human eyes. *Exp Eye Res.* 1971;12(3):275–281.
9. Bleiman BS, Schwartz AL. Paradoxical intraocular pressure response to pilocarpine. A proposed mechanism and treatment. *Arch Ophthalmol.* 1979;97(7):1305–1306.
10. Gaasterland D, Kupfer C, Ross K. Studies of aqueous humor dynamics in man. IV. Effects of pilocarpine upon measurements in young normal volunteers. *Invest Ophthalmol.* 1975;14(11):848–853.
11. Robbins R, Galin MA. Effect of osmotic agents on the vitreous body. *Arch Ophthalmol.* 1969;82(5):694–699.
12. Krohn DL, Breitfeller JM. Transcorneal flux of topical pilocarpine to the human aqueous. *Am J Ophthalmol.* 1979;87(1):50–56.
13. Asseff CF, Weisman RL, Podos SM, et al. Ocular penetration of pilocarpine in primates. *Am J Ophthalmol.* 1973;75(2):212–215.
14. Drance SM, Nash PA. The dose response of human intraocular pressure to pilocarpine. *Can J Ophthalmol.* 1971;6(1):9–13.
15. Drance SM, Bensted M, Schulzer M. Pilocarpine and intraocular pressure. Duration of effectiveness of 4 percent and 8 percent pilocarpine instillation. *Arch Ophthalmol.* 1974;91(2):104–106.
16. Harris LS, Galin MA. Effect of ocular pigmentation on hypotensive response to pilocarpine. *Am J Ophthalmol.* 1971;72(5):923–925.
17. Lazare R, Horlington M. Pilocarpine levels in the eyes of rabbits following topical application. *Exp Eye Res.* 1975;21(3):281–287.
18. Zimmerman TJ, Sharir M, Nardin GF, et al. Therapeutic index of pilocarpine, carbachol, and timolol with nasolacrimal occlusion. *Am J Ophthalmol.* 1992;114(1):1–7.
19. March WF, Stewart RM, Mandell AI, et al. Duration of effect of pilocarpine gel. *Arch Ophthalmol.* 1982;100(8):1270–1271.
20. Goldberg I, Ashburn FS Jr, Kass MA, et al. Efficacy and patient acceptance of pilocarpine gel. *Am J Ophthalmol.* 1979;88(5):843–846.
21. Johnson DH, Epstein DL, Allen RC, et al. A one-year multicenter clinical trial of pilocarpine gel. *Am J Ophthalmol.* 1984;97(6):723–729.
22. Smolen VF, Clevenger JM, Williams EJ, et al. Biphasic availability of ophthalmic carbachol. I. Mechanisms of cationic polymer- and surfactant-promoted miotic activity. *J Pharm Sci.* 1973;62(6):958–961.
23. Wolter-Czerwinska H, Nowak A. Comparison of pilocarpine and carbacholine following administration of the drug [in Polish]. *Klin Oczna.* 1973;43(7):785–788.
24. Ruiz RS, Rhem MN, Prager TC. Effects of carbachol and acetylcholine on intraocular pressure after cataract extraction. *Am J Ophthalmol.* 1989;107(1):7–10.
25. Hollands RH, Drance SM, House PH, et al. Control of intraocular pressure after cataract extraction. *Can J Ophthalmol.* 1990;25(3):128–132.
26. Virno M, Cantore P, Bietti C, et al. Oral glycerol in ophthalmology: a valuable new method for the reduction of intraocular pressure. *Am J Ophthalmol.* 1963;55:1133–1142.
27. O'Keeffe M, Nabil M. The use of mannitol in intraocular surgery. *Ophthalmic Surg.* 1983;14(1):55–56.
28. Smith EW, Drance SM. Reduction of human intraocular pressure with intravenous mannitol. *Arch Ophthalmol.* 1962;68:734–737.
29. Kini MM, Dahl AA, Roberts CR, et al. Echothiophate, pilocarpine, and open-angle glaucoma. *Arch Ophthalmol.* 1973;89(3):190–192.
30. Uusitalo RJ, Palkama A. Efficacy and safety of timolol/pilocarpine combination drops in glaucoma patients. *Acta Ophthalmol.* 1994;72(4):496–504.
31. Ellis PP, Wu PY, Riegel M. Aqueous humor pilocarpine and timolol levels after instillation of the single drug or in combination. *Invest Ophthalmol Vis Sci.* 1991;32(3):520–522.
32. Greco JJ, Kelman CD. Systemic pilocarpine toxicity in the treatment of angle closure glaucoma. *Ann Ophthalmol.* 1973;5(1):57–59.
33. Reyes PF, Dwyer BA, Schwartzman RJ, et al. Mental status changes induced by eye drops in dementia of the Alzheimer type. *J Neurol Neurosurg Psychiatry.* 1987;50(1):113–115.
34. Granstrom PA, Norell S. Visual ability and drug regimen: relation to compliance with glaucoma therapy. *Acta Ophthalmol.* 1983;61(2):206–219.
35. Abramson DH, Franzen LA, Coleman DJ. Pilocarpine in the presbyope. Demonstration of an effect on the anterior chamber and lens thickness. *Arch Ophthalmol.* 1973;89(2):100–102.

36. Webster AR, Luff AJ, Canning CR, et al. The effect of pilocarpine on the glaucomatous visual field. *Br J Ophthalmol.* 1993;77(11):721–725.

37. Pape LG, Forbes M. Retinal detachment and miotic therapy. *Am J Ophthalmol.* 1978;85(4):558–566.

38. Beasley H, Fraunfelder FT. Retinal detachments and topical ocular miotics. *Ophthalmology.* 1979;86(1):95–98.

39. Schuman JS, Hersh P, Kylstra J. Vitreous hemorrhage associated with pilocarpine. *Am J Ophthalmol.* 1989;108(3):333–334.

40. Garlikov RS, Chenoweth RG. Macular hole following topical pilocarpine. *Ann Ophthalmol.* 1975;7(10):1313–1316.

41. Benedict WL, Shami M. Impending macular hole associated with topical pilocarpine. *Am J Ophthalmol.* 1992;114(6):765–766.

42. Levene RZ. Uniocular miotic therapy. *Trans Sect Ophthalmol Am Acad Ophthalmol Otolaryngol.* 1975;79(2):OP376–OP380.

43. Johnson DH, Kenyon KR, Epstein DL, et al. Corneal changes during pilocarpine gel therapy. *Am J Ophthalmol.* 1986;101(1):13–15.

44. Massry GG, Assil KK. Pilocarpine-associated allograft rejection in postkeratoplasty patients. *Cornea.* 1995;14(2):202–205.

45. Birnbaum DB, Hull DS, Green K, et al. Effect of carbachol on rabbit corneal endothelium. *Arch Ophthalmol.* 1987;105(2):253–255.

46. Zimmerman TJ, Dukar U, Nardin GF, et al. Carbachol dose response. *Am J Ophthalmol.* 1989;108(4):456–457.

47. Mori M, Araie M, Sakurai M, et al. Effects of pilocarpine and tropicamide on blood–aqueous barrier permeability in man. *Invest Ophthalmol Vis Sci.* 1992;33(2):416–423.

48. Tauber J, Melamed S, Foster CS. Glaucoma in patients with ocular cicatricial pemphigoid. *Ophthalmology.* 1989;96(1):33–37.

49. Fiore PM, Jacobs IH, Goldberg DB. Drug-induced pemphigoid. A spectrum of diseases [review]. *Arch Ophthalmol.* 1987;105(12):1660–1663.

50. Schwab IR, Linberg JV, Gioia VM, et al. Foreshortening of the inferior conjunctival fornix associated with chronic glaucoma medications. *Ophthalmology.* 1992;99(2):197–202.

51. Jackson WB. Differentiating conjunctivitis of diverse origins [review]. *Surv Ophthalmol.* 1993;38(suppl):91–104.

52. Grabie MT, Gipstein RM, Adams DA, et al. Contraindications for mannitol in aphakic glaucoma. *Am J Ophthalmol.* 1981;91(2):265–267.

53. Miyake K, Miyake Y, Maekubo K. Increased aqueous flare as a result of a therapeutic dose of mannitol in humans. *Graefes Arch Clin Exp Ophthalmol.* 1992;230(2):115–118.

54. Oakley DE, Ellis PP. Glycerol and hyperosmolar nonketotic coma. *Am J Ophthalmol.* 1976;81(4):469–472.

33

Neuroprotection and Other Investigational Antiglaucoma Drugs

The primary goal of glaucoma therapy is to stop the loss of retinal ganglion cells (RGCs) by rescuing injured cells or regenerating new, functional cells to replace those that are lost. The classes of drugs discussed in the preceding chapters are used to reduce intraocular pressure (IOP), arguably the most important known risk factor for glaucomatous optic neuropathy. Although reducing IOP is often efficacious, in many cases achieving an appropriate target IOP for an individual patient may not halt progression. Over the past decades, our knowledge of neuronal function has greatly increased—and, along with it, the broader therapeutic concept of "neuroprotection." Medically speaking, this notion includes many classes of agents whose principal function is to protect RGCs utilizing approaches in addition to modulating IOP. In this chapter, the following topics are covered: investigational antiglaucoma drugs, immunomodulation, gene- and cell-based treatments, and drug delivery.

INVESTIGATIONAL ANTIGLAUCOMA DRUGS

In the late 1970s, neuroprotection was introduced as a concept that surrounding neurons are vulnerable to secondary neuronal degeneration adjacent to the area of ischemic stroke (1). Although some clinical and experimental evidence provided proof of concept for pharmacologic intervention to protect the brain tissue from ischemic insults, the use of calcium channel antagonists and agents that decrease the impact of excitatory amino acids in acute stroke has not been systematically evaluated in clinical studies (2,3).

In glaucoma, lowering the IOP has been validated by clinical trials as a neuroprotective approach to slow progression of glaucomatous optic neuropathy (see Chapter 29). Non–IOP-based approaches have also been described earlier, such as diphenylhydantoin (4). Currently, no glaucoma treatments approved by the U.S. Food and Drug Administration (FDA) are non-IOP (or neuroprotective) based, in part because the end points for efficacy in the past were based on pressure lowering. However, an interdisciplinary dialogue has been initiated to establish evidence-based guidelines for evaluating clinical trial end points for non–IOP-based treatment interventions (5).

In this section, the discussion is focused on IOP-based and non–IOP-based drugs that are being tested in registered clinical trials (www.clinicaltrials.gov/ct2/home) with the exception of cannabinoids. These include anecortave, cannabinoids, cellular cytoskeleton modulators, cellular signaling pathways, memantine, nitric oxide synthase (NOS) inhibitors, prostanoid agents, and rho kinase inhibitors.

Anecortave

Anecortave, an angiostatic steroid without glucocorticoid activity, has been evaluated for its therapeutic potential for glaucoma and age-related macular degeneration (6–8). Although there was promising IOP-lowering effect for the anterior justascleral depot injection of anecortave acetate in phase II and early phase III clinical trials (6–9), it is no longer being pursued for glaucoma treatment indications.

Cannabinoids

The role of marijuana for medical purposes continues to be controversial and complex. In the United States, marijuana is a Schedule I-controlled substance and is illegal under federal law. There is growing public support for its medicinal use and 14 U.S. states have legalized medical marijuana. Containing more than 460 active chemicals and over 60 unique cannabinoids, marijuana has the purported use for severe nausea and vomiting from chemotherapy, weight loss associated with debilitating illnesses like HIV infection and cancer, spasticity secondary to neurologic diseases, pain syndromes, and glaucoma (10). In addition, there are endogenous bioactive lipid compounds, called endocannabinoids, which have been implicated in physiologic functions, both in the central and peripheral nervous systems and in peripheral organs (11). The pharmacology of the cannabinoids includes the cannabinoid (CB) receptors type 1 and type 2, or CB1 and CB2, respectively, transporters, and enzymes that break down these molecules (12). The CB1 receptor is present in the ciliary body of rat and human (13,14).

The evidence for its use for glaucoma is based on the observation that smoking marijuana lowers IOP (15). The primary active ingredient in marijuana, tetrahydrocannabinol (THC), effectively lowered IOP when given orally or intravenously, but appeared to have no effect on topical application in humans (16–18). However in a monkey model of glaucoma, topical application of WIN 55212-2, a cannabinoid selective agonist for the cannabinoid type 1 receptor (CB1), lowered IOP by decreasing aqueous humor flow (19). Marijuana has also been shown to decrease aqueous humor flow in humans (20). In a rat model of glaucoma, weekly injections of THC lowered IOP in the episcleral vessel cauterized eye, but not the contralateral untreated eye, and attenuated the loss of ganglion cell death (21).

The acute systemic side effects include tachycardia, hypotension, and euphoria, and long-term adverse effects include pulmonary fibrosis and impaired neurologic behavior and performance (10). Ocular side effects associated with marijuana inhalation include conjunctival hyperemia, a slight miosis, and reduced tear production (22). In particular, the most disturbing

438

adverse reaction is systemic hypotension, which may be associated with reduced perfusion of the optic nerve head and could be detrimental in protecting against progressive glaucomatous optic atrophy (23). These side effects of the cannabinoids thus far tested in humans seriously limit their usefulness in the treatment of glaucoma.

Cellular Cytoskeletal Modulators

Ethacrynic acid is a prototype agent in this drug class. It is a sulfhydryl-reactive diuretic that has been shown to markedly change actin, alpha-actinin, vinculin, and vimentin in cultured trabecular meshwork cells (24), which is thought to alter trabecular meshwork shape as the main mechanism of action for lowering IOP. In monkeys, intracameral injection of this agent increased aqueous outflow (25) and lowered IOP but it also caused corneal edema (26). However, in human clinical trials, although there was IOP reduction, there were concerns of corneal toxicity and trabecular meshwork toxicity (27–29). These latter limitations precluded the clinical application of ethacrynic acid in the management of glaucoma.

Latrunculins are part of a family of natural toxins produced by a marine sponge Latrunculia and have been investigated for their potential therapeutic use due to disrupting the actin cytoskeleton (30). Topical application of latrunculin B lowers IOP in monkeys by increasing outflow facility and does not adversely affect the cornea (31). Histologic features of the treated monkey eye showed the following changes: loss of microfilament integrity in trabecular meshwork cells on the collagen beams; changes in cytoplasmic projections; reorganization of intermediate filaments in Schlemm canal inner wall cells; and massive "ballooning" of the juxtacanalicular region (32). There were no other apparent effects in the trabecular meshwork, and the corneal endothelium was unchanged. Based on these apparently selective effects on the trabecular meshwork, the compound INS115644 is now in clinical trials.

Other Cellular Signaling Pathways

Among this broad category, there is a clinical trial of an angiotensin II receptor antagonist, olmesartan (DE-092), currently being tested in Japan to determine safety and efficacy for lowering IOP. Components of the renin–angiotensin system are expressed in the eye (33), which is the rationale for testing the efficacy of such agents to lower IOP.

Another agent in clinical trials in Japan is lomerizine (DE-090), which is a calcium channel blocker that is currently approved for treating migraines. There has been long-standing interest in the potential use of calcium channel blockers for glaucoma based on the physiologic role of these channels in cardiovascular physiology (34). Several older studies have shown a favorable effect of calcium channel blockers in slight improvement or lack of progression in visual fields over various times of follow-up from patients with normal-tension glaucoma compared with similar groups not receiving such medication (35,36). In a recent randomized study of nilvadipine (2 mg twice daily) treatment versus placebo, nilvadipine-treated patients

with normal-tension glaucoma showed a slightly slow visual field progression compared with placebo-treated patients over 3 years (37). Of interest, the posterior choroidal circulation increased in treated patients, which supports the potential to improve vascular perfusion to the optic nerve head. Also, there was no significant change from baseline or intergroup difference was seen in blood pressure or pulse rate. Currently, however, the level of evidence at this time, as well as the potential serious systemic side effects of calcium channel blockers, does not support the use of this class of drugs for the routine management of glaucoma.

Neurotrophins are peptides that have an important role in the development and maintenance of various neuronal populations (38). In the adult human retina, there are neural progenitor cells that can be induced to differentiate into neuronal phenotypes with basic fibroblast growth factor (39). In models of glaucoma, obstruction to retrograde transport of neurotrophins at the optic nerve head results in the deprivation of neurotrophic support to RGCs, which contributes to apoptotic cell death (40). There was a recent report of beneficial effects of nerve growth factor eye drops with reduced RGC death in a rat model of glaucoma treated for 7 weeks and "long lasting improvements" in psychofunctional and electrofunctional tests in humans with glaucoma treated for 3 months (41). The results of this study should be interpreted with caution since the number of participants was small and follow-up testing was performed only 6 months after baseline testing. Other clinical trials have shown that visual field performance can fluctuate considerably and individual test locations exhibit both short- and long-term sensitivity variations (42). Additional guarded enthusiasm is based on a previous study showing that nerve growth factor was not effective in delaying RGC death because the protective effect is mediated through only one of the receptors, the prosurvival TrkA receptor, and not proapoptotic p75 receptor (43). In other retinal diseases, nerve growth factor was not very effective compared with ciliary neurotrophic factor, brain-derived neurotrophic factor, glia-derived neurotrophic factor, and others with development in gene-modulated protein therapy or gene transfer (44).

Memantine

Memantine is an N-methyl-D-aspartate (NMDA) receptor antagonist (45); it is used for the treatment of Parkinson disease, vascular dementia, and Alzheimer disease (46). The NMDA receptor is an ion channel that is activated once glutamate and the coagonist, glycine, bind to the receptor complex, allowing extracellular calcium to enter the cell. In normal physiologic conditions, the NMDA receptor has an important role in neurophysiologic processes, such as memory. However, excessive activation of the NMDA signaling cascade leads to "excitotoxicity" wherein intracellular calcium overloads neurons and causes cell death through apoptosis, which is also known as "programmed cell death." The cellular consequences of this excess calcium include activation of destructive pathways in the mitochondria, stimulation of nitric oxide production resulting from activation of calcium-dependent NOS (see next section), and stimulation of certain mitogen-activated protein kinases.

The concept of excitotoxicity in relation to glaucoma was based on the observation that subcutaneous glutamate injections caused inner retinal damage (47). However, there is controversy on the presence of glutamate in the vitreous as an indication of excess levels in animal models of glaucoma (48,49) and in patients with glaucoma (50,51). After completing phase III clinical trial in the United States, memantine did meet glaucoma end points of efficacy (52).

Nitric Oxide

Nitric oxide is a gaseous second messenger molecule that is highly reactive, short lived, and readily traverses the plasma membrane (53). The expression of nitric oxide is regulated by three different forms of NOS—endothelial NOS (eNOS), neuronal NOS (nNOS), and inducible NOS (iNOS). The expression and distribution of the various NOS isoforms have been examined and reviewed in the eye (54). The full role of nitric oxide in the eye is not completely understood, but it appears to have a physiologic role in aqueous humor dynamics, ocular blood flow, retinal function, and optic nerve function (55,56). In an experimental rat model of glaucoma with high IOP for 6 months, the optic nerves showed features compatible with damage characterized by pallor, cupping, and ganglion cell loss (57). After 6 months of treatment with aminoguanidine, a selective inhibitor of iNOS, the optic nerves appeared normal, and there was less ganglion cell loss despite elevated IOP. This study was the first to demonstrate that excess nitric oxide generated by iNOS in optic nerve astrocytes and microglia was associated with optic nerve damage. However, these preclinical studies have not led to the development of selective iNOS inhibitors as a neuroprotective approach in the management of glaucoma (58). These same investigators also demonstrated that upregulation and activation of the epidermal growth factor receptor is a common, regulatory pathway that triggers quiescent astrocytes into reactive astrocytes in response to neural injuries in the optic nerve (59). They suggest that targeting these receptors by using a tyrosine kinase inhibitor could present an alternative approach for the treatment of neurodegenerations that involve reactive astrocytes.

Prostanoid Agents

Two agents in this drug class are in clinical trials. Tafluprost (DE-085) has been launched for clinical use to treat glaucoma in Japan and Europe and is currently in clinical trials in the United States (60). Tafluprost is a synthetic prostaglandin $F_{2\alpha}$-agonist derivative with a fully preservative-free formulation (61). In a randomized, double-masked, parallel-group, 12-week phase III study, tafluprost, 0.0015%, once daily ($n = 96$) or vehicle ($n = 89$) was administered as adjunctive therapy to timolol, 0.5%, twice daily for 6 weeks, after which all patients received tafluprost for 6 weeks. IOP measurements were at 08:00, 10:00, and 16:00 at baseline, and weeks 2, 4, 6, and 12 (62). At week 6, the change from baseline in diurnal IOP ranged from -5.49 to -5.82 mm Hg. The overall treatment difference

between tafluprost and vehicle was -1.49 mm Hg (upper 95% confidence limit, -0.66; $P < 0.001$, intention-to-treat population, repeated measurements of the analysis of covariance model). At week 12, the change from baseline ranged from -6.22 to -6.79 mm Hg in the tafluprost group. Patients switched from vehicle to tafluprost achieved a similar decrease in IOP to those who received tafluprost throughout the study (group difference at 12 weeks, -0.09 mm Hg; $P = 0.8$).

Another agent that was in phase II clinical trials is PF-03187207, which is a nitric oxide–donating prostaglandin analog. However, since this agent did not achieve significantly greater IOP lowering compared with latanoprost, it was not pursued for further clinical trial testing.

Rho Kinase Inhibitors

There are two types of Rho kinases, ROCK1 and ROCK2, which are serine–threonine kinases that are downstream effectors of Rho GTPase (63). They regulate smooth muscle contraction in a calcium-independent manner. By targeting ROCK activity in the aqueous humor outflow pathway with selective inhibitors, aqueous humor drainage through the trabecular meshwork is increased, leading to a decrease in IOP. Several ROCK inhibitors (INS117548, DE-104, and RKI 983) are in clinical trials. Targeting the Rho GTPase–ROCK pathway with selective inhibitors represents a novel therapeutic approach aimed at lowering IOP.

IMMUNOMODULATION

In general, our appreciation of the complexities of the immune system with respect to detriment in the pathogenesis of some neurologic diseases, such as multiple sclerosis, and also as a potential therapeutic approach in treating or modifying the disease is improving (64). The immunomodulator interferon-β decreases the relapse of this disease, but there are clear variations in response to this treatment (65). Several vaccination approaches are being investigated using T cells and DNA-based vaccines (66,67).

There is some clinical evidence to suggest that the immune system may play a role in glaucoma. In a group of 67 patients with normal-tension glaucoma, 30% reported an immune-related disease, compared with only 8% in a control group (68). Other experimental clinical studies have shown the presence of serum autoantibodies that cross-react with glycosaminoglycans, heat shock proteins, and rhodopsin in patients with glaucoma, which may increase the susceptibility of the optic nerve to damage (69–71). It has been proposed that small chemical molecules or epitopes, which may include several amino acids, polysaccharides, and modified lipids, are similar biologically between organisms and infectious agents. These shared epitopes can result in immune cross-reactivity called "molecular mimicry" (72), which results in disease, such as experimental autoimmune uveitis (73).

It has been proposed that the immune system plays a key role in the ability of the optic nerve and the retina to withstand glaucoma (74). The mechanism involves recruitment of both innate and adaptive immune cells that together create a protective niche to halt progression. If the spontaneous immune response were insufficient, then a booster immunization with the appropriate antigen at specific timing and predetermined optimal dosing may be developed as a therapeutic vaccination for glaucoma. A recent study in a rat model of acute increase in IOP provided the proof of concept that there is a therapeutic window for protection against death of RGCs by vaccination with glatiramer acetate (Cop-1) and compared with brimonidine or MK-801, which is an NMDA receptor antagonist (75). After an acute transient rise of IOP by infusing normal saline, 0.9%, into the anterior chamber for 1 hour, ganglion cell survival was assessed 1 week and 2 weeks later and showed a 23% decrease at 1 week and 7% further decrease after the second week. Vaccination with Cop-1 on the day of the insult prevented 50% of the IOP-induced RGC loss. Similar neuroprotection was achieved by daily intraperitoneal injections of brimonidine, but not with MK-801.

GENE-BASED AND CELL-BASED TREATMENTS

There are exciting early results with the use of one subretinal injection of adeno-associated virus to replace the defective gene in a study of 12 patients, aged 8 to 44 years, with RPE65-associated Leber congenital amaurosis (76). At 2 years of follow-up, all patients showed sustained improvement in subjective and objective measurements of vision (i.e., dark adaptometry, pupillometry, electroretinography, nystagmus, and ambulatory behavior), with the greatest improvement noted in children, all of whom gained ambulatory vision. With our present understanding of the genetic basis of glaucoma, there is no genotype–phenotype of glaucoma that is comparable to Leber congenital amaurosis. Thus, as an alternative to "replacing a defective gene," targeting a tissue, such as the trabecular meshwork, to enhance function is being considered (77,78).

Another approach is a cell-based treatment, such as T-cell injections to protect the optic nerve or through stem cells with the goal to replace defective trabecular meshwork cells and ganglion cells (79–82).

DRUG DELIVERY

Another approach, to deal with challenges of adherence to multiple dosing of glaucoma medications (83) throughout the day, is with drug delivery. Formulating delivery of mitomycin C on a glaucoma drainage device has recently been studied as a means to improve the surgical outcome by decreasing scarring (84). Using the drainage implant as a drug reservoir, which may be refilled as needed, is also being investigated to provide a fixed and sustained release of glaucoma medication into the eye (85). Another alternative, currently being tested in clinical trials, involves the use of impregnated nasolacrimal plugs containing glaucoma medication.

KEY POINTS

- The burden of proof for potential neuroprotective agents is considerable given that reproducible and measurable differences in clinical end points—that is, visual fields or optic disc—must be shown for treated patients compared with patients randomly assigned to placebo.
- New drug classes, such as the rho kinase inhibitors, show promise to provide a different mechanism of action to lower IOP.
- Perhaps in the future combination drug therapies will not only target IOP reduction but also directly protect the optic nerve from pressure-independent mechanisms of glaucomatous optic neuropathy.

REFERENCES

1. Astrup J, Symon L, Branston NM. Cortical evoked potential and extracellular K+ and H+ at critical levels of brain ischemia. *Stroke.* 1977;8(1):51–57.
2. Fieschi C, Argentino C, Toni D. Calcium antagonists in ischemic stroke. *J Cardiovasc Pharmacol.* 1988;12(suppl 6):S83–S85.
3. Andine P, Lehmann A, Ellren K, et al. The excitatory amino acid antagonist kynurenic acid administered after hypoxic-ischemia in neonatal rats offers neuroprotection. *Neurosci Lett.* 1988;90(1–2):208–212.
4. Becker B, Stamper RL, Asseff C, et al. Effect of diphenylhydantoin on glaucomatous field loss: a preliminary report. *Trans Am Acad Ophthalmol Otolaryngol.* 1972;76(2):412–422.
5. Weinreb RN, Kaufman PL. The glaucoma research community and FDA look to the future: a report from the NEI/FDA CDER Glaucoma Clinical Trial Design and Endpoints Symposium. *Invest Ophthalmol Vis Sci.* 2009;50(4):1497–1505.
6. Robin AL, Clark AF, Covert DW, et al. Anterior juxtascleral delivery of anecortave acetate in eyes with primary open-angle glaucoma: a pilot investigation. *Am J Ophthalmol.* 2009;147(1):45–50.e2.
7. Prata TS, Tavares IM, Mello PA, et al. Hypotensive effect of juxtascleral administration of anecortave acetate in different types of glaucoma. *J Glaucoma.* 2009. Dec 30 [Epub ahead of print].
8. Clark AF. Mechanism of action of the angiostatic cortisene anecortave acetate. *Surv Ophthalmol.* 2007;52(suppl 1):S26–S34.
9. Robin AL, Suan EP, Sjaarda RN, et al. Reduction of intraocular pressure with anecortave acetate in eyes with ocular steroid injection-related glaucoma. *Arch Ophthalmol.* 2009;127(2):173–178.
10. Seamon MJ, Fass JA, Maniscalco-Feichtl M, al. Medical marijuana and the developing role of the pharmacist. *Am J Health Syst Pharm.* 2007;64(10):1037–1044.
11. Pacher P, Batkai S, Kunos G. The endocannabinoid system as an emerging target of pharmacotherapy. *Pharmacol Rev.* 2006;58(3):389–462.
12. Karanian DA, Bahr BA. Cannabinoid drugs and enhancement of endocannabinoid responses: strategies for a wide array of disease states. *Curr Mol Med.* 2006;6(6):677–684.
13. Porcella A, Casellas P, Gessa GL, et al. Cannabinoid receptor CB1 mRNA is highly expressed in the rat ciliary body: implications for the antiglaucoma properties of marihuana. *Brain Res Mol Brain Res.* 1998;58(1–2):240–245.
14. Straiker AJ, Maguire G, Mackie K, et al. Localization of cannabinoid CB1 receptors in the human anterior eye and retina. *Invest Ophthalmol Vis Sci.* 1999;40(10):2442–2448.
15. Hepler RS, Frank IR. Marihuana smoking and intraocular pressure. *JAMA.* 1971;217(10):1392.
16. Tiedeman JS, Shields MB, Weber PA, et al. Effect of synthetic cannabinoids on elevated intraocular pressure. *Ophthalmology.* 1981;88(3):270–277.
17. Purnell WD, Gregg JM. Delta(9)-tetrahydrocannabinol, euphoria and intraocular pressure in man. *Ann Ophthalmol.* 1975;7(7):921–923.
18. Jay WM, Green K. Multiple-drop study of topically applied 1% delta 9-tetrahydrocannabinol in human eyes. *Arch Ophthalmol.* 1983;101(4):591–593.

19. Chien FY, Wang RF, Mittag TW, et al. Effect of WIN 55212-2, a cannabinoid receptor agonist, on aqueous humor dynamics in monkeys. *Arch Ophthalmol.* 2003;121(1):87–90.

20. Zhan GL, Camras CB, Palmberg PF, et al. Effects of marijuana on aqueous humor dynamics in a glaucoma patient. *J Glaucoma.* 2005;14(2):175–177.

21. Crandall J, Matragoon S, Khalifa YM, et al. Neuroprotective and intraocular pressure-lowering effects of (−)Delta9-tetrahydrocannabinol in a rat model of glaucoma. *Ophthalmic Res.* 2007;39(2):69–75.

22. Green K. Marihuana and the eye. *Invest Ophthalmol.* 1975;14(4):261–263.

23. Gaasterland DE. Efficacy in glaucoma treatment—the potential of marijuana. *Ann Ophthalmol.* 1980;12(4):448, 450.

24. Erickson-Lamy K, Schroeder A, Epstein DL. Ethacrynic acid induces reversible shape and cytoskeletal changes in cultured cells. *Invest Ophthalmol Vis Sci.* 1992;33(9):2631–2840.

25. Epstein DL, Freddo TF, Bassett-Chu S, et al. Influence of ethacrynic acid on outflow facility in the monkey and calf eye. *Invest Ophthalmol Vis Sci.* 1987;28(12):2067–2075.

26. Tingey DP, Ozment RR, Schroeder A, et al. The effect of intracameral ethacrynic acid on the intraocular pressure of living monkeys. *Am J Ophthalmol.* 1992;113(6):706–711.

27. Melamed S, Kotas-Neumann R, Barak A, et al. The effect of intracamerally injected ethacrynic acid on intraocular pressure in patients with glaucoma. *Am J Ophthalmol.* 1992;113(5):508–512.

28. Tingey DP, Schroeder A, Epstein MP, et al. Effects of topical ethacrynic acid adducts on intraocular pressure in rabbits and monkeys. *Arch Ophthalmol.* 1992;110(5):699–702.

29. Johnson DH, Tschumper RC. Ethacrynic acid: outflow effects and toxicity in human trabecular meshwork in perfusion organ culture. *Curr Eye Res.* 1993;12(5):385–396.

30. Allingham JS, Klenchin VA, Rayment I. Actin-targeting natural products: structures, properties and mechanisms of action. *Cell Mol Life Sci.* 2006;63(18):2119–2134.

31. Okka M, Tian B, Kaufman PL. Effects of latrunculin B on outflow facility, intraocular pressure, corneal thickness, and miotic and accommodative responses to pilocarpine in monkeys. *Trans Am Ophthalmol Soc.* 2004;102:251–257; discussion 257–259.

32. Sabanay I, Tian B, Gabelt BT, et al. Latrunculin B effects on trabecular meshwork and corneal endothelial morphology in monkeys. *Exp Eye Res.* 2006;82(2):236–246.

33. Vaajanen A, Luhtala S, Oksala O, et al. Does the renin-angiotensin system also regulate intra-ocular pressure? *Ann Med.* 2008;40(6):418–427.

34. Belardetti F, Zamponi GW. Linking calcium-channel isoforms to potential therapies. *Curr Opin Investig Drugs.* 2008;9(7):707–715.

35. Netland PA, Chaturvedi N, Dreyer EB. Calcium channel blockers in the management of low-tension and open-angle glaucoma. *Am J Ophthalmol.* 1993;115(5):608–613.

36. Tomita G, Niwa Y, Shinohara H, et al. Changes in optic nerve head blood flow and retrobular hemodynamics following calcium-channel blocker treatment of normal-tension glaucoma. *Int Ophthalmol.* 1999;23(1):3–10.

37. Koseki N, Araie M, Tomidokoro A, et al. A placebo-controlled 3-year study of a calcium blocker on visual field and ocular circulation in glaucoma with low-normal pressure. *Ophthalmology.* 2008;115(11):2049–2057.

38. Hagg T. From neurotransmitters to neurotrophic factors to neurogenesis. *Neuroscientist.* 2009;15(1):20–27.

39. Mayer EJ, Carter DA, Ren Y, et al. Neural progenitor cells from postmortem adult human retina. *Br J Ophthalmol.* 2005;89(1):102–106.

40. Johnson EC, Guo Y, Cepurna WO, et al. Neurotrophin roles in retinal ganglion cell survival: lessons from rat glaucoma models. *Exp Eye Res.* 2009;88(4):808–815.

41. Lambiase A, Aloe L, Centofanti M, et al. Experimental and clinical evidence of neuroprotection by nerve growth factor eye drops: implications for glaucoma. *Proc Natl Acad Sci USA.* 2009. Aug 3 [Epub ahead of print].

42. Spry PG, Johnson CA. Identification of progressive glaucomatous visual field loss. *Surv Ophthalmol.* 2002;47(2):158–713.

43. Shi Z, Birman E, Saragovi HU. Neurotrophic rationale in glaucoma: a TrkA agonist, but not NGF or a p75 antagonist, protects retinal ganglion cells in vivo. *Dev Neurobiol.* 2007;67(7):884–894.

44. Thanos C, Emerich D. Delivery of neurotrophic factors and therapeutic proteins for retinal diseases. *Expert Opin Biol Ther.* 2005;5(11):1443–1152.

45. Rammes G, Danysz W, Parsons CG. Pharmacodynamics of memantine: an update. *Curr Neuropharmacol.* 2008;6(1):55–78.

46. Kavirajan H. Memantine: a comprehensive review of safety and efficacy. *Expert Opin Drug Saf.* 2009;8(1):89–109.

47. Lucas DR, Newhouse JP. The toxic effect of sodium L-glutamate on the inner layers of the retina. *AMA Arch Opthalmol.* 1957;58(2):193–201.

48. Brooks DE, Garcia GA, Dreyer EB, et al. Vitreous body glutamate concentration in dogs with glaucoma. *Am J Vet Res.* 1997;58(8):864–867.

49. Carter-Dawson L, Crawford ML, Harwerth RS, et al. Vitreal glutamate concentration in monkeys with experimental glaucoma. *Invest Ophthalmol Vis Sci.* 2002;43(8):2633–2637.

50. Dreyer EB, Zurakowski D, Schumer RA, et al. Elevated glutamate levels in the vitreous body of humans and monkeys with glaucoma. *Arch Ophthalmol.* 1996;114(3):299–305.

51. Honkanen RA, Baruah S, Zimmerman MB, et al. Vitreous amino acid concentrations in patients with glaucoma undergoing vitrectomy. *Arch Ophthalmol.* 2003;121(2):183–188.

52. Danesh-Meyer HV, Levin LA. Neuroprotection: extrapolating from neurologic diseases to the eye. *Am J Ophthalmol.* 2009;148(2):186–191.e2.

53. Bryan NS, Bian K, Murad F. Discovery of the nitric oxide signaling pathway and targets for drug development. *Front Biosci.* 2009;14:1–18.

54. Chiou GC. Review: effects of nitric oxide on eye diseases and their treatment. *J Ocul Pharmacol Ther.* 2001;17(2):189–198.

55. Carreiro S, Anderson S, Gukasyan HJ, et al. Correlation of in vitro and in vivo kinetics of nitric oxide donors in ocular tissues. *J Ocul Pharmacol Ther.* 2009;25(2):105–112.

56. Garcia-Campos J, Villena A, Diaz F, et al. Morphological and functional changes in experimental ocular hypertension and role of neuroprotective drugs. *Histol Histopathol.* 2007;22(12):1399–1411.

57. Neufeld AH, Sawada A, Becker B. Inhibition of nitric-oxide synthase 2 by aminoguanidine provides neuroprotection of retinal ganglion cells in a rat model of chronic glaucoma. *Proc Natl Acad Sci USA.* 1999;96(17):9944–9948.

58. Neufeld AH, Das S, Vora S, et al. A prodrug of a selective inhibitor of inducible nitric oxide synthase is neuroprotective in the rat model of glaucoma. *J Glaucoma.* 2002;11(3):221–225.

59. Liu B, Chen H, Johns TG, et al. Epidermal growth factor receptor activation: an upstream signal for transition of quiescent astrocytes into reactive astrocytes after neural injury. *J Neurosci.* 2006;26(28):7532–7540.

60. Hamacher T, Airaksinen J, Saarela V, et al. Efficacy and safety levels of preserved and preservative-free tafluprost are equivalent in patients with glaucoma or ocular hypertension: results from a pharmacodynamics analysis. *Acta Ophthalmol Suppl (Oxf).* 2008;242:14–19.

61. Uusitalo H, Kaarniranta K, Ropo A. Pharmacokinetics, efficacy and safety profiles of preserved and preservative-free tafluprost in healthy volunteers. *Acta Ophthalmol Suppl (Oxf).* 2008;242:7–13.

62. Egorov E, Ropo A. Adjunctive use of tafluprost with timolol provides additive effects for reduction of intraocular pressure in patients with glaucoma. *Eur J Ophthalmol.* 2009;19(2):214–222.

63. Rao VP, Epstein DL. Rho GTPase/Rho kinase inhibition as a novel target for the treatment of glaucoma. *BioDrugs.* 2007;21(3):167–177.

64. Weiner HL. The challenge of multiple sclerosis: how do we cure a chronic heterogeneous disease? *Ann Neurol.* 2009;65(3):239–348.

65. Bertolotto A, Gilli F. Interferon-beta responders and non-responders. A biological approach. *Neurol Sci.* 2008;29(suppl 2):S216–S217.

66. Vandenbark AA, Abulafia-Lapid R. Autologous T-cell vaccination for multiple sclerosis: a perspective on progress. *BioDrugs.* 2008;22(4):265–273.

67. Stuve O, Cravens PD, Eagar TN. DNA-based vaccines: the future of multiple sclerosis therapy? *Expert Rev Neurother.* 2008;8(3):351–360.

68. Cartwright MJ, Grajewski AL, Friedberg ML, et al. Immune-related disease and normal-tension glaucoma. A case-control study. *Arch Ophthalmol.* 1992;110(4):500–502.

69. Tezel G, Edward DP, Wax MB. Serum autoantibodies to optic nerve head glycosaminoglycans in patients with glaucoma. *Arch Ophthalmol.* 1999;117(7):917–924.

70. Tezel G, Seigel GM, Wax MB. Autoantibodies to small heat shock proteins in glaucoma. *Invest Ophthalmol Vis Sci.* 1998;39(12):2277–2287.

71. Wax MB, Tezel G, Saito I, et al. Anti-Ro/SS-A positivity and heat shock protein antibodies in patients with normal-pressure glaucoma [see comments]. *Am J Ophthalmol.* 1998;125(2):145–157.

72. Elde NC, Malik HS. The evolutionary conundrum of pathogen mimicry. *Nat Rev Microbiol.* 2009;7(11):787–797.

73. Caspi R. Autoimmunity in the immune privileged eye: pathogenic and regulatory T cells. *Immunol Res.* 2008;42(1–3):41–50.

74. Schwartz M, London A. Erratum to: Immune maintenance in glaucoma: boosting the body's own neuroprotective potential. *J Ocul Biol Dis Infor.* 2009;2(3):104–108.

75. Ben Simon GJ, Bakalash S, Aloni E, et al. A rat model for acute rise in intraocular pressure: immune modulation as a therapeutic strategy. *Am J Ophthalmol.* 2006;141(6):1105–1111.

76. Maguire AM, High KA, Auricchio A, et al. Age-dependent effects of RPE65 gene therapy for Leber's congenital amaurosis: a phase 1 dose-escalation trial. *Lancet.* 2009;374(9701):1597–1605.

77. Barraza RA, Rasmussen CA, Loewen N, et al. Prolonged transgene expression with lentiviral vectors in the aqueous humor outflow pathway of nonhuman primates. *Hum Gene Ther.* 2009;20(3):191–200.

78. Liu X, Rasmussen CA, Gabelt BT, et al. Gene therapy targeting glaucoma: where are we? *Surv Ophthalmol.* 2009;54(4):472–486.

79. Bakalash S, Shlomo GB, Aloni E, et al. T-cell-based vaccination for morphological and functional neuroprotection in a rat model of chronically elevated intraocular pressure. *J Mol Med.* 2005;83(11):904–916.

80. Kelley MJ, Rose AY, Keller KE, et al. Stem cells in the trabecular meshwork: present and future promises. *Exp Eye Res.* 2009;88(4):747–751.

81. Qiu F, Jiang H, Xiang M. A comprehensive negative regulatory program controlled by Brn3b to ensure ganglion cell specification from multipotential retinal precursors. *J Neurosci.* 2008;28(13):3392–3403.

82. Ohta K, Ito A, Tanaka H. Neuronal stem/progenitor cells in the vertebrate eye. *Dev Growth Differ.* 2008;50(4):253–259.

83. Tsai JC. A comprehensive perspective on patient adherence to topical glaucoma therapy. *Ophthalmology.* 2009;116(11 suppl):S30–S36.

84. Sahiner N, Kravitz DJ, Qadir R, et al. Creation of a drug-coated glaucoma drainage device using polymer technology: in vitro and in vivo studies. *Arch Ophthalmol.* 2009;127(4):448–453.

85. Lo R, Li PY, Saati S, et al. A passive MEMS drug delivery pump for treatment of ocular diseases. *Biomed Microdevices.* 2009. Apr 25 [Epub ahead of print].

34

Anatomic Principles of Glaucoma Surgery

All laser and incisional surgical procedures for glaucoma are designed to reduce the intraocular pressure (IOP) by increasing the rate of aqueous humor outflow or reducing aqueous production. The involved anatomy, therefore, is the anterior ocular structures related to aqueous outflow and the portions of the ciliary body associated with aqueous inflow. To properly perform any of the operations that make up the armamentarium of glaucoma surgery, the surgeon must be familiar with both the internal and external aspects of these structures. In this chapter, we consider these portions of the ocular anatomy as they relate to glaucoma surgery.

AN OVERVIEW OF THE ANATOMY

The structures involved in aqueous humor dynamics—that is, aqueous production and aqueous outflow—are in immediate proximity to each other in the periphery of the anterior ocular segment. The interrelationship between these structures is considered in Chapter 1 with a stepwise construction of a schematic model that may be summarized as follows.

At the junction between the cornea and the sclera is the transitional zone of connective tissue known as the limbus. On the inner surface of the limbus, extending for 360 degrees, is a depression, referred to as the scleral sulcus. The anterior margin of this sulcus slopes gradually into the peripheral cornea, while the posterior margin contains a lip of connective tissue called the scleral spur. This spur might be thought of as the dividing point between the structures of aqueous outflow anteriorly and those of aqueous production posteriorly. The trabecular meshwork attaches in part to the anterior side of the scleral spur and extends forward to blend into the sloping anterior wall of the scleral sulcus, which converts the sulcus into the Schlemm canal. The bulk of aqueous humor in the anterior chamber flows through the trabecular meshwork to the Schlemm canal, from where it leaves the eye via intrascleral channels and episcleral veins.

The ciliary body inserts into the posterior portion of the scleral spur. This is actually the only firm attachment of the ciliary body, with the remaining surfaces between the sclera and the ciliary body creating a potential space, referred to as the supraciliary space. The ciliary processes, the actual site of aqueous production, occupy the innermost and anteriormost portion of the ciliary body. The iris inserts into the ciliary body just anterior to the ciliary processes. Consequently, a peripheral iridectomy, as performed during glaucoma filtering surgery, often allows visualization of two to four ciliary processes. The insertion of the iris is usually such that a portion of the anterior ciliary body remains gonioscopically visible between the iris root and scleral spur. This is referred to as the ciliary body band, the physical entrance to the uveoscleral outflow pathway. The remainder of the trabecular meshwork—that is, the portion not inserted to the scleral spur—attaches to this band and to the peripheral iris.

INTERNAL ANATOMY

Ciliary Body

Most of the ciliary body is located posterior to the iris (**Fig. 34.1**) and cannot be directly visualized except in unusual circumstances, such as with marked iris retraction or absence of portions of the iris. The anterior 2 to 3 mm of the ciliary body, the pars plicata, is thicker than the posterior portion and contains the radial ridges of the ciliary processes. The latter are the site of aqueous production and the target of cyclodestructive procedures. In those unusual circumstances in which they can be visualized directly (by using cycloscopy), direct treatment with laser transpupillary cyclophotocoagulation or endoscopic visualization may be possible. When direct visualization is not

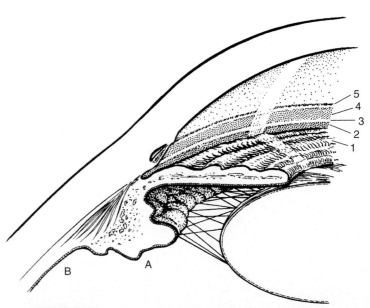

Figure 34.1 Internal anatomy. The ciliary body is located just posterior to the iris and is divided into the pars plicata (*A*) and the pars plana (*B*). The remaining internal structures can be seen by gonioscopy and include *1*, iris; *2*, ciliary body band; *3*, scleral spur; *4*, trabecular meshwork; *5*, Schwalbe line.

possible, an indirect, transscleral route can be used for cyclodestruction, requiring the use of external landmarks (discussed later in this chapter). The posterior 4 mm of the ciliary body is the thinner pars plana, which must also be approached by using external landmarks.

Structures Visualized by Gonioscopy

The following structures in the anterior chamber can be visualized by gonioscopic examination and are involved in several laser and incisional glaucoma surgical procedures.

Iris

The iris is the posteriormost structure of the anterior chamber angle. It is helpful to remember that the peripheral portion of the iris is thinner than the more central iris, which makes it, among other reasons, the preferred site for a laser iridotomy. Other anatomic considerations related to optimum laser iridotomy sites are iris crypts, or thinner areas of stroma that may be easier to penetrate. In addition, areas of increased pigmentation, such as iris freckles, may improve the absorption of laser energy in lightly pigmented eyes when using argon laser. It is generally preferred to place the iridotomy so that it is fully covered by the upper lid, to minimize the side effect of intermittent glare (1). However, peripheral iridotomies can result in symptomatic glare in any position.

Ciliary Body Band

The ciliary body band is located just anterior to the root of the iris; it typically has a dark gray or brown appearance on gonioscopic examination. The width of this band varies considerably from one patient to the next. Eyes with myopia often have a wide band, and those with hyperopia a narrow band. Surgeons should avoid confusing the pigmented ciliary body band with the trabecular meshwork in patients with lightly pigmented meshwork, especially when interpreting the depth of the anterior chamber angle. This is particularly relevant when performing laser trabeculoplasty. The patient usually lets the surgeon know when the latter mistake is made, because the ciliary body contains many nerve endings and is sensitive to the application of laser energy.

Scleral Spur

The scleral spur is seen gonioscopically as a white line just anterior to the ciliary body band. In some patients, visualization of the spur may be obscured because of variable degrees of high iris process insertion (but discontinuous; continuous areas of high iris insertion are peripheral anterior synechiae) or heavy pigment dispersion. This was the principal site of surgery with a cyclodialysis procedure, an operation of historical interest, in which an aqueous outflow pathway in the suprachoroidal space was constructed by separating ciliary body from the scleral spur. In the early stages of neovascular glaucoma, new vessels may be seen extending across the scleral spur from the iris and ciliary body to the trabecular meshwork. The vessels can be obliterated at this site with laser applications

in a procedure called goniophotocoagulation, which is also rarely used today.

Trabecular Meshwork

Just anterior to the scleral spur is the functional portion of the trabecular meshwork, the portion adjacent to the Schlemm canal through which the aqueous humor drains. This portion of the meshwork is demarcated gonioscopically by the presence of variable amounts of pigment. Because this pigment is presumably carried to the meshwork from uveal tissue by the aqueous humor flow, it is typically light in young individuals and varies considerably among individuals later in life according to the amount of intraocular pigment release. In some patients, especially with pathologic states such as the pigment dispersion syndrome and exfoliation syndrome, the meshwork is heavily pigmented. In other individuals, the meshwork may be so lightly pigmented that it is hard to see, which can lead to the incorrect diagnosis of a narrow, or even closed, anterior chamber angle. In some of these cases, blood reflux into the Schlemm canal or iris processes, which typically extends to the meshwork, may help identify this structure.

It is this pigmented portion of the trabecular meshwork to which the laser energy should be applied during argon laser trabeculoplasty, which delivers its energy within a 50-μm spot. However, there is another, less pigmented portion of the meshwork just anterior to the functional, pigmented portion. When performing argon laser trabeculoplasty, overlapping the laser beam between the pigmented and nonpigmented portions of the meshwork—that is, along the anterior border of the pigmented portion—may help reduce the complications of transient postoperative IOP rise and peripheral anterior synechia formation. Selective laser trabeculoplasty delivers its energy in a 400-μm spot; with this procedure, centering the spot over the entire trabecular meshwork is preferable.

When performing trabeculectomy ab interno, the scleral spur and trabecular meshwork must be clearly identified to initially penetrate through the trabecular meshwork into the Schlemm canal. If one penetrates posterior to the scleral spur, the probe will enter the suprachoroidal space, resulting in a substantially increased risk of complications.

Schwalbe Line

The Schwalbe line is the anteriormost structure in the anterior chamber angle and represents the junction between the nonpigmented portion of the trabecular meshwork and the peripheral cornea. In most individuals, a portion of this junction is represented by a small ridge. This is an important landmark when performing a goniotomy, in that the internal incision in that operation is made just posterior to the Schwalbe line. The structure may be difficult to visualize gonioscopically, unless there has been a moderate degree of pigment dispersion, in which case there may be a buildup of pigment along the anterior side of the ridge, especially inferiorly. Care must be taken to avoid confusing this pigmented line with the trabecular meshwork when performing laser trabeculoplasty. In other cases in which pigmentation is minimal, the location of the Schwalbe line can be established gonioscopically to help determine the depth of the peripheral anterior chamber. A fine beam of light from the slitlamp can be seen reflecting from both the anterior and posterior surfaces of the peripheral cornea. As the clear portion of the peripheral cornea approaches the Schwalbe line, it is replaced externally by opaque limbal tissue, which causes the two beams to converge at the Schwalbe line, providing a useful way for determining the location of this structure.

EXTERNAL ANATOMY

Anterior Limbus

On the external surface of the eye, the anterior boundary of the limbus is defined as the termination of the Bowman membrane, which is approximately 0.5 mm anterior to the insertion of the conjunctiva and Tenon capsule (**Fig. 34.2**). This has been referred to as the corneolimbal junction, or the apparent or anterior limbus. It is important to note that the conjunctiva inserts more anteriorly in the superior and inferior quadrants. Consequently, the limbus is wider in these quadrants, ranging between 1 and 1.5 mm, and gradually tapers to the narrowest width in the nasal and temporal quadrants, where the range is between 0.3 and 0.5 mm (2). In performing glaucoma filtering surgery, some surgeons choose to take advantage of the wider areas of the limbus by placing the surgical site at the 12-o'clock position. When performing surgery that involves the ciliary

body, such as a cyclodestructive procedure or a pars plana incision, the surgeon should remember that these structures are slightly more posterior in relation to the apparent limbus in the superior and inferior quadrants.

Conjunctiva and Tenon Capsule

The conjunctiva and Tenon capsule cover the limbus. The Tenon capsule is firmly attached to the connective tissue of the limbus approximately 0.5 to 1.0 mm posterior to the insertion of the conjunctiva, which creates a potential space between the anterior conjunctiva and Tenon capsule tissue and the limbal connective tissue. If the surgeon wishes to obtain maximum exposure of the limbus when preparing a limbus-based conjunctival flap, it is necessary to dissect this adherence between the Tenon capsule and the limbal tissue. Such a technique is not recommended for filtering surgery with use of adjunctive antimetabolites, because the resulting filtering bleb may be too thin. The adhesions between conjunctiva and the Tenon capsule are moderately firm, so that sharp dissection is required to dissect between these two structures when preparing the conjunctival flap. The adhesions between the Tenon capsule and the underlying limbus and sclera posteriorly are less firm, and these structures can often be separated with blunt dissection. With the current trabeculectomy techniques, adequate anterior dissection is possible under the partial-thickness scleral flap without dissecting the insertion of the Tenon capsule. It is also preferable, especially when performing filtering surgery with

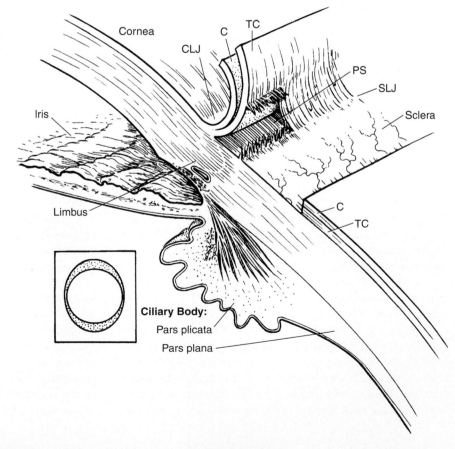

Figure 34.2 External anatomy. On the external surface, the limbus is bounded posteriorly by the sclerolimbal junction (*SLJ*) and anteriorly by the corneolimbal junction (*CLJ*). The width of the limbus varies from a maximum superiorly to a minimum on the sides (*inset*) due to the relative insertion of the conjunctiva (*C*). The Tenon capsule (*TC*) is firmly attached to limbal connective tissue approximately 0.5 mm behind the conjunctival insertion, creating a potential space (*PS*). Cyclodestructive procedures should be placed over the pars plicata, usually 1.0 to 1.5 mm posterior to the corneolimbal junction, whereas a posterior sclerotomy should be made through the pars plana, approximately 3 to 4 mm posterior to the corneolimbal junction.

an adjunctive antimetabolite, to leave this adhesion intact to avoid creating a filtering bleb that is too thin at the limbus.

Posterior Limbus

When the conjunctiva and Tenon capsule have been reflected, the posterior boundary of the limbus can be seen. This has been referred to as the sclerolimbal junction, or the surgical or posterior limbus. It is identified as the junction of the opaque white sclera posteriorly and the translucent bluish-gray limbus anteriorly. This boundary of the limbus is more useful than the anterior limbus in glaucoma surgery because it helps identify the location of the deeper structures of the anterior chamber angle. The scleral spur, for example, is located just posterior to the sclerolimbal junction and the Schlemm canal and therefore would be found just anterior to this landmark. In performing a trabeculotomy ab externo, a radial scratch incision across the sclerolimbal junction should reveal the Schlemm canal in the posterior portion of the gray zone. When performing a trabeculectomy, a circumferential incision beneath the partial-thickness scleral flap at the corneolimbal junction enters the anterior chamber just in front of the trabecular meshwork. By extending the dissection posteriorly with radial incisions to the sclerolimbal junction, a flap of deep limbal tissue is created that can be reflected to expose the anterior chamber angle structures and can then be excised along the scleral spur. If the latter incision is mistakenly made more posteriorly, the ciliary body may be damaged, resulting in brisk bleeding. A fistula that is too posterior is also at risk for obstruction by uveal tissue, hence the importance of correctly identifying the external landmarks during glaucoma filtering surgery.

The vasculature of the limbus originates primarily from the anterior ciliary arteries (3). The anterior ciliary arteries enter the ciliary body behind the scleral spur in locations corresponding to the positions of the rectus muscle tendons. These vessels should be avoided when possible during surgery to minimize excessive bleeding. Because the ciliary body cannot usually be visualized internally, external landmarks must be used when performing surgical procedures associated with these structures. In performing cyclodestructive procedures, which involve the pars plicata, it was once suggested that the destructive element, for example, the cryoprobe, should be placed 2 to 3 mm behind the corneolimbal junction, allowing for the previously discussed variation in this landmark (2). In most eyes, however, using this location would result in entry into the eye that is posterior to the pars plicata. This may not have been significant with the earlier cyclodestructive procedures in which the area of tissue destruction was so broad. With transscleral laser cyclophotocoagulation, however, the zone of tissue destruction is more precise, and a placement of the laser beam 1.5 mm behind the corneolimbal junction superiorly and inferiorly and 1.0 mm temporally and nasally is most likely to reach the pars plicata. Some probes, such as the G probe (Iridex Corporation, Mountain View, CA), are designed with a footplate that is placed at the limbus, and the energy is delivered posteriorly, approximating the correct location. When making a pars plana incision, as during a posterior sclerotomy for malignant glaucoma or when draining a suprachoroidal detachment or hemorrhage, the incision should be made 3 mm (in aphakic or pseudophakic eyes) to 4 mm (in phakic eyes) behind the corneolimbal junction.

KEY POINTS

- Laser and incisional surgical procedures for glaucoma are directed at the anatomic structures associated with aqueous inflow, that is, the ciliary body, and aqueous outflow, which includes the iris and the trabecular meshwork and related outflow pathways.
- For successful glaucoma surgery, it is necessary to be familiar with these structures by direct internal visualization through slitlamp and gonioscopic examination, and by their relationship to the external aspects of the limbal connective tissue and the overlying conjunctiva and Tenon capsule.

REFERENCES

1. Spaeth GL, Idowu O, Seligsohn A, et al. The effects of iridotomy size and position on symptoms following laser peripheral iridotomy. *J Glaucoma.* 2005;14(5):364–367.
2. Sugar HS. Surgical anatomy of glaucoma. *Surv Ophthalmol.* 1968;13:143.
3. Van Buskirk EM. The anatomy of the limbus. *Eye (Lond).* 1989; 3(pt 2):101.

35

Principles of Laser Surgery
for Glaucoma

The introduction of laser (i.e., light amplification by stimulated emission of radiation) therapy was a significant advance in the surgical treatment of glaucoma during the second half of the 20th century. The concept of using light energy to alter the structure of intraocular tissues, however, actually preceded the development of laser technology. Meyer-Schwickerath (1), beginning in the late 1940s, pioneered this field of ocular surgery, first using focused sunlight and later the xenon-arc photocoagulator. Although the latter technique was useful for certain retinal disorders, xenon-arc photocoagulation for the treatment of glaucoma never gained clinical acceptance.

In 1960, Maiman (2) described the first laser that used a ruby crystal stimulated by a flash lamp to emit red laser light at a wavelength of 694 nm. It was the development of the continuous-wave argon laser, near the end of that decade, that brought on a virtual explosion of laser applications for ocular diseases. Since the first report of argon laser use for ocular disease in the late 1960s, numerous wavelengths arising from different energy-emitting sources have been tried. Lasers are now used to treat various forms of glaucoma, and today it is the most commonly used mode of glaucoma surgery (3–6).

This chapter briefly reviews the physical and biologic aspects of laser therapy. The application of these principles to the treatment of specific forms of glaucoma is considered in subsequent chapters.

BASIC PRINCIPLES OF LASERS

When light is shined on a metal surface in a vacuum, it may free electrons from that surface. These electrons can be detected as a current flowing in the vacuum to an electrode. Only certain wavelengths can cause photoemission of electrons. In 1917, Albert Einstein wrote "Zur Quantum Theorie der Strahlung" (the quantum theory of radiation), in which he speculated that light consists of photons, each with discrete quantum of energy proportional to its wavelength. For an electron to be freed from the metal surface, it would need a photon with enough energy to overcome the energy that bound it to the atom. His theory formed the basis of laser technology.

When atoms absorb energy, called "pumping," they are "excited" from a lower to a higher energy level. When a substance (e.g., gas, liquid, or a semiconducting material) is excited by energy, it emits light in all directions. The sources of energy used to excite the lasing medium typically include electricity from a power supply or flash lamps, or the energy from another laser. If more atoms are in the excited state than in the unexcited state, population inversion is said to exist. Under such circumstances, photons with energy equal to the difference between the two levels of excitation have an enhanced probability of stimulating the atoms to decay back to their lower energy level by emitting photons, a process called stimulated emission. The emitted photons stimulate the emission of more photons, leading to a chain reaction.

If this system is enclosed between two mirrors, the photons bounce back and forth, creating multiple stimulated emissions of light, or light amplification. The mirrors form an optical cavity, which, in addition to amplifying the light, creates a parallel beam and acts as a resonator to limit the number of wavelengths. When the light amplification is sufficient, some photons are allowed to leave the cavity in the form of a laser beam through a partially permeable mirror (**Fig. 35.1**).

The laser beam can be delivered as a continuous wave or in a pulsed mode. In the latter situation, the energy is concentrated and delivered in a very short period of time, which can be accomplished in one of two ways. With one technique, called Q-switching, light is not allowed to travel back and forth in the cavity until maximum population inversion is reached. This is accomplished with an electronic shutter or misalignment of the mirrors. When the shutter is opened or the mirrors are aligned, stimulated emission and light amplification occur suddenly, and the energy is released in a pulse of a few to tens of nanoseconds. In the other form of pulsed delivery, called mode-locking, the energy is also released after achieving maximum population inversion, but different modes of light are synchronized, creating peaks of energy, which are emitted in tens of nanoseconds as a chain of pulses, each of which lasts a few tens of picoseconds. To provide some appreciation for the brevity of these exposures, it has been noted that the ratio between the duration of a Q-switched laser pulse and a conventional continuous-wave argon laser exposure is roughly the same as the ratio between the argon exposure and a human lifetime (6).

PROPERTIES OF LASER ENERGY

Light emitted by a laser differs from normal "white" light in several ways.

Coherence

Unlike the photons in a light bulb, which are emitted randomly, the resonator effect of the laser cavity causes the photons to be synchronized or coherent—that is, in phase with each other in time and space.

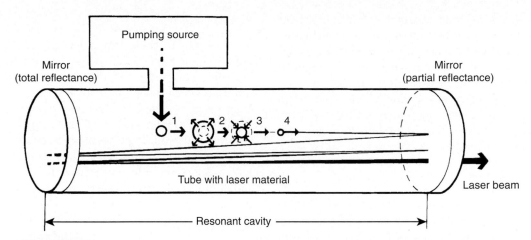

Figure 35.1 Schematic of laser system. Laser material is placed in a tube between two mirrors. When an energy source is pumped into the tube, atoms in the laser material (*1*) are excited to a higher energy level (*2*). In the excited state, atoms have an enhanced probability of being stimulated by photons to decay back to the lower energy level (*3*) by emitting photons (*4*). The emitted photons bounce between the mirrors, stimulating other excited atoms, until sufficient light amplification is achieved, at which time the light is allowed to leave the cavity as a laser beam.

Collimation (Directionality)

Because light amplification occurs only for photons that are aligned with the mirrors, a nearly parallel beam, in which all the waves travel in the same direction, is produced, as opposed to the diverging beam of an incandescent lamp. Although limited divergence occurs with all laser beams, it is minimal enough that a small focal spot can be created when the light is delivered through an optical system.

Monochromacy

Because the photons are emitted through the release of energy between two defined levels of the atom, the resulting light has only one discrete wavelength. In contrast, ordinary white light is a combination of many different wavelengths.

High Intensity

The light amplification of a laser can produce a beam with significantly more intensity than that of the sun.

LASER-INDUCED TISSUE INTERACTIONS

The tissue effects produced by laser surgery are of three types: thermal, ionizing, and photochemical (7).

Thermal Effects

In this situation, the absorption of laser energy by the target tissue produces temperatures high enough to induce chemical changes that can cause local inflammation and scarring (photocoagulation) or to vaporize intracellular and extracellular fluids, creating an incision in the tissue (photovaporization).

Factors influencing the laser thermal effect include (a) wavelength of the incident light, (b) duration of exposure, and (c) amount of light energy per area of exposure. Melanin, the pigment of most target tissues in glaucoma laser surgery, has a peak absorption in the blue-green portion of the visible spectrum. Therefore, lasers with wavelengths between 400 and 600 nm are most useful for these procedures, and the argon laser is the prototype photocoagulator.

The heat generated by the absorption of laser energy is dissipated by the surrounding tissue. A short exposure time and a high-energy level and area reduce heat conduction, which causes tissue temperatures to reach the critical boiling point, producing gas bubbles with tissue disruption and photovaporization through a microexplosion. This reaction can be used to create holes in ocular tissues, as with laser iridotomy. At lower energy levels, photocoagulation may produce contraction of collagen, which is the mechanism of pupilloplasty and iridoplasty, and possibly of laser trabeculoplasty.

Ionizing Effects

If intense laser energy is focused into a very small area for a very short period of time, a reaction occurs that is independent of pigment absorption and is referred to as photodisruption. An instantaneous electric field is generated, which strips electrons from target atoms, producing a gaseous state called plasma (6). As ionized atoms of plasma recombine with free electrons, photons with a wide range of energies are emitted, producing a spark of incoherent white light. Associated shock and pressure waves create additional mechanical damage to target tissues, resulting in a reaction that can disrupt both pigmented and nonpigmented structures. Thermal effects are also involved in the mechanism of photodisruption (8).

The Nd:YAG (neodymium:yttrium–aluminum–garnet) laser is the most commonly used photodisruptor. The pulse may be Q-switched or mode-locked, both of which have been shown to produce the same size of rupture in polyethylene membranes (8). The main clinical use has been for the disruption, or cutting, of relatively transparent anterior segment structures, most notably the posterior lens capsule. For glaucoma surgery, the primary application of the Q-switched Nd:YAG laser is the creation of iridotomies. Nd:YAG lasers can also be used in a pulsed thermal or continuous-wave mode for transscleral cyclophotocoagulation.

Photochemical Effects

The target tissue in this laser-induced effect is volatilized (vaporized) by short-pulsed ultraviolet radiation (photoablation). Some tissues, such as tumors, can be photosensitized with hematoporphyrin or other photosensitizing agent and selectively destroyed with laser energy of a specific wavelength (photodynamic therapy or photoradiation).

LASER DELIVERY SYSTEMS

Most laser units use a slitlamp biomicroscope, in which a system of fiber optics or mirrors in an articulated arm direct the laser beam from the laser tube, through the slitlamp, and into the patient's eye. Various types of contact lenses are normally used during laser surgery with slitlamp delivery. Some contain mirrors to direct the laser beam into the anterior chamber angle, and others incorporate convex lenses to concentrate the light energy on the iris. Other laser delivery systems use contact probes attached to the fiber optics, which allows application of laser energy to the ocular tissues by external placement of the probe on the eye or by aiming directly at internal ocular structures with the probe tip in the eye. By using a fiber-optic camera and fiber-optic delivery, it is also possible to deliver laser energy (diode) endoscopically.

For lasers in the visual spectrum, an aiming beam of attenuated laser energy can be used to allow positioning and focusing of the laser beam on the target tissue. For lasers with wavelengths outside the visual spectrum, an additional laser such as a helium–neon, or semiconductor diode, with wavelengths of 633 and 640 nm, respectively, is used as the aiming beam. A foot pedal or finger trigger is used to release the full laser energy, producing the tissue alteration. The variables on the control units of most laser systems include spot size (usually expressed in microns), exposure duration (expressed in tenths of seconds, milliseconds, microseconds, or nanoseconds), and energy (joules or millijoules) or power (watts or milliwatts). Energy in joules equals power in watts times duration in seconds.

SPECIFIC LASERS FOR GLAUCOMA SURGERY

Lasers differ primarily according to the medium in which the atoms exist that produce the stimulated emission of photons. The lasers used most commonly for glaucoma surgery are argon, Nd:YAG, and semiconductor diode, although experience with many other lasers has also been reported.

Argon Lasers

The medium in these instruments is argon gas, which is pumped by an electrical discharge. The wavelengths are in the blue (488-nm) and green (514-nm) portions of the visible spectrum, which are optimum for absorption by melanin. Most argon lasers operate in the continuous-wave mode and have maximum power levels of 2 to 6 watts. Units are also available, however, that produce pulses of approximately 100 microseconds with powers of 20 to 50 watts. The latter instruments achieve full power only as needed, which reduces heat buildup and improves energy efficiency.

Nd:YAG Lasers

In these instruments, the neodymium atoms are embedded in a crystal of yttrium–aluminum–garnet (YAG) and are pumped by a xenon flash lamp. The laser wavelength is in the near-infrared (1064-nm) range, although it can be made a visible-light emitter by frequency doubling or an ultraviolet emitter by frequency tripling (7). Nd:YAG lasers can be operated in the continuous-wave mode to provide a photocoagulation effect but are more commonly used with pulsed delivery, by using Q-switching or mode-locking, to allow photodisruption. The selective laser uses spectrum of the wavelength that is selectively absorbed by a pigment in the tissue. The laser destroys melanin in the tissue (e.g., trabecular meshwork), while minimizing thermal injury to surrounding structures. The mechanism is based on the principle of selective photothermolysis (9), developed in the Wellman Laboratory by Parrish and Anderson in the early 1980s. This principle is used in selective laser trabeculoplasty (10).

Semiconductor Diode Lasers

Two light-emitting diodes are used in this system to produce a wavelength in the near-infrared spectrum (800 to 820 nm). Solid-state construction allows compact size, durability, and low maintenance. The wavelength, between that of the argon and Nd:YAG lasers, provides better scleral penetration than the argon and better absorption by melanin than the Nd:YAG lasers, making it useful for transscleral cyclophotocoagulation (11). Diode lasers can also be operated in the red range of the visible spectrum (640 nm), in which case they are used as an aiming beam.

Other Lasers

Other lasers are being developed and evaluated for ocular surgery. Among these are the dye lasers, which use a solution of complex organic dyes, such as rhodamine, and can produce monochromatic wavelengths at relatively high-output powers through a large range of the visible spectrum. This allows the selection of a wavelength that would be most highly absorbed by the target tissue, thereby minimizing the transmittal of laser energy through the ocular media (12). Carbon dioxide lasers in the infrared spectrum (10,600 nm) have been used in the continuous-wave mode to cut tissue by vaporization with very little coagulation necrosis, whereas excimer lasers in the ultraviolet range (193 to 248 nm) are being evaluated in the pulsed mode to cut tissue with no visible necrosis (13). The ruby laser in the visible spectrum (694 nm) can produce photoablation with high-energy pulses, and the krypton laser in the yellow–red wavelength can be used for photocoagulation. The helium–neon laser in the red wavelength is, as previously noted, used as an aiming beam in many laser systems that operate at nonvisible wavelengths (7).

LASER SAFETY

Although the properties of laser energy make lasers ideal tools for the surgical manipulation of tissues, they also pose serious hazards, including electric shock, direct laser burns, explosions, and fires. Probably, the most common and serious health hazard, however, is accidental exposure of the retina, either directly or from reflected laser light.

The following classification of lasers is generally accepted regarding hazards (14). Class I: Do not emit hazardous levels. Class II: Visible-light lasers that are safe for momentary viewing but should not be stared into continuously; an example is the aiming beam of ophthalmic lasers, or laser pointers. Class III: Unsafe for even momentary viewing, requiring procedural controls and safety equipment. Class IV: Also pose a significant fire and skin hazard; most therapeutic laser beams used in ocular surgery are in this class.

During glaucoma laser surgery, the patient has the greatest risk of injury from accidental exposure of the retina or lens. The risk to the corneal endothelium has been evaluated with specular microscopy 1 year after laser trabeculoplasty or iridotomy; some investigators have found a significant increase in cell size and endothelial cell loss (15,16), but others have found no significant changes (17,18).

The surgeon is theoretically protected during each exposure of therapeutic laser energy in most slitlamp delivery systems by a built-in filter. There is some evidence, however, that subtle, but definite, alterations in color vision can be seen in ophthalmic laser surgeons who are exposed chronically to argon blue light (19,20). Because there is no apparent clinical advantage to blue-green wavelengths in ophthalmic surgery, it is advisable to use green-only whenever possible.

Aside from the patient and the surgeon, the individuals at greatest risk for retinal burns are other personnel in the laser room during the treatment whose eyes may be exposed to reflected laser light. One study with argon lasers and various contact lenses indicated that a hazard can exist for a bystander at the side of the slitlamp who is exposed to unattenuated back reflections of the treatment beam within 1 m of the contact lens (21). To minimize this hazard, only antireflective-coated contact lenses should be used, ancillary personnel should wear protective goggles or look away from the laser when it is in use, and access to the laser room should be limited to necessary individuals during the treatment.

KEY POINTS

- Lasers operate on the principle that excited atoms can be stimulated to emit photons, resulting in a markedly amplified light that possesses the unique properties of coherence, collimation, monochromacy, and high intensity.
- The nature of this light allows precise alteration of tissues by thermal effects (photocoagulation and photovaporization), ionizing effects (photodisruption), and photochemical effects (photoablation and photodynamic therapy or photoradiation).
- The tissue interactions, especially the photocoagulation and photodisruption, are used in a wide variety of glaucoma surgical procedures.

REFERENCES

1. Meyer-Schwickerath G. *Light Coagulation.* [Translated by Drance SM]. St. Louis, MO: CV Mosby; 1960.
2. Maiman TH. Stimulated optical radiation in ruby. *Nature.* 1960;187:493–494.
3. Peyman GA, Raichand M, Zeimer RC. Ocular effects of various laser wavelengths [review]. *Surv Ophthalmol.* 1984;28:391–404.
4. Belcher CD III. *Photocoagulation for Glaucoma and Anterior Segment Disease.* Baltimore, MD: Williams & Wilkins; 1984.
5. Schwartz L, Spaeth G. *Laser Therapy of the Anterior Segment: A Practical Approach.* Thorofare, NJ: Slack; 1984.
6. Mainster MA, Sliney DH, Belcher CD III, et al. Laser photodisruptors: damage mechanisms, instrument design and safety. *Ophthalmology.* 1983;90:973–991.
7. Lasers in medicine and surgery [review]. Council on Scientific Affairs. *JAMA.* 1986;256:900–907.
8. Vogel A, Hentschel W, Holzfuss J, et al. Cavitation bubble dynamics and acoustic transient generation in ocular surgery with pulsed neodymium: YAG lasers. *Ophthalmology.* 1986;93:1259–1269.
9. Anderson RR, Parrish JA. Selective photothermolysis: precise microsurgery by selective absorption of pulsed radiation. *Science.* 1983;220:524–527.
10. Latina MA, Park C. Selective targeting of trabecular meshwork cells: in vitro studies of pulsed and CW laser interactions. *Exp Eye Res.* 1995;60:359–371.
11. Schuman JS, Jacobson JJ, Puliafito CA, et al. Experimental use of semiconductor diode laser in contact transscleral cyclophotocoagulation in rabbits. *Arch Ophthalmol.* 1990;108:1152–1157.
12. L'Esperance FA Jr. Clinical photocoagulation with the organic dye laser: a preliminary communication. *Arch Ophthalmol.* 1985;103:1312–1316.
13. Gibson KF, Kernohan WG. Lasers in medicine—a review. *J Med Eng Technol.* 1993;17:51–57.
14. Sliney DH, Wolbarsht ML. *Safety with Lasers and Other Optical Sources: A Comprehensive Handbook.* New York, NY: Plenum Press; 1980.
15. Hong C, Kitazawa Y, Tanishima T. Influence of argon laser treatment of glaucoma on corneal endothelium. *Jpn J Ophthalmol.* 1983;27:567–574.
16. Wu SC, Jeng S, Huang SC, et al. Corneal endothelial damage after neodymium:YAG laser iridotomy. *Ophthalmic Surg Lasers.* 2000;31:411–416.
17. Thoming C, Van Buskirk EM, Samples JR. The corneal endothelium after laser therapy for glaucoma. *Am J Ophthalmol.* 1987;103:518–522.
18. Schwenn O, Sell F, Pfeiffer N, et al. Prophylactic Nd:YAG-laser iridotomy versus surgical iridectomy: a randomized, prospective study. *Ger J Ophthalmol.* 1995;4:374–379.
19. Arden GB, Berninger T, Hogg CR, et al. A survey of color discrimination in German ophthalmologists: changes associated with the use of lasers and operating microscopes. *Ophthalmology.* 1991;98:567–575.
20. Berninger TA, Canning CR, Gunduz K, et al. Using argon laser blue light reduces ophthalmologists' color contrast sensitivity: argon blue and surgeons' vision. *Arch Ophthalmol.* 1989;107:1453–1458.
21. Sliney DH, Mainster MA. Potential laser hazards to the clinician during photocoagulation. *Am J Ophthalmol.* 1987;103:758–760.

36

Surgery of the Anterior Chamber Angle and Iris

In this chapter, we consider the laser and incisional operations that are designed to reduce the intraocular pressure (IOP) through increased aqueous outflow by treating specific structures of the anterior chamber angle and the iris. (Filtration procedures and glaucoma drainage-device surgery, which involve not only the anterior chamber angle but also limbal and external ocular tissues, are considered in Chapters 38 and 39, respectively; procedures for children are discussed in Chapter 40.)

LASER TRABECULOPLASTY

Historical Background

In 1961, Zweng and Flocks (1) introduced the concept of applying light energy to the anterior chamber angle for the treatment of glaucoma. Using the xenon-arc photocoagulator of Meyer-Schwickerath (discussed later in this chapter), they selectively coagulated the filtration angles of cats, dogs, and monkeys and reported subsequent lowering of the IOP. Histopathologic examination of the treated tissue revealed fragmentation of the trabecular lamellae, atrophy of ciliary muscle, and destruction of ciliary processes. Little more was said about this technique, however, until more than a decade later, when several investigators revived the concept by using the light energy of the laser. Yet another decade of investigative work would elapse before the operation would achieve widespread clinical popularity.

In the early 1970s, reports began to appear from several parts of the world, most notably from Krasnov (2) in Russia, Hager (3) in Germany, Demailly and associates (4) in France, and Worthen and Wickham (5) in the United States, regarding attempts to improve aqueous outflow by creating holes in the trabecular meshwork with laser energy. Although trabecular perforations were achieved, they eventually closed in most cases due to fibrosis, and IOP reduction was usually temporary. The value of laser treatment to the trabecular meshwork came under further question when, in 1975, Gaasterland and Kupfer (6) reported that experimental glaucoma could be produced by applying argon laser energy to the meshwork of rhesus monkeys. The following year, however, Ticho and Zauberman (7) noted that long-term reduction in IOP occurred in some patients despite the lack of permanent trabecular openings. This led to a new concept in laser trabecular therapy in which lower energy levels were used to photocoagulate, rather than to penetrate, portions of the meshwork. In 1979, Wise and Witter (8) described the first successful protocol of what has become known as laser trabeculoplasty. Their preliminary work was corroborated in 1981 (9–11).

In the subsequent years, many different energy sources producing different wavelengths of laser light, such as krypton (red [647.1 nm] or yellow [568.2 nm] wavelengths), Nd:YAG (neodymium:yttrium–aluminum–garnet) (continuous-wave [1064 nm] and frequency-double Q-switched [532 nm]), and diode (840 nm), have been studied for laser trabeculoplasty (12–20). At the time of publication, the only other laser that has attained popularity is the frequency-doubled Nd:YAG laser, otherwise known as selective laser trabeculoplasty (SLT).

Theories of Mechanism

Argon Laser Trabeculoplasty

Tonographic studies indicate that argon laser trabeculoplasty (ALT) reduces IOP by improving the facility of outflow (12, 21–24), while showing no significant influence on aqueous production on fluorophotometric investigations (23,25,26). Although fluorescein leakage into the anterior chamber is seen during the first week after trabeculoplasty, suggesting a breakdown in the blood–aqueous barrier, it is gone within 1 month and does not seem to be a factor in the long-term effect of this procedure (27).

The mechanism of improved aqueous outflow facility by ALT is uncertain. Wise and Witter (8) originally postulated that the thermal energy produced by pigment absorption of laser light caused shrinkage of collagen in the trabecular lamellae. They believed that the subsequent shortening of the treated meshwork might enlarge existing spaces between two treatment sites or expand the Schlemm canal by pulling the meshwork centrally. Laboratory studies have provided partial support for this theory but have also suggested alternative or additional mechanisms of action.

Light and electron microscopic and immunohistochemical evaluations of trabecular meshwork from normal and glaucomatous human eyes, obtained hours to weeks after ALT, revealed disruption of trabecular beams, fibrinous material, and necrosis of occasional cells, followed by shrinkage of the collagenous components of the meshwork and accumulation of fibronectin in the aqueous drainage channels (28–33). Surviving endothelial cells near the laser lesions showed phagocytic and migratory activity (29,30). Specimens obtained several months after therapy had partial or total occlusion of intertrabecular spaces by a monocellular layer (28,30,31). These observations were thought to support the theories of heat-induced shrinkage of collagen in the trabecular lamellae with possible stretching of the meshwork between two treatment sites and fibronectin-mediated attachment of trabecular beams supporting an adhesive tightening of the trabecular components (31).

Studies with monkeys have provided similar observations to those noted in humans, with some additional insight into the mechanism of ALT. Within the first few hours, there is disruption of the trabecular beams and coagulative necrosis with accumulation of debris in the juxtacanalicular region (34). As with human eyes, surviving trabecular endothelial cells are noted to have increased phagocytic activity with removal of tissue debris and increased cell division (34,35). By 1 month, the treated regions are flat with collapsed beams and are covered with an endothelial layer (36). The latter is more likely to occur when the laser energy is applied to the anterior portion of the trabecular meshwork (37). Perfusion with ferritin shows lack of flow through the treated meshwork, with diversion of flow through the adjacent nonlasered meshwork, which becomes structurally altered to compensate for the overload of flow (38). It has also been suggested that concomitant collagen degeneration and loss of trabecular cells may widen the intertrabecular spaces with improved outflow (39). However, light and electron microscopic studies of the trabecular meshwork and the inner wall of the Schlemm canal 3 to 17 months after 360-degree trabeculoplasty in monkeys revealed no significant difference from untreated eyes (40). Whether the human eye has similar reparative capacity is unclear, but this and other studies suggest that alternative or additional mechanisms to the mechanical theory must account for the long-term benefit of laser trabeculoplasty.

Studies of human autopsy eyes treated with ALT revealed a significant reduction in the trabecular cell density and an increase in radioactive sulfate incorporation into the extracellular matrix of laser-treated eyes (41). The latter findings have also been reported with human trabecular tissue treated with ALT before trabeculectomy and subsequently studied with radioactive leucine (31), and in cat eyes that were studied in vivo with radioactive thymidine following trabeculoplasty (42,43). Studies with a human corneoscleral organ culture system indicate that ALT causes an early trabecular endothelial cell division in the anterior meshwork, with migration of the new cells to repopulate the burn sites over the next few weeks (44,45).

It has been postulated that ALT eliminates some trabecular cells, which may stimulate the remaining cells to produce a different composition of extracellular matrix with improved outflow properties (41–43). This hypothesis is further supported by demonstration of induction of matrix metalloproteinases in response to laser trabeculoplasty (46–48). The matrix metalloproteinases are the enzymes that normally break down the extracellular matrix to maintain normal turnover of the trabecular meshwork (49). Manipulation of activity of these enzymes has been demonstrated in perfused human anterior segment organ culture to increase outflow facility with increasing matrix metalloproteinases (50). Evaluation of two members of the matrix metalloproteinases family, stromelysin and gelatinase B, after ALT of anterior segment organ cultures also supports the hypothesis that extracellular matrix turnover is important in the regulation of aqueous humor outflow. An

increase of stromelysin expression has been demonstrated in the juxtacanalicular region of the meshwork in response to laser trabeculoplasty (47). This would be expected to degrade trabecular proteoglycans, a presumed source of outflow resistance in the juxtacanalicular meshwork. If reduced juxtacanalicular extracellular matrix turnover is responsible for the reduction in aqueous humor outflow, an increase in stromelysin in this specific area of the meshwork should increase the outflow (47).

Additional studies have been designed to identify factors that mediate the matrix metalloproteinases response to ALT. Matrix metalloproteinases expression was increased by adding recombinant interleukin-1α in human anterior segment organ cultures and tumor necrosis factor-α in porcine trabecular meshwork (50,51). Expression of stromelysin was partially blocked by either interleukin-1 receptor antagonist or tumor necrosis factor-α–blocking antibodies (48).

Although the precise mechanism of ALT still remains only partially understood, an initial mechanical injury appears to trigger activation of unique signaling pathways resulting in cellular response and tissue remodeling, leading to an improved outflow (52).

Selective Laser Trabeculoplasty

In 1995, Latina and Park reported that the energy of a Q-switched, frequency-doubled Nd:YAG laser would preferentially be absorbed by pigmented trabecular meshwork cells, in culture (53), called an SLT (54,55). The laser selectively targets pigmented trabecular meshwork cells without causing structural damage to nonpigmented cells. Experimental study on the trabecular meshwork from human autopsy eyes after SLT revealed no coagulative damage or disruption of the corneoscleral or uveal trabecular beams (32). The only evidence of laser tissue interaction with SLT was cracking of intracytoplasmic pigment granules and disruption of trabecular endothelial cells, suggesting that it may potentially be a repeatable procedure (32). Evaluation of the trabecular meshwork after ALT revealed crater formation in the uveal meshwork at the junction of the pigmented and nonpigmented trabecular meshwork, with coagulative damage at the base and along the edge of craters, disruption of the collagen beams, fibrinous exudate, lysis of endothelial cells, and nuclear and cytoplasmic debris (32). However, in another study, the mechanical damage observed after low-power ALT and SLT was similar, with both lasers producing disruption of trabecular beams, cellular debris, and fragmentation of endothelium (33). The similarity of changes in the trabecular meshwork produced by both lasers may explain their similar IOP-lowering responses (33).

The impact of 360-degree SLT on free oxygen radicals and antioxidant enzymes of the aqueous humor has been evaluated in rabbits. Concentrations of lipid peroxide in the aqueous humor of the treated eyes were significantly higher than those in the untreated eyes until the 7th day (56). Glutathione S-transferase levels were significantly decreased between 12 hours and 7 days after the trabeculoplasty, suggesting that free oxygen radicals are formed in the pigmented trabecular meshwork during SLT and may be responsible for the inflammatory complications of this procedure (56).

Basic Techniques

Instruments

The original laser unit for trabeculoplasty is the continuous-wave argon laser. It has traditionally been operated in the blue-green, biochromatic wavelength spectrum (454.5 to 528.7 nm). No differences were noted in the postoperative IOP course or incidence of complications when compared with the use of green, monochromatic laser light (514.5 nm) (57). As noted in the previous chapter, however, green-only argon light may be safer for the surgeon with regard to an influence on color vision. The Q-switched Nd:YAG laser has only one wavelength setting, at 532 nm.

A contact lens with a mirror for visualization of the anterior chamber angle (gonioprism) is used in trabeculoplasty. As with all contact lenses for laser application, it should have an antireflection coating on the front surface. A standard Goldmann-type three-mirror lens, in which one mirror is inclined at 59 degrees for gonioscopy, or a single-mirror gonioscopy lens can be used (**Fig. 36.1**). Both, however, have the slight disadvantage of requiring rotation of the lens to view all quadrants of the anterior chamber angle. This disadvantage can be eliminated by using the Thorpe four-mirror gonioscopy lens, in which all mirrors are inclined at 62 degrees, or the Ritch trabeculoplasty laser lens, in which two mirrors are inclined at 59 degrees for viewing the inferior quadrants and two at 64 degrees for viewing the superior angle (58,59). In the latter lens, a 17-diopter (D) planoconvex button lens over two mirrors provides 1.4× magnification, reducing a 50-μm laser spot to 35 μm, which may be particularly useful, because a 50-μm spot size with most argon lasers produces a burn in excess of 70 μm (60). A double-mirror gonioscopic lens has also been developed to facilitate the visualization of the anterior chamber angle (61). The Latina lens was specifically designed for SLT and has a single mirror at a 63-degree angle; it has a 1.0× magnification to maintain the 400-μm spot size.

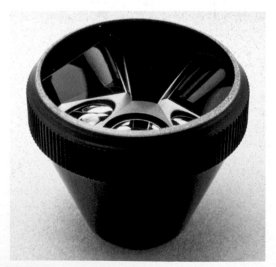

Figure 36.1 The Goldmann-type three-mirror lens, modified with antireflection coating, is a commonly used gonioprism for visualizing the anterior chamber angle and for use in performing laser trabeculoplasty.

Gonioscopic Considerations

Successful laser trabeculoplasty requires accurate identification and treatment of the trabecular meshwork. The surgeon must, therefore, have a detailed knowledge of the anterior chamber angle anatomy and its many variations. The basic aspects of this subject are discussed in Chapters 2 and 34; additional features that are pertinent to laser trabeculoplasty are considered here.

Two variations of the anterior chamber angle that may interfere with accurate laser application to the trabecular meshwork are (a) the degree of pigmentation and (b) the width of the chamber angle. With regard to pigmentation, some angles are so diffusely pigmented from the ciliary body band to the Schwalbe line that the exact location of the meshwork is obscured. This is usually most marked in the inferior quadrants, and a careful inspection of all quadrants before starting treatment usually discloses the functional position of the meshwork in some areas, which can then be used as a guide in locating the meshwork in the remainder of the angle. At the opposite extreme, the trabecular meshwork in some angles is so lightly pigmented that it is hard to see. In some cases, iris processes, which normally extend to the meshwork, may be a useful indicator. Identification of the ciliary body band or Schwalbe line may also help determine the relative position of the meshwork.

A narrow anterior chamber angle can lead to improper placement of the laser burns or may prohibit performing trabeculoplasty. If the peripheral iris obscures the visualization of the meshwork, a heavily pigmented Schwalbe line may be mistaken for the meshwork. Rotating the contact lens in relation to the eye, by asking the patient to look in the direction of the mirror being used, often provides a deeper view into the angle, enhancing visualization of the meshwork. Care must be taken with this maneuver, however, not to distort the size and shape of the aiming beam. If positioning of the contact lens is not sufficient to expose the meshwork, the chamber angle may be deepened by applying low-energy laser burns to the peripheral iris, a technique called iridoplasty or gonioplasty (discussed later in this chapter). If the angle is still too narrow, a laser iridotomy (also discussed later in this chapter) should be performed, and the trabeculoplasty should be done at a later date.

Original Protocol

The original protocol of Wise and Witter (8) has remained the standard approach to ALT against which variations in technique have been evaluated. A 25× magnification in the slitlamp delivery system usually provides an optimum balance between detail and field of view. Argon laser settings of 0.1-second duration exposure and 50-μm beam diameter have remained constant through most variations in protocol. One study compared durations of 0.2 to 0.1 second and found no advantage to the former (62). The most commonly used power levels range between 700 and 1500 mW, with an average of 1000 mW. A survey by the American Society of Cataract and Refractive Surgery in 1999 indicated that most general ophthalmologists use a duration of 0.1 second and a spot size of 50 μm, and that 39% of the respondents use initial power between 501 and

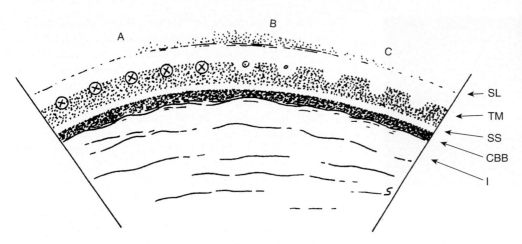

Figure 36.2 Placement of laser burns *(A)* along anterior portion of trabecular meshwork *(TM)*. Desired visual result is depigmentation of the treatment site *(B,C)* or a small gas bubble *(B)*. *SL*, Schwalbe line; *SS*, scleral spur; *CBB*, ciliary body band; *I*, iris.

799 mW and 41% use 800 to 1000 mW (63). One study evaluated powers ranging from 100 to 1000 mW and found that power of more than 500 mW gave the maximum success rates (64). The power should be adjusted to produce a depigmentation spot or a small gas bubble at the treatment site (**Fig. 36.2**). This response is influenced by the amount of pigment in the trabecular meshwork. With a heavily pigmented meshwork, a lower power level may be sufficient, whereas lightly pigmented meshworks require higher levels. In a retrospective study, the decrease of IOP was greater in the eyes in which ALT was a primary therapy and was not influenced by the power level (65). The initial IOP response to ALT in patients with glaucoma associated with exfoliation syndrome was greater than in patients with chronic open-angle glaucoma (COAG) (66,67), although the long-term outcome was similar (66). A preoperative IOP higher than 31 mm Hg and visual field defect and light pigmentation of the trabecular meshwork were found to be predictive of ALT failure (67).

Originally, ALT laser burns were applied onto or immediately posterior to the pigmented band of the trabecular meshwork, with approximately 100 applications evenly spaced around the full 360 degrees of the meshwork (8). Complications associated with this basic protocol, however, led to variations in technique. We consider, first, the complications and how they are managed and, then, the variations in technique that have been used to minimize the complications.

With SLT, a total of approximately 50 to 70 adjacent, nonoverlapping spots are placed over 180 degrees of the trabecular meshwork, with energy ranging from 0.5 to 1.2 mJ per pulse, set to prevent bubble formation. Typically, the power is titrated until the appearance of tiny air bubbles are released from the site of the laser burn, termed "champagne bubbles." After the bubbles are seen, the power is slightly reduced to eliminate their appearance.

Alternative Protocols with Argon Laser

The parameter evaluated most extensively has been the total number of laser applications and the amount of trabecular meshwork treated. Applying 25 burns to 90% of the meshwork is less effective than protocols with larger amounts of treatment (68,69). However, the application of 50 burns to 180 degrees or 360 degrees has a similar effect on IOP reduction as treatment of 100 burns to 360 degrees of the meshwork (69–71). In one such study, the eyes receiving 50 applications over 180 or 360 degrees had a lower probability of requiring subsequent filtering surgery than those receiving 100 applications over 360 degrees (72). A two-stage protocol, in which treatment of the full 360-degree circumference is divided into two sessions, 1 month apart, had the same IOP reduction as the full treatment in one session (73). With the latter technique, most of the pressure reduction is achieved with the first stage of therapy, although some patients may have minimal benefit from the first stage and yet a substantial pressure reduction after the second stage (74). The main advantage of the lower number of laser applications during a single session is a reduction in the transient IOP rise in the immediate postoperative period (69–71,73–77). In one study, however, the frequency and magnitude of postlaser IOP increase were the same in groups receiving 360-degree treatment in one or two stages (78). The long-term outcome does not appear to be influenced by which quadrants are treated first. One study randomly assigned patients into initial inferior versus superior halves and found no significant difference between the two groups (72).

Another variation from the basic protocol that appears to minimize the complication of early posttreatment IOP rise is the placement of the laser applications along the anterior portion of the pigmented meshwork (**Fig. 36.3**) (69,71,77). An anterior placement of the laser burns also reduces the complication of peripheral anterior synechiae (79,80). It may, however, increase the potential complication of cellular proliferation from the corneal endothelium over the trabecular meshwork (37).

Complications and Postoperative Management

Transient IOP elevation in the immediate postoperative period is the most serious early complication of ALT (75,76,81–84). In most cases, the pressure rise is mild and lasts less than 24 hours, causing no long-term problems. In some patients, however, the elevation is marked and sustained and can lead to further loss of vision, especially in eyes with advanced visual field loss before trabeculoplasty. The IOP rise occurs within 2 hours after treatment in most cases, although some eyes may not develop an increase until 4 to 7 hours after therapy (82,83). Postoperative

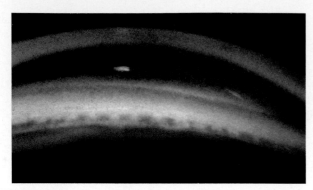

Figure 36.3 Gonioscopic view of patient following argon laser trabeculoplasty. Note the typical blanched lesions of the pigmented trabecular meshwork, which may persist for several days.

management, therefore, should include a pressure check within the first few hours after the procedure. Patients who have a significant early postoperative pressure rise or who have advanced glaucomatous damage may require an IOP check the following day. However, a pressure rise on the first postoperative day is uncommon, with only 4.2% having a rise greater than 3 mm Hg in one study, and seeing most patients in 1 to 3 weeks postoperatively is considered reasonable (85). With SLT, approximately 25% of patients had a transient IOP elevation of 5 to 6 mm Hg (54,86,87), and in one study, some patients had an IOP elevation of more than 10 mm Hg (88).

Histopathologic studies suggest that the mechanism of posttrabeculoplasty pressure rise after ALT is an inflammatory reaction, with fibrinous material and tissue debris in the meshwork (28,34,89,90). Laboratory studies in bovine eyes indicate that the trabecular meshwork can contract in response to endothelin-1, which may be a mechanism in the immediate posttrabeculoplasty IOP elevation (91,92). This hypothesis is supported by the finding of an increased concentration of endothelin-1 in the aqueous humor of rabbit eyes after ALT (93–95).

The main patient characteristic associated with the transient pressure rise is meshwork pigmentation (84). Two patients with exfoliation syndrome had a delayed IOP rise during the first postlaser month, associated with inflammatory precipitates on the trabecular meshwork (96). It should also be noted that eyes with active inflammation are at a high risk for marked IOP rise after ALT, and the operation is contraindicated in these eyes.

Iritis is a common early posttrabeculoplasty complication. In one study, by using a laser flare-cell meter, 49% of 71 eyes showed significant inflammation, which peaked 2 days after treatment (97). The inflammation was significantly more frequent in eyes with exfoliation syndrome or pigmentary glaucoma than in those with COAG. Postoperative iritis is usually mild and transient and is easily controlled with a brief postoperative course of topical corticosteroids. A typical protocol for postoperative management of ALT includes prednisolone, 1%, fluorometholone, 0.1%, or the equivalent four times daily for 5 days. Pretreatment with topical steroids or nonsteroidal anti-inflammatory agents (98–101) has been shown to reduce posttrabeculoplasty inflammation but had no effect on the postoperative IOP elevation (102,103). There is no definite consensus on the posttrabeculoplasty anti-inflammatory regimen following SLT. Various protocols, ranging from use of topical prednisolone acetate, 1%, to use of a topical nonsteroidal anti-inflammatory agent, to use of no anti-inflammatory agents, have been used. However, a greater anterior chamber reaction was seen after the SLT than after ALT in one study (104).

The formation of peripheral anterior synechiae is also a common complication of trabeculoplasty (79). These are typically small and tented, corresponding to the location of the laser applications. Alterations of corneal endothelium after ALT may include a significant increase in cell size (105), although another study showed no statistically significant changes (106). The formation of peripheral anterior synechiae after SLT is rare.

The most serious late-posttrabeculoplasty complication is, at the present time, more theoretical than real. Histopathologic studies, as previously described, show changes in the trabecular meshwork, including an endothelial layer over the inner surface (**Fig. 36.4**), which could eventually lead to an increase in

Figure 36.4 Scanning electron microscopic view of trabeculectomy specimen from eye with failed argon laser trabeculoplasty showing endothelial growth over portions of the intertrabecular spaces (arrows).

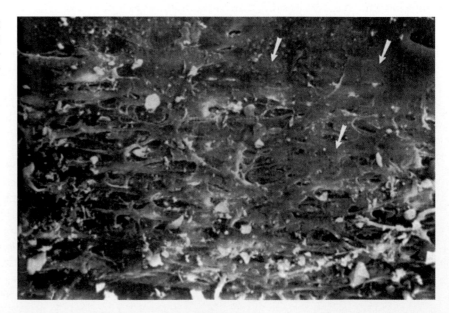

resistance to aqueous outflow (28–30,36,37). One retrospective study evaluated ALT specimens treated with one or more ALT procedures before trabeculectomy and found that eyes treated with argon laser had an increased incidence of membrane formation in the chamber angle. Half of the specimens had a cellular and collagenous membrane covering the entire trabecular meshwork, which was more common in eyes in which more ALT procedures were performed (107). Whether these structural changes eventually make the glaucoma more difficult to control has never been proven, despite more than 30 years of experience. There is, however, a limit to the amount of laser treatment that an eye can tolerate, and the success is time limited in nearly all patients, as discussed later in this chapter. There has also been concern that laser trabeculoplasty might interfere with the success rate of subsequent filtering surgery, causing a higher rate of encapsulation in eyes with previous ALT (108), although this did not appear to be the case in another study (109).

Pharmacologic Control of Increased Pressure

Topical application of the α_2-adrenergic agonist apraclonidine, 1%, at 1 hour before and immediately after laser trabeculoplasty was shown to have a marked effect on minimizing the postoperative pressure rise (110). When compared with eyes treated with pilocarpine, 4%, timolol, 0.5%, dipivefrin, 0.1%, or acetazolamide, 250 mg, each given 1 hour before and immediately after trabeculoplasty, only 3% of apraclonidine-treated eyes had IOP increases greater than 5 mm Hg, in contrast to 33%, 32%, 38%, and 39%, respectively, with the other treatments (111). A single drop of apraclonidine 15 minutes before or immediately after the laser treatment is as effective as the two doses, and apraclonidine, 0.5%, is as effective as 1% (112–115). This has now become a standard part of laser trabeculoplasty for most surgeons. So profound is the benefit of apraclonidine that treatment in two sessions of 180 degrees each may no longer be necessary to avoid the transient IOP rise. In one study, 360-degree trabeculoplasty with perioperative apraclonidine had the same early postoperative IOP course as the 180% treatment without apraclonidine (116). However, caution is advised for patients on long-term α_2-adrenergic agonist therapy, in which case the apraclonidine may be less effective.

The selective α_2-adrenergic agonist brimonidine, 0.5%, has been shown to effectively control the postlaser pressure rise when given either before or after the laser surgery (117,118). Brimonidine, 0.2%, has also been found to be as effective as apraclonidine, 1.0%, in preventing IOP spikes after ALT (119).

Pilocarpine, 4%, alone immediately after ALT was also shown to be effective in minimizing the IOP elevation (120). In a randomized trial, apraclonidine, 1%, was not effective in preventing the IOP spikes in patients on long-term apraclonidine (121). Pilocarpine, 4%, was only slightly less effective in patients on long-term pilocarpine therapy and was at least as effective as apraclonidine, 1%, in post-ALT IOP spike prophylaxis. Another study found that adding pilocarpine to apraclonidine therapy further reduced the incidence of postoperative pressure rise (122). Pilocarpine, therefore, can be considered as a first choice for prevention of posttrabeculoplasty IOP spike, especially in patients treated with apraclonidine (121) or possibly with other α_2-adrenergic agonists.

Acetazolamide was also shown to reduce the IOP rise following ALT in one study (123), although, as previously noted, it is less effective than apraclonidine (111). As discussed previously, neither corticosteroids (98), nor the prostaglandin synthetase inhibitors indomethacin or flurbiprofen, significantly influenced the postoperative IOP (99,100,124,125). One study showed that patients receiving topical indomethacin had higher pressures after 1 month than those receiving a placebo (124). Prostaglandin synthetase inhibitors also appear to have no influence on the postoperative iritis (100,126).

Results

Short-Term Intraocular Pressure Control

Most reports show that useful IOP reduction is achieved in approximately 85% of eyes treated with ALT (8–11,22,75,127). Some eyes may have a pressure drop within the first few hours after treatment, although days or weeks are usually required to achieve the full response to ALT and SLT, with further IOP reduction rarely occurring beyond 1 month. The magnitude of the final pressure reduction averages 6 to 9 mm Hg, which is usually insufficient to allow discontinuation of all medical therapy, although the medication can occasionally be reduced or eliminated (128). One study suggested that pilocarpine may lose its effectiveness after ALT (129), and it may be advisable to re-evaluate the efficacy of any miotic treatment approximately 1 month after the laser treatment. However, a later study showed no difference between the IOP-lowering effect of pilocarpine, 1%, before and after ALT (130).

The IOP reduction after the SLT ranged from 3 to 18 mm Hg (86). Six months after 180-degree SLT, the mean IOP reduction was 4.4 mm Hg, with a success rate of 64.6%. An elevated preoperative IOP was the significant determinant for success, whereas age, sex, history of ALT, and trabecular meshwork pigmentation were not significantly related to success (87). When the trabecular meshwork was treated 360 degrees with the SLT, the IOP was reduced in all eyes by approximately 40% at 6 weeks after the treatment (88). In a prospective study, 50 eyes were treated with SLT, with the mean IOP reduction of approximately 5 mm Hg at 1, 3, 6, and 12 months (131). In another clinical trial of 10 eyes treated with SLT, the IOP was reduced only slightly less in the exfoliative glaucoma than in the COAG (132). In a randomized trial, patients with previously failed ALT had a better IOP reduction with the selective laser than with a repeated argon laser (104). IOP lowering during the first 6 months after the SLT was similar to that of ALT and appears to diminish over the first year of follow-up (133).

Factors Affecting IOP Response

Many factors influence the IOP response to ALT. Eyes with a higher pretreatment IOP tend to have a greater decrease in IOP (134), but a pretreatment IOP greater than 30 mm Hg has been associated with a higher frequency of failure (135,136), whereas eyes with pressures closer to the target IOP may obtain useful pressure reduction after trabeculoplasty (137–139).

Another significant factor influencing IOP response to ALT is the type of glaucoma. A particularly favorable response is obtained with COAG, exfoliation syndrome, and pigmentary glaucoma (21,127,134,135,140–143). Success in the latter two conditions is most likely related to the favorable influence of increased trabecular meshwork pigmentation (144). In pigmentary glaucoma, younger patients appear to have a more sustained pressure reduction than older patients with the same condition do (142,143). Some clinicians have noted that eyes with darkly pigmented trabecular meshwork are at greater risk for an immediate IOP spike following SLT (145). In these eyes, decreasing the power of the SLT is generally recommended.

Other forms of glaucoma that respond to ALT, although less well than those noted earlier, include open-angle glaucoma in aphakia or pseudophakia and angle-closure glaucoma after an iridotomy (140,146). Although eyes that have had multiple operations generally do not do well with ALT (141), those with a single failed trabeculectomy may obtain useful pressure reduction after the laser surgery (147). Other forms of glaucoma that do not respond well to ALT include glaucoma associated with uveitis, angle-recession glaucoma, and congenital or juvenile glaucoma (140,141).

Some investigators believe that young age has an unfavorable effect on the results of laser trabeculoplasty (127,136,148), although one study showed no effect of age (135). As previously noted, young patients with pigmentary glaucoma appear to do better than older patients with the same condition (142,143).

Race may influence the results of laser trabeculoplasty (149). In the Advanced Glaucoma Intervention Study (AGIS), eyes were randomly assigned to an ALT–trabeculectomy–trabeculectomy sequence or a trabeculectomy–ALT–trabeculectomy sequence. The initial report from this randomized clinical trial recommended the initial use of the ALT for all black patients (150). However, a later report from the AGIS provided only a weak suggestion that an initial trabeculoplasty delays the progression of glaucoma more effectively in black patients than in white patients (151).

Long-Term Intraocular Pressure Control

A major question regarding the results of laser trabeculoplasty is how long the IOP reduction will last. Although a high percentage of patients show an initial favorable reduction in IOP, most patients gradually lose this effect (152–159). Failure is most common in the first year, with reported rates of 19% to 23%, and thereafter failure occurs at a rate of 5% to 9% per year (157,159). As a result, approximately half of the patients will have lost the benefit of the initial trabeculoplasty by 5 years, and two thirds within 10 years, after the procedure (159).

Repeated Trabeculoplasty

If a successful IOP reduction is never achieved after 360-degree ALT, further argon laser treatment is generally not thought to be indicated. When an initial good response to treatment, lasting for approximately 1 year or more, was followed by a return to higher pressures, repeated trabeculoplasty was once common

practice. However, most studies have shown a much lower success rate with repeated ALT than with the initial treatment, in the range of one third to one half (158,160–166). In one long-term study, success rates with repeated ALT were 35% at 6 months, 21% at 12 months, 11% at 24 months, and 5% at 48 months (166). Although one study suggested that the ALT can be repeated with good results (167), most surgeons no longer recommend repeated ALT. Some studies have noted a higher incidence of transient IOP rise after repeated ALT (160,161,166), and it is probably advisable to perform these in two stages of 180 degrees each, if a repeated procedure is attempted.

SLT caused more significant IOP lowering in patients with previously failed ALT compared with repeated ALT in a randomized trial (104). Repeated SLT may be almost as effective as initial SLT based on a single retrospective study (168). Repeated SLT, after either initial SLT or initial ALT, may become accepted practice, although further long-term experience is needed. Because of the greater preservation of trabecular meshwork with SLT, it has been suggested that SLT may be less likely to interfere with future incisional surgery (169).

Indications

Laser trabeculoplasty may be indicated in the treatment of those forms of open-angle glaucoma in which favorable responses have been reported, including COAG, exfoliation syndrome, pigmentary glaucoma, and open-angle glaucoma in aphakia or pseudophakia. The IOP-lowering effect was more pronounced in pseudophakic than aphakic eyes, and in eyes that had extracapsular surgery rather than intracapsular surgery (170). ALT was also preferred to cyclocryotherapy for the initial treatment of patients with uncontrolled glaucoma after a penetrating keratoplasty (171).

During the first decade of experience with ALT, the procedure was used as a supplement to maximum tolerable medical therapy, and studies have shown it to be effective in this regard (75,172). The rationale for this approach was based not only on the risk for early postoperative complications, especially the transient pressure rise, but also on the concern that eyes treated with laser trabeculoplasty might eventually become more difficult to control than if they had been left on medical therapy. The histopathologic studies showing proliferation of a cellular layer over the trabecular meshwork have given reason to seriously consider this theoretical complication (28,30,36,37). Nevertheless, short-term and long-term studies of ALT for open-angle glaucoma suggest that the procedure may be a safe and effective initial treatment of glaucoma (172–179).

In a multicenter clinical trial (the Glaucoma Laser Trial), 271 patients with newly diagnosed open-angle glaucoma were randomly assigned to initial ALT in one eye and timolol, 0.5%, in the other eye, with the same stepped regimen of additional medical therapy in either eye as required (178). During the first 2 years of follow-up, the laser-treated eyes had a slightly lower mean IOP of 1 to 2 mm Hg, although more than half of these eyes eventually required the addition of one or more medications. In a follow-up study of 203 of these patients, with a mean duration of 7 years, eyes initially treated with laser trabeculoplasty had 1.2–mm Hg greater reduction in IOP, 0.6-dB greater improvement in visual field, and slightly less optic nerve head deterioration (179). Although these findings suggest that initial treatment with ALT is at least as efficacious as initial treatment with topical medications that were available at the time of the study, medical therapy is still more commonly used in North America, particularly with the newer, more efficient IOP-lowering topical medications.

A shorter-term study comparing SLT and a topical prostaglandin, latanoprost, found that the two therapies were equally effective over 1 year (180,181). Randomized, controlled trials comparing treatment of 180 degrees of trabecular meshwork with ALT versus SLT showed no difference regarding effectiveness of IOP lowering up to 5 years (182,183). However, most clinicians treat 360 degrees of trabecular meshwork with SLT at one time. Some support in the literature indicates that 360 degrees is more effective than 180 degrees (181,184). Furthermore, a second treatment of the trabecular meshwork using SLT after SLT or ALT as the first laser trabeculoplasty is effective (168,185).

LASER IRIDOTOMY

Historical Background

In 1956, Meyer-Schwickerath (186) first reported the use of light energy to create a hole in the iris. Using the xenon-arc photocoagulator, he and others found that a peripheral iridotomy could be produced, but that the amount of heat required damaged the cornea and the lens (186,187). With the introduction of lasers in the 1960s, investigation of this treatment modality continued, primarily with ruby lasers (188–191). However, as with laser trabeculoplasty, laser iridotomy became clinically practical after the advent of argon laser technology in the 1970s. By the mid-1970s, several reports of successful argon laser iridotomy appeared in the literature (192–195), and by the end of that decade, laser iridotomy had replaced incisional iridectomy as the surgical procedure of choice for angle-closure glaucomas. During the 1980s, continued study of laser iridotomy techniques led to the popular use of the Nd:YAG laser for this operation.

Techniques

The basic principle of laser iridotomy is the creation of a hole in the peripheral iris with an argon or Nd:YAG laser, which allows equalization of the pressure between the posterior and anterior chambers, deepening of the anterior chamber, and opening of the anterior chamber angle.

Instruments

Several different types of lasers and surgical techniques can be used to create an iridotomy. The unit most commonly used in the early days of laser surgery was the continuous-wave argon laser (192–201). Other lasers were also shown to be effective for creating iridotomies, including the pulsed argon laser and the krypton laser (197,202,203). However, the pulsed Nd:YAG laser subsequently gained popularity and is the most commonly used unit for creating laser iridotomies today (204–211). A portable Nd:YAG laser is effective for use in remote geographic areas (212). Other lasers have also been evaluated for performing iridotomies. Those units and the relative merits of the argon versus Nd:YAG laser iridotomies are considered later in this chapter.

A contact lens is helpful in performing a laser iridotomy, because it (a) keeps the lids separated, (b) minimizes corneal epithelial burns by acting as a heat sink, and (c) provides some control of eye movement. In addition, convex-surfaced contact lenses have been designed to increase the power density on the iris (213–215). The most commonly used is the Abraham iridotomy lens, which has a 66-D planoconvex button bonded to the front surface of the contact lens (**Fig. 36.5**) (213). This lens doubles the laser-beam diameter at the level of the cornea, while reducing it to approximately one half of the original size on the iris, which reduces the power density at the cornea to one fourth of the original level and increases it on the iris by a factor of four. Another contact lens, the Wise iridotomy–sphincterotomy lens, has a 103-D optical button decentered at

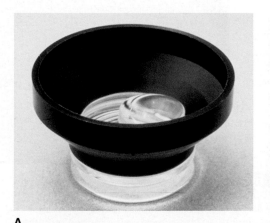
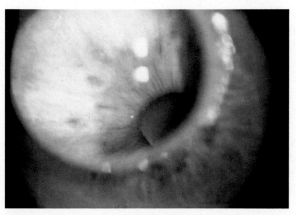

A   **B**

Figure 36.5   **A:** Abraham contact lens with planoconvex button bonded to front surface for laser iridotomy. **B:** Slitlamp view of an iris magnified with the Abraham iridotomy lens.

2.5 mm, which further reduces the iris focal spot and increases the energy density (215). These principles have their greatest application with the argon laser, although the same contact lenses are also useful with the Nd:YAG laser.

With all lasers and contact lenses, a high magnification (e.g., 40×) should be used in the slitlamp delivery system.

Preoperative Medication

Topical pilocarpine may be instilled before the procedure, which helps to maximally thin and stretch the peripheral iris. If the patient presents with an acute attack of angle-closure glaucoma, it is best to break the attack medically, if possible, and maintain the patient on medication to allow clearing of any corneal edema and to facilitate constriction of the pupil. If significant iritis persists after breaking the attack, it may be advisable to use topical steroids for 24 to 48 hours before proceeding with the laser surgery. However, if the attack does not respond to medical therapy, laser iridotomy (or iridoplasty or pupilloplasty, as discussed later in this chapter) may be effective in breaking the attack (216).

In nearly all cases, only topical anesthesia, such as proparacaine, 0.5%, is required. Only rarely is a retrobulbar injection needed for a patient who has nystagmus or is uncooperative. It has become a standard practice among most surgeons to also use topical apraclonidine to reduce the risk for a postoperative IOP rise (217). In the original studies, apraclonidine, 1%, was instilled 45 to 60 minutes before and immediately after the procedure (218), although a single postoperative drop of apraclonidine, 0.5%, has been shown to be as effective as the 1% concentration in preventing IOP elevation (114).

Selection of Treatment Site

Any quadrant of the iris can be used to create the laser iridotomy, although our preference is between 11 and 1 o'clock if the opening will be entirely covered by the lid, and otherwise temporally. The reason for this is to avoid the iridotomy in a location where the lid margin bisects the iridotomy, as this can result in monocular optical symptoms such as transient ghosting of images, blurring, shadows, halos, glare, crescents, or a horizontal line (219,220). When argon laser iridotomy is performed, the 12-o'clock position is usually avoided, because gas bubbles may collect in that area and interfere with completion of the procedure. One exception to the selection of a superior iris quadrant is the patient with silicone oil in an aphakic eye, in which case the iridotomy should be placed inferiorly to avoid blockage by the oil, which rises to the top of the eye.

Whichever quadrant is used, the slitlamp should always be positioned so that the laser beam is directed away from the macula. The iridotomy is usually placed between the middle and peripheral thirds of the iris. However, if this is not feasible, because of peripheral corneal haze or close proximity between peripheral iris and cornea, a more central location can be used, as long as it is peripheral to the sphincter muscle.

Several features of the iris may facilitate creation of the iridotomy. An area of thin iris or a large crypt is usually easier to penetrate. In lightly pigmented eyes, a local area of increased pigmentation, such as a freckle, may improve absorption of argon laser energy. In addition, the radially arranged white collagen strands in the stroma can be very difficult to penetrate, especially with argon laser, and selecting a treatment site where two strands are more widely separated is helpful (221). The collagen strands may also contain radial vessels, which should be avoided with Nd:YAG laser iridotomy.

Techniques with Continuous-Wave Argon Laser

Several basic techniques have been advocated for producing iridotomies with the continuous-wave argon laser. The "hump" technique involves first creating a localized elevation of the iris with a large-diameter, low-energy burn, and then penetrating the hump with small, intense burns (222). In the "drumhead" technique, large-diameter, low-energy burns are placed around the intended treatment site to put the iris on stretch, and that area is then penetrated with small, high-energy burns (198,223). A third, and probably the most commonly used, approach goes directly to penetrating burns (197,200,201). This last technique may be modified by using multiple short-duration burns (224,225). None of these approaches, however, is ideal for all situations, and it is best to tailor the iridotomy technique primarily according to the color of the iris. For irides of any color, the argon laser settings are first selected for the iris stroma and then adjusted for the pigment epithelium.

Medium Brown Iris

This is the easiest iris to penetrate with continuous-wave argon laser, and the following method represents one technique to use in these patients. Protocols for irides of other colors are modifications of this basic technique.

Argon laser settings of 0.1- to 0.2-second duration, 50-μm spot size, and 700 to 1500 mW (average, 1000 mW) are initially used to create a crater in the iris stroma. The first few applications may produce gas bubbles, which usually float up away from the treatment site (**Fig. 36.6**). If the bubble does not move, it can be dislodged by going through it with the next laser

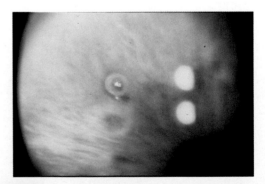

Figure 36.6 Argon laser was used to create a crater in the stroma of this medium brown iris. Gas bubbles (shown) can form with the first few laser applications; they usually float away from the treatment site but can be dislodged by subsequent laser applications, if necessary.

application or by placing the beam adjacent to the bubble. A cluster of several contiguous burns is used to produce a stromal crater of approximately 500 μm in diameter. Additional laser applications are then placed in the bed of the crater until the pigment epithelial layer is reached, as evidenced by a cloud of pigment.

When most of the stroma in the crater has been eliminated and only pigment epithelium remains, the laser intensity should be reduced to clean away the remaining tissue. Typical settings for this stage of the procedure are 100 μm and 500 to 700 mW, or 50 μm and 200 to 600 mW, with a duration of 0.1 to 0.2 second. Higher-intensity burns at this stage of the treatment may dislodge adjacent pigment epithelium, creating a "cascade phenomenon," which causes further obstruction of the iridotomy. These same settings can be used for irides of other colors because the pigment epithelial layer is similar in all eyes.

This two-stage technique for argon laser iridotomy in the medium brown iris normally takes 30 to 60 laser applications to create a patent iridotomy.

Dark Brown Iris

A laser iridotomy is more difficult to achieve in these eyes, partially because of the thick, dense stroma. Standard initial settings (as described previously) often produce a black char in the stromal crater, making the site resistant to further penetration. One way to minimize this complication and achieve a patent iridotomy in the dark brown iris is to use multiple short-duration burns, called the "chipping" technique (222,224,226). The important feature of this modification is the short exposure time of 0.02 to 0.05 second, with standard settings of 50 μm and 700 to 1500 mW. With this approach, minute fragments of stroma are "chipped away," often requiring 200 to 300 applications to penetrate the stroma. Once the pigment epithelial layer is reached, the settings should be changed to the lower intensity level, as described for the medium brown iris, to complete the procedure.

Blue Iris

These eyes can also be difficult with argon laser iridotomy because the lightly pigmented stroma does not absorb laser light sufficiently to produce a burn through this portion of the iris. The pigment epithelium near the treatment site may be dislodged, leaving intact stroma that is impermeable to aqueous flow. Some surgeons prefer a two-stage approach, in which settings of 500 μm and 200 to 300 mW are first used to create a local tan-colored area of increased stromal density, followed by penetration burns of 50 μm, 500 to 700 mW, and 0.1 second to create a full-thickness hole in the stroma (227). Others have suggested a direct approach, using settings of 50 μm, 1000 to 1500 mW, and a prolonged duration of 0.5 second, which usually burns a hole through the stroma in two to three applications (221,226). With either technique, the settings should then be changed to those described for the medium brown iris to penetrate or remove the remaining pigment epithelium from the iridotomy site.

Techniques with Nd:YAG Laser

As previously noted, Nd:YAG is now the most commonly used technique for laser iridotomy. The extremely high energy levels and short exposure times of these lasers electromechanically disrupt tissue, independent of pigment absorption and the thermal effect. As a result, they are particularly useful in creating iridotomies in light blue irides but are effective in all eyes. The technique usually involves simultaneous perforation of the iris stroma and pigment epithelium with energy levels in the range of 5 to 15 mJ (204–211). The pulse duration is fixed for each instrument, in the range of 12 nanoseconds, but the number of pulses per burst can be adjusted in most units, with surgeons generally preferring 1 to 3 pulses per burst. The spot size is also fixed, although some units provide a choice between a single focal point and multiple focal points, with the latter creating a larger lesion. Because the wavelength of the Nd:YAG laser is beyond the visible spectrum, a helium–neon or diode laser beam is typically used for focusing on the iris. With instruments that allow a selected separation between the focal points of the two laser beams, the setting should be such that they are coincident when performing a laser iridotomy.

The standard technique uses the same criteria as for argon laser iridotomy in selecting the iris site, although it is often possible to place the iridotomy more peripherally with the Nd:YAG laser. The latter is desirable, among other reasons, to avoid injuring the lens. When selecting the treatment site, attention should be given to avoid any apparent iris vessels, because these are more likely to bleed with Nd:YAG than with argon laser surgery. A patent iridotomy can often be created with a single laser application, and rarely are more than two or three required, especially in blue or light brown eyes. However, the iridotomy may be smaller than those produced with an argon laser (**Fig. 36.7A,B**). Cases have been reported of acute angle-closure glaucoma in eyes with patent, but small, Nd:YAG laser iridotomies, and it has been suggested that an iridotomy should be at least 150 to 200 μm in diameter (228). The iridotomy may change in shape and position and occasionally in area after dilatation (229), and it is good practice to make it large enough initially but also to check it after dilatation. If there is doubt regarding the size of the iridotomy during the procedure and it is difficult to enlarge it, creating more than one iridotomy is advisable.

Several variations in technique have been described. One uses both the argon and Nd:YAG lasers by first creating a stromal crater with short-duration argon laser burns and then penetrating the iris with low-energy, single-pulse Nd:YAG applications (230–232). This has an advantage of minimizing bleeding by first coagulating iris vessels. It is especially useful in eyes with thick, dark iris stroma, in which the Nd:YAG laser energy may cause considerable disruption and dispersion of stromal tissue before penetrating the iris. Another technique involves multiple low-energy (1.0 to 1.7 mJ) applications in a line across the radial iris fibers to create an iridotomy of larger, more controllable size, which was thought to be safer than a similar approach with the argon laser or the standard, higher-energy Nd:YAG technique (233,234). Iridotomies have also been created experimentally

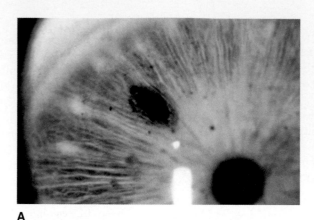 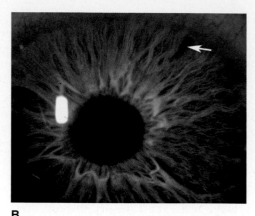

A   **B**

Figure 36.7   **A:** Argon laser iridotomy with patency demonstrated by visualization of anterior lens capsule. **B:** Typical appearance of peripheral iridotomy created with an Nd:YAG laser.

with the transscleral application of longer-duration thermal Nd:YAG laser burns via a fiber-optic system (235).

Techniques with Other Lasers

Pulsed Argon Laser

This instrument emits laser energy in a chain of very short pulses, rather than in a continuous wave, which vaporizes the absorbing tissue with minimal heat loss and destruction to the surrounding area. These features provide some advantage over continuous-wave argon lasers for producing iridotomies in that more energy is used in penetrating the iris, with less distortion and disruption of the surrounding tissue (202).

The basic technique is similar to that for continuous-wave argon laser iridotomy. The settings, however, differ considerably for the pulsed argon laser unit. The perforating mode is used, and the power setting is 20 to 25 W. The usual parameters are 50 μm, 0.2 second, and 300 pulses/sec, adjusted according to tissue response (the individual pulse is fixed at 128 microseconds). With these settings, the number of exposures to achieve an iridotomy varies from 2 to 250, depending on the type of iris (202).

Neodymium: Yttrium Lithium Fluoride (Nd:YLF) Laser

This 1053-nm laser can create iridotomies of precise size and shape with minimal thermal damage to the surrounding tissue because of low energy per pulse levels, with a short pulse duration in picoseconds, and a high repetition rate. Optimal settings, established in a series of cadaver eyes, included a rectangular cutting pattern of 0.3 × 0.3 mm, 500-μm cutting depth, 50-μm spot separation, and 200 to 400 pulses/sec (236,237).

Semiconductor Diode Laser

As noted in Chapter 35, the semiconductor diode laser has several distinct advantages over other lasers, including the small, portable size, the solid-state construction, which provides durability and relatively low maintenance requirements, and the need for only a standard electric outlet and no water cooling. With a wavelength of approximately 805 nm and operation in the continuous-wave mode, the mechanism of iridotomy is like that of the argon laser—that is, absorption by melanin,

resulting in photocoagulation, rather than the electromechanical disruption of the Nd:YAG and Nd:YLF lasers. In rabbit studies and preliminary clinical trials, the settings and the clinical and histopathologic results were all similar to those noted in this chapter for the argon laser (238–240).

Other Lasers

As noted previously, the krypton laser was found to be effective in creating iridotomies (203). A Q-switched ruby laser was also found in monkey studies to be suitable for producing iridotomies (241), and dye lasers have been used clinically to create iridotomies with a single pulse (242). The continuous-wave, frequency-doubled Nd:YAG laser with a wavelength of 532 nm, pumped by a diode laser, successfully created patent iridotomies in rabbit eyes with the thermal damage zones comparable to the argon laser (243).

Results of Argon and Nd:YAG Laser Iridotomies

When laser iridotomy is performed for an acute angle closure, the IOP decreases and remains stable without requiring additional surgery in approximately two thirds of white patients and half of Asian patients (201,244–246). The difference may be explained by mechanisms other than pupillary block, such as changes in the angle morphologic characteristics, a longer duration, and severity of the attack (245,247).

In chronic angle-closure glaucoma, despite widening of the angle in 73% to 97% of eyes (246,248), eyes that have optic disc and visual field damage require filtering surgery in approximately half of the patients, despite the presence of a patent iridotomy (249,250). The outcomes appear to be similar among white and Asian patients (250). The effect of iridotomy on one eye is predictive of the effect on the fellow eye (248).

Prophylactic laser iridotomy prevented IOP elevation in 88.8% of fellow eyes in patients with acute angle closure within 4 years of follow-up and is recommended for the treatment of fellow eyes of patients with acute angle closure (250,251). However, because some of the fellow eyes may experience IOP elevation within 6 to 12 months, despite the presence of a patent iridotomy, close follow-up is recommended (245,252).

Comparison of Argon and Nd:YAG Laser Iridotomies

Histologic studies have shown that iridotomies created with an argon laser have more extensive early edema and tissue destruction at the margins of the treatment site than iridotomies created with the Nd:YAG laser, in which the lesions are more circumscribed with limited tissue alterations at the margins (202,209,211,253). However, freeze-frame analysis of high-speed cinematography in ox eyes showed particles traveling over 8 mm from the Nd:YAG treatment site at speeds in excess of 20 km/h (210), and the shock waves affected the trabecular meshwork and corneal endothelium of monkey eyes when the Nd:YAG application was within 0.8 mm of the limbus (254).

Argon and Nd:YAG laser iridotomies were compared in human autopsy eyes using a high-magnification video recording system that allowed real-time observation of the posterior iris during the laser procedures (255). With argon laser iridotomy, gradual mounding up of iris pigment epithelium occurred with each successive energy application before final penetration. In contrast, Nd:YAG laser iridotomy caused a complete disruption and dispersal of the pigment epithelium with a single pulse of energy. These observations may explain the tendency for argon laser iridotomies to become obstructed with pigment epithelium, which is rarely seen with Nd:YAG laser iridotomies.

In clinical comparisons of the two surgical approaches, the Nd:YAG laser iridotomies had the disadvantage of frequent bleeding, although this usually stops spontaneously or by applying pressure to the eye with the contact lens and rarely leads to significant complications (206,207,256,257). Disadvantages of argon laser iridotomy, on the other hand, include more iritis, pupillary distortion, and late closure of the iridotomy. When an iridotomy could not be created with the argon laser, a patent iridotomy was be achieved in all eyes with the Nd:YAG laser in single sessions (258). Nd:YAG laser iridotomies, in general, require considerably fewer total applications, with a marked reduction in total energy delivery, compared with argon laser iridotomies.

Prevention and Management of Complications

As with laser trabeculoplasty, a transient IOP rise and a mild anterior uveitis are common early postoperative complications. Other potential complications include closure of the iridotomy, corneal damage, hyphema, cataract formation, retinal burns, malignant glaucoma, and monocular blurring.

Transient Intraocular Pressure Rise

This is one of the most common serious complications in the early period after argon or Nd:YAG laser iridotomy (259,260). It was reported in 24% of the eyes undergoing Nd:YAG iridotomy (246). The IOP rise is caused by reduced outflow facility, with an actual decrease in aqueous production (261). A biphasic IOP response has been seen in rabbits, in which the initial IOP rise of 0.5 to 2 hours' duration is followed by a prolonged IOP reduction lasting 6 to 24 hours (262). Studies in rabbits also suggest that this pressure response is related to a release of prostaglandin and prostaglandin-like substances into the aqueous with a breakdown in the blood–aqueous barrier and an accumulation of blood plasma and fibrin in the anterior chamber angle (262–268). A histopathologic study in monkey revealed a rapid accumulation of particulate debris in the angle (269), which may also contribute to the transient IOP elevation.

Clinically, the risk for a transient IOP rise was found in one study to be related to the total energy delivered, but not to the presence of chronic angle-closure glaucoma (260), whereas another study found no correlation with total laser energy but did find that the preoperative outflow facility was directly related to the maximum postoperative IOP elevation (261). As previously noted, 1 drop of apraclonidine, 0.5% to 1%, 1 hour before or immediately after the laser surgery has a profound effect on minimizing this complication (114,218).

Pretreatment with latanoprost was associated with an increase in IOP within the first 2 hours following iridotomy (270). This was likely due to the short time interval between drug instillation and laser treatment, which prevents the medication from achieving its peak effect and limits the effectiveness of latanoprost as a prophylactic medication in anterior segment laser surgery (270).

Anterior Uveitis

Some degree of transient iritis occurs after laser iridotomy in all eyes, which is associated with the blood–aqueous barrier breakdown noted in animal studies (264,266–268). Topical steroids for the first 3 to 5 postoperative days are sufficient to control this mild complication in most cases. In rare cases, however, an eye may have a marked inflammation, sometimes occurring days or weeks after the procedure, with associated hypopyon (271,272). Granulomatous endophthalmitis was reported following laser iridotomy, associated with several large tears in the anterior lens capsule of a blind eye with a mature cataract (272). A case of prolonged iritis with transient cystoid macular edema has also been described (273), and two cases have been reported in which postoperative inflammation and long-term miotic therapy were thought to be responsible for occlusion of the pupil with a pigmented pseudomembrane (274).

Closure of Iridotomy

The iridotomy may close during the first few weeks, especially with argon laser iridotomy, due to accumulation of pigment granules and debris. It may be advisable, therefore, to continue use of pilocarpine for the first 4 to 6 postoperative weeks. If the iridotomy remains patent, stopping use of the miotic after this time is usually safe, unless it is needed to control a chronic pressure elevation. Some authors suggested that a mydriatic provocative test should be used after stopping use of the miotic to confirm the functional reliability of the iridotomy (201). Late closure is rare with Nd:YAG laser iridotomies. In one series of 200 cases, the two late closures were in eyes with preexisting chronic uveitis (275).

As discussed earlier, the minimum diameter of a laser iridotomy that is needed to prevent further attacks of angle-closure glaucoma is yet to be determined and probably differs from one patient to the next. Cases have been reported in which angle closure recurred despite patent but small iridotomies, and as previously noted, a minimum diameter of 150 to 200 μm has been recommended (228,276). In some eyes following argon laser surgery, the laser iridotomy spontaneously enlarges over months or years (277), although this should not be relied on in borderline situations, in which case the opening should be further enlarged.

Patency of the iridotomy is best confirmed by visualizing anterior lens capsule or vitreous face through the opening (Fig. 36.7A). Transillumination can also be used, although this is sometimes misleading, especially with a blue iris, in which dislodged pigment epithelium can produce a transillumination defect despite an intact overlying stroma, which is impermeable to aqueous flow.

Corneal Damage

Focal epithelial and endothelial burns of the cornea are not uncommon when larger amounts of laser energy are used, although these usually heal quickly with no apparent sequelae. In monkey eyes, laser iridotomy was not associated with significant endothelial cell damage (278). In several clinical trials, pachymetry has revealed no significant difference in corneal thickness before and after laser iridotomy (279–281). Specular microscopic studies have been less conclusive, however, with some showing no significant difference in endothelial cell count (279,280), whereas others have revealed a loss of endothelial cells or an increase in cell size (105,281–283). Generalized corneal decompensation has been reported in several series, nearly all of which involved argon laser iridotomy (283–287). This often begins with focal corneal edema overlying the iridotomy site, followed by generalized corneal decompensation, which may not appear until months to years after the laser surgery. These cases frequently require penetrating keratoplasty, histology of which typically reveals abnormalities characteristic of Fuchs endothelial corneal dystrophy (285,287). Factors that may predispose to this complication include episodes of angle-closure glaucoma with pressure elevations and inflammation, cornea guttata, diabetes, and high total laser energy (284–287). Descemet membrane detachment after laser iridotomy was also reported (288).

Hyphema

As previously noted, a small amount of bleeding from the iridotomy site is common following Nd:YAG laser iridotomy but is rarely serious (204–208). Persistent bleeding from the treatment site can usually be stopped by applying pressure to the eye with the contact lens for a few seconds to a minute. Hyphemas are uncommon after argon laser iridotomies but may occur (289,290), especially in eyes with rubeosis iridis or uveitis.

Cataract Formation

Focal anterior lens opacities are common beneath an iridotomy produced with argon laser energy (206,208,291). Most of these are nonprogressive, although reduced visual acuity due to cataract progression has been documented (291). The rate of progression is similar to that following incisional surgical iridectomy (201), and a clear cause-and-effect relationship between either surgical approach and cataracts has not been established. Lens changes are much less common with Nd:YAG laser iridotomies (206–208), although capsular damage with rare cataract formation has been reported (292–294). In two rabbit studies, no lens damage was seen with either argon or Nd:YAG laser iridotomy, even when additional laser applications were placed through patent iridotomies (295,296). A study in monkeys, however, suggested a threshold for lens damage with Nd:YAG laser iridotomy, with no damage at 6 mJ or less and one to two pulses per burst, but local damage with higher energies or three pulses per burst (297).

Retinal Injuries

Most visual function studies have shown no adverse effect from argon laser iridotomy (298), and the same is presumably true for Nd:YAG laser iridotomy. One study, however, did reveal static perimetric and fluorescein angiographic evidence of focal retinal damage in the quadrant of treatment 6 months after argon laser iridotomy (299). Retinal damage is best minimized by always aiming the laser beam toward peripheral retina. Failure to do so may result in serious retinal burns, and acute permanent loss of vision due to inadvertent foveal photocoagulation during argon laser iridotomy has been reported (300). Macular injuries from an Nd:YAG iridotomy have also been reported (301). The final visual acuity in these cases depends on the distance between the injury and the fovea (301). The risk is also reduced but not eliminated by using an Abraham lens (302). One case of temporary bilateral serous choroidal and nonrhegmatogenous retinal detachment following Nd:YAG laser iridotomy has also been reported (303).

Malignant Glaucoma

Cases of possible malignant glaucoma have also been reported following laser iridotomy for acute or chronic angle-closure glaucoma (304–307), one of which was a simultaneous bilateral case 4 weeks after bilateral laser iridotomy (308).

Monocular Blurring

If the iridotomy is not fully covered by the upper lid, the patient may report monocular blurring, diplopia, or "ghost images." Diplopia, or "ghost images," may occur when the upper lid and associated tear film bisect the light path through the patent iridotomy. In some patients, diplopia, often alleviated when the lid is lifted away from the eye, may result despite an iridotomy that is well covered by the upper eyelid. This may result from a prism-like effect of the tear meniscus along the margin of the upper eyelid. If tinted glasses or sunglasses fail to relieve symptoms, a cosmetic contact lens can be helpful in unusually symptomatic cases. Some investigators report that diplopia occurs less frequently when the iridotomy is placed in the horizontal axis (3- or 9-o'clock positions) (309).

LASER PERIPHERAL IRIDOPLASTY (GONIOPLASTY)

There are times in which a patent iridotomy may fail to relieve angle closure, as with a microphthalmic or nanophthalmic eye, the swelling (e.g., sulfonamide-induced uveal effusion) or forward rotation of the ciliary body (i.e., plateau iris syndrome), or the presence of peripheral anterior synechiae. In each of these situations, the anterior chamber angle may be opened by applying low-energy argon laser contraction burns to the peripheral iris. The procedure has been referred to as laser peripheral iridoplasty, gonioplasty, or peripheral iris retraction.

Mechanisms of Action

The mechanism of action is a tightening of the peripheral iris, which pulls it posteriorly from the trabecular meshwork. The histopathology of eyes treated with peripheral iridoplasty revealed contraction furrow formation, proliferation of fibroblast-like cells, collagen deposition on the iris surface, denaturation of stromal collagen, and coagulative necrosis of blood vessels in the anterior two thirds of the iris stroma (310). These findings are believed to suggest that the immediate, short-term mechanism of peripheral iridoplasty is heat shrinkage of collagen, whereas the long-term effects may be related to contraction of a fibroblastic membrane. The observation of coagulative necrosis of iris blood vessels also provides a note of caution that overtreatment may lead to iris necrosis.

Techniques

Suggested argon laser settings for peripheral iridoplasty vary considerably, with ranges of 50- to 500-µm spot size, 0.5-second duration, and 150 to 1000 mW of power (217,311–313). In general, however, a laser application of relatively large area, long duration, and low power is preferable, and reasonable initial settings are 200 µm, 0.2 second, and 400 mW. The power or duration should be increased if no contraction is produced but reduced if pigment liberation is produced by the laser application. The recommended number of applications also varies. Approximately 10 to 15 burns are usually applied to peripheral iris in each quadrant, and additional applications can be placed in a row adjacent to the first burns if necessary (**Fig. 36.8**). It is usually advisable to treat no more than 180 degrees of an angle in a single session. Gonioplasty with a diode laser was also reported for the treatment of chronic angle-closure glaucoma and acute angle closure (314,315).

The most commonly used technique for applying the laser burns is with a Goldmann three-mirror or single-mirror goniolens, which causes the laser beam to strike the iris tangentially. It is important with this technique to ensure that a portion of the laser beam does not strike exposed angle structures. An alternative is to apply the laser burns directly through peripheral cornea, which is usually best done through the flat surface of a laser contact lens (e.g., peripheral Abraham lens). When using this technique, the spot size should be larger and the power lower than with the tangential approach, because the direct approach creates smaller burns with higher energy per unit area.

Indications

As noted earlier, peripheral iridoplasty may be useful in opening a functionally closed anterior chamber angle, as with pupillary block glaucoma, when corneal edema prevents

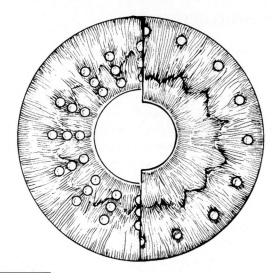

Figure 36.8 Laser peripheral iridoplasty *(right)* deepens the anterior chamber angle with low-energy contraction burns to the peripheral iris, while laser pupilloplasty *(left)* dilates the pupil with low-energy contraction burns to the more central iris.

adequate laser energy delivery to create an iridotomy (217,316,317). In other cases, a patent iridotomy may fail to relieve the angle closure because of "crowding" of the angle, as with a small, microphthalmic or nanophthalmic eye; an eye with plateau iris; iris cysts; or forward rotation of the ciliary body due to various mechanisms, including retinal detachment surgery (318–320). Laser peripheral iridoplasty has been successful in opening the anterior chamber angle in many of these cases. Another reason for failure of a patent iridotomy is the presence of extensive peripheral anterior synechiae. Gonioplasty can open the angle in some of these cases if the laser energy is applied to the base of the synechiae (311,312). The success rate is higher if the duration of synechial closure is short. It has been suggested that gonioscopy should be performed immediately after an iridotomy for pupillary block glaucoma and for any synechial closure (311). However, success has also been reported after several years of synechial closure (312). Another reported indication for gonioplasty is to open areas of persistent or recurrent synechial closure after incisional goniosynechialysis (313). In addition, peripheral iridoplasty can be used to deepen the anterior chamber angle to facilitate laser trabeculoplasty.

Complications

Peripheral iridoplasty may be complicated by further elevation of the IOP. This is usually transient, but it may be chronic if the outflow structures are further compromised by the laser applications. A mild, transient iritis is a consistent finding and should be treated with several days of topical steroid therapy. Other potential complications include corneal endothelial burns, distortion of the pupil, and focal iris atrophy.

LASER PUPILLOPLASTY

Laser pupilloplasty is a technique by which the pupil can be partially dilated by applying contraction burns near the pupillary portion of the iris. Suggested argon laser settings are 200 to 500 μm, 0.2 to 0.5 second, and 200 to 500 mW (217). Several rows of laser energy are applied to the sphincter portion of the iris, starting at the pupillary border and working peripherally. One technique is to use a smaller spot size near the pupillary border and then enlarge the spot size for more peripheral burns. The contraction of stroma with each application tents the pupil in the direction of the treatment site. Radial rows of contraction burns can be applied for 360 degrees to create symmetric pupillary dilatation or in one quadrant to create focal dilatation (Fig. 36.8).

One indication for laser pupilloplasty is as another alternative treatment of pupillary block when a laser iridotomy is not possible, as with a cloudy cornea. It is an especially useful technique for pupillary block glaucoma in aphakia or pseudophakia (321–323). By peaking the pupil in one quadrant, the iris may be retracted away from an area of vitreous contact or beyond a point of apposition with the intraocular lens implant, thereby reestablishing communication between the anterior and posterior chambers. This usually works only when the amount of lens–iris contact is minimal, because the degree of pupillary retraction is small. When pupilloplasty is not effective in these cases, combined therapy with peripheral iridoplasty may be effective (217).

Pupilloplasty may also be used to dilate a chronically constricted pupil, although the amount of dilatation is usually small and often temporary. The procedure in this situation may be complicated by a significant IOP rise. Transient iritis is also a consistent complication and should be treated with several days of topical steroid therapy.

IRIS SPHINCTEROTOMY

A technique has been described in which the pupil can be enlarged, reshaped, or repositioned by making a linear cut across the iris with an argon laser set at 0.01 to 0.05 second, 50 μm, and 1.5 W, allowing the intrinsic tension of the iris to spread the cut apart (324). A pupil can be also "created" by opening pupillary membranes with the Nd:YAG laser (325).

INCISIONAL IRIDECTOMY

Laser Iridotomy versus Incisional Iridectomy

The incisional surgical iridectomy is one of the safest, most effective operations for glaucoma. For the laser iridotomy to replace it as the procedure of choice, however, significant advantages had to be demonstrated. Long-term follow-up studies have shown that laser iridotomies are similar to the incisional procedures in terms of efficacy and safety (201,244, 326,327). However, in treatment of acute angle closure, filtering surgery is more likely to be required after laser iridotomy than after incisional peripheral iridectomy, particularly after longer duration of the angle-closure attack (328).

Laser iridotomy has become the procedure of choice for most cases of angle-closure glaucoma. There are situations, however, when the incisional approach is still required. Some patients cannot sit at the slitlamp or cooperate sufficiently for laser therapy. At other times, the cornea may be too cloudy or the iris may be too close to the cornea to allow laser iridotomy. There is also the rare case in which a patent iridotomy cannot be achieved with laser treatment, or in which the opening repeatedly closes postoperatively. The latter is particularly common in eyes with marked uveitis. For these reasons, the surgeon must still be familiar with the time-honored procedure of incisional iridectomy.

Techniques

Peripheral Iridectomy

Basic Technique

In the technique described by Chandler (329), a small conjunctival flap is prepared in one of the superior quadrants with either a fornix or a limbus base. A 3- to 4-mm incision is made into the anterior chamber, beginning approximately 1 to 1.5 mm behind the corneolimbal junction (**Fig. 36.9**).

If the iris prolapses, it is lifted up with iris forceps and a small section is excised using iris scissors that are held parallel to the limbus. If the iris does not spontaneously come through the limbal opening, a slight pressure on the posterior margin of the incision may cause the prolapse. Factors that may prevent the peripheral iris from prolapsing through the limbal incision include (a) inaccurate placement of the incision, (b) a hypotonus eye, (c) peripheral anterior synechiae, (d) a hole elsewhere in the iris, and (e) ciliary–iridial processes (attachments between the posterior peripheral iris and the ciliary body).

When iris prolapse cannot be achieved, the iris is grasped with forceps and brought up through the incision to make the iridectomy. The iris is then repositioned by a gentle stroking action across the cornea in a direction away from the incision, using a blunt instrument, such as a muscle hook.

In closing the wound, a single suture may be placed through both the limbal wound and the conjunctiva if a fornix-based flap was used. With a limbus-based flap, closure of the conjunctiva alone may be sufficient, if the limbal incision was beveled slightly to achieve spontaneous apposition.

Modifications

Some surgeons prefer to make the incision into the anterior chamber through clear cornea adjacent to the corneolimbal junction (330–332). The main advantage is that the undamaged conjunctiva remains available for future filtering surgery if required. The incision is usually placed perpendicular to the limbus to reach peripheral iris, and suture closure is generally necessary. However, some surgeons believe suturing is not essential (330), especially if the incision is beveled posteriorly (332).

Another modification of the peripheral iridectomy is transfixation, in which the anterior chamber is entered at the limbus with a narrow blade, which is then passed across the anterior segment of the eye, piercing first the peripheral iris and then the iris near the sphincter muscle. This approach has been

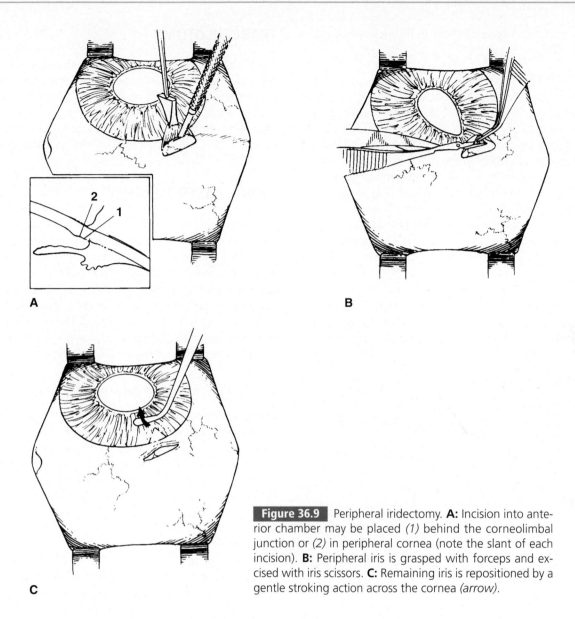

Figure 36.9 Peripheral iridectomy. **A:** Incision into anterior chamber may be placed *(1)* behind the corneolimbal junction or *(2)* in peripheral cornea (note the slant of each incision). **B:** Peripheral iris is grasped with forceps and excised with iris scissors. **C:** Remaining iris is repositioned by a gentle stroking action across the cornea *(arrow)*.

favored by some surgeons for the management of iris bombé in an inflamed eye, in the hope that it would reduce the danger of hemorrhage. However, one study showed that a conventional peripheral iridectomy does not have a greater incidence of bleeding (333).

A procedure called pigment vacuum iridectomy was described for phakic refractive lens implantation, in which the stromal layer is initially removed by surgical excision, and the pigment layer is removed by gentle vacuum aspiration with a 25-gauge cannula to ensure a proper basal iridectomy (334).

Sector Iridectomy

A sector iridectomy may have advantages over a peripheral iridectomy in some situations. Such situations include the need to enlarge the optical opening, to minimize total posterior synechiae, and to provide a better view of the fundus when retinal disease is suspected. In the technique described by King and Wadsworth (335), a limbal incision larger than that for the peripheral iridectomy is required so that the iris can be grasped within 1 to 2 mm of the pupillary margin and brought well out

through the wound. A radial cut is then made across the iris at one side of the exposed portion, the iris is torn at its root, and a second incision is made across the other side of the exposed tissue. This creates a truly basal iridectomy. An alternative approach is to grasp the midperipheral iris, withdraw it until the pupillary margin is exposed, and excise the tissue with a single cut.

Prevention and Management of Complications

Intraoperative Complications

Hemorrhage

Cut edges of the iris normally do not bleed. However, hemorrhage may occur, especially if inflammation or neovascularization is present. To minimize bleeding in the latter situations, the use of bipolar cauterization of the iris surface before cutting the iridectomy has been suggested (336,337). Brisk bleeding is especially likely to occur if the ciliary body is inadvertently cut. Hemorrhage from either iris or ciliary body can usually be stopped by placing a large air bubble in the anterior chamber for several minutes.

Incomplete Iridectomy

It is possible to cut only the stroma of the iris, leaving intact pigment epithelium, which prevents a successful operation. This complication should be avoided at the time of surgery by checking the iridectomy specimen for the dark pigment epithelium and by noting transillumination through the iridectomy if there is any doubt about its patency. If the complication is discovered postoperatively, it is best managed by penetrating the epithelial layer with the argon laser (338). Low energy settings of 300 to 400 mW, with a 100-μm spot size and a 0.1-second duration of exposure, are sufficient in most cases, and the pigment epithelium is usually eliminated with a few applications.

Injury to the Lens

Injury to the lens or disruption of the lens zonules with possible dislocation of the lens and vitreous loss should be avoided by gentle surgical manipulation. Intralenticular hemorrhage has also been reported as a rare complication of iridectomy (339).

Postoperative Complications
Intraocular Pressure Elevation

If the central anterior chamber is flat and the IOP is elevated, malignant (ciliary block) glaucoma should be suspected. This is an uncommon complication, with only one such case encountered in one series of 155 eyes (340). However, the consequences can be devastating. (The management of this situation is discussed in Chapter 26.) An incomplete iridectomy is another cause of high pressure and a flat anterior chamber, with the distinguishing feature from malignant glaucoma being more central anterior chamber depth with a bombé configuration of the iris. This situation can be managed (as described previously) by completing the iridotomy with the argon laser. A formed anterior chamber and patent iridectomy with an elevated pressure suggest that chronic obstruction of the trabecular meshwork may be present. The latter should initially be managed with IOP-lowering medications, although laser trabeculoplasty or a filtering procedure may be required if medical therapy is inadequate.

Hyphema

Hyphemas should be handled conservatively with elevation of the head and limited activity.

Cataract Formation

Cataracts. The frequency with which peripheral iridectomies lead to cataract formation is somewhat controversial. However, several studies indicate that some degree of lenticular opacity occurs in up to half of cases with an acute angle-closure glaucoma attack and in one third of eyes treated prophylactically (341–344). The mechanism of this complication is uncertain, although the frequency increases with age.

Endophthalmitis

As with any intraocular procedure, infection is a potential complication.

TRABECULOTOMY

The basic principle of this operation is the creation of an opening in the trabecular meshwork to establish a direct communication between the anterior chamber and the Schlemm canal. It is generally performed with incisional surgical techniques, although laser techniques are also being evaluated. (Trabeculotomy in children is discussed in detail in Chapter 40.)

CANAL-BASED SURGERY

There has long been an interest in enhancing aqueous drainage such that the formation of a subconjunctival bleb is not necessary. At the time of this publication, two procedures were gaining popularity in the United States. Canaloplasty uses an ab externo approach, whereas thermal ablation of the trabecular meshwork using the Trabectome has an ab interno approach. Many other procedures presented are of largely historical interest but demonstrate that the fundamental concepts behind canaloplasty and Trabectome have been investigated for several decades.

Incisional Trabeculotomy

In 1960, Burian (345) and Smith (346) independently described techniques for incising the trabecular meshwork from an ab externo approach. The procedure was modified by Harms and Dannheim (347), who reported success in adults as well as children, although the primary application of trabeculotomy has been with the management of childhood glaucomas (348) (discussed in detail in Chapter 40).

Basic Technique

The following technique, described by McPherson (349), encompasses aspects of the procedures developed by Allen and Burian (350) and Harms and Dannheim (347).

A conjunctival flap is prepared, and a partial-thickness scleral flap is dissected. A radial incision is then made across the sclerolimbal junction until the Schlemm canal is entered. One arm of a McPherson, or a Harms, trabeculotome is threaded into the Schlemm canal, using the other, parallel arm as a guide (**Fig. 36.10**). The trabeculotome is then rotated so that the arm within the canal tears through trabecular meshwork into the anterior chamber. The same procedure is then performed on the other side of the radial incision. The scleral and conjunctival flaps are closed in the same manner as for filtering procedures.

A trabeculotome can also be introduced into the Schlemm canal through an external collecting channel for better localization (351). A modified trabeculotome, corresponding to corneal diameters of 10, 12, and 14 mm, has been described (352).

Variations
Suture Trabeculotomy

In this technique, originally described by Smith (346), a nylon or Prolene suture is threaded into the Schlemm canal for 360 degrees, or between incisions 180 degrees apart, and the exposed ends are pulled taut, causing the suture to rupture

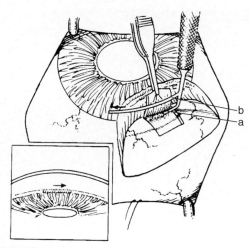

Figure 36.10 Trabeculotomy. The internal arm *(a)* of a trabeculotome is threaded into the Schlemm canal, using the external, parallel arm *(b)* as a guide; *inset* shows the gonioscopic appearance of the internal arm as it moves through the canal *(arrow)*.

through the trabecular meshwork into the anterior chamber (353). A suture trabeculotomy can be transformed into a traditional trabeculotomy at any time (354).

Combined Trabeculotomy–Trabeculectomy

If the Schlemm canal cannot be located with certainty, the procedure can be converted to a trabeculectomy by removing a block of deep limbal tissue beneath the scleral flap. In addition, the two procedures can be combined by first performing the trabeculotomy and then creating the fistula beneath the scleral flap. In some situations, such as with the Sturge–Weber syndrome, in which the exact mechanism of the glaucoma is uncertain (see Chapter 21), the combined procedure may offer the best chance of success (355–360). Bilateral combined trabeculotomy–trabeculectomy and trabeculotomy in combination with deep sclerectomy have been reported (361,362). Combined trabeculotomy–trabeculectomy may be particularly useful in eyes with corneal opacification (363).

Combined Trabeculotomy–Cataract Surgery

Cataract surgery can be combined with trabeculotomy in patients with coexisting glaucoma and cataract to reduce the occurrence of flat anterior chamber (364–368). However, in low-tension glaucoma, the combination may not always sufficiently lower the IOP (369). Combined trabeculotomy–cataract surgery also appears more likely to reduce IOP in patients who are 70 years of age or older (370). Although hypotony is seen infrequently, hyphema may often occur; it was seen in 20% of the eyes in one retrospective study (369). However, the combination of phacoemulsification with trabeculotomy appears to decrease the frequency of hyphema, compared with trabeculotomy alone (371). IOP spikes of more than 30 mm Hg, probably related to hyphema, have been reported in 10% to 25% of eyes (369–371). Combined phacoemulsification and trabeculotomy in the eyes with exfoliation syndrome achieved similar results (372).

Trabeculotomy and viscocanalostomy combined with phacoemulsification achieved similar postoperative pressures. The eyes in the viscocanalostomy group had better postoperative visual acuity, but the incidence of postoperative fibrin reaction and perforations of the Descemet membrane was less common after trabeculotomy (373).

Combined Trabeculotomy–Sinusotomy

Combined trabeculotomy and sinusotomy (procedure for externalization of the Schlemm canal) was suggested to obtain lower IOP than after trabeculotomy alone. In one study, the mean IOP was 15.6 mm Hg after the combined procedure and 17.8 mm Hg after trabeculotomy alone at the end of the first postoperative year (374). However, in another study, sinusotomy did not play an important role in IOP control in combined trabeculotomy and sinusotomy in patients with juvenile glaucoma, compared with trabeculotomy alone (375). The eyes treated with nonpenetrating trabeculectomy with sinusotomy and trabeculotomy had significantly lower IOP than those treated with nonpenetrating trabeculectomy with sinusotomy but without trabeculotomy (376).

Ab Interno Goniotrabeculotomy

Ab interno goniotrabeculotomy creates a surgical incision of the iridocorneal angle to establish a direct communication between the aqueous humor of the anterior chamber and the Schlemm canal (377–380). In a randomized trial, this procedure was compared with trabeculectomy with adjunct mitomycin C in adult patients with open-angle glaucoma. At the end of follow-up, more than 80% of patients in each group had an IOP of 14 mm Hg or lower, although fewer postoperative complications occurred in the goniotrabeculotomy group (381).

Miscellaneous Variations

Electrocautery has been used in modified trabeculotomies by insulating all sides of the probe except that exposed to the trabecular meshwork (382–384). By burning an opening in the meshwork, fibrotic closure of the severed edges is thought to be avoided. Other experimental types of trabeculotomy used aqueous veins to localize the Schlemm canal by threading a probe through a large vein and into the canal or by forcing air into a vein, which causes multiple ruptures in the meshwork (385,386). The trabeculectome, an instrument that excises a strip of trabecular meshwork as it is pulled along the anterior chamber angle by a probe in the Schlemm canal, has also been developed (387). A segment of the trabecular meshwork and internal wall of the Schlemm canal can also be removed ab interno by using retinal forceps to create a direct communication between the anterior chamber and the Schlemm canal (388,389). The 308-nm excimer laser can also be used for ablation of the trabecular meshwork, allowing only a very small amount of collateral thermal damage at the boundaries of the ablation zone (390).

Complications

If the Schlemm canal is not properly identified, a false passage may be created into either the anterior chamber or the supraciliary space, resulting in the creation of a cyclodialysis and

Figure 36.11 Intraoperative images of a Trabectome procedure showing a direct view of the angle using a modified Swan–Ganz lens and the tip of the device (**A**). The tip of the device is inserted into the Schlemm canal, and thermal energy is used to ablate the trabecular meshwork. The exposed posterior wall of the Schlemm canal can be seen to the right of the probe (**B**).

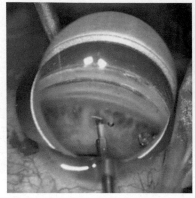 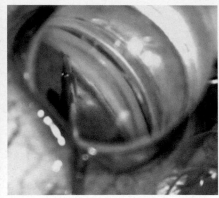

A **B**

possible hyphema. If the Schlemm canal cannot be identified, the procedure can be converted to a trabeculectomy. When the probe is rotated into the anterior chamber, it may strip the Descemet membrane if it is too far anterior or damage the iris or lens if it is too far posterior. As with all intraocular glaucoma procedures, postoperative bleeding and infection are potential complications.

Ab Interno Trabeculectomy: Trabectome

Ab interno trabeculectomy refers to the removal of trabecular meshwork tissue from an internal approach. Several different techniques have been described, such as trabeculopuncture, goniophotoablation, laser trabecular ablation, and goniocurretage. All of these procedures, including use of the Trabectome, are variations of goniotomy, which is incision (without removal) of the trabecular meshwork allowing for direct communication between the anterior chamber and the Schlemm canal. Through a temporal clear corneal approach, a probe is inserted through trabecular meshwork and into the Schlemm canal. Thermal ablation is used to remove the nasal trabecular meshwork and internal wall of the Schlemm canal for 60 to 140 degrees (**Fig. 36.11**).

Initial clinical results were first published in 1995 (391). To date, the published data have been from consecutive case series as an independent procedure or combined with cataract extraction. The largest series described a lowering of IOP from 25.7 ± 7.7 mm Hg to 16.6 ± 4.0 mm Hg with concurrent reduction in the number of antiglaucoma medications from 2.9 to 1.2 at 2 years. Kaplan–Meier survival analysis, with failure defined as IOP greater than 21 mm Hg with or without medications and not reduced by 20% on two consecutive visits or repeated surgery, demonstrated a success rate of approximately 70% at 24 months. Transient hyphema as a result of reflux bleeding from collecting channels is common but temporary. Sustained hypotony does not occur, and vision-threatening complications are rare (392). When ab interno trabeculectomy was combined with cataract surgery, the IOP decreased from a mean of 20.0 ± 6.3 mm Hg to 15.5 ± 2.9 mm Hg at 1 year with a concurrent decrease in the number of antiglaucoma medications from 2.7 to 1.4 (393).

Canaloplasty

Using an external transconjunctival approach, a cutdown to the Schlemm canal is made to unroof the outer wall of the Schlemm canal, and a flexible microcatheter is used to circumferentially inject viscoelastic agent to dilate the Schlemm canal (**Fig. 36.12A,B**). A 10-0 or 9-0 Prolene suture is tied under tension within the Schlemm canal. The inner sclera flap is removed, and the outer scleral flap is then closed. Because the trabecular meshwork and Descemet membrane are left intact, this is not considered a penetrating procedure.

The exact mechanism of IOP lowering is unknown, but it is believed that the combination of the dilatation and chronic stretch of the trabecular meshwork induced by the Prolene suture increases the aqueous outflow. In addition, transudation of aqueous through the Descemet window into the intrascleral lake may create an intrascleral bleb with fluid diffusing through the scleral or into the uvea and suprachoroidal space. The results of canaloplasty are partially dependent on the degree of outflow resistance within either the Schlemm canal or episcleral veins (394). The initial clinical results were first published in 2007 (395). To date, the published data have been from consecutive case series as an independent procedure or combined with cataract extraction. As a stand-alone procedure, canaloplasty reduced IOP from approximately 23.2 ± 4.0 mm Hg to 16.3 ± 3.7 mm Hg and decreased the number of antiglaucoma medications used from 2.0 ± 0.8 to 0.6 ± 0.8 at 24 months of follow-up (396). When combined with phacoemulsification cataract extraction, the IOP decreased from 24 to 14 mm Hg at 1 year, with a decrease of 1.3 antiglaucoma medications (397). Transient IOP elevations and Descemet detachments can occur, but long-term vision-threatening complications are rare.

Laser Trabeculotomy (Trabeculopuncture)

The earliest efforts to treat glaucoma by the application of laser energy to the trabecular meshwork were attempts to create holes through the trabecular meshwork into the Schlemm canal (2–5,7). This approach lost popularity because of early failures and the subsequent enthusiasm for

Figure 36.12 Intraoperative images of canaloplasty. **A:** Initial surgical dissection showing the outer and inner corneoscleral flaps. Underneath the inner flap is the exposed inner wall of the Schlemm canal and Descemet window *(left image)*. **B:** The tip of the intracanalicular catheter *(left image)* that has a fiber-optic red light that can be visualized through the sclera as it traverses through the Schlemm canal when the microscope lights are dimmed *(center image)*. Appearance of the Descemet window after amputation of the inner corneoscleral flap creating the intrascleral space for aqueous drainage *(right image)*.

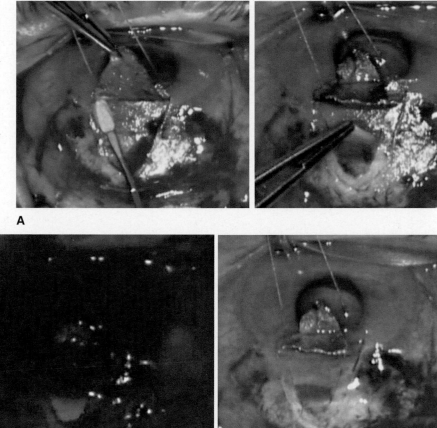

laser trabeculoplasty, although advances in the technology of pulsed lasers have led to a re-evaluation of laser trabeculotomy, or trabeculopuncture.

In laboratory studies with monkeys, the Q-switched ruby laser did not produce persistent penetration to the Schlemm canal (398). With Q-switched Nd:YAG lasers, holes were created in the trabecular meshwork but were soon sealed by proliferation of corneal endothelium and scar tissue (399,400). Laboratory studies with human ocular tissue have shown that pulsed Nd:YAG lasers at energy levels between 3 and 6 mJ can produce discrete lesions in the Schlemm canal with minimal damage to adjacent structures (401,402). In human autopsy eyes, energy levels of 30 mJ produced openings in the trabecular meshwork of approximately 100 μm in diameter (403). A similar technique was used in four human eyes treated within 18 hours of enucleation, which produced irregular craters of 150 to 300 μm in the meshwork, with denuding of endothelial cells and deposition of debris in the adjacent trabecular and corneal tissues (404).

Early clinical experience with laser trabeculotomy has provided variable results. In one series of eight eyes of six patients with juvenile glaucoma, pressure control was achieved in six eyes (75%) with a mean follow-up of 6 months (405). The most effective technique in this study was to make two confluent trabeculotomies of 1 clock-hour each in extent. Nd:YAG laser trabeculopuncture may have value in patients with angle-recession glaucoma. In one series, the probability of success at 1 year was calculated at 90%, compared with 27% with ALT (406). In another study, however, the success rate at a mean of 12 months was only 42% with Nd:YAG laser trabeculopuncture (407).

Laser trabecular ablation with an erbium-doped YAG (Er:YAG) laser, focused into a single-crystal sapphire optical fiber, was shown to increase outflow in human cadaver eyes. Even so, the thermal damage induced by the pulsed Er:YAG laser appears to be less than that of other laser modalities, and histopathologic analysis revealed the presence of thermal damage at all energy levels (408).

Trabeculodialysis

In this technique, the trabecular meshwork is scraped from the scleral sulcus with the flat side of a goniotomy blade. This technique may be especially useful in glaucoma associated with inflammation, presumably because the trabecular tissue is friable and easily scraped away in these cases (409,410). A histologic study has shown that this operation works by establishing a communication between the anterior chamber and Schlemm canal (410).

Comparison of Goniotomy and Trabeculotomy

The techniques, complications, and results of goniotomy, which is limited primarily to the management of childhood glaucomas, are discussed in Chapter 40. However, a comparison of trabeculotomy and goniotomy follows.

Results

Reported success with trabeculotomy and goniotomy is similar, ranging from approximately 70% to 90%, although it may be that fewer repeated procedures are required with trabeculotomy than with goniotomy (411–420). The two surgical approaches appear to provide equally good results in the hands of experienced surgeons (421).

Glaucoma in Juveniles and Adults

Although trabeculotomy and goniotomy are used primarily for glaucomas in childhood, some success has been reported with trabeculotomy in juveniles and adults. In a series of 16 eyes of 11 patients with juvenile glaucoma, ranging in age between 10 and 45 years, trabeculotomy maintained an IOP of 21 mm Hg or less in 88% during a mean follow-up of 7 years (422). In a retrospective study on adult patients, the final success probability at 5 years after trabeculotomy was 56% for the open-angle glaucoma and 73.5% for the exfoliation syndrome (423). In adults with open-angle glaucoma randomly assigned to either trabeculotomy or trabeculectomy with adjunctive mitomycin C, the probability of success at 1 year was 86% and 84%, respectively, and the only significant difference was less frequent complications in the trabeculotomy group (424). Retrospective study of 29 eyes with aniridic glaucoma showed that in 10 of 12 eyes, with trabeculotomy as the initial surgery, good visual acuity and IOP control were maintained within 9.5 years of follow-up (425). Surgical results of external trabeculotomy for steroid-induced glaucoma remain effective for a long time (426).

OTHER PROCEDURES OF THE ANTERIOR CHAMBER ANGLE

Cyclodialysis

Cyclodialysis, as an operation for glaucoma, was described by Heine (427) in 1905. It was used as an alternative to filtering surgery, especially in aphakic eyes or in combination with cataract extraction. The procedure has lost popularity in recent years because of unpredictable results and availability of newer, better surgical techniques.

Theories of Mechanism

Cyclodialysis involves the separation of the ciliary body from the scleral spur, which creates a direct communication between the anterior chamber and the suprachoroidal space. An increase in pressure-dependent uveoscleral outflow and reduced aqueous production, due to an alteration in the ciliary body anatomy, may play a role in a successful cyclodialysis procedure (428–435).

Techniques

An incision is made through conjunctiva and Tenon capsule approximately 8 mm from the corneolimbal junction, usually in a superior quadrant between the insertions of two rectus muscles. A 3- to 4-mm full-thickness scleral incision, 4 to 6 mm from the anatomic limbus, is then made parallel to the limbus. A cyclodialysis spatula is inserted through the scleral incision and into the supraciliary space and advanced until the tip enters the anterior chamber. Movements of the spatula tip are then made to separate about one third of the ciliary body from the scleral spur. After withdrawal of the spatula, only the conjunctiva is closed (427,436).

Implants of various materials have been inserted into the cyclodialysis cleft to keep it open (437–439). The injection of air or sodium hyaluronate into the anterior chamber has been advocated as a means of holding the cleft open during the early postoperative period (440–442). A technique called iridocycloretraction, in which scleral pedicles are folded forward into a cyclodialysis cleft to maintain a patent cyclodialysis cleft, has been described (443–445).

Complications

Hemorrhage is a frequent complication during cyclodialysis. Improper position of the spatula can cause several complications, such as stripping of the Descemet membrane, corneal damage, tearing the ciliary body or iris, lens injury, and possible vitreous loss. At any time after surgery, a sudden, marked increase in IOP may occur, which is thought to be due to closure of the cyclodialysis cleft.

Hypotony is a common complication of cyclodialysis. The primary clinical interest in cyclodialysis in recent years has been in techniques to treat the inadvertent cyclodialysis that may result from injury or surgical trauma with subsequent hypotony. Penetrating cyclodiathermy or cyclocryotherapy to "wall off" the cleft may correct the problem, but the results are highly unpredictable. The application of argon laser energy into the cyclodialysis cleft has been reported to successfully close the cleft in some cases (446,447). Successful laser settings include 0.1 to 0.2 second, 50 to 100 μm, and 300 to 700 mW. In especially difficult cases, powers of 2 to 3 W have been used (447). The latter technique usually requires retrobulbar anesthesia, whereas topical anesthesia is typically sufficient for the lower power settings. Contiguous laser burns are applied to all exposed scleral and uveal surfaces of the cleft for approximately 50 burns. Successful closure of a cyclodialysis cleft with sutures has also been described and may be the procedure of choice when the argon laser therapy has failed (448,449).

Goniosynechialysis

Campbell and Vela (450) reported a procedure for synechial angle-closure glaucoma. The technique involves deepening the anterior chamber with sodium hyaluronate and separating the synechiae from the trabecular meshwork with an irrigating cyclodialysis spatula under direct gonioscopic visualization. The procedure has also been employed during penetrating keratoplasty, by using a dental mirror to visualize the anterior chamber angle (451). The primary value of the procedure is thought to be for patients in whom the synechiae have not been present for a prolonged period. In one study of 15 patients with synechial angle-closure glaucoma, goniosynechialysis alone or in combination with other surgical procedures was associated with a reduction in mean IOP from 40 to 14 mm Hg (452). Goniosynechialysis combined with laser peripheral iridoplasty and phacoemulsification was found to be an effective treatment of synechial chronic angle-closure glaucoma and cataract (314,453). In a series of 70 eyes with angle-closure glaucoma that did not respond to laser or incisional iridectomy, goniosynechialysis maintained an IOP below 20 mm Hg in 87% of aphakic eyes, but in only 42% of phakic eyes (454). It has also been reported that successful goniosynechialysis was achieved in five of seven patients with a Q-switched Nd:YAG laser (455). Ultrasonographic biomicroscopy was found to be useful in demonstrating successful restoration of an anterior chamber angle after goniosynechialysis (456).

Goniophotocoagulation

Simmons and associates (457,458) described a form of laser treatment for use in the early open-angle stages of neovascular glaucoma. The purpose of the procedure is to eliminate new vessels in the anterior chamber angle by direct laser photocoagulation. The technique involves the application of argon laser energy to the vessels as they cross the scleral spur to arborize on the trabecular meshwork. The customary laser settings are 0.2 second, 150 μm, and power sufficient to blanch and constrict the vessels (usually 100 to 800 mW) (458).

Although this technique is rarely used today, it was considered effective in the rubeosis stage to prevent progression of angle neovascularization with subsequent angle closure and intractable glaucoma (459). It has been used in conjunction with panretinal photocoagulation, especially when the latter was not successful or when the retinal therapy was not possible or advisable. In the more advanced, florid open-angle stage of neovascular glaucoma, however, goniophotocoagulation should not be used, because it may cause hemorrhage or accelerated closure of the anterior chamber angle.

Trabecular Aspiration

An irrigation–aspiration device has been described for the removal of pigment and exfoliation material from the trabecular meshwork in eyes with glaucoma associated with the exfoliation syndrome (460–463). Its use has been reported before, in combination with, and after cataract extraction and as a primary surgical procedure (462,464–467), with significant IOP reduction resulting in all groups. ALT before trabecular aspiration reduces the IOP-lowering effect of this procedure (460).

Eyes with pigment dispersion syndrome responded better to trabecular aspiration than did those with pigmentary glaucoma in a clinical trial, although trabecular aspiration failed to

achieve long-term pressure control in either of the two groups (468). Patients with exfoliative glaucoma undergoing phacoemulsification were randomly assigned to trabecular aspiration or trabeculectomy, with the success rate lower for the trabecular aspiration group (462,463). Trabecular aspiration causes only a short-term reduction of IOP in patients with exfoliative glaucoma, limited to a few weeks in most patients. This effect was attributed to a continuous production and release of exfoliative material (460); therefore, trabecular aspiration does not appear to be a long-term solution in the management of exfoliative glaucoma (467).

KEY POINTS

■ Laser trabeculoplasty involves the application of evenly spaced photocoagulation burns to all or part of the trabecular meshwork.
  • This typically decreases the IOP by improving aqueous outflow through mechanisms not yet fully understood.
  • The most serious known complication is an early, transient rise in ocular tension, which can be minimized with topical medication use.
  • Many patients lose the ocular hypotensive effect with time, and repeated trabeculoplasty is less effective than the initial procedure.
  • A modification, SLT, may, with further experience, prove to have advantages over traditional trabeculoplasty.
■ Laser iridotomies have become the procedure of choice for the surgical management of angle-closure glaucomas and can be achieved with continuous-wave or pulsed lasers.
  • Techniques vary with the type of laser and the color of the iris.
  • Complications include transient IOP elevation, uveitis, and burns of the cornea, lens, or retina.
  • In some situations, laser iridotomies are impossible to achieve, in which case incisional iridectomies are still required.
  • Laser energy can also be used to treat certain types of angle-closure glaucoma by mechanically flattening the peripheral iris (iridoplasty or gonioplasty) or dilating the pupil (pupilloplasty).
■ Cyclodialysis, which involves the separation of the ciliary body from the scleral spur, was once used to treat glaucoma, but the primary clinical interest today is treatment of inadvertent cyclodialyses with hypotony.
■ Other reported surgical procedures of the anterior chamber angle include goniosynechialysis for synechial angle-closure glaucoma, goniophotocoagulation for neovascular glaucoma, and trabecular aspiration for the exfoliation syndrome.

REFERENCES

1. Zweng HC, Flocks M. Experimental photocoagulation of the anterior chamber angle. A preliminary report. *Am J Ophthalmol.* 1961;52: 163–165.

2. Krasnov MM. Laser puncture of the anterior chamber angle in glaucoma (a preliminary report) [in Russian]. *Vestn Oftalmol*. 1972;3:27–31.

3. Hager H. Special microsurgical interventions. 2. First experiences with the argon laser apparatus 800 [in German]. *Klin Monbl Augenheilkd*. 1973;162(4):437–450.

4. Demailly P, Haut J, Bonnet-Boutier M, et al. Trabeculotomy with argon laser (preliminary note) [in French]. *Bull Soc Ophtalmol Fr*. 1973; 73(2):259–264.

5. Worthen DM, Wickham MG. Argon laser trabeculotomy. *Trans Am Acad Ophthalmol Otolaryngol*. 1974;78(2):OP371–OP375.

6. Gaasterland D, Kupfer C. Experimental glaucoma in the rhesus monkey. *Invest Ophthalmol*. 1974;13(6):455–457.

7. Ticho U, Zauberman H. Argon laser application to the angle structures in the glaucomas. *Arch Ophthalmol*. 1976;94(1):61–64.

8. Wise JB, Witter SL. Argon laser therapy for open-angle glaucoma. A pilot study. *Arch Ophthalmol*. 1979;97(2):319–322.

9. Wise JB. Long-term control of adult open angle glaucoma by argon laser treatment. *Ophthalmology*. 1981;88(3):197–202.

10. Schwartz AL, Whitten ME, Bleiman B, et al. Argon laser trabecular surgery in uncontrolled phakic open angle glaucoma. *Ophthalmology*. 1981;88(3):203–212.

11. Wilensky JT, Jampol LM. Laser therapy for open angle glaucoma. *Ophthalmology*. 1981;88(3):213–217.

12. Schrems W, Sold J, Krieglstein GK, et al. Demonstration of the tonographic effect in YAG chronic [in German]. *Klin Monbl Augenheilkd*. 1985;187(3):170–172.

13. Spurny RC, Lederer CM Jr. Krypton laser trabeculoplasty. A clinical report. *Arch Ophthalmol*. 1984;102(11):1626–1628.

14. Makabe R. Comparative krypton and argon laser trabeculoplasty [in German]. *Klin Monbl Augenheilkd*. 1986;189(2):118–120.

15. McMillan TA, Stewart WC, Legler UF, et al. Comparison of diode and argon laser trabeculoplasty in cadaver eyes. *Invest Ophthalmol Vis Sci*. 1994;35(2):706–710.

16. McHugh D, Marshall J, Ffytche TJ, et al. Ultrastructural changes of human trabecular meshwork after photocoagulation with a diode laser. *Invest Ophthalmol Vis Sci*. 1992;33(9):2664–2671.

17. McHugh D, Marshall J, Ffytche TJ, et al. Diode laser trabeculoplasty (DLT) for primary open angle glaucoma and ocular hypertension. *Br J Ophthalmol*. 1990;74(12):743–747.

18. Moriarty AP, McHugh JD, Ffytche TJ, et al. Long-term follow-up of diode laser trabeculoplasty for primary open-angle glaucoma and ocular hypertension. *Ophthalmology*. 1993;100(11):1614–1618.

19. Moriarty AP, McHugh JD, Spalton DJ, et al. Comparison of the anterior chamber inflammatory response to diode and argon laser trabeculoplasty using a laser flare meter. *Ophthalmology*. 1993;100(8):1263–1267.

20. Brancato R, Carassa R, Trabucchi G. Diode laser compared with argon laser for trabeculoplasty. *Am J Ophthalmol*. 1991;112(1):50–55.

21. Pohjanpelto P. Argon laser treatment of the anterior chamber angle for increased intraocular pressure. *Acta Ophthalmol*. 1981;59(2):211–220.

22. Lichter PR. Argon laser trabeculoplasty. *Trans Am Ophthalmol Soc*. 1982;80:288–301.

23. Brubaker RF, Liesegang TJ. Effect of trabecular photocoagulation on the aqueous humor dynamics of the human eye. *Am J Ophthalmol*. 1983;96(2):139–147.

24. Merte HJ, von Denffer H, Hirsch B. Aqueous humor outflow capacity after argon laser trabeculoplasty. Preliminary report [in German]. *Klin Monbl Augenheilkd*. 1985;186(3):220–223.

25. Araie M, Yamamoto T, Shirato S, et al. Effects of laser trabeculoplasty on the human aqueous humor dynamics: a fluorophotometric study. *Ann Ophthalmol*. 1984;16(6):540–542, 544.

26. Yablonski ME, Cook DJ, Gray J. A fluorophotometric study of the effect of argon laser trabeculoplasty on aqueous humor dynamics. *Am J Ophthalmol*. 1985;99(5):579–582.

27. Feller DB, Weinreb RN. Breakdown and reestablishment of blood-aqueous barrier with laser trabeculoplasty. *Arch Ophthalmol*. 1984;102(4):537–538.

28. Rodrigues MM, Spaeth GL, Donohoo P. Electron microscopy of argon laser therapy in phakic open-angle glaucoma. *Ophthalmology*. 1982;89(3):198–210.

29. Alexander RA, Grierson I. Morphological effects of argon laser trabeculoplasty upon the glaucomatous human meshwork. *Eye (Lond)*. 1989;3(6):719–726.

30. Alexander RA, Grierson I, Church WH. The effect of argon laser trabeculoplasty upon the normal human trabecular meshwork. *Graefes Arch Clin Exp Ophthalmol*. 1989;227(1):72–77.

31. Babizhayev MA, Brodskaya MW, Mamedov NG, et al. Clinical, structural and molecular phototherapy effects of laser irradiation on the trabecular meshwork of human glaucomatous eyes. *Graefes Arch Clin Exp Ophthalmol*. 1990;228(1):90–100.

32. Kramer TR, Noecker RJ. Comparison of the morphologic changes after selective laser trabeculoplasty and argon laser trabeculoplasty in human eye bank eyes. *Ophthalmology*. 2001;108(4):773–779.

33. Cvenkel B, Hvala A, Drnovsek-Olup B, et al. Acute ultrastructural changes of the trabecular meshwork after selective laser trabeculoplasty and low power argon laser trabeculoplasty. *Lasers Surg Med*. 2003;33(3):204–208.

34. Melamed S, Pei J, Epstein DL. Short-term effect of argon laser trabeculoplasty in monkeys. *Arch Ophthalmol*. 1985;103(10):1546–1552.

35. Dueker DK, Norberg M, Johnson DH, et al. Stimulation of cell division by argon and Nd:YAG laser trabeculoplasty in cynomolgus monkeys. *Invest Ophthalmol Vis Sci*. 1990;31(1):115–124.

36. Melamed S, Pei J, Epstein DL. Delayed response to argon laser trabeculoplasty in monkeys. Morphological and morphometric analysis. *Arch Ophthalmol*. 1986;104(7):1078–1083.

37. van der Zypen E, Fankhauser F. Ultrastructural changes of the trabecular meshwork of the monkey (*Macaca speciosa*) following irradiation with argon laser light. *Graefes Arch Clin Exp Ophthalmol*. 1984;221(6): 249–261.

38. Melamed S, Epstein DL. Alterations of aqueous humour outflow following argon laser trabeculoplasty in monkeys. *Br J Ophthalmol*. 1987;71(10):776–781.

39. van der Zypen E, Fankhauser F, England C, et al. Morphology of the trabecular meshwork within monkey (*Macaca speciosa*) eyes after irradiation with the free-running Nd:YAG laser. *Ophthalmology*. 1987;94(2):171–179.

40. Kee C, Pickett JP, Dueker DK, et al. Argon laser trabeculoplasty and pilocarpine effects on outflow facility in the cynomolgus monkey. *J Glaucoma*. 1995;4(5):334–343.

41. Van Buskirk EM, Pond V, Rosenquist RC, et al. Argon laser trabeculoplasty. Studies of mechanism of action. *Ophthalmology*. 1984;91(9): 1005–1010.

42. Kimpel MW, Johnson DH. Factors influencing in vivo trabecular cell replication as determined by 3H-thymidine labelling; an autoradiographic study in cats. *Curr Eye Res*. 1992;11(4):297–306.

43. Bylsma SS, Samples JR, Acott TS, et al. DNA replication in the cat trabecular meshwork after laser trabeculoplasty in vivo. *J Glaucoma*. 1994;3(1):36–43.

44. Bylsma SS, Samples JR, Acott TS, et al. Trabecular cell division after argon laser trabeculoplasty. *Arch Ophthalmol*. 1988;106(4):544–547.

45. Acott TS, Samples JR, Bradley JM, et al. Trabecular repopulation by anterior trabecular meshwork cells after laser trabeculoplasty. *Am J Ophthalmol*. 1989;107(1):1–6.

46. Parshley DE, Bradley JM, Samples JR, et al. Early changes in matrix metalloproteinases and inhibitors after in vitro laser treatment to the trabecular meshwork. *Curr Eye Res*. 1995;14(7):537–544.

47. Parshley DE, Bradley JM, Fisk A, et al. Laser trabeculoplasty induces stromelysin expression by trabecular juxtacanalicular cells. *Invest Ophthalmol Vis Sci*. 1996;37(5):795–804.

48. Bradley JM, Anderssohn AM, Colvis CM, et al. Mediation of laser trabeculoplasty-induced matrix metalloproteinase expression by IL-1beta and TNFalpha. *Invest Ophthalmol Vis Sci*. 2000;41(2):422–430.

49. Alexander JP, Samples JR, Van Buskirk EM, et al. Expression of matrix metalloproteinases and inhibitor by human trabecular meshwork. *Invest Ophthalmol Vis Sci*. 1991;32(1):172–180.

50. Bradley JM, Vranka J, Colvis CM, et al. Effect of matrix metalloproteinases activity on outflow in perfused human organ culture. *Invest Ophthalmol Vis Sci*. 1998;39(13):2649–2658.

51. Alexander JP, Acott TS. Involvement of the Erk-MAP kinase pathway in TNFalpha regulation of trabecular matrix metalloproteinases and TIMPs. *Invest Ophthalmol Vis Sci*. 2003;44(1):164–169.

52. Van Buskirk EM. Pathophysiology of laser trabeculoplasty. *Surv Ophthalmol*. 1989;33(4):264–272.

53. Latina MA, Park C. Selective targeting of trabecular meshwork cells: in vitro studies of pulsed and CW laser interactions. *Exp Eye Res*. 1995;60(4):359–371.

54. Latina MA, Sibayan SA, Shin DH, et al. Q-switched 532-nm Nd:YAG laser trabeculoplasty (selective laser trabeculoplasty): a multicenter, pilot, clinical study. *Ophthalmology*. 1998;105(11):2082–2088; discussion 2089–2090.

55. Sanfilippo P. A review of argon and selective laser trabeculoplasty as primary treatments of open-angle glaucoma. *Clin Exp Optom.* 1999;82(6):225–229.

56. Guzey M, Vural H, Satici A, et al. Increase of free oxygen radicals in aqueous humour induced by selective Nd:YAG laser trabeculoplasty in the rabbit. *Eur J Ophthalmol.* 2001;11(1):47–52.

57. Smith J. Argon laser trabeculoplasty: comparison of bichromatic and monochromatic wavelengths. *Ophthalmology.* 1984;91(4):355–360.

58. Dieckert JP, Mainster MA, Ho PC. Contact lenses for laser applications. *Ophthalmology.* 1983;(suppl):55–62.

59. Ritch R. A new lens for argon laser trabeculoplasty. *Ophthalmic Surg.* 1985;16(5):331–332.

60. Wise JB. Errors in laser spot size in laser trabeculoplasty. *Ophthalmology.* 1984;91(2):186–190.

61. Iwasaki N, Takagi T, Lewis JM, et al. The double-mirror gonioscopic lens for surgery of the anterior chamber angle. *Arch Ophthalmol.* 1997;115(10):1333–1335.

62. Blondeau P, Roberge JF, Asselin Y. Long-term results of low power, long duration laser trabeculoplasty. *Am J Ophthalmol.* 1987;104(4):339–342.

63. Brown RH, Shingleton BJ, Johnstone M, et al. Glaucoma laser treatment parameters and practices of ASCRS members—1999 survey. American Society of Cataract and Refractive Surgery. *J Cataract Refract Surg.* 2000;26(5):755–765.

64. Rouhiainen H, Terasvirta M. The laser power needed for optimum results in argon laser trabeculoplasty. *Acta Ophthalmol.* 1986;64(3):254–257.

65. Rouhiainen H, Leino M, Terasvirta M. The effect of some treatment variables on long-term results of argon laser trabeculoplasty. *Ophthalmologica.* 1995;209(1):21–24.

66. Threlkeld AB, Hertzmark E, Sturm RT, et al. Comparative study of the efficacy of argon laser trabeculoplasty for exfoliation and primary open-angle glaucoma. *J Glaucoma.* 1996;5(5):311–316.

67. Odberg T, Sandvik L. The medium and long-term efficacy of primary argon laser trabeculoplasty in avoiding topical medication in open angle glaucoma. *Acta Ophthalmol Scand.* 1999;77(2):176–181.

68. Wilensky JT, Weinreb RN. Low-dose trabeculoplasty. *Am J Ophthalmol.* 1983;95(4):423–426.

69. Schwartz LW, Spaeth GL, Traverso C, et al. Variation of techniques on the results of argon laser trabeculoplasty. *Ophthalmology.* 1983;90(7):781–784.

70. Weinreb RN, Ruderman J, Juster R, et al. Influence of the number of laser burns administered on the early results of argon laser trabeculoplasty. *Am J Ophthalmol.* 1983;95(3):287–292.

71. Lustgarten J, Podos SM, Ritch R, et al. Laser trabeculoplasty. A prospective study of treatment variables. *Arch Ophthalmol.* 1984;102(4):517–519.

72. Grayson D, Chi T, Liebmann J, et al. Initial argon laser trabeculoplasty to the inferior vs superior half of trabecular meshwork. *Arch Ophthalmol.* 1994;112(4):446–447.

73. Heijl A. One- and two-session laser trabeculoplasty. A randomized, prospective study. *Acta Ophthalmol.* 1984;62(5):715–724.

74. Klein HZ, Shields MB, Ernest JT. Two-stage argon laser trabeculoplasty in open-angle glaucoma. *Am J Ophthalmol.* 1985;99(4):392–395.

75. Thomas JV, Simmons RJ, Belcher CD III. Argon laser trabeculoplasty in the presurgical glaucoma patient. *Ophthalmology.* 1982;89(3):187–197.

76. Weinreb RN, Ruderman J, Juster R, et al. Immediate intraocular pressure response to argon laser trabeculoplasty. *Am J Ophthalmol.* 1983;95(3):279–286.

77. Kitazawa Y, Yamamoto T, Shirato S, et al. The technic of argon laser trabeculoplasty and its results [in German]. *Klin Monbl Augenheilkd.* 1984;184(4):274–277.

78. Elsas T, Johnsen H, Brevik TA. The immediate pressure response to primary laser trabeculoplasty—a comparison of one- and two-stage treatment. *Acta Ophthalmol.* 1989;67(6):664–668.

79. Rouhiainen HJ, Terasvirta ME, Tuovinen EJ. Peripheral anterior synechiae formation after trabeculoplasty. *Arch Ophthalmol.* 1988;106(2):189–191.

80. Traverso CE, Greenidge KC, Spaeth GL. Formation of peripheral anterior synechiae following argon laser trabeculoplasty. A prospective study to determine relationship to position of laser burns. *Arch Ophthalmol.* 1984;102(6):861–863.

81. Hoskins HD Jr, Hetherington J Jr, Minckler DS, et al. Complications of laser trabeculoplasty. *Ophthalmology.* 1983;90(7):796–799.

82. Krupin T, Kolker AE, Kass MA, et al. Intraocular pressure the day of argon laser trabeculoplasty in primary open-angle glaucoma. *Ophthalmology.* 1984;91(4):361–365.

83. Frucht J, Bishara S, Ticho U. Early intraocular pressure response following laser trabeculoplasty. *Br J Ophthalmol.* 1985;69(10):771–773.

84. The Glaucoma Laser Trial Research Group. The Glaucoma Laser Trial. I. Acute effects of argon laser trabeculoplasty on intraocular pressure. *Arch Ophthalmol.* 1989;107(8):1135–1142.

85. Mittra RA, Allingham RR, Shields MB. Follow-up of argon laser trabeculoplasty: is a day-one postoperative IOP check necessary? *Ophthalmic Surg Lasers.* 1995;26(5):410–413.

86. Kajiya S, Hayakawa K, Sawaguchi S. Clinical results of selective laser trabeculoplasty. *Jpn J Ophthalmol.* 2000;44(5):574–575.

87. Kano K, Kuwayama Y, Mizoue S, et al. Clinical results of selective laser trabeculoplasty [in Japanese]. *Nippon Ganka Gakkai Zasshi.* 1999;103(8):612–616.

88. Lanzetta P, Menchini U, Virgili G. Immediate intraocular pressure response to selective laser trabeculoplasty. *Br J Ophthalmol.* 1999;83(1):29–32.

89. Greenidge KC, Rodrigues MM, Spaeth GL, et al. Acute intraocular pressure elevation after argon laser trabeculoplasty and iridectomy: a clinicopathologic study. *Ophthalmic Surg.* 1984;15(2):105–110.

90. Koss MC, March WF, Nordquist RE, et al. Acute intraocular pressure elevation produced by argon laser trabeculoplasty in the cynomolgus monkey. *Arch Ophthalmol.* 1984;102(11):1699–1703.

91. Wiederholt M, Dorschner N, Groth J. Effect of diuretics, channel modulators and signal interceptors on contractility of the trabecular meshwork. *Ophthalmologica.* 1997;211(3):153–160.

92. Hollo G. Membrane formation in the chamber angle after failure of argon laser trabeculoplasty. *Br J Ophthalmol.* 2000;84(6):673–674.

93. Hollo G, Lakatos P. Increase of endothelin-1 concentration in aqueous humour induced by argon laser trabeculoplasty in the rabbit. A preliminary study. *Acta Ophthalmol Scand.* 1998;76(3):289–293.

94. Hollo G, Lakatos P, Vargha P. Immediate increase in aqueous humour endothelin 1 concentration and intra-ocular pressure after argon laser trabeculoplasty in the rabbit. *Ophthalmologica.* 2000;214(4):292–295.

95. Guzey M, Vural H, Satici A. Endothelin-1 increase in aqueous humour caused by frequency-doubled Nd:YAG laser trabeculoplasty in rabbits. *Eye (Lond).* 2001;15(6):781–785.

96. Fiore PM, Melamed S, Epstein DL. Trabecular precipitates and elevated intraocular pressure following argon laser trabeculoplasty. *Ophthalmic Surg.* 1989;20(10):697–701.

97. Mermoud A, Pittet N, Herbort CP. Inflammation patterns after laser trabeculoplasty measured with the laser flare meter. *Arch Ophthalmol.* 1992;110(3):368–370.

98. Ruderman JM, Zweig KO, Wilensky JT, et al. Effects of corticosteroid pretreatment on argon laser trabeculoplasty. *Am J Ophthalmol.* 1983;96(1):84–89.

99. Weinreb RN, Robin AL, Baerveldt G, et al. Flurbiprofen pretreatment in argon laser trabeculoplasty for primary open-angle glaucoma. *Arch Ophthalmol.* 1984;102(11):1629–1632.

100. Pappas HR, Berry DP, Partamian L, et al. Topical indomethacin therapy before argon laser trabeculoplasty. *Am J Ophthalmol.* 1985;99(5):571–575.

101. Herbort CP, Mermoud A, Schnyder C, et al. Anti-inflammatory effect of diclofenac drops after argon laser trabeculoplasty. *Arch Ophthalmol.* 1993;111(4):481–483.

102. Shin DH, Frenkel RE, David R, et al. Effect of topical anti-inflammatory treatment on the outcome of laser trabeculoplasty. The Fluorometholone-Laser Trabeculoplasty Study Group. *Am J Ophthalmol.* 1996;122(3):349–354.

103. Kim YY, Glover BK, Shin DH, et al. Effect of topical anti-inflammatory treatment on the long-term outcome of laser trabeculoplasty. Fluorometholone-Laser Trabeculoplasty Study Group. *Am J Ophthalmol.* 1998;126(5):721–723.

104. Damji KF, Shah KC, Rock WJ, et al. Selective laser trabeculoplasty v argon laser trabeculoplasty: a prospective randomised clinical trial. *Br J Ophthalmol.* 1999;83(6):718–722.

105. Hong C, Kitazawa Y, Tanishima T. Influence of argon laser treatment of glaucoma on corneal endothelium. *Jpn J Ophthalmol.* 1983;27(4):567–574.

106. Traverso C, Cohen EJ, Groden LR, et al. Central corneal endothelial cell density after argon laser trabeculoplasty. *Arch Ophthalmol.* 1984;102(9):1322–1324.

107. Koller T, Sturmer J, Reme C, et al. Membrane formation in the chamber angle after failure of argon laser trabeculoplasty: analysis of risk factors. *Br J Ophthalmol.* 2000;84(1):48–53.

108. Schwartz AL, Van Veldhuisen PC, Gaasterland DE, et al. The Advanced Glaucoma Intervention Study (AGIS): 5. Encapsulated bleb after initial trabeculectomy. *Am J Ophthalmol.* 1999;127(1):8–19.

109. Schoenleber DB, Bellows AR, Hutchinson BT. Failed laser trabeculoplasty requiring surgery in open-angle glaucoma. *Ophthalmic Surg.* 1987;18(11):796–799.

110. Robin AL, Pollack IP, House B, et al. Effects of ALO 2145 on intraocular pressure following argon laser trabeculoplasty. *Arch Ophthalmol.* 1987;105(5):646–650.

111. Robin AL. Argon laser trabeculoplasty medical therapy to prevent the intraocular pressure rise associated with argon laser trabeculoplasty. *Ophthalmic Surg.* 1991;22(1):31–37.

112. Birt CM, Shin DH, Reed SY, et al. One vs. two doses of 1.0% apraclonidine for prophylaxis of intraocular pressure spike after argon laser trabeculoplasty. *Can J Ophthalmol.* 1995;30(5):266–269.

113. Holmwood PC, Chase RD, Krupin T, et al. Apraclonidine and argon laser trabeculoplasty. *Am J Ophthalmol.* 1992;114(1):19–22.

114. Rosenberg LF, Krupin T, Ruderman J, et al. Apraclonidine and anterior segment laser surgery. Comparison of 0.5% versus 1.0% apraclonidine for prevention of postoperative intraocular pressure rise. *Ophthalmology.* 1995;102(9):1312–1318.

115. Threlkeld AB, Assalian AA, Allingham RR, et al. Apraclonidine 0.5% versus 1% for controlling intraocular pressure elevation after argon laser trabeculoplasty. *Ophthalmic Surg Lasers.* 1996;27(8):657–660.

116. Allf BE, Shields MB. Early intraocular pressure response to laser trabeculoplasty 180 degrees without apraclonidine versus 360 degrees with apraclonidine. *Ophthalmic Surg.* 1991;22(9):539–542.

117. David R, Spaeth GL, Clevenger CE, et al. Brimonidine in the prevention of intraocular pressure elevation following argon laser trabeculoplasty. *Arch Ophthalmol.* 1993;111(10):1387–1390.

118. The Brimonidine-ALT Study Group. Effect of brimonidine 0.5% on intraocular pressure spikes following 360% argon laser trabeculoplasty. *Ophthalmic Surg Lasers.* 1995;26(5):404–409.

119. Barnes SD, Campagna JA, Dirks MS, et al. Control of intraocular pressure elevations after argon laser trabeculoplasty: comparison of brimonidine 0.2% to apraclonidine 1.0%. *Ophthalmology.* 1999;106(10):2033–2037.

120. Ofner S, Samples JR, van Buskirk EM. Pilocarpine and the increase in intraocular pressure after trabeculoplasty. *Am J Ophthalmol.* 1984;97(5):647–649.

121. Ren J, Shin DH, Chung HS, et al. Efficacy of apraclonidine 1% versus pilocarpine 4% for prophylaxis of intraocular pressure spike after argon laser trabeculoplasty. *Ophthalmology.* 1999;106(6):1135–1139.

122. Dapling RB, Cunliffe IA, Longstaff S. Influence of apraclonidine and pilocarpine alone and in combination on post laser trabeculoplasty pressure rise. *Br J Ophthalmol.* 1994;78(1):30–32.

123. Metcalfe TW, Etchells DE. Prevention of the immediate intraocular pressure rise following argon laser trabeculoplasty. *Br J Ophthalmol.* 1989;73(8):612–616.

124. Gelfand YA, Wolpert M. Effects of topical indomethacin pretreatment on argon laser trabeculoplasty: a randomised, double-masked study on black South Africans. *Br J Ophthalmol.* 1985;69(9):668–672.

125. Tuulonen A. The effect of topical indomethacin on acute pressure elevation of laser trabeculoplasty in capsular glaucoma. *Acta Ophthalmol.* 1985;63(2):245–249.

126. Hotchkiss ML, Robin AL, Pollack IP, et al. Nonsteroidal anti-inflammatory agents after argon laser trabeculoplasty. A trial with flurbiprofen and indomethacin. *Ophthalmology.* 1984;91(8):969–976.

127. Forbes M, Bansal RK. Argon laser goniophotocoagulation of the trabecular meshwork in open-angle glaucoma. *Trans Am Ophthalmol Soc.* 1981;79:257–275.

128. Pollack IP, Robin AL, SaxH. The effect of argon laser trabeculoplasty on the medical control of primary open-angle glaucoma. *Ophthalmology.* 1983;90(7):785–789.

129. Quaranta L, Ripandelli G, Manni GL, et al. Hypotensive effect of pilocarpine after argon laser trabeculoplasty. *J Glaucoma.* 1992;1(4):233–236.

130. Teus MA, Castejon MA, Calvo MA, et al. Ocular hypotensive effect of pilocarpine before and after argon laser trabeculoplasty. *Acta Ophthalmol Scand.* 1997;75(5):503–506.

131. Gracner T. Intraocular pressure response to selective laser trabeculoplasty in the treatment of primary open-angle glaucoma. *Ophthalmologica.* 2001;215(4):267–270.

132. Gracner T. Intraocular pressure response of capsular glaucoma and primary open-angle glaucoma to selective Nd:YAG laser trabeculoplasty: a prospective, comparative clinical trial. *Eur J Ophthalmol.* 2002;12(4):287–292.

133. Cvenkel B. One-year follow-up of selective laser trabeculoplasty in open-angle glaucoma. *Ophthalmologica.* 2004;218(1):20–25.

134. Brooks AM, Gillies WE. Do any factors predict a favourable response to laser trabeculoplasty? *Aust J Ophthalmol.* 1984;12(2):149–153.

135. Tuulonen A, Airaksinen PJ, Kuulasmaa K. Factors influencing the outcome of laser trabeculoplasty. *Am J Ophthalmol.* 1985;99(4):388–391.

136. The AGIS Investigators. The Advanced Glaucoma Intervention Study (AGIS): 11. Risk factors for failure of trabeculectomy and argon laser trabeculoplasty. *Am J Ophthalmol.* 2002;134(4):481–498.

137. Strasser G, Stelzer R. Laser trabeculoplasty in low-tension glaucoma [in German]. *Klin Monbl Augenheilkd.* 1983;183(6):507–508.

138. Schwartz AL, Perman KI, Whitten M. Argon laser trabeculoplasty in progressive low-tension glaucoma. *Ann Ophthalmol.* 1984;16(6):560–562, 566.

139. Sharpe ED, Simmons RJ. Argon laser trabeculoplasty as a means of decreasing intraocular pressure from "normal" levels in glaucomatous eyes. *Am J Ophthalmol.* 1985;99(6):704–707.

140. Robin AL, Pollack IP. Argon laser trabeculoplasty in secondary forms of open-angle glaucoma. *Arch Ophthalmol.* 1983;101(3):382–384.

141. Lieberman MF, Hoskins HD Jr, Hetherington J Jr. Laser trabeculoplasty and the glaucomas. *Ophthalmology.* 1983;90(7):790–795.

142. Lunde MW. Argon laser trabeculoplasty in pigmentary dispersion syndrome with glaucoma. *Am J Ophthalmol.* 1983;96(6):721–725.

143. Ritch R, Liebmann J, Robin A, et al. Argon laser trabeculoplasty in pigmentary glaucoma. *Ophthalmology.* 1993;100(6):909–913.

144. Rouhiainen HJ, Terasvirta ME, Tuovinen EJ. The effect of some treatment variables on the results of trabeculoplasty. *Arch Ophthalmol.* 1988;106(5):611–613.

145. Harasymowycz PJ, Papamatheakis DG, Latina M, et al. Selective laser trabeculoplasty (SLT) complicated by intraocular pressure elevation in eyes with heavily pigmented trabecular meshworks. *Am J Ophthalmol.* 2005;139(6):1110–1113.

146. Dreyer EB, Gorla M. Laser trabeculoplasty in the pseudophakic patient. *J Glaucoma.* 1993;2(4):313–315.

147. Fellman RL, Starita RJ, Spaeth GL, et al. Argon laser trabeculoplasty following failed trabeculectomy. *Ophthalmic Surg.* 1984;15(3):195–198.

148. Safran MJ, Robin AL, Pollack IP. Argon laser trabeculoplasty in younger patients with primary open-angle glaucoma. *Am J Ophthalmol.* 1984;97(3):292–295.

149. Krupin T, Patkin R, Kurata FK, et al. Argon laser trabeculoplasty in black and white patients with primary open-angle glaucoma. *Ophthalmology.* 1986;93(6):811–816.

150. The AGIS Investigators. The Advanced Glaucoma Intervention Study (AGIS): 4. Comparison of treatment outcomes within race. Seven-year results. *Ophthalmology.* 1998;105(7):1146–1164.

151. The AGIS Investigators. The Advanced Glaucoma Intervention Study (AGIS): 9. Comparison of glaucoma outcomes in black and white patients within treatment groups. *Am J Ophthalmol.* 2001;132(3):311–320.

152. Grinich NP, Van Buskirk EM, Samples JR. Three-year efficacy of argon laser trabeculoplasty. *Ophthalmology.* 1987;94(7):858–861.

153. Schwartz AL, Kopelman J. Four-year experience with argon laser trabecular surgery in uncontrolled open-angle glaucoma. *Ophthalmology.* 1983;90(7):771–780.

154. Tuulonen A, Niva AK, Alanko HI. A controlled five-year follow-up study of laser trabeculoplasty as primary therapy for open-angle glaucoma. *Am J Ophthalmol.* 1987;104(4):334–338.

155. Shingleton BJ, Richter CU, Bellows AR, et al. Long-term efficacy of argon laser trabeculoplasty. *Ophthalmology.* 1987;94(12):1513–1518.

156. Ticho U, Nesher R. Laser trabeculoplasty in glaucoma. Ten-year evaluation. *Arch Ophthalmol.* 1989;107(6):844–846.

157. Spaeth GL, Baez KA. Argon laser trabeculoplasty controls one third of cases of progressive, uncontrolled, open angle glaucoma for 5 years. *Arch Ophthalmol.* 1992;110(4):491–494.

158. Spiegel D, Wegscheider E, Lund OE. Argon laser trabeculoplasty: long-term follow-up of at least 5 years. *Ger J Ophthalmol.* 1992;1(3–4):156–158.

159. Shingleton BJ, Richter CU, Dharma SK, et al. Long-term efficacy of argon laser trabeculoplasty. A 10-year follow-up study. *Ophthalmology.* 1993;100(9):1324–1329.

160. Starita RJ, Fellman RL, Spaeth GL, et al. The effect of repeating full-circumference argon laser trabeculoplasty. *Ophthalmic Surg.* 1984;15(1):41–43.

161. Brown SV, Thomas JV, Simmons RJ. Laser trabeculoplasty re-treatment. *Am J Ophthalmol.* 1985;99(1):8–10.

162. Richter CU, Shingleton BJ, Bellows AR, et al. Retreatment with argon laser trabeculoplasty. *Ophthalmology.* 1987;94(9):1085–1089.

163. Messner D, Siegel LI, Kass MA, et al. Repeat argon laser trabeculoplasty. *Am J Ophthalmol.* 1987;103(1):113–115.

164. Grayson DK, Camras CB, Podos SM, et al. Long-term reduction of intraocular pressure after repeat argon laser trabeculoplasty. *Am J Ophthalmol.* 1988;106(3):312–321.

165. Weber PA, Burton GD, Epitropoulos AT. Laser trabeculoplasty retreatment. *Ophthalmic Surg.* 1989;20(10):702–706.

166. Feldman RM, Katz LJ, Spaeth GL, et al. Long-term efficacy of repeat argon laser trabeculoplasty. *Ophthalmology.* 1991;98(7):1061–1065.

167. Garcia GS, Garcia DS. Is it useful to repeating trabeculoplasty? [in Spanish]. *Arch Soc Esp Oftalmol.* 2000;75(12):803–806.

168. Hong BK, Winer JC, Martone JF, et al. Repeat selective laser trabeculoplasty. *J Glaucoma.* 2009;18(3):180–183.

169. Latina MA, Tumbocon JA. Selective laser trabeculoplasty: a new treatment option for open angle glaucoma. *Curr Opin Ophthalmol.* 2002;13(2):94–96.

170. Schwartz AL, Wilson MC, Schwartz LW. Efficacy of argon laser trabeculoplasty in aphakic and pseudophakic eyes. *Ophthalmic Surg Lasers.* 1997;28(3):215–218.

171. Van Meter WS, Allen RC, Waring GO III, et al. Laser trabeculoplasty for glaucoma in aphakic and pseudophakic eyes after penetrating keratoplasty. *Arch Ophthalmol.* 1988;106(2):185–188.

172. Sherwood MB, Lattimer J, Hitchings RA. Laser trabeculoplasty as supplementary treatment for primary open angle glaucoma. *Br J Ophthalmol.* 1987;71(3):188–191.

173. Thomas JV, El-Mofty A, Hamdy EE, et al. Argon laser trabeculoplasty as initial therapy for glaucoma. *Arch Ophthalmol.* 1984;102(5):702–703.

174. Rosenthal AR, Chaudhuri PR, Chiapella AP. Laser trabeculoplasty primary therapy in open-angle glaucoma. A preliminary report. *Arch Ophthalmol.* 1984;102(5):699–701.

175. Migdal C, Hitchings R. Primary therapy for chronic simple glaucoma the role of argon laser trabeculoplasty. *Trans Ophthalmol Soc UK.* 1985;104(1):62–66.

176. Tuulonen A, Koponen J, Alanko HI, et al. Laser trabeculoplasty versus medication treatment as primary therapy for glaucoma. *Acta Ophthalmol.* 1989;67(3):275–280.

177. Elsas T, Johnsen H. Long-term efficacy of primary laser trabeculoplasty. *Br J Ophthalmol.* 1991;75(1):34–37.

178. The Glaucoma Laser Trial Research Group. The Glaucoma Laser Trial (GLT). 2. Results of argon laser trabeculoplasty versus topical medicines. *Ophthalmology.* 1990;97(11):1403–1413.

179. The Glaucoma Laser Trial Research Group. The Glaucoma Laser Trial (GLT) and glaucoma laser trial follow-up study: 7. Results. *Am J Ophthalmol.* 1995;120(6):718–731.

180. McIlraith I, Strasfeld M, Colev G, et al. Selective laser trabeculoplasty as initial and adjunctive treatment for open-angle glaucoma. *J Glaucoma.* 2006;15(2):124–130.

181. Nagar M, Ogunyomade A, O'Brart DP, et al. A randomised, prospective study comparing selective laser trabeculoplasty with latanoprost for the control of intraocular pressure in ocular hypertension and open angle glaucoma. *Br J Ophthalmol.* 2005;89(11):1413–1417.

182. Damji KF, Bovell AM, Hodge WG, et al. Selective laser trabeculoplasty versus argon laser trabeculoplasty: results from a 1-year randomised clinical trial. *Br J Ophthalmol.* 2006;90(12):1490–1494.

183. Juzych MS, Chopra V, Banitt MR, et al. Comparison of long-term outcomes of selective laser trabeculoplasty versus argon laser trabeculoplasty in open-angle glaucoma. *Ophthalmology.* 2004;111(10):1853–1859.

184. Prasad N, Murthy S, Dagianis JJ, et al. A comparison of the intervisit intraocular pressure fluctuation after 180 and 360 degrees of selective laser trabeculoplasty (SLT) as a primary therapy in primary open angle glaucoma and ocular hypertension. *J Glaucoma.* 2009;18(2):157–160.

185. Birt CM. Selective laser trabeculoplasty retreatment after prior argon laser trabeculoplasty: 1-year results. *Can J Ophthalmol.* 2007;42(5):715–719.

186. Meyer-Schwickerath G. Experiments with light-coagulation of the retina and iris [in German]. *Doc Ophthalmol Proc Ser.* 1956;10:91–118.

187. Hogan MJ, Schwartz A. Experimental photocoagulation of the iris of guinea pigs: a pilot study. *Am J Ophthalmol.* 1960;49:629–630.

188. Flocks M, Zweng HC. Laser coagulation of ocular tissues. *Arch Ophthalmol.* 1964;72:604–611.

189. Snyder WB. Laser coagulation of the anterior segment. 1. Experimental laser iridotomy. *Arch Ophthalmol.* 1967;77(1):93–98.

190. Hallman DL, Perkins ES, Watts GK, et al. Laser irradiation of the anterior segment of the eye—rabbit eyes. *Exp Eye Res.* 1968;7(4):481–486.

191. Hallman VL, Perkins ES, Watts GK, et al. Laser irradiation of the anterior segment of the eye. II. Monkey eyes. *Exp Eye Res.* 1969;8(1):1–4.

192. Khuri CH. Argon laser iridectomies. *Am J Ophthalmol.* 1973;76(4):490–493.

193. L'Esperance FA Jr, James WA Jr. Argon laser photocoagulation of iris abnormalities. *Trans Sect Ophthalmol Am Acad Ophthalmol Otolaryngol.* 1975;79(2):OP321–OP339.

194. Abraham RK, Miller GL. Outpatient argon laser iridectomy for angle closure glaucoma: a two-year study. *Trans Sect Ophthalmol Am Acad Ophthalmol Otolaryngol.* 1975;79(3 pt 2):OP529–OP537.

195. Anderson DR, Forster RK, Lewis ML. Laser iridotomy for aphakic pupillary block. *Arch Ophthalmol.* 1975;93(5):343–346.

196. Pollack IP, Patz A. Argon laser iridotomy: an experimental and clinical study. *Ophthalmic Surg.* 1976;7(1):22–30.

197. Pollack IP. Use of argon laser energy to produce iridotomies. *Trans Am Ophthalmol Soc.* 1979;77:674–706.

198. Podos SM, Kels BD, Moss AP, et al. Continuous wave argon laser iridectomy in angle-closure glaucoma. *Trans Am Ophthalmol Soc.* 1979;77:51–62.

199. Yassur Y, Melamed S, Cohen S, et al. Laser iridotomy in closed-angle glaucoma. *Arch Ophthalmol.* 1979;97(10):1920–1921.

200. Pollack IP. Use of argon laser energy to produce iridotomies. *Ophthalmic Surg.* 1980;11(8):506–515.

201. Quigley HA. Long-term follow-up of laser iridotomy. *Ophthalmology.* 1981;88(3):218–224.

202. Schwartz LW, Rodrigues MM, Spaeth GL, et al. Argon laser iridotomy in the treatment of patients with primary angle-closure or pupillary block glaucoma: a clinicopathologic study. *Ophthalmology.* 1978;85(3):294–309.

203. Yassur Y, David R, Rosenblatt I, et al. Iridotomy with red krypton laser. *Br J Ophthalmol.* 1986;70(4):295–297.

204. Latina MA, Puliafito CA, Steinert RR, et al. Experimental iridotomy with the Q-switched neodymium-YAG laser. *Arch Ophthalmol.* 1984;102(8):1211–1213.

205. Klapper RM. Q-switched neodymium:YAG laser iridotomy. *Ophthalmology.* 1984;91(9):1017–1021.

206. Robin AL, Pollack IP. A comparison of neodymium: YAG and argon laser iridotomies. *Ophthalmology.* 1984;91(9):1011–1016.

207. McAllister JA, Schwartz LW, Moster M, et al. Laser peripheral iridectomy comparing Q-switched neodymium YAG with argon. *Trans Ophthalmol Soc UK.* 1985;104(1):67–69.

208. Pollack IP, Robin AL, Dragon DM, et al. Use of the neodymium:YAG laser to create iridotomies in monkeys and humans. *Trans Am Ophthalmol Soc.* 1984;82:307–328.

209. Rodrigues MM, Spaeth GL, Moster M, et al. Histopathology of neodymium:YAG laser iridectomy in humans. *Ophthalmology.* 1985;92(12):1696–1700.

210. Vernon SA, Cheng H. Freeze frame analysis on high speed cinematography of Nd/YAG laser explosions in ocular tissues. *Br J Ophthalmol.* 1986;70(5):321–325.

211. Goldberg MF, Tso MO, Mirolovich M. Histopathological characteristics of neodymium-YAG laser iridotomy in the human eye. *Br J Ophthalmol.* 1987;71(8):623–628.

212. Robin AL, Arkell S, Gilbert SM, et al. Q-switched neodymium-YAG laser iridotomy. A field trial with a portable laser system. *Arch Ophthalmol.* 1986;104(4):526–530.

213. Abraham RK. Protocol for single-session argon laser iridectomy for angle-closure glaucoma. *Int Ophthalmol Clin.* 1981;21(1):145–166.

214. Schirmer KE. One-piece contact lens for laser iridotomy at iris base by argon and Nd:YAG laser. *Ophthalmologica.* 1990;200(1):7–9.

215. Wise JB, Munnerlyn CR, Erickson PJ. A high-efficiency laser iridotomy-sphincterotomy lens. *Am J Ophthalmol.* 1986;101(5):546–553.

216. Ritch R. Argon laser treatment for medically unresponsive attacks of angle-closure glaucoma. *Am J Ophthalmol.* 1982;94(2):197–204.

217. Lewis R, Perkins TW, Gangnon R, et al. The rarity of clinically significant rise in intraocular pressure after laser peripheral iridotomy with apraclonidine. *Ophthalmology.* 1998;105(12):2256–2259.

218. Krupin T, Stank T, Feitl ME. Apraclonidine pretreatment decreases the acute intraocular pressure rise after laser trabeculoplasty or iridotomy. *J Glaucoma.* 1992;1(2):79–86.

219. Murphy PH, Trope GE. Monocular blurring. A complication of YAG laser iridotomy. *Ophthalmology.* 1991;98(10):1539–1542.

220. Spaeth GL, Idowu O, Seligsohn A, et al. The effects of iridotomy size and position on symptoms following laser peripheral iridotomy. *J Glaucoma.* 2005;14(5):364–367.

221. Hoskins HD, Migliazzo CV. Laser iridectomy—a technique for blue irises. *Ophthalmic Surg.* 1984;15(6):488–490.

222. Abraham RK. Procedure for outpatient argon laser iridectomies for angle-closure glaucoma. *Int Ophthalmol Clin.* 1976;16(4):1–14.

223. Harrad RA, Stannard KP, Shilling JS. Argon laser iridotomy. *Br J Ophthalmol.* 1985;69(5):368–372.

224. Yamamoto T, Shirato S, Kitazawa Y. Argon laser iridotomy in angle-closure glaucoma: a comparison of two methods. *Jpn J Ophthalmol.* 1982;26(4):387–396.

225. Mandelkorn RM, Mendelsohn AD, Olander KW, et al. Short exposure times in argon laser iridotomy. *Ophthalmic Surg.* 1981;12(11):805–809.

226. Kolker AE. Techniques of argon laser iridectomy. *Trans Am Ophthalmol Soc.* 1984;82:302–306.

227. Stetz D, Smith H Jr, Ritch R. A simplified technique for laser iridectomy in blue irides. *Am J Ophthalmol.* 1983;96(2):249–251.

228. Fleck BW. How large must an iridotomy be? *Br J Ophthalmol.* 1990;74(10):583–588.

229. Fleck BW, Fairley E, Wright E. A photometric study of the effect of pupil dilatation on Nd:YAG laser iridotomy area. *Br J Ophthalmol.* 1992;76(11):678–680.

230. Damerow A, Utermann D. Combined thermal-photodisruptive iridotomy using the argon and neodymium:YAG laser [in German]. *Klin Monbl Augenheilkd.* 1989;195(2):61–67.

231. Goins K, Schmeisser E, Smith T. Argon laser pretreatment in Nd:YAG iridotomy. *Ophthalmic Surg.* 1990;21(7):497–500.

232. Ho T, Fan R. Sequential argon-YAG laser iridotomies in dark irides. *Br J Ophthalmol.* 1992;76(6):329–331.

233. Wise JB. Large iridotomies by the linear incision technique using the neodymium:YAG laser at low energy levels. A study using cynomolgus monkeys. *Ophthalmology.* 1987;94(1):82–86.

234. Wise JB. Low-energy linear-incision neodymium:YAG laser iridotomy versus linear-incision argon laser iridotomy. A prospective clinical investigation. *Ophthalmology.* 1987;94(12):1531–1537.

235. Rol P, Kwasniewska S, van der Zypen E, et al. Transscleral iridotomy using a neodymium:YAG laser operated both with standard equipment and an optical fiber system—a preliminary report: Part I—Optical system and biomicroscopic results. *Ophthalmic Surg.* 1987;18(3):176–182.

236. Oram O, Gross RL, Severin TD, et al. Picosecond neodymium:yttrium lithium fluoride (Nd:YLF) laser peripheral iridotomy. *Am J Ophthalmol.* 1995;119(4):408–414.

237. Frangie JP, Park SB, Aquavella JV. Peripheral iridotomy using Nd:YLF laser. *Ophthalmic Surg.* 1992;23(3):220–221.

238. Jacobson JJ, Schuman JS, el Koumy H, et al. Diode laser peripheral iridectomy. *Int Ophthalmol Clin.* 1990;30(2):120–122.

239. Emoto I, Okisaka S, Nakajima A. Diode laser iridotomy in rabbit and human eyes. *Am J Ophthalmol.* 1992;113(3):321–327.

240. Schuman JS, Puliafito CA, Jacobson JJ. Semiconductor diode laser peripheral iridotomy. *Arch Ophthalmol.* 1990;108(9):1207–1208.

241. Bonney CH, Gaasterland DE. Low-energy, Q-switched ruby laser iridotomies in *Macaca mulatta. Invest Ophthalmol Vis Sci.* 1979;18(3):278–287.

242. Bass MS, Cleary CV, Perkins ES, et al. Single treatment laser iridotomy. *Br J Ophthalmol.* 1979;63(1):29–30.

243. Abreu MM, Sierra RA, Netland PA. Diode laser-pumped, frequency-doubled neodymium: YAG laser peripheral iridotomy. *Ophthalmic Surg Lasers.* 1997;28(4):305–310.

244. Robin AL, Pollack IP. Argon laser peripheral iridotomies in the treatment of primary angle closure glaucoma. Long-term follow-up. *Arch Ophthalmol.* 1982;100(6):919–923.

245. Aung T, Ang LP, Chan SP, et al. Acute primary angle-closure: long-term intraocular pressure outcome in Asian eyes. *Am J Ophthalmol.* 2001;131(1):7–12.

246. Hsiao CH, Hsu CT, Shen SC, et al. Mid-term follow-up of Nd:YAG laser iridotomy in Asian eyes. *Ophthalmic Surg Lasers Imaging.* 2003;34(4):291–298.

247. Gazzard G, Friedman DS, Devereux JG, et al. A prospective ultrasound biomicroscopy evaluation of changes in anterior segment morphology after laser iridotomy in Asian eyes. *Ophthalmology.* 2003;110(3):630–638.

248. Thomas R, Arun T, Muliyil J, et al. Outcome of laser peripheral iridotomy in chronic primary angle closure glaucoma. *Ophthalmic Surg Lasers.* 1999;30(7):547–553.

249. Alsagoff Z, Aung T, Ang LP, et al. Long-term clinical course of primary angle-closure glaucoma in an Asian population. *Ophthalmology.* 2000;107(12):2300–2304.

250. Rosman M, Aung T, Ang LP, et al. Chronic angle-closure with glaucomatous damage: long-term clinical course in a North American population and comparison with an Asian population. *Ophthalmology.* 2002;109(12):2227–2231.

251. Saw SM, Gazzard G, Friedman DS. Interventions for angle-closure glaucoma: an evidence-based update. *Ophthalmology.* 2003;110(10):1869–1878; quiz 1878–1879, 1930.

252. Ang LP, Aung T, Chew PT. Acute primary angle closure in an Asian population: long-term outcome of the fellow eye after prophylactic laser peripheral iridotomy. *Ophthalmology.* 2000;107(11):2092–2096.

253. Rodrigues MM, Streeten B, Spaeth GL, et al. Argon laser iridotomy on primary angle closure or pupillary block glaucoma. *Arch Ophthalmol.* 1978;96(12):2222–2230.

254. Richardson TM, Brown SV, Thomas JV, et al. Shock-wave effect on anterior segment structures following experimental neodymium:YAG laser iridectomy. *Ophthalmology.* 1985;92(10):1387–1395.

255. Prum BE Jr, Shields SR, Shields MB, et al. *In vitro* videographic comparison of argon and Nd:YAG laser iridotomy. *Am J Ophthalmol.* 1991;111(5):589–594.

256. Moster MR, Schwartz LW, Spaeth GL, et al. Laser iridectomy. A controlled study comparing argon and neodymium:YAG. *Ophthalmology.* 1986;93(1):20–24.

257. Del Priore LV, Robin AL, Pollack IP. Neodymium:YAG and argon laser iridotomy. Long-term follow-up in a prospective, randomized clinical trial. *Ophthalmology.* 1988;95(9):1207–1211.

258. Robin AL, Pollack IP. Q-switched neodymium-YAG laser iridotomy in patients in whom the argon laser fails. *Arch Ophthalmol.* 1986;104(4):531–535.

259. Krupin T, Stone RA, Cohen BH, et al. Acute intraocular pressure response to argon laser iridotomy. *Ophthalmology.* 1985;92(7):922–926.

260. Taniguchi T, Rho SH, Gotoh Y, et al. Intraocular pressure rise following Q-switched neodymium:YAG laser iridectomy. *Ophthalmol Laser Ther.* 1987;2:99.

261. Wetzel W. Ocular aqueous humor dynamics after photodisruptive laser surgery procedures. *Ophthalmic Surg.* 1994;25(5):298–302.

262. Sugiyama K, Kitazawa Y, Kawai K, et al. Biphasic intraocular pressure response to Q-switched Nd:YAG laser irradiation of the iris and the apparent mediatory role of prostaglandins. *Exp Eye Res.* 1990;51(5):531–536.

263. Gailitis R, Peyman GA, Pulido J, et al. Prostaglandin release following Nd:YAG iridotomy in rabbits. *Ophthalmic Surg.* 1986;17(8):467–469.

264. Joo CK, Kim JH. Prostaglandin E in rabbit aqueous humor after Nd-YAG laser photodisruption of iris and the effect of topical indomethacin pretreatment. *Invest Ophthalmol Vis Sci.* 1992;33(5):1685–1689.

265. Weinreb RN, Weaver D, Mitchell MD. Prostanoids in rabbit aqueous humor: effect of laser photocoagulation of the iris. *Invest Ophthalmol Vis Sci.* 1985;26(8):1087–1092.

266. Sanders DR, Joondeph B, Hutchins R, et al. Studies on the blood-aqueous barrier after argon laser photocoagulation of the iris. *Ophthalmology.* 1983;90(2):169–174.

267. Schrems W, van Dorp HP, Wendel M, et al. The effect of YAG laser iridotomy on the blood aqueous barrier in the rabbit. *Graefes Arch Clin Exp Ophthalmol.* 1984;221(4):179–181.

268. Tawara A, Inomata H. Histological study on transient ocular hypertension after laser iridotomy in rabbits. *Graefes Arch Clin Exp Ophthalmol.* 1987;225(2):114–122.

269. Robin AL, Pollack IP, Quigley HA, et al. Histologic studies of angle structures after laser iridotomy in primates. *Arch Ophthalmol.* 1982;100(10):1665–1670.

270. Liu CJ, Cheng CY, Chiang SC, et al. Use of latanoprost to reduce acute intraocular pressure rise following neodymium:Yag laser iridotomy. *Acta Ophthalmol Scand.* 2002;80(3):282–286.

271. Cohen JS, Bibler L, Tucker D. Hypopyon following laser iridotomy. *Ophthalmic Surg.* 1984;15(7):604–606.

272. Margo CE, Lessner A, Goldey SH, et al. Lens-induced endophthalmitis after Nd:YAG laser iridotomy. *Am J Ophthalmol.* 1992;113(1):97–98.

273. Choplin NT, Bene CH. Cystoid macular edema following laser iridotomy. *Ann Ophthalmol.* 1983;15(2):172–173.

274. Geyer O, Mayron Y, Rothkoff L, et al. Pigmented pupillary pseudomembranes as a complication of argon laser iridotomy. *Ophthalmic Surg.* 1991;22(3):162–164.

275. Schwartz LW, Moster MR, Spaeth GL, et al. Neodymium-YAG laser iridectomies in glaucoma associated with closed or occludable angles. *Am J Ophthalmol.* 1986;102(1):41–44.

276. Brainard JO, Landers JH, Shock JP. Recurrent angle closure glaucoma following a patent 75-micron laser iridotomy: a case report. *Ophthalmic Surg.* 1982;13(12):1030–1032.

277. Sachs SW, Schwartz B. Enlargement of laser iridotomies over time. *Br J Ophthalmol.* 1984;68(8):570–573.

278. Hirst LW, Robin AL, Sherman S, et al. Corneal endothelial changes after argon-laser iridotomy and panretinal photocoagulation. *Am J Ophthalmol.* 1982;93(4):473–481.

279. Smith J, Whitted P. Corneal endothelial changes after argon laser iridotomy. *Am J Ophthalmol.* 1984;98(2):153–156.

280. Panek WC, Lee DA, Christensen RE. Effects of argon laser iridotomy on the corneal endothelium. *Am J Ophthalmol.* 1988;105(4):395–397.

281. Panek WC, Lee DA, Christensen RE. The effects of Nd:YAG laser iridotomy on the corneal endothelium. *Am J Ophthalmol.* 1991;111(4):505–507.

282. Marraffa M, Marchini G, Pagliarusco A, et al. Ultrasound biomicroscopy and corneal endothelium in Nd:YAG-laser iridotomy. *Ophthalmic Surg Lasers.* 1995;26(6):519–523.

283. Wu SC, Jeng S, Huang SC, et al. Corneal endothelial damage after neodymium:YAG laser iridotomy. *Ophthalmic Surg Lasers.* 2000;31(5):411–416.

284. Schwartz AL, Martin NF, Weber PA. Corneal decompensation after argon laser iridectomy. *Arch Ophthalmol.* 1988;106(11):1572–1574.

285. Zabel RW, MacDonald IM, Mintsioulis G. Corneal endothelial decompensation after argon laser iridotomy. *Can J Ophthalmol.* 1991;26(7): 367–373.

286. Jeng S, Lee JS, Huang SC. Corneal decompensation after argon laser iridectomy—a delayed complication. *Ophthalmic Surg.* 1991;22(10): 565–569.

287. Wilhelmus KR. Corneal edema following argon laser iridotomy. *Ophthalmic Surg.* 1992;23(8):533–537.

288. Liu DT, Lai JS, Lam DS. Descemet membrane detachment after sequential argon-neodymium:YAG laser peripheral iridotomy. *Am J Ophthalmol.* 2002;134(4):621–622.

289. Hodes BL, Bentivegna JF, Weyer NJ. Hyphema complicating laser iridotomy. *Arch Ophthalmol.* 1982;100(6):924–925.

290. Rubin L, Arnett J, Ritch R. Delayed hyphema after argon laser iridectomy. *Ophthalmic Surg.* 1984;15(10):852–853.

291. Yamamoto T, Shirato S, Kitazawa Y. Treatment of primary angle-closure glaucoma by argon laser iridotomy: a long-term follow-up. *Jpn J Ophthalmol.* 1985;29(1):1–12.

292. Welch DB, Apple DJ, Mendelsohn AD, et al. Lens injury following iridotomy with a Q-switched neodymium-YAG laser. *Arch Ophthalmol.* 1986;104(1):123–125.

293. Wollensak G, Eberwein P, Funk J. Perforation rosette of the lens after Nd:YAG laser iridotomy. *Am J Ophthalmol.* 1997;123(4):555–557.

294. Berger CM, Lee DA, Christensen RE. Anterior lens capsule perforation and zonular rupture after Nd:YAG laser iridotomy. *Am J Ophthalmol.* 1989;107(6):674–675.

295. Seedor JA, Greenidge KC, Dunn MW. Neodymium:YAG laser iridectomy and acute cataract formation in the rabbit. *Ophthalmic Surg.* 1986; 17(8):478–482.

296. Higginbotham EJ, Ogura Y. Lens clarity after argon and neodymium-YAG laser iridotomy in the rabbit. *Arch Ophthalmol.* 1987;105(4): 540–541.

297. Gaasterland DE, Rodrigues MM, Thomas G. Threshold for lens damage during Q-switched Nd:YAG laser iridotomy. A study of rhesus monkey eyes. *Ophthalmology.* 1985;92(11):1616–1623.

298. Anderson DR, Knighton RW, Feuer WJ. Evaluation of phototoxic retinal damage after argon laser iridotomy. *Am J Ophthalmol.* 1989;107(4): 398–402.

299. Karmon G, Savir H. Retinal damage after argon laser iridotomy. *Am J Ophthalmol.* 1986;101(5):554–560.

300. Berger BB. Foveal photocoagulation from laser iridotomy. *Ophthalmology.* 1984;91(9):1029–1033.

301. Thach AB, Lopez PF, Snady-McCoy LC, et al. Accidental Nd:YAG laser injuries to the macula. *Am J Ophthalmol.* 1995;119(6):767–773.

302. Bongard B, Pederson JE. Retinal burns from experimental laser iridotomy. *Ophthalmic Surg.* 1985;16(1):42–44.

303. Karjalainen K, Laatikainen L, Raitta C. Bilateral nonrhegmatogenous retinal detachment following neodymium-YAG laser iridotomies. *Arch Ophthalmol.* 1986;104(8):1134.

304. Brooks AM, Harper CA, Gillies WE. Occurrence of malignant glaucoma after laser iridotomy. *Br J Ophthalmol.* 1989;73(8):617–620.

305. Robinson A, Prialnic M, Deutsch D, et al. The onset of malignant glaucoma after prophylactic laser iridotomy. *Am J Ophthalmol.* 1990; 110(1):95–96.

306. Cashwell LF, Martin TJ. Malignant glaucoma after laser iridotomy. *Ophthalmology.* 1992;99(5):651–658.

307. Small KM, Maslin KF. Malignant glaucoma following laser iridotomy. *Aust NZ J Ophthalmol.* 1995;23(4):339–341.

308. Aminlari A, Sassani JW. Simultaneous bilateral malignant glaucoma following laser iridotomy. *Graefes Arch Clin Exp Ophthalmol.* 1993; 231(1):12–14.

309. Kiage D, Damji KF. Laser surgery for glaucoma. *Tech Ophthalmol.* 2008;6(3):76–82.

310. Sassani JW, Ritch R, McCormick S, et al. Histopathology of argon laser peripheral iridoplasty. *Ophthalmic Surg.* 1993;24(11):740–745.

311. Weiss HS, Shingleton BJ, Goode SM, et al. Argon laser gonioplasty in the treatment of angle-closure glaucoma. *Am J Ophthalmol.* 1992;114(1): 14–18.

312. Wand M. Argon laser gonioplasty for synechial angle closure. *Arch Ophthalmol.* 1992;110(3):363–367.

313. Tanihara H, Nagata M. Argon-laser gonioplasty following goniosynechialysis. *Graefes Arch Clin Exp Ophthalmol.* 1991;229(6):505–507.

314. Lai JS, Tham CC, Chua JK, et al. Efficacy and safety of inferior 180 degrees goniosynechialysis followed by diode laser peripheral iridoplasty in the treatment of chronic angle-closure glaucoma. *J Glaucoma.* 2000;9(5):388–391.

315. Lai JS, Tham CC, Chua JK, et al. Immediate diode laser peripheral iridoplasty as treatment of acute attack of primary angle closure glaucoma: a preliminary study. *J Glaucoma.* 2001;10(2):89–94.

316. Lam DS, Lai JS, Tham CC, et al. Argon laser peripheral iridoplasty versus conventional systemic medical therapy in treatment of acute primary angle-closure glaucoma: a prospective, randomized, controlled trial. *Ophthalmology.* 2002;109(9):1591–1596.

317. Lai JS, Tham CC, Chua JK, et al. Laser peripheral iridoplasty as initial treatment of acute attack of primary angle-closure: a long-term follow-up study. *J Glaucoma.* 2002;11(6):484–487.

318. Kimbrough RL, Trempe CS, Brockhurst RJ, et al. Angle-closure glaucoma in nanophthalmos. *Am J Ophthalmol.* 1979;88(3 pt 2):572–579.

319. Caronia RM, Sturm RT, Fastenberg DM, et al. Bilateral secondary angle-closure glaucoma as a complication of anticoagulation in a nanophthalmic patient. *Am J Ophthalmol.* 1998;126(2):307–309.

320. Burton TC, Folk JC. Laser iris retraction for angle-closure glaucoma after retinal detachment surgery. *Ophthalmology.* 1988;95(6):742–748.

321. Patti JC, Cinotti AA. Iris photocoagulation therapy of aphakic pupillary block. *Arch Ophthalmol.* 1975;93(5):347–348.

322. Theodossiadis G. A new argon-laser-approach for the management of aphakic pupillary block [in German]. *Klin Monbl Augenheilkd.* 1976;169(2):153–158.

323. Theodossiadis GP. Pupilloplasty in aphakic and pseudophakic pupillary block glaucoma. *Trans Ophthalmol Soc UK.* 1985;104(2):137–141.

324. Wise JB. Iris sphincterotomy, iridotomy, and synechiotomy by linear incision with the argon laser. *Ophthalmology.* 1985;92(5):641–645.

325. Vangelova A. ND YAG laser impact for creating a pupil [in Bulgarian]. *Khirurgiia (Sofiia).* 2001;57(1–2):59–61.

326. Go FJ, Akiba Y, Yamamoto T, et al. Argon laser iridotomy and surgical iridectomy in treatment of primary angle-closure glaucoma. *Jpn J Ophthalmol.* 1984;28(1):36–46.

327. Salmon JF. Long-term intraocular pressure control after Nd-YAG laser iridotomy in chronic angle-closure glaucoma. *J Glaucoma.* 1993;2(4): 291–296.

328. Buckley SA, Reeves B, Burdon M, et al. Acute angle closure glaucoma: relative failure of YAG iridotomy in affected eyes and factors influencing outcome. *Br J Ophthalmol.* 1994;78(7):529–533.

329. Chandler PA. Peripheral Iridectomy. *Arch Ophthalmol.* 1964;72:804–807.

330. Weene LE. Self-sealing incision for peripheral iridectomy. *Ophthalmic Surg.* 1978;9(6):64–66.

331. Freeman LB, Ridgway AE. Peripheral iridectomy via a corneal section: a follow-up study. *Ophthalmic Surg.* 1979;10(5):53–57.

332. Ahmad N. Transcorneal peripheral iridectomy. *Ophthalmic Surg.* 1980;11(2):124–127.

333. Curran RE. Surgical management of iria bombe. *Arch Ophthalmol.* 1973;90(6):464–465.

334. Hoffer KJ. Pigment vacuum iridectomy for phakic refractive lens implantation. *J Cataract Refract Surg.* 2001;27(8):1166–1168.

335. King JH, Wadsworth JAC. *An Atlas of Ophthalmic Surgery.* Philadelphia, PA: JB Lippincott; 1970.

336. Kass MA, Hersh SB, Albert DM. Experimental iridectomy with bipolar microcautery. *Am J Ophthalmol.* 1976;81(4):451–454.

337. Hersh SB, Kass MA. Iridectomy in rubeosis iridis. *Ophthalmic Surg.* 1976;7(1):19–21.

338. Tessler HH, Peyman GA, Huamonte F, et al. Argon laser iridotomy in incomplete peripheral iridectomy. *Am J Ophthalmol.* 1975;79(6):1051–1052.

339. Feibel RM, Bigger JF, Smith ME. Intralenticular hemorrhage following iridectomy. *Arch Ophthalmol.* 1972;87(1):36–38.

340. Go FJ, Kitazawa Y. Complications of peripheral iridectomy in primary angle-closure glaucoma. *Jpn J Ophthalmol.* 1981;25:222.

341. Sugar HS. Cataract formation and refractive changes after surgery for angle-closure glaucoma. *Am J Ophthalmol.* 1970;69(5):747–749.

342. Floman N, Berson D, Landau L. Peripheral iridectomy in closed angle glaucoma—late complications. *Br J Ophthalmol.* 1977;61(2):101–104.

343. Godel V, Regenbogen L. Cataractogenic factors in patients with primary angle-closure glaucoma after peripheral iridectomy. *Am J Ophthalmol.* 1977;83(2):180–184.

344. Krupin T, Mitchell KB, Johnson MF, et al. The long-term effects of iridectomy for primary acute angle-closure glaucoma. *Am J Ophthalmol.* 1978;86(4):506–509.

345. Burian HM. A case of Marfan's syndrome with bilateral glaucoma. With description of a new type of operation for developmental glaucoma (trabeculotomy ab externo). *Am J Ophthalmol.* 1960;50:1187–1192.

346. Smith R. A new technique for opening the canal of Schlemm. Preliminary report. *Br J Ophthalmol.* 1960;44:370–373.

347. Harms H, Dannheim R. Trabeculotomy results and problems. In: MacKensen G, ed. *Microsurgery in Glaucoma*. Basel, Switzerland: S Karger; 1970:121.

348. Meyer G, Schwenn O, Pfeiffer N, et al. Trabeculotomy in congenital glaucoma. *Graefes Arch Clin Exp Ophthalmol*. 2000;238(3):207–213.

349. McPherson SD Jr. Results of external trabeculotomy. *Am J Ophthalmol*. 1973;76(6):918–920.

350. Allen L, Burian HM. Trabeculotomy ab externo. A new glaucoma operation: technique and results of experimental surgery. *Am J Ophthalmol*. 1962;53:19–26.

351. Kong L, Yang S, Kong Z. Treatment of congenital glaucoma with trabeculotomy [in Chinese]. *Zhonghua Yan Ke Za Zhi*. 1997;33(3):169–172.

352. Filous A, Brunova B. Results of the modified trabeculotomy in the treatment of primary congenital glaucoma. *J AAPOS*. 2002;6(3):182–186.

353. Beck AD, Lynch MG. 360 degrees trabeculotomy for primary congenital glaucoma. *Arch Ophthalmol*. 1995;113(9):1200–1202.

354. Gloor BR. Risks of 360 degree suture trabeculotomy [in German]. *Ophthalmologe*. 1998;95(2):100–103.

355. Board RJ, Shields MB. Combined trabeculotomy-trabeculectomy for the management of glaucoma associated with Sturge-Weber syndrome. *Ophthalmic Surg*. 1981;12(11):813–817.

356. Irkec M, Kiratli H, Bilgic S. Results of trabeculotomy and guarded filtration procedure for glaucoma associated with Sturge-Weber syndrome. *Eur J Ophthalmol*. 1999;9(2):99–102.

357. Mandal AK. Primary combined trabeculotomy-trabeculectomy for early-onset glaucoma in Sturge-Weber syndrome. *Ophthalmology*. 1999;106(8):1621–1627.

358. Rothkoff L, Blumenthal M, Biedner B. Trabeculotomy in late onset congenital glaucoma. *Br J Ophthalmol*. 1979;63(1):38–39.

359. Elder MJ. Combined trabeculotomy-trabeculectomy compared with primary trabeculectomy for congenital glaucoma. *Br J Ophthalmol*. 1994;78(10):745–748.

360. Mandal AK, Naduvilath TJ, Jayagandan A. Surgical results of combined trabeculotomy-trabeculectomy for developmental glaucoma. *Ophthalmology*. 1998;105(6):974–982.

361. Mandal AK, Bhatia PG, Gothwal VK, et al. Safety and efficacy of simultaneous bilateral primary combined trabeculotomy-trabeculectomy for developmental glaucoma. *Indian J Ophthalmol*. 2002;50(1):13–19.

362. Luke C, Dietlein TS, Jacobi PC, et al. Combined deep sclerectomy and trabeculotomy in congenital glaucoma with complications [in German]. *Ophthalmologe*. 2003;100(3):230–233.

363. Mullaney PB, Selleck C, Al-Awad A, et al. Combined trabeculotomy and trabeculectomy as an initial procedure in uncomplicated congenital glaucoma. *Arch Ophthalmol*. 1999;117(4):457–460.

364. Honjo M, Tanihara H, Negi A, et al. Trabeculotomy ab externo, cataract extraction, and intraocular lens implantation: preliminary report. *J Cataract Refract Surg*. 1996;22(5):601–606.

365. Kubota T, Touguri I, Onizuka N, et al. Phacoemulsification and intraocular lens implantation combined with trabeculotomy for open-angle glaucoma and coexisting cataract. *Ophthalmologica*. 2003;217(3):204–207.

366. Tanito M, Ohira A, Chihara E. Surgical outcome of combined trabeculotomy and cataract surgery. *J Glaucoma*. 2001;10(4):302–308.

367. Bloomberg LB. Modified trabeculotomy/trabeculotomy with no-stitch cataract surgery. *J Cataract Refract Surg*. 1996;22(1):14–22.

368. Tanihara H, Honjo M, Inatani M, et al. Trabeculotomy combined with phacoemulsification and implantation of an intraocular lens for the treatment of primary open-angle glaucoma and coexisting cataract. *Ophthalmic Surg Lasers*. 1997;28(10):810–817.

369. Hoffmann E, Schwenn O, Karallus M, et al. Long-term results of cataract surgery combined with trabeculotomy. *Graefes Arch Clin Exp Ophthalmol*. 2002;240(1):2–6.

370. Tanito M, Ohira A, Chihara E. Factors leading to reduced intraocular pressure after combined trabeculotomy and cataract surgery. *J Glaucoma*. 2002;11(1):3–9.

371. Inatani M, Tanihara H, Muto T, et al. Transient intraocular pressure elevation after trabeculotomy and its occurrence with phacoemulsification and intraocular lens implantation. *Jpn J Ophthalmol*. 2001;45(3):288–292.

372. Honjo M, Tanihara H, Inatani M, et al. Phacoemulsification, intraocular lens implantation, and trabeculotomy to treat exfoliation syndrome. *J Cataract Refract Surg*. 1998;24(6):781–786.

373. Tanito M, Park M, Nishikawa M, et al. Comparison of surgical outcomes of combined viscocanalostomy and cataract surgery with combined trabeculotomy and cataract surgery. *Am J Ophthalmol*. 2002;134(4):513–520.

374. Mizoguchi T, Nagata M, Matsumura M, et al. Surgical effects of combined trabeculotomy and sinusotomy compared to trabeculotomy alone. *Acta Ophthalmol Scand*. 2000;78(2):191–195.

375. Kubota T, Takada Y, Inomata H. Surgical outcomes of trabeculotomy combined with sinusotomy for juvenile glaucoma. *Jpn J Ophthalmol*. 2001;45(5):499–502.

376. Ogawa T, Dake Y, Saitoh AK, et al. Improved nonpenetrating trabeculectomy with trabeculotomy. *J Glaucoma*. 2001;10(5):429–435.

377. Tailor U. Sulla incisione dell'angolo irideo (Contribuzione alla cura del glaucoma). *Ann Ophthalmol*. 1891;20:117.

378. De Vincentiis C. Sulla cosidetta "sclerotomia" interna. In: Pasquale V, ed. *Lavori Della Clinica Oculistica Dell' Università Di Napoli*. Napoli; 1894:227–235.

379. Bietti GB, Quaranta CA. Surgical indications for goniotomy [in French]. *Annee Ther Clin Ophthalmol*. 1967;18:291–321.

380. Bietti GB, Quaranta CA. Indications for and results of irido-corneal angle incision. (Goniotomy, goniotrabeculotomy or trabeculectomy). *Trans Ophthalmol Soc NZ*. 1968;20(suppl):20.

381. Quaranta L, Hitchings RA, Quaranta CA. Ab-interno goniotrabeculotomy versus mitomycin C trabeculectomy for adult open-angle glaucoma: a 2-year randomized clinical trial. *Ophthalmology*. 1999;106(7):1357–1362.

382. Moses RA. Electrocautery puncture of the trabecular meshwork in enucleated human eyes. *Am J Ophthalmol*. 1971;72(6):1094–1096.

383. Maselli E, Sirellini M, Pruneri F, et al. Diathermo—trabeculotomy ab externo. A new technique for opening the canal of Schlemm. *Br J Ophthalmol*. 1975;59(9):516–517.

384. Maselli E, Galantino G, Pruneri F, et al. Diathermo-trabeculotomy ab externo: indications and long-term results. *Br J Ophthalmol*. 1977;61(11):675–676.

385. Bonnet M, Schiffer HP. Trabeculotomy ab externo: localization of Schlemm's canal through catheterization of an aqueous-humor vein [in German]. *Klin Monbl Augenheilkd*. 1972;161(5):563–566.

386. Jocson VL. Air trabeculotomy. *Am J Ophthalmol*. 1975;79(1):107–111.

387. Skjaerpe F. Selective trabeculectomy. A report of a new surgical method for open angle glaucoma. *Acta Ophthalmol*. 1983;61(4):714–727.

388. Soltau JB, Mohay J, Shafranov G, et al. Internal glaucoma surgery: a pilot study. *Invest Ophthalmol Vis Sci*. 2000;41(suppl):S579.

389. Ferrari E, Bandello F, Ortolani F, et al. Ab-interno trabeculo-canalectomy: surgical approach and histological examination. *Eur J Ophthalmol*. 2002;12(5):401–405.

390. Walker R, Specht H. Theoretical and physical aspects of excimer laser trabeculotomy (ELT) ab interno with the AIDA laser with a wave length of 308 mm [in German]. *Biomed Tech (Berl)*. 2002;47(5):106–110.

391. Minckler DS, Baerveldt G, Alfaro MR, et al. Clinical results with the Trabectome for treatment of open-angle glaucoma. *Ophthalmology*. 2005;112(6):962–967. Erratum in: *Ophthalmology*. 2005;112(9):1540.

392. Minckler D, Mosaed S, Dustin L, et al. Trabectome (trabeculectomy-internal approach): additional experience and extended follow-up. *Trans Am Ophthalmol Soc*. 2008;106:149–159; discussion 159–160.

393. Francis BA, Minckler D, Dustin L, et al. Combined cataract extraction and trabeculotomy by the internal approach for coexisting cataract and open-angle glaucoma: initial results. *J Cataract Refract Surg*. 2008;34(7):1096–1103.

394. Grieshaber MC, Pienaar A, Olivier J, et al. Clinical evaluation of the aqueous outflow system in primary open-angle glaucoma for canaloplasty. *Invest Ophthalmol Vis Sci*. 2010;51(3):1498–1504.

395. Lewis RA, von Wolff K, Tetz M, et al. Canaloplasty: circumferential viscodilation and tensioning of Schlemm's canal using a flexible microcatheter for the treatment of open-angle glaucoma in adults: interim clinical study analysis. *J Cataract Refract Surg*. 2007;33(7):1217–1226.

396. Lewis RA, von Wolff K, Tetz M, et al. Canaloplasty: circumferential viscodilation and tensioning of Schlemm canal using a flexible microcatheter for the treatment of open-angle glaucoma in adults: two-year interim clinical study results. *J Cataract Refract Surg*. 2009;35(5):814–824.

397. Shingleton B, Tetz M, Korber N. Circumferential viscodilation and tensioning of Schlemm canal (canaloplasty) with temporal clear corneal phacoemulsification cataract surgery for open-angle glaucoma and visually significant cataract: one-year results. *J Cataract Refract Surg*. 2008;34(3):433–440.

398. Gaasterland DE, Bonney CH III, Rodrigues MM, et al. Long-term effects of Q-switched ruby laser on monkey anterior chamber angle. *Invest Ophthalmol Vis Sci*. 1985;26(2):129–135.

399. van der Zypen E, Fankhauser F. The ultrastructural features of laser trabeculopuncture and cyclodialysis. Problems related to successful treatment of chronic simple glaucoma. *Ophthalmologica.* 1979;179(4): 189–200.

400. Melamed S, Pei J, Puliafito CA, et al. Q-switched neodymium-YAG laser trabeculopuncture in monkeys. *Arch Ophthalmol.* 1985;103(1):129–133.

401. Dutton GN, Cameron SA, Allan D, et al. Parameters for neodymium-YAG laser trabeculotomy: an in-vitro study. *Br J Ophthalmol.* 1987;71(10):782–786.

402. Dutton GN, Allan D, Cameron SA. Pulsed neodymium-YAG laser trabeculotomy: energy requirements and replicability. *Br J Ophthalmol.* 1989;73(3):177–181.

403. Venkatesh S, Lee WR, Guthrie S, et al. An in-vitro morphological study of Q-switched neodymium/YAG laser trabeculotomy. *Br J Ophthalmol.* 1986;70(2):89–96.

404. Lee WR, Dutton GN, Cameron SA. Short-pulsed neodymium-YAG laser trabeculotomy. An *in vivo* morphological study in the human eye. *Invest Ophthalmol Vis Sci.* 1988;29(11):1698–1707.

405. Melamed S, Latina MA, Epstein DL. Neodymium:YAG laser trabeculopuncture in juvenile open-angle glaucoma. *Ophthalmology.* 1987;94(2):163–170.

406. Fukuchi T, Iwata K, Sawaguchi S, et al. Nd:YAG laser trabeculopuncture (YLT) for glaucoma with traumatic angle recession. *Graefes Arch Clin Exp Ophthalmol.* 1993;231(10):571–576.

407. Melamed S, Ashkenazi I, Gutman I, et al. Nd:YAG laser trabeculopuncture in angle-recession glaucoma. *Ophthalmic Surg.* 1992;23(1):31–35.

408. McHam ML, Eisenberg DL, Schuman JS, et al. Erbium:YAG laser trabecular ablation with a sapphire optical fiber. *Exp Eye Res.* 1997;65(2): 151–155.

409. Haas J. Goniotomy in aphakia. In: Welsh R, ed. *The Second Report on Cataract Surgery.* Miami, FL: Miami Educational Press; 1971:551.

410. Herschler J, Davis EB. Modified goniotomy for inflammatory glaucoma. Histologic evidence for the mechanism of pressure reduction. *Arch Ophthalmol.* 1980;98(4):684–687.

411. Promesberger H, Busse H, Mewe L. Findings and surgical therapy in congenital glaucoma [in German]. *Klin Monbl Augenheilkd.* 1980; 176(1):186–190.

412. McPherson SD Jr, McFarland D. External trabeculotomy for developmental glaucoma. *Ophthalmology.* 1980;87(4):302–305.

413. Luntz MH, Livingston DG. Trabeculotomy ab externo and trabeculectomy in congenital and adult-onset glaucoma. *Am J Ophthalmol.* 1977;83(2):174–179.

414. Gregersen E, Kessing SV. Congenital glaucoma before and after the introduction of microsurgery. Results of "macrosurgery"1943–1963 and of microsurgery (trabeculotomy/ectomy) 1970–1974. *Acta Ophthalmol.* 1977;55(3):422–430.

415. Luntz MH. Congenital, infantile, and juvenile glaucoma. *Ophthalmology.* 1979;86(5):793–802.

416. Dannheim R, Haas H. Visual acuity and intraocular pressure after surgery in congenital glaucoma [in German]. *Klin Monbl Augenheilkd.* 1980;177(3):296–303.

417. Quigley HA. Childhood glaucoma: results with trabeculotomy and study of reversible cupping. *Ophthalmology.* 1982;89(3):219–226.

418. McPherson SD Jr, Berry DP. Goniotomy vs external trabeculotomy for developmental glaucoma. *Am J Ophthalmol.* 1983;95(4):427–431.

419. Kiefer G, Schwenn O, Grehn F. Correlation of postoperative axial length growth and intraocular pressure in congenital glaucoma—a retrospective study in trabeculotomy and goniotomy. *Graefes Arch Clin Exp Ophthalmol.* 2001;239(12):893–899.

420. Olsen KE, Huang AS, Wright MM. The efficacy of goniotomy/trabeculotomy in early-onset glaucoma associated with the Sturge-Weber syndrome. *J AAPOS.* 1998;2(6):365–368.

421. Anderson DR. Trabeculotomy compared to goniotomy for glaucoma in children. *Ophthalmology.* 1983;90(7):805–806.

422. Kjer B, Kessing SV. Trabeculotomy in juvenile primary open-angle glaucoma. *Ophthalmic Surg.* 1993;24(10):663–668.

423. Tanihara H, Negi A, Akimoto M, et al. Surgical effects of trabeculotomy ab externo on adult eyes with primary open angle glaucoma and exfoliation syndrome. *Arch Ophthalmol.* 1993;111(12):1653–1661.

424. Chihara E, Nishida A, Kodo M, et al. Trabeculotomy ab externo: an alternative treatment in adult patients with primary open-angle glaucoma. *Ophthalmic Surg.* 1993;24(11):735–739.

425. Adachi M, Dickens CJ, Hetherington J Jr, et al. Clinical experience of trabeculotomy for the surgical treatment of aniridic glaucoma. *Ophthalmology.* 1997;104(12):2121–2125.

426. Honjo M, Tanihara H, Inatani M, et al. External trabeculotomy for the treatment of steroid-induced glaucoma. *J Glaucoma.* 2000;9(6):483–485.

427. Heine L. Die Cyklodialyse, eine neue Glaucomoperation. *Deutsche Med Wehnschr.* 1905;31:825.

428. Bill A. The routes for bulk drainage of aqueous humour in rabbits with and without cyclodialysis. *Doc Ophthalmol.* 1966;20:157–169.

429. Suguro K, Toris CB, Pederson JE. Uveoscleral outflow following cyclodialysis in the monkey eye using a fluorescent tracer. *Invest Ophthalmol Vis Sci.* 1985;26(6):810–813.

430. Toris CB, Pederson JE. Effect of intraocular pressure on uveoscleral outflow following cyclodialysis in the monkey eye. *Invest Ophthalmol Vis Sci.* 1985;26(12):1745–1749.

431. Pederson JE, Gaasterland DE, MacLellan HM. Experimental ciliochoroidal detachment. Effect on intraocular pressure and aqueous humor flow. *Arch Ophthalmol.* 1979;97(3):536–541.

432. Barkan O. Cyclodialysis: its mode of action. Histologic observations in a case of glaucoma in which both eyes were successfully treated by cyclodialysis. *Arch Ophthal.* 1950;43(5):793–803.

433. Chandler PA, Maumenee AE. A major cause of hypotony. *Am J Ophthalmol.* 1961;52:609–618.

434. Auricchio G. Findings on the mechanism of action of cyclodialysis [in Italian]. *Boll Ocul.* 1956;35(6):401–411.

435. Gills JP Jr, Paterson CA, Paterson ME. Action of cyclodialysis utilizing an implant studied by manometry in a human eye. *Exp Eye Res.* 1967;6(2):75–78.

436. Ascher KW. Some details of the technique of cyclodialysis. *Am J Ophthalmol.* 1960;50:1207–1215.

437. Gills JP Jr. Cyclodialysis implants. *South Med J.* 1967;60(7):692–695.

438. Portney GL. Silicone elastomer implantation cyclodialysis. A negative report. *Arch Ophthalmol.* 1973;89(1):10–12.

439. Streeten BW, Belkowitz M. Experimental hypotony with silastic. *Arch Ophthalmol.* 1967;78(4):503–511.

440. Miller RD, Nisbet RM. Cyclodialysis with air injection in black patients. *Ophthalmic Surg.* 1981;12(2):92–94.

441. Haisten MW, Guyton JS. Cyclodialysis with air injection; technique and results in ninety-four consecutive operations. *Arch Ophthalmol.* 1958;59(4):507–514.

442. Alpar JJ. Sodium hyaluronate (Healon) in cyclodialysis. *CLAO J.* 1985;11(3):201–204.

443. Krasnov MM. Iridocyclo-retraction in narrow-angle glaucoma. *Br J Ophthalmol.* 1971;55(6):389–395.

444. Aviner Z. Modified Krasnov's iridocycloretraction for aphakic glaucoma. *Ann Ophthalmol.* 1975;7(6):859–861.

445. Nesterov AP, Kolesnikova LN. Filtering iridocycloretraction in chronic closed-angle glaucoma. *Am J Ophthalmol.* 1985;99(3):340–342.

446. Partamian LG. Treatment of a cyclodialysis cleft with argon laser photocoagulation in a patient with a shallow anterior chamber. *Am J Ophthalmol.* 1985;99(1):5–7.

447. Ormerod LD, Baerveldt G, Sunalp MA, et al. Management of the hypotonous cyclodialysis cleft. *Ophthalmology.* 1991;98(9):1384–1393.

448. Best W, Hartwig H. Traumatic cyclodialysis and its treatment [in German]. *Klin Monbl Augenheilkd.* 1977;170(6):917–922.

449. Tate GW Jr, Lynn JR. A new technique for the surgical repair of cyclodialysis induced hypotony. *Ann Ophthalmol.* 1978;10(9):1261–1268.

450. Campbell DG, Vela A. Modern goniosynechialysis for the treatment of synechial angle-closure glaucoma. *Ophthalmology.* 1984;91(9): 1052–1060.

451. Weiss JS, Waring GO III. Dental mirror for goniosynechialysis during penetrating keratoplasty. *Am J Ophthalmol.* 1985;100(2):331–332.

452. Shingleton BJ, Chang MA, Bellows AR, et al. Surgical goniosynechialysis for angle-closure glaucoma. *Ophthalmology.* 1990;97(5):551–556.

453. Teekhasaenee C, Ritch R. Combined phacoemulsification and goniosynechialysis for uncontrolled chronic angle-closure glaucoma after acute angle-closure glaucoma. *Ophthalmology.* 1999;106(4):669–674; discussion 674–675.

454. Tanihara H, Nishiwaki K, Nagata M. Surgical results and complications of goniosynechialysis. *Graefes Arch Clin Exp Ophthalmol.* 1992;230(4): 309–313.

455. Senn P, Kopp B. Nd:YAG laser synechiolysis in glaucoma due to iridocorneal angle synechiae [in German]. *Klin Monbl Augenheilkd.* 1990;196(4):210–213.

456. Canlas OA, Ishikawa H, Liebmann JM, et al. Ultrasound biomicroscopy before and after goniosynechialysis. *Am J Ophthalmol.* 2001;132(4):570–571.

457. Simmons RJ, Dueker DK, Kimbrough RL, et al. Goniophotocoagulation for neovascular glaucoma. *Trans Sect Ophthalmol Am Acad Ophthalmol Otolaryngol.* 1977;83(1):80–89.

458. Simmons RJ, Deppermann SR, Dueker DK. The role of goniophotocoagulation in neovascularization of the anterior chamber angle. *Ophthalmology.* 1980;87(1):79–82.

459. Lee PF. Goniophotocoagulation in the management of rubeosis iridis. *Lasers Surg Med.* 1981;1(3):215–220.

460. Jacobi PC, Dietlein TS, Krieglstein GK. Bimanual trabecular aspiration in exfoliation glaucoma: an alternative in nonfiltering glaucoma surgery. *Ophthalmology.* 1998;105(5):886–894.

461. Georgopoulos GT, Chalkiadakis J, Livir-Rallatos G, et al. Combined clear cornea phacoemulsification and trabecular aspiration in the treatment of pseudoexfoliative glaucoma associated with cataract. *Graefes Arch Clin Exp Ophthalmol.* 2000;238(10):816–821.

462. Jacobi PC, Dietlein TS, Krieglstein GK. Comparative study of trabecular aspiration vs trabeculectomy in glaucoma triple procedure to treat exfoliation glaucoma. *Arch Ophthalmol.* 1999;117(10):1311–1318.

463. Jacobi PC, Dietlein TS, Krieglstein GK. The risk profile of trabecular aspiration versus trabeculectomy in glaucoma triple procedure. *Graefes Arch Clin Exp Ophthalmol.* 2000;238(7):545–551.

464. Jacobi PC, Krieglstein GK. Trabecular aspiration: clinical results of a new surgical approach to improve trabecular facility in glaucoma capsulare. *Ophthalmic Surg.* 1994;25(9):641–645.

465. Jacobi PC, Engels B, Dietlein TS, et al. Effect of trabecular aspiration on early intraocular pressure rise after cataract surgery. *J Cataract Refract Surg.* 1997;23(6):923–929.

466. Jacobi PC, Krieglstein GK. Trabecular aspiration. A new mode to treat exfoliation glaucoma. *Invest Ophthalmol Vis Sci.* 1995;36(11):2270–2276.

467. Grub M, Mielke J, Rohrbach JM, et al. Trabecular aspiration in pseudoexfoliative glaucoma—surgery to primarily reduce intraocular pressure [in German]. *Klin Monbl Augenheilkd.* 2002;219(5):353–357.

468. Jacobi PC, Dietlein TS, Krieglstein GK. Effect of trabecular aspiration on intraocular pressure in pigment dispersion syndrome and pigmentary glaucoma. *Ophthalmology.* 2000;107(3):417–421.

Principles of Incisional Surgery

37

A division between laser surgery for glaucoma and the more traditional glaucoma operations is becoming more and more artificial. The latter surgical category was originally distinguished by the term "conventional surgery," although laser techniques have now become the more conventional forms of surgery for glaucoma, prompting the need to reconsider the terminology. "Invasive surgery" is not a satisfactory alternative, because invading the eye with a laser beam can cause just as much tissue alteration as invading it with a knife. The term "incisional surgery," as used in this text, is not fully satisfactory either, because some of the newer laser procedures include incisional techniques. The fact is that as laser technology continues to expand, the day may come when all glaucoma surgery will include laser instruments. For these reasons, the chapters that follow combine laser and incisional procedures under general surgical categories, and this chapter, although it pertains primarily to incisional techniques, actually relates to both disciplines of glaucoma surgery.

WOUND HEALING

The incision of any tissue is followed by a complex process that attempts to heal the wound. The desire in most operations is to achieve complete, strong wound healing. For the glaucoma surgeon who is performing a filtering procedure, however, excessive wound healing can be a detriment, leading to failure of the operation. This chapter considers general aspects of wound healing. (Specifics related to filtering surgery and measures to prevent excessive scarring are discussed in Chapter 38.)

Wound healing is typically considered to occur in three phases: inflammation, proliferation, and remodeling. However, it may help to think of this complex, and only partially understood, process in four overlapping phases: (a) clot phase, (b) proliferative phase, (c) granulation phase, and (d) collagen phase.

Clot Phase

Almost immediately after a tissue incision, blood vessels constrict and leak blood cells, platelets, and plasma proteins, which include fibrinogen, fibronectin, and plasminogen. In addition, blood-vessel rupture stimulates platelet aggregation and activation of various tissue growth factors, which are chemotactic to inflammatory cells, stimulating the intrinsic coagulation cascade [1–4]. As a result, these blood elements clot to form a gel-like fibrin–fibronectin matrix [1,5].

Proliferative Phase

Inflammatory cells, including monocytes and macrophages, along with fibroblasts and new capillaries, migrate into the clot within a few days after the surgery. In a rabbit model of filtering surgery, fibroblasts were seen to migrate from episcleral tissue, epimysium of the superior rectus, and subconjunctival connective tissue [6], and in a monkey model, they were proliferating along the walls of the limbal fistula by day 6 [7]. By using the incorporation of tritiated thymidine as a marker of cell division to study the time course of cellular proliferation after filtering surgery in monkeys, incorporation was detected as early as 24 hours postoperatively, peaked in 5 days, and returned to baseline by day 11 [8]. Angiogenesis, or proliferation of new blood vessels, also takes place during this phase [9].

Granulation Phase

As the fibrin–fibronectin clot is degraded by inflammatory cells, the fibroblasts begin to synthesize fibronectin, interstitial collagens, and glycosaminoglycans to form young fibrovascular connective tissue, or granulation tissue [5]. In the rabbit model, granulation tissue was seen in the fistula by the third day [6], whereas in the monkey model, it was lining the fistula by at least day 10 [7].

Collagen Phase

Procollagen is synthesized intracellularly by fibroblasts [10], and it is then secreted into the extracellular spaces, where it undergoes biochemical transformation into tropocollagen. Approximately 2 weeks after surgery, the tropocollagen molecules aggregate into immature soluble collagen fibrils, and over the next few months undergo cross-linking to form mature collagen. The amount of collagen in the wound is the result of collagen synthesis and degradation. The degradation process is controlled by the family of proteolytic enzymes, called matrix metalloproteinases [11–15]. Although the matrix metalloproteinases have been found in healthy subconjunctival tissues and aqueous humor [16–18], their elevated levels have been associated with more aggressive scarring in the eye [19]. Eventually, blood vessels are partially reabsorbed, and fibroblasts largely disappear, probably by apoptosis [20], leaving a collagenous scar with scattered fibroblasts and blood vessels [5].

ANESTHESIA

Although most laser procedures require only topical anesthesia, incisional surgery and some glaucoma laser operations require local anesthesia. General anesthesia is usually reserved for children or adults in whom cooperation or other considerations do not permit surgery under local anesthesia.

Local Anesthesia

Retrobulbar Injection

Commonly used injectable anesthetics include lidocaine, bupivacaine, and mepivacaine. When compared on the basis of induced lid akinesia, these three agents were found to be similar with regard to onset (less than 6 minutes) and depth of anesthesia, whereas bupivacaine had the longest duration of effect (up to 6 hours, compared with 90 minutes for mepivacaine and 15 to 30 minutes for lidocaine) (21). In an evaluation of combined agents, bupivacaine, 0.5%, lidocaine, 2%, and 1:100,000 epinephrine were more effective in producing lid and globe akinesia than bupivacaine alone or the two anesthetics without epinephrine (22). Bupivacaine alone was slower in producing anesthesia but was more effective in producing akinesia than the two anesthetics combined without epinephrine. The three combinations were similar with regard to frequency of pain during a 30-minute operation and the need for analgesia 6 hours postoperatively.

Epinephrine may enhance the effect of local anesthetics, presumably by minimizing systemic spread from the injection site by its vasoconstrictive action. However, it may also impose an additional risk in glaucomatous eyes by reducing vascular perfusion to an already compromised optic nerve head. Another supplement to local anesthesia that does appear to be safe and effective is hyaluronidase, which serves to improve local tissue spread within the injection site by breaking down the connective tissue ground substances. In recent years, however, hyaluronidase has become difficult to obtain commercially.

Although retrobulbar and orbicularis anesthesia were traditionally given as separate injections, it was shown that the retrobulbar injection alone provides adequate facial akinesia, because of the decreased stimulus for orbicularis contraction in the vast majority of cases (23). For the retrobulbar injection, an Atkinson needle has the advantages of being short and blunt, both of which help avoid retrobulbar hemorrhage (24). An injection of 3 to 5 cc of a 50:50 mixture of 0.75% bupivacaine and 2% to 4% lidocaine with hyaluronidase, if available, usually provides adequate anesthesia and akinesia. Complications of retrobulbar anesthesia may include retrobulbar hemorrhage, extraocular muscle injury, perforation of the eye globe, and optic nerve injury. Firm pressure to the globe for 30 seconds after the injection may also help minimize retrobulbar hemorrhage by tamponading any small, bleeding vessel.

Other Types of Local Anesthesia

Some surgeons prefer to avoid the risks associated with retrobulbar anesthesia by using peribulbar (transconjunctival injection near the equator of the globe without entering the muscle cone), sub-Tenon (more anterior placement near the surgical site), subconjunctival, or topical anesthesia (25–29). The last three methods may be the safest of these approaches in patients with glaucoma, because both retrobulbar and peribulbar injections can cause significant IOP elevations (30,31). In a study of 104 eyes with and without glaucoma receiving retrobulbar or peribulbar anesthesia for intraocular surgery, the 40 eyes with glaucoma had higher and more persistent increases in IOP (30). One minute after injection, the IOP was 10 mm Hg or more above baseline in 35% of the glaucomatous eyes, and 20 mm Hg or more in 10%. The mean IOP elevation after 5 minutes was greater with retrobulbar anesthesia, although ocular compression significantly reduced the IOP at 5 minutes.

A reported technique for sub-Tenon anesthesia involves the injection of lidocaine, 2%, over the superior, medial, and lateral rectus muscles in conjunction with a lid block and standard sedative (32). In a randomized trial comparing this approach with retrobulbar anesthesia, the sub-Tenon anesthesia required a smaller volume of local anesthetic, less additional anesthesia, and less postoperative analgesia (32).

Subconjunctival anesthesia by using a 1- to 2-mL injection of 1:1 mixture of mepivacaine, 2%, and bupivacaine, 0.75%, in the superotemporal quadrant was found to be an effective alternative to peribulbar anesthesia for trabeculectomy (33).

Topical anesthesia appears to provide optimal conditions for the surgeon and similar amounts of patient comfort, compared with retrobulbar anesthesia (28,29); however, in another study, patients who experienced both topical anesthesia and retrobulbar block appeared to prefer the retrobulbar anesthesia (34). The techniques can be combined by starting the conjunctival incision under topical anesthesia, followed by sub-Tenon or even retrobulbar delivery by following the sclera plane posteriorly with a blunt irrigating cannula.

Adjuncts to Local Anesthesia

Although general anesthesia is not commonly used in glaucoma surgery, it is advisable to routinely use the assistance of an anesthesiologist or anesthetist to monitor the patient's vital signs and to provide adjunctive medications. The latter may include short-acting analgesics, such as propofol and fentanyl citrate, and short-acting central nervous system depressants, such as midazolam HCl, for sedation. The addition of alfentanil to midazolam has also been shown to be advantageous (35). Remifentanil is another, relatively new, ultrashort-acting opioid that can be rapidly titrated and individualized for various levels of surgical interventions. Although it is expensive, and respiratory depression and postoperative nausea are considerations, studies have shown that respiratory depression with remifentanil is mild, and remifentanil sedation for retrobulbar blocks appeared to be superior to sedation with propofol (36). A combination of remifentanil and propofol has provided excellent relief of pain and anxiety with the fewest adverse effects (37,38).

In addition, ultrashort-acting barbiturate anesthetics such as methohexital sodium (Brevital) can be administered intravenously to provide a few minutes of sleep while the retrobulbar injection is being given.

BASIC TECHNIQUES AND INSTRUMENTS

Eyelid Separation

Good exposure of the surgical field is critical to a successful glaucoma operation. This begins with the selection of an appropriate eyelid speculum. Instruments are available in a wide range of designs, each with certain advantages and disadvantages. A desirable speculum, however, is one that not only separates the eyelids but also lifts them from the globe and allows the surgeon to adjust the degree of lid separation. Lateral canthotomy may also be performed to improve exposure in selected eyes.

Traction Sutures

Because most glaucoma surgery is performed in the superior quadrants, the next step toward good exposure is to rotate the eye down, which is usually accomplished with a traction (or bridle) suture. A traditional technique is the superior rectus traction suture, in which a 4-0 silk suture is passed transconjunctivally beneath the muscles and then attached to the head of the surgical drape with a clamp (**Fig. 37.1**). Potential complications with this approach include subconjunctival hemorrhage, conjunctival defects, scleral perforation, patient discomfort, and postoperative ptosis. A corneal traction suture, in which a 7-0 silk or polyglactin (e.g., Vicryl) suture on a cutting needle (i.e., S-29 for silk sutures) is passed through approximately three-fourths thickness, superior, peripheral cornea and attached to the drape over the cheek (**Fig. 37.2**), provides good exposure while eliminating the foregoing complications (39,40). However, it can distort the cornea and anterior chamber when the eye is soft.

Hemostasis

As noted earlier in this chapter, bleeding is the first step in the wound healing process, which can lead to excessive, detrimental scarring especially in glaucoma filtering surgery. It is desirable, therefore, in all surgical procedures to minimize bleeding. It is helpful to stop use of anticoagulants, such as aspirin, nonsteroidal anti-inflammatory drugs, and sodium warfarin (Coumadin), if possible, before surgery. During surgery, the surgeon should try

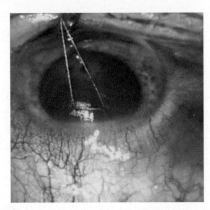

Figure 37.2 Eye rotated down by corneal traction suture and attached to surgical drape over cheek.

to avoid large vessels, such as the anterior ciliary arteries near the insertions of the rectus muscles. When bleeding does occur, it should be continuously flushed from the surgical site with a gentle stream of balanced salt solution. Small bleeders may eventually close spontaneously, although most require cauterization. An ideal cautery unit for glaucoma surgery is a small-diameter, tapered, blunt, bipolar cautery instrument (41) (**Fig. 37.3**). This provides adequate cauterization of episcleral bleeders without excessive tissue charring or tissue contraction and can be used at lower energy levels to cauterize intraocular bleeding as from the ciliary body or iris.

Tissue Handling

Most glaucoma surgery is performed on the extraocular tissues of the anterior ocular segment. Gentle handling of these tissues is essential to avoid tearing the conjunctiva or cutting more tissue than necessary, which can also increase the risks of excessive scarring. When possible, it is best to grasp the Tenon capsule and avoid direct contact of the instrument with the conjunctiva. When it is necessary to grasp the conjunctiva, it should be done with smooth-tipped (nontoothed) forceps to avoid piercing or tearing the conjunctiva. When dissecting conjunctiva, it is best to use a blunt dissecting instrument, when possible, and to cut tissue with scissors or a blade only when necessary. (Details regarding

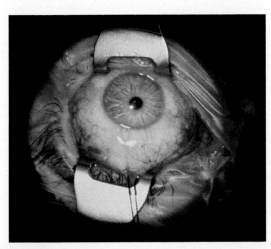

Figure 37.1 Eye rotated down by superior rectus traction suture and attached to head of surgical drape.

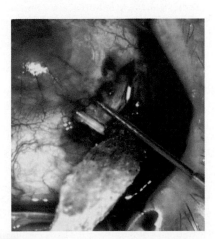

Figure 37.3 Cauterization of sclera with tapered, blunt tip, bipolar cautery instrument.

specific instruments for the various surgical procedures are provided in the following chapters that deal with those operations.)

Suturing

To minimize excessive inflammatory reaction and subsequent scarring, select suture material with the least tendency to induce tissue reaction. For corneoscleral suturing, 9-0 or 10-0 nylon on a fine, cutting needle can be effective; however, manually removing nonabsorbable nylon sutures in the postoperative period is often necessary. For the conjunctiva, however, polyglycolic acid or polyglactin sutures are nearly as nonreactive as nylon and have the advantage of being biodegradable. It is also important to use a needle that will not tear or leave a large hole in the conjunctiva. Fine, tapered, noncutting, or vascular needles are useful for closing conjunctival tissues.

KEY POINTS

- The wound healing process after the incision of a tissue includes clot formation, cellular proliferation, granulation tissue formation, and the synthesis and maturation of collagen.
- Most incisional glaucoma surgery is performed under local anesthesia, with agents such as lidocaine and bupivacaine.
- Epinephrine, as a supplement, is usually avoided because of the risk to the optic nerve head, although hyaluronidase may be useful as a tissue-spreading factor.
- Basic techniques and instruments for incisional glaucoma surgery include attention to good surgical exposure with an appropriate eyelid speculum and traction suture, adequate hemostasis, gentle wound handling, and the proper suture and needle for wound closure.

REFERENCES

1. Chang L, Crowston JG, Cordeiro MF, et al. The role of the immune system in conjunctival wound healing after glaucoma surgery [review]. *Surv Ophthalmol.* 2000;45:49–68.
2. Bennett NT, Schultz GS. Growth factors and wound healing: biochemical properties of growth factors and their receptors [review]. *Am J Surg.* 1993;165:728–737.
3. Postlethwaite AE, Smith GN, Mainardi CL, et al. Lymphocyte modulation of fibroblast function in vitro: stimulation and inhibition of collagen production by different effector molecules. *J Immunol.* 1984;132:2470–2477.
4. Kaplan AP. Hageman factor-dependent pathways: mechanism of initiation and bradykinin formation. *Fed Proc.* 1983;42:3123–3127.
5. Skuta GL, Parrish RK. Wound healing in glaucoma filtering surgery [review]. *Surv Ophthalmol.* 1987;32:149–170.
6. Miller MH, Grierson I, Unger WI, et al. Wound healing in an animal model of glaucoma fistulizing surgery in the rabbit. *Ophthalmic Surg.* 1989;20:350–357.
7. Desjardins DC, Parrish RK, Folberg R, et al. Wound healing after filtering surgery in owl monkeys. *Arch Ophthalmol.* 1986;104:1835–1839.
8. Jampel HD, McGuigan LJ, Dunkelberger GR, et al. Cellular proliferation after experimental glaucoma filtration surgery. *Arch Ophthalmol.* 1988;106:89–94.
9. Li J, Zhang YP, Kirsner RS. Angiogenesis in wound repair: angiogenic growth factors and the extracellular matrix. *Microsc Res Tech.* 2003;60:107–114.
10. Lorena D, Uchio K, Costa AM, et al. Normal scarring: importance of myofibroblasts. *Wound Repair Regen.* 2002;10:86–92.
11. Parsons SL, Watson SA, Brown PD, et al. Matrix metalloproteinases. *Br J Surg.* 1997;84:160–166.
12. Daniels JT, Occleston NL, Crowston JG, et al. Understanding and controlling the scarring response: the contribution of histology and microscopy [review]. *Microsc Res Tech.* 1998;42:317–333.
13. Porter RA, Brown RA, Eastwood M, et al. Ultrastructural changes during contraction of collagen lattices by ocular fibroblasts. *Wound Repair Regen.* 1998;6:157–166.
14. Agren MS, Jorgensen LN, Andersen M, et al. Matrix metalloproteinase 9 level predicts optimal collagen deposition during early wound repair in humans. *Br J Surg.* 1998;85:68–71.
15. Khaw PT, Chang L, Wong TT, et al. Modulation of wound healing after glaucoma surgery [review]. *Curr Opin Ophthalmol.* 2001;12:143–148.
16. Kawashima Y, Saika S, Yamanaka O, et al. Immunolocalization of matrix metalloproteinases and tissue inhibitors of metalloproteinases in human subconjunctival tissues. *Curr Eye Res.* 1998;17:445–451.
17. Ando H, Twining SS, Yue BY, et al. MMPs and proteinase inhibitors in the human aqueous humor. *Invest Ophthalmol Vis Sci.* 1993;34:3541–3548.
18. Huang SH, Adamis AP, Wiederschain DG, et al. Matrix metalloproteinases and their inhibitors in aqueous humor. *Exp Eye Res.* 1996;62:481–490.
19. Wong TT, Mead AL, Khaw PT. Matrix metalloproteinase inhibition modulates postoperative scarring after experimental glaucoma filtration surgery. *Invest Ophthalmol Vis Sci.* 2003;44:1097–1103.
20. Desmouliere A, Redard M, Darby I, et al. Apoptosis mediates the decrease in cellularity during the transition between granulation tissue and scar. *Am J Pathol.* 1995;146:56–66.
21. Parrish RK, Spaeth GL, Poryzees EM, et al. Evaluation of local anesthesia agents using a new force-sensitive lid speculum. *Ophthalmic Surg.* 1983;14:575–578.
22. Vettese T, Breslin CW. Retrobulbar anesthesia for cataract surgery: comparison of bupivacaine and bupivacaine/lidocaine combinations. *Can J Ophthalmol.* 1985;20:131–134.
23. Martin SR, Baker SS, Muenzler WS. Retrobulbar anesthesia and orbicularis akinesia. *Ophthalmic Surg.* 1986;17:232–233.
24. Atkinson WS. Retrobulbar injection of anesthetic within the muscle cone (cone injection). *Arch Ophthalmol.* 1936;16:494–503.
25. Hansen EA, Mein CE, Mazzoli R. Ocular anesthesia for cataract surgery: a direct sub-Tenon's approach. *Ophthalmic Surg.* 1990;21:696–699.
26. Ritch R, Liebmann JM. Sub-Tenon's anesthesia for trabeculectomy. *Ophthalmic Surg.* 1992;23:502–504.
27. Smith R. Cataract extraction without retrobulbar anaesthetic injection. *Br J Ophthalmol.* 1990;74:205–207.
28. Zabriskie NA, Ahmed II, Crandall AS, et al. A comparison of topical and retrobulbar anesthesia for trabeculectomy. *J Glaucoma.* 2002;11:306–314.
29. Ahmed II, Zabriskie NA, Crandall AS, et al. Topical versus retrobulbar anesthesia for combined phacotrabeculectomy: prospective randomized study. *J Cataract Refract Surg.* 2002;28:631–638.
30. O'Donoghue E, Batterbury M, Lavy T. Effect on intraocular pressure of local anaesthesia in eyes undergoing intraocular surgery. *Br J Ophthalmol.* 1994;78:605–607.
31. Bowman R, Liu C, Sarkies N. Intraocular pressure changes after peribulbar injections with and without ocular compression. *Br J Ophthalmol.* 1996;80:394–397.
32. Buys YM, Trope GE. Prospective study of sub-Tenon's versus retrobulbar anesthesia for inpatient and day-surgery trabeculectomy. *Ophthalmology.* 1993;100:1585–1589.
33. Azuara-Blanco A, Moster MR, Marr BP. Subconjunctival versus peribulbar anesthesia in trabeculectomy: a prospective, randomized study. *Ophthalmic Surg Lasers.* 1997;28:896–899.
34. Boezaart A, Berry R, Nell M. Topical anesthesia versus retrobulbar block for cataract surgery: the patients' perspective. *J Clin Anesth.* 2000;12:58–60.
35. McHardy FE, Fortier J, Chung F, et al. A comparison of midazolam, alfentanil and propofol for sedation in outpatient intraocular surgery. *Can J Anaesth.* 2000;47:211–214.
36. Boezaart AP, Berry RA, Nell ML, et al. A comparison of propofol and remifentanil for sedation and limitation of movement during periretrobulbar block. *J Clin Anesth.* 2001;13:422–426.
37. Holas A, Krafft P, Marcovic M, et al. Remifentanil, propofol or both for conscious sedation during eye surgery under regional anaesthesia. *Eur J Anaesthesiol.* 1999;16:741–748.
38. Rewari V, Madan R, Kaul HL, et al. Remifentanil and propofol sedation for retrobulbar nerve block. *Anaesth Intensive Care.* 2002;30:433–437.
39. Conklin JD, Goins KM, Smith TJ. Corneal traction suture in trabeculectomy [letter]. *Ophthalmic Surg.* 1991;22:494.
40. Cohen SW. Corneal traction suture [letter]. *Ophthalmic Surg.* 1988;19:371.
41. Shields MB. Evaluation of a tapered, blunt, bipolar cautery tip for trabeculectomy. *Ophthalmic Surg.* 1994;25:54–56.

Filtering Surgery

38

The incisional operation most frequently used for chronic forms of glaucoma, especially in adults, is commonly referred to as a filtering procedure. Although several variations for this surgical procedure have been described, all filtering operations share the same basic mechanism of action and general surgical principles. We first consider these aspects and then discuss specific filtration techniques and potential complications.

MECHANISMS OF ACTION

Drainage Fistula

The basic mechanism of all filtering procedures is the creation of an opening, or fistula, at the limbus, which allows a direct communication between the anterior chamber and subconjunctival space. This fistula bypasses the trabecular meshwork, Schlemm canal, and collecting channels. From the subconjunctival spaces, aqueous is absorbed by surrounding tissues or crosses the conjunctival epithelium and drains with tears through the nasolacrimal duct.

Filtering Bleb

Most, but not all, successful glaucoma filtering procedures are characterized by an elevation of the conjunctiva at the surgical site, which is commonly referred to as a filtering bleb. The clinical appearance and function of these blebs vary considerably with regard to extent, elevation, and vascularity (1,2). The blebs that are most often associated with good intraocular pressure (IOP) control have decreased vascularity with numerous microcysts in the epithelium and are either low and diffuse or more circumscribed and elevated (3) (**Fig. 38.1**).

The histologic appearance of both functioning and failed filtering blebs consists of normal epithelium with no encircling-type junctions between the cells that would limit fluid flow (3). The subepithelial connective tissue may contain viable activated fibrocytes (4), and the histologic appearance at this level correlates better with bleb status than does that of the epithelium, in that functioning blebs have loosely arranged tissue with histologically clear spaces, whereas the failed blebs have dense collagenous connective tissue (3). Change in morphology and a decrease in the number of epithelial and goblet cells have been found in conjunctival epithelium overlying thin cystic blebs (5).

Routes of Aqueous Drainage

Studies have suggested that aqueous in the filtering bleb usually filters through the conjunctiva and mixes with the tear film or is absorbed by vascular or perivascular conjunctival tissue (6–10). Less commonly, a filtering procedure may be associated with IOP control in the absence of an apparent filtering bleb. This is more common when the fistula is covered by a partial-thickness scleral flap (trabeculectomy), and suggested mechanisms of aqueous drainage in these cases include flow through (a) lymphatic vessels near the scarred margins of the surgical area; (b) atypical, newly incorporated aqueous veins; and (c) normal aqueous veins (6,10). Preservation of the aqueous drainage route beneath the scleral flap, as seen on ultrasound biomicroscopy, appears to correlate with the development of a filtering bleb following trabeculectomy (11,12).

BASIC TECHNIQUES OF FILTERING SURGERY

The various types of filtering surgery differ primarily according to the method used to create the drainage fistula. The other aspects of the operation are basically the same for all filtering procedures and are discussed first before specific fistulizing techniques are considered.

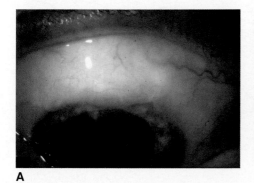

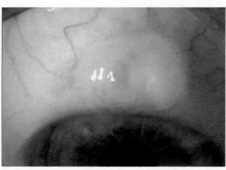

Figure 38.1 Types of functioning filtering blebs. **A:** Low, diffuse bleb. **B:** Discrete, elevated bleb. Note that both are avascular.

A   B

Figure 38.2 Bridle suture.

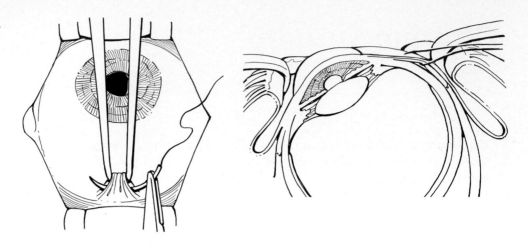

Traction Sutures

Good surgical exposure is critical to the successful outcome of a filtering procedure. In most cases, this requires the use of a traction suture. The two most common techniques are (a) a superior rectus traction suture (**Fig. 38.2**) and (b) a clear cornea traction suture (**Fig. 38.3**). With the former technique, the globe is rotated down, and the superior rectus muscle is grasped with forceps, through conjunctiva, 10 to 15 mm behind the limbus. A 4-0 silk suture is then passed through conjunctiva and around the muscle beneath the tips of the forceps, and the suture is attached to the head of the surgical drape. With the clear cornea technique, a 7-0 polyglactin or silk suture is passed to a corneal depth of approximately three-fourths thickness, 1 mm from the limbus with a bite width of 4 to 5 mm, and is then attached to the drape over the cheek. The rectus suture has the potential disadvantages of a subconjunctival hemorrhage or a hole in the conjunctiva that may leak postoperatively. The corneal suture is preferred by most surgeons but may distort the cornea and anterior chamber during the surgery. Additional Tenon traction sutures have been suggested to help in visualization and surgical access during filtering procedures (13).

Limbal Stab Incision (Paracentesis Site)

Some surgeons create a paracentesis, which consists of a self-sealing, beveled incision into the anterior chamber at the limbus, usually temporally at the horizontal meridian, or in the inferior-temporal quadrant, as a route for injecting fluid at the end of the procedure. This can be done with a tapered, pointed knife, or number 75 blade before entering anterior chamber under the scleral flap. If antifibrosis agents (discussed later in this chapter) are to be used, however, it may be best to wait until after that step of the operation, to avoid a route for potential entry of the drug into the anterior chamber.

Preparation of the Conjunctival Flap

Preparation of the conjunctival flap is a critical step in all filtering procedures, in that the most common cause of failure is scarring of the filtering bleb. Although techniques differ among surgeons, meticulous detail with minimal tissue damage and bleeding is essential.

Position of the Flap

Some surgeons elect to make the flap at the 12-o'clock position to take advantage of the wider limbus in this area. Others prefer

Figure 38.3 Corneal traction suture.

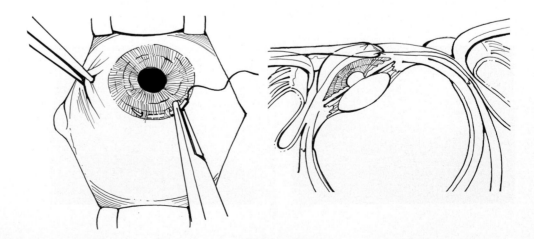

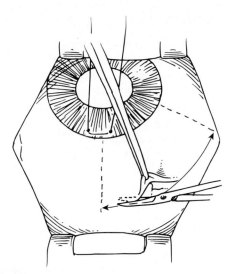

Figure 38.4   Incision through conjunctiva in preparation of a limbus-based conjunctival flap.

one of the superior quadrants, leaving the adjacent quadrant available for future surgery if required. The inferior quadrant was used in the past when previous ocular surgery resulted in scarring of conjunctiva in the superior quadrants (14). However, the latter technique is associated with an increased risk for endophthalmitis and should be avoided (15).

Limbus-Based versus Fornix-Based Flap

Conjunctival flaps for glaucoma filtering surgery have traditionally been limbus based—that is, with the initial incision in the fornix (**Fig. 38.4**). More recently, a fornix-based flap has gained favor (**Fig. 38.5**), particularly in association with a trabeculectomy (16–18). Several studies have compared limbus- and fornix-based conjunctival flaps in association with trabeculectomy and reported similar success rates, whether used in combination with cataract surgery or as a separate procedure (19–28). However, one investigative team found slightly better postoperative IOP control with the limbus-based flap (29), whereas others found better pressure control

and more diffuse blebs with the fornix-based flaps (17,30). One retrospective study found cystic leaking blebs only in eyes with limbus-based flaps (24).

Surgeons differ on this aspect of filtering surgery, with some preferring the relative ease and improved surgical exposure of the fornix-based flap and others preferring the tighter wound closure that may be achieved with the limbus-based flaps. One circumstance in which a fornix-based conjunctival flap is especially useful is when such a flap was used previously, as during an extracapsular cataract or scleral buckling surgery, leaving a band of scar tissue at the limbus. In these cases, it is difficult to dissect a limbus-based flap sufficiently anteriorly without creating holes in the conjunctiva. A preferable alternative is to excise the band of scar tissue and pull the new edge of the conjunctival flap down to peripheral cornea.

Management of Tenon Capsule

There is some controversy regarding the value of removing all or a portion of Tenon capsule, the main source of fibroblasts in the area of the conjunctival flap. Two studies revealed no difference in postoperative IOP control between eyes with excision of the capsular tissue and those in which it was left partially or totally intact (31,32). For this reason, many surgeons routinely preserve Tenon capsule by dissecting between the capsule and episclera when preparing the conjunctival flap. This may be especially important when using adjunctive antifibrosis agents, to avoid excessively thin or leaking filtering blebs in the late postoperative course. Sub-Tenon space also appears to be the best cleavage plane for aqueous drainage because there is less scarring and subsequently less resistance to flow (33). Modified fornix-based techniques have been described, such as small incision trabeculectomy and microtrabeculectomy (34–36), by using 2.5- to 3-mm conjunctival peritomy within 2 mm of the limbal area and avoiding Tenon capsule. Other surgeons excise variable amounts of Tenon capsule when it appears to be unusually thick, as in young patients. This can be accomplished by dissecting between the conjunctiva and Tenon capsule and then excising the capsule from the episclera. An alternative approach

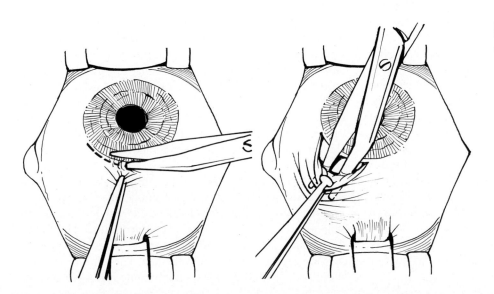

Figure 38.5   Incision through conjunctiva in preparation of a fornix-based conjunctival flap.

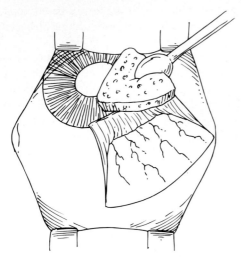

Figure 38.6 | Retraction of conjunctival flap over the cornea.

is to dissect Tenon capsule from underlying episclera, strip a portion of the capsule from the conjunctiva with gentle traction, and then excise the exposed portion of capsular tissue.

With all techniques, blunt dissection is used when possible to avoid bleeding, and sharp dissection is used only when required. Gentle handling of the conjunctiva is essential at all times, and nontoothed conjunctival forceps are preferable to avoid tearing or crushing the conjunctiva. During the fistulizing part of the operation, it is important to keep the conjunctival flap moist and to minimize handling of the tissue. With a limbus-based flap, this can be conveniently accomplished by reflecting the flap over the cornea with a surgical sponge (**Fig. 38.6**) or nontoothed forceps. When manipulating the conjunctiva–Tenon capsule flap, it is best to grasp the capsule and avoid touching the conjunctiva.

Use of Viscoelastic Agents

The injection of a viscoelastic agent (e.g., sodium hyaluronate) into the anterior chamber at the completion of the filtering procedure did not reduce the incidence of postoperative flat anterior chambers in most studies (37–39). However, injecting the agent through a paracentesis incision at the outset of a trabeculectomy procedure was associated with a lower incidence of this complication (40,41), presumably by avoiding intraoperative hypotony and the subsequent suprachoroidal effusion that may initiate the cascade of events leading to a shallow anterior chamber. Others have supported this finding and noted that the technique also tends to minimize intraoperative bleeding (42) but not postoperative hyphema or postoperative corneal endothelial cell loss (43,44). Complications of intracameral viscoelastics include iris prolapse during surgery and a higher early postoperative IOP, for which the preoperative use of pilocarpine, 2%, and a slightly less tight closure of the scleral flap were recommended (41,44). Injection of dense viscoelastics, such as Healon or Healon 5, into the anterior chamber may be used as a temporary solution for postoperative flat anterior chambers (45–47).

Peripheral Iridectomy

A peripheral iridectomy is a routine part of all standard filtering procedures and is usually made after the fistula has been prepared (48). However, if the iris prolapses into the limbal wound, it is generally best to make the iridectomy and then complete the fistula. The iridectomy should extend beyond the margins of sclerectomy to avoid obstruction of the fistula by the peripheral iris. The technique for the incisional peripheral iridectomy is discussed in Chapter 36.

Complications of the surgical iridectomy itself can include inflammation, hyphema, and iridodialysis. It is preferable not to make the iris incision too close to the iris root for concern of incising the ciliary body and inducing significant bleeding. Some surgeons omit the peripheral iridectomy in patients who have pseudophakia or undergo a combined trabeculectomy with cataract surgery using a small-clear corneal incision. This is especially true in cases where there is a deep anterior chamber and the risk of iris incarceration into the sclerectomy is low. In one study, patients with and without peripheral iridectomy had similar postoperative vision and IOP control (49,50).

Closure of the Conjunctival Flap

Watertight closure of the conjunctival flap is also a critical aspect of any filtering procedure, because a leaking wound may lead to a persistently flat bleb or anterior chamber, or both. This can lead to failure of the filtering bleb to develop properly. A fine absorbable suture, such as 10-0 polyglycolic acid or polyglactin, on a tapered, vascular needle is desirable, because it minimizes leakage at the suture sites and excessive tissue reaction. For closure of a limbus-based flap, a running suture with close bites provides the tightest closure. When Tenon capsule has been preserved, a double running closure, first of Tenon tissue, and then conjunctiva, may increase the chances of tight wound closure (**Fig. 38.7**) (51). Alternatively, several interrupted sutures that close Tenon capsule may be used to approximate the wound edges before running closure. This is especially important when adjunctive antifibrosis agents are used.

A running suture can also be placed along the limbus for fornix-based flaps, especially when a small edge of conjunctiva is retained adjacent to the limbus (52). Various techniques have been described for placing a running mattress suture at the limbus, which provides tight wound closure and is especially useful when adjunctive antifibrosis agents are used (52–54). In other situations, surgeons find it adequate to use a single interrupted suture at one or both ends of the conjunctival flap (18,55) (Fig. 38.7), which stretches the conjunctiva tightly over peripheral cornea.

If a paracentesis is made at the outset, balanced salt solution, or a viscoelastic, by using a cannula on a syringe, may be injected into the anterior chamber via that incision at two stages during the completion of the procedure. The first of these is after suturing the scleral flap in a trabeculectomy to ensure appropriate flow around the flap. The anterior chamber should deepen and the eye should become slightly firm before

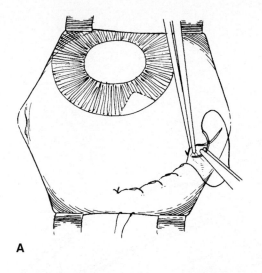

A

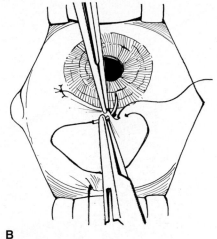

B

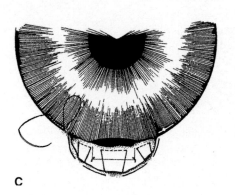

C

Figure 38.7 **A:** Closure of conjunctival flap with running suture. (From Shields MB. Trabeculectomy vs. full-thickness filtering operation for control of glaucoma. *Ophthalmic Surg.* 1980;11:498, with permission.) **B:** Closure of fornix-based conjunctival flap. **C:** Closure of fornix-based conjunctival flap—Wise closure. (From Ng PW, Yeung BY, Yick DW, et al. Fornix-based trabeculectomy with Wise's suture technique in Chinese patients. *Ophthalmology.* 2000;107:2310–2313, with permission.)

fluid begins to flow around the flap edges. If the flow is too brisk and the chamber collapses, more sutures should be added. Conversely, sutures may need to be loosened if the eye remains too firm. The second stage of fluid injection is after closure of the conjunctival flap. This should deepen the anterior chamber and create a sustained elevation of the bleb, thereby demonstrating patency of the fistula and watertight closure of the conjunctival incision. Some surgeons examine the conjunctival closure for bleb leaks by coating the bleb surface with fluorescein at the end of the case.

POSTOPERATIVE MANAGEMENT

Topical mydriatic–cycloplegics may be used for the first 2 to 3 weeks to help maintain the anterior chamber depth, particularly in patients with phakic eyes and those with postoperative hypotony. Some investigators feel that these agents may also reduce postoperative inflammation (56). Topical antibiotics are used routinely for 7 to 10 days. Use of topical corticosteroids decreases conjunctival scarring and is associated with higher success rates with trabeculectomy. They are typically used for 4 to 6 weeks, although some surgeons use low-dose topical corticosteroids indefinitely. (The effect of postoperative corticosteroid use is discussed in more detail later in the chapter.)

FISTULIZING TECHNIQUES

There are two basic types of fistulas: (a) those which extend through the full thickness of the limbal tissue and (b) those which are covered by a partial-thickness scleral flap. During the first half of the 20th century, the former technique was used exclusively. The concept of a guarded fistula (trabeculectomy) began to gain popularity in the 1970s. With the advent of adjunctive antifibrosis agents and laser suture lysis, the full-thickness procedures lost favor compared with conventional trabeculectomy surgery and are now primarily of historical interest.

Partial-Thickness Fistulas (Trabeculectomy)

The standard full-thickness filtering procedures were often complicated by excessive aqueous filtration, which led to a high incidence of prolonged flat anterior chambers, associated with corneal decompensation, synechiae formation, and cataracts. In addition, the filtering blebs often became thin and were susceptible to rupture, creating the danger of endophthalmitis. One way to minimize these complications is to place a partial-thickness scleral flap over the fistula. This concept was suggested by Sugar (57) in 1961 but was popularized by the 1968 report of Cairns (58). Both authors referred to the technique as a trabeculectomy, and this remains the most commonly used technique for filtering surgery today.

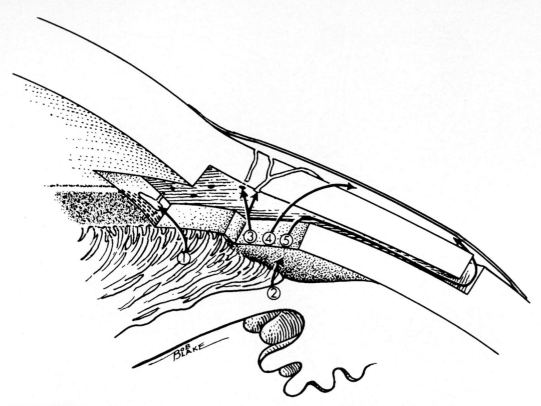

Figure 38.8 Possible routes of aqueous humor flow associated with a trabeculectomy: *1*, Aqueous flow into cut ends of Schlemm canal (rare); *2*, cyclodialysis (if tissue is dissected posterior to scleral spur); *3*, filtration through outlet channels in scleral flap; *4*, filtration through connective tissue substance of scleral flap; *5*, filtration around the margins of the scleral flap.

Theories of Mechanism

It was originally thought that aqueous might flow into the cut ends of Schlemm canal (58). Subsequent studies, however, showed fibrotic closure of the canal at its cut ends in monkey and human (59,60) eyes, and the presence of Schlemm canal in the "trabeculectomy" specimen did not correlate with the outcome of the procedure (61–63). Furthermore, it was noted that most successful cases had a filtering bleb, and the amount of fluorescein-stained aqueous in the filtration area correlated with the success of the procedure (64), suggesting that external filtration was the principal mode of IOP reduction. The outer layers of limbus and anterior sclera do not differ ultrastructurally from the inner layers in a way that might predispose to increased passage of aqueous (65). Perfusion studies of human autopsy eyes, in which a trabeculectomy was created and the margins of the scleral flap were sealed with adhesive, did show a significant flow through the scleral flap (66). Fluorescein angiographic studies of eyes with successful trabeculectomies showed the primary route of external filtration to be around the margins of the scleral flap (67). It may be that external filtration occurs around or through the scleral flap, depending on how tightly the flap is sutured or the thickness of the scleral flap. Use of antimetabolites often leads to alterations of the scleral flap ranging from a complete melt to a minimal decrease of integrity. Other contributors to the outflow resistance are the surface area of the bleb available for diffusion and the quality of the conjunctiva overlying the bleb (i.e., thin and avascular,

or thicker with only decreased vascularity) (**Fig. 38.8**). Other possible mechanisms of IOP reduction by trabeculectomy include cyclodialysis, if the fistula extends posterior to scleral spur (59), or aqueous outflow through newly developed aqueous veins, lymphatic vessels, or normal aqueous veins (68,69).

Basic Trabeculectomy Technique

With the trabeculectomy technique (**Fig. 38.9**), the margins of the scleral flap, adjacent to the corneolimbal junction, are outlined first with light cautery and then with partial-thickness scleral incisions. The original technique described by Cairns involved a 5 × 5-mm square, but numerous variations in size and shape of the scleral flap have been described, as discussed later in this section. A lamellar flap, hinged at the limbus, is then dissected forward until at least 1 mm of the bluish-gray zone of the peripheral cornea is exposed. It is difficult to precisely determine the relative thickness of the scleral flap, but in general, it should be one-half to two-thirds sclera thickness.

The fistula is begun by first entering the anterior chamber with a knife just behind the hinge of the scleral flap, and then widening the incision with the knife or scissors to within approximately 0.5 mm of the scleral flap margins. Radial incisions are then extended posteriorly on either end of the initial incision for 1 mm, and the resulting flap of deep limbal tissue is reflected until the angle structures can be visualized, and the tissue is excised with scissors along the scleral spur. Today most surgeons prefer using a scleral punch (described later).

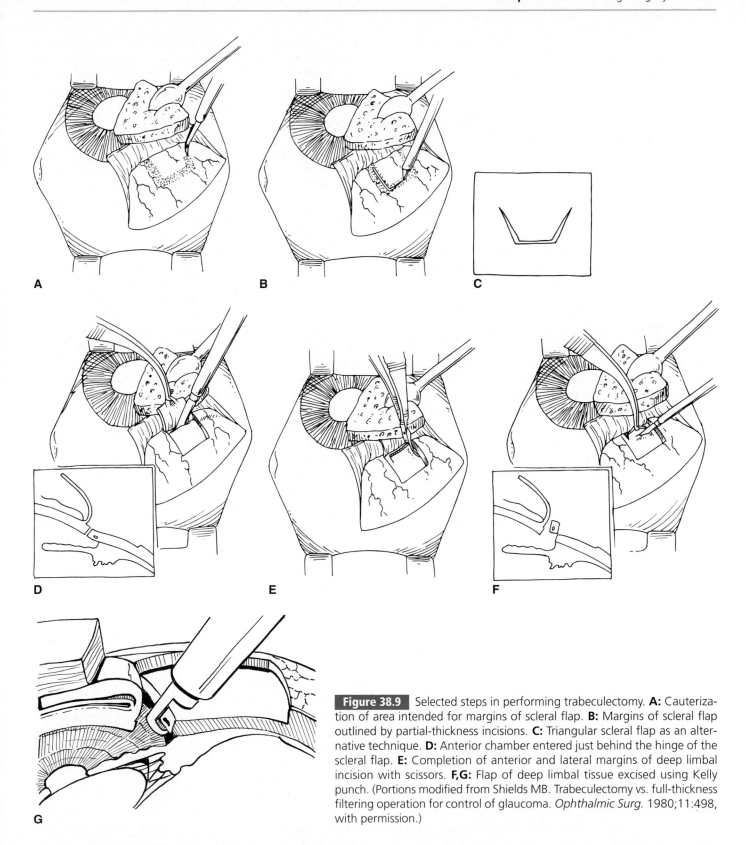

Figure 38.9 Selected steps in performing trabeculectomy. **A:** Cauterization of area intended for margins of scleral flap. **B:** Margins of scleral flap outlined by partial-thickness incisions. **C:** Triangular scleral flap as an alternative technique. **D:** Anterior chamber entered just behind the hinge of the scleral flap. **E:** Completion of anterior and lateral margins of deep limbal incision with scissors. **F,G:** Flap of deep limbal tissue excised using Kelly punch. (Portions modified from Shields MB. Trabeculectomy vs. full-thickness filtering operation for control of glaucoma. *Ophthalmic Surg.* 1980;11:498, with permission.)

After making a peripheral iridectomy, the scleral flap is approximated with 10-0 nylon sutures. Some surgeons prefer to approximate the scleral flap loosely with two sutures at the posterior corners to promote filtration around the margins of the flap. Others prefer tighter closure at the posterior corners and sometimes use additional sutures to avoid the complications of hypotony and a flat anterior chamber. However, loose and tight closures did not differ significantly within 3 months postoperatively in one study (70). Closure that achieves mild-to-moderate resistance to aqueous flow, thus maintaining anterior chamber depth, is optimal. It is especially important when using adjunctive antifibrosis agents, because these eyes are much more susceptible to excessive filtration and hypotony. Most surgeons prefer to achieve tighter scleral wound closure, with the plan to lyse sutures postoperatively with an argon or diode laser, if necessary, using specially designed lenses (71–74). An alternative to laser suture lysis is the use of releasable sutures, which can be removed, as required, at the slitlamp. Several effective techniques for releasable sutures have been described (75–78). As noted earlier, the scleral flap can be tested for adequate flow resistance before closing the conjunctival flap by injecting balanced salt solution into the anterior chamber via a paracentesis.

Modifications in Technique

The numerous variations of the guarded filtering procedure that have been reported primarily involve modifications in the scleral flap or in the fistulizing technique.

Variations in the Scleral Flap

Rather than making a square flap, some surgeons prefer a triangular (79), semicircular (80), or trapezoid shape. There is no apparent advantage of one shape over another with regard to long-term success. Some surgeons attempt to influence the degree of postoperative filtration by modifying the scleral flap. It has been suggested, for example, that the thickness of the flap correlates with the final IOP, in that thinner flaps provide greater filtration and lower pressures (81). Other variations in surgical technique have included attempts to enhance filtration around the flap by applying light cautery to the lateral margins (67), omitting all sutures for the scleral flap (82), or excising the distal 2 mm of the flap (82). These techniques predate the era of antifibrosis agents, however, and should be avoided when such adjunctive therapy is used. Placement of amniotic membrane under the scleral flap and suturing it with 10-0 nylon has been suggested for prevention of postoperative adhesion of conjunctiva and sclera in patients with whom the risk for failure is high (83). Another variation in creating the scleral flap involves the scleral tunnel technique, as has been used with phacoemulsification (84). The sides of the tunnel are then incised with scissors to create the flap.

Variations in the Fistulizing Technique

Watson (85,86) modified Cairns's basic technique by starting the dissection of the tissue block posteriorly over ciliary body, separating it from the underlying structure, and excising it at Schwalbe line. Other techniques to create the fistula beneath a scleral flap include trephinations, sclerectomies, thermal sclerostomies, and sclerostomies with a carbon dioxide laser (80,87–91). Most surgeons use a Kelly Descemet membrane punch or Crozafon–De Laage punch to excise limbal tissue sections from the posterior lip of the initial incision beneath the scleral flap (92,93).

Modifications for Neovascular Glaucoma

As discussed in Chapter 19, intraocular surgery in eyes with neovascular glaucoma is often complicated by intraoperative hyphema. One trabeculectomy variation to minimize this risk includes excision of a large trabecular segment, partial nonpenetrating cyclodiathermy in the scleral bed, and partial ablation of abnormal iris vessels with a wide sector iridectomy (94). Glaucoma drainage-device surgery and diode laser cyclophotocoagulation are increasingly considered to be the treatments of choice for this disorder (95), and they are discussed in other chapters.

The optimum approach to filtering surgery in eyes with neovascular glaucoma, however, is to precede it with an intravitreal injection of anti–vascular endothelial growth factor (anti-VEGF) agent or panretinal photocoagulation, when possible, which often reduces neovascularization, decreasing the likelihood or degree of postoperative hyphema regardless of the surgical treatment used.

Trabeculectomy for neovascular glaucoma often fails because of scarring of the filtering bleb; therefore, the use of mitomycin C (MMC) and 5-fluorouracil (5-FU) has been advocated in those eyes. One study classified two thirds of eyes after panretinal photocoagulation followed by trabeculectomy with MMC as surgical success after 2 years of follow-up (96). Another study did not find that differences in the MMC concentration or application time affected postoperative IOP or complication rates (97). The number of successful surgeries was 71% at 1 month and decreased to 29% after 1 year. Postoperative needling, in conjunction with intraoperative MMC use and postoperative intrableb 5-FU injection, was found efficacious and saved further surgery in some intractable cases (98). Regression of rubeosis, sometimes seen after trabeculectomy with MMC, has been suggested to be a pharmacologic side effect of MMC and not necessarily the effect of IOP lowering alone (99). In a preliminary study, trabeculectomy 1 month after use of intravitreal bevacizumab resulted in a decrease in anterior segment neovascularization and fewer complications (100). Even if an anti-VEGF agent is used, the effects of these agents are temporary, and further injections or panretinal photocoagulation may be needed for long-term control of neovascularization.

Modifications for Previous Intraocular Surgery

The fornix-based conjunctival flap, as previously discussed (16–18,26), is particularly useful in eyes that have had previous intraocular surgery involving the conjunctiva—for example, when a fornix-based conjunctival flap has been used during a cataract procedure. The conjunctiva in these eyes is usually tightly scarred down to episclera near the limbus, making preparation of a limbus-based flap difficult. When using a fornix-based flap, it is probably best to suture the lateral margins of the scleral flap to promote drainage posteriorly. An anterior vitrectomy may also be required if loose vitreous is in the anterior chamber or presents at the iridectomy site. Nonpenetrating trabeculectomy was once advocated for glaucoma in aphakia (101). However, early results from the Tube versus Trabeculectomy study indicate that implantation of glaucoma drainage devices may be a better alternative for these cases (102).

Use of antimetabolites for trabeculectomy in pseudophakic eyes may improve the success rate. However, in aphakic and pseudophakic eyes of children, after congenital cataract

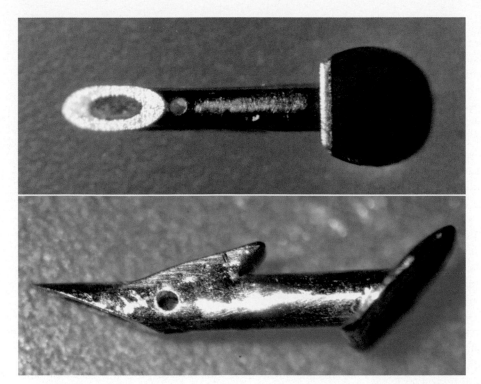

Figure 38.10 R-50 model of Ex-PRESS mini glaucoma shunt (actual length, approximately 400 microns.

surgery, trabeculectomy was successful in only one third of patients, regardless of whether MMC was used during the surgery (103). Implantation of glaucoma drainage devices has been gaining broader acceptance in these challenging cases.

Adjunctive Devices

The Ex-PRESS mini glaucoma shunt (**Fig. 38.10**) is a stainless steel device that was originally developed to be implanted subconjunctivally through the limbus, providing direct communication between the anterior chamber and subconjunctival space, resembling a full-thickness procedure, relying upon the intrinsic resistance of the device. Although successful in lowering IOP, procedures using this device had high complication rates, and as a result, surgeons began implanting the shunt device beneath a partial-thickness scleral flap (104,105). The technique of implantation and indications of use resemble those of trabeculectomy (i.e., a guarded filtration procedure), aside from the absence of an iridectomy. In a retrospective comparison with trabeculectomies, implantation with Ex-PRESS mini glaucoma shunts achieved similar IOP control but had a lower rate of early postoperative hypotony (106).

Wound Healing

The most common cause of failure in glaucoma filtering surgery is scarring of the filtering bleb (107). The increased amount of collagen in the failed blebs suggests that proliferation of fibroblasts with associated production of collagen and glycosaminoglycans is important in the response to filtering surgery (3). However, as discussed in Chapter 37, wound healing is a complex process with several phases, and it is likely that bleb failure in filtering surgery involves many of these factors and certain unique characteristics of the glaucomatous eye. Newer antifibrotic agents and drug delivery systems are under development in an effort to improve efficacy and safety.

Influence of Aqueous Humor on Wound Healing

Aqueous humor normally slows or fails to support the growth of conjunctival fibroblasts in tissue culture (108–110). A possible explanation is that aqueous contains one or more inhibitory factors for fibroblast proliferation. Cell culture studies have shown that the high concentration of ascorbic acid, normally present in aqueous humor, is cytotoxic to dividing human Tenon capsule fibroblasts, which may contribute to the development of a successful filtering bleb (111). Aqueous humor also contains a wide variety of growth factors, which maintain the normal function of ocular tissues in health and have a significant role in abnormal states and wound healing (112). Transforming growth factor-β (TGF-β), a potent modulator of tissue repair, is in human aqueous and plays a role in the healing process after glaucoma filtering surgery (113). Contrary to the influence of primary aqueous humor, aqueous obtained shortly after intraocular surgery or mixed with 20% desiccated embryo extract does promote proliferation of fibroblasts (110,114). Secondary aqueous humor has also been shown to stimulate the proliferation of cultured corneal endothelial cells (115). In addition, aqueous humor has chemoattractant activity for ocular fibroblasts, and this activity is significantly greater in eyes with previously failed glaucoma surgery (116). Therefore, components of normal aqueous humor and alterations in some glaucoma patients are likely to influence both success and failure of the filtering bleb.

Other Factors Affecting Wound Healing

Numerous studies have suggested that young age and African heritage adversely influence the outcomes of glaucoma filtering surgery. The explanation for these observations is not clear. Histologic studies of conjunctival specimens obtained before trabeculectomy in patients with chronic open-angle glaucoma (COAG) showed no significant influence of age or ethnicity on conjunctival factors that might relate to surgical outcome (117,118). A more significant influence may be chronic topical glaucoma medical therapy before trabeculectomy. Some studies have identified long-term topical combination therapy as a risk factor for failure of trabeculectomy (119,120), although one study that compared success rates before and after the introduction of topical β-blockers did not indicate that the preoperative use of topical medication influenced the outcome of surgery (121). Histologic studies of conjunctiva from patients after long-term topical glaucoma medical therapy revealed a significant degree of subclinical inflammation (122,123), although one study could only correlate the number of goblet cells with successful outcomes (124). Conjunctival impression cytology correlated significant degrees of metaplasia with the number of glaucoma medications used (125). One clinical study, however, indicated that stopping topical adrenergic therapy and adding use of topical corticosteroids 1 month before surgery was associated with a decrease in the number of conjunctival fibroblasts and inflammatory cells and an improvement in the success rate of trabeculectomy (126). Another study suggested that a high number of conjunctival goblet cells may be a predictor of lower IOP after trabeculectomy without use of antimetabolites (127). The number of conjunctival fibroblasts and inflammatory cells increases after previous ocular surgery involving the conjunctiva, possibly causing an increased risk of trabeculectomy failure (128).

Antifibrotic Agents

Corticosteroids

Considerable attention has been given to measures—primarily medication use—that may prevent bleb failure by modulating the wound healing process. The first of these to be used clinically were the corticosteroids. Tissue culture studies of human Tenon capsule fibroblasts have shown that both corticosteroids and nonsteroidal anti-inflammatory drugs inhibit cell attachment and proliferation (129,130). Clinical investigations have confirmed the efficacy of topical corticosteroids, although no additional benefit was achieved with systemic steroids (131,132). It has also been suggested that subconjunctival triamcinolone before filtering surgery may improve the success rate (133). Despite the benefit of corticosteroids, the incidence of bleb failure remains high with certain types of glaucoma (e.g., glaucoma in aphakia and pseudophakia and neovascular glaucoma), which has prompted the search for additional agents to modify wound healing.

5-Fluorouracil

5-FU was the first drug to be studied extensively as an adjunct to corticosteroids in the control of wound healing following trabeculectomy. This pyrimidine analog antimetabolite, which blocks DNA synthesis through the inhibition of thymidylate synthesis, has been shown to inhibit fibroblast proliferation in cell cultures (134,135). The subconjunctival injection of 5-FU after filtering surgery significantly improved bleb formation in monkeys and improved the rate of success in difficult clinical cases (136–138). A subsequent multicenter, randomized clinical trial of 213 patients with glaucoma in aphakia or pseudophakia or a previous failed filter in a phakic eye confirmed the ability of 5-FU to improve the success rate of filtering surgery in these high-risk cases (139,140). However, the protocol required twice-daily subconjunctival injections of 5-mg 5-FU for 7 days and then once daily for 7 more days. In addition, serious complications included conjunctival wound leaks and corneal epithelial defects in the early postoperative course, plus an increased risk for late-onset bleb leakage (139,140). Therefore, lower effective doses, alternative delivery systems, and alternative agents have been sought.

Success has been reported with daily injections of 5-mg 5-FU for 7 to 14 days (141–143), which probably represents the most common range of dosages in current use. In one study of patients with COAG and "secondary" glaucoma or refractory glaucoma, the average total dose of 5-FU was 36.5, 36.0, and 49.5 mg, respectively, and the probability of IOP control below 16 mm Hg with 5-year follow-up was 77.9%, 66.8%, and 26.9%, respectively (143). Adjunctive use of 5-FU increases the success rate of trabeculectomy in eyes undergoing initial filtering surgery, patients younger than 40 years, infants, and patients requiring extremely low IOPs (144–148). However, the complication rate is higher than in trabeculectomy without 5-FU, and caution is advised, especially with initial surgery (140). There is a high risk of failure in patients with neovascular glaucoma (149). The treatment is believed to be most effective if started prophylactically on the first postoperative day, although success has been reported with starting 3 to 15 days postoperatively when signs of impending bleb failure are noted (150,151). Several clinical trials have shown that 5-FU is also beneficial when used intraoperatively, usually on a surgical sponge soaked in 25 to 50 mg/mL of the drug and applied to the surgical site for 5 minutes (152–156). The type of sponge can also affect the intraocular tissue levels of 5-FU delivered (157).

Mitomycin C

Use of MMC was reported by Chen (158) in 1983 to enhance the IOP-lowering efficacy of trabeculectomy when applied intraoperatively in eyes at high risk for surgical failure. MMC is an antineoplastic antibiotic isolated from *Streptomyces caespitosus*. Tissue culture studies of human Tenon capsule fibroblasts revealed almost complete inhibition of fibroblast proliferation (159), the degree of which correlated with the outcome of filtering surgery (160). When compared with 5-FU, the effect on rabbit fibroblast proliferation was much more prolonged with MMC (161). 5-FU was toxic to cultured mouse fibroblasts while sparing bovine vascular endothelial cells, whereas MMC was cytotoxic for both cell types (162). Intraoperative application of

MMC in rabbits significantly prolonged bleb duration after glaucoma filtering surgery (163). Subsequent clinical trials supported the benefit of MMC use as an adjunct to trabeculectomy (164), and randomized comparisons with postoperative use of subconjunctival 5-FU generally showed intraoperative use of MMC to have superior IOP-lowering efficacy after trabeculectomy (165–169). MMC has been shown to enhance the success rate of trabeculectomy for refractory glaucoma in black patients, in glaucoma associated with uveitis, in congenital and developmental glaucoma, in normal-tension glaucoma, and in primary, uncomplicated trabeculectomies (170–176). A retrospective study has shown that primary trabeculectomy with MMC maintained an IOP level of 15 mm Hg or less in more than 80% of patients after 1 year and in 60% after 6 years, suggesting that the use of MMC may be justified in primary trabeculectomies in patients with severe glaucoma (177). However, care must be exercised with the use of adjunctive MMC, especially in the primary, uncomplicated cases, because of the significant incidence of serious complications.

Although adjunctive use of MMC is less likely to cause the postoperative complications that are typically associated with 5-FU, such as corneal epithelial toxicity and wound leaks (165–168), it is associated with other complications that can be even more serious. The most significant of these is hypotony maculopathy, in which prolonged IOP reduction is associated with disc edema, vascular tortuosity, and chorioretinal folds in the macular area, potentially producing marked reduction in visual acuity (178). The main cause of the hypotony is excessive filtration, and histologic studies of excised overfiltering blebs have revealed an irregular epithelium and a largely acellular subepithelium of loosely arranged connective tissue (179–181). However, another mechanism of hypotony may be aqueous hyposecretion, in that one enucleated human eye revealed disruption of the ciliary body epithelium beneath the site of MMC application (181). Other potential complications, as suggested by animal studies, include anterior chamber reaction and corneal endothelial toxicity if the MMC gains entry into the eye (182,183). (The management of these complications is discussed later in the chapter.) The following modifications in technique may minimize the complications.

In early protocols, a sponge soaked in MMC, 0.5 mg/mL, was applied to the subconjunctival tissues for 5 minutes. Subsequent attempts to reduce the risk of hypotony have included reduced concentrations and exposure times (179,184). It has also been suggested that adjustment of exposure time according to each patient's risk of excessive fibrosis may enhance the balance between successful IOP control and incidence of complications (179). Some retrospective studies suggested that MMC, 0.2 mg/mL, applied for 2 minutes may be as effective as higher doses but may be associated with few complications (184,185). However, the optimum protocol has yet to be established.

Various sponges have been advocated as vehicles for MMC, including Merocel and various microsurgical sponges, and it may be that manipulating the size or shape of the sponge can influence the effect of the MMC (186–188). One study suggested that placing the sponge beneath the scleral flap rather than over intact episclera may improve the success rate without increasing complications (177,189). In rabbits, irrigating the ocular tissues with balanced salt solution after removal of the sponge substantially reduced intraocular diffusion of MMC (190).

In an experimental model, irrigation reduced the MMC concentration only in the external half of the sclera, leaving the deep intrascleral concentrations unchanged (191), suggesting that a lower-dose MMC application without irrigation may be a rational approach (192). Intraoperative application of MMC without touching the conjunctiva or Tenon capsule was ineffective in inhibiting the development of thin, avascular blebs in eyes undergoing primary trabeculectomy (193).

Other Antifibrotic Agents

Alternative agents that have been evaluated as antiproliferative drugs include cytosine arabinoside, bleomycin, rapamycin, doxorubicin, daunorubicin, 5-fluorouridine, 5'-monophosphate, 5-fluoroorotate, heparin, Taxol, cytochalasin-B, colchicine, immunotoxins, and interferon-α-2b (134,194–207). Suramin, a substance that inhibits the action of growth factors, was evaluated in rabbits and in humans in a prospective study (208,209). The use of suramin had fewer complications, compared with use of MMC, with similar success rates, suggesting that it may become an alternative to antimetabolite therapy in glaucoma surgery (209). Beta irradiation also inhibited fibroblast proliferation in tissue culture and delayed wound healing in rabbits (210–212). In a preliminary clinical trial, beta irradiation did not improve the results of trabeculectomies (213), although a study of patients aged 18 years or younger with congenital glaucoma suggested a beneficial effect on the prognosis of trabeculectomy (214). Amniotic membrane transplantation or subconjunctival perfluoropropane (C3F8) gas has been suggested as a safer alternative to MMC (215–217).

In addition to drugs that influence fibroblast proliferation, agents have also been evaluated that will alter other phases of the wound healing process. For example, tissue plasminogen activator, which causes localized fibrinolysis, γ-interferon and calcium ionophores, which inhibit collagen biosynthesis, and β-aminopropionitrile and d-penicillamine, which inhibit cross-linking of collagen, have shown promise in in vitro and in vivo studies (218–227). Perioperative injection of bevacizumab has also shown promise to decrease conjunctival scarring and vascularity (228,229).

TGF-β is a potent stimulant of scarring, and it has been identified as an important component of wound healing, particularly in the conjunctival scarring response (230). It has been found in human aqueous and appears to play a role in the healing process after glaucoma filtering surgery (113). Inhibition of TGF-β appears to be a more physiologic approach to wound healing modulation (231,232).

Although subconjunctival administration of a TGF-β_2 antibody in the postoperative period improved the outcome of glaucoma surgery in an animal model and appeared more efficacious than 5-FU without some of the side effects (233), a randomized, controlled trial of CAT-152, a monoclonal antibody

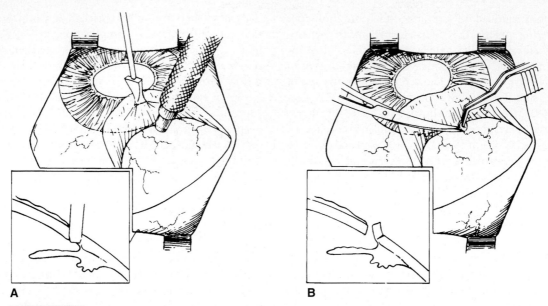

A   **B**

Figure 38.11 Limboscleral trephination. **A:** Trephine button partially excised by tilting the trephine anteriorly. **B:** Completion of excision by cutting posterior attachment with scissors.

against TGF-β_2, was no more effective than placebo and required frequent subconjunctival injections in the postoperative period (234). Tranilast (N-3′,4′-dimethoxycinnamoyl-anthranilic acid), a drug with antikeloid and antiscarring properties, inhibits TGF-β_1 secretion and therefore could be a promising drug to prevent scarring after glaucoma filtration surgery (235–237).

In the future, combinations of agents may be administered according to the various phases of the wound healing process to prevent bleb failure.

Earlier Full-Thickness Fistulas

Sclerectomy

The original type of limbal fistula, which has been largely replaced by trabeculectomy with or without adjunctive use of antifibrosis agents, involves the creation of a direct opening through the full thickness of the limbal tissue. The fistula may be created by using various techniques.

In 1906, LaGrange (238) described a technique in which a full-thickness limbal incision was made, and a piece of tissue was then excised from the anterior lip of the wound to create a limbal fistula. Holth (239) modified this procedure 3 years later by performing the sclerectomy with a punch. However, the sclerectomy technique that became most popular in the mid-20th century was the posterior lip sclerectomy described by Iliff and Haas (240).

Trephination

In 1909, Elliot (241) and Fergus (242) described a glaucoma filtering procedure in which the fistula was created with a small trephine placed just behind the corneolimbal junction. Elliot (243) later modified the technique by splitting the peripheral cornea and placing the trephine more anteriorly (sclerocorneal trephining). However, this modification produced a thinner

filtering bleb with an increased chance of late infection, and Sugar (244) advocated a return to the original, more posterior placement of the trephine, which he called limboscleral trephination (or trepanation) (245) (**Fig. 38.11**).

Thermal Sclerostomy (Scheie Procedure)

In 1924, Preziosi (246) described a filtering technique in which a limbal fistula was created by entering the anterior chamber angle with an electrocautery instrument. Scheie (247) later described a procedure that also used cautery but differed from the operation described by Preziosi in that a limbal scratch incision was first made, and the cautery was then used to retract the wound edges, thereby creating the fistula.

The thermal sclerostomy technique (**Fig. 38.12**) involves application of light cautery to the sclera in a 1 × 5-mm area behind the corneolimbal junction. A 5-mm limbal scratch incision is then made through the cauterized area, perpendicular to the scleral surface, and cautery is applied to the lips of the incision until the wound edges separate by at least 1 mm.

The escape of aqueous from the limbal incision may interfere with the application of cautery, which can be partially avoided by stopping the initial scratch incision just before it enters the anterior chamber, applying cautery, and then completing the incision (248). In addition, bipolar cautery can be effectively used in the wet field. Another modification is to place a temporary suture across the fistula to avoid an early flat anterior chamber (249).

Iridencleisis

This procedure differs from the other forms of full-thickness filtering surgery in that a wedge of iris is incarcerated into the limbal incision to maintain a patent channel for aqueous outflow (250). This was once a popular procedure, but it lost favor partly because of the suspicion that the associated incidence of

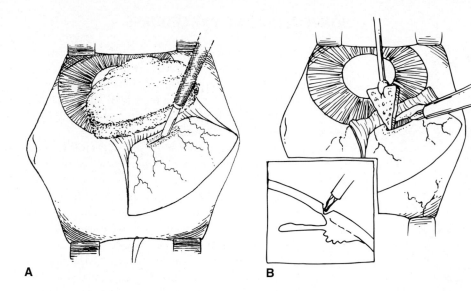

Figure 38.12 Thermal sclerostomy. **A:** Limbal incision created (may initially be partial or full thickness). **B:** Application of cautery to the lips of the incision to separate the wound edges. A partial-thickness incision is then extended into the anterior chamber and cautery is applied to the depths of the wound.

sympathetic ophthalmia was higher than with other filtering procedures. Although this fear was unsubstantiated, the operation never regained popularity.

Laser and Other Sclerostomy Techniques

Laser Sclerostomy Ab Externo

Laser energy has also been used to create the fistula, most of which are full thickness. This can be performed from an ab externo or ab interno approach. The argon laser has been studied for the former approach (251), although the holmium laser, also referred to as THC:YAG (thulium, holmium, and chromium-doped yttrium aluminum garnet crystal) laser, has undergone the most extensive evaluation for laser sclerostomy ab externo (252–267). The laser operates in the near-infrared region, with a wavelength of 2100 nm. A right-angle exit of the laser beam from the tip of the fiberoptic probe allows subconjunctival advancement of the probe from a small conjunctival incision to the limbus where the fistula is created.

Rabbit studies supported the feasibility of the holmium procedure (252,253), and preliminary clinical trials provided encouraging short-term results (254,255). Longer follow-up, however, revealed estimated probabilities of success of approximately 65% at 1 year, 57% at 30 months, 44% at 2 years, and 36% at 4 years (256–259).

However, higher incidences of hypotony (due to the full-thickness nature of the fistula), choroidal detachments, and iris incarcerations, along with a progressing rate of failure, make this procedure less effective than trabeculectomy for long-term pressure control (266,267). Other lasers that have been evaluated for laser sclerostomy ab externo include a giant-pulsed (up to 200 W of peak power at pulses of 20 or 40 milliseconds) neodymium:yttrium–aluminum–garnet (Nd:YAG), a picosecond Nd:YLF (yttrium lithium fluoride) 1053-nm laser, a semiconductor diode laser, and a 193-nm excimer laser (268–273). The sclerostomies created with diode laser (260) have been associated with heat coagulation damage and disruption of scleral collagen. Pulsed laser has also been associated with

thermal and mechanical damage (261). A continuous-wave, mid-infrared diode laser system appears to be superior to pulsed lasers (261). Excimer lasers have also been used in a modified trabeculectomy to precisely remove scleral tissue overlying the Schlemm canal, leaving the trabecular meshwork intact (274–276), and in a modified nonpenetrating filtering surgery to perform trabeculodissection under a scleral flap through the Schlemm canal and the juxtacanalicular trabecular meshwork (277). The approach of using lasers for an ab externo approach for laser sclerostomy has been largely abandoned.

Laser Sclerostomy Ab Interno

In addition to creating full-thickness fistulas with laser energy from the external approach, lasers and other instruments have been evaluated to create sclerostomies ab interno (i.e., from the anterior chamber to the subconjunctival space). The main theoretical advantage of this technique is that it requires no dissection of the conjunctiva, which is elevated before creating the sclerostomy with a fluid injection over the surgical site, thereby reducing the risk of scarring and bleb failure. The first attempt at laser sclerostomy ab interno was made with a Q-switched Nd:YAG laser, focused into the anterior chamber angle through a special gonioprism (278–280). This was shown to be effective in creating a sclerostomy but required very high levels of energy. Subsequent modifications involved staining the sclera with methylene blue dye by iontophoresis and using a pulsed dye laser with a wavelength of 660 nm, which is maximally absorbed by methylene blue (281–283). In a prospective study in rabbits, internal sclerostomy made by a pulsed dye laser appeared to have similar efficacy in lowering IOP as a posterior lip sclerectomy (284).

Other attempts at laser sclerostomy ab interno have used contact laser probes, the tip of which is introduced into the anterior chamber via a limbal incision 180 degrees from the sclerostomy site. The tip is passed across the anterior chamber to the trabecular meshwork, where the sclerostomy is created (**Fig. 38.13**). This technique has been evaluated with continuous-wave Nd:YAG lasers; high-energy argon blue-green laser;

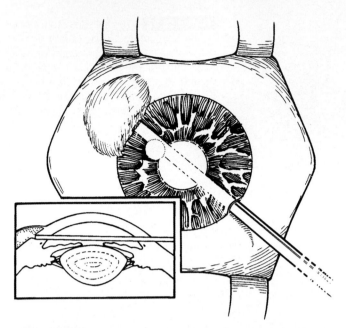

Figure 38.13 Internal sclerostomy. A laser fiberoptic probe tip or automated trephine is inserted into the anterior chamber through a limbal stab incision and is used to create a full-thickness fistula beneath elevated conjunctiva 180 degrees from the entry site.

and excimer, erbium, diode, and Nd:YLF lasers (285–294). An intraocular endoscope has been suggested for use with an erbium:YAG laser for precise location of the sclerostomy and to reduce scarring at the filtering site (295). Rabbit studies of Nd:YAG, holmium, and erbium lasers indicate that increasing wavelengths are associated with decreasing thermal damage around the sclerostomy, which would theoretically decrease subconjunctival scarring and filtration failure (296,297). Excimer laser trabeculectomy ab interno performed on rabbit eyes produced permanent openings into the Schlemm canal through trabecular meshwork, reducing the outflow resistance (298). In human eyes with glaucoma, openings created in the trabecular meshwork with an excimer laser allow an open communication between the anterior chamber and Schlemm canal. The minimal trauma to the eye of this procedure makes other types of glaucoma surgery possible if needed in the future (299).

Despite the general interest and potential advantages of these approaches, they have not gained favor among glaucoma surgeons. This may largely be because most of these surgeries are full-thickness procedures, with the attendant risks of hypotony, shallow anterior chambers, and choroidal effusions.

Other Internal Sclerostomy Techniques

Internal sclerostomies have also been successfully performed with an automated trephine, and bipolar cautery and diathermy probes (300–303). Other instruments and techniques will probably be evaluated in the future as this promising approach to glaucoma filtering surgery continues to evolve. Internal sclerostomy techniques have not been widely accepted to date and currently compete with trabeculectomy ab interno (Trabectome) and trabecular bypass shunts.

NONPENETRATING PROCEDURES

Krasnov (304) described a procedure called sinusotomy, in which a strip of sclera is excised to expose a portion of Schlemm canal. It is unclear whether the benefit of this operation is from relieving obstruction of the scleral outlet channels or from relieving the collapse of Schlemm canal (305,306), or whether it is just another filtration technique.

A technique called nonpenetrating trabeculectomy carries the subscleral dissection of deep limbal tissue down to the Schlemm canal but leaves the trabecular meshwork intact (101). This was thought to be especially advantageous in aphakic eyes and was reported to have fewer postoperative complications than a standard trabeculectomy did in the phakic eye (307). The technique was modified by using the Nd:YAG laser postoperatively to perforate the meshwork at the surgical site (308,309). More recent reports have suggested that nonpenetrating surgery has advantages over conventional trabeculectomy by not entering the anterior chamber; avoiding iridectomy; and limiting early postoperative hypotony, shallow anterior chambers, hyphema, and choroidal effusions.

More recently described nonpenetrating surgery is currently divided into two techniques. The first, called deep sclerectomy, is based on the original description by Krasnov (304,310) and was later modified by Kozlov (311). A Descemet window is created, which allows aqueous to escape the anterior chamber and drain subconjunctivally, forming a low-filtering bleb. The addition of a collagen implant in the scleral bed has been advocated to help maintain the scleral drainage (311–313). The second technique, called viscocanalostomy, also requires deep scleral dissection and a filtering window. The outflow, however, appears to rely on the patency of aqueous exit channels, hypothetically achieved by identifying and dilating Schlemm canal by using high-density viscoelastic. The superficial scleral flap is sutured down tightly, minimizing subconjunctival aqueous outflow and bleb formation (314). However, subconjunctival drainage appears to be an important component of these procedures, in that blebs have been reported to be clearly visible after deep sclerectomy and in many cases of viscocanalostomy (315). The mechanism of action appears to be increasing permeability of the inner wall of Schlemm canal and the formation of an intrascleral lake (316–318).

In a phase I study, a 193-nm photopolishing scanning excimer laser was used to achieve the deep dissection required to perform a "nonpenetrating laser trabeculodissection" under a scleral flap through the Schlemm canal and the juxtacanalicular trabecular meshwork. The scleral flap was closed loosely, and MMC was used intraoperatively. A good filtering bleb was achieved with substantial reduction in the IOP (277). Another study has also shown that an excimer laser may be an effective modification of nonpenetrating filtering surgery and may be easier to perform (319). Even though the nonpenetrating surgery may have fewer complications, it appears to be less effective in achieving low levels of IOP control when compared with conventional trabeculectomy. Randomized, controlled trials comparing viscocanalostomy and trabeculectomy have found no differences; however, to date studies have had only small sample sizes, leaving the general applicability of this result in question (320,321).

Canaloplasty, a modification of earlier nonpenetrating surgeries, has recently been advocated. In this procedure, Schlemm canal is exposed and vasodilation is performed similar to those described earlier. A microcatheter is used to cannulate Schlemm canal throughout its circumference. A nonabsorbable tensioning suture is placed within the Schlemm canal, stretching the canal and improving aqueous egress through the episcleral venous system. Initial results are promising. A multicenter trial reported reductions in IOP from a baseline of 23.6 mm Hg to 16.3 mm Hg in patients having canaloplasty alone (322).

PREVENTION AND MANAGEMENT OF COMPLICATIONS

The following complications may occur with any filtering procedure, although some operations and techniques appear to provide certain advantages over others. We first consider the complications in general and then compare the merits of the various filtering procedures. It is helpful to think of these complications in three phases: intraoperative, early postoperative, and late postoperative.

Intraoperative Complications

Tearing or Buttonholing the Conjunctival Flap

The conjunctiva may be inadvertently torn or cut during preparation or closure of the flap. A buttonhole was reported in 3% of fornix-based conjunctival flaps in one series (323). This complication can be minimized by gentle handling of the tissues as outlined earlier in this chapter. When it does occur, it may be possible to close the Tenon conjunctival defect by using 10-0 nylon mattress suture on a round, tapered, noncutting needle (324,325). When 10-0 polyglycolic acid or polyglactin sutures are used, they have the advantage of being absorbable. With small holes, the tissue can be puckered together with a figure-of-8 or mattress suture, whereas a large tear may require a running suture. Tissue adhesive and light bipolar cautery may also be used to close small holes (326), but these methods are less reliable than suturing. Small leaks may close spontaneously or with the application of a large bandage contact lens.

Hemorrhage

Episcleral bleeding is particularly common in patients who have been on long-term antiglaucoma medications. It can be managed with irrigation or light cautery and should be under control before the anterior chamber is entered. Once inside the eye, inadvertent cutting of the ciliary body may cause brisk bleeding. Cauterization is difficult in these cases, although the intraocular, bipolar units at a low setting are usually effective. Alternative management involves gentle, sustained pressure over the fistula with a sponge or a large air bubble in the anterior chamber. A choroidal or expulsive hemorrhage is a particularly devastating complication that usually results from sudden reduction in the IOP with rupture of a large choroidal vessel. Risk factors for intraoperative suprachoroidal hemorrhage include high preoperative pressure, generalized atherosclerosis, and elevated intraoperative pulse (327,328). The most important step in the management of these cases is immediate closure of the fistula. Some surgeons make a scleral incision in the inferior-temporal quadrant to allow the blood to drain from this site until it stops spontaneously, although the value of this approach has not been substantiated.

Choroidal Effusion

This complication may occur intraoperatively during glaucoma filtering surgery, especially in eyes with prominent episcleral vessels, as in patients with Sturge–Weber syndrome (329), nanophthalmos, or any condition associated with elevated episcleral venous pressure. The suprachoroidal fluid in patients with Sturge–Weber syndrome contains little protein (18% of plasma concentration), suggesting that a pressure differential drives fluid and small molecules from choroidal capillaries into extravascular spaces (330). This complication is usually recognized by a sudden shallowing of the anterior chamber during the operation or by the rotation of ciliary processes through the iridectomy and into the surgical fistula. If severe, it can be managed by making a scleral incision 3 to 5 mm posterior to the limbus to release the suprachoroidal fluid (329). Placement of posterior sclerotomies before or after trabeculectomy should be considered for surgical patients in whom this complication is likely to occur, such as those with nanophthalmos or Sturge–Weber syndrome.

Other Intraoperative Complications

Vitreous loss may occur during creation of the fistula or iridectomy because of rupture of the lens zonules and hyaloid membrane, which usually results from excessive manipulation. The vitreous should be carefully removed from the surgical site with sponges and scissors or, where visualization permits, a vitrectomy instrument. Lens injury may remain limited to the surgical site if it is small, whereas larger injuries may cause gradual widespread extension or acute cataract formation, occasionally with severe inflammation (331). Stripping of Descemet membrane during glaucoma surgery, with subsequent corneal edema, has also been reported (332). The scleral flap may be inadvertently torn from its limbal hinge, in which case it can be reattached with 10-0 nylon mattress sutures or, if the flap is too thin, replaced with donor sclera or a pericardial (Tutoplast) graft (333,334). Alternatively, a new site for the scleral flap may be chosen.

Early Postoperative Complications

During the first few days or weeks after a filtering procedure, the most common complications are IOPs that are too low (hypotony) or too high. In either case, the anterior chamber may be shallow to flat or deep. Physicians should know the mechanisms that can lead to the resulting four categories of complications and how these complications can be managed.

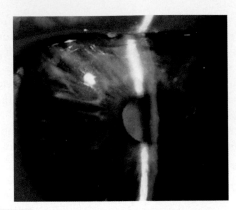

Figure 38.14 Slitlamp appearance of shallow anterior chamber in early postoperative period following a trabeculectomy showing iridocorneal touch with separation between cornea and lens.

Hypotony and Flat Anterior Chamber

A low, often nonrecordable IOP is not uncommon during the early postoperative period and is typically associated with a shallow anterior chamber. The anterior chamber is usually shallowest on postoperative day 2 or 3 and gradually deepens over the next 2 weeks (335). It is important to distinguish between a shallow anterior chamber with iridocorneal touch and a flat anterior chamber with cornea–lens touch, because the management and prognosis differ significantly (336). In the former situation, the cornea is typically clear and the iris stroma has not been flattened by the gentle touch with the cornea (**Fig. 38.14**). In most of these eyes, the anterior chamber deepens spontaneously with time and requires no special management beyond the usual postoperative care. The prolonged shallow anterior chamber may be associated with a reduced corneal endothelial cell count (337) and peripheral anterior synechia formation (338). However, these sequelae do not usually influence the long-term outcome and must be weighed against the risk of interfering with the bleb function by premature intervention. If the shallow chamber persists beyond the first week or two, measures to reform the anterior chamber are usually indicated. With a truly flat anterior chamber, in which the cornea is swollen, usually as a result of direct lens–cornea contact, and the iris stroma is flattened, immediate postoperative management is required to avoid a poor result.

As in all cases, the best way to deal with a potential complication is to take steps to avoid it. Careful closure of scleral flap to reduce the likelihood of postoperative overfiltration and meticulous conjunctival closure (as discussed earlier) are two such steps to avoid a flat anterior chamber. Other measures (also discussed earlier) are the injection of a viscoelastic into the anterior chamber (45–47,339) or use of a combination of a long-acting gas and a viscoelastic material (340). Most studies have shown that these measures do not reduce the incidence of flat anterior chambers when injected at the end of the filtering procedure (37,38), although deepening the anterior chamber with sodium hyaluronate at the beginning of the operation and maintaining the chamber depth throughout the procedure may result in deeper chambers postoperatively (40,41).

When hypotony and a flat anterior chamber do occur, the first step is to determine the cause and then take the appropriate corrective steps. These causes and their management are considered here.

Conjunctival Defect

If there is an obvious hole in the conjunctival flap or a leak at the wound edge, it may be possible to achieve spontaneous closure with a pressure patch (**Fig. 38.15**). A fusiform-shaped cotton ball can be placed over the lid in the area of the fistula and held in place with the gauze pads to act as a tamponade. If this type of pressure dressing is used, the patient should be directed to look straight ahead, because the Bell phenomenon of sleep may place the tamponade over the center of the cornea. Examination 1 to 2 hours later (the pressure patch is usually left on from morning until evening) often reveals closure of the defect and reformation of the anterior chamber. If the leaking defect persists, however, a large-diameter (17 to 22 mm) therapeutic soft contact lens can be effective. If patching with a contact lens is not successful, repairing the leak with cyanoacrylate tissue adhesive or autologous fibrin glue has been described (341–344). If the leak is small, temporarily tapering topical corticosteroids to allow increased fibrosis can be effective. Other cases may require suturing of the defect or, when the defect is large, constructing a new conjunctival flap from tissue posterior to the defect or free conjunctival autografts. Injections of autologous fibrinogen concentrate inside a bleb have been used to treat persistent hypotony after MMC-augmented trabeculectomy, with improvement of macular edema and visual acuity and preservation of a functioning trabeculectomy (345).

Excessive Filtration

In other cases, there may be no apparent conjunctival defect or wound leak, but overfiltration may occur as a result of loose scleral flap closure or an exceptionally large filtering bleb. It is in this regard that trabeculectomies offer a significant advantage over full-thickness filtering procedures, since the protective scleral flap reduces the likelihood of excessive filtration. However, with the advent of antimetabolite adjunctive therapy, there is a tendency for increased flow of aqueous around the scleral flap and through the conjunctival bleb, and overfiltration has become a more common early postoperative complication. Antimetabolites in and of themselves do not cause hypotony but allow it to persist by inhibiting the natural fibrotic response, thus reducing aqueous outflow resistance to a level insufficient to produce a more physiologic IOP. To minimize this risk, some surgeons choose to increase the protective aspect of a trabeculectomy by using multiple nylon sutures to create a tighter closure of the scleral flap. Sutures can be selectively cut postoperatively with a laser if filtration is inadequate. Other surgeons prefer to secure the scleral flap with releasable sutures, which can be removed postoperatively as needed (75–78,346).

If the early postoperative period is complicated by excessive filtration associated with a quiet bleb, a flat anterior chamber, and corneal decompensation, the first step is to decrease the frequency of postoperative topical corticosteroid administration. Firm patching of the eye with a bandage contact lens or

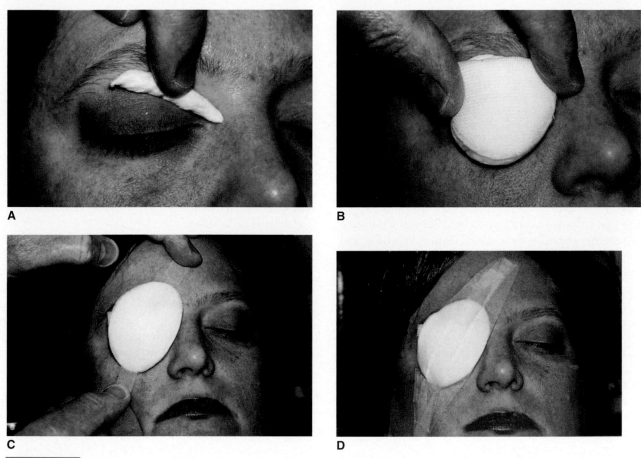

Figure 38.15 Pressure patch technique for eye with flat anterior chamber due to excessive filtration in early postoperative period. **A:** Fusiform-shaped cotton ball placed over upper lid in location corresponding to surgical fistula. **B:** Folded eye pad placed just below brow. **C:** Second, open eye pad positioned. **D:** Multiple strips of tape applied with moderate tension.

other tamponading device may be used. If the chamber depth cannot be maintained after several days, and especially if corneal decompensation is present, surgical intervention is usually indicated. It is generally necessary to deepen the anterior chamber with a viscoelastic substance. Air, perfluoropropane, and sulfur hexafluoride have also been used (347,348). However, the air and gases are more toxic than balanced salt solution or viscoelastics and can cause cataract formation (348–350). A study with rabbits, however, suggests that 15% perfluoropropane or 50% sulfur hexafluoride is no more toxic than air and may be beneficial and relatively safe in reforming persistently flat anterior chambers (350).

Serous Choroidal Detachments

Anterior chamber deepening alone may not be sufficient if large choroidal detachments are also present. Fluid commonly collects in the suprachoroidal space in hypotonus eyes. Hypotony is generally thought to contribute to the mechanism of choroidal detachments, although additional factors, such as inflammation and venous congestion, also appear to be important (351). The fluid in the detachments is high in protein (67% of plasma concentration), suggesting that a pressure differential causes fluid with small- and medium-sized protein molecules to pass from choroidal capillaries to extravascular spaces

(330,352). The choroidal detachment apparently prolongs the hypotony by reducing aqueous production and possibly by increasing uveoscleral outflow.

Most serous choroidal detachments resolve spontaneously when the IOP rises during the first few postoperative days or weeks. Typically, choroidal effusions resolve after IOP rises above 7 to 9 mm Hg. If limited in size and duration, they do not interfere with the long-term outcome of trabeculectomy surgery, and it is usually only necessary to drain them when they are associated with a persistent flat anterior chamber or when a choroidal hemorrhage is suspected. The technique involves draining the suprachoroidal fluid through one or more sclerotomies in the inferior quadrants and deepening the anterior chamber with a balanced salt solution or viscoelastic.

Much less commonly, a serous retinal detachment may occur after glaucoma filtering surgery, presumably by a mechanism similar to that for choroidal detachments (353). In most cases, these also resolve spontaneously, although the patient may not regain full preoperative visual acuity.

Hypotony and Deep Anterior Chamber

A lower-than-normal IOP in the first week or two after trabeculectomy usually does not constitute a complication, as long as there are no related problems, such as wound leak, excessive inflammation, flat anterior chamber, or posterior pole abnormality. If the hypotony persists, however, it can lead to one of the more serious complications, referred to as hypotony maculopathy. The typical fundus findings include fine macular striae radiating from the fovea, often with more extensive choroidal folds and tortuous retinal vessels and occasional disc swelling, but no evidence of vascular leakage. The visual acuity can be markedly reduced. The maculopathy does not develop in all patients with subnormal IOP; risk factors for this complication include young age, myopia, and the preoperative use of carbonic anhydrase inhibitors (354,355). The hypotony can occur with any filtering surgery technique, although the risk is increased with the use of adjunctive antimetabolites.

The best approach is prevention by minimizing the use of antimetabolites and using tight wound closure. When the complication does occur, it is difficult to treat. Standard measures, such as pressure patching or the application of trichloroacetic acid or cryotherapy to the bleb, are rarely effective, especially when antimetabolites have been used. Oversized bandage contact lenses have been helpful in the management of early hypotony (356). Some success has been reported with the injection of autologous blood into the bleb or around the bleb, or a combination of autologous blood injection and bleb compression sutures (**Fig. 38.16**) (357–365). However, some studies have not found the results of autologous blood injection to be favorable (366,367), and reported complications have included a markedly raised IOP, corneal blood staining, loss of vision, delayed hyphema, and intravitreal blood (368–372).

When these measures are not successful in managing hypotony maculopathy, surgical revision is indicated. Surgical approaches include conjunctival compression sutures, resuturing the scleral flap, and patch grafting with donor sclera or preserved pericardium (373–377). Another effective technique is to excise the filtering bleb, undermine adjacent conjunctiva, and pull it down to the limbus to create a new filtering bleb (179). More recently, an approach involving placement of transconjunctival sutures through the scleral flap has been described (378). It is unclear how long an eye can tolerate

hypotony maculopathy before the visual loss is irreversible, but return of good vision has been reported when the overfiltration was reversed within 6 months of the onset of the complication (375).

Elevated Intraocular Pressure and Flat Anterior Chamber

An elevated IOP with a flat anterior chamber in the early postoperative course suggests one of three mechanisms: (a) aqueous misdirection syndrome (also known as malignant [ciliary block] glaucoma), (b) an incomplete iridectomy with pupillary block, or (c) a delayed suprachoroidal hemorrhage. Although the diagnosis and management of these conditions are discussed in Chapter 26, here are a few additional details regarding the delayed hemorrhage.

Delayed Suprachoroidal Hemorrhages

Patients with delayed suprachoroidal hemorrhages after filtering surgery typically present during the first few postoperative days with severe pain, occasional nausea, and a marked reduction in vision. The IOP is usually elevated, the anterior chamber is shallow or flat, and large choroidal detachments, often with central apposition, are present. On the basis of retrospective studies, the complication is uncommon, occurrin in approximately 2% of most large series (379–383). However, in a prospective study involving ultrasonographic evaluation of 158 patients after filtering surgery, delayed suprachoroidal hemorrhage was detected in 11 patients (7%), suggesting that most cases go clinically unrecognized (384). One large retrospective study showed a slightly higher incidence (2.9%) of delayed suprachoroidal hemorrhages with all filtering procedures, but the relative incidence varied depending on the type of procedure (385). In one study, delayed suprachoroidal hemorrhage occurred in 1.5% of trabeculectomies without antimetabolite, 2.4% of trabeculectomies with antimetabolite, 2.8% of implantations of valved glaucoma drainage devices, and 7.1% of implantations of nonvalved glaucoma drainage devices (385). In addition, the incidence goes up considerably with certain risk factors, especially in the presence of aphakia

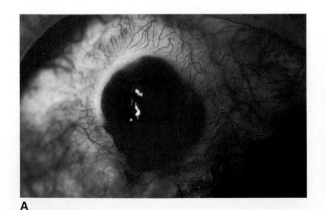

A

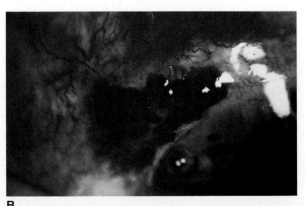

B

Figure 38.16 The injection of autologous blood to manage a leaking or overfiltering bleb. Blood is withdrawn from a vein in the patient's arm; after replacing the needle with a 30-in. gauge, the needle is passed beneath the conjunctiva, adjacent to the bleb, then into the bleb, and the bleb is filled with the blood, as shown in **A** and **B**. One complication of the procedure is the extension of the blood into the anterior chamber, which can be minimized by injecting viscoelastic into the anterior chamber.

or previous vitrectomy (379–382,384). In one series of 305 filtering procedures, the overall incidence of delayed suprachoroidal hemorrhage was 1.6%, but this rose to 13% in aphakic eyes and to 33% of aphakic, vitrectomized eyes (381).

High-frequency ultrasonography in eyes with suprachoroidal hemorrhage may show high reflectivity in the inner space of a choroidal detachment, with the ciliary processes and iris anteriorly displaced due to the ciliary detachment and forward pressure of the anterior vitreous (386). Not all cases require surgical correction, and in those that do, it is best to wait until the clotted blood has lysed. In one series monitored by echography, the mean time for clot lysis was 14 days, and the mean duration of central retinal apposition was 15 days (387). The visual outcome of patients with delayed suprachoroidal hemorrhages is poor and is worse with associated retinal detachment and 360-degree suprachoroidal hemorrhage (385). The latter findings constitute indications for surgical intervention, along with kissing choroidal detachments, vitreous incarceration, and vitreoretinal adhesions (388–390). Surgical intervention is usually limited to drainage of the hemorrhage through anterior sclerostomies, with vitrectomy reserved for vitreous incarceration or vitreoretinal adhesions (389,390). In most cases, drainage of choroidal blood must wait 7 to 10 days for the clot to liquify.

Delayed suprachoroidal hemorrhage after viscocanalostomy has also been reported, suggesting that the risk of suprachoroidal hemorrhage may not be completely eliminated even with nonpenetrating glaucoma procedures (391).

Elevated Intraocular Pressure and Deep Anterior Chamber

An elevated IOP with a deep anterior chamber indicates inadequate filtration, most often due to a tight scleral flap or obstruction of the fistula by iris, ciliary processes, lens, blood, or vitreous. A tight flap is treated by laser suture lysis. Creating an adequate fistula and iridectomy can prevent the most common causes of obstruction. When faced with a high pressure and deep anterior chamber, the possibility of obstruction of the fistula should first be evaluated by gonioscopy. If iris or ciliary processes are obstructing the fistula, it may be possible to retract the tissue with the application of low-energy argon laser therapy or by Nd:YAG laser disruption. If the internal obstruction cannot be eliminated with laser therapy, it is usually necessary to revise the filter.

When the fistula is thought to be obstructed by scar tissue along the margins of the scleral flap but a filtering bleb is still present, internal bleb revision may be useful. In the operating room, an incision is made through peripheral cornea 90 to 180 degrees from the fistula. Viscoelastic may be injected to maintain a deep anterior chamber. A cyclodialysis spatula is passed through the incision and into the fistula to elevate the scleral flap and break adhesions along the margins with a sweeping action of the spatula. 5-FU should probably be used postoperatively to reduce subsequent scarring of the fistula. If fistula obstruction is not found, attention must then be given to bleb failure, which (as discussed earlier) is the most common cause of failure in glaucoma filtering surgery (107). Distinction must be made between a failing bleb and an encapsulated bleb.

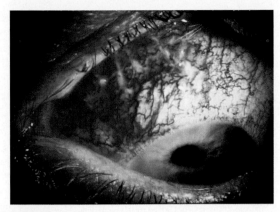

Figure 38.17 Typical appearance of a failing filtering bleb, characterized by a low-to-flat, heavily vascularized conjunctiva.

Management of the Failing Bleb

The filtering bleb in these cases is typically low to flat and heavily vascularized with no microcysts (**Fig. 38.17**). The risk for failure is high unless immediate, aggressive steps are taken. Corticosteroid therapy should be increased, typically consisting of prednisolone acetate, 1%, every 1 to 2 hours, occasionally with the addition of subconjunctival steroids. Scleral flap sutures should be lysed or removed in the case of releasable sutures. Tissue plasminogen activator may be injected subconjunctivally or in the anterior chamber when blood or fibrin is present in the aqueous outflow pathway (392,393). As previously noted, subconjunctival 5-FU may also be effective even if started several days after the surgery (150). Anti-VEGF therapy may prove to be beneficial but is investigational at the time of this publication.

Intermittent application of digital pressure can be used to expand the subconjunctival space by forcing aqueous into it. This may be performed by applying steady pressure with the index finger to the inferior sclera through the lower lid for approximately 15 seconds. Applying pressure with the index finger or a Q-tip through the upper lid behind the bleb, with the patient looking down, allows visualization of the bleb during the procedure. If the digital pressure lowers the tension and expands the bleb, certain reliable patients may be instructed to perform the digital pressure through the lower lid at home several times each day. A modification of digital pressure, after trabeculectomy, involves pressing an anesthetic-moistened applicator beside the edge of the scleral flap (394). If the IOP cannot be lowered by digital pressure, the next step is usually laser suture lysis or removal of a releasable suture (395–400). Laser suture lysis or removal, by acutely lowering the IOP, may be associated with complications common to glaucoma surgery, including hypotony, flat anterior chamber, external aqueous leak, malignant glaucoma, iris incarceration, and excessive filtering blebs (72,401). Most of these complications resolve with appropriate management (discussed previously) (72).

The argon laser is the most commonly used procedure for suture lysis, with typical settings of 50 μm, 0.1-second duration, and 250 to 1000 mW of power. Other lasers may also be effective, including krypton and diode, and a laser lens holder has been developed for performing diode laser suture lysis in children under anesthesia (397,402). Suture lysis is performed through the conjunctiva, which is compressed with a corner of a four-mirror goniolens or with a specially designed Hoskins lens or Ritch lens to improve visualization of scleral flap sutures. After one suture had been lysed, the status of the eye should be reassessed and IOP remeasured with and without digital pressure. If the bleb has reformed and the IOP has decreased, the patient can be examined the next day. If no effect is seen within 1 hour, a second suture lysis or removal may be considered. Longer time from surgery to laser suture lysis is associated with decreased IOP-lowering effect. In general, laser suture lysis is best performed within the first 3 weeks of surgery; beyond that time, responses are often inadequate.

If suture lysis or release is ineffective, or if a blood or fibrin clot appears to be obstructing the fistula, intracameral tissue plasminogen activator may be beneficial (392). The recommended intracameral dose is 6 to 12.5 µg. A subconjunctival dose of tissue plasminogen activator can be used to free a scleral flap closed by blood and fibrin in the early postoperative period (403).

When these measures fail, use of glaucoma drug should be resumed. Revision of a flat, vascularized bleb has a low chance of success but can be tried. In most cases, a repeated filtering procedure with adjunctive MMC or 5-FU or implantation of a glaucoma drainage device will eventually be required.

Encapsulated Filtering Bleb

These blebs, which have also been called Tenon capsule cysts and high bleb phase, are characterized by a highly elevated, smooth-domed bleb with large vessels but intervening avascular spaces and no microcysts (**Fig. 38.18**). It is typical to see a patent sclerostomy on gonioscopy. Movement of the conjunctiva reveals a second, stationary set of vessels beneath the conjunctiva, which is in the layer of fibrous tissue that lines the bleb. It is important to distinguish this type of bleb from the typical failing bleb, as previously discussed. Both are associated with an elevated IOP and deep anterior chamber in the early postoperative period, but the prognosis and management differ considerably.

Encapsulated blebs are common, occurring in 3.6% to 28% of eyes (404–409), typically developing within the first 2 months after the surgery. Long-term topical glaucoma therapy may be a risk factor for failure of trabeculectomy (119,120), and it has been associated with increased inflammation of the conjunctiva and Tenon capsule after filtering surgery (410). Reports are conflicting regarding the influence of argon laser trabeculoplasty (404,411,412). In the Advanced Glaucoma Intervention Study, encapsulated blebs were found in 18.5% of eyes after previously failed argon laser trabeculoplasty and in 14.5% of eyes without previous laser procedure, but the difference was not statistically significant (408). Higher frequencies of encapsulated bleb have been reported in males and in patients undergoing trabeculectomy alone versus trabeculectomy combined with cataract surgery (408,413,414). Adjunctive 5-FU may reduce the incidence of encapsulated blebs (415). Use of MMC was suggested to increase it, on the basis of a 29% incidence in one series (413), although other studies have not confirmed that finding (409,416). Encapsulation appears to develop more often (33% to 44%) in eyes with congenital and juvenile glaucoma (407).

In managing the encapsulated bleb, the physician should be aware that most begin functioning well within a few months (409). It is generally agreed that the mainstay of treatment is to resume the use of glaucoma medication until the improvement occurs (417). Opinions differ, however, on whether steroids and digital pressure should be used. One study suggested that prolonged steroid therapy may actually increase the incidence of encapsulated blebs (418), and digital pressure may further reduce aqueous flow through the encapsulated bleb by compressing the subconjunctival layer of tissue (406). Some surgeons prefer early needling (discussed later) of the encapsulated bleb. However, because this is more invasive and may be associated with severe complications, most surgeons believe that medical treatment with digital pressure should be used as the initial treatment in eyes with encapsulated blebs (419).

Blebs that do not respond to conservative medical management may be restored surgically. One such technique is called needling, in which a 25- to 30-gauge needle is passed beneath the conjunctiva about 5 to 10 mm from the bleb, is used to balloon up the conjunctiva, and is then passed into the bleb to puncture and incise the fibrous episcleral tissue (420). An effective modification is to inject 5 mg of 5-FU (0.5 cc of 10 mg/mL, or 0.1 cc of 50 mg/mL) subconjunctivally at the time of the needling (421–425), although higher doses should be avoided because they can cause corneal endothelial toxicity (426). Subconjunctival injection of MMC at the time of the needling has also been advocated (427–429). A more involved, but possibly more definitive, technique is to dissect the conjunctiva from the fibrous tissue, completely excise the latter, and resuture the conjunctiva (430).

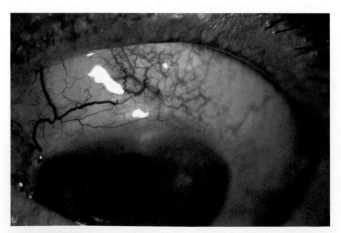

Figure 38.18 Typical appearance of an encapsulated bleb, characterized by an elevated, smooth-domed conjunctiva with large vessels but intervening avascular areas and no microcysts.

Other Early Postoperative Complications

Uveitis and Hyphema

Anterior uveitis is seen to some degree in the early postoperative period in all patients. It is routinely managed with topical corticosteroids and a mydriatic–cycloplegic. When the inflammation is excessive (3 + cell and flare, or fibrinoid iritis), increasing the frequency of steroid administration to every hour or two is usually sufficient; only rarely is stronger anti-inflammatory therapy required. Hyphema is less common and is usually managed conservatively, with elevation of the head and limited activity. The incidence of postoperative hyphema appears to be reduced by placing the sclerostomy anterior to scleral spur (431). Some surgeons place the sclerostomy in clear cornea anterior to the Schwalbe line, which essentially eliminates bleeding from the angle tissues, although iris bleeding from an iridectomy is still a risk.

Dellen

Dellen adjacent to large filtering blebs may occur in the early or late postoperative period. Most heal uneventfully with tear film replacements or bandage contact lens. Corneal ulcers can complicate dell formation if not adequately treated (432). Persistent dellen formation or discomfort from overhanging blebs may require surgical revision.

Loss of Central Vision

Loss of central vision ("snuff out" syndrome) may occur after glaucoma filtering surgery. Most studies have shown this to be uncommon (433–437). In one study, snuff out occurred in 4 of 508 eyes (0.8%) (436). Risk factors included older age, preoperative macular splitting in the visual field, and hypotony. Although a small central island or split fixation is not considered to be a contraindication to glaucoma filtering surgery (433–437), these patients appear to be at greater risk of losing central vision postoperatively (438). The patient should be informed of the risk, and efforts should be made to minimize postoperative extremes in IOP.

Ocular Decompression Retinopathy

Ocular decompression retinopathy is a term that was used to describe eyes of patients who developed intraretinal hemorrhages immediately after trabeculectomies (439–444). An especially high preoperative IOP with sudden decompression and alteration in the configuration of the lamina cribrosa may lead to retinal vein obstruction and cause this complication. This may occur more commonly in children.

Late Postoperative Complications

Late Failure of Filtration

The most common late complication of any filtering procedure is eventual failure to maintain a low IOP. This may develop within months to years after an initially successful operation. It is hard to predict on the basis of the appearance of the bleb which eyes will ultimately experience failure, although

persistent inflammation, along with preoperative and postoperative factors that predispose to an inflammatory response, appears to play an important role.

The mechanism of late bleb failure may be closure of the fistula, although it is more commonly related to fibrosis of the scleral flap or scarring of the conjunctival portion of the bleb. A histopathologic study of failed blebs revealed a marked inflammatory response, abundant fibroblasts, and deposition of new collagen in the first few months after surgery (445). In eyes with failure in the later postoperative period, a hypocellular capsule of fibrous tissue lined by a thick layer of fibrin was seen beneath relatively normal conjunctiva and Tenon capsule.

These cases rarely respond to digital pressure or pharmacologic agents to suppress inflammation or fibrosis. When the pressure cannot be controlled medically and the bleb appears to be encapsulated, it may be possible to revise the bleb surgically by using the techniques described earlier.

When clinical evaluation suggests that the procedure has failed because of closure of the fistula by membranous tissue, it may be possible to re-establish patency by incising the tissue with a knife or needle through an ab externo or ab interno approach. It may also be possible to remove the obstructing element with laser surgery. Argon laser treatment has been reported to be effective for this purpose when the membrane is pigmented (446,447), while pulsed Nd:YAG lasers have been used successfully to eliminate nonpigmented tissue from the fistula or to loosen or penetrate the scleral flap through the fistula (448–452). These techniques, however, are usually only successful in eyes with previously well-established filtering blebs, in which failure has occurred abruptly and the bleb is still moderately elevated.

When the aforementioned measures are ineffective in re-establishing a failed filtering procedure, it is usually necessary to revise the bleb with incisional surgery, to repeat the operation in the other superior quadrant with use of adjunctive MMC or 5-FU, or to consider performing glaucoma drainage-device surgery. Revision is usually more successful when dealing with encapsulated blebs rather than those that are flat and scarred down to underlying episclera (453).

A Leaking Filtering Bleb

A bleb wall that has become too thin may rupture, leading to loss of the anterior chamber and possible endophthalmitis (**Fig. 38.19**). Blebs with a large avascular area are at increased risk for leaks (454). Severe coughing, for example, is a potential cause of late posttrabeculectomy bleb leaks (455). Small, focal cystic blebs under tension are also thought to be at increased risk for leaks.

Bleb leaks seem to occur more often after full-thickness procedures or when antimetabolites are used (456). Transconjunctival oozing and point leak at least 3 months after trabeculectomy with use of 5-FU or MMC occurred in 11.9% and 2.0%, respectively, in one series (457). Oozing was significantly more common after use of 5-FU than MMC, and point leak was associated with a larger avascular area. The defects are usually small, and the Seidel test is often helpful in confirming the

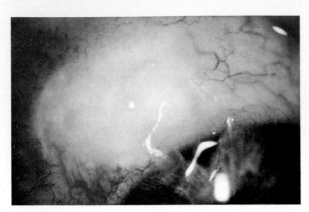

Figure 38.19 Leaking of a filtering bleb, associated with a shallow to flat anterior chamber and low IOP. This slitlamp photograph shows an eye with an avascular, thin-walled filtering bleb, which was found to be leaking near the limbus.

leak (**Fig. 38.20**). If the leak is small, aqueous suppressants and observation alone may be sufficient. In some cases, the defect will close beneath a soft bandage contact lens (458), which can be left in place for a few weeks. Coverage with a topical antibiotic is advisable during the course of treatment for bleb leaks.

Some leaks can be sealed with cyanoacrylate glue (341) or autologous fibrin glue (459). When these measures fail, surgical revision of the leaking bleb may be required (460). Results of a retrospective analysis of patients with late bleb leaks suggest that bleb revision is associated with more successful outcomes and less serious intraocular infections than in those managed more conservatively (461). Bleb revision techniques include resection of the bleb and creation of a new conjunctival flap posterior to the defect or a rotational conjunctival flap to cover the defect (461,462). When there is insufficient conjunctiva for a flap, autologous conjunctival grafts can be obtained from the fornix and placed over existing de-epithelialized leaking blebs (463).

A retrospective analysis of various surgical techniques for bleb revision demonstrated a high success rate with few postoperative complications, and it was suggested that choosing different techniques for specific clinical situations may enhance the success of surgical bleb revision (464). Histologic examination of 10 leaking filtering blebs revealed an epithelial tract running from the surface of the bleb to the episclera in eight cases, and it was suggested that the bleb should be excised before bringing down the new flap to prevent epithelial downgrowth (465). Autologous Tenon and partial-thickness scleral patch grafts have been found adequate, safe, and effective for closing excessively draining fistulas (466). Bleb excision and repair of the scleral defect with a full-thickness scleral graft, followed by coverage with the advancement of a conjunctival flap or by a free conjunctival autograft, have also been useful for the treatment of leaks in association with full-thickness scleral defects (467).

Amniotic membrane transplantation has been considered as a substitute for conjunctiva in the revision of glaucoma filtration blebs (468–470). Although a prospective, randomized clinical trial failed to support the value of amniotic membrane transplantation (471), the simplicity of the technique may make it useful in certain clinical situations (472).

Bleb-Related Infections

Infection after glaucoma filtering surgery is rare in the early postoperative period but tends to occur months or years after the surgery. It typically begins as a bleb infection (blebitis), in which the bleb is white and surrounded by intense conjunctival injection (**Fig. 38.21**). There are usually variable degrees of anterior chamber reaction, but the vitreous is clear (473). Bleb-related endophthalmitis is characterized by the addition of vitreous involvement. The two forms of bleb-related infection are clinically distinct, with different presentations, prognoses, and outcomes. Although blebitis is considered a limited form of bleb-related infection in which inflammation is limited to the bleb and the surrounding conjunctiva, with or without cells in the anterior chamber, bleb-related endophthalmitis is the virulent form of bleb-related infection with rapidly worsening vision, redness, and pain with diffuse conjunctival injection. When associated with endophthalmitis, blebs usually have a white "milky" appearance, with or without epithelial defects; fibrin or hypopyon is usually seen in the anterior chamber; and vitritis is present (**Fig. 38.22**) (474,475).

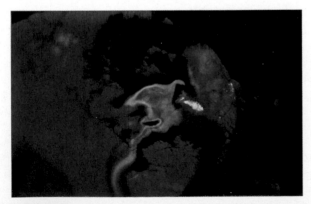

Figure 38.20 Leakage from the filtering bleb can be clearly documented by using the Seidel test: Fluorescein is applied to the area in question and observed at the slitlamp with a cobalt blue light; leaking aqueous will be seen as bright yellow fluid flowing from the leaking site.

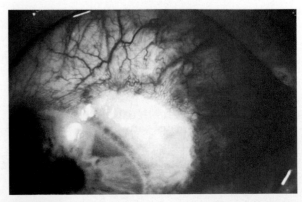

Figure 38.21 Slitlamp view of an eye with early bleb infection (blebitis), with characteristic intense conjunctival injection around a whitish bleb.

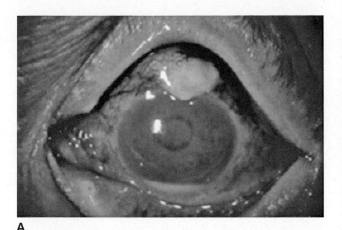
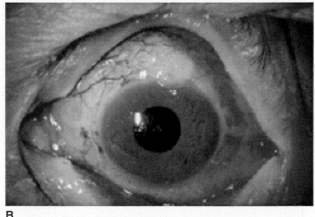

A   **B**

Figure 38.22 Bleb-associated endophthalmitis occurring 2 years after glaucoma filtering surgery. **A:** Marked purulence of the bleb, hypopyon, and fibrin in the pupil. Visual acuity was reduced to hand motion. The patient was treated with a vitreous tap and injected with intravitreal antibiotics. **B:** Coagulase-negative staphylococcus was isolated from the vitreous. Final visual acuity was 20/400 because advanced glaucomatous disease limited visual recovery. (From Scott IU, Flynn HW Jr., Han DP. Endophthalmitis: categories, management and prevention. In: Tasman W, Jaeger EA, eds. *Duane's Clinical Ophthalmology*. Vol 6. Philadelphia:Lippincott, Williams & Wilkins;chap 64.)

Blebitis

Incidence

A record review has found that the incidence of delayed-onset, bleb-related infection after trabeculectomy with antiproliferative treatment is similar to that after trabeculectomy without antimetabolites: 1.1% to 1.3% (476). Bleb-related infection was reported to develop an average of 3.1 years after trabeculectomy (476).

Risk Factors

Early, chronic, intermittent bleb leaks are risk factors for the bleb-related infection (477). Increased axial length, conjunctivitis, upper respiratory infection, winter season (477), intraoperative use of MMC, and antibiotic use after the postoperative period have also been associated with an increased risk for bleb-related infection (478).

Treatment

Blebitis usually responds well to intensive topical antibiotic treatment, returning visual acuity and IOP to preinfection levels (474,479). Most patients with blebitis are treated as outpatients. With prompt, aggressive therapy at this stage, the prognosis for visual recovery is much better than for fulminant endophthalmitis. Prophylactic antibiotic use is not recommended for patients with filtering surgery. A survey of American Glaucoma Society members, published in 2001, has shown that methods of the managing blebitis continue to differ among specialists. More than two thirds do not ask their patients to keep topical antibiotics in their homes for early symptoms of blebitis but prefer to examine a patient with symptoms of blebitis within 1 hour of an onset of symptoms, or as soon as possible. Most glaucoma specialists prescribe a topical fluoroquinolone, alone or in combination with one or two other antibiotics, as the initial empirical treatment of isolated blebitis. Twenty-one percent choose a combination of fortified topical

agents, usually including a fortified aminoglycoside, vancomycin, or cephalosporin. Only a minority of patients use an oral antibiotic in cases of blebitis, and approximately two thirds use topical corticosteroids in conjunction with antibiotic treatment. Most glaucoma specialists perform surgical bleb revision in eyes with a persistently leaking bleb (480). Oral fluoroquinolones have good vitreous penetration and may be considered in the treatment of blebitis or endophthalmitis (481).

Prognosis

With aggressive treatment, blebitis has much better prognosis for visual recovery than endophthalmitis does (473). In one retrospective study, the majority of patients who developed blebitis retained their preinfection visual acuity (475).

Bleb-Related Endophthalmitis

Bleb-related endophthalmitis is usually associated with a thin-walled filtering bleb. Bleb-related endophthalmitis is a virulent form of bleb-related infection with a poor visual prognosis despite aggressive immediate treatment with topical, systemic, and intravitreal antibiotic administration combined with core vitrectomy (474).

Early Postoperative Endophthalmitis

Differentiation of early (approximately first 3 months) versus late endophthalmitis is based not only on the time of onset but also on the pathogenesis. A retrospective analysis of 1100 consecutive trabeculectomies revealed an incidence of fewer than 0.1% for early and 0.2% for late endophthalmitis (482). The 7- to 10-year incidence of early endophthalmitis has been reported to be 0.05% to 0.09% for overall intraocular surgery, with higher rates of 0.12% to 0.2% for glaucoma procedures and 0.11% for combined cataract and glaucoma surgery. However, visual acuity outcomes were better with glaucoma surgery than with other types of surgery (483,484). Another retrospective analysis from a large referral eye center showed that, in early endophthalmitis, *Staphylococcus epidermidis* was isolated from vitreous culture in 4 of 6 cases, whereas in late endophthalmitis, this organism was isolated in only 1 of 27 cases (479).

Incidence

The incidence of endophthalmitis in one study was the same with thermal sclerostomy and trabeculectomy (485). In a retrospective review of primary trabeculectomy with MMC and laser suture lysis, bleb leak occurred in 14.6% of eyes, blebitis occurred in 5.7% of eyes, and endophthalmitis occurred in 0.8% of eyes during 1 to 3 years of follow-up (486). The incidence of endophthalmitis per year was 1.3% after trabeculectomy with MMC in another retrospective review. The 5-year probability of developing a bleb leak, blebitis, or endophthalmitis was 17.9%, 6.3%, and 7.5%, respectively. An isolated bleb leak seems to be a relatively benign condition, in that three fourths resolved with office-based methods (487). In a retrospective analysis of trabeculectomy performed with adjunctive use of MMC, 2.1% of patients developed bleb-associated endophthalmitis, an average of 18 months after the surgery. The incidence of bleb-related endophthalmitis was significantly greater after inferior trabeculectomy than after superior trabeculectomy. The cumulative incidence was 13% for inferior limbal blebs and 1.6% for superior limbal blebs. *Streptococcus sanguis* and *Haemophilus influenzae* were the most frequently found organisms. The incidence of bleb-related endophthalmitis is higher with adjunctive antimetabolites than the reported rate in eyes undergoing filtering surgery without the use of antifibrotic agents (0.2% to 1.5%) (488). In a retrospective review of trabeculectomies with adjunctive use of MMC, the overall incidence of bleb-related endophthalmitis was 2.6% (489).

Risk Factors

The increased use of adjunctive antimetabolites in trabeculectomy has caused an increased concern about the risk of bleb-related endophthalmitis (490), although reports show that use of antifibrotic agents is not always associated with an increased risk of bleb-related endophthalmitis (476,491). Other risk factors for bleb-related infections include an inferior or nasally located bleb, presence of a high bleb or blepharitis, development of a late-onset bleb leak, diabetes mellitus (492), chronic antibiotic use, and performance of a trabeculectomy alone versus a combined procedure. Glaucoma procedures that provide the lowest IOP are often those that predispose to bleb-related infections (493). Contact lens use may increase the risk of bleb-associated infection (478). The risk of endophthalmitis in eyes with filtering blebs makes it imperative that any evidence of external infection, such as conjunctivitis, be treated aggressively.

Causative Organisms

The most common causative organisms of delayed-onset bleb-associated endophthalmitis are *Streptococcus* and *Staphylococcus* species and *H. influenzae* (488,494–499). Staphylococcal species may be associated with better visual outcomes (499). The infection may rapidly progress over a few days (496), and despite successful treatment of the infection, visual outcomes

are generally poor (495). *Moraxella* species, *Acremonium filamentous* fungi, *Neisseria meningitidis*, *Pseudomonas aeruginosa*, and *Aspergillus niger* have been reported as causes of delayed-onset endophthalmitis in patients with filtering blebs (500–510).

Clinicopathologic Features

Common pathologic features of the eyes enucleated for endophthalmitis include inflammation involving the anterior segment, lens, and choroid, with one eye showing evidence of focal granulomatous uveitis (496). In one case-control study, eyes with endophthalmitis had hypopyon, cells in the anterior vitreous cavity, or a positive vitreous biopsy sampling result. The risk of endophthalmitis is increased if vitrectomy is performed in conjunction with glaucoma surgery (511). In a significant number of patients, prodromal signs or symptoms were documented by ophthalmologists days or weeks before the blebitis or endophthalmitis was diagnosed (475).

Treatment

As noted previously, most of these cases are caused by virulent organisms, such as gram-negative rods and streptococci, which require prompt, aggressive management (512). When vitreous involvement is present or suspected, a recommended approach is to establish the diagnosis with aqueous and vitreous aspirates and then to begin treatment with high-dose, broad-spectrum parenteral and periocular antibiotics, such as gentamicin and cefazolin, and intravitreal antibiotics, such as vancomycin and gentamicin—with adjustment of the treatment, if necessary, according to culture and sensitivity results (512–515). In the Endophthalmitis Vitrectomy Study, which involved endophthalmitis after cataract surgery or secondary intraocular lens implantation, a vitrectomy (rather than a vitreous tap or biopsy) was beneficial only in eyes with initial light perception vision, and the use of systemic antibiotics had no benefit (516). Corticosteroid therapy should also be used after antibiotic therapy has been established. However, the results of the Endophthalmitis Vitrectomy Study cannot be simply projected to the posttrabeculectomy endophthalmitis because of the difference in pathogenesis and spectrum of organisms (479).

Prognosis

Despite successful treatment of the infection, visual outcomes are generally poor (495). Patients in whom endophthalmitis develops after trabeculectomy do poorly, even with aggressive medical and surgical intervention.

Cataracts

Patients undergoing glaucoma surgery are at increased risk for the development and progression of cataracts, which are reported to occur in approximately one third of eyes after filtering surgery (433,517). The mechanism of this complication is uncertain, but possible factors include (a) patient's age, (b) duration of miotic therapy, (c) surgical manipulation, (d) postoperative iritis, (e) prolonged flat anterior chamber, and (f) nutritional changes (517–519).

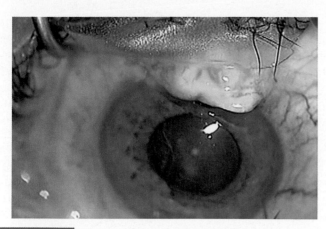

Figure 38.23 Excessive filtering bleb extending over cornea as a late complication of glaucoma filtering surgery.

In the Advanced Glaucoma Intervention Study, a trabeculectomy increased the risk for cataract development by 78%, compared with those who did not have a trabeculectomy. The risk decreased to 47% when the glaucoma surgery was uncomplicated, and it approximately doubled with complications, such as marked inflammation and a flat anterior chamber (520). In the Collaborative Interventional Glaucoma Study, cataract extraction was required more often (521).

Overhanging Filtering Blebs

In some cases, a large bleb may gradually extend down over the cornea, possibly because of the effect of eyelid movements (**Fig. 38.23**). These blebs can be bothersome to the patient, especially when overhanging the cornea. In some cases, these can be reduced by applying argon laser energy to the bleb (522), whereas others require incisional surgical correction by lifting the bleb from the cornea with an iris spatula, excising it near the limbus, and suturing the free edges (523). Excision of the excessive bleb near the limbus does not lead to a bleb leak and generally does not require suturing (524,525). Bleb window cryopexy has also been reported to be an effective treatment for selected patients with large, symptomatic, overhanging blebs (526).

Spontaneous Hyphema

Spontaneous hyphema may occur weeks to years after filtering surgery (527). The bleeding may come from one of the cut ends of Schlemm canal or from abnormal vessels near the internal portion of the fistula (528,529). Argon laser photocoagulation can be effective if the source of bleeding can be visualized.

Hypotony and Ciliochoroidal Detachment

Hypotony and ciliochoroidal detachment may occur at any time after a filtering procedure. Some may be chronic and recurrent, and inflammation is frequently present (530,531). Other apparent risk factors include drugs that can incite ocular inflammation and aqueous suppressants (530,532). Management in these cases involves discontinuing use of the responsible drugs and initiating aggressive anti-inflammatory therapy. Cataracts are common with this condition, and cataract extraction may be associated with resolution of the choroidal detachments (530). Tearing of the retinal pigment epithelium can be a sequela of hypotony and choroidal or serous retinal detachment after glaucoma surgery (533).

Corneal Changes

Patients with glaucoma appear to have a decreased corneal endothelial cell count, particularly when exfoliation is present or when patients are taking three or more glaucoma medications (534,535). Corneal endothelial cell count has been shown to be further reduced after glaucoma filtering surgery, which is influenced by early postoperative iridocorneal touch but not by the use of adjunctive MMC (536,537). However, severe endothelial damage after trabeculectomy with MMC was reported in two eyes with pre-existing cornea guttata (538). The trabeculectomy procedure can also alter corneal topography, although it may be undetectable without topographic analysis and usually does not persist (539,540). Limbal stem cell deficiency can also occur in patients receiving 5-FU after trabeculectomy, which can be treated with amniotic membrane transplantation. However, for total limbal stem cell deficiency, limbal transplantation has been suggested as an alternative to restore the corneal surface (541).

Eyelid Changes

Upper eyelid retraction after glaucoma filtering surgery was described in two patients and was thought to result from the adrenergic effect of aqueous humor on Müller muscle (542). Ptosis has also been reported after trabeculectomy in 6% to 12% of patients and was not significantly affected by combined cataract surgery, type of conjunctival flap, or previous ocular surgery (543). Ptosis may be related to surgical trauma to the levator muscle and adjacent tissue.

Sympathetic Ophthalmia

Sympathetic ophthalmia after glaucoma surgery is a rare complication. Studies suggest that this is unrelated to the type of operation, but rather to the preoperative condition of the eye, in that it occurs more commonly when operating on a blind, painful eye or after a uveal trauma (544,545).

OUTCOMES OF FILTERING PROCEDURES

Trabeculectomy versus Full-Thickness Procedures

As previously noted, most surgeons prefer some form of trabeculectomy rather than a full-thickness procedure. Studies that have specifically compared trabeculectomies and full-thickness operations have shown both types of procedures to have similar glaucoma control (546,547). Some surveys suggested slightly better IOP control with full-thickness procedures (67,548–552), although these studies were done before the advent of adjunctive antimetabolite therapy. In general, the IOP results were similar to those that had been previously described for various full-thickness procedures, with variable reductions in the incidence of complications (553–558).

Long-Term Outcomes with Trabeculectomy

Several studies in the late 1970s and 1980s reported outcomes after various forms of trabeculectomy. More recent studies, with up to 12 years of follow-up, have shown a gradual decline in the probability of successful IOP control over time, although the actual numbers vary considerably (559–561). In one study of 75 patients followed up for 6 to 12 years, IOP control of 21 mm Hg or less was achieved in 90% at 5 years and the final visit (559), whereas in another study of 43 eyes with COAG, 67% maintained an IOP below 21 mm Hg during a 7- to 10-year follow-up (560). Yet a third study, in which success was defined as an IOP of 20 mm Hg or less and a minimum reduction of 20%, revealed a probability of success after a single operation of 48% and 40% at 3 and 5 years, respectively (561). Of greater significance are visual field outcomes. One study of 54 patients revealed further loss of visual field in 28% during the first 5 years (562), whereas another study of 239 patients followed up for up to 10 years revealed progressive glaucomatous damage in 25%, 30%, 43%, and 58% at 1, 2, 5, and 10 years, respectively (563). Consistent with previous reports, the reported incidence of cataract formation ranged from 22% to 78% (520,559–561). For uncertain reasons, when primary trabeculectomies were performed in both eyes of patients, encapsulated blebs and hypotony occurred slightly more frequently in the second operated eye, despite a similar clinical course (564).

Trabeculectomy versus Nonpenetrating Procedures

Nonpenetrating procedures may reduce the complication rate, but they do not typically achieve IOPs as low as trabeculectomy does. In a randomized trial comparing viscocanalostomy and trabeculectomy without intraoperative use of antimetabolites, trabeculectomy provided only slightly better IOP control after 2 years (320). Other studies have also found that trabeculectomy is more effective than viscocanalostomy in reducing the IOP, whereas viscocanalostomy has a lower incidence of complications (565–567). Trabeculectomy also decreases the IOP more than the nonpenetrating deep sclerectomy technique does, although the complication rate again seems to be lower with the latter procedure (568). Deep sclerectomy may be combined with phacoemulsification (569), achieving an IOP reduction similar to that achieved with phacoemulsification combined with trabeculectomy, but with lower complication rates (570).

Deep sclerectomy with collagen implantation provided pressure results similar to those with trabeculectomy but with a lower rate of early postoperative complications (571,572). One study has shown that when a deep sclerectomy is complicated by perforation of the trabeculo-Descemet membrane, the long-term success rate is similar to that of trabeculectomy, but the likelihood of immediate postoperative complications, such as hypotony and hyphema, is increased (573).

Outcomes in High-Risk Populations

For most filtering procedures, glaucoma control is generally thought to be poorer among black patients than white patients, although this has not been substantiated in all studies. With trabeculectomies, success rates in black patients have mostly been in the same range as those for white patients (574–578), although in some series standard trabeculectomies were successful in fewer than 75% of black patients (82,579,580). The difference in outcome, if it truly exists, may be explained by an increase in macrophages and fibroblasts and a decrease in mast cells and goblet cells in the conjunctiva at the time of filtering surgery, compared with white patients (580). Some surgeons have noted improved pressure control in black patients when the trabeculectomy technique is modified to enhance filtration around the scleral flap (82,581). Comparative studies of trabeculectomies and full-thickness filtering procedures in black populations have given conflicting results (552,582–584).

Children, when compared with adults, generally have worse outcomes with filtering procedures (585), including trabeculectomies (586–588). In one study, trabeculectomy was no better than other procedures for advanced pediatric glaucomas (589), although the results are probably different with the addition of adjunctive antimetabolite therapy. Patients aged 15 to 40 years have outcomes similar to those in older patients (590), unless additional risk factors are present (591). A retrospective analysis of primary trabeculectomy has shown that primary infantile glaucoma had a better outcome than secondary developmental glaucoma, and that the visual outcome depends on early and sustained control of IOP and aggressive treatment of the amblyopia (592).

In patients with glaucoma after congenital cataract surgery, trabeculectomy controlled IOP in only slightly more than one third of aphakic eyes after 3 years, regardless of MMC use (103). A retrospective review revealed that with trabeculectomies in children with aphakia, aniridia, anterior segment dysgenesis, and other secondary glaucomas, IOP control and stabilization of visual acuity and optic disc appearance were achieved in 51% of eyes (593).

Aphakia is another factor that adversely affects all types of filtering procedures, including trabeculectomies (594,595). Patients with advanced COAG also have a worse outcome than the general glaucoma population, with approximately one third requiring a second operation within 3 years (596). In all these types of high-risk cases, however, the use of adjunctive antimetabolite therapy appears to generally improve the surgical outcome.

KEY POINTS

- Glaucoma filtering procedures lower the IOP by creating a limbal fistula through which aqueous humor drains into a subconjunctival space and subsequently filters through the conjunctiva to the tear film or is absorbed by surrounding tissues.
- The standard filtering techniques use common principles regarding preparation of the conjunctival flap and the iridectomy. They differ primarily according to the method of creating the fistula, with the earlier procedures using a full-thickness fistula and the technique most commonly used today incorporating a guarded fistula beneath a partial-thickness scleral flap (trabeculectomy).

- Considerable attention has been given to the pharmacologic modulation of wound healing to minimize bleb failure.
- Complications may be encountered during filtering operations (e.g., tearing the conjunctival flap, hemorrhage, and choroidal effusion) and in the early postoperative period (e.g., hypotony, pressure elevation, uveitis, and hemorrhage) or late postoperative course (e.g., bleb failure, bleb leak, endophthalmitis, and cataracts).

REFERENCES

1. Picht G, Grehn F. Classification of filtering blebs in trabeculectomy: biomicroscopy and functionality. *Curr Opin Ophthalmol.* 1998;9(2):2–8.
2. Cantor LB, Mantravadi A, WuDunn D, et al. Morphologic classification of filtering blebs after glaucoma filtration surgery: the Indiana Bleb Appearance Grading Scale. *J Glaucoma.* 2003;12(3):266–271.
3. Addicks EM, Quigley HA, Green WR, et al. Histologic characteristics of filtering blebs in glaucomatous eyes. *Arch Ophthalmol.* 1983;101(5): 795–798.
4. Hutchinson AK, Grossniklaus HE, Brown RH, et al. Clinicopathologic features of excised mitomycin filtering blebs. *Arch Ophthalmol.* 1994;112(1):74–79.
5. Kim JW. Conjunctival impression cytology of the filtering bleb. *Korean J Ophthalmol.* 1997;11(1):25–31.
6. Benedikt O. The effect of filtering operations [in German]. *Klin Monatsbl Augenheilkd.* 1977;170(1):10–19.
7. Powers TP, Stewart WC, Stroman GA. Ultrastructural features of filtration blebs with different clinical appearances. *Ophthalmic Surg Lasers.* 1996;27(9):790–794.
8. Kronfeld FC. The chemical demonstration of transconjunctival passage of aqueous after antiglaucomatous operations. *Am J Ophthalmol.* 1952;35(5:2):38–45.
9. Galin MA, Baras I, McLean JM. How does a filtering bleb work? *Trans Am Acad Ophthalmol Otolaryngol.* 1965;69(6):1082–1091.
10. Teng CC, Chi HH, Katzin HM. Histology and mechanism of filtering operations. *Am J Ophthalmol.* 1959;47(1, pt 1):16–33.
11. Jinza K, Saika S, Kin K, et al. Relationship between formation of a filtering bleb and an intrascleral aqueous drainage route after trabeculectomy: evaluation using ultrasound biomicroscopy. *Ophthalmic Res.* 2000; 32(5):240–243.
12. Avitabile T, Russo V, Uva MG, et al. Ultrasound-biomicroscopic evaluation of filtering blebs after laser suture lysis trabeculectomy. *Ophthalmologica.* 1998;212(suppl 1):17–21.
13. Hill RA. Tenon's traction sutures: an aid for trabeculectomy and aqueous drainage device implantation. *J Glaucoma.* 2002;11(6):529–530.
14. Vesti E, Raitta C. Trabeculectomy at the inferior limbus. *Acta Ophthalmol.* 1992;70(2):220–224.
15. Caronia RM, Liebmann JM, Friedman R, et al. Trabeculectomy at the inferior limbus. *Arch Ophthalmol.* 1996;114(4):387–391.
16. Luntz MH. Trabeculectomy using a fornix-based conjunctival flap and tightly sutured scleral flap. *Ophthalmology.* 1980;87(10):985–989.
17. Brincker P, Kessing SV. Limbus-based versus fornix-based conjunctival flap in glaucoma filtering surgery. *Acta Ophthalmol.* 1992;70(5):641–644.
18. Faggioni R. Trabeculectomy with conjunctival flap in the fornix: 12 months' follow-up [in German]. *Klin Monatsbl Augenheilkd.* 1983; 182(5):385–386.
19. Kozobolis VP, Siganos CS, Christodoulakis EV, et al. Two-site phacotrabeculectomy with intraoperative mitomycin-C: fornix- versus limbus-based conjunctival opening in fellow eyes. *J Cataract Refract Surg.* 2002; 28(10):1758–1762.
20. Shingleton BJ, Chaudhry IM, O'Donoghue MW, et al. Phacotrabeculectomy: limbus-based versus fornix-based conjunctival flaps in fellow eyes. *Ophthalmology.* 1999;106(6):1152–1155.
21. Tezel G, Kolker AE, Kass MA, et al. Comparative results of combined procedures for glaucoma and cataract: II. Limbus-based versus fornix-based conjunctival flaps. *Ophthalmic Surg Lasers.* 1997;28(7):551–557.
22. Berestka JS, Brown SV. Limbus- versus fornix-based conjunctival flaps in combined phacoemulsification and mitomycin C trabeculectomy surgery. *Ophthalmology.* 1997;104(2):187–196.
23. Lemon LC, Shin DH, Kim C, et al. Limbus-based vs fornix-based conjunctival flap in combined glaucoma and cataract surgery with adjunctive mitomycin C. *Am J Ophthalmol.* 1998;125(3):340–345.
24. el Sayyad F, el-Rashood A, Helal M, et al. Fornix-based versus limbus-based conjunctival flaps in initial trabeculectomy with postoperative 5-fluorouracil: four-year follow-up findings. *J Glaucoma.* 1999;8(2):124–128.
25. Auw-Haedrich C, Funk J, Boemer TG. Long-term results after filtering surgery with limbus-based and fornix-based conjunctival flaps. *Ophthalmic Surg Lasers.* 1998;29(7):575–580.
26. Shuster JN, Krupin T, Kolker AE, et al. Limbus- v fornix-based conjunctival flap in trabeculectomy. A long-term randomized study. *Arch Ophthalmol.* 1984;102(3):361–362.
27. Traverso CE, Tomey KF, Antonios S. Limbal- vs fornix-based conjunctival trabeculectomy flaps. *Am J Ophthalmol.* 1987;104(1):28–32.
28. Grehn F, Mauthe S, Pfeiffer N. Limbus-based versus Fornix-based conjunctival flap in filtering surgery. A randomized prospective study. *Int Ophthalmol.* 1989;13(1–2):139–143.
29. Reichert R, Stewart W, Shields MB. Limbus-based versus fornix-based conjunctival flaps in trabeculectomy. *Ophthalmic Surg.* 1987;18(9): 672–676.
30. Agbeja AM, Dutton GN. Conjunctival incisions for trabeculectomy and their relationship to the type of bleb formation—a preliminary study. *Eye.* 1987;1(6):738–743.
31. Miller KN, Blasini M, Shields MB, et al. A comparison of total and partial tenonectomy with trabeculectomy. *Am J Ophthalmol.* 1991;111(3):323–326.
32. Kapetansky FM. Trabeculectomy, or trabeculectomy plus tenectomy: a comparative study. *Glaucoma.* 1980;2:451–453.
33. Zigiotti GL, Savini G, De Caro R, et al. The features of Tenon's capsule at the limbus. *Ital J Anat Embryol.* 1997;102(1):5–11.
34. Lerner SF. Small incision trabeculectomy avoiding Tenon's capsule. A new procedure for glaucoma surgery. *Ophthalmology.* 1997;104(8): 1237–1241.
35. Das JC, Sharma P, Chaudhuri Z, et al. Small incision trabeculectomy: experiences with this new procedure for glaucoma surgery in Indian eyes. *Acta Ophthalmol Scand.* 2001;79(4):394–398.
36. Ophir A. Mini-trabeculectomy without radial incisions. *Am J Ophthalmol.* 1999;127(2):212–213.
37. Hung SO. Role of sodium hyaluronate (Healonid) in triangular flap trabeculectomy. *Br J Ophthalmol.* 1985;69(1):46–50.
38. Teekhasaenee C, Ritch R. The use of PhEA 34c in trabeculectomy. *Ophthalmology.* 1986;93(4):487–491.
39. Vesti E, Raitta C. A review of the outcome of trabeculectomy in open-angle glaucoma. *Ophthalmic Surg Lasers.* 1997;28(2):128–132.
40. Wand M. Viscoelastic agent and the prevention of post-filtration flat anterior chamber. *Ophthalmic Surg.* 1988;19(7):523–524.
41. Wand M. Intraoperative intracameral viscoelastic agent in the prevention of postfiltration flat anterior chamber. *J Glaucoma.* 1994;3(2):101–105.
42. Raitta C, Vesti E. The effect of sodium hyaluronate on the outcome of trabeculectomy. *Ophthalmic Surg.* 1991;22(3):145–149.
43. Raitta C, Lehto I, Puska P, et al. A randomized, prospective study on the use of sodium hyaluronate (Healon) in trabeculectomy. *Ophthalmic Surg.* 1994;25(8):536–539.
44. Barak A, Alhalel A, Kotas R, et al. The protective effect of early intraoperative injection of viscoelastic material in trabeculectomy. *Ophthalmic Surg.* 1992;23(3):206–209.
45. Osher RH, Cionni RJ, Cohen JS. Re-forming the flat anterior chamber with Healon. *J Cataract Refract Surg.* 1996;22(4):411–415.
46. Hoffman RS, Fine IH, Packer M. Stabilization of flat anterior chamber after trabeculectomy with Healon5. *J Cataract Refract Surg.* 2002; 28(4):712–714.
47. Gutierrez-Ortiz C, Moreno-Lopez M. Healon5 as a treatment option for recurrent flat anterior chamber after trabeculectomy. *J Cataract Refract Surg.* 2003;29(4):635.
48. Freedman J. Iridectomy technique in trabeculectomy. *Ophthalmic Surg.* 1978;9(2):45–47.
49. Shingleton BJ, Chaudhry IM, O'Donoghue MW. Phacotrabeculectomy: peripheral iridectomy or no peripheral iridectomy? *J Cataract Refract Surg.* 2002;28(6):998–1002.
50. Manners TD, Mireskandari K. Phacotrabeculectomy without peripheral iridectomy. *Ophthalmic Surg Lasers.* 1999;30(8):631–635.
51. Parrish RK II, Schiffman JC, Feuer WJ, et al. Fluorouracil Filtering Surgery Study Group. Prognosis and risk factors for early postoperative wound leaks after trabeculectomy with and without 5-fluorouracil. *Am J Ophthalmol.* 2001;132(5):633–640.
52. Liss RP, Scholes GN, Crandall AS. Glaucoma filtration surgery: new horizontal mattress closure of conjunctival incision. *Ophthalmic Surg.* 1991;22(5):298–300.
53. Wise JB. Mitomycin-compatible suture technique for fornix-based conjunctival flaps in glaucoma filtration surgery. *Arch Ophthalmol.* 1993;111(7):992–997.

54. Ng PW, Yeung BY, Yick DW, et al. Fornix-based trabeculectomy with Wise's suture technique in Chinese patients. *Ophthalmology.* 2000;107(12): 2310–2313.

55. Ng PW, Yeung BY, Yick DW, et al. Fornix-based trabeculectomy using the 'anchoring' corneal suture technique. *Clin Experiment Ophthalmol.* 2003;31(2):133–137.

56. Orengo-Nania S, El-Harazi SM, Oram O, et al. Effects of atropine on anterior chamber depth and anterior chamber inflammation after primary trabeculectomy. *J Glaucoma.* 2000;9(4):303–310.

57. Sugar HS. Experimental trabeculectomy in glaucoma. *Am J Ophthalmol.* 1961;51:623–627.

58. Cairns JE. Trabeculectomy. Preliminary report of a new method. *Am J Ophthalmol.* 1968;66(4):673–679.

59. Rich AM, McPherson SD. Trabeculectomy in the owl monkey. *Ann Ophthalmol.* 1973;5(10):1082–1088.

60. Spencer WH. Symposium: microsurgery of the outflow channels. Histologic evaluation of microsurgical glaucoma techniques. *Trans Am Acad Ophthalmol Otolaryngol.* 1972;76(2):389–397.

61. Schmitt H. Histological examination on disks obtained by goniotrephining with scleral flap [in German]. *Klin Monatsbl Augenheilkd.* 1975; 167(3):372–376.

62. Taylor HR. A histologic survey of trabeculectomy. *Am J Ophthalmol.* 1976;82(5):733–735.

63. Lalive d'Epinay S, Remé C, Witmer R. Influence of different topographical locations of trabeculectomy specimens on regulation of intraocular pressure and the quality of the filtering bleb [in German]. *Klin Monatsbl Augenheilkd.* 1983;182(5):387–390.

64. Linnér E. Aqueous outflow pathways following trabeculectomy [in German]. *Klin Monatsbl Augenheilkd.* 1989;195(11):291–293.

65. Shields MB, Shelburne JD, Bell SW. The ultrastructure of human limbal collagen. *Invest Ophthalmol Vis Sci.* 1977;16(9):864–866.

66. Shields MB, Bradbury MJ, Shelburne JD, et al. The permeability of the outer layers of limbus and anterior sclera. *Invest Ophthalmol Vis Sci.* 1977;16(9):866–869.

67. Shields MB. Trabeculectomy vs full-thickness filtering operation for control of glaucoma. *Ophthalmic Surg.* 1980;11(8):498–505.

68. Benedikt O. The mode of action of trabeculectomy [in German]. *Klin Monatsbl Augenheilkd.* 1975;167(5):679–685.

69. Benedikt O. Demonstration of aqueous outflow patterns of normal and glaucomatous human eyes through the injection of fluorescein solution in the anterior chamber [in German]. *Albrecht Von Graefes Arch Klin Exp Ophthalmol.* 1976;199(1):45–67.

70. Bluestein EC, Stewart WC. Tight versus loose scleral flap closure in trabeculectomy surgery. *Doc Ophthalmol.* 1993;84(4):379–385.

71. Melamed S, Ashkenazi I, Glovinski J, et al. Tight scleral flap trabeculectomy with postoperative laser suture lysis. *Am J Ophthalmol.* 1990; 109(3):303–309.

72. Macken P, Buys Y, Trope GE. Glaucoma laser suture lysis. *Br J Ophthalmol.* 1996;80(5):398–401.

73. Hoskins HD Jr, Migliazzo C. Management of failing filtering blebs with the Argon laser. *Ophthalmic Surg.* 1984;15(9):731–733.

74. Ritch R, Potash SD, Liebmann JM. A new lens for argon laser suture lysis. *Ophthalmic Surg.* 1994;25(2):126–127.

75. Johnstone MA, Wellington DP, Ziel CJ. A releasable scleral-flap tamponade suture for guarded filtration surgery. *Arch Ophthalmol.* 1993; 111(3):398–403.

76. Hsu CT, Yarng SS. A modified removable suture in trabeculectomy. *Ophthalmic Surg.* 1993;24(9):579–584; discussion 84–85.

77. Kolker AE, Kass MA, Rait JL. Trabeculectomy with releasable sutures. *Arch Ophthalmol.* 1994;112(1):62–66.

78. Maberley D, Apel A, Rootman DS. Releasable "U" suture for trabeculectomy surgery. *Ophthalmic Surg.* 1994;25(4):251–255.

79. Clemente P. Goniotrepanation with triangular scleral flap [in German]. *Klin Monatsbl Augenheilkd.* 1980;177(4):455–458.

80. Dellaporta A. Experiences with trepano-trabeculectomy. *Trans Sect Ophthalmol Am Acad Ophthalmol Otolaryngol.* 1975;79(2):OP362–OP371.

81. David R, Sachs U. Quantitative trabeculectomy. *Br J Ophthalmol.* 1981;65(7):457–459.

82. Welsh NH. Trabeculectomy with fistula formation in the African. *Br J Ophthalmol.* 1972;56(1):32–36.

83. Fujishima H, Shimazaki J, Shinozaki N, et al. Trabeculectomy with the use of amniotic membrane for uncontrollable glaucoma. *Ophthalmic Surg Lasers.* 1998;29(5):428–431.

84. Schumer RA, Odrich SA. A scleral tunnel incision for trabeculectomy. *Am J Ophthalmol.* 1995;120(4):528–530.

85. Watson PG. Surgery of the glaucomas. *Br J Ophthalmol.* 1972;56(3):299–306.

86. Watson PG, Barnett F. Effectiveness of trabeculectomy in glaucoma. *Am J Ophthalmol.* 1975;79(5):831–845.

87. Hollwich F, Fronimopoulos J, Junemann G, et al. Indication, technique and results of goniotrephining with scleral flap in primary chronic glaucoma [in German]. *Klin Monatsbl Augenheilkd.* 1973;163(5):513–517.

88. Papst W, Brunke R. Goniotrepanation as a second fistulizing procedure [in German]. *Klin Monatsbl Augenheilkd.* 1980;176(6):915–921.

89. Smith BF, Schuster H, Seidenberg B. Subscleral sclerectomy: a double-flap operation for glaucoma. *Am J Ophthalmol.* 1971;71(4):884–888.

90. Schimek RA, Williamson WR. Trabeculectomy with cautery. *Ophthalmic Surg.* 1977;8(1):35–39.

91. Beckman H, Fuller TA. Carbon dioxide laser scleral dissection and filtering procedure for glaucoma. *Am J Ophthalmol.* 1979;88(1):73–77.

92. Suzuki R. Trabeculectomy with a Kelly Descemet membrane punch. *Ophthalmologica.* 1997;211(2):93–94.

93. Sandvig KU. Results of a combined procedure for cataract and glaucoma, using Crozafon-De Laage punch. *Acta Ophthalmol Scand.* 1999;77(1): 88–90.

94. Lee PF, Shihab ZM, Fu YA. Modified trabeculectomy: a new procedure for neovascular glaucoma. *Ophthalmic Surg.* 1980;11(3):181–185.

95. Sivak-Callcott JA, O'Day DM, Gass JD, et al. Evidence-based recommendations for the diagnosis and treatment of neovascular glaucoma. *Ophthalmology.* 2001;108(10):1767–1776; quiz 1777, 1800.

96. Mandal AK, Majji AB, Mandal SP, et al. Mitomycin-C-augmented trabeculectomy for neovascular glaucoma. A preliminary report. *Indian J Ophthalmol.* 2002;50(4):287–293.

97. Hyung SM, Kim SK. Mid-term effects of trabeculectomy with mitomycin C in neovascular glaucoma patients. *Korean J Ophthalmol.* 2001;15(2): 98–106.

98. Ophir A, Porges Y. Needling with intra-bleb 5 fluorouracil for intractable neovascular glaucoma. *Ophthalmic Surg Lasers.* 2000;31(1):38–42.

99. Gaspar AZ, Flammer J, Hendrickson P. Regression of rubeosis iridis after trabeculectomy combined with mitomycin-C. *Ophthalmic Surg Lasers.* 1996;27(8):709–712.

100. Kitnarong N, Chindasub P, Metheetrairut A. Surgical outcome of intravitreal bevacizumab and filtration surgery in neovascular glaucoma. *Adv Ther.* 2008;25(5):438–443.

101. Zimmerman TJ, Kooner KS, Ford VJ, et al. Effectiveness of nonpenetrating trabeculectomy in aphakic patients with glaucoma. *Ophthalmic Surg.* 1984;15(1):44–50.

102. Gedde SJ, Schiffman JC, Feuer WJ, et al. Treatment outcomes in the tube versus trabeculectomy study after one year of follow-up. *Am J Ophthalmol.* 2007;143(1):9–22.

103. Mandal AK, Bagga H, Nutheti R, et al. Trabeculectomy with or without mitomycin-C for paediatric glaucoma in aphakia and pseudophakia following congenital cataract surgery. *Eye.* 2003;17(1):53–62.

104. Dahan E, Carmichael TR. Implantation of a miniature glaucoma device under a scleral flap. *J Glaucoma.* 2005;14(2):98–102.

105. Wamsley S, Moster MR, Rai S, et al. Results of the use of the Ex-PRESS miniature glaucoma implant in technically challenging, advanced glaucoma cases: a clinical pilot study. *Am J Ophthalmol.* 2004;138(6): 1049–1051.

106. Maris PJ Jr, Ishida K, Netland PA. Comparison of trabeculectomy with Ex-PRESS miniature glaucoma device implanted under scleral flap. *J Glaucoma.* 2007;16(1):14–19.

107. Maumenee AE. External filtering operations for glaucoma: the mechanism of function and failure. *Trans Am Ophthalmol Soc.* 1960;58:319–328.

108. Kornblueth W, Tenenbaum E. The inhibitory effect of aqueous humor on the growth of cells in tissue cultures. *Am J Ophthalmol.* 1956;42(1):70–74.

109. Herschler J, Claflin AJ, Fiorentino G. The effect of aqueous humor on the growth of subconjunctival fibroblasts in tissue culture and its implications for glaucoma surgery. *Am J Ophthalmol.* 1980;89(2):245–249.

110. Radius RL, Herschler J, Claflin A, et al. Aqueous humor changes after experimental filtering surgery. *Am J Ophthalmol.* 1980;89(2):250–254.

111. Jampel HD. Ascorbic acid is cytotoxic to dividing human Tenon's capsule fibroblasts. A possible contributing factor in glaucoma filtration surgery success. *Arch Ophthalmol.* 1990;108(9):1323–1325.

112. Tripathi RC, Borisuth NSC, Tripathi BJ. Growth factors in the aqueous humor and their therapeutic implications in glaucoma and anterior segment disorders of the human eye. *Drug Dev Res.* 1991;22(1):1–23.

113. Jampel HD, Roche N, Stark WJ, et al. Transforming growth factor-beta in human aqueous humor. *Curr Eye Res.* 1990;9(10):963–969.

114. Albrink WS, Wallace AC. Aqueous humor as a tissue culture nutrient. *Proc Soc Exp Biol Med.* 1951;77(4):754–758.

115. Ledbetter SR, Hatchell DL, O'Brien WJ. Secondary aqueous humor stimulates the proliferation of cultured bovine corneal endothelial cells. *Invest Ophthalmol Vis Sci.* 1983;24(5):557–562.

116. Joseph JP, Grierson I, Hitchings RA. Chemotactic activity of aqueous humor. A cause of failure of trabeculectomies? *Arch Ophthalmol.* 1989;107(1):69–74.

117. Gwynn DR, Stewart WC, Hennis HL, et al. The influence of age upon inflammatory cell counts and structure of conjunctiva in chronic open-angle glaucoma. *Acta Ophthalmol.* 1993;71(5):691–695.

118. McMillan TA, Stewart WC, Hennis HL, et al. Histologic differences in the conjunctiva of black and white glaucoma patients. *Ophthalmic Surg.* 1992;23(11):762–765.

119. Lavin MJ, Wormald RP, Migdal CS, et al. The influence of prior therapy on the success of trabeculectomy. *Arch Ophthalmol.* 1990;108(11):1543–1548.

120. Broadway DC, Grierson I, O'Brien C, et al. Adverse effects of topical antiglaucoma medication. II. The outcome of filtration surgery. *Arch Ophthalmol.* 1994;112(11):1446–1454.

121. Johnson DH, Yoshikawa K, Brubaker RF, et al. The effect of long-term medical therapy on the outcome of filtration surgery. *Am J Ophthalmol.* 1994;117(2):139–148.

122. Broadway DC, Grierson I, O'Brien C, et al. Adverse effects of topical antiglaucoma medication. I. The conjunctival cell profile. *Arch Ophthalmol.* 1994;112(11):1437–1445.

123. Baudouin C, Garcher C, Haouat N, et al. Expression of inflammatory membrane markers by conjunctival cells in chronically treated patients with glaucoma. *Ophthalmology.* 1994;101(3):454–460.

124. Gwynn DR, Stewart WC, Pitts RA, et al. Conjunctival structure and cell counts and the results of filtering surgery. *Am J Ophthalmol.* 1993;116(4):464–468.

125. Brandt JD, Wittpenn JR, Katz LJ, et al. Conjunctival impression cytology in patients with glaucoma using long-term topical medication. *Am J Ophthalmol.* 1991;112(3):297–301.

126. Broadway DC, Grierson I, Sturmer J, et al. Reversal of topical antiglaucoma medication effects on the conjunctiva. *Arch Ophthalmol.* 1996;114(3):262–267.

127. Arici MK, Demircan S, Topalkara A, et al. Effect of conjunctival structure and inflammatory cell counts on intraocular pressure after trabeculectomy. *Ophthalmologica.* 1999;213(6):371–375.

128. Broadway DC, Grierson I, Hitchings RA. Local effects of previous conjunctival incisional surgery and the subsequent outcome of filtration surgery. *Am J Ophthalmol.* 1998;125(6):805–818.

129. Nguyen KD, Lee DA. Effect of steroids and nonsteroidal antiinflammatory agents on human ocular fibroblast. *Invest Ophthalmol Vis Sci.* 1992;33(9):2693–2701.

130. Sun R, Gimbel HV, Liu S, et al. Effect of diclofenac sodium and dexamethasone on cultured human Tenon's capsule fibroblasts. *Ophthalmic Surg Lasers.* 1999;30(5):382–388.

131. Starita RJ, Fellman RL, Spaeth GL, et al. Short- and long-term effects of postoperative corticosteroids on trabeculectomy. *Ophthalmology.* 1985;92(7):938–946.

132. Araujo SV, Spaeth GL, Roth SM, et al. A ten-year follow-up on a prospective, randomized trial of postoperative corticosteroids after trabeculectomy. *Ophthalmology.* 1995;102(12):1753–1759.

133. Giangiacomo J, Dueker DK, Adelstein E. The effect of preoperative subconjunctival triamcinolone administration on glaucoma filtration. I. Trabeculectomy following subconjunctival triamcinolone. *Arch Ophthalmol.* 1986;104(6):838–841.

134. Blumenkranz MS, Claflin A, Hajek AS. Selection of therapeutic agents for intraocular proliferative disease. Cell culture evaluation. *Arch Ophthalmol.* 1984;102(4):598–604.

135. Khaw PT, Ward S, Porter A, et al. The long-term effects of 5-fluorouracil and sodium butyrate on human Tenon's fibroblasts. *Invest Ophthalmol Vis Sci.* 1992;33(6):2043–2052.

136. Gressel MG, Parrish RK II, Folberg R. 5-Fluorouracil and glaucoma filtering surgery. I. An animal model. *Ophthalmology.* 1984;91(4):378–383.

137. Heuer DK, Parrish RK II, Gressel MG, et al. 5-Fluorouracil and glaucoma filtering surgery. II. A pilot study. *Ophthalmology.* 1984;91(4):384–394.

138. Heuer DK, Parrish RK II, Gressel MG, et al. 5-Fluorouracil and glaucoma filtering surgery. III. Intermediate follow-up of a pilot study. *Ophthalmology.* 1986;93(12):1537–1546.

139. The Fluorouracil Filtering Surgery Study Group. Fluorouracil Filtering Surgery Study one-year follow-up. *Am J Ophthalmol.* 1989;108(6):625–635.

140. The Fluorouracil Filtering Surgery Study Group. Three-year follow-up of the Fluorouracil Filtering Surgery Study. *Am J Ophthalmol.* 1993;115(1):82–92.

141. Weinreb RN. Adjusting the dose of 5-fluorouracil after filtration surgery to minimize side effects. *Ophthalmology.* 1987;94(5):564–570.

142. Ruderman JM, Welch DB, Smith MF, et al. A randomized study of 5-fluorouracil and filtration surgery. *Am J Ophthalmol.* 1987;104(3):218–224.

143. Araie M, Shoji N, Shirato S, et al. Postoperative subconjunctival 5-fluorouracil injections and success probability of trabeculectomy in Japanese: results of 5-year follow-up. *Jpn J Ophthalmol.* 1992;36(2):158–168.

144. Goldenfeld M, Krupin T, Ruderman JM, et al. 5-Fluorouracil in initial trabeculectomy. A prospective, randomized, multicenter study. *Ophthalmology.* 1994;101(6):1024–1029.

145. Whiteside-Michel J, Liebmann JM, Ritch R. Initial 5-fluorouracil trabeculectomy in young patients. *Ophthalmology.* 1992;99(1):7–13.

146. Bansal RK, Gupta A. 5-Fluorouracil in trabeculectomy for patients under the age of 40 years. *Ophthalmic Surg.* 1992;23(4):278–280.

147. Zalish M, Leiba H, Oliver M. Subconjunctival injection of 5-fluorouracil following trabeculectomy for congenital and infantile glaucoma. *Ophthalmic Surg.* 1992;23(3):203–205.

148. Wilson RP, Steinmann WC. Use of trabeculectomy with postoperative 5-fluorouracil in patients requiring extremely low intraocular pressure levels to limit further glaucoma progression. *Ophthalmology.* 1991;98(7):1047–1052.

149. Tsai JC, Feuer WJ, Parrish RK II, et al. 5-Fluorouracil filtering surgery and neovascular glaucoma. Long-term follow-up of the original pilot study. *Ophthalmology.* 1995;102(6):887–892; discussion 892–893.

150. Krug JH Jr, Melamed S. Adjunctive use of delayed and adjustable low-dose 5-fluorouracil in refractory glaucoma. *Am J Ophthalmol.* 1990;109(4):412–418.

151. Hefetz L, Keren T, Naveh N. Early and late postoperative application of 5-fluorouracil following trabeculectomy in refractory glaucoma. *Ophthalmic Surg.* 1994;25(10):715–719.

152. Smith MF, Sherwood MB, Doyle JW, et al. Results of intraoperative 5-fluorouracil supplementation on trabeculectomy for open-angle glaucoma. *Am J Ophthalmol.* 1992;114(6):737–741.

153. Egbert PR, Williams AS, Singh K, et al. A prospective trial of intraoperative fluorouracil during trabeculectomy in a black population. *Am J Ophthalmol.* 1993;116(5):612–616.

154. Cunliffe IA, Longstaff S. Intra-operative use of 5-fluorouracil in glaucoma filtering surgery. *Acta Ophthalmol.* 1993;71(6):739–743.

155. Feldman RM, Dietze PJ, Gross RL, et al. Intraoperative 5-fluorouracil administration in trabeculectomy. *J Glaucoma.* 1994;3(4):302–307.

156. Sidoti PA, Choi JC, Morinelli EN, et al. Trabeculectomy with intraoperative 5-fluorouracil. *Ophthalmic Surg Lasers.* 1998;29(7):552–561.

157. Wilkins MR, Occleston NL, Kotecha A, et al. Sponge delivery variables and tissue levels of 5-fluorouracil. *Br J Ophthalmol.* 2000;84(1):92–97.

158. Chen CW. Enhanced intraocular pressure controlling effectiveness of trabeculectomy by local application of mitomycin-C. *Trans Asia Pac Acad Ophthalmol.* 1983;9:172–177.

159. Jampel HD. Effect of brief exposure to mitomycin C on viability and proliferation of cultured human Tenon's capsule fibroblasts. *Ophthalmology.* 1992;99(9):1471–1476.

160. Madhavan HN, Rao SB, Vijaya L, et al. In vitro sensitivity of human Tenon's capsule fibroblasts to mitomycin C and its correlation with outcome of glaucoma filtration surgery. *Ophthalmic Surg.* 1995;26(1):61–67.

161. Khaw PT, Doyle JW, Sherwood MB, et al. Prolonged localized tissue effects from 5-minute exposures to fluorouracil and mitomycin C. *Arch Ophthalmol.* 1993;111(2):263–267.

162. Smith S, D'Amore PA, Dreyer EB. Comparative toxicity of mitomycin C and 5-fluorouracil in vitro. *Am J Ophthalmol.* 1994;118(3):332–337.

163. Bergstrom TJ, Wilkinson WS, Skuta GL, et al. The effects of subconjunctival mitomycin-C on glaucoma filtration surgery in rabbits. *Arch Ophthalmol.* 1991;109(12):1725–1730.

164. Palmer SS. Mitomycin as adjunct chemotherapy with trabeculectomy. *Ophthalmology.* 1991;98(3):317–321.

165. Skuta GL, Beeson CC, Higginbotham EJ, et al. Intraoperative mitomycin versus postoperative 5-fluorouracil in high-risk glaucoma filtering surgery. *Ophthalmology.* 1992;99(3):438–444.

166. Katz GJ, Higginbotham EJ, Lichter PR, et al. Mitomycin C versus 5-fluorouracil in high-risk glaucoma filtering surgery. Extended follow-up. *Ophthalmology.* 1995;102(9):1263–1269.

167. Kitazawa Y, Kawase K, Matsushita H, et al. Trabeculectomy with mitomycin. A comparative study with fluorouracil. *Arch Ophthalmol.* 1991;109(12):1693–1698.

168. Lamping KA, Belkin JK. 5-Fluorouracil and mitomycin C in pseudophakic patients. *Ophthalmology.* 1995;102(1):70–75.

169. Palanca-Capistrano AM, Hall J, Cantor LB, et al. Long-term outcomes of intraoperative 5-fluorouracil versus intraoperative mitomycin C in primary trabeculectomy surgery. *Ophthalmology.* 2009;116(2):185–190.

170. Mermoud A, Salmon JF, Murray AD. Trabeculectomy with mitomycin C for refractory glaucoma in blacks. *Am J Ophthalmol.* 1993;116(1):72–78.

171. Prata JA Jr, Neves RA, Minckler DS, et al. Trabeculectomy with mitomycin C in glaucoma associated with uveitis. *Ophthalmic Surg.* 1994;25(9):616–620.

172. Susanna R Jr, Oltrogge EW, Carani JC, et al. Mitomycin as adjunct chemotherapy with trabeculectomy in congenital and developmental glaucomas. *J Glaucoma.* 1995;4(3):151–157.

173. Yamamoto T, Ichien M, Suemori-Matsushita H, et al. Trabeculectomy for normal-tension glaucoma [in Japanese]. *Nippon Ganka Gakkai Zasshi.* 1994;98(6):579–583.

174. Costa VP, Moster MR, Wilson RP, et al. Effects of topical mitomycin C on primary trabeculectomies and combined procedures. *Br J Ophthalmol.* 1993;77(11):693–697.

175. Mirza GE, Karakucuk S, Dogan H, et al. Filtering surgery with mitomycin-C in uncomplicated (primary open angle) glaucoma. *Acta Ophthalmol.* 1994;72(2):155–161.

176. Kupin TH, Juzych MS, Shin DH, et al. Adjunctive mitomycin C in primary trabeculectomy in phakic eyes. *Am J Ophthalmol.* 1995;119(1):30–39.

177. Beckers HJ, Kinders KC, Webers CA. Five-year results of trabeculectomy with mitomycin C. *Graefes Arch Clin Exp Ophthalmol.* 2003;241(2):106–110.

178. Costa VP, Wilson RP, Moster MR, et al. Hypotony maculopathy following the use of topical mitomycin C in glaucoma filtration surgery. *Ophthalmic Surg.* 1993;24(6):389–394.

179. Shields MB, Scroggs MW, Sloop CM, et al. Clinical and histopathologic observations concerning hypotony after trabeculectomy with adjunctive mitomycin C. *Am J Ophthalmol.* 1993;116(6):673–683.

180. Mietz H, Brunner R, Addicks K, et al. Histopathology of an avascular filtering bleb after trabeculectomy with mitomycin-C. *J Glaucoma.* 1993;2(4):266–270.

181. Nuyts RM, Felten PC, Pels E, et al. Histopathologic effects of mitomycin C after trabeculectomy in human glaucomatous eyes with persistent hypotony. *Am J Ophthalmol.* 1994;118(2):225–237.

182. Derick RJ, Pasquale L, Quigley HA, et al. Potential toxicity of mitomycin C. *Arch Ophthalmol.* 1991;109(12):1635.

183. Morrow GL, Stein RM, Heathcote JG, et al. Ocular toxicity of mitomycin C and 5-fluorouracil in the rabbit. *Can J Ophthalmol.* 1994;29(6):268–273.

184. Megevand GS, Salmon JF, Scholtz RP, et al. The effect of reducing the exposure time of mitomycin C in glaucoma filtering surgery. *Ophthalmology.* 1995;102(1):84–90.

185. Casson R, Rahman R, Salmon JF. Long term results and complications of trabeculectomy augmented with low dose mitomycin C in patients at risk for filtration failure. *Br J Ophthalmol.* 2001;85(6):686–688.

186. Bank A, Allingham RR. Application of mitomycin C during filtering surgery. *Am J Ophthalmol.* 1993;116(3):377–379.

187. Shin DH, Reed SY, Swords RC, et al. Cellulose sponge punch for controlled mitomycin application. *Arch Ophthalmol.* 1994;112(12):1624–1625.

188. Flynn WJ, Carlson DW, Bifano SL. Mitomycin trabeculectomy: the microsurgical sponge difference. *J Glaucoma.* 1995;4(2):86–90.

189. Prata JA Jr, Minckler DS, Baerveldt G, et al. Site of mitomycin-C application during trabeculectomy. *J Glaucoma.* 1994;3(4):296–301.

190. Prata JA Jr, Minckler DS, Koda RT. Effects of external irrigation on mitomycin-C concentration in rabbit aqueous and vitreous humor. *J Glaucoma.* 1995;4(1):32–35.

191. Vass C, Georgopoulos M, El Menyawi I, et al. Intrascleral concentration vs depth profile of mitomycin-C after episcleral application: impact of irrigation. *Exp Eye Res.* 2000;70(2):139–143.

192. Georgopoulos M, Vass C, Vatanparast Z. Impact of irrigation in a new model for in vitro diffusion of mitomycin-C after episcleral application. *Curr Eye Res.* 2002;25(4):221–225.

193. Susanna R Jr, Costa VP, Malta RF, et al. Intraoperative mitomycin-C without conjunctival and Tenon's capsule touch in primary trabeculectomy. *Ophthalmology.* 2001;108(6):1039–1042.

194. Litin BS, Kwong EM, Jones MA, et al. Effect of antineoplastic drugs on cell proliferation—individually and in combination. *Ophthalmic Surg.* 1985;16(1):34–39.

195. Lee DA, Goodwin LT Jr, Panek WC, et al. Effects of cytosine arabino side-impregnated bioerodible polymers on glaucoma filtration surgery in rabbits. *J Glaucoma.* 1993;2(2):96–100.

196. Chu JL, Shields SR, Netland PA. Enhancement of filtration surgery with cytosine arabinoside and reversal of toxicity with 2'-deoxycytidine. *Curr Eye Res.* 1994;13(11):839–843.

197. Sakamoto T, Oshima Y, Sakamoto M, et al. Electroporation and bleomycin in glaucoma-filtering surgery. *Invest Ophthalmol Vis Sci.* 1997;38(13):2864–2868.

198. Salas-Prato M, Assalian A, Mehdi AZ, et al. Inhibition by rapamycin of PDGF- and bFGF-induced human tenon fibroblast proliferation *in vitro.* *J Glaucoma.* 1996;5(1):54–59.

199. Saika S, Ooshima A, Yamanaka O, et al. In vitro effects of doxorubicin and mitomycin C on human Tenon's capsule fibroblasts. *Ophthalmic Res.* 1997;29(2):91–102.

200. Xu Y, Yang GH, Gin WM, et al. Effect of subconjunctival daunorubicin on glaucoma surgery in rabbits. *Ophthalmic Surg.* 1993;24(6):382–388.

201. Skuta GL, Assil K, Parrish RK II, et al. Filtering surgery in owl monkeys treated with the antimetabolite 5-fluorouridine 5'-monophosphate entrapped in multivesicular liposomes. *Am J Ophthalmol.* 1987;103(5):714–716.

202. Alvarado JA. The use of a liposome-encapsulated 5-fluoroorotate for glaucoma surgery: I. Animal studies. *Trans Am Ophthalmol Soc.* 1989;87:489–514.

203. Del Vecchio PJ, Bizios R, Holleran LA, et al. Inhibition of human scleral fibroblast proliferation with heparin. *Invest Ophthalmol Vis Sci.* 1988;29(8):1272–1276.

204. Joseph JP, Grierson I, Hitchings RA. Taxol, cytochalasin B and colchicine effects on fibroblast migration and contraction: a role in glaucoma filtration surgery? *Curr Eye Res.* 1989;8(2):203–215.

205. Wilkerson M, Fulcher S, Shields MB, et al. Inhibition of human subconjunctival fibroblast proliferation by immunotoxin. *Invest Ophthalmol Vis Sci.* 1992;33(7):2293–2298.

206. Gillies M, Su T, Sarossy M, et al. Interferon-alpha 2b inhibits proliferation of human Tenon's capsule fibroblasts. *Graefes Arch Clin Exp Ophthalmol.* 1993;231(2):118–121.

207. Gillies MC, Brooks AM, Young S, et al. A randomized phase II trial of interferon-alpha2b versus 5-fluorouracil after trabeculectomy. *Aust N Z J Ophthalmol.* 1999;27(1):37–44.

208. Akman A, Bilezikci B, Kucukerdonmez C, et al. Suramin modulates wound healing of rabbit conjunctiva after trabeculectomy: comparison with mitomycin C. *Curr Eye Res.* 2003;26(1):37–43.

209. Mietz H, Krieglstein GK. Suramin to enhance glaucoma filtering procedures: a clinical comparison with mitomycin. *Ophthalmic Surg Lasers.* 2001;32(5):358–369.

210. Nevarez JA, Parrish RK II, Heuer DK, et al. The effect of beta irradiation on monkey Tenon's capsule fibroblasts in tissue culture. *Curr Eye Res.* 1987;6(5):719–723.

211. Khaw PT, Ward S, Grierson I, et al. Effect of beta radiation on proliferating human Tenon's capsule fibroblasts. *Br J Ophthalmol.* 1991;75(10):580–583.

212. Miller MH, Grierson I, Unger WG, et al. The effect of topical dexamethasone and preoperative beta irradiation on a model of glaucoma fistulizing surgery in the rabbit. *Ophthalmic Surg.* 1990;21(1):44–54.

213. Miller MH, Joseph NH, Wishart PK, et al. Lack of beneficial effect of intensive topical steroids and beta irradiation of eyes undergoing repeat trabeculectomy. *Ophthalmic Surg.* 1987;18(7):508–512.

214. Miller MH, Rice NS. Trabeculectomy combined with beta irradiation for congenital glaucoma. *Br J Ophthalmol.* 1991;75(10):584–590.

215. Demir T, Turgut B, Akyol N, et al. Effects of amniotic membrane transplantation and mitomycin C on wound healing in experimental glaucoma surgery. *Ophthalmologica.* 2002;216(6):438–442.

216. Lu DW, Tai MC, Chiang CH. Subconjunctival retention of C3F8 gas increased the success rates of trabeculectomy in young people. *J Ocul Pharmacol Ther.* 1997;13(3):235–242.

217. Wong HT, Seah SK. Augmentation of filtering blebs with perfluoropropane gas bubble: an experimental and pilot clinical study. *Ophthalmology.* 1999;106(3):545–549.

218. Fourman S, Vaid K. Effects of tissue plasminogen activator on glaucoma filter blebs in rabbits. *Ophthalmic Surg.* 1989;20(9):663–667.

219. Fourman S, Wiley L. Tissue plasminogen activator modifies healing of glaucoma filtering surgery in rabbits. *Ophthalmic Surg.* 1991;22(12):718–723.

220. Ozment RR, Liaw ZC, Latina MA. The use of tissue plasminogen activator in experimental filtration surgery. *Ophthalmic Surg.* 1992;23(1):22–30.

221. Latina MA, Belmonte SJ, Park C, et al. Gamma-interferon effects on human fibroblasts from Tenon's capsule. *Invest Ophthalmol Vis Sci.* 1991;32(10):2806–2815.

222. Lee YC, Park MH, Baek NH. Effect of gamma-interferon on fibroblast proliferation and collagen synthesis after glaucoma filtering surgery in white rabbits. *Korean J Ophthalmol.* 1991;5(2):59–67.

223. Nguyen KD, Hoang AT, Lee DA. Transcriptional control of human Tenon's capsule fibroblast collagen synthesis in vitro by gamma-interferon. *Invest Ophthalmol Vis Sci.* 1994;35(7):3064–3070.

224. Assil KK, Saperstein D, Weinreb RN, et al. Inhibition of collagen synthesis in human episcleral fibroblasts by calcium ionophore a23187. *J Glaucoma.* 1995;4(1):41–44.

225. McGuigan LJ, Mason RP, Sanchez R, et al. D-penicillamine and beta-aminopropionitrile effects on experimental filtering surgery. *Invest Ophthalmol Vis Sci.* 1987;28(10):1625–1629.

226. Fourman S. Effects of aminopropionitrile on glaucoma filter blebs in rabbits. *Ophthalmic Surg.* 1988;19(9):649–652.

227. McGuigan LJ, Cook DJ, Yablonski ME. Dexamethasone, D-penicillamine, and glaucoma filter surgery in rabbits. *Invest Ophthalmol Vis Sci.* 1986;27(12):1755–1757.

228. Grewal DS, Jain R, Kumar H, et al. Evaluation of subconjunctival bevacizumab as an adjunct to trabeculectomy a pilot study. *Ophthalmology.* 2008;115(12):2141–2145.e2.

229. Coote MA, Ruddle JB, Qin Q, et al. Vascular changes after intra-bleb injection of bevacizumab. *J Glaucoma.* 2008;17(7):517–518.

230. Cordeiro MF. Beyond Mitomycin: TGF-beta and wound healing. *Prog Retin Eye Res.* 2002;21(1):75–89.

231. Cordeiro MF, Reichel MB, Gay JA, et al. Transforming growth factor-beta1, -beta2, and -beta3 in vivo: effects on normal and mitomycin C-modulated conjunctival scarring. *Invest Ophthalmol Vis Sci.* 1999;40(9):1975–1982.

232. Cordeiro MF. Role of transforming growth factor beta in conjunctival scarring. *Clin Sci.* 2003;104(2):181–187.

233. Mead AL, Wong TT, Cordeiro MF, et al. Evaluation of anti-TGF-beta2 antibody as a new postoperative anti-scarring agent in glaucoma surgery. *Invest Ophthalmol Vis Sci.* 2003;44(8):3394–3401.

234. Khaw P, Grehn F, Hollo G, et al. A phase III study of subconjunctival human antitransforming growth factor beta (2) monoclonal antibody (CAT-152) to prevent scarring after first-time trabeculectomy. *Ophthalmology.* 2007;114(10):1822–1830.

235. Ochiai H, Ochiai Y, Chihara E. Tranilast inhibits TGF- A1 secretion without affecting its mRNA levels in conjunctival cells. *Kobe J Med Sci.* 2001;47(5):203–209.

236. Chihara E, Dong J, Ochiai H, et al. Effects of tranilast on filtering blebs: a pilot study. *J Glaucoma.* 2002;11(2):127–133.

237. Oshima T, Kurosaka D, Kato K, et al. Tranilast inhibits cell proliferation and collagen synthesis by rabbit corneal and Tenon's capsule fibroblasts. *Curr Eye Res.* 2000;20(4):283–286.

238. LaGrange F. Iridectomie et sclerectomie combinees dans le traitement du glaucome chronique. Procede nouveau pour l'etablissement de la cicatrice filtrante [in French]. *Arch d'Opht.* 1906;26:481.

239. Holth S. Sclerectomie avec la pince emporte-piece dans le glaucome, de preference apres incision a la pique [in French]. *Ann d'Ocul.* 1909;142:1.

240. Iliff CE, Haas JS. Posterior lip sclerectomy. *Am J Ophthalmol.* 1962;54:688–693.

241. Elliot RH. A preliminary note on a new operative procedure for the establishment of a filtering cicatrix in the treatment of glaucoma. *Ophthalmoscope.* 1909;7:804–806.

242. Fergus F. Treatment of glaucoma by trephining. *Br Med J.* 1909;2:983–984.

243. Elliot RH. *Sclero-Corneal Trephining in the Operative Treatment of Glaucoma* London: George Pulman and Sons; 1913.

244. Sugar HS. Limboscleral trephination. *Am J Ophthalmol.* 1961;52:29–36.

245. Sugar HS. Limbal trepanation: fourteen years' experience. *Ann Ophthalmol.* 1975;7(10):1399–1404.

246. Preziosi CL. The electro-cautery in the treatment of glaucoma. *Br J Ophthalmol.* 1924;8(9):414–417.

247. Scheie HG. Retraction of scleral wound edges as a fistulizing procedure for glaucoma. *Trans Am Acad Ophthalmol Otolaryngol.* 1958;62(6):803–811.

248. Viswanathan B, Brown IA. Peripheral iridectomy with scleral cautery for glaucoma. *Arch Ophthalmol.* 1975;93(1):34–35.

249. Shaffer RN, Hetherington HD Jr, Hoskins HD Jr. Guarded thermal sclerostomy. *Am J Ophthalmol.* 1971;72(4):769–772.

250. Gess LA, Koeth E, Gralle I. Trabeculectomy with iridencleisis. *Br J Ophthalmol.* 1985;69(12):881–885.

251. Litwin RL. Successful argon laser sclerostomy for glaucoma. *Ophthalmic Surg.* 1979;10(7):22–24.

252. Hoskins HD Jr, Iwach AG, Drake MV, et al. Subconjunctival THC:YAG laser limbal sclerostomy ab externo in the rabbit. *Ophthalmic Surg.* 1990;21(8):589–592.

253. Onda E, Jikihara S, Kitazawa Y, et al. Determination of an appropriate laser setting for THC-YAG laser sclerostomy ab externo in rabbits. *Ophthalmic Surg.* 1992;23(3):198–202.

254. Hoskins HD Jr, Iwach AG, Vassiliadis A, et al. Subconjunctival THC:YAG laser thermal sclerostomy. *Ophthalmology.* 1991;98(9):1394–1399; discussion 1399–1400.

255. Saheb NE. Short-term results of holmium laser sclerostomy in patients with uncontrolled glaucoma. *Can J Ophthalmol.* 1993;28(7):317–319.

256. Iwach AG, Hoskins HD Jr, Drake MV, et al. Subconjunctival THC:YAG ("holmium") laser thermal sclerostomy ab externo. A one-year report. *Ophthalmology.* 1993;100(3):356–365; discussion 365–366.

257. Bonomi L, Perfetti S, Marraffa M, et al. Subconjunctival THC:YAG laser sclerostomy for the treatment of glaucoma: preliminary data. *Ophthalmic Surg.* 1993;24(5):300–303.

258. Iwach AG, Hoskins HD Jr, Drake MV, et al. Update of the subconjunctival THC:YAG (holmium) laser sclerostomy ab externo clinical trial: 30-month report. *Ophthalmic Surg.* 1994;25(1):13–21.

259. Iwach AG, Hoskins HD Jr, Mora JS, et al. Update on the subconjunctival THC:YAG (holmium) laser sclerostomy ab externo clinical trial: a 4-year report. *Ophthalmic Surg Lasers.* 1996;27(10):823–831.

260. Rodrigues M, Shelton K, Glaser E, et al. Histologic effect of diode laser sclerostomy in human cadaver eyes. *Ophthalmic Surg Lasers.* 1998;29(9):758–761.

261. Brinkmann R, Droge G, Schroer F, et al. Ablation dynamics in laser sclerostomy ab externo by means of pulsed lasers in the mid-infrared spectral range. *Ophthalmic Surg Lasers.* 1997;28(10):853–865.

262. Feldman RM, Oram O, Gross RL, et al. Histopathologic characteristics of failed holmium laser sclerostomy. *Am J Ophthalmol.* 1993;116(6):766–767.

263. Wang TH, Hung PT, Ho TC. THC:YAG laser sclerostomy with mitomycin subconjunctival injection in rabbits. *J Ocul Pharmacol.* 1992;8(4):325–332.

264. Wetzel W, Scheu M. Laser sclerostomy ab externo using mid infrared lasers. *Ophthalmic Surg.* 1993;24(1):6–12.

265. McHam ML, Eisenberg DL, Schuman JS, et al. Erbium:YAG laser sclerectomy with a sapphire optical fiber. *Ophthalmic Surg Lasers.* 1997;28(1):55–58.

266. Jacobi PC, Dietlein TS, Krieglstein GK. Prospective study of ab externo erbium:YAG laser sclerostomy in humans. *Am J Ophthalmol.* 1997;123(4):478–486.

267. Spiegel D, Wetzel W, Birngruber R. Ab externo erbium YAG laser sclerostomy versus conventional trabeculectomy. Treatment of glaucoma patients [in German]. *Ophthalmologe.* 1998;95(8):537–541.

268. Barak A, Rosner M, Solomon A, et al. Use of the giant-pulse Nd:YAG laser for abexterno sclerostomy in rabbits and humans. *Ophthalmic Surg.* 1995;26(1):68–72.

269. Cooper HM, Schuman JS, Puliafito CA, et al. Picosecond neodymium: yttrium lithium fluoride laser sclerectomy. *Am J Ophthalmol.* 1993;115(2):221–224.

270. Park SB, Kim JC, Aquavella JV. Nd:YLF laser sclerostomy. *Ophthalmic Surg.* 1993;24(2):118–120.

271. Karp CL, Higginbotham EJ, Griffin EO. Adjunctive use of transconjunctival mitomycin-C in ab externo diode laser sclerostomy surgery in rabbits. *Ophthalmic Surg.* 1994;25(1):22–27.

272. Allan BD, van Saarloos PP, Cooper RL, et al. 193-nm excimer laser sclerostomy using a modified open mask delivery system in rhesus monkeys with experimental glaucoma. *Graefes Arch Clin Exp Ophthalmol.* 1993;231(11):662–666.

273. Allan BD, van Saarloos PP, Cooper RL, et al. 193 nm excimer laser sclerostomy in pseudophakic patients with advanced open angle glaucoma. *Br J Ophthalmol.* 1994;78(3):199–205.

274. Seiler T, Kriegerowski M, Bende T, et al. Partial external trabeculectomy [in German]. *Klin Monatsbl Augenheilkd.* 1989;195(4):216–220.

275. Brooks AM, Samuel M, Carroll N, et al. Excimer laser filtration surgery. *Am J Ophthalmol.* 1995;119(1):40–47.

276. Walker R, Specht H. Theoretical and physical aspects of excimer laser trabeculotomy (ELT) ab interno with the AIDA laser with a wave length of 308 mm [in German]. *Biomed Tech.* 2002;47(5):106–110.

277. O'Donnell FE Jr, Santos BA, Overby J. Laser trabeculodissection with a photopolishing scanning excimer laser. *Ophthalmic Surg Lasers.* 2000;31(6):508–511.

278. March WF, Gherezghiher T, Koss MC, et al. Experimental YAG laser sclerostomy. *Arch Ophthalmol.* 1984;102(12):1834–1836.

279. March WF, Gherezghiher T, Koss MC, et al. Histologic study of a neodymium-YAG laser sclerostomy. *Arch Ophthalmol.* 1985;103(6):860–863.

280. Gherezghiher T, March WF, Koss MC, et al. Neodymium-YAG laser sclerostomy in primates. *Arch Ophthalmol.* 1985;103(10):1543–1545.

281. Latina MA, Dobrogowski M, March WF, et al. Laser sclerostomy by pulsed-dye laser and goniolens. *Arch Ophthalmol.* 1990;108(12):1745–1750.

282. Latina MA, Melamed S, March WF, et al. Gonioscopic ab interno laser sclerostomy. A pilot study in glaucoma patients. *Ophthalmology.* 1992;99(11):1736–1744.

283. Melamed S, Solomon A, Neumann D, et al. Internal sclerostomy using laser ablation of dyed sclera in glaucoma patients: a pilot study. *Br J Ophthalmol.* 1993;77(3):139–144.

284. Rabowsky JH, Dukes AJ, Lee DA. Gonioscopic laser sclerostomy versus filtration surgery in a rabbit model. *Eye.* 1997;11(6):830–837.

285. Federman JL, Wilson RP, Ando F, et al. Contact laser: thermal sclerostomy ab interna. *Ophthalmic Surg.* 1987;18(10):726–727.
286. Higginbotham EJ, Kao G, Peyman G. Internal sclerostomy with the Nd:YAG contact laser versus thermal sclerostomy in rabbits. *Ophthalmology.* 1988;95(3):385–390.
287. Javitt JC, O'Connor SS, Wilson RP, et al. Laser sclerostomy ab interno using a continuous wave Nd:YAG laser. *Ophthalmic Surg.* 1989;20(8):552–556.
288. Wilson RP, Javitt JC. Ab interno laser sclerostomy in aphakic patients with glaucoma and chronic inflammation. *Am J Ophthalmol.* 1990;110(2):178–184.
289. Jaffe GJ, Mieler WF, Radius RL, et al. Ab interno sclerostomy with a high-powered argon endolaser. Clinicopathologic correlation. *Arch Ophthalmol.* 1989;107(8):1183–1185.
290. Adachi M, Ohya T, Hirata Y, et al. Internal sclerostomy with a high-powered argon laser [in Japanese]. *Nippon Ganka Gakkai Zasshi.* 1991;95(7):657–662.
291. Berlin MS, Rajacich G, Duffy M, et al. Excimer laser photoablation in glaucoma filtering surgery. *Am J Ophthalmol.* 1987;103(5):713–714.
292. Shields SR, Netland PA, Chu JL, et al. Transcorneal erbium laser sclerostomy: towards a guarded laser sclerostomy technique. *J Glaucoma.* 1995;4(6):391–397.
293. Karp CL, Higginbotham EJ, Edward DP, et al. Diode laser surgery. Ab interno and ab externo versus conventional surgery in rabbits. *Ophthalmology.* 1993;100(10):1567–1573.
294. Oram O, Gross RL, Severin TD, et al. Gonioscopic ab interno Nd:YLF laser sclerostomy in human cadaver eyes. *Ophthalmic Surg.* 1995;26(2):136–138.
295. Mizota A, Takasoh M, Kobayashi K, et al. Internal sclerostomy with the Er:YAG laser using a gradient-index (GRIN) endoscope. *Ophthalmic Surg Lasers.* 2002;33(3):214–220.
296. Ozler SA, Hill RA, Andrews JJ, et al. Infrared laser sclerostomies. *Invest Ophthalmol Vis Sci.* 1991;32(9):2498–2503.
297. Hill RA, Ozler SA, Baerveldt G, et al. Ab-interno neodymium:YAG versus erbium:YAG laser sclerostomies in a rabbit model. *Ophthalmic Surg.* 1992;23(3):192–197.
298. Huang S, Yu M, Feng G, et al. Histopathological study of trabeculum after excimer laser trabeculectomy ab interno. *Yan Ke Xue Bao.* 2001;17(1):11–15.
299. Vogel M, Lauritzen K. Selective excimer laser ablation of the trabecular meshwork. Clinical results [in German]. *Ophthalmologe.* 1997;94(9):665–667.
300. Brown RH, Denham DB, Bruner WE, et al. Internal sclerectomy for glaucoma filtering surgery with an automated trephine. *Arch Ophthalmol.* 1987;105(1):133–136.
301. Brown RH, Lynch MG, Denham DB, et al. Internal sclerectomy with an automated trephine for advanced glaucoma. *Ophthalmology.* 1988;95(6):728–734.
302. Au YK, Reynolds MD, Chadalavada R, et al. Bipolar cautery and internal thermal sclerostomy in a rabbit model. *Ophthalmic Surg.* 1992;23(3):188–191.
303. Brown SV, Higginbotham EJ, Griffin EO, et al. Ab-interno sclerostomy using a goniodiathermy instrument. *Ophthalmic Surg.* 1994;25(2):112–116.
304. Krasnov MM. Externalization of Schlemm's canal (sinusotomy) in glaucoma. *Br J Ophthalmol.* 1968;52(2):157–161.
305. Nesterov AP. Role of the blockade of Schlemm's canal in pathogenesis of primary open-angle glaucoma. *Am J Ophthalmol.* 1970;70(5):691–696.
306. Ellingsen BA, Grant WM. Trabeculotomy and sinusotomy in enucleated human eyes. *Invest Ophthalmol.* 1972;11(1):21–28.
307. Zimmerman TJ, Kooner KS, Ford VJ, et al. Trabeculectomy vs. nonpenetrating trabeculectomy: a retrospective study of two procedures in phakic patients with glaucoma. *Ophthalmic Surg.* 1984;15(9):734–740.
308. Weber PA, Keates RH, Opremcek EM, et al. Two-stage Neodymium-YAG laser trabeculotomy. *Ophthalmic Surg.* 1983;14(7):591–594.
309. Hara T. Deep sclerectomy with Nd:YAG laser trabeculotomy ab interno: two-stage procedure. *Ophthalmic Surg.* 1988;19(2):101–106.
310. Krasnov MM. Symposium: microsurgery of the outflow channels. Sinusotomy. Foundations, results, prospects. *Trans Am Acad Ophthalmol Otolaryngol.* 1972;76(2):368–374.
311. Kozlova T, Zagorski ZF, Rakowska E. A simplified technique for non-penetrating deep sclerectomy. *Eur J Ophthalmol.* 2002;12(3):188–192.
312. Chiou AG, Mermoud A, Underdahl JP, et al. An ultrasound biomicroscopic study of eyes after deep sclerectomy with collagen implant. *Ophthalmology.* 1998;105(4):746–750.
313. Sanchez E, Schnyder CC, Sickenberg M, et al. Deep sclerectomy: results with and without collagen implant. *Int Ophthalmol.* 1996;20(1–3):157–162.
314. Stegmann R, Pienaar A, Miller D. Viscocanalostomy for open-angle glaucoma in black African patients. *J Cataract Refract Surg.* 1999;25(3):316–322.
315. Khaw PT, Wells AP, Lim KS. Surgery for glaucoma. *Br J Ophthalmol.* 2003;87(4):517.
316. Tamm ER, Carassa RG, Albert DM, et al. Viscocanalostomy in rhesus monkeys. *Arch Ophthalmol.* 2004;122(12):1826–1838.
317. Carassa RG, Bettin P, Fiori M, et al. Viscocanalostomy: a pilot study. *Eur J Ophthalmol.* 1998;8(2):57–61.
318. Roters S, Luke C, Jonescu-Cuypers CP, et al. Ultrasound biomicroscopy and its value in predicting the long term outcome of viscocanalostomy. *Br J Ophthalmol.* 2002;86(9):997–1001.
319. Maldonado-Bas A, Maldonado-Junyent A. Filtering glaucoma surgery using an excimer laser. *J Cataract Refract Surg.* 2001;27(9):1402–1409.
320. Carassa RG, Bettin P, Fiori M, et al. Viscocanalostomy versus trabeculectomy in white adults affected by open-angle glaucoma: a 2-year randomized, controlled trial. *Ophthalmology.* 2003;110(5):882–887.
321. Yalvac IS, Sahin M, Eksioglu U, et al. Primary viscocanalostomy versus trabeculectomy for primary open-angle glaucoma: three- year prospective randomized clinical trial. *J Cataract Refract Surg.* 2004;30(10):2050–2057.
322. Lewis RA, von Wolff K, Tetz M, et al. Canaloplasty: circumferential viscodilation and tensioning of Schlemm canal using a flexible microcatheter for the treatment of open-angle glaucoma in adults: two-year interim clinical study results. *J Cataract Refract Surg.* 2009;35(5):814–824.
323. Levkovitch-Verbin H, Goldenfeld M, Melamed S. Fornix-based trabeculectomy with mitomycin-C. *Ophthalmic Surg Lasers.* 1997;28(10):818–822.
324. Brown SV. Management of a partial-thickness scleral-flap buttonhole during trabeculectomy. *Ophthalmic Surg.* 1994;25(10):732–733.
325. Petursson GJ, Fraunfelder FT. Repair of an inadvertent buttonhole or leaking filtering bleb. *Arch Ophthalmol.* 1979;97(5):926–927.
326. Awan KJ, Spaeth PG. Use of isobutyl-2-cyanoacrylate tissue adhesive in the repair of conjunctival fistula in filtering procedures for glaucoma. *Ann Ophthalmol.* 1974;6(8):851–853.
327. The Fluorouracil Filtering Surgery Study Group. Risk factors for suprachoroidal hemorrhage after filtering surgery. *Am J Ophthalmol.* 1992;113(5):501–507.
328. Speaker MG, Guerriero PN, Met JA, et al. A case-control study of risk factors for intraoperative suprachoroidal expulsive hemorrhage. *Ophthalmology.* 1991;98(2):202–209.
329. Bellows AR, Chylack LT Jr, Epstein DL, et al. Choroidal effusion during glaucoma surgery in patients with prominent episcleral vessels. *Arch Ophthalmol.* 1979;97(3):493–497.
330. Bellows AR, Chylack LT Jr, Hutchinson BT. Choroidal detachment. Clinical manifestation, therapy and mechanism of formation. *Ophthalmology.* 1981;88(11):1107–1115.
331. Swan KC, Lindgren TW. Unintentional lens injury in glaucoma surgery. *Trans Am Ophthalmol Soc.* 1980;78:55–69.
332. Kozart DM, Eagle RC Jr. Stripping of Descemet's membrane after glaucoma surgery. *Ophthalmic Surg.* 1981;12(6):420–423.
333. Riley SF, Smith TJ, Simmons RJ. Repair of a disinserted scleral flap in trabeculectomy. *Ophthalmic Surg.* 1993;24(5):349–350.
334. Riley SF, Lima FL, Smith TJ, et al. Using donor sclera to create a flap in glaucoma filtering procedures. *Ophthalmic Surg.* 1994;25(2):117–118.
335. Kao SF, Lichter PR, Musch DC. Anterior chamber depth following filtration surgery. *Ophthalmic Surg.* 1989;20(5):332–336.
336. Stewart WC, Shields MB. Management of anterior chamber depth after trabeculectomy. *Am J Ophthalmol.* 1988;106(1):41–44.
337. Fiore PM, Richter CU, Arzeno G, et al. The effect of anterior chamber depth on endothelial cell count after filtration surgery. *Arch Ophthalmol.* 1989;107(11):1609–1611.
338. Phillips CI, Clark CV, Levy AM. Posterior synechiae after glaucoma operations: aggravation by shallow anterior chamber and pilocarpine. *Br J Ophthalmol.* 1987;71(6):428–432.
339. Salvo EC Jr, Luntz MH, Medow NB. Use of viscoelastics post-trabeculectomy: a survey of members of the American Glaucoma Society. *Ophthalmic Surg Lasers.* 1999;30(4):271–275.
340. Kurtz S, Leibovitch I. Combined perfluoropropane gas and viscoelastic material injection for anterior chamber reformation following trabeculectomy. *Br J Ophthalmol.* 2002;86(11):1225–1227.
341. Zalta AH, Wieder RH. Closure of leaking filtering blebs with cyanoacrylate tissue adhesive. *Br J Ophthalmol.* 1991;75(3):170–173.
342. Graham SL, Goldberg I. Cyanoacrylate adhesive closure of wound leaks following fornix-based trabeculectomy with adjunct 5-fluorouracil. *J Glaucoma.* 1993;2(4):297–302.

343. Graham SL, Murray B, Goldberg I. Closure of fornix-based posttrabeculectomy conjunctival wound leaks with autologous fibrin glue. *Am J Ophthalmol.* 1992;114(2):221–222.

344. Asrani SG, Wilensky JT. Management of bleb leaks after glaucoma filtering surgery. Use of autologous fibrin tissue glue as an alternative. *Ophthalmology.* 1996;103(2):294–298.

345. Yieh FS, Lu DW, Wang HL, et al. The use of autologous fibrinogen concentrate in treating ocular hypotony after glaucoma filtration surgery. *J Ocul Pharmacol Ther.* 2001;17(5):443–448.

346. Cohen JS, Osher RH. Releasable suture in filtering and combined procedures. In: Sheilds MB, Pollack IP, Kolker AE, eds. *Perspectives in Glaucoma: Transactions of the First Scientific Meeting of the American Glaucoma Society.* Thorofare, NJ: Slack; 1988:157.

347. Stewart RH, Kimbrough RL. A method of managing flat anterior chamber following trabeculectomy. *Ophthalmic Surg.* 1980;11(6):382–383.

348. Franks WA, Hitchings RA. Intraocular gas injection in the treatment of cornea-lens touch and choroidal effusion following fistulizing surgery. *Ophthalmic Surg.* 1990;21(12):831–834.

349. Asamoto A, Yablonski ME. Posttrabeculectomy anterior subcapsular cataract formation induced by anterior chamber air. *Ophthalmic Surg.* 1993;24(5):314–319.

350. Lee DA, Wilson MR, Yoshizumi MO, et al. The ocular effects of gases when injected into the anterior chamber of rabbit eyes. *Arch Ophthalmol.* 1991;109(4):571–575.

351. Brubaker RF, Pederson JE. Ciliochoroidal detachment. *Surv Ophthalmol.* 1983;27(5):281–289.

352. Chylack LT Jr, Bellows AR. Molecular sieving in suprachoroidal fluid formation in man. *Invest Ophthalmol Vis Sci.* 1978;17(5):420–427.

353. Lavin M, Franks W, Hitchings RA. Serous retinal detachment following glaucoma filtering surgery. *Arch Ophthalmol.* 1990;108(11):1553–1555.

354. Stamper RL, McMenemy MG, Lieberman MF. Hypotonous maculopathy after trabeculectomy with subconjunctival 5-fluorouracil. *Am J Ophthalmol.* 1992;114(5):544–553.

355. Seah SK, Prata JA Jr, Minckler DS, et al. Hypotony following trabeculectomy. *J Glaucoma.* 1995;4(2):73–79.

356. Smith MF, Doyle JW. Use of oversized bandage soft contact lenses in the management of early hypotony following filtration surgery. *Ophthalmic Surg Lasers.* 1996;27(6):417–421.

357. Wise JB. Treatment of chronic postfiltration hypotony by intrableb injection of autologous blood. *Arch Ophthalmol.* 1993;111(6):827–830.

358. Nuyts RM, Greve EL, Geijssen HC, et al. Treatment of hypotonous maculopathy after trabeculectomy with mitomycin C. *Am J Ophthalmol.* 1994;118(3):322–331.

359. Leen MM, Moster MR, Katz LJ, et al. Management of overfiltering and leaking blebs with autologous blood injection. *Arch Ophthalmol.* 1995;113(8):1050–1055.

360. Smith MF, Magauran RG III, Betchkal J, et al. Treatment of postfiltration bleb leaks with autologous blood. *Ophthalmology.* 1995;102(6):868–871.

361. Chen PP, Palmberg PF, Culbertson WW, et al. Management of overfiltering and leaking blebs with autologous blood injection. *Arch Ophthalmol.* 1996;114(5):633–634.

362. Doyle JW, Smith MF, Garcia JA, et al. Injection of autologous blood for bleb leaks in New Zealand white rabbits. *Invest Ophthalmol Vis Sci.* 1996;37(11):2356–2361.

363. Okada K, Tsukamoto H, Masumoto M, et al. Autologous blood injection for marked overfiltration early after trabeculectomy with mitomycin C. *Acta Ophthalmol Scand.* 2001;79(3):305–308.

364. Haynes WL, Alward WL. Combination of autologous blood injection and bleb compression sutures to treat hypotony maculopathy. *J Glaucoma.* 1999;8(6):384–387.

365. Morgan JE, Diamond JP, Cook SD. Remodelling the filtration bleb. *Br J Ophthalmol.* 2002;86(8):872–875.

366. Choudhri SA, Herndon LW, Damji KF, et al. Efficacy of autologous blood injection for treating overfiltering or leaking blebs after glaucoma surgery. *Am J Ophthalmol.* 1997;123(4):554–555.

367. Burnstein A, WuDunn D, Ishii Y, et al. Autologous blood injection for late-onset filtering bleb leak. *Am J Ophthalmol.* 2001;132(1):36–40.

368. Siegfried CJ, Grewal RK, Karalekas D, et al. Marked intraocular pressure rise complicating intrableb autologous blood injection. *Arch Ophthalmol.* 1996;114(4):492–493.

369. Ayyala RS, Urban RC Jr, Krishnamurthy MS, et al. Corneal blood staining following autologous blood injection for hypotony maculopathy. *Ophthalmic Surg Lasers.* 1997;28(10):866–868.

370. Lu DW, Azuara-Blanco A, Katz LJ. Severe visual loss after autologous blood injection for mitomycin-C-associated hypotonous maculopathy. *Ophthalmic Surg Lasers.* 1997;28(3):244–245.

371. Flynn WJ, Rosen WJ, Campbell DG. Delayed hyphema and intravitreal blood following intrableb autologous blood injection after trabeculectomy. *Am J Ophthalmol.* 1997;124(1):115–116.

372. Ellong A, Mvogo CE, Bella-Hiag AL, et al. Autologous blood injections for treating hypotonies after trabeculectomy [in French]. *Sante.* 2001;11(4):273–276.

373. Zacchei AC, Palmberg PF, Mendosa A, et al. Compression sutures: a new treatment for leaking or painful filtering blebs [abstract 2032]. *Invest Ophthalmol Vis Sci.* 1996;37(4):S444.

374. Chen PP, Takahashi Y, Leen MM, et al. The effects of compression sutures on filtering blebs in rabbit eyes. *Ophthalmic Surg Lasers.* 1999;30(3):216–220.

375. Cohen SM, Flynn HW Jr, Palmberg PF, et al. Treatment of hypotony maculopathy after trabeculectomy. *Ophthalmic Surg Lasers.* 1995;26(5):435–441.

376. Haynes WL, Alward WL. Rapid visual recovery and long-term intraocular pressure control after donor scleral patch grafting for trabeculectomy-induced hypotony maculopathy. *J Glaucoma.* 1995;4(3):200–201.

377. Clune MJ, Shin DH, Olivier MM, et al. Partial-thickness scleral-patch graft in revision of trabeculectomy. *Am J Ophthalmol.* 1993;115(6):818–820.

378. Maruyama K, Shirato S. Efficacy and safety of transconjunctival scleral flap resuturing for hypotony after glaucoma filtering surgery. *Graefes Arch Clin Exp Ophthalmol.* 2008;246(12):1751–1756.

379. Gressel MG, Parrish RK II, Heuer DK. Delayed nonexpulsive suprachoroidal hemorrhage. *Arch Ophthalmol.* 1984;102(12):1757–1760.

380. Ruderman JM, Harbin TS Jr, Campbell DG. Postoperative suprachoroidal hemorrhage following filtration procedures. *Arch Ophthalmol.* 1986;104(2):201–205.

381. Givens K, Shields MB. Suprachoroidal hemorrhage after glaucoma filtering surgery. *Am J Ophthalmol.* 1987;103(5):689–694.

382. Canning CR, Lavin M, McCartney AC, et al. Delayed suprachoroidal haemorrhage after glaucoma operations. *Eye.* 1989;3(pt 3):327–331.

383. Chu TG, Green RL. Suprachoroidal hemorrhage. *Surv Ophthalmol.* 1999;43(6):471–486.

384. Rockwood EJ, Kalenak JW, Plotnik JL, et al. Prospective ultrasonographic evaluation of intraoperative and delayed postoperative suprachoroidal hemorrhage from glaucoma filtering surgery. *J Glaucoma.* 1995;4(1):16–24.

385. Tuli SS, WuDunn D, Ciulla TA, et al. Delayed suprachoroidal hemorrhage after glaucoma filtration procedures. *Ophthalmology.* 2001;108(10):1808–1811.

386. Okamoto F, Yamamoto N, Iguchi A, et al. High-frequency ultrasonographic imaging in suprachoroidal hemorrhage after filtering surgery. *Ophthalmic Surg Lasers Imaging.* 2003;34(3):259–262.

387. Chu TG, Cano MR, Green RL, et al. Massive suprachoroidal hemorrhage with central retinal apposition. A clinical and echographic study. *Arch Ophthalmol.* 1991;109(11):1575–1581.

388. Reynolds MG, Haimovici R, Flynn HW Jr, et al. Suprachoroidal hemorrhage. Clinical features and results of secondary surgical management. *Ophthalmology.* 1993;100(4):460–465.

389. Le Mer Y, Renard Y, Allagui M. Secondary management of suprachoroidal hemorrhages. *Graefes Arch Clin Exp Ophthalmol.* 1993;231(6):351–353.

390. Freeman WR, Schneiderman TE, Weinreb RN, et al. Hemorrhagic choroidal detachment with anterior vitreoretinal adhesions. *Ophthalmic Surg.* 1991;22(11):670–675.

391. Cheema RA, Choong YF, Algawi KD. Delayed suprachoroidal hemorrhage following viscocanalostomy. *Ophthalmic Surg Lasers Imaging.* 2003;34(3):209–211.

392. Lundy DC, Sidoti P, Winarko T, et al. Intracameral tissue plasminogen activator after glaucoma surgery. Indications, effectiveness, and complications. *Ophthalmology.* 1996;103(2):274–282.

393. Smith MF, Doyle JW. Use of tissue plasminogen activator to revive blebs following intraocular surgery. *Arch Ophthalmol.* 2001;119(6):809–812.

394. Traverso CE, Greenidge KC, Spaeth GL, et al. Focal pressure: a new method to encourage filtration after trabeculectomy. *Ophthalmic Surg.* 1984;15(1):62–65.

395. Pappa KS, Derick RJ, Weber PA, et al. Late argon laser suture lysis after mitomycin C trabeculectomy. *Ophthalmology.* 1993;100(8):1268–1271.

396. Haynes WL, Alward WL, McKinney JK. Low-energy argon laser suture lysis after trabeculectomy. *Am J Ophthalmol.* 1994;117(6):800–801.

397. Beck AD, Lynch MG, Noe R, et al. The use of a new laser lens holder for performing suture lysis in children. *Arch Ophthalmol.* 1995;113(2):140–141.

398. Morinelli EN, Sidoti PA, Heuer DK, et al. Laser suture lysis after mitomycin C trabeculectomy. *Ophthalmology.* 1996;103(2):306–314.

399. Singh J, Bell RW, Adams A, et al. Enhancement of post trabeculectomy bleb formation by laser suture lysis. *Br J Ophthalmol.* 1996;80(7):624–627.

400. Morris DA, Peracha MO, Shin DH, et al. Risk factors for early filtration failure requiring suture release after primary glaucoma triple procedure with adjunctive mitomycin. *Arch Ophthalmol.* 1999;117(9):1149–1154.

401. Bardak Y, Cuypers MH, Tilanus MA, et al. Ocular hypotony after laser suture lysis following trabeculectomy with mitomycin C. *Int Ophthalmol.* 1997;21(6):325–330.

402. Mudgil AV, To KW, Balachandran RM, et al. Relative efficacy of the argon green, argon blue-green, and krypton red lasers for 10-0 nylon subconjunctival laser suture lysis. *Ophthalmic Surg Lasers.* 1999;30(7):560–564.

403. Piltz JR, Starita RJ. The use of subconjunctivally administered tissue plasminogen activator after trabeculectomy. *Ophthalmic Surg.* 1994;25(1):51–53.

404. Feldman RM, Gross RL, Spaeth GL, et al. Risk factors for the development of Tenon's capsule cysts after trabeculectomy. *Ophthalmology.* 1989;96(3):336–341.

405. Sherwood MB, Spaeth GL, Simmons ST, et al. Cysts of Tenon's capsule following filtration surgery. Medical management. *Arch Ophthalmol.* 1987;105(11):1517–1521.

406. Scott DR, Quigley HA. Medical management of a high bleb phase after trabeculectomies. *Ophthalmology.* 1988;95(9):1169–1173.

407. Richter CU, Shingleton BJ, Bellows AR, et al. The development of encapsulated filtering blebs. *Ophthalmology.* 1988;95(9):1163–1168.

408. Schwartz AL, Van Veldhuisen PC, Gaasterland DE, et al. The Advanced Glaucoma Intervention Study (AGIS): 5. Encapsulated bleb after initial trabeculectomy. *Am J Ophthalmol.* 1999;127(1):8–19.

409. Mandal AK. Results of medical management and mitomycin C-augmented excisional bleb revision for encapsulated filtering blebs. *Ophthalmic Surg Lasers.* 1999;30(4):276–284.

410. Sherwood MB, Grierson I, Millar L, et al. Long-term morphologic effects of antiglaucoma drugs on the conjunctiva and Tenon's capsule in glaucomatous patients. *Ophthalmology.* 1989;96(3):327–335.

411. Ignjatovic Z, Misailovic K, Kuljaca Z. Encapsulated filtering blebs—incidence and methods of treatment [in Serbian]. *Srp Arh Celok Lek.* 2001;129(11–12):296–299.

412. Schoenleber DB, Bellows AR, Hutchinson BT. Failed laser trabeculoplasty requiring surgery in open-angle glaucoma. *Ophthalmic Surg.* 1987;18(11):796–799.

413. Campagna JA, Munden PM, Alward WL. Tenon's cyst formation after trabeculectomy with mitomycin C. *Ophthalmic Surg.* 1995;26(1):57–60.

414. Gutierrez Diaz E, Montero Rodriguez M, Julve San Martin A, et al. Incidence of encapsulated bleb after filtering surgery [in Spanish]. *Arch Soc Esp Oftalmol.* 2001;76(5):279–284.

415. Oh Y, Katz LJ, Spaeth GL, et al. Risk factors for the development of encapsulated filtering blebs. The role of surgical glove powder and 5-fluorouracil. *Ophthalmology.* 1994;101(4):629–634.

416. Azuara-Blanco A, Bond JB, Wilson RP, et al. Encapsulated filtering blebs after trabeculectomy with mitomycin-C. *Ophthalmic Surg Lasers.* 1997;28(10):805–809.

417. Shingleton BJ, Richter CU, Bellows AR, et al. Management of encapsulated filtration blebs. *Ophthalmology.* 1990;97(1):63–68.

418. Loftfield K, Ball SF. Filtering bleb encapsulation increased by steroid injection. *Ophthalmic Surg.* 1990;21(4):282–287.

419. Costa VP, Correa MM, Kara-Jose N. Needling versus medical treatment in encapsulated blebs. A randomized, prospective study. *Ophthalmology.* 1997;104(8):1215–1220.

420. Pederson JE, Smith SG. Surgical management of encapsulated filtering blebs. *Ophthalmology.* 1985;92(7):955–958.

421. Ewing RH, Stamper RL. Needle revision with and without 5-fluorouracil for the treatment of failed filtering blebs. *Am J Ophthalmol.* 1990;110(3):254–259.

422. Hodge W, Saheb N, Balazsi G, et al. Treatment of encapsulated blebs with 30-gauge needling and injection of low-dose 5-fluorouracil. *Can J Ophthalmol.* 1992;27(5):233–236.

423. Shin DH, Juzych MS, Khatana AK, et al. Needling revision of failed filtering blebs with adjunctive 5-fluorouracil. *Ophthalmic Surg.* 1993;24(4):242–248.

424. Allen LE, Manuchehri K, Corridan PG. The treatment of encapsulated trabeculectomy blebs in an out-patient setting using a needling technique and subconjunctival 5-fluorouracil injection. *Eye.* 1998;12(1):119–123.

425. Gracia Garcia-Miguel T, Gutierrez Diaz E, Montero Rodriguez M, et al. Management of encapsulated blebs after glaucoma drainage device surgery [in Spanish]. *Arch Soc Esp Oftalmol.* 2002;77(8):429–433.

426. Mazey BJ, Siegel MJ, Siegel LI, et al. Corneal endothelial toxic effect secondary to fluorouracil needle bleb revision. *Arch Ophthalmol.* 1994;112(11):1411.

427. Mardelli PG, Lederer CM Jr, Murray PL, et al. Slitlamp needle revision of failed filtering blebs using mitomycin C. *Ophthalmology.* 1996;103(11):1946–1955.

428. Iwach AG, Delgado MF, Novack GD, et al. Transconjunctival mitomycin-C in needle revisions of failing filtering blebs. *Ophthalmology.* 2003;110(4):734–742.

429. Ben-Simon GJ, Glovinsky Y. Needle revision of failed filtering blebs augmented with subconjunctival injection of mitomycin C. *Ophthalmic Surg Lasers Imaging.* 2003;34(2):94–99.

430. Van Buskirk EM. Cysts of Tenon's capsule following filtration surgery. *Am J Ophthalmol.* 1982;94(4):522–527.

431. Konstas AG, Jay JL. Modification of trabeculectomy to avoid postoperative hyphema. The 'guarded anterior fistula' operation. *Br J Ophthalmol.* 1992;76(6):353–357.

432. Soong HK, Quigley HA. Dellen associated with filtering blebs. *Arch Ophthalmol.* 1983;101(3):385–387.

433. O'Connell EJ, Karseras AG. Intraocular surgery in advanced glaucoma. *Br J Ophthalmol.* 1976;60(2):124–131.

434. Lawrence GA. Surgical treatment of patients with advanced glaucomatous field defects. *Arch Ophthalmol.* 1969;81(6):804–807.

435. Lichter PR, Ravin JG. Risks of sudden visual loss after glaucoma surgery. *Am J Ophthalmol.* 1974;78(6):1009–1013.

436. Costa VP, Smith M, Spaeth GL, et al. Loss of visual acuity after trabeculectomy. *Ophthalmology.* 1993;100(5):599–612.

437. Martinez JA, Brown RH, Lynch MG, et al. Risk of postoperative visual loss in advanced glaucoma. *Am J Ophthalmol.* 1993;115(3):332–337.

438. Aggarwal SP, Hendeles S. Risk of sudden visual loss following trabeculectomy in advanced primary open-angle glaucoma. *Br J Ophthalmol.* 1986;70(2):97–99.

439. Fechtner RD, Minckler D, Weinreb RN, et al. Complications of glaucoma surgery. Ocular decompression retinopathy. *Arch Ophthalmol.* 1992;110(7):965–968.

440. Cordido Carballido M, Alvarez Martinez E, Lopez Rodriguez I, et al. Ocular decompression retinopathy after trabeculectomy [in Spanish]. *Arch Soc Esp Oftalmol.* 2002;77(6):331–334.

441. Karadimas P, Papastathopoulos KI, Bouzas EA. Decompression retinopathy following filtration surgery. *Ophthalmic Surg Lasers.* 2002;33(2):175–176.

442. Danias J, Rosenbaum J, Podos SM. Diffuse retinal hemorrhages (ocular decompression syndrome) after trabeculectomy with mitomycin C for neovascular glaucoma. *Acta Ophthalmol Scand.* 2000;78(4):468–469.

443. Suzuki R, Nakayama M, Satoh N. Three types of retinal bleeding as a complication of hypotony after trabeculectomy. *Ophthalmologica.* 1999;213(2):135–138.

444. Dudley DF, Leen MM, Kinyoun JL, et al. Retinal hemorrhages associated with ocular decompression after glaucoma surgery. *Ophthalmic Surg Lasers.* 1996;27(2):147–150.

445. Hitchings RA, Grierson I. Clinico pathological correlation in eyes with failed fistulizing surgery. *Trans Ophthalmol Soc U K.* 1983;103(pt 1):84–88.

446. Ticho U, Ivry M. Reopening of occluded filtering blebs by argon laser photocoagulation. *Am J Ophthalmol.* 1977;84(3):413–418.

447. Van Buskirk EM. Reopening filtration fistulas with the argon laser. *Am J Ophthalmol.* 1982;94(1):1–3.

448. Latina MA, Rankin GA. Internal and transconjunctival neodymium:YAG laser revision of late failing filters. *Ophthalmology.* 1991;98(2):215–221.

449. Praeger DL. The reopening of closed filtering blebs using the neodymium:YAG laser. *Ophthalmology.* 1984;91(4):373–377.

450. Dailey RA, Samples JR, Van Buskirk EM. Reopening filtration fistulas with the neodymium-YAG laser. *Am J Ophthalmol.* 1986;102(4):491–495.

451. Oh Y, Katz LJ. Indications and technique for reopening closed filtering blebs using the Nd:YAG laser—a review and case series. *Ophthalmic Surg.* 1993;24(9):617–622.

452. Cohn HC, Whalen WR, Aron-Rosa D. YAG laser treatment in a series of failed trabeculectomies. *Am J Ophthalmol.* 1989;108(4):395–403.

453. Durcan FJ, Cioffi GA, Van Buskirk EM. Same-site revision of failed filtering blebs. *J Glaucoma.* 1992;1(1):2–6.

454. Hu CY, Matsuo H, Tomita G, et al. Clinical characteristics and leakage of functioning blebs after trabeculectomy with mitomycin-C in primary glaucoma patients. *Ophthalmology.* 2003;110(2):345–352.

455. Shaikh A, Ahmado A, James B. Severe cough: a cause of late bleb leak. *J Glaucoma.* 2003;12(2):181–183.

456. Loane ME, Galanopoulos A. The surgical management of leaking filtering blebs. *Curr Opin Ophthalmol.* 1999;10(2):121–125.

457. Matsuo H, Tomidokoro A, Suzuki Y, et al. Late-onset transconjunctival oozing and point leak of aqueous humor from filtering bleb after trabeculectomy. *Am J Ophthalmol.* 2002;133(4):456–462.

458. Blok MD, Kok JH, van Mil C, et al. Use of the Megasoft Bandage Lens for treatment of complications after trabeculectomy. *Am J Ophthalmol.* 1990;110(3):264–268.

459. Gammon RR, Prum BE Jr, Avery N, et al. Rapid preparation of small-volume autologous fibrinogen concentrate and its same day use in bleb leaks after glaucoma filtration surgery. *Ophthalmic Surg Lasers.* 1998;29(12):1010–1012.

460. Myers JS, Yang CB, Herndon LW, et al. Excisional bleb revision to correct overfiltration or leakage. *J Glaucoma.* 2000;9(2):169–173.

461. Burnstein AL, WuDunn D, Knotts SL, et al. Conjunctival advancement versus nonincisional treatment for late-onset glaucoma filtering bleb leaks. *Ophthalmology.* 2002;109(1):71–75.

462. Hamard P, Tazartes M, Ayed T, et al. Prognostic outcome of leaking filtering blebs reconstruction with rotational conjunctival flaps [in French]. *J Fr Ophtalmol.* 2001;24(5):482–490.

463. Miyazawa D, Kondo T. Free conjunctival autograft harvested from the fornix for repair of leaking blebs. *Br J Ophthalmol.* 2000;84(4):440–441.

464. Wadhwani RA, Bellows AR, Hutchinson BT. Surgical repair of leaking filtering blebs. *Ophthalmology.* 2000;107(9):1681–1687.

465. Sinnreich Z, Barishak R, Stein R. Leaking filtering blebs. *Am J Ophthalmol.* 1978;86(3):345–349.

466. Morris DA, Ramocki JM, Shin DH, et al. Use of autologous Tenon's capsule and scleral patch grafts for repair of excessively draining fistulas with leaking filtering blebs. *J Glaucoma.* 1998;7(6):417–419.

467. Kosmin AS, Wishart PK. A full-thickness scleral graft for the surgical management of a late filtration bleb leak. *Ophthalmic Surg Lasers.* 1997;28(6):461–468.

468. Zhong Y, Zhou Y, Wang K. Effect of amniotic membrane on filtering bleb after trabeculectomy in rabbit eyes [in Chinese]. *Yan Ke Xue Bao.* 2000;16(2):73–76, 83.

469. Barton K, Budenz DL, Khaw PT, et al. Glaucoma filtration surgery using amniotic membrane transplantation. *Invest Ophthalmol Vis Sci.* 2001;42(8):1762–1768.

470. Kee C, Hwang JM. Amniotic membrane graft for late-onset glaucoma filtering leaks. *Am J Ophthalmol.* 2002;133(6):834–835.

471. Budenz DL, Barton K, Tseng SC. Amniotic membrane transplantation for repair of leaking glaucoma filtering blebs. *Am J Ophthalmol.* 2000;130(5):580–588.

472. Lin HY, Wu KY. Tentative surgical repair of leaking filtering bleb with amniotic membrane transplantation—a case report. *Kaohsiung J Med Sci.* 2001;17(9):495–498.

473. Brown RH, Yang LH, Walker SD, et al. Treatment of bleb infection after glaucoma surgery. *Arch Ophthalmol.* 1994;112(1):57–61.

474. Ayyala RS, Bellows AR, Thomas JV, et al. Bleb infections: clinically different courses of "blebitis" and endophthalmitis. *Ophthalmic Surg Lasers.* 1997;28(6):452–460.

475. Poulsen EJ, Allingham RR. Characteristics and risk factors of infections after glaucoma filtering surgery. *J Glaucoma.* 2000;9(6):438–443.

476. Mochizuki K, Jikihara S, Ando Y, et al. Incidence of delayed onset infection after trabeculectomy with adjunctive mitomycin C or 5-fluorouracil treatment. *Br J Ophthalmol.* 1997;81(10):877–883.

477. Ashkenazi I, Melamed S, Avni I, et al. Risk factors associated with late infection of filtering blebs and endophthalmitis. *Ophthalmic Surg.* 1991;22(10):570–574.

478. Jampel HD, Quigley HA, Kerrigan-Baumrind LA, et al. Risk factors for late-onset infection following glaucoma filtration surgery. *Arch Ophthalmol.* 2001;119(7):1001–1008.

479. Ciulla TA, Beck AD, Topping TM, et al. Blebitis, early endophthalmitis, and late endophthalmitis after glaucoma-filtering surgery. *Ophthalmology.* 1997;104(6):986–995.

480. Reynolds AC, Skuta GL, Monlux R, et al. Management of blebitis by members of the American Glaucoma Society: a survey. *J Glaucoma.* 2001;10(4):340–347.

481. Fiscella RG, Nguyen TK, Cwik MJ, et al. Aqueous and vitreous penetration of levofloxacin after oral administration. *Ophthalmology.* 1999;106(12):2286–2290.

482. Katz LJ, Cantor LB, Spaeth GL. Complications of surgery in glaucoma. Early and late bacterial endophthalmitis following glaucoma filtering surgery. *Ophthalmology.* 1985;92(7):959–963.

483. Aaberg TM Jr, Flynn HW Jr, Schiffman J, et al. Nosocomial acute-onset postoperative endophthalmitis survey. A 10-year review of incidence and outcomes. *Ophthalmology.* 1998;105(6):1004–1010.

484. Eifrig CW, Flynn HW Jr, Scott IU, et al. Acute-onset postoperative endophthalmitis: review of incidence and visual outcomes (1995–2001). *Ophthalmic Surg Lasers.* 2002;33(5):373–378.

485. Freedman J, Gupta M, Bunke A. Endophthalmitis after trabeculectomy. *Arch Ophthalmol.* 1978;96(6):1017–1018.

486. Bindlish R, Condon GP, Schlosser JD, et al. Efficacy and safety of mitomycin-C in primary trabeculectomy: five-year follow-up. *Ophthalmology.* 2002;109(7):1336–1341; discussion 1341–1342.

487. DeBry PW, Perkins TW, Heatley G, et al. Incidence of late-onset bleb-related complications following trabeculectomy with mitomycin. *Arch Ophthalmol.* 2002;120(3):297–300.

488. Greenfield DS, Suner IJ, Miller MP, et al. Endophthalmitis after filtering surgery with mitomycin. *Arch Ophthalmol.* 1996;114(8):943–949.

489. Higginbotham EJ, Stevens RK, Musch DC, et al. Bleb-related endophthalmitis after trabeculectomy with mitomycin C. *Ophthalmology.* 1996;103(4):650–656.

490. Ticho U, Ophir A. Late complications after glaucoma filtering surgery with adjunctive 5-fluorouracil. *Am J Ophthalmol.* 1993;115(4):506–510.

491. Solomon A, Ticho U, Frucht-Pery J. Late-onset, bleb-associated endophthalmitis following glaucoma filtering surgery with or without antifibrotic agents. *J Ocul Pharmacol Ther.* 1999;15(4):283–293.

492. Lehmann OJ, Bunce C, Matheson MM, et al. Risk factors for development of post-trabeculectomy endophthalmitis. *Br J Ophthalmol.* 2000;84(12):1349–1353.

493. Mac I, Soltau JB. Glaucoma-filtering bleb infections. *Curr Opin Ophthalmol.* 2003;14(2):91–94.

494. Kangas TA, Greenfield DS, Flynn HW Jr, et al. Delayed-onset endophthalmitis associated with conjunctival filtering blebs. *Ophthalmology.* 1997;104(5):746–752.

495. Song A, Scott IU, Flynn HW Jr, et al. Delayed-onset bleb-associated endophthalmitis: clinical features and visual acuity outcomes. *Ophthalmology.* 2002;109(5):985–991.

496. Beck AD, Grossniklaus HE, Hubbard B, et al. Pathologic findings in late endophthalmitis after glaucoma filtering surgery. *Ophthalmology.* 2000;107(11):2111–2114.

497. Akova YA, Bulut S, Dabil H, et al. Late bleb-related endophthalmitis after trabeculectomy with mitomycin C. *Ophthalmic Surg Lasers.* 1999;30(2):146–151.

498. Strmen P, Hlavackova K, Ferkova S, et al. Endophthalmitis after intraocular interventions [in German]. *Klin Monatsbl Augenheilkd.* 1997;211(4):245–249.

499. Waheed S, Ritterband DC, Greenfield DS, et al. New patterns of infecting organisms in late bleb-related endophthalmitis: a ten year review. *Eye.* 1998;12(6):910–915.

500. Lobue TD, Deutsch TA, Stein RM. *Moraxella nonliquefaciens* endophthalmitis after trabeculectomy. *Am J Ophthalmol.* 1985;99(3):343–345.

501. Berrocal AM, Scott IU, Miller D, et al. Endophthalmitis caused by *Moraxella* species. *Am J Ophthalmol.* 2001;132(5):788–790.

502. Laukeland H, Bergh K, Bevanger L. Posttrabeculectomy endophthalmitis caused by *Moraxella nonliquefaciens. J Clin Microbiol.* 2002;40(7):2668–2770.

503. Lipman RM, Deutsch TA. Late-onset *Moraxella catarrhalis* endophthalmitis after filtering surgery. *Can J Ophthalmol.* 1992;27(5):249–250.

504. Wang MX, Shen DJ, Liu JC, et al. Recurrent fungal keratitis and endophthalmitis. *Cornea.* 2000;19(4):558–560.

505. Saperstein DA, Bennett MD, Steinberg JP, et al. Exogenous *Neisseria meningitidis* endophthalmitis. *Am J Ophthalmol.* 1997;123(1):135–136.

506. Phillips WB II, Wong TP, Bergren RL, et al. Late onset endophthalmitis associated with filtering blebs. *Ophthalmic Surg.* 1994;25(2):88–91.

507. Del Piero E, Pennett M, Leopold I. *Pseudomonas cepacia* endophthalmitis. *Ann Ophthalmol.* 1985;17(12):753–756.

508. Eifrig CW, Scott IU, Flynn HW Jr, et al. Endophthalmitis caused by *Pseudomonas aeruginosa. Ophthalmology.* 2003;110(9):1714–1717.

509. Lebowitz D, Gurses-Ozden R, Rothman RF, et al. Late-onset bleb-related panophthalmitis with orbital abscess caused by *Pseudomonas stutzeri. Arch Ophthalmol.* 2001;119(11):1723–1725.

510. Krzystolik MG, Ciulla TA, Topping TM, et al. Exogenous *Aspergillus niger* endophthalmitis in a patient with a filtering bleb. *Retina.* 1997;17(5):461–462.

511. Coleman AL, Yu F, Greenland S. Factors associated with elevated complication rates after partial-thickness or full-thickness glaucoma surgical procedures in the United States during 1994. *Ophthalmology.* 1998;105(7):1165–1169.

512. Mandelbaum S, Forster RK, Gelender H, et al. Late onset endophthalmitis associated with filtering blebs. *Ophthalmology.* 1985;92(7):964–972.

513. Kanski JJ. Treatment of late endophthalmitis associated with filtering blebs. *Arch Ophthalmol.* 1974;91(5):339–343.

514. Stern GA, Engel HM, Driebe WT Jr. The treatment of postoperative endophthalmitis. Results of differing approaches to treatment. *Ophthalmology.* 1989;96(1):62–67.

515. Olk RJ, Bohigian GM. The management of endophthalmitis: diagnostic and therapeutic guidelines including the use of vitrectomy. *Ophthalmic Surg.* 1987;18(4):262–267.

516. Endophthalmitis Vitrectomy Study Group. Results of the Endophthalmitis Vitrectomy Study. A randomized trial of immediate vitrectomy and of intravenous antibiotics for the treatment of postoperative bacterial endophthalmitis. *Arch Ophthalmol.* 1995;113(12):1479–1496.

517. Sugar HS. Postoperative cataract in successfully filtering glaucomatous eyes. *Am J Ophthalmol.* 1970;69(5):740–746.

518. Chauvaud D, Clay-Fressinet C, Pouliquen Y, et al. Opacification of the crystalline lens after trabeculectomy. Study of 95 cases [in French]. *Arch Ophthalmol (Paris).* 1976;36(5):379–386.

519. Vesti E. Development of cataract after trabeculectomy. *Acta Ophthalmol.* 1993;71(6):777–781.

520. The AGIS Investigators. The Advanced Glaucoma Intervention Study: 8. Risk of cataract formation after trabeculectomy. *Arch Ophthalmol.* 2001;119(12):1771–1779.

521. Musch DC, Gillespie BW, Niziol LM, et al. Cataract extraction in the collaborative initial glaucoma treatment study: incidence, risk factors, and the effect of cataract progression and extraction on clinical and quality-of-life outcomes. *Arch Ophthalmol.* 2006;124(12):1694–1700.

522. Fink AJ, Boys-Smith JW, Brear R. Management of large filtering blebs with the argon laser. *Am J Ophthalmol.* 1986;101(6):695–699.

523. Scheie HG, Guehl JJ III. Surgical management of overhanging blebs after filtering procedures. *Arch Ophthalmol.* 1979;97(2):325–326.

524. Lanzl IM, Katz LJ, Shindler RL, et al. Surgical management of the symptomatic overhanging filtering bleb. *J Glaucoma.* 1999;8(4):247–249.

525. La Borwit SE, Quigley HA, Jampel HD. Bleb reduction and bleb repair after trabeculectomy. *Ophthalmology.* 2000;107(4):712–718.

526. El-Harazi SM, Fellman RL, Feldman RM, et al. Bleb window cryopexy for the management of oversized, misplaced blebs. *J Glaucoma.* 2001;10(1):47–50.

527. Harris LS, Galin MA. Delayed spontaneous hyphema following successful sclerotomy with cautery in three patients. *Am J Ophthalmol.* 1971;72(2):458–459.

528. Namba H. Blood reflux into anterior chamber after trabeculectomy. *Jpn J Ophthalmol.* 1983;27:616–625.

529. Wilensky JT. Late hyphema after filtering surgery for glaucoma. *Ophthalmic Surg.* 1983;14(3):227–228.

530. Berke SJ, Bellows AR, Shingleton BJ, et al. Chronic and recurrent choroidal detachment after glaucoma filtering surgery. *Ophthalmology.* 1987;94(2):154–162.

531. Burney EN, Quigley HA, Robin AL. Hypotony and choroidal detachment as late complications of trabeculectomy. *Am J Ophthalmol.* 1987;103(5):685–688.

532. Vela MA, Campbell DG. Hypotony and ciliochoroidal detachment following pharmacologic aqueous suppressant therapy in previously filtered patients. *Ophthalmology.* 1985;92(1):50–57.

533. Laatikainen L, Syrdalen P. Tearing of retinal pigment epithelium after glaucoma surgery. *Graefes Arch Clin Exp Ophthalmol.* 1987;225(4):308–310.

534. Gagnon MM, Boisjoly HM, Brunette I, et al. Corneal endothelial cell density in glaucoma. *Cornea.* 1997;16(3):314–318.

535. Inoue K, Okugawa K, Oshika T, et al. Morphological study of corneal endothelium and corneal thickness in exfoliation syndrome. *Jpn J Ophthalmol.* 2003;47(3):235–239.

536. Smith DL, Skuta GL, Lindenmuth KA, et al. The effect of glaucoma filtering surgery on corneal endothelial cell density. *Ophthalmic Surg.* 1991;22(5):251–255.

537. Pastor SA, Williams R, Hetherington J, et al. Corneal endothelial cell loss following trabeculectomy with mitomycin C. *J Glaucoma.* 1993;2(2):112–113.

538. Fukuchi T, Hayakawa Y, Hara H, et al. Corneal endothelial damage after trabeculectomy with mitomycin C in two patients with glaucoma with cornea guttata. *Cornea.* 2002;21(3):300–304.

539. Rosen WJ, Mannis MJ, Brandt JD. The effect of trabeculectomy on corneal topography. *Ophthalmic Surg.* 1992;23(6):395–398.

540. Hugkulstone CE. Changes in keratometry following trabeculectomy. *Br J Ophthalmol.* 1991;75(4):217–218.

541. Pires RT, Chokshi A, Tseng SC. Amniotic membrane transplantation or conjunctival limbal autograft for limbal stem cell deficiency induced by 5-fluorouracil in glaucoma surgeries. *Cornea.* 2000;19(3):284–287.

542. Putterman AM, Urist MJ. Upper eyelid retraction after glaucoma filtering procedures. *Ann Ophthalmol.* 1975;7(2):263–266.

543. Song MS, Shin DH, Spoor TC. Incidence of ptosis following trabeculectomy: a comparative study. *Korean J Ophthalmol.* 1996;10(2):97–103.

544. Shammas HF, Zubyk NA, Stanfield TF. Sympathetic uveitis following glaucoma surgery. *Arch Ophthalmol.* 1977;95(4):638–641.

545. Scherer V, Schmidbauer J, Kasmann-Kellner B, et al. Increased glare and distorted vision. Sympathetic ophthalmia after glaucoma surgery with uveal trauma [in German]. *Ophthalmologe.* 2000;97(12):896–897.

546. Drance SM, Vargas E. Trabeculectomy and thermosclerectomy: a comparison of two procedures. *Can J Ophthalmol.* 1973;8(3):413–415.

547. Lewis RA, Phelps CD. Trabeculectomy v thermosclerostomy. A five-year follow-up. *Arch Ophthalmol.* 1984;102(4):533–536.

548. Spaeth GL, Joseph NH, Fernandes E. Trabeculectomy: a reevaluation after three years and a comparison with Scheie's procedure. *Trans Sect Ophthalmol Am Acad Ophthalmol Otolaryngol.* 1975;79(2):OP349–OP361.

549. Spaeth GL, Poryzees E. A comparison between peripheral iridectomy with thermal sclerostomy and trabeculectomy: a controlled study. *Br J Ophthalmol.* 1981;65(11):783–789.

550. Watkins PH Jr, Brubaker RF. Comparison of partial-thickness and full-thickness filtration procedures in open-angle glaucoma. *Am J Ophthalmol.* 1978;86(6):756–761.

551. Blondeau P, Phelps CD. Trabeculectomy vs thermosclerostomy. A randomized prospective clinical trial. *Arch Ophthalmol.* 1981;99(5):810–816.

552. Wilson MR. Posterior lip sclerectomy vs trabeculectomy in West Indian blacks. *Arch Ophthalmol.* 1989;107(11):1604–1608.

553. Wilson P. Trabeculectomy: long-term follow-up. *Br J Ophthalmol.* 1977;61(8):535–538.

554. D'Ermo F, Bonomi L, Doro D. A critical analysis of the long-term results of trabeculectomy. *Am J Ophthalmol.* 1979;88(5):829–835.

555. Zaidi AA. Trabeculectomy: a review and 4-year follow-up. *Br J Ophthalmol.* 1980;64(6):436–439.

556. Jerndal T, Lundstrom M. 330 trabeculectomies. A long time study (3–5 1/2 years). *Acta Ophthalmol.* 1980;58(6):947–956.

557. Mills KB. Trabeculectomy: a retrospective long-term follow-up of 444 cases. *Br J Ophthalmol.* 1981;65(11):790–795.

558. Inaba Z. Long-term results of trabeculectomy in the Japanese: an analysis by life-table method. *Jpn J Ophthalmol.* 1982;26(4):361–373.

559. Popovic V, Sjostrand J. Long-term outcome following trabeculectomy: I Retrospective analysis of intraocular pressure regulation and cataract formation. *Acta Ophthalmol.* 1991;69(3):299–304.

560. Akafo SK, Goulstine DB, Rosenthal AR. Long-term post trabeculectomy intraocular pressures. *Acta Ophthalmol.* 1992;70(3):312–316.

561. Nouri-Mahdavi K, Brigatti L, Weitzman M, et al. Outcomes of trabeculectomy for primary open-angle glaucoma. *Ophthalmology.* 1995;102(12):1760–1769.

562. Popovic V, Sjostrand J. Long-term outcome following trabeculectomy: II Visual field survival. *Acta Ophthalmol.* 1991;69(3):305–309.

563. Tornqvist G, Drolsum LK. Trabeculectomies. A long-term study. *Acta Ophthalmol.* 1991;69(4):450–454.

564. Mietz H, Jacobi PC, Welsandt G, et al. Trabeculectomies in fellow eyes have an increased risk of tenon's capsule cysts. *Ophthalmology.* 2002;109(5):992–997.

565. Kobayashi H, Kobayashi K, Okinami S. A comparison of the intraocular pressure-lowering effect and safety of viscocanalostomy and trabeculectomy with mitomycin C in bilateral open-angle glaucoma. *Graefes Arch Clin Exp Ophthalmol.* 2003;241(5):359–366.

566. Jonescu-Cuypers C, Jacobi P, Konen W, et al. Primary viscocanalostomy versus trabeculectomy in white patients with open-angle glaucoma: a randomized clinical trial. *Ophthalmology.* 2001;108(2):254–258.

567. O'Brart DP, Rowlands E, Islam N, et al. A randomised, prospective study comparing trabeculectomy augmented with antimetabolites with a viscocanalostomy technique for the management of open angle glaucoma uncontrolled by medical therapy. *Br J Ophthalmol.* 2002;86(7):748–754.

568. Chiselita D. Non-penetrating deep sclerectomy versus trabeculectomy in primary open-angle glaucoma surgery. *Eye.* 2001;15(pt 2):197–201.

569. Di Staso S, Taverniti L, Genitti G, et al. Combined phacoemulsification and deep sclerectomy vs phacoemulsification and trabeculectomy. *Acta Ophthalmol Scand Suppl.* 2000;(232):59–60.

570. Gianoli F, Schnyder CC, Bovey E, et al. Combined surgery for cataract and glaucoma: phacoemulsification and deep sclerectomy compared with phacoemulsification and trabeculectomy. *J Cataract Refract Surg.* 1999;25(3):340–346.

571. Ambresin A, Shaarawy T, Mermoud A. Deep sclerectomy with collagen implant in one eye compared with trabeculectomy in the other eye of the same patient. *J Glaucoma.* 2002;11(3):214–220.

572. Mermoud A, Schnyder CC, Sickenberg M, et al. Comparison of deep sclerectomy with collagen implant and trabeculectomy in open-angle glaucoma. *J Cataract Refract Surg.* 1999;25(3):323–331.

573. Sanchez E, Schnyder CC, Mermoud A. Comparative results of deep sclerectomy transformed to trabeculectomy and classical trabeculectomy [in French]. *Klin Monatsbl Augenheilkd.* 1997;210(5):261–264.

574. Freedman J, Shen E, Ahrens M. Trabeculectomy in a Black American glaucoma population. *Br J Ophthalmol.* 1976;60(8):573–574.

575. Ferguson JG Jr, Macdonald R Jr. Trabeculectomy in blacks: a two-year follow-up. *Ophthalmic Surg.* 1977;8(6):41–43.

576. David R, Freedman J, Luntz MH. Comparative study of Watson's and Cairns's trabeculectomies in a Black population with open angle glaucoma. *Br J Ophthalmol.* 1977;61(2):117–119.

577. BenEzra D, Chirambo MC. Trabeculectomy. *Ann Ophthalmol.* 1978; 10(8):1101–1105.

578. Stewart WC, Reid KK, Pitts RA. The results of trabeculectomy surgery in African-American versus white glaucoma patients. *J Glaucoma.* 1993; 2(4):236–240.

579. Miller RD, Barber JC. Trabeculectomy in black patients. *Ophthalmic Surg.* 1981;12(1):46–50.

580. Broadway D, Grierson I, Hitchings R. Racial differences in the results of glaucoma filtration surgery: are racial differences in the conjunctival cell profile important? *Br J Ophthalmol.* 1994;78(6):466–475.

581. Thommy CP, Bhar IS. Trabeculectomy in Nigerian patients with open-angle glaucoma. *Br J Ophthalmol.* 1979;63(9):636–642.

582. Sandford-Smith JH. The surgical treatment of open-angle glaucoma in Nigerians. *Br J Ophthalmol.* 1978;62(5):283–286.

583. Bakker NJ, Manku SI. Trabeculectomy versus Scheie's operation: a comparative retrospective study in open-angle glaucoma in Kenyans. *Br J Ophthalmol.* 1979;63(9):643–645.

584. Kietzman B. Glaucoma surgery in Nigerian eyes: a five-year study. *Ophthalmic Surg.* 1976;7(4):52–58.

585. Cadera W, Pachtman MA, Cantor LB, et al. Filtering surgery in childhood glaucoma. *Ophthalmic Surg.* 1984;15(4):319–322.

586. Stewart RH, Kimbrough RL, Bachh H, et al. Trabeculectomy and modifications of trabeculectomy. *Ophthalmic Surg.* 1979;10(1):76–80.

587. Kolozsvari L. Trabeculectomy in buphthalmos [in German]. *Klin Monatsbl Augenheilkd.* 1983;183(6):503–506.

588. Gressel MG, Heuer DK, Parrish RK II. Trabeculectomy in young patients. *Ophthalmology.* 1984;91(10):1242–1246.

589. Beauchamp GR, Parks MM. Filtering surgery in children: barriers to success. *Ophthalmology.* 1979;86(1):170–180.

590. Costa VP, Katz LJ, Spaeth GL, et al. Primary trabeculectomy in young adults. *Ophthalmology.* 1993;100(7):1071–1076.

591. Sturmer J, Broadway DC, Hitchings RA. Young patient trabeculectomy. Assessment of risk factors for failure. *Ophthalmology.* 1993;100(6): 928–939.

592. O'Reilly J, Lanigan B, O'Keefe M. Long-term visual results following primary trabeculectomy for infantile glaucoma. *Acta Ophthalmol Scand.* 2001;79(5):472–475.

593. Wallace DK, Plager DA, Snyder SK, et al. Surgical results of secondary glaucomas in childhood. *Ophthalmology.* 1998;105(1):101–111.

594. Levene RZ. Glaucoma filtering surgery factors that determine pressure control. *Trans Am Ophthalmol Soc.* 1984;82:282–301.

595. Heuer DK, Gressel MG, Parrish RK II, et al. Trabeculectomy in aphakic eyes. *Ophthalmology.* 1984;91(9):1045–1051.

596. Salmon JF. The role of trabeculectomy in the treatment of advanced chronic angle-closure glaucoma. *J Glaucoma.* 1993;2(4):285–290.

39

Glaucoma Drainage-Device Surgery

In an attempt to maintain patency of a drainage fistula in glaucoma filtering operations, a wide variety of foreign materials have been implanted in the eye, extending from the anterior chamber to a subconjunctival space. These were once referred to as setons, because the implants consisted of solid structures, such as threads, wires, or hairs, that were placed in a wound to form a drainage, permitting aqueous to run alongside the surface of the inserted material. These procedures were uniformly unsuccessful in maintaining a patent fistula. Most devices use tubes that drain aqueous out of the eye to external reservoirs and have been clinically beneficial. This chapter reviews the most commonly used drainage implant devices, the surgical techniques of implantation, the complications and

their management, and the comparative merits and indications for this group of glaucoma surgical procedures.

PHYSIOLOGY OF DRAINAGE IMPLANTS

Most current drainage implant devices (**Fig. 39.1**) have the same basic design, which typically consists of a silicone tube that extends from the anterior chamber (or, in some cases, the vitreous cavity) to a plate, disc, or encircling element beneath conjunctiva and Tenon capsule. The edge of the external plate has a ridge, through which the distal end of the tube inserts onto the upper surface of the plate. The ridge decreases

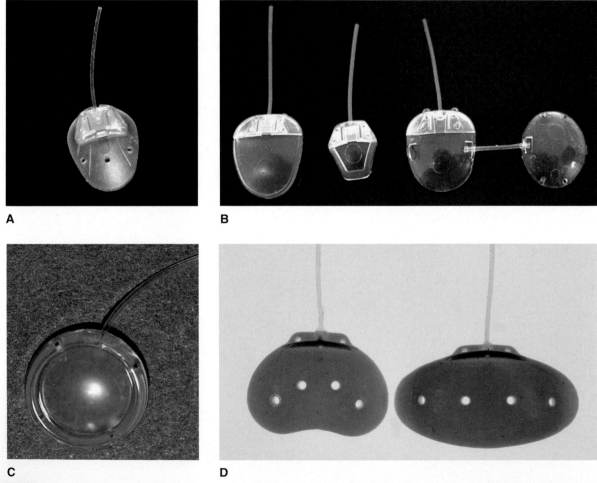

A

B

C

D

Figure 39.1　Examples of glaucoma drainage devices. **A:** Ahmed FP-7 (silicone). **B:** Ahmed S2 (polypropylene; image shown at *left*), S3 pediatric (polypropylene; *middle*), and B1 (polypropylene—double plate; *right*). **C:** Single-plate Molteno device. **D:** Baerveldt 250 mm^2 (*left*) and 350 mm^2 (*right*).

the risk for obstruction of the posterior opening of the tube with the surrounding tissue and fibrous capsule. The plates of the glaucoma drainage devices have large surface areas and promote the formation of the filtering bleb posteriorly, near the equator.

The mechanism by which drainage implant devices control the intraocular pressure (IOP) relates to a fibrous capsule that forms a filtering bleb around the external portion of the draining device and, to some degree, the surface area of the implant plate. The morphology of this filtering bleb differs from that of the blebs seen after trabeculectomy.

After insertion of the drainage device, a thin collagenous capsule, surrounded by a granulomatous reaction, is present at 1 month. The granulomatous reaction resolves after 4 months, capsule thickness remains relatively stable, and the collagen stroma becomes less compact. The fibrous capsule matures over time and becomes thinner after 6 months in rabbit eyes (1). Although the bleb histology in the rabbit model is similar to that of humans and other primates, the eventual development of a fibroblastic inner lining in the rabbit model differs from that in humans, in whom the inner lining remains only as a meshwork of collagen-like bundles at some areas of the inner bleb wall (1,2). Even though the filtering bleb around the implant is lined with a thick layer of connective tissue, microcystic spaces within that layer, seen on light and electron microscopy, may serve as the channels for aqueous drainage (2). Studies of monkey eyes with single-plate Molteno implants indicate that the capsule functions by a passive mechanism, shunting the flow of aqueous humor to the surrounding orbital tissues (3). All surfaces of the fibrous capsule contribute to filtration, which is consistent with echographic studies in human eyes that reveal bleb formation on both sides of the plate in successful cases (4). Histopathologic study of human eyes enucleated 2 to 6 years after Molteno implant surgery revealed patent tubes with no appreciable anterior chamber reaction and minimal inflammatory reaction in the outer layers of the bleb wall (5).

Measurement of the flow resistance using modified Baerveldt plates in rabbits showed a direct relationship between the surface area of the implants and the filtering capacity of their surrounding capsule (6). At the same time, reduction of the bleb diameter decreases surface tension on the bleb, capsular fibrosis, and thickness, which increases the effectiveness of the filtering surface (7,8).

Drainage devices with open tubes are likely to be complicated by early postoperative hypotony and therefore require temporary closure with a ligature or stent. The vast majority of glaucoma drainage devices develop an elevated IOP in the weeks to months after implantation as a result of capsule formation around the implant plate. This is frequently termed the hypertensive phase (9,10).

The filtering bleb may fail after surgery due to the increased thickness of fibrous capsule around the drainage implant. Movement of the drainage plate against the scleral surface may be the mechanism of glaucoma implant failure resulting from the stimulation of the low-level wound healing response, increased collagen scar formation, and increased fibrous capsule thickness (11).

IMPLANT DESIGNS

Performance of similar drainage devices can vary significantly, depending on the standards in manufacturing. This causes a wide range of clinical outcomes and indicates a strong need for enhanced quality-control procedures in the device-manufacturing process (12). The glaucoma drainage devices also differ according to the size, shape, and materials from which the external component and tube are constructed. External portions of glaucoma drainage devices are made from materials that prevent fibroblast adherence. Different materials may influence the amount of inflammation in surrounding tissues. Polypropylene, used in some Ahmed and Molteno implants, may produce more inflammation than the silicone used in Baerveldt, Krupin, and Ahmed devices. Flexible plates caused less inflammation in the subconjunctival space of rabbit eyes than in the rigid ones (13,14).

Alternative materials, such as hydroxylapatite (15) and expanded polytetrafluoroethylene (16,17), that increase vascularization of the fibrous capsule around the plate, may offer a theoretical advantage by enhancing the efficacy, decreasing the capsule size, and increasing the functional lifetime of the implant (15).

One of the most fundamental design differences, however, is whether the device has an open, unobstructed drainage tube or one that contains a pressure-regulating valve. Baerveldt, Molteno, and Schocket implants are examples of open-tube implants. Ahmed and Krupin implants are designed to have a flow-restricting valve mechanism.

Open-Tube Drainage Devices

Baerveldt Implant

The unique feature of this series of popular nonvalved drainage implants is the large surface area of the plates, which are designed in such a way that they can be easily implanted through a one-quadrant conjunctival incision. A silicone tube is attached to a soft barium-impregnated silicone plate with a surface area of 250 mm^2 (20 mm × 13 mm) or 350 mm^2 (32 mm × 14 mm) (18). In an 18-month prospective study, the 350-mm^2 implant had a similar rate of success but lower risk for complications than did the 500-mm^2 model (19), which is no longer available.

The plate is typically positioned under the rectus muscle insertions, typically in the superotemporal quadrant (**Fig. 39.2**). The Baerveldt plate has fenestrations that allow growth of fibrous tissue through the plate, serving to reduce the height of the bleb, which reduces the risk for diplopia and helps secure the implant (19). A fibrous capsule forms after the first 3 to 6 postoperative weeks into which fluid can drain and from which fluid can be absorbed by the surrounding tissues.

After a previously failed trabeculectomy or cataract surgery, Baerveldt drainage devices were found to be more likely to control IOP, compared with trabeculectomy, but at the cost of greater ocular motility disturbances after 1 year of follow-up in a randomized, controlled trial (20,21). In retrospective

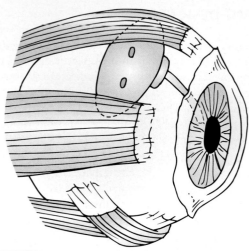

Figure 39.2 Baerveldt implant is positioned under the superior and temporal rectus muscles.

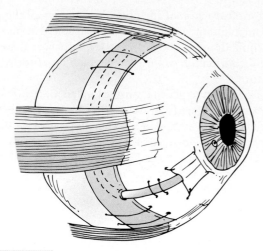

Figure 39.3 Schocket glaucoma drainage device.

case–control or consecutive case series, a 350-mm^2 Baerveldt implant had lowered IOP by a similar amount as a double-plate Molteno implant or Ahmed implant (discussed later) in patients with uncontrolled, complicated glaucoma (22–24). In a retrospective study, the 350-mm^2 implant maintained IOP below 21 mm Hg in 87% of the eyes, compared with 70% with the 500-mm^2 implant after 3 years (25). The success rate declined to 79% in the 350-mm^2 group and to 66% in the 500-mm^2 group after 5 years. The rate of complications was similar between the two groups, but complications occurred slightly more often in the 500-mm^2 group (25). Retrospective studies are limited by selection bias and may not detect small or mild differences.

Molteno Implant

This is the prototype drainage implant device and has had the longest and most extensive clinical experience since Molteno introduced it in 1969 (26). The original design consists of a single plate of thin acrylic with a diameter of 13 mm and an area of 135 mm^2. A silicone tube with an external diameter of 0.62 mm and an internal diameter of 0.30 mm connects to the upper surface of the plate. The plate has a thickened rim, which is perforated to allow suturing to the sclera.

Subsequent modifications addressed various problems encountered with the original design. Success rates with single-plate Molteno implantation for glaucomas with poor surgical prognoses (aphakic or pseudophakic eyes, prior failed filters, neovascular glaucoma, and patient age younger than 3 years) ranged from 25% to 46% in one study but rose to 40% to 71% with implantation of a second plate (27). A double-plate Molteno implant combines two plates, one of which is attached to the silicone tube in the anterior chamber, whereas a second tube connects the two plates, giving an increased surface area of 270 mm^2 (28). In a randomized trial comparing single-plate and double-plate implants, the latter provided better IOP control but was associated with a greater risk for complications, most of which were related to hypotony (29). Another modification, which addresses the problem of hypotony, is the dual-chamber, single-plate implant, in which a V-shaped "pressure

ridge" on the upper surface of the plate encases an area of 10.5 mm^2 around the opening of the silicone tube (30). In concept, the pressure ridge and overlying Tenon capsule regulate the flow of aqueous into the main bleb cavity during the early postoperative period, thereby minimizing excessive filtration and hypotony. The validity of this concept was supported in one study of 40 consecutive patients (31), but the ridge effect was found to be unpredictable in a more recent study (32). A third-generation implant, named Molteno 3, has a bowl-shaped structure on the implant plate immediately at the opening tube. It is designed to function as a biologic valve by limiting the available area of filtration during times of low aqueous production. To date, no data on the effectiveness of the Molteno 3, which is available with plate sizes of 175 and 230 mm^2, have been published.

Schocket Tube Shunt

Schocket and associates (33,34) developed a technique in which a silicone, or silastic, tube is extended from the anterior chamber to a 360-degree encircling silicone band, as used in retinal detachment repair (**Fig. 39.3**), which functioned in developing the reservoir for aqueous drainage. Modifications have included insertion of the tube into a band extending for only 90 degrees beneath two rectus muscles or into the preexisting encircling band in eyes with glaucoma after scleral buckling surgery (35,36). A long Krupin–Denver valve implant (discussed later under "Krupin Implants") has also been used in combination with a 180-degree scleral band (37).

Two randomized trials compared Schocket tube shunts with double-plate Molteno implants. Although the Schocket shunt typically provides a larger surface area of the reservoir than the Molteno implants do, the latter provided lower final IOP in both studies (38,39).

Flow-Restricted Drainage Devices

Little resistance is offered to aqueous outflow until the plate becomes encapsulated. The incorporation of a valve mechanism in implants seems to decrease early postoperative hypotony by

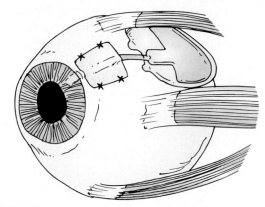

Figure 39.4 Ahmed glaucoma drainage device.

providing resistance to the flow and therefore regulating the pressure within a desired range.

Ahmed Glaucoma Valve

The Ahmed glaucoma valve implant is one of the most commonly used flow-restricted implants in difficult glaucomas. In this valved drainage implant design, a silicone tube is connected to a silicone sheet valve, which is held in a polypropylene body (40) (**Fig. 39.4**). The body of the S2 and FP-7 models has a surface area of 184 mm^2 (16 mm × 13 mm) and is 1.9 mm thick; the reservoir plate of the S2 model is made from polymethylmethacrylate, whereas that of the FP-7 model is made from silicone. A small retrospective comparison suggested that the FP-7 model may lower IOP at 1 year more than the S2 model does (41). The valve mechanism consists of two thin silicone elastomer membranes, 8 mm long and 7 mm wide, which allows one-way regulation of the flow with a goal of keeping the IOP between 8 and 10 mm Hg in the early postoperative period. A second plate can be connected to the reservoir plate and implanted in a second quadrant to increase the surface area by 180 mm^2. These plates are made from both silicone and polypropylene, models FX1 and B1, respectively, to connect to corresponding valved plate FP-7 or S2. Furthermore, a smaller valved implant of 96 mm^2 is available and made from silicone (FP-8) or polypropylene (S3).

The inlet cross section of the chamber is wider than the outlet, which offers a theoretical small pressure differential between the anterior chamber and subconjunctival space, which is claimed to enable the valve to remain open even when only a small difference in pressure exists. However, no definitive proof of this has been given, and application of the Bernoulli equation (flow rate of a fluid is inversely proportional to pressure of the fluid) to the parameters that exist within the physiologic IOP range shows that the Bernoulli effect is almost nonexistent in either the Ahmed glaucoma valve chamber or the Krupin eye valve (discussed later). Calculations indicate that there is no significant pressure drop across the "valves" and that the critical site for pressure drop is at the capsule surrounding the glaucoma implants (42).

One study evaluated obstruction to aqueous flow with the Ahmed implant. The obstructions were separated into tube-related and capsule- or valve-related obstructions. The Ahmed implant, as with other implants, has a hypertensive phase, which is a transient phase of low capsule permeability seen at 4 to 8 weeks postoperatively. The authors also introduced the concept of the "no-touch zone" on the Ahmed glaucoma valve, which is the area of the implant covering the chamber with the silicone leaflets. If the implant is grasped with forceps along the center line, it may separate the valve cover from the implant. The external pressure on the valve chamber can cause a defect in closure of the valve with consequent early postoperative hypotony and fibrovascular membrane ingrowth between the leaflets (43). This may lead to a failure of the valve due to adhesion of the valve membranes (44).

In a retrospective review, the double-plate Molteno implant with mitomycin C was more likely than the Ahmed drainage device with mitomycin C to result in an IOP lower than 15 mm Hg (45). Success rates at 1 year were 80% for the Molteno implant, 39% for the Krupin eye valve with disc, and 35% for the Ahmed drainage device. However, the Ahmed device was less likely to cause complications requiring another surgery (45).

Krupin Implants

In 1976, Krupin and associates introduced the concept of a one-way valve that opens at a predetermined IOP level to avoid the early postoperative complications of excessive drainage and hypotony (46). The original Krupin–Denver valve was composed of an internal Supramid tube cemented to an external silastic tube (46). The valve effect was created by making slits in the closed external end of the silastic tube, designed to open at an IOP between 9 and 11 mm Hg. The tube was short, extending only a few millimeters subconjunctivally, and had no external plate. Although preliminary experience was encouraging (47,48), fibrosis eventually closed the subconjunctival portion of the valved tube (49), which led to failure in most cases.

In a subsequent technique, a long Krupin–Denver drainage tube, with the same one-way valve design, was attached to a 180-degree Schocket-type scleral explant, as previously described (37). This led to development of the Krupin eye valve with disc, which is the design in current use. A silastic tube is attached to an oval silastic disc, conformed to the curvature of the globe, 13 mm × 18 mm, with side walls that are 1.75 mm high (50). The valve at the distal end of the tube is the same design as in the earlier Krupin implants and is manometrically calibrated to open at pressures between 10 and 12 mm Hg. In the newer design of the Krupin implant, the valve lies inside the rim of the plate at its insertion and, as such, is exposed directly to the subconjunctival tissues (51). A review of 113 patients with the Krupin eye valve with disc implants identified 8 patients with primary valve malfunction requiring surgical revision, which involved manipulation, replacement of the valve, and amputation of the valve. Transient postoperative hypotony was noted in three patients, and chronic hypotony with loss of light perception in one patient. One explanted valve was examined and found to have partially fused leaflets, possibly related to the sterilization process and prolonged storage before implantation (51).

Other Drainage Devices

The Ex-PRESS glaucoma drainage device is a more recently introduced implant, but it differs significantly from the aforementioned devices. The other implants have the basic design of a silicone tube that connects an intraocular space, most commonly the anterior chamber, with a subconjunctivally located reservoir plate, whereas this reservoir plate allows for the development of a delimited potential space and the formation of a fibrous capsule to create the resistance to outflow. The Ex-PRESS device does not have a reservoir plate, is implanted under a traditional trabeculectomy flap, and is subject to all of the considerations of a trabeculectomy (see Chapter 38).

At the time of publication, two other drainage devices are under investigation for approval in the United States. The Solx Gold Shunt (Solx Inc., Waltham, MA) is made from 24-karat gold and works to connect the anterior chamber and suprachoroidal space. Although the device is implanted by using an ab externo approach, no subconjunctival drainage occurs (i.e., no bleb). Effectiveness data have yet to be published. The iStent trabecular microbypass stent (Glaukos Corporation, Laguna Hills, CA) is a stainless-steel stent with a lumen that is implanted from an ab interno approach. The device traverses the trabecular meshwork and drains aqueous from the anterior chamber into the Schlemm canal, enhancing aqueous drainage (52). According to early studies, the iStent appears to lower IOP in chronic open-angle glaucoma as a stand-alone procedure and when used in conjunction with cataract extraction (53,54).

IN VITRO COMPARISON OF DEVICES

The Krupin, Baerveldt, Ahmed, and OptiMed implants were compared at physiologic flow rates in vitro and in vivo in rabbits (55). With all devices, opening pressures were higher in vivo than in vitro because of tissue-induced resistance around the explant. Pressures with all devices dropped to 0 mm Hg after conjunctival wound disruption. In air, the Krupin and Ahmed implants had opening pressures of 7.2 and 9.2 mm Hg and closing pressures of 3.9 and 5.2 mm Hg, respectively. The OptiMed implant had the highest resistance values, with IOPs of 19.6 mm Hg, compared with 7.5 mm Hg with the Ahmed implant in vivo. The resistance was similar for the Baerveldt, Krupin, and Molteno dual-chamber devices implanted in vivo. Both Ahmed and Krupin valves functioned as flow-restricting devices, rather than true valves at the flow rates studied, but did not close after initial perfusion with fluid. Neither the Ahmed nor Krupin device had demonstrable opening or closing pressures in balanced salt solution. In another comparative study, the Joseph implants provided slightly lower IOPs and had significantly fewer failures than did the Schocket devices, although the Molteno implants provided the lowest pressures at 12 months among eyes with successful IOP control (56).

Resistance and pressure responses of the OptiMed, Krupin, and Ahmed drainage devices were compared by using a 30-gauge cannula as a simple resistor to determine whether the devices function as true valves. Resistance remained relatively constant for the Krupin and OptiMed implants, whereas the Ahmed offered a variable resistance over a range of flow rates and pressures between 12 and 15 mm Hg. The Ahmed device functioned as a valve that closely regulated pressure within a desired range by decreasing or increasing resistance as a function of flow (57).

SURGICAL TECHNIQUES

Basic Principles

Although certain variations of surgical techniques are required for implantation of the different implant designs, the basic surgical principles apply in general to all glaucoma drainage devices.

Adequate surgical exposure is dependent on proper placement of a traction suture. A 6-0 polyglactin (Vicryl) or silk traction suture on a spatulated needle is placed through superficial cornea near the superior limbus and attached to the drape beneath the eye.

A fornix-based conjunctival–Tenon capsule flap is created, usually in the superotemporal quadrant, to expose the scleral bed (**Fig. 39.5A**). The flap is slightly elevated to allow for blunt dissection between Tenon and episclera with blunt Westcott

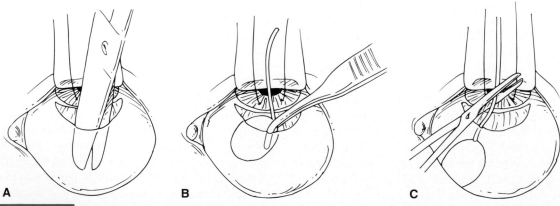

A **B** **C**

Figure 39.5 **A:** Creation of subconjunctival space in the superotemporal quadrant. **B:** Insertion of plate into subconjunctival space. **C:** Cutting the tube to the appropriate length.

scissors. Radial relaxing incisions on one or both sides of the conjunctival flap can improve surgical exposure. A muscle hook is then used to isolate the two rectus muscles on either side of the surgical site.

Whenever possible, the superonasal quadrant should be avoided, especially with the larger plate designs, to reduce the risk for strabismus (discussed later) (58). The Ahmed drainage device, when placed in the superonasal quadrant, has also been shown to come within 1 mm of the optic nerve (59).

With Ahmed valved implants, balanced salt solution must be irrigated through the tube using 27-gauge cannula, before the insertion into the anterior chamber, to ensure that the valve opens properly.

The external plate is then tucked posteriorly into the sub-Tenon space (**Fig. 39.5B**) and is sutured to sclera with nonabsorbable 9-0 Prolene or nylon sutures through the anterior positional holes of the plate, with the anterior border at 8 to 10 mm posterior to the limbus. Variations of this technique are required for different plate designs. Implants with plates of larger circumferential dimensions, such as the Baerveldt, should be tucked under adjacent rectus muscles, whereas Schocket-type designs require dissection of one or more additional quadrants, depending on the extent of the encircling band. In the case of the Ahmed device, which has larger anteroposterior dimensions, extending the anterior border of the plate more than 8 mm behind the limbus is not advisable. However, it is advisable to have the reservoir plates at least 5 to 6 mm posterior to the limbus to prevent conjunctival erosion over the plate (**Fig. 39.6**).

With nonvalved devices, restriction of aqueous flow to avoid severe early postoperative hypotony can be achieved by using a two-stage implantation technique, in which the external plate is placed in the subconjunctival space without inserting the tube into the anterior chamber. The tube is inserted 6 to 8 weeks later, after the fibrous capsule has formed around the external plate (60–62). A more popular technique is to occlude the tube by a ligature of 6-0, 7-0, or 8-0 Vicryl before inserting

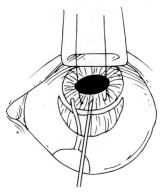

Figure 39.7 Entering the anterior chamber through the limbal area with a 23-gauge or a 22-gauge needle parallel to the iris plane.

it into the anterior chamber. Injection of a balanced salt solution with a 30-gauge cannula into the tube helps to confirm that the tube is totally occluded. This procedure prevents any drainage of aqueous until 4 to 6 weeks after the operation when the Vicryl suture dissolves, allowing aqueous to drain into the preformed capsule. This technique provides the advantage over the two-stage technique of avoiding a second operation (63). Various tube ligatures and stents have been used to minimize postoperative hypotony (as discussed later under "Complications: Prevention and Management").

The tube is then cut, bevel up, to permit its extension 2 to 3 mm into the anterior chamber (**Fig. 39.5C**). Before the tube is inserted into the anterior chamber, a limbal area is cauterized to prevent bleeding from the insertion. A paracentesis can be made inferotemporally to allow placement of a small amount of viscoelastic in the anterior chamber. It is best to maintain the anterior chamber at a normal depth and avoid displacing iris posteriorly in order to assess the true position of the implant tube in the anterior chamber.

The anterior chamber is then entered through the cauterized limbal area with a 23-gauge or a 22-gauge needle, parallel to the iris plane (**Fig. 39.7**). The needle creates a watertight seal, preventing leakage around the tube and thus reducing the risk for postoperative hypotony (64). The angle at which the needle enters the anterior chamber is critical, because it is important that the tube, which will pass through this needle track, is positioned between cornea and iris, without touching the cornea.

The tube is then inserted into the anterior chamber via the needle track; there are specially designed tube-insertion forceps, but these generally are not necessary (**Fig. 39.8**). The tube can be secured to the sclera by using a nonabsorbable suture, such as 9-0 Prolene or nylon, but this step is also optional. Contact of the tube with the iris does not seem to cause any clinically noticeable problems, although tube occlusion by the iris and a distortion of the pupil have been reported (65,66). The anterior chamber may need to be deepened with balanced salt solution, or viscoelastic, via the paracentesis, and the tube is checked for proper position in the anterior chamber.

The tube may occasionally erode through both sclera and overlying conjunctiva at the limbus. To avoid this potential complication, most surgeons suture a rectangle of preserved

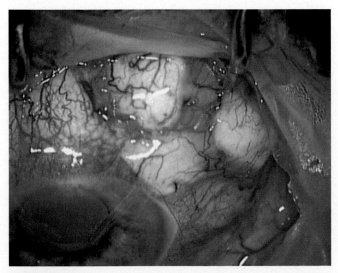

Figure 39.6 Exposed plate of an Ahmed glaucoma drainage device that was placed too close to the limbus.

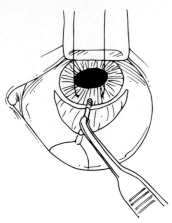

Figure 39.8 Tube insertion into the anterior chamber via the needle track, using nontoothed or specially designed tube-insertion forceps.

donor tissue of approximately 5 mm × 7 mm over the tube at the limbus (67) (**Fig. 39.9**). Processed pericardium (Tutoplast), donor sclera, dura, and fascia lata are available commercially for this purpose. It is also possible to use autologous sclera or to place the tube under a partial-thickness scleral flap, similar to a trabeculectomy procedure.

The conjunctiva is then sutured back to its original position using Vicryl sutures. Subconjunctival steroids and antibiotics are injected at the completion of the procedure in a quadrant away from the surgical site. The basic postoperative management is the same as that described in Chapter 38 for filtering surgery, using topical steroid–antibiotic and mydriatic–cycloplegic preparations for the first several weeks.

Modifications of Basic Technique

Sometimes the conjunctiva is scarred at the limbus, making conjunctival dissection impossible without destroying much of the conjunctival tissue. In this case, the initial conjunctival incision may be made approximately 8 mm from the limbus to create a limbal-based conjunctival flap. Another option is to use the inferotemporal or a superonasal quadrant.

Various occlusion ligatures include a posteriorly placed suture, a releasable suture, and an anterior chamber tube

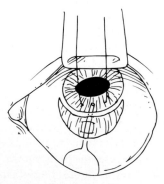

Figure 39.9 Suturing of donor sclera or other patch material over the tube area at the limbus.

ligature. A 5-0 nylon suture can be threaded into the tube at the plate end and secured with one or two absorbable sutures around the tube (68,69). The exposed end of the nylon suture is positioned subconjunctivally near the limbus for subsequent removal. Biodegradable stents, such as collagen lacrimal plugs or 4-0 chromic suture, have also been evaluated, but they have been less satisfactory because they do not always dissolve (70,71). The internal and external occlusion techniques may be combined. For example, a 5-0 nylon or 3-0 Supramid internal occlusion suture is placed, along with an external Vicryl ligature around the tube. The internal stent is then pulled without difficulty in the office treatment room (68).

Using a clear corneal graft, tied with 8-0 nylon, instead of the pericardium or scleral graft to cover the outer portion of the tube provides the view of the tube with the suture for postoperative laser suture lysis (72).

As an alternative to the use of a preserved tissue, an autologous, partial-thickness scleral patch graft crafted from the sclera adjacent to the tube has been described. No complications were reported in the study, but the risk for perforation of the globe exists during the dissection of the flap, and this may not be a good choice in the eyes with high myopia or with scleritis (73).

Some surgeons combine stent occlusion (**Fig. 39.10**) with longitudinal slits in the tube to provide early IOP control (74), and a laboratory study indicated that a slit valve of 2.0 mm appears to provide an opening pressure of approximately 10 mm Hg (75). Using the 350-mm² Baerveldt implant, the role of fenestrations in the tube and antimetabolites was studied in controlling IOP in the early postoperative period. An occlusive 7-0 Vicryl suture was placed just anterior to the plate, followed by a through-and-through penetration of the tube with a standard 15-degree blade in longitudinal orientation just anterior to the ligature. The IOP was elevated at day 21 because of fibrotic blockage of the fenestrations before the ligature dissolved, but the pressure was well controlled by antiglaucoma medication use or laser suture lysis of the 7-0 Vicryl occlusion suture. The use of antimetabolites did not improve the outcome (76).

Another potential complication, as with all filtration procedures, is failure due to excessive fibrosis. In a rabbit study that compared intraoperative use of mitomycin C, 0.5 mg/mL for 5 minutes, with implantation of 200-mm² Baerveldt implants, the mitomycin C–treated eyes had lower IOPs and higher perfusion rates at 2, 4, and 6 weeks (77). In one retrospective study, implantation of Ahmed glaucoma drainage devices combined with the use of mitomycin C achieved lower postoperative IOP, with fewer glaucoma medications and similar complication rates compared with Ahmed devices implanted without antimetabolites (78). However, three retrospective studies of Baerveldt and Molteno implants and a randomized trial with Baerveldt implants did not show any benefit to using intraoperative mitomycin C (76,79–81). At the present time, the preponderance of evidence indicates that use of antimetabolites in conjunction with glaucoma drainage-device surgery incurs little benefit.

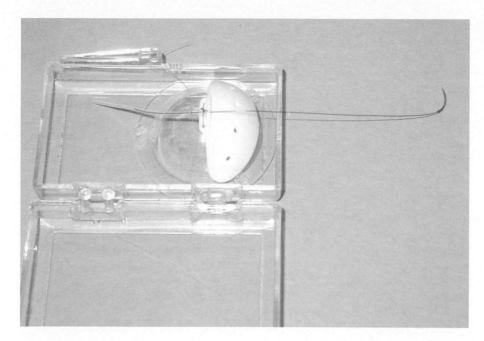

Figure 39.10 Example of a Baerveldt 350-mm² implant in which a 5-0 nylon stent suture is placed and a 7-0 polyglactin suture is tied around the silicone tube, constricting it occlusively around the stent suture. The needle of the 5-0 nylon suture allows for easy externalization and placement under the bulbar conjunctiva.

Special Situations

Pars Plana Insertion

In aphakic (or possibly pseudophakic) eyes in which a vitrectomy has been performed, the tube can be inserted through a pars plana incision into the vitreous cavity. The pars plana tube shunts are usually used when placing the tube into anterior chamber is impossible or undesirable or when a need for pars plana vitrectomy coexists. A Hoffman elbow has been designed for pars plana insertion, and excellent results were demonstrated with the Baerveldt implant following pars plana vitrectomy and fluid–gas exchange. A mean postoperative IOP of 14 mm Hg with an average of 0.6 glaucoma medications was reported in one study (82). The pars plana insertion has the advantage of keeping the tube away from the cornea (especially after penetrating keratoplasty [PKP]) and iris and of reducing the risk for epithelial downgrowth. It is especially important in eyes with corneal grafts. Repositioning of the glaucoma drainage device from the anterior chamber into the vitreous cavity after pars plana vitrectomy for anterior segment complications, such as corneal decompensation, or recurrent tube erosion, is another option (83).

Preexisting Scleral Buckle

The treatment of a retinal detachment may be associated with postoperative glaucoma. The presence of the scleral buckle presents a special challenge in cases in which IOP cannot be controlled medically. Conjunctival scarring caused by retinal surgery can significantly decrease the success of trabeculectomy, even with the use of antimetabolites. Cyclodestructive procedures can be used, but they are unpredictable and may cause significant complications. Glaucoma drainage devices are a useful option to control IOP in such eyes, although the presence of scleral buckle makes placement of the plate challenging.

When a scleral buckle has been placed in the eye for more than 3 months, a silicone tube can be inserted into the anterior cham-

ber, with the distal end introduced into the fibrous capsule of the preexisting scleral buckle, which serves as an external reservoir for aqueous drainage. Because the buckle is already encapsulated, no ligation of the tube to restrict the flow is necessary. In one study, the IOP was successfully controlled in 85% of patients (36).

Long Krupin–Denver valved implants with a flow restrictor at the distal end of the tube can further decrease the chances of postoperative hypotony in eyes with scleral buckle. If the scleral buckle was placed more recently than 3 months and the fibrous capsule has not formed yet, a smaller Baerveldt implant can be used, and the "wings" of the device sometimes need to be trimmed to position the plate underneath the existing scleral band. The fibrous capsule then is expected to grow around the buckle and the Baerveldt implant (84).

Successful insertion of a Baerveldt drainage device behind or over a preexisting scleral buckle, or in the segment without retinal hardware, has been described. Excising the capsule overlying the band allows continuous encapsulation of the band and Baerveldt plate to achieve greater IOP reduction. After 1 year, IOP control was achieved without medications in 78% of patients with 350-mm² plates, but in only 29% of patients with 250-mm² plates (85).

Preexisting Corneal Graft

Glaucoma after PKP remains a difficult management issue. PKP often causes additional damage to the angle, inducing peripheral anterior synechiae formation, with further impediment to aqueous outflow. Control of post-PKP glaucoma is complicated by the need to preserve graft clarity for visual function. When medical management fails, if the angle is open and grossly normal, argon laser trabeculoplasty may be an option. If further intervention is indicated, a glaucoma drainage device, in eyes with good visual potential, is recommended. For eyes with poor visual potential (or for patients who cannot undergo surgery), transscleral cyclophotocoagulation may be a better option (86).

However, placement of glaucoma drainage devices in the anterior chamber may be complicated by tube–cornea touch and endothelial decompensation, particularly after corneal transplantation. Only 70% and 55% of the corneal grafts survived at 2 and 3 years, respectively, after insertion of glaucoma drainage devices into the anterior chamber (87). A retrospective review of simultaneous PKP and Ahmed glaucoma drainage-device implantation showed 92% and 50% graft success and 92% and 86% IOP control at 1 and 3 years, respectively (88).

Pars plana insertion is a reasonable option for patients who have undergone PKP or in whom PKP is anticipated, despite the need for a complete pars plana vitrectomy. The pars plana approach avoids complications related to limbal tube placement and offers better corneal graft survival, but the incidence of posterior segment complications may be higher for pars plana insertion (89).

Implantation of the tube through the ciliary sulcus is another alternative to anterior chamber angle placement in pseudophakic or aphakic eyes with refractory glaucoma and a high risk for corneal decompensation, or eyes with a shallow anterior chamber or extensive synechial angle closure. Positioning of the tube under the iris may be particularly advantageous in the presence of an anterior chamber intraocular lens, because the tube would not disturb the lens. This procedure is contraindicated in phakic eyes because of a possible injury to the crystalline lens (90).

COMPLICATIONS: PREVENTION AND MANAGEMENT

Hypotony

Until the fibrous capsule has developed around the external plate to regulate aqueous flow, the open, nonvalved drainage devices, as noted earlier, provide very low resistance to flow, and hypotony in the early postoperative course with nonvalved implants is a serious complication. By far the best way to prevent this potential complication is by temporarily obstructing the tube lumen. Many techniques have been described to achieve this goal. Basic techniques include suture ligation of the tube, as previously described; temporary occlusion of the tube lumen with a stent; two-stage implantation; or use of a valved implant. Early postoperative hypotony was found in fewer than 10% of patients after Ahmed glaucoma drainage-device surgery (9,91). If early postoperative hypotony happens in combination with a flat anterior chamber, then injection of dense viscoelastic into the anterior chamber and close observation in the first 24 hours may be helpful. If the flat chamber and hypotony reoccur, then removal of the tube from the anterior chamber is recommended to prevent corneal decompensation with planning to reposition the tube into the anterior chamber within the next few days.

Late hypotony from glaucoma drainage-device implantation is usually treated with permanent occlusion of the proximal tube or removal of the tube from the anterior chamber, which permanently removes the effect of the entire implant. Permanent ligation of the tube to the distal plate of double-plate Molteno implant has the advantage of reducing, but not completely eliminating, the effect of the implant (92).

Elevated Intraocular Pressure

Glaucoma drainage-device procedures can also be complicated by elevated IOP in the early or the late postoperative period. Before the ligature around the tube dissolves, there may be a transient elevation of the IOP. It can be prevented by combining a trabeculectomy without mitomycin C with the drainage device, or it can be managed medically. Within the first 7 to 10 days after surgery, a hypotensive phase may present with low IOP, conjunctival and corneal edema, and congestion of conjunctival blood vessels in tissues covering the plate of the implant. This may be followed by a second, hypertensive phase, which is characterized by IOP elevation associated with the formation of the capsule. In this phase, the edema disappears and fibrous tissue develops in the deepest layers of the bleb. During the first 1 to 4 weeks of this phase, the bleb wall becomes congested, causing the IOP elevation. Congestion and inflammation subsequently subside, with IOP reduction and stabilization over the next 3 to 6 months. The hypertensive phase portends a poor prognosis for IOP control (9,93).

Elevated IOP in the early postoperative period may be due to obstruction of the tube by fibrin, blood, iris, vitreous membranes, or silicone oil (**Fig. 39.11**). This was observed in 11% of eyes after implantation of an Ahmed glaucoma drainage device (91), with iris and fibrinous membranes being the most common tissues responsible for blockage (30.8% each), followed by a neovascular membrane, a fibrinous strand, and an iridocorneal endothelial membrane. Iridectomy at the site of the tube ostium has been recommended to prevent iris plugging the tube ostium (94) but requires a larger incision. Nd:YAG laser membranectomy was effective for reopening blocked glaucoma tube shunts and maintaining the patency over time in 84.6% of the

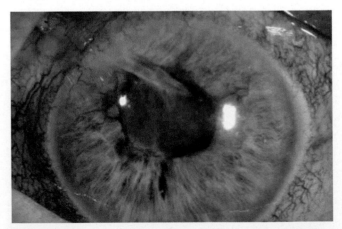

Figure 39.11 Occlusion of a glaucoma drainage device by fibrin in a patient with neovascular glaucoma. (From Junk AK, Katz LJ. Tube shunts for refractory glaucomas. In: Tasman W, Jaeger EA, eds. *Duane's Clinical Ophthalmology*. Vol 6. Lippincott Williams & Wilkins; 2007:chap 17.)

eyes in one retrospective study, but recurrence of the blockage occurred in 53.8% of eyes within the first 11 weeks. Postlaser complications included moderate anterior chamber reaction, hyphema, corneal edema, pressure spike, and a shallow anterior chamber (95). Distal tube occlusion by fibrous tissue has been reported after placement of glaucoma drainage devices in the fibrous capsule around a preexisting scleral buckle (36,56,96).

Reported techniques to open the occluded tube include irrigation of the tube with balanced salt solution using a 30-gauge cannula through a paracentesis incision, the use of Nd:YAG or neodymium-doped yttrium lithium fluoride to open occluded tubes, and the intracameral injection of tissue plasminogen activator (0.1 cc of 5 to 13 μg) to dissolve a fibrin clot (97–101).

Late IOP elevation, especially when the intraocular portion of the tube appears to be patent, is usually due to an excessively thick fibrous capsule. Needling revision can improve function of the encapsulated drainage implant. It is more successful when the drainage device has a larger surface area, although the risk for severe complications, including endophthalmitis, exists (102).

When needling is unsuccessful after a few attempts, removing a portion of the encapsulated bleb beneath the conjunctiva may be beneficial. In a retrospective study assessing 95 eyes (of 79 consecutive patients) that underwent a single-stage Molteno implantation, 14 eyes (of 12 patients) developed recurrence of the encapsulated bleb. With a mean follow-up of 30 months, the mean IOP after capsule excision was significantly lower than the preoperative IOP, achieving a 75% success rate (103).

Topical corticosteroid therapy can cause IOP elevation despite the presence of a functioning glaucoma drainage device (104).

Migration, Extrusion, and Erosion

Tube migration may occur after glaucoma drainage-device procedures (105). If the tube is not adequately secured to the sclera, it may migrate posteriorly out of the anterior chamber, which may require repositioning of the tube and securing it to the sclera with additional 9-0 Prolene sutures. Anterior migration of the tube can occur due to the dislocation of the external plate.

In pediatric patients, the tube may retract out of the anterior chamber or even erode through the cornea (106–109). Extrusion of the implant was the most common reason for repeated surgery in children who received an Ahmed glaucoma drainage device (110). This may occur as the eye grows, requiring repositioning of the tube from the original site (111). The tube may also need to be repositioned when it is blocked by the cornea, iris, or vitreous (64). If the tube end is too short to allow for repositioning, a silastic sleeve or silastic extension tube may be used (112). A 22-gauge angiocatheter and a piece of pediatric lacrimal tubing, with a 0.3-mm internal diameter and 0.64-mm external diameter, may be used for this purpose (113).

Avulsion of an implant after blunt trauma may force the tube against the cornea, causing corneal melting and requiring explantation of the implant and possibly corneal grafting. Placing the connecting tube of a double-plate Molteno

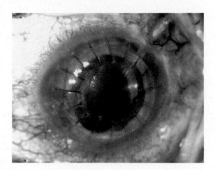

Figure 39.12 Exposed silicone tube posterior to the limbus in a patient with a Baerveldt glaucoma implant device. The patient had undergone penetrating keratoplasty and implantation of a glaucoma drainage device for treatment of essential iris atrophy.

implant under the superior rectus muscle might decrease the risk for shunt avulsion after trauma (114).

Erosion of the silicone tube through the overlying conjunctiva is a recognized complication of glaucoma drainage devices (**Fig. 39.12**). A partial-thickness scleral flap does not prevent erosion of the tube, and (as previously described) the tube and fistula site should be covered with preserved sclera, dura, fascia lata, or pericardium. However, pericardial graft thinning, melting, and conjunctival erosion despite the patch graft have occurred (115–117).

If a scleral graft is too thick, it may elevate the limbal conjunctiva enough to produce dellen formation. Conversely, a thin scleral patch graft may predispose the tube to erosion. In addition, immune reactions resulting in scleral melting have been reported (118). The use of preserved sclera also has the disadvantages of dependence on eye bank supplies, precluding its use in emergency cases; possibly greater cost; and concerns about infectious disease transmission, despite donor screening (119,120). Studies using polymerase chain reaction have shown evidence of the human immunodeficiency virus (HIV) genome in sclera obtained from HIV-1–seropositive donors, despite treatment with heat, alcohol, or formalin, but not after irradiation (120).

Solvent-preserved cadaver pericardium (Tutoplast) offers several advantages, including availability, lower cost, uniformity in size and tissue quality, and enhanced sterility. A dehydration process leaves the graft devoid of antigenic stimuli yet preserves the tissue's inherent strength and flexibility (121). Tissue sterilization is achieved through the treatment with organic solvents followed by low-dose radiation, which inactivates bacteria, fungi, and viruses, including HIV and Creutzfeldt–Jakob disease virus (120,122,123).

Thin (0.25 mm) polytetrafluoroethylene patches were well tolerated in rabbit eyes and may be an alternative to donor sclera for reinforcement in glaucoma drain surgery (124).

If the plate of an implant migrates toward the medial rectus muscle insertion, myositis may develop. This was reported to resolve after removal of the implant (125).

Endophthalmitis

As mentioned previously, endophthalmitis may develop after needling of the implant (102).

Recurrent *Propionibacterium acnes* endophthalmitis has been reported after surgical revision of a Molteno drainage device, based on a positive culture of anterior chamber needle aspirate. The response to repeated intraocular vancomycin injections was poor, and explantation of the device was required to achieve complete resolution of the infection. Reinsertion of the drainage device into the anterior chamber resulted in recurrence of the infection (126).

Removal of the glaucoma drainage device in cases of endophthalmitis may be necessary to remove the contaminated foreign body. Early postoperative endophthalmitis after placement of a glaucoma drainage device may be successfully treated by immediate removal of the implant and surgical management of the infection, with subsequent placement of a new device (127).

Endophthalmitis may also occur in the late postoperative course. Exposure of the tube seems to be a major risk factor for these infections. Surgical revision with a patch graft in all cases in which a tube is exposed is indicated to prevent this potentially devastating complication (128).

Sterile endophthalmitis was also described approximately 1 month after discontinuation of postoperative corticosteroid therapy (129).

Visual Loss

In one series of 41 patients after Molteno device implantation, the incidence of reduced visual acuity was 22%, with hypotony and shallow anterior chambers being the most commonly associated events (130). Other reported mechanisms of visual loss include retinal detachment, vitreous hemorrhage, cystoid macular edema, and operating microscope–induced retinal phototoxicity (130–134). These complications often occurred despite successful control of IOP.

Corneal Decompensation and Graft Failure

The causes of corneal decompensation and graft failure in eyes with glaucoma drainage devices are not completely clear but may be related to the retrograde flow from the encapsulated reservoir to the anterior chamber. Serial corneal endothelial cell counts in 19 patients after uneventful Molteno device implantation revealed slight, clinically insignificant progressive cell loss (135). Tube–cornea touch is another cause of corneal decompensation. In one study of Ahmed glaucoma drainage-device implantation in pediatric patients, cornea–tube contact occurred in 18.5% (136). When the tube–cornea contact is seen, removal of the tube from the anterior chamber, shortening of the tube, and subsequent reinsertion may be necessary. Because this technique may require extensive revision with possible complications, a simpler technique was described for trimming the silicone tube in situ (137).

In one retrospective review, corneal edema developed on average after 21 months in 50% of patients after Molteno drainage-device implantation, and in 6.7% after multiple eye surgeries, including a trabeculectomy, but not after the trabeculectomy alone (138). In another study, when corneal complications thought to be unrelated to the implant were excluded from the definition of failure in a cohort of patients with Ahmed drainage devices with a mean follow-up for 30.5 months, only 21.5% of the eyes experienced failure, and cumulative probabilities of success at 1, 2, 3, and 4 years were 87%, 82%, 76%, and 76%, respectively. However, when corneal decompensation and corneal graft failure were included in the definition of failure, 43% of the eyes were considered to have experienced failure, decreasing cumulative probabilities of success at 1, 2, 3, and 4 years to 76%, 68%, 54%, and 45%, respectively. These corneal problems may be secondary to the underlying ocular condition or to the drainage device itself (139). Phosphorylcholine polymer coating of the glaucoma drainage devices was suggested to reduce the rate of corneal endothelial failure (140).

A comparative study showed that although implantation of an additional glaucoma drainage device provided better IOP control than with tube repositioning, the most common complication with this approach was corneal edema (141). Another study showed that device replacement after initial drainage-device failure has high corneal morbidity, reaching a corneal decompensation rate of 36% (142). However, an IOP less than 21 mm Hg or 20% reduction in IOP after the second tube procedure was achieved in 86.4% with a 3-year follow-up.

Diplopia and Ocular Motility Disturbance

As previously noted, devices with larger plates, especially when implanted in the superonasal quadrant, can interrupt extraocular muscle function and cause strabismus and diplopia (58). Characteristic patterns are exotropia, hypertropia, or limitation of ocular rotations (143–147), although a Brown superior oblique tendon-like syndrome has also been described (58,148,149). Whereas the complication is usually associated with the larger plates, such as the 350-mm^2 Baerveldt drainage device and the Krupin eye valve with disc (143,145–148), it may also occur with smaller plates, such as the single-plate or double-plate Molteno implants, especially in children (144). Corrective measures may require removal of the device, replacement with a device that has a smaller plate, or transfer of the device to the superotemporal quadrant, which usually relieves the diplopia (143).

In one study, postoperative motility disturbance, including acquired Brown syndrome, superior oblique palsy, and lateral rectus palsy, developed in 11 of 24 eyes (24%) more than 6 months after implantation of a double-plate Molteno drainage device, although this may resolve spontaneously with time (149). Surgical treatment may require several interventions but can be successful (150).

Other Complications

Epithelial downgrowth is an uncommon but potential risk, especially with tubes inserted at the limbus. It can cause failure of the implant function; corneal decompensation; and, when associated with the formation of a true Tenon cyst, significant cosmetic deformity and motility disturbance (151).

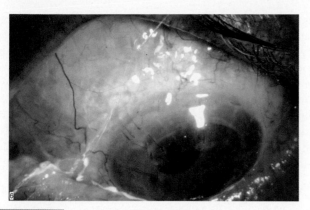

Figure 39.13 Appearance of silicone subconjunctival silicone oil extravasation through a Baerveldt drainage device.

Epithelial invasion into the fibrous capsule with persistent aqueous leak was described in four patients during the early postoperative course following Baerveldt drainage-device implantation (152). All reported cases of epithelial ingrowth occurred in previously operated eyes. In advanced cases of epithelial downgrowth associated with secondary glaucoma, the combination of a glaucoma drainage device and PKP may be indicated to maintain useful vision (153).

Sterile hypopyon has been reported after removal of 4-0 chromic suture stents (154).

Silicone oil drainage from the vitreous cavity to the subconjunctival space through a Molteno drainage device was reported in an eye with an anterior chamber Molteno implant, lensectomy, vitrectomy, and intravitreal silicone oil injection (155). This complication can occur with any device implanted in the superior quadrants (**Fig. 39.13**). A glaucoma drainage device may thus be inappropriate in eyes with intravitreal silicone oil.

Some patients may develop an irregular pupil years after implantation of a silicone drainage device because the iris root may adhere to the tube (66). However, placing the intraocular portion of the silicone tube away from the cornea is more important to minimize corneal endothelial loss, because contact with the iris stromal root does not typically cause significant problems (66).

Globe perforation can occur while suturing the plate to the sclera, causing retinal detachment or vitreous hemorrhage. The risk is greater in buphthalmic or highly myopic eyes with thin sclera. Implantation under the scleral buckle may be complicated by scleral perforation at the site of severe ectasia underlying the previous buckle (152).

Retinal complications with glaucoma drainage devices include retinal detachment, suprachoroidal hemorrhage, choroidal effusions, and vitreous hemorrhages. The most common risk factors for suprachoroidal hemorrhage (**Fig. 39.14**) are older age, postoperative choroidal effusions, low IOP immediately after the tube opened, hypertension, or atherosclerosis. Complete ligation of the proximal part of open-tube design with a 7-0 Vicryl suture, testing for watertightness before placing the tube in the anterior chamber, may decrease the rate of retinal complications (64). In one study with Baerveldt devices, the median onset of a postoperative retinal complication was 12.5 days, with 10 patients (83%) experiencing complications within 35 days. Serous choroidal effusions usually resolve spontaneously. Serious retinal complications were distributed evenly among patients with Krupin eye valves with discs and Molteno and Baerveldt devices (156).

OUTCOMES AND INDICATIONS

Long-Term Outcomes

Outcome studies have been reported for the most commonly used glaucoma drainage devices. The following data were derived from long-term follow-ups (usually a mean of 12 months or more) of overall study populations in which success was typically defined as a low-end cutoff of 5 to 6 mm Hg and a high-end cutoff of 21 to 22 mm Hg with or without medication use. In trials with Molteno implants, the success rates were 73% to 74% with a mean or minimum follow-up of 18 months and 57% with a mean follow-up of 43 to 44 months

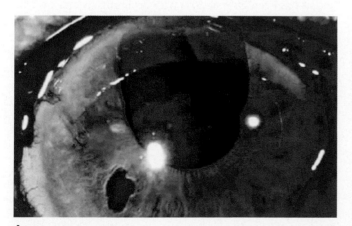

A

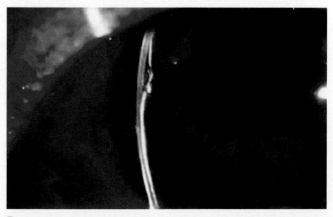

B

Figure 39.14 Slitlamp photograph. **A:** Massive suprachoroidal hemorrhage after glaucoma drainage-device implantation. The tube with an intraluminal suture in place can be seen in the anterior chamber. **B:** Slit-beam illumination reveals a flat anterior chamber. (From Azuara-Blanco A, Katz LJ. Prevention and management of complications of glaucoma surgery. In: Tasman W, Jaeger EA, eds. *Duane's Clinical Ophthalmology.* Vol 6. Lippincott Williams & Wilkins; 2007:chap 24.)

(157–160). A success rate of 76% was reported in eyes with uveitic glaucoma and a follow-up of 5 to 10 years (161). A study of 82 black patients treated with Molteno implants and followed up for a mean of 30 months reported a similar success rate of 72% (162). Survival analysis in a retrospective study showed that failure was most common in the first postoperative year, and variables associated with a significantly increased risk for failure were pseudophakia and neovascular glaucoma. Postoperative IOP tended to be lower after double-plate than after single-plate implantation. Outcomes with Molteno drainage devices did not significantly differ on the basis of age, sex, race, previous PKP, or previous conjunctival surgery (159).

With Schocket-type drainage devices, reported success rates were 91% with a mean follow-up of 10 months and 81% with a 17.5-month mean follow-up (35,163) but fell to 30% at 36 months in one study using life tables (164).

Reported success with Baerveldt implants was 93% and 88% for 350-mm^2 and 500-mm^2 drainage devices, respectively, after 18 months (19), although other studies reported 71% to 72% success with a minimum of 6 months, a mean of 13.6 months, and 2 years of follow-up (165–167).

Studies involving the Krupin eye valve and disc revealed 6-month and 12-month success rates of 84% and 66%, respectively (168), whereas another group found an 80% success rate with a mean follow-up of 25 months (44). Studies of the Ahmed drainage device revealed success rates of 77% to 87% at 1-year follow-up and 75% success rate at 2-year follow-up (9,40,91). The visual acuity improved or remained within one Snellen line of the preoperative value in 62% to 78% of the various studies, which is undoubtedly influenced by the relative proportion of glaucoma types in each study.

Success tends to be somewhat lower in pediatric populations. Ahmed glaucoma drainage-device surgery implantation in children was reported to have cumulative probabilities of success of 77.9% at 12 months and 60.6% at 24 months (169), which is similar to those of other implants when used in a pediatric population (110). Another study showed that 6 months after glaucoma drainage-device surgery in the management of childhood glaucoma, the IOP was controlled in 72.2% with or without use of glaucoma medication, decreasing to 44.4% after 2 or more years (170). Although 38.9% remained within one line of preoperative vision or improved, 27.8% lost light perception. Most children required additional surgical procedures to control IOP or manage drainage device–related complications. The limited success rate in this study, the relatively high complication rate, and the need for frequent surgical intervention suggest caution regarding the prognosis of glaucoma drainage-device surgery in children with glaucoma.

Indications

Traditionally, glaucoma drainage-device surgery is reserved for patients in whom trabeculectomy with adjunctive antimetabolite therapy has either failed or is thought to have a very low chance of success, and in whom there is still a reasonable potential for vision. The Tube Versus Trabeculectomy study has shown an advantage with drainage-device implantation compared with repeated trabeculectomy. Some surgeons are exploring the possible role as a primary surgical procedure. Other traditional indications include young patients; individuals with neovascular glaucoma, glaucoma associated with uveitis, severe conjunctival scarring, refractory pediatric glaucoma, or glaucoma in aphakia or pseudophakia; and patients with other prior surgery, such as vitreoretinal surgery and PKP. Success rates vary with the different patient characteristics and underlying disorders.

Young Patients

As previously noted, glaucoma drainage-device surgery in the pediatric population (1 month to 13 years), as with any surgery for childhood glaucoma, is more problematic than in adults. Nevertheless, success rates of 55% to 95% have been reported, with no definite advantage among Molteno, Baerveldt, and Ahmed implants (107,171–174).

Drainage-device implantation may be especially useful in children with juvenile rheumatoid arthritis and uveitic glaucoma and with glaucoma associated with the Sturge–Weber syndrome (61,65,175,176). In the latter situation, an advantage of glaucoma drainage devices over trabeculectomy with antimetabolites is the reduced risk for expulsive hemorrhage associated with marked IOP reduction. Glaucoma drainage devices have also been shown to succeed in children after cycloablation (136). Complications of drainage-device implantation in children include tube malposition, flat anterior chamber, tube obstruction by iris or vitreous, cataract, cornea–tube touch, choroidal detachment, corneal edema, and corneal abrasion (65,171).

Neovascular Glaucoma

Glaucoma drainage-device surgery has been successful in some eyes with neovascular glaucoma (177), although the success declines with time. In one study, the success rate with Molteno implants was 62.1% at 1 year, declining to 10.3% at 5 years (178). Reported success with the Baerveldt and Ahmed implants has been 60% to 80% with declining success over time and a generally lower success rate than with other forms of glaucoma (91,179). Better outcomes in the eyes with neovascular glaucoma have been reported with glaucoma drainage-device surgery than with noncontact cyclophotocoagulation (180,181). Prospective comparison of Ahmed drainage implant and contact diode and endoscopic cyclophotocoagulation found no significant differences in the success rate at 24 months (182,183).

Uveitic Glaucoma

Ahmed drainage devices have been shown to be a safe alternative in high-risk patients with uncontrolled uveitic glaucoma who have had multiple previous ocular surgeries (184,185). Success may be enhanced by preoperative and long-term postoperative immunotherapy. The most common complications are encapsulated bleb (**Fig. 39.15**), transient hypotony, and hyphema. Hypotony may occur less frequently in patients with uveitis with the use of valved versus nonvalved devices.

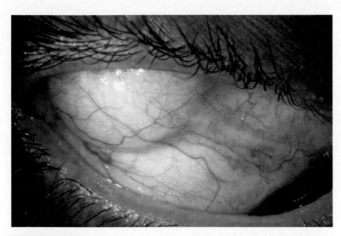

Figure 39.15 Bleb encapsulation of a glaucoma drainage device, producing elevated IOP in the late postoperative period. (From Junk AK, Katz LJ. Tube shunts for refractory glaucomas. In: Tasman W, Jaeger EA, eds. *Duane's Clinical Ophthalmology*. Vol 6. Lippincott Williams & Wilkins; 2007:chap 17.)

Severe Conjunctival Scarring and Previous Ocular Surgery

A failed trabeculectomy, especially when the conjunctiva is scarred down in both superior quadrants, could be an indication for a glaucoma drainage-device procedure. In addition, other types of ocular surgery may cause such conjunctival scarring that an implant will have a better chance than a trabeculectomy. Both Molteno and Baerveldt drainage devices have been effective for glaucomas associated with aphakia or pseudophakia (186,187). The Molteno device has also been used with some success in eyes with epithelial downgrowth (188). Molteno and Schocket devices have been used in association with pars plana vitrectomy in eyes with vitreoretinal disorders and in eyes following PKP (189–191). The Molteno device and the Ahmed device have also been used with success in eyes with prior cyclodestructive therapy (136,192).

Aniridia

Medical and surgical therapy may not always be efficient in controlling IOP in aniridia. Molteno drainage devices and the Ahmed drainage device have been used in these patients (193,194). In a retrospective review, implantation of a glaucoma drainage device in patients with aniridia had a success rate of 88% after 1 year (195), reducing the IOP from 35 to 15 mm Hg, with most of the eyes having improved or unchanged visual acuity.

Comparison with Alternative Procedures

In patients with glaucomas associated with a high risk for surgical failure, the surgeon usually must choose among a filtering operation with adjunctive antimetabolites, a glaucoma drainage-device procedure, or a cyclodestructive operation. Aside from the Tube Versus Trabeculectomy study, similar results have been reported with implantation of a single-plate Molteno device and trabeculectomy without use of an adjunctive antimetabolite (196), or trabeculectomy with postoperative 5-fluorouracil (197), whereas trabeculectomy with

intraoperative mitomycin C provided significantly greater IOP reduction (198). In each of these studies, the types of complications differed between the two procedures (as previously discussed), but they tended to be more frequent with the glaucoma drainage-device operations. However, a randomized comparison of Ahmed drainage devices and trabeculectomy with mitomycin C found no difference in the rate of complications, although the IOP was better controlled in the trabeculectomy group during the first year (199). After 3 years, the results were similar in both groups (200).

Glaucoma drainage devices provide better IOP control in eyes with advanced uncontrolled glaucoma than cyclophotocoagulation, but they more often require repeated surgery and have a higher rate of complications, including vision loss (201). The two procedures were similar in one series of eyes with PKP, although a trend toward more graft failure, hypotony, and visual loss occurred with the laser surgery (202). As mentioned previously, in eyes with neovascular glaucoma, Ahmed drainage devices provide IOP control at 12 to 24 months similar to that achieved with contact or endoscopic cyclophotocoagulation.

KEY POINTS

- Glaucoma drainage devices have been successful in controlling IOP since the development of tubes that drain into subconjunctival reservoirs created by external plates.
- Implant designs differ according to the size and the shape of the external plate and whether the tube is open (Molteno, Schocket, and Baerveldt) or valved (Krupin and Ahmed).
- The basic surgical technique involves implantation of one end of the tube in the anterior chamber, with the other attached to the plate near the equator. A fibrous capsule develops around the plate, which regulates the aqueous flow.
- Complications include hypotony, elevated IOP, ocular motility disturbance, and loss of visual acuity.
- Indications for glaucoma drainage-device surgery include previous failed filters, young age, neovascular glaucoma, glaucoma associated with uveitis, and glaucomas after cataract extraction or other types of ocular surgery.

REFERENCES

1. Lloyd MA, Baerveldt G, Nguyen QH, et al. Long-term histologic studies of the Baerveldt implant in a rabbit model. *J Glaucoma*. 1996;5(5):334–339.
2. Philipp W, Klima G, Miller K. Clinicopathological findings 11 months after implantation of a functioning aqueous-drainage silicone implant. *Graefes Arch Clin Exp Ophthalmol*. 1990;228(5):481–486.
3. Wilcox MJ, Minckler DS, Ogden TE. Pathophysiology of artificial aqueous drainage in primate eyes with Molteno implants. *J Glaucoma*. 1994;3(2):140–151.
4. Lloyd MA, Minckler DS, Heuer DK, et al. Echographic evaluation of glaucoma shunts. *Ophthalmology*. 1993;100(6):919–927.
5. Rubin B, Chan CC, Burnier M, et al. Histopathologic study of the Molteno glaucoma implant in three patients. *Am J Ophthalmol*. 1990;110(4):371–379.
6. Prata JA Jr, Santos RC, LaBree L, et al. Surface area of glaucoma implants and perfusion flow rates in rabbit eyes. *J Glaucoma*. 1995;4(4):274–280.

7. Kadri OA, Wilcox MJ. Surface tension controls capsule thickness and collagen orientation in glaucoma shunt devices. *Biomed Sci Instrum.* 2001;37:257–262.

8. Wilcox MJ, Barad JP, Wilcox CC, et al. Performance of a new, low-volume, high-surface area aqueous shunt in normal rabbit eyes. *J Glaucoma.* 2000;9(1):74–82.

9. Ayyala RS, Zurakowski D, Smith JA, et al. A clinical study of the Ahmed glaucoma valve implant in advanced glaucoma. *Ophthalmology.* 1998;105(10):1968–1976.

10. Molteno AC, Dempster AG. Methods of controlling bleb fibrosis around draining implants. In: Mills KB, ed. *Glaucoma: Proceedings of the Fourth International Symposium of the Northern Eye Institute, Manchester, UK, 14–16 July 1988.* Oxford: Pergamon Press; 1989:192–211.

11. Jacob JT, Burgoyne CF, McKinnon SJ, et al. Biocompatibility response to modified Baerveldt glaucoma drains. *J Biomed Mater Res.* 1998;43(2):99–107.

12. Porter JM, Krawczyk CH, Carey RF. In vitro flow testing of glaucoma drainage devices. *Ophthalmology.* 1997;104(10):1701–1707.

13. Ayyala RS, Harman LE, Michelini-Norris B, et al. Comparison of different biomaterials for glaucoma drainage devices. *Arch Ophthalmol.* 1999;117(2):233–236.

14. Ayyala RS, Michelini-Norris B, Flores A, et al. Comparison of different biomaterials for glaucoma drainage devices: part 2. *Arch Ophthalmol.* 2000;118(8):1081–1084.

15. Pandya AD, Rich C, Eifrig DE, et al. Experimental evaluation of a hydroxylapatite reservoir tube shunt in rabbits. *Ophthalmic Surg Lasers.* 1996;27(4):308–314.

16. Boswell CA, Noecker RJ, Mac M, et al. Evaluation of an aqueous drainage glaucoma device constructed of ePTFE. *J Biomed Mater Res.* 1999;48(5):591–595.

17. Kim S, Kim Y, Choi S, et al. Clinical experience of e-PTFE membrane implant surgery for refractory glaucoma. *Br J Ophthalmol.* 2003;87(1):63–70.

18. Lloyd MA, Baerveldt G, Heuer DK, et al. Initial clinical experience with the Baerveldt implant in complicated glaucomas. *Ophthalmology.* 1994;101(4):640–650.

19. Lloyd MA, Baerveldt G, Fellenbaum PS, et al. Intermediate-term results of a randomized clinical trial of the 350- versus the 500-mm^2 Baerveldt implant. *Ophthalmology.* 1994;101(8):1456–1463; discussion 1463–1464.

20. Gedde SJ, Schiffman JC, Feuer WJ, et al. Treatment outcomes in the tube versus trabeculectomy study after one year of follow-up. *Am J Ophthalmol.* 2007;143(1):9–22.

21. Rauscher FM, Gedde SJ, Schiffman JC, et al. Motility disturbances in the tube versus trabeculectomy study during the first year of follow-up. *Am J Ophthalmol.* 2009;147(3):458–466.

22. Smith MF, Doyle JW, Sherwood MB. Comparison of the Baerveldt glaucoma implant with the double-plate Molteno drainage implant. *Arch Ophthalmol.* 1995;113(4):444–447.

23. Syed HM, Law SK, Nam SH, et al. Baerveldt-350 implant versus Ahmed valve for refractory glaucoma: a case-controlled comparison. *J Glaucoma.* 2004;13(1):38–45.

24. Tsai JC, Johnson CC, Kammer JA, et al. The Ahmed shunt versus the Baerveldt shunt for refractory glaucoma II: longer-term outcomes from a single surgeon. *Ophthalmology.* 2006;113(6):913–917.

25. Britt MT, LaBree LD, Lloyd MA, et al. Randomized clinical trial of the 350-mm^2 versus the 500-mm^2 Baerveldt implant: longer term results: is bigger better? *Ophthalmology.* 1999;106(12):2312–2318.

26. Molteno AC. New implant for drainage in glaucoma. Clinical trial. *Br J Ophthalmol.* 1969;53(9):606–615.

27. Lloyd MA, Sedlak T, Heuer DK, et al. Clinical experience with the single-plate Molteno implant in complicated glaucomas. Update of a pilot study. *Ophthalmology.* 1992;99(5):679–687.

28. Molteno AC. The optimal design of drainage implants for glaucoma. *Trans Ophthalmol Soc N Z.* 1981;33:39–41.

29. Heuer DK, Lloyd MA, Abrams DA, et al. Which is better? One or two? A randomized clinical trial of single-plate versus double-plate Molteno implantation for glaucomas in aphakia and pseudophakia. *Ophthalmology.* 1992;99(10):1512–1519.

30. Molteno AC. The dual chamber single plate implant—its use in neovascular glaucoma. *Aust N Z J Ophthalmol.* 1990;18(4):431–436.

31. Freedman J. Clinical experience with the Molteno dual-chamber single-plate implant. *Ophthalmic Surg.* 1992;23(4):238–241.

32. Gerber SL, Cantor LB, Sponsel WE. A comparison of postoperative complications from pressure-ridge Molteno implants versus Molteno implants with suture ligation. *Ophthalmic Surg Lasers.* 1997;28(11):905–910.

33. Schocket SS, Lakhanpal V, Richards RD. Anterior chamber tube shunt to an encircling band in the treatment of neovascular glaucoma. *Ophthalmology.* 1982;89(10):1188–1194.

34. Schocket SS, Nirankari VS, Lakhanpal V, et al. Anterior chamber tube shunt to an encircling band in the treatment of neovascular glaucoma and other refractory glaucomas. A long-term study. *Ophthalmology.* 1985;92(4):553–562.

35. Omi CA, De Almeida GV, Cohen R, et al. Modified Schocket implant for refractory glaucoma. Experience of 55 cases. *Ophthalmology.* 1991;98(2):211–214.

36. Sidoti PA, Minckler DS, Baerveldt G, et al. Aqueous tube shunt to a pre-existing episcleral encircling element in the treatment of complicated glaucomas. *Ophthalmology.* 1994;101(6):1036–1043.

37. Krupin T, Ritch R, Camras CB, et al. A long Krupin-Denver valve implant attached to a 180 degrees scleral explant for glaucoma surgery. *Ophthalmology.* 1988;95(9):1174–1180.

38. Smith MF, Sherwood MB, McGorray SP. Comparison of the double-plate Molteno drainage implant with the Schocket procedure. *Arch Ophthalmol.* 1992;110(9):1246–1250.

39. Wilson RP, Cantor L, Katz LJ, et al. Aqueous shunts. Molteno versus Schocket. *Ophthalmology.* 1992;99(5):672–676; discussion 676–678.

40. Coleman AL, Hill R, Wilson MR, et al. Initial clinical experience with the Ahmed glaucoma valve implant. *Am J Ophthalmol.* 1995;120(1):23–31.

41. Hinkle DM, Zurakowski D, Ayyala RS. A comparison of the polypropylene plate Ahmed glaucoma valve to the silicone plate Ahmed glaucoma flexible valve. *Eur J Ophthalmol.* 2007;17(5):696–701.

42. Lee VW. Glaucoma "valves"—truth versus myth. *Ophthalmology.* 1998;105(4):567–568.

43. Hill RA, Pirouzian A, Liaw L. Pathophysiology of and prophylaxis against late Ahmed glaucoma valve occlusion. *Am J Ophthalmol.* 2000;129(5):608–612.

44. Feldman RM, El-Harazi SM, Villanueva G. Valve membrane adhesion as a cause of Ahmed glaucoma valve failure. *J Glaucoma.* 1997;6(1):10–12.

45. Taglia DP, Perkins TW, Gangnon R, et al. Comparison of the Ahmed glaucoma valve, the Krupin eye valve with disk, and the double-plate Molteno implant. *J Glaucoma.* 2002;11(4):347–353.

46. Krupin T, Podos SM, Becker B, et al. Valve implants in filtering surgery. *Am J Ophthalmol.* 1976;81(2):232–235.

47. Krupin T, Kaufman P, Mandell A, et al. Filtering valve implant surgery for eyes with neovascular glaucoma. *Am J Ophthalmol.* 1980;89(3):338–343.

48. Krupin T, Kaufman P, Mandell AI, et al. Long-term results of valve implants in filtering surgery for eyes with neovascular glaucoma. *Am J Ophthalmol.* 1983;95(6):775–782.

49. Folberg R, Hargett NA, Weaver JE, et al. Filtering valve implant for neovascular glaucoma in proliferative diabetic retinopathy. *Ophthalmology.* 1982;89(3):286–289.

50. The Krupin Eye Valve Filtering Surgery Study Group. Krupin eye valve with disk for filtration surgery. *Ophthalmology.* 1994;101(4):651–658.

51. Burchfield JC, Kass MA, Wax MB. Primary valve malfunction of the Krupin eye valve with disk. *J Glaucoma.* 1997;6(3):152–156.

52. Bahler CK, Smedley GT, Zhou J, et al. Trabecular bypass stents decrease intraocular pressure in cultured human anterior segments. *Am J Ophthalmol.* 2004;138(6):988–994.

53. Spiegel D, Garcia-Feijoo J, Garcia-Sanchez J, et al. Coexistent primary open-angle glaucoma and cataract: preliminary analysis of treatment by cataract surgery and the iStent trabecular micro-bypass stent. *Adv Ther.* 2008;25(5):453–464.

54. Spiegel D, Wetzel W, Haffner DS, et al. Initial clinical experience with the trabecular micro-bypass stent in patients with glaucoma. *Adv Ther.* 2007;24(1):161–170.

55. Prata JA Jr, Mermoud A, LaBree L, et al. In vitro and in vivo flow characteristics of glaucoma drainage implants. *Ophthalmology.* 1995;102(6):894–904.

56. Lavin MJ, Franks WA, Wormald RP, et al. Clinical risk factors for failure in glaucoma tube surgery. A comparison of three tube designs. *Arch Ophthalmol.* 1992;110(4):480–485.

57. Francis BA, Cortes A, Chen J, et al. Characteristics of glaucoma drainage implants during dynamic and steady-state flow conditions. *Ophthalmology.* 1998;105(9):1708–1714.

58. Prata JA Jr, Minckler DS, Green RL. Pseudo-Brown's syndrome as a complication of glaucoma drainage implant surgery. *Ophthalmic Surg.* 1993;24(9):608–611.

59. Leen MM, Witkop GS, George DP. Anatomic considerations in the implantation of the Ahmed glaucoma valve. *Arch Ophthalmol.* 1996;114(2):223–224.

60. Billson F, Thomas R, Aylward W. The use of two-stage Molteno implants in developmental glaucoma. *J Pediatr Ophthalmol Strabismus.* 1989; 26(1):3–8.

61. Budenz DL, Sakamoto D, Eliezer R, et al. Two-staged Baerveldt glaucoma implant for childhood glaucoma associated with Sturge–Weber syndrome. *Ophthalmology.* 2000;107(11):2105–2110.

62. Molteno AC, Van Biljon G, Ancker E. Two-stage insertion of glaucoma drainage implants. *Trans Ophthalmol Soc N Z.* 1979;31:17–26.

63. Molteno AC, Polkinghorne PJ, Bowbyes JA. The vicryl tie technique for inserting a draining implant in the treatment of secondary glaucoma. *Aust N Z J Ophthalmol.* 1986;14(4):343–354.

64. Nguyen QH, Budenz DL, Parrish RK II. Complications of Baerveldt glaucoma drainage implants. *Arch Ophthalmol.* 1998;116(5):571–575.

65. Valimaki J, Airaksinen PJ, Tuulonen A. Molteno implantation for secondary glaucoma in juvenile rheumatoid arthritis. *Arch Ophthalmol.* 1997;115(10):1253–1256.

66. Fuller JR, Molteno AC, Bevin TH. Iris creep producing correctopia in response to Molteno implants. *Arch Ophthalmol.* 2001;119(2):304.

67. Krebs DB, Liebmann JM, Ritch R, et al. Late infectious endophthalmitis from exposed glaucoma setons. *Arch Ophthalmol.* 1992;110(2):174–175.

68. Latina MA. Single stage Molteno implant with combination internal occlusion and external ligature. *Ophthalmic Surg.* 1990;21(6):444–446.

69. Susanna R Jr. Modifications of the Molteno implant and implant procedure. *Ophthalmic Surg.* 1991;22(10):611–613.

70. Stewart W, Feldman RM, Gross RL. Collagen plug occlusion of Molteno tube shunts. *Ophthalmic Surg.* 1993;24(1):47–48.

71. Ball SF, Herrington RG. Long-term retention of chromic occlusion suture in glaucoma seton tubes. *Arch Ophthalmol.* 1993;111(2):169.

72. Rojanapongpun P, Ritch R. Clear corneal graft overlying the seton tube to facilitate laser suture lysis. *Am J Ophthalmol.* 1996;122(3):424–425.

73. Aslanides IM, Spaeth GL, Schmidt CM, et al. Autologous patch graft in tube shunt surgery. *J Glaucoma.* 1999;8(5):306–309.

74. Sherwood MB, Smith MF. Prevention of early hypotony associated with Molteno implants by a new occluding stent technique. *Ophthalmology.* 1993;100(1):85–90.

75. Brooks SE, Dacey MP, Lee MB, et al. Modification of the glaucoma drainage implant to prevent early postoperative hypertension and hypotony: a laboratory study. *Ophthalmic Surg.* 1994;25(5):311–316.

76. Trible JR, Brown DB. Occlusive ligature and standardized fenestration of a Baerveldt tube with and without antimetabolites for early postoperative intraocular pressure control. *Ophthalmology.* 1998;105(12):2243–2250.

77. Prata JA Jr, Minckler DS, Mermoud A, et al. Effects of intraoperative mitomycin-C on the function of Baerveldt glaucoma drainage implants in rabbits. *J Glaucoma.* 1996;5(1):29–38.

78. Kook MS, Yoon J, Kim J, et al. Clinical results of Ahmed glaucoma valve implantation in refractory glaucoma with adjunctive mitomycin C. *Ophthalmic Surg Lasers.* 2000;31(2):100–106.

79. Irak I, Moster MR, Fontanarosa J. Intermediate-term results of Baerveldt tube shunt surgery with mitomycin C use. *Ophthalmic Surg Lasers Imaging.* 2004;35(3):189–196.

80. Lee D, Shin DH, Birt CM, et al. The effect of adjunctive mitomycin C in Molteno implant surgery. *Ophthalmology.* 1997;104(12):2126–2135.

81. Cantor L, Burgoyne J, Sanders S, et al. The effect of mitomycin C on Molteno implant surgery: a 1-year randomized, masked, prospective study. *J Glaucoma.* 1998;7(4):240–246.

82. Luttrull JK, Avery RL, Baerveldt G, et al. Initial experience with pneumatically stented Baerveldt implant modified for pars plana insertion for complicated glaucoma. *Ophthalmology.* 2000;107(1):143–149; discussion 149–150.

83. Joos KM, Lavina AM, Tawansy KA, et al. Posterior repositioning of glaucoma implants for anterior segment complications. *Ophthalmology.* 2001;108(2):279–284.

84. Smith MF, Doyle JW, Fanous MM. Modified aqueous drainage implants in the treatment of complicated glaucomas in eyes with pre-existing episcleral bands. *Ophthalmology.* 1998;105(12):2237–2242.

85. Scott IU, Gedde SJ, Budenz DL, et al. Baerveldt drainage implants in eyes with a preexisting scleral buckle. *Arch Ophthalmol.* 2000;118(11):1509–1513.

86. Doyle JW, Smith MF. Glaucoma after penetrating keratoplasty. *Semin Ophthalmol.* 1994;9(4):254–257.

87. Kwon YH, Taylor JM, Hong S, et al. Long-term results of eyes with penetrating keratoplasty and glaucoma drainage tube implant. *Ophthalmology.* 2001;108(2):272–278.

88. Al-Torbak A. Graft survival and glaucoma outcome after simultaneous penetrating keratoplasty and Ahmed glaucoma valve implant. *Cornea.* 2003;22(3):194–197.

89. Sidoti PA, Mosny AY, Ritterband DC, et al. Pars plana tube insertion of glaucoma drainage implants and penetrating keratoplasty in patients with coexisting glaucoma and corneal disease. *Ophthalmology.* 2001;108(6):1050–1058.

90. Rumelt S, Rehany U. Implantation of glaucoma drainage implant tube into the ciliary sulcus in patients with corneal transplants. *Arch Ophthalmol.* 1998;116(5):685–687.

91. Huang MC, Netland PA, Coleman AL, et al. Intermediate-term clinical experience with the Ahmed glaucoma valve implant. *Am J Ophthalmol.* 1999;127(1):27–33.

92. Taglia DP, Perkins TW. Permanent ligation of double-plate Molteno implant distal tube to control late hypotony. *Arch Ophthalmol.* 1999;117(9):1244–1245.

93. Nouri-Mahdavi K, Caprioli J. Evaluation of the hypertensive phase after insertion of the Ahmed glaucoma valve. *Am J Ophthalmol.* 2003; 136(6):1001–1008.

94. Molteno AC, Van Rooyen MM, Bartholomew RS. Implants for draining neovascular glaucoma. *Br J Ophthalmol.* 1977;61(2):120–125.

95. Singh K, Eid TE, Katz LJ, et al. Evaluation of Nd:YAG laser membranectomy in blocked tubes after glaucoma tube-shunt surgery. *Am J Ophthalmol.* 1997;124(6):781–786.

96. Sherwood MB, Joseph NH, Hitchings RA. Surgery for refractory glaucoma. Results and complications with a modified Schocket technique. *Arch Ophthalmol.* 1987;105(4):562–569.

97. Krawitz PL. Treatment of distal occlusion of Krupin eye valve with disk using cannular flush. *Ophthalmic Surg.* 1994;25(2):102–104.

98. Fiore PM, Melamed S. Use of neodymium: YAG laser to open an occluded molteno tube. *Ophthalmic Surg.* 1989;20(5):373–374.

99. Oram O, Gross RL, Severin TD, et al. Opening an occluded Molteno tube with the picosecond neodymium-yttrium lithium fluoride laser. *Arch Ophthalmol.* 1994;112(8):1023.

100. Pastor SA, Schumann SP, Starita RJ, et al. Intracameral tissue plasminogen activator: management of a fibrin clot occluding a Molteno tube. *Ophthalmic Surg.* 1993;24(12):853–854.

101. Sidoti PA, Morinelli EN, Heuer DK, et al. Tissue plasminogen activator and glaucoma drainage implants. *J Glaucoma.* 1995;4(4):258–262.

102. Chen PP, Palmberg PF. Needling revision of glaucoma drainage device filtering blebs. *Ophthalmology.* 1997;104(6):1004–1010.

103. Valimaki J, Tuulonen A, Airaksinen PJ. Capsule excision after failed Molteno surgery. *Ophthalmic Surg Lasers.* 1997;28(5):382–386.

104. Mermoud A, Salmon JF. Corticosteroid-induced ocular hypertension in draining Molteno single-plate implants. *J Glaucoma.* 1993;2(1): 32–36.

105. Cantor LB. Tube migration after glaucoma shunt procedure. *Am J Ophthalmol.* 1989;108(3):334–335.

106. Munoz M, Tomey KF, Traverso C, et al. Clinical experience with the Molteno implant in advanced infantile glaucoma. *J Pediatr Ophthalmol Strabismus.* 1991;28(2):68–72.

107. Netland PA, Walton DS. Glaucoma drainage implants in pediatric patients. *Ophthalmic Surg.* 1993;24(11):723–729.

108. Al-Torbak A, Edward DP. Transcorneal tube erosion of an Ahmed valve implant in a child. *Arch Ophthalmol.* 2001;119(10):1558–1559.

109. Maki JL, Nesti HA, Shetty RK, et al. Transcorneal tube extrusion in a child with a Baerveldt glaucoma drainage device. *J AAPOS.* 2007; 11(4):395–397.

110. Coleman AL, Smyth RJ, Wilson MR, et al. Initial clinical experience with the Ahmed glaucoma valve implant in pediatric patients. *Arch Ophthalmol.* 1997;115(2):186–191.

111. Billson F, Thomas R, Grigg J. Resiting Molteno implant tubes. *Ophthalmic Surg Lasers.* 1996;27(9):801–803.

112. Kooner KS. Repair of Molteno implant during surgery. *Am J Ophthalmol.* 1994;117(5):673.

113. Smith MF, Doyle JW. Results of another modality for extending glaucoma drainage tubes. *J Glaucoma.* 1999;8(5):310–314.

114. Liu SM, Su J, Hemady RK. Corneal melting after avulsion of a Molteno shunt plate. *J Glaucoma.* 1997;6(6):357–358.

115. Raviv T, Greenfield DS, Liebmann JM, et al. Pericardial patch grafts in glaucoma implant surgery. *J Glaucoma.* 1998;7(1):27–32.

116. King AJ, Azuara-Blanco A. Pericardial patch melting following glaucoma implant insertion. *Eye (Lond).* 2001;15(pt 2):236–237.

117. Lama PJ, Fechtner RD. Tube erosion following insertion of a glaucoma drainage device with a pericardial patch graft. *Arch Ophthalmol.* 1999;117(9):1243–1244.

118. Brandt JD. Patch grafts of dehydrated cadaveric dura mater for tube-shunt glaucoma surgery. *Arch Ophthalmol.* 1993;111(10):1436–1439.

119. Tanji TM, Lundy DC, Minckler DS, et al. Fascia lata patch graft in glaucoma tube surgery. *Ophthalmology.* 1996;103(8):1309–1312.

120. Seiff SR, Chang JS Jr, Hurt MH, et al. Polymerase chain reaction identification of human immunodeficiency virus-1 in preserved human sclera. *Am J Ophthalmol.* 1994;118(4):528–530.

121. Hinton R, Jinnah RH, Johnson C, et al. A biomechanical analysis of solvent-dehydrated and freeze-dried human fascia lata allografts. A preliminary report. *Am J Sports Med.* 1992;20(5):607–612.

122. Simonds RJ, Holmberg SD, Hurwitz RL, et al. Transmission of human immunodeficiency virus type 1 from a seronegative organ and tissue donor. *N Engl J Med.* 1992;326(11):726–732.

123. Diringer H, Braig HR. Infectivity of unconventional viruses in dura mater. *Lancet.* 1989;1(8635):439–440.

124. Jacob T, LaCour OJ, Burgoyne CF, et al. Expanded polytetrafluoroethylene reinforcement material in glaucoma drain surgery. *J Glaucoma.* 2001;10(2):115–120.

125. Oh KT, Alward WL, Kardon RH. Myositis associated with a Baerveldt glaucoma implant. *Am J Ophthalmol.* 1999;128(3):375–376.

126. Fanous MM, Cohn RA. Propionibacterium endophthalmitis following Molteno tube repositioning. *J Glaucoma.* 1997;6(4):201–202.

127. Perkins TW. Endophthalmitis after placement of a Molteno implant. *Ophthalmic Surg.* 1990;21(10):733–734.

128. Gedde SJ, Scott IU, Tabandeh H, et al. Late endophthalmitis associated with glaucoma drainage implants. *Ophthalmology.* 2001;108(7):1323–1327.

129. Heher KL, Lim JI, Haller JA, et al. Late-onset sterile endophthalmitis after Molteno tube implantation. *Am J Ophthalmol.* 1992;114(6):771–772.

130. Melamed S, Cahane M, Gutman I, et al. Postoperative complications after Molteno implant surgery. *Am J Ophthalmol.* 1991;111(3):319–322.

131. Huna R, Melamed S, Hirsh A, et al. Retinal detachment adherent to posterior chamber IOL after Molteno implant surgery. *Ophthalmic Surg.* 1990;21(12):854–856.

132. Lotufo DG. Postoperative complications and visual loss following Molteno implantation. *Ophthalmic Surg.* 1991;22(11):650–656.

133. Waterhouse WJ, Lloyd MA, Dugel PU, et al. Rhegmatogenous retinal detachment after Molteno glaucoma implant surgery. *Ophthalmology.* 1994;101(4):665–671.

134. Kramer T, Brown R, Lynch M, et al. Molteno implants and operating microscope-induced retinal phototoxicity. A clinicopathologic report. *Arch Ophthalmol.* 1991;109(3):379–383.

135. McDermott ML, Swendris RP, Shin DH, et al. Corneal endothelial cell counts after Molteno implantation. *Am J Ophthalmol.* 1993;115(1):93–96.

136. Englert JA, Freedman SF, Cox TA. The Ahmed valve in refractory pediatric glaucoma. *Am J Ophthalmol.* 1999;127(1):34–42.

137. Asrani S, Herndon L, Allingham RR. A newer technique for glaucoma tube trimming. *Arch Ophthalmol.* 2003;121(9):1324–1326.

138. Zalloum JN, Ahuja RM, Shin D, et al. Assessment of corneal decompensation in eyes having undergone molteno shunt procedures compared to eyes having undergone trabeculectomy. *CLAO J.* 1999;25(1):57–60.

139. Topouzis F, Coleman AL, Choplin N, et al. Follow-up of the original cohort with the Ahmed glaucoma valve implant. *Am J Ophthalmol.* 1999;128(2):198–204.

140. Lim KS. Corneal endothelial cell damage from glaucoma drainage device materials. *Cornea.* 2003;22(4):352–354.

141. Shah AA, WuDunn D, Cantor LB. Shunt revision versus additional tube shunt implantation after failed tube shunt surgery in refractory glaucoma. *Am J Ophthalmol.* 2000;129(4):455–460.

142. Burgoyne JK, WuDunn D, Lakhani V, et al. Outcomes of sequential tube shunts in complicated glaucoma. *Ophthalmology.* 2000;107(2):309–314.

143. Cardakli UF, Perkins TW. Recalcitrant diplopia after implantation of a Krupin valve with disc. *Ophthalmic Surg.* 1994;25(4):256–258.

144. Christmann LM, Wilson ME. Motility disturbances after Molteno implants. *J Pediatr Ophthalmol Strabismus.* 1992;29(1):44–48.

145. Frank JW, Perkins TW, Kushner BJ. Ocular motility defects in patients with the Krupin valve implant. *Ophthalmic Surg.* 1995;26(3):228–232.

146. Munoz M, Parrish RK II. Strabismus following implantation of Baerveldt drainage devices. *Arch Ophthalmol.* 1993;111(8):1096–1099.

147. Smith SL, Starita RJ, Fellman RL, et al. Early clinical experience with the Baerveldt 350-mm² glaucoma implant and associated extraocular muscle imbalance. *Ophthalmology.* 1993;100(6):914–918.

148. Ball SF, Ellis GS Jr, Herrington RG, et al. Brown's superior oblique tendon syndrome after Baerveldt glaucoma implant. *Arch Ophthalmol.* 1992;110(10):1368.

149. Dobler-Dixon AA, Cantor LB, Sondhi N, et al. Prospective evaluation of extraocular motility following double-plate Molteno implantation. *Arch Ophthalmol.* 1999;117(9):1155–1160.

150. Roizen A, Ela-Dalman N, Velez FG, et al. Surgical treatment of strabismus secondary to glaucoma drainage device. *Arch Ophthalmol.* 2008;126(4):480–486.

151. Rhee DJ, Casuso LA, Rosa RH Jr, et al. Motility disturbance due to true Tenon cyst in a child with a Baerveldt glaucoma drainage implant. *Arch Ophthalmol.* 2001;119(3):440–442.

152. Sidoti PA, Minckler DS, Baerveldt G, et al. Epithelial ingrowth and glaucoma drainage implants. *Ophthalmology.* 1994;101(5):872–875.

153. Costa VP, Katz LJ, Cohen EJ, et al. Glaucoma associated with epithelial downgrowth controlled with Molteno tube shunts. *Ophthalmic Surg.* 1992;23(12):797–800.

154. Ball SF, Loftfield K, Scharfenberg J. Molteno rip-cord suture hypopyon. *Ophthalmic Surg.* 1990;21(6):407–411; discussion 411–412.

155. Hyung SM, Min JP. Subconjunctival silicone oil drainage through the Molteno implant. *Korean J Ophthalmol.* 1998;12(1):73–75.

156. Law SK, Kalenak JW, Connor TB Jr, et al. Retinal complications after aqueous shunt surgical procedures for glaucoma. *Arch Ophthalmol.* 1996;114(12):1473–1480.

157. Airaksinen PJ, Aisala P, Tuulonen A. Molteno implant surgery in uncontrolled glaucoma. *Acta Ophthalmol.* 1990;68(6):690–694.

158. Price FW Jr, Wellemeyer M. Long-term results of Molteno implants. *Ophthalmic Surg.* 1995;26(2):130–135.

159. Broadway DC, Iester M, Schulzer M, et al. Survival analysis for success of Molteno tube implants. *Br J Ophthalmol.* 2001;85(6):689–695.

160. Mills RP, Reynolds A, Emond MJ, et al. Long-term survival of Molteno glaucoma drainage devices. *Ophthalmology.* 1996;103(2):299–305.

161. Molteno AC, Sayawat N, Herbison P. Otago glaucoma surgery outcome study: long-term results of uveitis with secondary glaucoma drained by Molteno implants. *Ophthalmology.* 2001;108(3):605–613.

162. Freedman J, Rubin B. Molteno implants as a treatment for refractory glaucoma in black patients. *Arch Ophthalmol.* 1991;109(10):1417–1420.

163. Spiegel D, Shrader RR, Wilson RP. Anterior chamber tube shunt to an encircling band (Schocket procedure) in the treatment of refractory glaucoma. *Ophthalmic Surg.* 1992;23(12):804–807.

164. Watanabe J, Sawaguchi S, Iwata K. Long-term results of anterior chamber tube shunt to an encircling band in the treatment of refractory glaucomas. *Acta Ophthalmol.* 1992;70(6):766–771.

165. Hodkin MJ, Goldblatt WS, Burgoyne CF, et al. Early clinical experience with the Baerveldt implant in complicated glaucomas. *Am J Ophthalmol.* 1995;120(1):32–40.

166. Siegner SW, Netland PA, Urban RC Jr, et al. Clinical experience with the Baerveldt glaucoma drainage implant. *Ophthalmology.* 1995;102(9):1298–1307.

167. Krishna R, Godfrey DG, Budenz DL, et al. Intermediate-term outcomes of 350-mm² Baerveldt glaucoma implants. *Ophthalmology.* 2001;108(3):621–626.

168. Fellenbaum PS, Almeida AR, Minckler DS, et al. Krupin disk implantation for complicated glaucomas. *Ophthalmology.* 1994;101(7):1178–1182.

169. Andreanos D, Papaconstantinou D, Georgopoulos G, et al. Ahmed valve in high-risk glaucoma surgery [in French]. *J Fr Ophtalmol.* 2001;24(1):60–63.

170. Eid TE, Katz LJ, Spaeth GL, et al. Long-term effects of tube-shunt procedures on management of refractory childhood glaucoma. *Ophthalmology.* 1997;104(6):1011–1016.

171. Djodeyre MR, Peralta Calvo J, Abelairas Gomez J. Clinical evaluation and risk factors of time to failure of Ahmed glaucoma valve implant in pediatric patients. *Ophthalmology.* 2001;108(3):614–620.

172. Fellenbaum PS, Sidoti PA, Heuer DK, et al. Experience with the Baerveldt implant in young patients with complicated Glaucomas. *J Glaucoma.* 1995;4(2):91–97.

173. Hill RA, Heuer DK, Baerveldt G, et al. Molteno implantation for glaucoma in young patients. *Ophthalmology.* 1991;98(7):1042–1046.

174. Nesher R, Sherwood MB, Kass MA, et al. Molteno implants in children. *J Glaucoma.* 1992;1(4):228–232.

175. Celebi S, Alagoz G, Aykan U. Ocular findings in Sturge–Weber syndrome. *Eur J Ophthalmol.* 2000;10(3):239–243.

176. Hamush NG, Coleman AL, Wilson MR. Ahmed glaucoma valve implant for management of glaucoma in Sturge–Weber syndrome. *Am J Ophthalmol.* 1999;128(6):758–760.

177. Ancker E, Molteno AC. Molteno drainage implant for neovascular glaucoma. *Trans Ophthalmol Soc U K.* 1982;102(pt 1):122–124.

178. Mermoud A, Salmon JF, Alexander P, et al. Molteno tube implantation for neovascular glaucoma. Long-term results and factors influencing the outcome. *Ophthalmology.* 1993;100(6):897–902.

179. Sidoti PA, Dunphy TR, Baerveldt G, et al. Experience with the Baerveldt glaucoma implant in treating neovascular glaucoma. *Ophthalmology.* 1995;102(7):1107–1118.

180. Chalam KV, Gandham S, Gupta S, et al. Pars plana modified Baerveldt implant versus neodymium:YAG cyclophotocoagulation in the management of neovascular glaucoma. *Ophthalmic Surg Lasers.* 2002;33(5):383–393.

181. Eid TE, Katz LJ, Spaeth GL, et al. Tube-shunt surgery versus neodymium:YAG cyclophotocoagulation in the management of neovascular glaucoma. *Ophthalmology.* 1997;104(10):1692–1700.

182. Lima FE, Magacho L, Carvalho DM, et al. A prospective, comparative study between endoscopic cyclophotocoagulation and the Ahmed drainage implant in refractory glaucoma. *J Glaucoma.* 2004;13(3): 233–237.

183. Yildirim N, Yalvac IS, Sahin A, et al. A comparative study between diode laser cyclophotocoagulation and the Ahmed glaucoma valve implant in neovascular glaucoma: a long-term follow-up. *J Glaucoma.* 2009; 18(3):192–196.

184. Da Mata A, Burk SE, Netland PA, et al. Management of uveitic glaucoma with Ahmed glaucoma valve implantation. *Ophthalmology.* 1999; 106(11):2168–2172.

185. Gil-Carrasco F, Salinas-VanOrman E, Recillas-Gispert C, et al. Ahmed valve implant for uncontrolled uveitic glaucoma. *Ocul Immunol Inflamm.* 1998;6(1):27–37.

186. Ancker E, Molteno AC. Surgical treatment of chronic aphakic glaucoma with the Molteno plastic implant [in German]. *Klin Monatsbl Augenheilkd.* 1980;177(3):365–370.

187. Varma R, Heuer DK, Lundy DC, et al. Pars plana Baerveldt tube insertion with vitrectomy in glaucomas associated with pseudophakia and aphakia. *Am J Ophthalmol.* 1995;119(4):401–407.

188. Fish LA, Heuer DK, Baerveldt G, et al. Molteno implantation for secondary glaucomas associated with advanced epithelial ingrowth. *Ophthalmology.* 1990;97(5):557–561.

189. Gandham SB, Costa VP, Katz LJ, et al. Aqueous tube-shunt implantation and pars plana vitrectomy in eyes with refractory glaucoma. *Am J Ophthalmol.* 1993;116(2):189–195.

190. McDonnell PJ, Robin JB, Schanzlin DJ, et al. Molteno implant for control of glaucoma in eyes after penetrating keratoplasty. *Ophthalmology.* 1988;95(3):364–369.

191. Sherwood MB, Smith MF, Driebe WT Jr, et al. Drainage tube implants in the treatment of glaucoma following penetrating keratoplasty. *Ophthalmic Surg.* 1993;24(3):185–189.

192. Wellemeyer ML, Price FW Jr. Molteno implants in patients with previous cyclocryotherapy. *Ophthalmic Surg.* 1993;24(6):395–398.

193. Wiggins RE Jr, Tomey KF. The results of glaucoma surgery in aniridia. *Arch Ophthalmol.* 1992;110(4):503–505.

194. Lee WB, Brandt JD, Mannis MJ, et al. Aniridia and Brachmann-de Lange syndrome: a review of ocular surface and anterior segment findings. *Cornea.* 2003;22(2):178–180.

195. Arroyave CP, Scott IU, Gedde SJ, et al. Use of glaucoma drainage devices in the management of glaucoma associated with aniridia. *Am J Ophthalmol.* 2003;135(2):155–159.

196. Hill RA, Nguyen QH, Baerveldt G, et al. Trabeculectomy and Molteno implantation for glaucomas associated with uveitis. *Ophthalmology.* 1993;100(6):903–908.

197. Bluestein EC, Stewart WC. Trabeculectomy with 5-fluorouracil vs single-plate Molteno implantation. *Ophthalmic Surg.* 1993;24(10): 669–673.

198. Sayyad FE, Helal M, Elsherif Z, et al. Molteno implant versus trabeculectomy with adjunctive introperative mitomycin-C in high-risk glaucoma patients. *J Glaucoma.* 1995;4(2):80–85.

199. Wilson MR, Mendis U, Smith SD, et al. Ahmed glaucoma valve implant vs trabeculectomy in the surgical treatment of glaucoma: a randomized clinical trial. *Am J Ophthalmol.* 2000;130(3):267–273.

200. Wilson MR, Mendis U, Paliwal A, et al. Long-term follow-up of primary glaucoma surgery with Ahmed glaucoma valve implant versus trabeculectomy. *Am J Ophthalmol.* 2003;136(3):464–470.

201. Noureddin BN, Wilson-Holt N, Lavin M, et al. Advanced uncontrolled glaucoma. Nd:YAG cyclophotocoagulation or tube surgery. *Ophthalmology.* 1992;99(3):430–436.

202. Ayyala RS, Pieroth L, Vinals AF, et al. Comparison of mitomycin C trabeculectomy, glaucoma drainage device implantation, and laser neodymium:YAG cyclophotocoagulation in the management of intractable glaucoma after penetrating keratoplasty. *Ophthalmology.* 1998;105(8): 1550–1556.

Medical and Surgical Treatments for Childhood Glaucomas

The successful treatment of childhood glaucoma presents many challenges, with control of intraocular pressure (IOP) as the first but not the only priority. The optimal treatment strategies for children often differ greatly from those for adults with glaucoma. Factors influencing decisions about therapy include those related not only to the type and severity of the glaucoma but also to the age and needs of the particular child.

MEDICAL THERAPY

Although surgical intervention is the primary treatment for primary congenital glaucoma and closed-angle glaucomas (e.g., secondary to cicatricial retinopathy of prematurity), medications are the initial and often the mainstay of therapy for juvenile open-angle glaucoma and other secondary glaucomas (e.g., such as those occurring in aphakia or with uveitis). Medications also play an important auxiliary role even in cases of congenital glaucoma, wherein they may help clear the cornea preoperatively to facilitate goniotomy and may help control IOP postoperatively until the success of surgical intervention has been determined. Medical therapy is also indicated in managing those difficult cases in which surgery poses particular risks or has incompletely controlled glaucoma (1). Besides inadequate IOP reduction, multiple factors conspire against the success of long-term medical therapy in childhood glaucomas: the difficulties with long-term adherence, adequate ascertainment of drug-induced side effects, and potential adverse systemic effects of protracted therapy, among others.

Many medications are now available for the reduction of IOP in patients with glaucoma. The Food and Drug Administration (FDA) initially approved all of them for use without requiring data on the safety and efficacy of these drugs in pediatric patients. Ongoing study of several major new drugs is currently being undertaken by several major pharmaceutical companies, under the supervision of the FDA. For example, a randomized, double-masked, 3-month trial compared dorzolamide, 2%, three times daily with timolol, 0.25% or 0.5%, once daily in patients younger than 6 years who had glaucoma; the study found both treatments to be relatively safe and effective (2). A similarly designed study, again conducted among children with glaucoma who were younger than 6, compared use of brinzolamide, 1%, twice a day with use of levobetaxolol, 0.5%, twice a day, and it demonstrated that both drugs were well tolerated and lowered IOP (3). Nonetheless, many of the commonly used glaucoma drugs still carry a warning that "safety and efficacy in pediatric patients have not been established." Furthermore, certain drugs, such as brimonidine, carry warnings about dangerous systemic side effects in infants and young children. Because eyedrops are not downsized for pediatric use and because the plasma volume of a small child is much smaller than that of an average adult counterpart, blood levels of glaucoma drugs can reach high levels in young children at doses recommended for use in adults (4). Even topical glaucoma medication must be used with careful forethought in children, particularly in those who are very small or with special considerations such as premature birth, asthma, or other cardiac or pulmonary problems.

Table 40.1 gives information pertaining to the suggested use of various glaucoma drugs specifically in infants and children with glaucoma. (Detailed information on the use and mechanisms of these medications is provided elsewhere in this text.)

Carbonic Anhydrase Inhibitors

Oral carbonic anhydrase inhibitors, primarily acetazolamide (Diamox), have effectively reduced elevated IOP in infants and children with primary infantile (and other types of) glaucoma for decades, often reducing the IOP about 20% to 35%. When administered orally with food or milk three or four times daily (total dosage, 10 to 20 mg/kg/day), acetazolamide is fairly well tolerated (1,5). Caregivers should be queried specifically about the occurrence of diarrhea, diminished energy levels, and loss of appetite in children on this therapy, as such effects would necessitate a dosage adjustment or discontinuation of use. Metabolic acidosis has also been reported in infants (6), in whom it may manifest as rapid breathing and may be somewhat ameliorated with oral sodium citrate and citric acid oral solution (Bicitra, 1 mEq/kg/day) (7).

The topical carbonic anhydrase inhibitor, dorzolamide (Trusopt), offers a viable alternative to acetazolamide for many patients. In a small crossover trial, 11 children whose glaucoma was controlled on topical β-blocker and oral acetazolamide switched from the oral acetazolamide to topical dorzolamide, three times daily, in the study eye. Mean IOP reduction with use of the topical agent was approximately 25%, compared with approximately 35% on acetazolamide (8). Although systemic side effects occurred commonly in patients receiving the acetazolamide, no adverse effects were noted with the use of topical dorzolamide. The addition of oral acetazolamide to topical dorzolamide has been reported to reduce IOP further than when either drug is used alone (9).

A second topical carbonic anhydrase inhibitor, brinzolamide (Azopt), has also been well tolerated by children, with IOP reduction similar to that obtained with use of dorzolamide

Table 40.1	Medications in Children with Glaucoma	
Medication Type	**Indications**	**Contraindications/Side Effects**
β-Blockers		
Nonselective Selective	First-line therapy for many, second-line for some older children Nonselective drugs more effective than selective drugs, but the latter are relatively safer in children with asthma	Systemic effects: bronchospasm, bradycardia. Avoid in premature or tiny infants, and in children with history of reactive airways. Start with 0.25% in smaller children
Carbonic Anhydrase Inhibitors		
Topical (dorzolamide, brinzolamide), twice- or thrice-daily dosing Oral (acetazolamide), 10–20 mg/kg/day, given twice to four times daily	First- or second-line in young children, add well to other classes Topical therapy better tolerated but not as effective; may use both if needed	Topical systemically safe May wish to avoid, or use as later option, in children with compromised corneas, especially with corneal transplant Dorzolamide stings Metabolic acidosis may occur with oral therapy
Miotics		
Echothiophate iodide Pilocarpine	Echothiophate rarely used, sometimes in aphakia; pilocarpine after angle surgery and sometimes with JOAG; less effective IOP reduction in congenital glaucoma	Systemic effects (echothiophate): sometimes diarrhea, warn about use of succinyl choline with echothiophate; (both) headache; both may induce myopic shift; possible proinflammatory effect (echothiophate)
Adrenergic Agonists		
Epinephrine compounds	Rarely used, limited effectiveness	Systemic effects: hypertension, tachycardia in small children
α₂-Agonists Apraclonidine, 0.5%	Helps during/after angle surgery; useful in the short term in infants and after corneal transplantation	Systemically safe; effect may wear off; rarely local allergy or red eye
Brimonidine (use lowest concentration, e.g., Alphagan P, 0.10%, in smaller children)	Use only in older children: second- or third-line therapy with JOAG, aphakia, older children with other glaucoma types	DO NOT USE IN INFANTS/SMALL CHILDREN < 40 lb (approx.), as may cause bradycardia, hypotension, hypothermia, hypotonia, apnea—especially if used with β-blocker
Prostaglandins and Similar Drugs		
Latanoprost, travoprost, bimatoprost	First-, second-, or third-line with JOAG; usually second- or third-line (after β-blockers and topical CAIs) in others	Systemically safe in children; long eyelashes will result (beware unilateral use); redness common (especially with bimatoprost); use caution with uveitic glaucoma

approx., approximately; CAI, carbonic anhydrase inhibitor; JOAG, juvenile open-angle glaucoma.

(Freedman SF, unpublished data). In one study of brinzolamide and levobunolol treatment in children with glaucoma younger than 6 years, both drugs were well tolerated, but brinzolamide was more effective in patients with glaucoma associated with systemic or ocular abnormalities than in patients with primary congenital glaucoma (3). The carbonic anhydrase inhibitors are useful for treating pediatric glaucoma and may be appropriate first- and second-line agents, respectively, when β-blocker use is contraindicated or inadequately effective (Table 40.1; also see the following text). (The combination of a topical carbonic anhydrase inhibitor [dorzolamide] with the β-blocker timolol is discussed further in the β-Blockers section.)

Miotics

The use of miotic drugs has largely been supplanted by that of newer medications. Cholinergic stimulators, often called miotics, have limited value in the treatment of childhood glaucoma. Eyes with congenital glaucoma often show poor IOP reduction to miotics, perhaps because of the abnormal insertion of the ciliary muscle into the trabecular meshwork (10,11). However, pilocarpine is often used to achieve and maintain miosis before and after goniotomy or trabeculotomy for congenital glaucoma (12,13). Stronger miotics, such as echothiophate iodide (phospholine iodide), have also been administered in infants, especially those with aphakic glaucoma, with less ocular irritation than that observed in adults (12). Echothiophate iodide therapy has sometimes been accompanied by diarrhea and requires extreme care in the concurrent use of succinyl choline for general anesthesia. Older children, if phakic, often experience severe visual blurring attributable to myopia induced by miotics. If they are necessary and effective in treating the glaucoma, miotics in these children may be better tolerated when the induced myopia is rendered stable, so that spectacles can compensate for it. When used in older children, higher concentrations (e.g., pilocarpine, 2% to 4%) may be useful (Table 40.1).

β-Adrenergic Antagonists (β-Blockers)

Topical β-blockers have been available for the treatment of glaucoma since the introduction of timolol in 1978. Several studies have examined the role of timolol in treating uncontrolled childhood glaucomas (4,14–18). In a study of 67 patients (100 eyes) with childhood glaucomas who began topical therapy with timolol before 18 years of age, 30 patients (40 eyes) experienced a mean IOP decrement of 21.3% and required no further surgery or medical therapy over a 2.5-year follow-up period (17). Most patients whose glaucoma stabilized on timolol did so using 0.25% twice daily, and all the patients with adverse reactions (10%) were using timolol, 0.5%. Only two patients discontinued use of timolol because of side effects—a 10-year-old who developed severe asthma and a 17-year-old with symptomatic bradycardia (17). The incidence of systemic side effects reported in these studies varied from 0% to 18% (4,14–18).

The most severe systemic adverse effects in children receiving topical timolol therapy have included acute asthma attacks, bradycardia, and apneic spells (the latter in neonates) (4,18–20). Plasma timolol levels measured in children using 0.25% timolol (ranging from 3.5 ng/mL in a 5-year-old to 34 ng/mL in a 3-week-old) vastly exceeded those in adults using 0.5% timolol (range, 0.34 to 2.45 ng/mL) (4). The use of punctal occlusion in adults further lowered mean 1-hour plasma timolol levels by 40% in the adult patients in this study (from 1.34 to 0.9 ng/mL). The high plasma timolol levels in children may be explained by a child's volume of distribution for the drug, which is much smaller than that of an adult.

When timolol is used in small children, treatment should always begin with 0.25% drops, excluding those children with a history of asthma or bradycardia. Topical β-blockers should be used with extreme caution in neonates, with particular attention to the possibility of apnea. It may be reasonable to observe children for adverse systemic effects for 1 to 2 hours in the office after an initial dose of β-blocker has been given before prescribing the β-blocker for outpatient use (16,20). Punctal occlusion, when feasible, should be performed by parents or other caretakers (16). There is anecdotal evidence that using timolol as Timoptic XE or timolol gel-forming solution, once daily, may result in lower plasma drug levels, compared with the same concentration of solution used twice daily.

There is little information available on the use of topical β-blockers other than timolol in the treatment of childhood glaucoma. A short-term, randomized, double-masked comparison of levobetaxolol and brinzolamide in children younger than 6 years demonstrated that both drugs were well tolerated and lowered IOP in this group. In children naïve to prior medication, levobetaxolol was more effective in primary congenital glaucoma than in glaucoma with associated ocular or systemic abnormalities (3). Based on experience in adults, betaxolol, as a relatively β-1–selective β-blocker, may be less susceptible to precipitating acute asthma attacks (which may present as coughing) than the nonselective β-blockers. The remaining nonselective β-blockers should be approached in a fashion similar to timolol regarding risks and probable efficacy. As in adults, β-blockers used in children often do have an additive effect to oral and topical carbonic anhydrase inhibitors in treating children with glaucoma (1,15).

Two combination preparations that include timolol, 0.5%, are currently available commercially in the United States. The first preparation, combining timolol, 0.5%, and dorzolamide, 2.0% (Cosopt, now also available as generic; used twice daily), is a potent IOP-reducing agent in older children, but it must be avoided in infants because of the relatively high concentration of timolol. The newer drug, Combigan, combines timolol, 0.5%, plus brimonidine, 0.2%; this potent agent must be used with caution in children and never in those for whom either ingredient alone would be contraindicated (see Adrenergic Agonists section; Table 40.1).

Topical β-blockers, despite their contraindication in some cases, still have an important role in treating children with glaucoma and are appropriate first-line drugs for many children (Table 40.1).

Adrenergic Agonists

Epinephrine compounds have been used in infants and children with glaucoma (21,22), but there are little published data to suggest optimal dosing schedules or the magnitude of the pressure decrement to be expected from these drugs. These drugs, furthermore, are relegated to secondary importance because of their potential for systemic toxicity (e.g., tachyarrhythmias, hypertension) and their ocular side effects (e.g., irritation, reactive hyperemia, adrenochrome deposits), together with their limited effectiveness. Topical dipivefrin (Propine), as an epinephrine prodrug, should theoretically have fewer systemic side effects in children than epinephrine does.

The two commercially available α_2-adrenergic agonists, apraclonidine and brimonidine, have a valid role in the treatment of pediatric glaucoma, although neither drug has been approved by the FDA for use in children. Apraclonidine (Iopidine, 0.5%) can be useful and well tolerated in the setting of angle surgery to minimize intraoperative hyphema (see later under Goniotomy) and may have a short-term role for treating infants who cannot tolerate β-blockers or who have had recent corneal transplantation (and in whom one therefore wishes to avoid topical carbonic anhydrase inhibitors). Wright and Freedman found an 8% incidence of side effects among 75 infants and children given apraclonidine, 0.5%, with lethargy reported in 3 children younger than 5 months of age (23).

Brimonidine (available as brimonidine, 0.2%, and Alphagan P, 0.10% and 0.15%) can be useful in reducing IOP in older children, but it must be used with extreme caution in younger children. Its use should be avoided altogether in infants and in small and underweight children, because of its propensity to cause severe systemic side effects. Topical brimonidine administration has caused bradycardia, hypotension, hypothermia, hypotonia, and apnea in infants, and severe somnolence in toddlers (24–26), especially when combined with topical β-blockers (27).

Brimonidine is rarely an appropriate first-line drug for children, except in selected older children with intolerance to β-blockers and carbonic anhydrase inhibitors. It may, however, be useful adjunctive therapy in those patients needing additional IOP reduction (Table 40.1).

The combination of brimonidine, 0.2%, and timolol, 0.5%, Combigan, is a potent drug (see the preceding text) that should not be used in children with contraindication to either of the component ingredients.

Prostaglandins

The prostaglandin-type drugs can prove useful in some selected cases of pediatric glaucoma, although published data are limited, and none of these drugs has received FDA approval for pediatric use. Latanoprost (Xalatan) has been useful in selected cases of pediatric glaucoma, particularly in patients with juvenile open-angle glaucoma and some patients with aphakia and port-wine stain–associated glaucoma; no serious systemic side effects have been reported (28–31). Travoprost (Travatan) has recently been reported to be well tolerated and effective at IOP reduction in selected patients with pediatric glaucoma (32). The prostaglandin drugs do induce growth of eyelashes in pediatric patients (29,30,33) (**Fig. 40.1**); surface redness, periocular skin pigmentation, and iris darkening have all been noted as well ((30); Freedman SF, unpublished data). Caution is advised if these drugs are used in children with uveitis, or with aphakia or pseudophakia (although reports of cystoid macular edema in pediatric cases are lacking at this time).

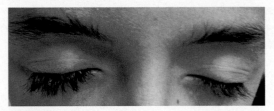

Figure 40.1 Long and thick eyelashes in both eyes of an 11-year-old boy who has taken latanoprost for treatment of mild aphakic glaucoma.

Prostaglandin-like agents do not yet seem appropriate as first-line treatment for children, except perhaps for selected cases of juvenile open-angle glaucoma with special risk for β-blocker use. These agents may play an important adjunctive role when IOP control is inadequate despite use of other medications already discussed (Table 40.1).

SURGICAL THERAPY

There are various surgical procedures available to treat children with glaucoma (**Table 40.2**). Although the appropriate intervention in some cases is clear and widely agreed on (e.g., angle surgery for congenital–infantile glaucoma [see later]), the optimal surgical algorithm is, in many cases, open to disagreement, even among experts who care for these children. One reason for this heterogeneity in surgical management undoubtedly relates to the challenges in performing surgery in children with refractory glaucoma. Even the anesthesia itself poses significant risks, especially in neonates. Many factors make the infant eye behave differently (usually in a more challenging way) from the adult eye during glaucoma surgery—a smaller palpebral fissure, less rigid and often thinned sclera and limbal tissue (especially in buphthalmic eyes), clouding of the cornea, and narrowness of the anterior chamber are a few. Postoperatively, it may be challenging to adequately protect the operated eye from accidental injury, to monitor for possible surgical complications and response to surgery, and to ensure adherence to medication regimens and recommended restriction of physical activity.

Often, it can be helpful to develop appropriate expectations on the part of the family ahead of the surgery; hence family members should be informed preoperatively of the multiple visits and additional anesthesias that may be needed postoperatively, and the likelihood that further surgery may be required to control the glaucoma. Often, the first examination under anesthesia can be immediately followed by the first indicated surgical procedure.

Angle Surgery

The introduction of angle surgery (first goniotomy and then trabeculotomy ab externo) drastically improved the previously poor prognosis for children with primary congenital–infantile glaucoma. Both goniotomy and trabeculotomy ab externo have their staunch advocates, but neither procedure has been

Table 40.2	Indications for Surgery in Childhood Glaucomas

I. ANGLE SURGERY
  A. GONIOTOMY (may repeat one or more times)
   1. Primary congenital/infantile open-angle glaucoma
   2. Other primary glaucomas (generally poorer success)
       a. Juvenile open-angle glaucoma
       b. Axenfeld–Rieger syndrome
       c. Lowe syndrome
       d. Neurofibromatosis
       e. Sturge–Weber syndrome
       f. Possible selected other types
   3. Selected secondary glaucomas
       a. Maternal rubella syndrome[a]
       b. Open-angle glaucoma occurring soon after congenital cataract surgery
       c. Glaucoma associated with chronic anterior uveitis (especially juvenile idiopathic arthritis-related uveitis in phakic eyes with mostly open angle)
   4. Possible treatment in aniridia with progressive angle closure[b]
  B. TRABECULOTOMY (may repeat one time)
   1. (Same as for goniotomy, but preferred in the presence of corneal opacification)
   2. Performed by some surgeons after two goniotomies have failed
   3. May be combined with trabeculectomy (see IIIA, below)
   4. Standard with trabeculotome vs. 360-degree modification

II. PERIPHERAL IRIDECTOMY
  (Secondary pupillary block glaucoma)

III. FILTRATION SURGERY
  A. COMBINED TRABECULOTOMY–TRABECULECTOMY
   1. When trabeculotomy cannot be completed (failure to cannulate Schlemm canal)
   2. Failed previous angle surgery (≤2 goniotomies and/or trabeculotomies)
  B. TRABECULECTOMY (usually with intraoperative mitomycin C)
   1. Any glaucoma in an eye with reasonable visual potential and unscarred conjunctiva after angle surgery has failed, with guaranteed faithful follow-up (not usually suggested for infants and aphakic eyes)
   2. Low likelihood of success with angle surgery (would sometimes favor IIIA, above)
  C. COMBINED CATARACT REMOVAL–TRABECULECTOMY
  (Not usually recommended)

IV. GLAUCOMA DRAINAGE-DEVICE (TUBE SHUNT) SURGERY
  A. Infants and aphakic eyes after failed angle surgery or if low likelihood of success
  B. Failed trabeculectomy with intraoperative mitomycin C and reasonable visual potential
  C. High risk for complications with filtration surgery (e.g., Sturge–Weber syndrome)
  D. High risk for failure with trabeculectomy from scarring (e.g., after multiple conjunctival surgeries)
  E. Consider simultaneous IPSILATERAL LATERAL RECTUS RECESSION (e.g., patient with exotropia and planned Baerveldt placement)
  F. COMBINED CATARACT REMOVAL–GLAUCOMA DRAINAGE-DEVICE SURGERY
  (Rare cases only [e.g., cataract and refractory glaucoma in older child with uveitic or traumatic glaucoma *and* quiet eye])

V. CYCLODESTRUCTIVE PROCEDURES
  A. TRANSSCLERAL CYCLOPHOTOCOAGULATION (Diode laser)
   1. Failed angle surgery (or angle surgery not possible) and minimal visual potential
   2. Failed trabeculectomy and/or glaucoma drainage-device surgery with poor central vision
   3. IOP too high after glaucoma drainage-device surgery with encapsulation but not blockage
   4. Anatomy precluding trabeculectomy or glaucoma drainage-device surgery (e.g., disorganized anterior segment after trauma, sclerocornea)
   5. In patients who are gravely ill, or when follow-up and postoperative care cannot be assured, or general anesthesia with intubation poses life-threatening risk
   6. High risk for complications with intraocular surgery (e.g., Sturge–Weber syndrome)
  B. ENDOSCOPIC CYCLOPHOTOCOAGULATION (Diode laser)
   1. May be considered for any patient in whom transscleral cycloablation would be reasonable, provided anatomy allows limbal or pars plana approach to ciliary processes (best in aphakic/pseudophakic eyes)
   2. May be appropriate after transscleral cyclophotocoagulation has failed to reduce IOP
   3. May be appropriate in cases needing cycloablation in whom risk of inflammation is high

Table 40.2	Indications for Surgery in Childhood Glaucomas (*Continued*)

C. CYCLOCRYOTHERAPY
    1. Usually not indicated, except where anatomic considerations make transscleral or endoscopic laser cyclophotocoagulation difficult or unlikely to succeed
    2. Repeat therapy in selected quadrants after previous cyclocryotherapy

[a]Rare outside of developing countries.
[b]Should be performed only by surgeons very comfortable with goniotomy, given unprotected lens.
IOP, intraocular pressure.

definitively proven better than the other for treating primary infantile glaucoma. These procedures are also useful in other selected cases of pediatric glaucoma (see later and **Table 40.3**).

With the aim of incising the uveal trabecular meshwork under direct visualization, goniotomy is the surgical procedure of choice in many cases of primary congenital glaucoma. Trabeculotomy ab externo (see the following text), an alternative procedure, is especially useful when corneal clouding prevents an optimal view of the angle structures by gonioscopy.

Goniotomy

In 1893, the Italian ophthalmologist Carlo de Vincentiis described a new operation that attempted to open Schlemm canal by incising the angle tissues (without visualization of the angle) (34). Because of a high complication rate and poor results in adults with chronic open-angle glaucoma, this operation was initially abandoned. With the advantage of clinical gonioscopy,

Otto Barkan modified the technique as an operation for primary congenital glaucoma in 1938, dubbing it "goniotomy" (Gk. *gonio*—angle and *tomein*—to cut) (35). This effective operation for congenital glaucoma dramatically improved the previously dismal prognosis for this condition (36). The technique for performing goniotomy has remained essentially unaltered for more than 50 years—a testament to the effectiveness and widespread use of this elegant, brief, conjunctival-sparing procedure as an initial intervention for primary congenital glaucoma (1). Although the aim of goniotomy is to open a route for aqueous humor to exit the anterior chamber into the Schlemm canal by removing obstructing tissue, the precise mechanism by which pressure reduction occurs remains obscure. Successful goniotomy does appear, however, to reduce the IOP by improving facility of aqueous outflow (37). Goniotomy enjoys its greatest success in the treatment of primary congenital glaucoma presenting between 3 and 12 months of

Table 40.3	Angle Surgery—Expected Beneficial Outcomes on Intraocular Pressure Control

Indication for Angle Surgery	**Outcome (% with Benefit)**
Primary congenital open-angle glaucoma	Very favorable (>75%)
Glaucoma with Rubinstein–Taybi syndrome, rubella	
Glaucoma secondary to chronic anterior uveitis	
Steroid-induced glaucoma	
Glaucoma with Axenfeld–Rieger syndrome	Possibly favorable (<50%)
Glaucoma with Lowe syndrome	
Congenital glaucoma in the newborn	
Glaucoma with iris hypoplasia	
Juvenile open-angle glaucoma	
Early-onset glaucoma after congenital cataract surgery	
Early-onset glaucoma with Sturge–Weber syndrome	
Congenital aniridic glaucoma[a]	
Later-onset glaucoma with Sturge–Weber syndrome	Unfavorable (<25%)
Glaucoma secondary to neurofibromatosis	
Acquired aniridic glaucoma	
Glaucoma with ectropion uveae	
Older child with open-angle glaucoma after cataract removal	

[a]Preventive—see Table 40.2.

age (1), but it may also be used in other primary developmental and secondary glaucomas, although with reduced success (1,37) (Table 40.3). Examples of these other primary glaucomas include juvenile open-angle glaucoma (38) and early-onset glaucomas associated with Sturge–Weber syndrome, neurofibromatosis, and Lowe syndrome. Several secondary glaucomas may respond favorably to goniotomy in some cases (7), including glaucoma complicating chronic anterior uveitis and selected cases of aphakic glaucoma presenting early after congenital cataract surgery (39,40). Goniotomy has been advocated as a prophylactic procedure in congenital aniridia before glaucoma develops, but its use in this setting is particularly technically challenging (41,42) (Table 40.3).

Preoperative medications should ideally be used for several days before planned goniotomy to maximally reduce the IOP and clear the cornea. Medications often used include oral acetazolamide or topical dorzolamide, together with apraclonidine, 0.5%, and judicious use of a topical β-blocker in selected cases. To produce miosis, pilocarpine, 1% or 2%, should be placed on the eye just before it undergoes surgery, to promote miosis and thereby aid in protecting the crystalline lens from

injury during the procedure. Acetylcholine chloride 1:100 (e.g., Miochol) may be injected into the anterior chamber if necessary to promote further miosis. Apraclonidine, 0.5%, may be applied to the eye just before surgery and may help decrease intraoperative bleeding.

Basic Technique

Goniotomy is performed by using a surgical goniolens and a goniotomy knife or needle (**Table 40.4; Fig. 40.2**) (43). There are several available types of goniolens, in addition to the round-domed Barkan goniolens, including the Lister modification, which includes irrigation, the Swan–Jacobs lens, which incorporates a handle, as well as the Hill goniolens and Khaw surgical goniolens, both of which allow the surgeon holding the lens also to fixate the globe. Numerous modifications of the Barkan goniotomy knife have been described, including attached fiber optics for intraocular illumination (44). A nontapered Swan knife (or needle–knife) enters the anterior chamber easily and cuts in either direction. Alternatively, a disposable 25-gauge needle attached to a syringe containing viscoelastic or Miochol may be used in place of a knife, allowing the

Table 40.4	Child-Specific Recommendations for Commonly Performed Surgical Procedures in Glaucoma

GONIOTOMY

1. Ensure adequate angle view: if corneal edema present, use aqueous suppressants before surgery, and topical sodium chloride, 5%, just prior to surgery; place goniotomy lens on mound of viscoelastic, tip microscope approximately 45 degrees from the vertical, tip child's head toward surgical side.

2. Stabilize globe and practice rotation: use locking forceps on Tenon insertion (usually 6 and 12 o'clock); use speculum with low profile, try globe rotation before entering eye.

3. Optimize wound entry: enter eye only one time using 25-gauge, 1.5-inch needle, making entry into peripheral cornea and parallel to iris; pass needle carefully over iris to engage anterior trabecular meshwork.

4. Perform effective trabecular meshwork incision: make incision superficial and into anterior trabecular meshwork, passing first one direction, then the other; assistant rotates globe while needle is *not* engaged in the meshwork.

5. Avoid injury to lens: constrict pupil with pilocarpine, 2%, before surgery; visualize tip of needle at all times and maintain plane parallel to iris for all movements.

6. Minimize bleeding: use apraclonidine, 0.5%, drops before incision; incise the trabecular meshwork only; remove the needle carefully over the iris and have assistant "relax" any pull on locking forceps at this time; prepare to push on entry site with forceps to minimize chamber collapse, refill with balanced salt and filtered air bubble; dissolvable 10-0 suture to close entry site securely.

TRABECULOTOMY

1. Optimize location: unless combined with trabeculectomy, place incision temporal or nasal and just above or below the horizontal to facilitate scleral flap and spare superior conjunctiva for possible later surgery.

2. Optimize incision and scleral flap: fornix-based conjunctival flap; triangular limbus-based scleral flap (thick enough to facilitate watertight closure); radial scratch incision to one side of base of flap (to allow a second cut-down, if needed).

3. Maximize chances of finding Schlemm canal: make radial incision gradually, watching for transverse fibers of canal, at sclerolimbal junction; watch for blood–aqueous reflux.

4. Minimize chance of false passage: confirm Schlemm canal location by passing a blunted 6-0 Prolene suture into the canal, either for 360-degree suture technique or to verify that suture remains parallel to limbus (not in anterior chamber or suprachoroidal space); four-mirror gonioprism can sometimes visualize suture in the canal; place and rotate metal trabeculotome (if used) gently and under direct view to avoid tearing iris or stripping Descemet membrane.

5. Secure wound and minimize bleeding: fill chamber with viscoelastic before pulling suture for 360-degree technique, and often after first trabeculotome pass before second pass in opposite direction; close scleral flap tightly with 10-0 Vicryl suture; close conjunctiva tightly with Vicryl suture.

Table 40.4	Child-Specific Recommendations for Commonly Performed Surgical Procedures in Glaucoma (*Continued*)

TRABECULECTOMY (USUALLY WITH MITOMYCIN C)

1. Optimize exposure and stabilization: place 7-0 Vicryl suture into peripheral cornea in two places opposite intended surgery (e.g., at about 10:30 and 2:30 o'clock for superior site), to avoid corneal suture into thin cornea superiorly where view may be obstructed.

2. Optimize incision and future bleb morphology: fornix-based conjunctival flap for most cases, except where cornea compromised, thin superior limbus expected, or high risk with flat chamber (e.g., aniridia).

3. Use of antimetabolite: mitomycin C usually indicated (except in older children, in whom 5-FU may be used intraoperatively and postoperatively); apply to broad area of uncut sclera and Tenon capsule, but keep away from conjunctival edges and cornea, concentration usually 0.2 to 0.4 mg/mL for 2 to 5 min.

4. Scleral flap preparation, sclerostomy, and iridectomy: cut fairly thick flap with hinge at limbus; rectangular (approximately 4 × 4 mm); enter under flap into cornea with supersharp blade (after paracentesis elsewhere); punch large (1 × 2 mm) anteriorly placed window; do not extend opening to edges of scleral flap hinge; make iridectomy; avoid ciliary processes if visualized.

5. Scleral flap closure: 10-0 nylon sutures at back corners of scleral flap; and two anterior releasable sutures buried into clear cornea (if feasible), titrated to adequate flow; buried knots.

6. Conjunctival closure and hypotony prevention: 8-0 Vicryl on vascular needle to close "wings" of fornix-based incision, with two horizontal 10-0 Vicryl mattress sutures between; same suture to close both Tenon and conjunctival layers separately in limbus-based incision; avoid covering releasable corneal portion of scleral flap sutures; fill chamber and bleb first with balanced salt then with Healon if left "leaky;" leave paracentesis for office refilling in older children.

GLAUCOMA DRAINAGE-DEVICE SURGERY (STEPS SPECIFIC TO CHILDREN)

1. Choice of incision: best to make fornix incision unless scarring or abnormal anatomy precludes; winged limbal incision if necessary.

2. Choice of implant and location: size the device to the eye (e.g., S2 or FP-7 Ahmed requires axial length at least 21 mm or must either trim back of plate or place it closer to limbus; valved implant if immediate pressure reduction needed, otherwise Baerveldt 250 mm^2 in most cases; superotemporal quadrant usual best location; suture plate 7 to 8 mm from limbus with 8-0 nylon suture.

3. Consider lateral rectus recession for exotropia noted at time of device placement: avoids need for later dissection near bleb.

4. Optimize tube position and placement: tube into anterior chamber in most cases, parallel to iris and as far back as practical to prevent exposure and corneal-tube touch, almost parallel to superior limbus rather than toward central pupil; use 30-gauge "finder" needle on viscoelastic before 23-gauge entry for tube; consider posterior chamber (over intraocular lens implant) or pars plana tube location in selected cases (need full vitrectomy if pars plana entry).

5. Wound closure and hypotony prevention: tube completely ligated (6-0 Vicryl) if nonvalved device; watertight closure (8-0 Vicryl running closure of both Tenon and conjunctiva if fornix incision vs. 8-0 Vicryl running closure of each wing, with "hood" onto cornea and central 10-0 Vicryl mattress sutures if limbal incision); chamber filled with viscoelastic unless tube ligated closed; optional venting slits in tubing for nonvalved device (made using 9-0 nylon needle).

6. Prophylaxis against the encapsulated bleb/high pressure phase: maintain anti-inflammatory treatment for several months (topical steroid then nonsteroidal agents) and use aqueous suppressants liberally to keep pressure low.

CYCLOABLATION

1. Optimal type of ablation: transscleral vs. endoscopic laser initially vs. cryotherapy rarely.

2. Limit treatment with transscleral and endoscopic laser to three quadrants to help avoid hypotony, vs. two quadrants with cyclocryotherapy.

3. Minimize excess inflammation: use adequate anti-inflammatory treatment and consider short oral steroid taper.

4. Minimize risk of phthisis: keep careful records of prior treatment, beware 360-degrees cumulative treatment.

5. Discuss limitations of treatment fully with parents to achieve mutual understanding of risks and alternatives.

Modified from Freedman SF, Johnston SC. Glaucoma in infancy and early childhood. In: Wilson ME, Saunders RA, Trivedi RH, eds. *Pediatric Ophthalmology: Current Thought and a Practical Guide*. Springer; 2009.

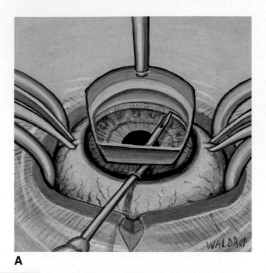 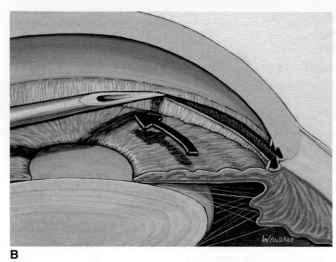

Figure 40.2 Goniotomy from temporal side, shown using a Barkan goniotomy lens and 25-gauge needle used as the goniotomy knife. **A:** Incision in anterior trabecular meshwork, shown beginning from right to left. **B:** Correct location and depth of the goniotomy incision.

anterior chamber to be deepened before incision and to be maintained on instrument removal (45,46). The author prefers the latter method, using only enough viscoelastic to ensure chamber maintenance on needle withdrawal. Enthusiastic use of the viscoelastic may acutely increase corneal edema by increasing IOP, thereby degrading the surgeon's view of the angle structures.

To perform goniotomy safely and effectively, corneal clarity must be sufficient to allow an adequate view of the angle structures. To this end, preoperative use of glaucoma medications and prompt application of sodium chloride, 5%, drops to the cornea under anesthesia may improve the angle view in borderline cases. Although corneal epithelial scraping has been described to facilitate an angle view for goniotomy, corneal stromal edema often persists after epithelial removal; in this setting trabeculotomy may be preferred (see Trabeculotomy). Alternatively, endoscopic visualization has been used for goniotomy in the setting of corneal opacification (47–49).

Goniotomy surgery can be performed with a binocular head loupe, although the operating microscope provides better visualization (and affords the assistant a view of the angle) (50). The surgeon usually sits opposite to the portion of the angle to be operated (i.e., to the temporal side of the patient for nasal goniotomy), with the patient's head slightly rotated away from the surgeon. Moody or other locking fixation forceps may be placed on the superior and inferior rectus muscles when a nasal or temporal goniotomy is planned. Alternatively, the globe can be adequately held by applying the locking forceps nearer to the limbus, at the level of the Tenon insertion, with less likelihood of acutely worsening corneal edema. Viscoelastic may be placed onto the central cornea just before the operating goniolens is placed and may be helpful in preventing the formation of air bubbles between the goniolens and the cornea. The goniotomy lens may be stabilized with a nontoothed fine forceps in the positioning holes of the lens, or it may be modified to include a handle.

The goniotomy knife or needle is placed through peripheral clear cornea 1 mm from the limbus, opposite to the midpoint

of the intended goniotomy, in a plane parallel to the iris. The knife or needle is guided over iris tissue (not pupil) to engage trabecular meshwork in its anterior third, just posterior to the Schwalbe line (Fig. 40.2A). A circumferential incision is then made for about 4 to 5 clock-hours (Fig. 40.2B), and the knife or needle is carefully and quickly withdrawn from the eye over iris tissue at all times. The incision should be superficial, with no grating or scraping sensation noted. A deeper cleft, with exposure of whiter tissue may be noted in the wake of the incision, with a widening of the angle, and a posterior movement of peripheral iris in some cases. The assistant may help the surgeon to extend the angle available to goniotomy by rotating the eye clockwise and counterclockwise at the surgeon's request. After knife (or needle) withdrawal, blood often egresses from the angle incision, stopping when the chamber is refilled with balanced salt solution; placing a sterile air bubble can assist in assessing the anterior chamber the next morning. A single suture of 10-0 Vicryl secures the corneal wound (37,51).

Postoperative treatment includes the use of topical antibiotic, steroid, and miotic agents. (Miotics are often omitted, however, in cases of uveitic glaucoma.) The baby's head should be kept elevated (a car seat works well for this), and the eye should be shielded for 1 to 2 nights, until any hyphema has settled. If bilateral goniotomies are needed, they may be performed in a single anesthesia session, as long as all instruments are sterilized or replaced; all drapes, gowns, and gloves are replaced; and the fellow eye is reprepared and draped in sterile fashion after the first procedure (52).

Mild to moderate hyphemas commonly occur after goniotomy, but they almost always clear rapidly without sequelae over several days. Other complications after goniotomy are rare and include iridodialysis, cyclodialysis, the appearance of small peripheral anterior synechiae in the incised angle, damage to the crystalline lens, and retinal detachment in eyes with high myopia (42,52).

The results of goniotomy should be evaluated weekly in the immediate postoperative period and are often evident by 3 to 6 weeks. Gonioscopy after successful goniotomy often reveals

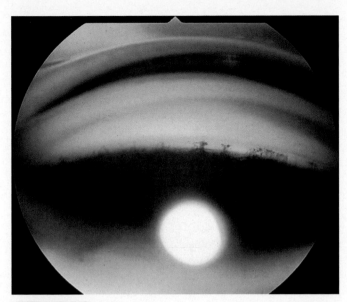

Figure 40.3 Cleft in angle after goniotomy, resulting in a widened angle to the right half of the gonioscopic view in a black infant with primary congenital glaucoma.

a widened angle in the previous incision site, with improved visibility of the ciliary band and scleral spur (**Fig. 40.3**). Scattered peripheral anterior synechiae may sometimes develop in the bed of the goniotomy and may even partly obscure a view of the incised angle. Because 4 to 5 clock-hours of angle tissue are incised with a single goniotomy, repeated procedures in untreated portions of the angle may enhance pressure control in selected cases. Goniotomy may fail to control infantile glaucoma in some instances because of improper placement and depth of the angle incision, or the obliteration of the incision by peripheral synechiae. In approximately 10% of cases, if the first two procedures have produced substantial but still inadequate IOP reduction, a third goniotomy procedure may help further lower the IOP (1).

The success of goniotomy in controlling glaucoma varies with the cause of the glaucoma. The best results—80% to more than 90% success after one to two procedures—are achieved in infants with primary congenital glaucoma presenting between 3 months and 1 year of age (1,53). Others report lower success of closer to 70% after one to two procedures (54). In one study of seven infants treated with two simultaneous goniotomies in one eye and a single goniotomy in the fellow eye, no significant differences were noted in the results (55). Success rates with goniotomy (and angle surgery in general) are much lower for cases of primary congenital–infantile glaucoma presenting at birth or after 12 months of age (success in these groups is usually about 30% to 50%) (1,37,53).

Procedures Related to Goniotomy (Historical Perspective)

Scheie reported a modification of goniotomy, goniopuncture, which involved passage of a goniotomy knife through the trabecular meshwork and sclera to the subconjunctival space after standard goniotomy (56,57). Scarring of the limbal incision limited the usefulness of goniopuncture.

The Nd:YAG (neodymium:yttrium–aluminum–garnet) laser has been used to perform trabeculopuncture by directing laser energy gonioscopically at the trabecular meshwork, to penetrate through to the Schlemm canal. Success was reported with this procedure in six of eight eyes with juvenile glaucoma over a 6-month follow-up period (58). A technique requiring a large limbal incision, direct goniotomy has also been described, but it has been superseded by trabeculotomy (see later) (59).

Trabeculodialysis, a modification of goniotomy in which the trabecular meshwork is scraped or retracted from the scleral sulcus after a standard goniotomy incision, has been effective in the treatment of children with glaucoma secondary to anterior uveitis (60% pressure control reported in a series of 23 such patients) (39). Goniotomy alone is also effective in these patients (37,40).

Argon laser trabeculoplasty is ineffective in the treatment of childhood glaucomas and is not feasible to perform in young patients (60,61).

Trabeculotomy Ab Externo

The surgical technique of trabeculotomy ab externo is performed by cannulating the Schlemm canal from an external approach and then tearing through the trabecular meshwork into the anterior chamber. This procedure thus creates a direct communication between the anterior chamber and Schlemm canal. Burian and Smith independently described trabeculotomy ab externo in 1960 as an alternative procedure to goniotomy (62,63). The initial technique was later modified by Harms, Dannheim, and McPherson (1). Success rates varying from 73% to 100% have been reported for this procedure in congenital glaucoma (1). In a series of 140 eyes (89 children) with developmental glaucoma treated with trabeculotomy surgery, overall success was 89% after an average follow-up of 9.5 years (64). While conjunctival scarring and a longer surgical duration are the salient disadvantages of trabeculotomy (compared with goniotomy), this procedure is little affected by an edematous or scarred cornea. (Additional comparison of these two angle procedures follows.)

Basic Technique

In the surgical technique described by McPherson (65), a limbal-based conjunctival flap and a partial-thickness triangular or rectangular scleral flap are created as for standard trabeculectomy (see Chapter 38). Most surgeons prefer to perform trabeculotomy under a small fornix-based conjunctival peritomy. Preoperative use of pilocarpine helps to induce miosis, and use of topical apraclonidine may reduce intraoperative bleeding. An inferotemporal approach for trabeculotomy is suggested (unless combined trabeculectomy is planned) to spare the superior quadrants for possible later filtration or other surgery.

A radial scratch incision is made in the bed of the scleral flap across the sclerolimbal junction. This scratch incision is gradually deepened under high magnification until the Schlemm canal is identified just anterior to the circumferential fibers of the scleral spur (near the posterior aspect of the limbal "gray zone"). Often a small amount of blood or aqueous humor refluxes through the cut ends of the Schlemm canal, and the internal wall of the canal appears slightly pigmented. At this point (or earlier, if preferred, or if the anterior chamber is inadvertently entered before the Schlemm canal is identified), a paracentesis should be made, with injection into the anterior chamber of a small amount of viscoelastic recommended. To confirm the identity of the canal, a 6-0 gauge suture (Prolene with a cautery-blunted tip is recommended) should thread easily to both the left and the right sides of the radial incision. If resistance is met, the suture may need to be repositioned, the radial incision deepened, or a second parallel radial incision made beneath the same scleral flap to assist in finding the Schlemm canal (the presence of the suture in Schlemm canal may sometimes be confirmed by gonioscopy by using a Zeiss four-mirror lens). After the canal has been located, the internal arm of a trabeculotome should be passed gently into the canal (to the right side first for a right-handed surgeon) as far as possible without meeting excessive resistance, and by using the parallel external arm as a guide (**Fig. 40.4A**). The internal arm is then gently rotated into the anterior chamber, with care to avoid entry into peripheral cornea or beneath the iris plane (Fig. 40.4B). Rotation of the trabeculotome into the anterior

chamber tears through the intervening trabecular meshwork and requires little force (**Fig. 40.4B, C**). Rotation should be halted once about 75% to 80% of the internal arm of the trabeculotome is visible in the anterior chamber. The anterior chamber may shallow slightly, and blood may egress from the torn trabecular meshwork and Schlemm canal as the trabeculotome is removed from the eye along its path of entry. In similar fashion, the trabeculotome should be placed into the left side of the radial incision and the procedure repeated to the left. Leaving a portion of intact trabecular meshwork underlying the radial incision into the Schlemm canal helps prevent prolapse of iris into the wound. The scleral flap is then sutured with 10-0 Vicryl. If a limbus-based conjunctival flap was used, the flap may be closed with a running suture of 8-0 Vicryl as for standard trabeculectomy (66). Alternatively, wing sutures of 10-0 Vicryl often suffice for watertight closure of a fornix-based conjunctival flap. Subconjunctival antibiotic and short-acting steroid may be given at the end of the surgery.

Postoperatively, patients are treated with topical antibiotics and steroids, together with low-dose pilocarpine for several weeks, as with goniotomy. Although hyphema occurs commonly after trabeculotomy, rarer complications include inadvertent filtering blebs, choroidal detachment, iridotomy,

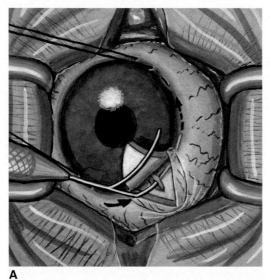

A

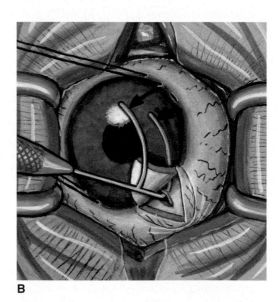

B

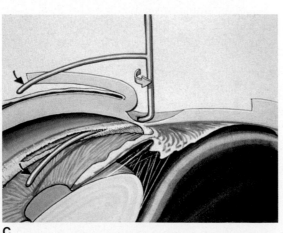

C

Figure 40.4 Trabeculotomy under a fornix-based conjunctival and partial-thickness scleral flap. Preferred inferotemporal approach is shown, using a traction suture at the limbus to help hold the eye in adduction. **A:** Placement of trabeculotome into the cut end of Schlemm canal to the right. **B:** Rotation of the trabeculotome into the anterior chamber, tearing through the intervening trabecular meshwork. **C:** View of internal arm of trabeculotome tearing through trabecular meshwork as the instrument is rotated into the anterior chamber.

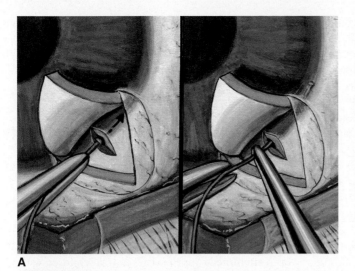
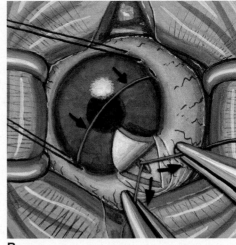

A

B

Figure 40.5 Trabeculotomy (360-degree modification using Prolene suture). Modification of trabeculotomy surgery (Fig. 40.4) in which the entire circumference of the Schlemm canal is cannulated with a 6-0 Prolene suture (blunted to have a small mushroom-shaped tip using disposable cautery) (**A**), and then both ends of the suture are pulled (**B**), resulting in 360-degree trabeculotomy.

damage to the lens, creation of a false passage into the anterior chamber or suprachoroidal space, and infection (66,67).

One proposed modification of trabeculotomy involves the use of a Prolene suture (6-0 gauge and with a cautery-blunted tip) to perform a 180- or 360-degree trabeculotomy at one surgery, using one or two external incisions into Schlemm canal (68,69). The early results of 360-degree trabeculotomy are similar to those reported for more conventional trabeculotomy procedures (which usually affect 100 to 120 degrees of the angle described earlier) (**Fig. 40.5**).

Complete 360-degree trabeculotomy has also been recently performed by using the lighted Schlemm canal probe (ITrack 250 microcatheter, IScience Interventional, Menlo Park, CA), which was initially developed for use in canaloplasty (**Fig. 40.6**) (see Chapter 36). In this procedure, the catheter is threaded into one cut end of the Schlemm canal (usually made slightly larger with a small radial cut by using a Vannas scissor), and its lighted tip allows easy monitoring of its trajectory around the circumference of the Schlemm canal. One can also visualize the catheter if it attempts to leave the canal through a collector channel. Occasionally, the catheter can be redirected in these cases, although usually the best chance of complete cannulation occurs in these cases by withdrawing and then replacing the catheter through the opposite cut end of Schlemm canal in the opposite direction. Small amounts of viscoelastic material can also be injected through the catheter tip as it is advanced. Early experience suggests that this procedure may be as effective as 360-degree suture trabeculotomy, although increased postoperative hyphema has been reported (Freedman SF, unpublished data).

The effects of trabeculotomy should be determined about 1 month after surgery. Trabeculotomy (unless 360-degree suture trabeculotomy was performed) may be repeated in a different portion of the angle if inadequate effect was noted after the first procedure.

Combined Trabeculotomy–Trabeculectomy

If Schlemm canal has not been successfully cannulated or if similar trabeculotomy procedures have previously failed to control the IOP, the trabeculotomy can be combined with a trabeculectomy by removal of a full-thickness block of limbal tissue in the bed of the scleral flap, followed by peripheral iridectomy as in standard trabeculectomy. Some surgeons advocate combined trabeculotomy–trabeculectomy as the first surgery for congenital glaucoma (70–72), whereas others note that this procedure works better than angle surgery alone for primary congenital glaucoma with more severe clinical presentation (73). For this combined surgery, the surgeon chooses a conjunctival incision

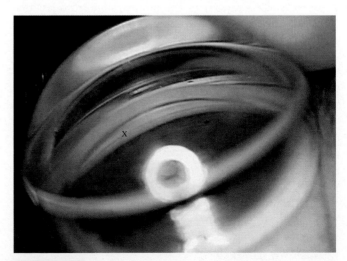

Figure 40.6 Cleft in angle created by 360-degree trabeculotomy with IScience endoscopic Schlemm canal probe, in 5-year-old with pseudophakia and glaucoma. (An "X" marks the whitish cleft that runs circumferentially around the entire circumference of the angle.)

site according to his or her preferred trabeculectomy technique (see the following text), and may apply an antimetabolite, such as mitomycin C, to the sclera at the site of intended scleral flap formation before dissection of the scleral flap (as described for adult trabeculectomy). If mitomycin C has been applied, it is advisable to ensure watertight closure of the Tenon and conjunctival layers with a vascular needle and absorbable suture, as for trabeculectomy (Chapter 38). Postoperative care should be as for pediatric trabeculectomy in this case (see Trabeculectomy). The mechanism of long-term pressure control in combined trabeculotomy–trabeculectomy (improved outflow of the trabecular–Schlemm canal pathway rather than filtration through the trabeculectomy site) has been debated, with no definitive agreement at this time.

When the exact mechanism of the glaucoma is uncertain, such as with early-onset glaucoma in the Sturge–Weber syndrome (see Chapter 20), a combined trabeculotomy–trabeculectomy procedure may offer higher success rate than either procedure separately (74), although the risks associated with intraocular surgery in eyes with choroidal hemangioma make simple angle surgery preferred by some surgeons for this condition.

Goniotomy versus Trabeculotomy

Each of these procedures has staunch advocates who espouse the advantages of one technique over the other (75–78). Reported success has been similarly high with both procedures in favorable cases of glaucoma (e.g., previously unoperated eyes with primary congenital glaucoma, with postnatal onset in the 1st year of life) and primary congenital glaucoma with mild clinical presentation (73,77,79,80). In a retrospective, comparative study by Mendicino, Beck, and colleagues, the success rate with 360-degree suture trabeculotomy was higher than that with goniotomy for primary congenital glaucoma (81).

If the cornea is clear, goniotomy has certain advantages over trabeculotomy: no conjunctival scarring, anatomic precision, less trauma to adjacent tissues, and shorter operating time. Reported success rates with goniotomy range from less than 80% to approximately 90%, although the procedure must be repeated in about one half of cases (1,79,80).

The reported success rates with trabeculotomy are basically the same as with goniotomy, although fewer repeated procedures may be required, especially if the suture modification of trabeculotomy facilitates opening the Schlemm canal for 360 degrees in one operative session (68,81). On the other hand, the microsurgeon experienced in adult glaucoma surgery may find trabeculotomy a more familiar procedure than goniotomy; moreover, trabeculotomy is not dependent on a clear cornea, and it can be converted directly to trabeculectomy if the Schlemm canal is not found or is inadequately cannulated (75–77).

Peripheral Iridectomy

Several types of pupillary block glaucoma occur in children. Although uncommon, pupillary block glaucoma occurring after cataract surgery may respond to peripheral iridectomy (with or without vitrectomy or synechialysis) (82,83).

Glaucoma associated with advanced cicatricial retinopathy of prematurity may similarly improve with iridectomy alone or coupled with lens removal (84). In these cases, peripheral iridectomy should proceed essentially as described for adults (see Chapter 36).

FILTERING SURGERY—TRABECULECTOMY

Filtering surgery is usually performed when goniotomy or trabeculotomy fails or—as is the case in some primary and many secondary glaucomas—is unlikely to succeed. This surgery should not be undertaken lightly in the child, as it removes permanently from use the child's native (albeit inadequately functioning) drainage system. Many such surgical procedures have been attempted over the years to treat children with glaucoma, including iridencleisis, cyclodiathermy, thermal sclerostomy (Scheie procedure), and standard trabeculectomy (1). Success rates were usually poor (in the 50% range, sometimes with multiple procedures), visual outcomes were limited, and rates of complication—which could include vitreous loss, scleral collapse, ectasia, retinal detachment, and endophthalmitis—were not insignificant (approximately 20%) (85–87). Poor outcome from trabeculectomy is most likely multifactorial, with contributing factors including low scleral rigidity, exuberant healing response, and enlargement of glaucomatous eyes with thinning and distortion of intraocular anatomy. Adding to these physiologic considerations are the challenges of postoperative management in children; the long-term risks of infection and eye injury; and possible visual loss from nonglaucomatous causes, such as amblyopia. By contrast, several authors have recently reported much higher rates of success by using primary trabeculectomy in children with glaucoma, mostly in congenital cases (88,89).

Intraoperative β-irradiation to the surgical site, used in Britain, was associated with improved success of standard trabeculectomy in that country. In a retrospective series of 66 eyes (in patients younger than 18 years with congenital glaucoma), Miller and Rice reported successful pressure control (IOP < 21 mm Hg) in roughly 40% of eyes after standard trabeculectomy, compared with greater than 65% after irradiation-augmented trabeculectomy. The authors found no complications attributable to the use of this low-dose β-irradiation (90).

Although subconjunctival 5-fluorouracil (5-FU) has been administered postoperatively in children after trabeculectomy, resulting in successful filtration, its administration usually requires multiple sequential anesthesias and is limited by corneal epithelial toxicity, as in adults (91,92).

The intraoperative use of mitomycin C has greatly enhanced the success of trabeculectomy in controlling glaucoma in adults at high risk for surgical failure (see Chapter 38) (93,94), presumably by limiting postoperative scarring by Tenon capsule and scleral fibroblasts. The use of mitomycin C–augmented trabeculectomy in children with refractory glaucoma seems to have improved the ability to reduce IOP; however, this increased "success" carries with it the sobering risks of late bleb infection (see later). Success rates vary from as high as 95% to much lower figures, some below 50% (92, 95–104). The reported success of mitomycin C–augmented trabeculectomy in children varies for numerous reasons, including differences in the method of defining and reporting success, the length of follow-up, the composition of the sample, and perhaps the surgical technique and postoperative management. Let us consider just a few of the more obvious examples. Mandal reported 95% success at last follow-up with this surgery in a group of mostly older patients with phakic eyes, although the duration of follow-up was fairly limited (95,96); subsequent success more recently reported by the same surgeon fell to 65% at 18 months, this time assessed by performing Kaplan–Meier life-table analysis (105). In a retrospective study of 114 children with congenital or developmental glaucoma, with a mean age slightly younger than 6 years, Giampani and colleagues reported 5-year success of mitomycin C–augmented trabeculectomy to be 51%, with endophthalmitis developing in eight eyes (5%) (106).

The success of mitomycin C–augmented trabeculectomy in children is much higher in those who are older and phakic. Hence several authors independently found young age and aphakia to be associated with poorer outcomes (92,101,103). Mitomycin C application has included concentrations ranging from 0.2 to 0.5 mg/mL, applied from between 2 and 5 minutes (92,95,98,99,101,102). To help titrate the postoperative filtration rate, Lynch and colleagues developed a probe tip (a modified Hoskins lens) for the diode laser (Iris Medical) that allows postoperative laser suture lysis of scleral flap sutures in the first 1 to 2 weeks after surgery during brief anesthesia (107). Others have used absorbable sutures (e.g., 10-0 Vicryl) or releasable sutures (see Chapter 38) in the trabeculectomy flap (Kenneth Nischal, MD, personal communication).

The response of very young children to mitomycin C–augmented trabeculectomy is extremely variable, with some patients scarring rapidly despite antifibrotic therapy and others developing hypotony with large avascular filtration blebs and even scleral ectasia. In addition to postoperative laser suture lysis and use of releasable scleral flap sutures, postoperative subconjunctival 5-FU may be used after trabeculectomy with mitomycin C to further retard healing and enhance filtration; this additional antifibrotic therapy did not enhance the success of mitomycin C–augmented trabeculectomy compared with other published series of similar cases (96,98,101).

Infants and children are subject to complications similar to those of adult patients. Hypotony, flat anterior chamber, choroidal detachment, decompression retinal and preretinal hemorrhages, and lens opacification have all been reported in pediatric cases (96–98,101). Most concerning, however, have been the cases of bleb-related infection, often associated with thin, avascular, and leaking blebs (**Fig. 40.7**), including cases of

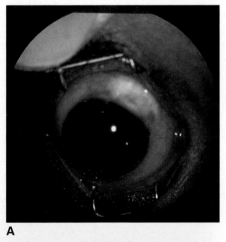

A

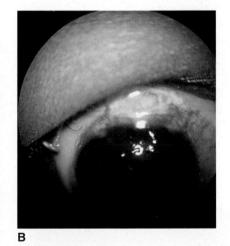

B

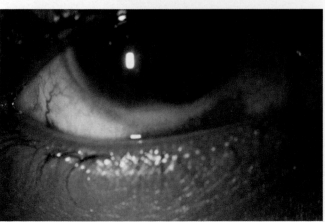

C

Figure 40.7 Bleb infection in a long-standing avascular and intermittently leaking filtering bleb. **A:** Thin, avascular filtering bleb 5 years after mitomycin C–augmented trabeculectomy in a child with congenital glaucoma. The eye intermittently had hypotony and a flat anterior chamber after apparently minimal trauma. **B:** Brisk positive Seidel test associated with the leaking filtering bleb and flat anterior chamber described above in A. **C:** Hypopyon and fibrin plague on the lens capsule in association with endophthalmitis from an infected filtering bleb, 1 year after the leak shown in B. The child had an upper respiratory infection at the same time. The infection responded to vigorous topical and intravitreal antibiotics, and subsequently the bleb was removed and a Baerveldt implant placed, with preservation of preinfection vision and a clear lens.

endophthalmitis with devastating visual loss in the operated eye (92,100,103,106,108,109). Given the nontrivial incidence of bleb-related infection in adults several years after trabeculectomy augmented by the use of antiproliferative drugs (110–112) (see Chapter 38), young children with filtering blebs must be watched very carefully for bleb leak and infection. Some glaucoma surgeons have tended toward alternatives to mitomycin C–augmented trabeculectomy in infants and very young children, partly on the basis of an assumed unacceptably high cumulative risk of bleb-related infection. An additional consideration regarding the exposure of a child's eye to mitomycin C relates to the potential long-term carcinogenic risk of using this potent alkylating agent (seen in rodents after systemic mitomycin C application) (113,114). Because we do not know the long-term ocular sequelae of topical mitomycin C application to the sclera and Tenon capsule of young children with glaucoma, caution is advised in repeating mitomycin C filters in children with glaucoma. One must weigh the potential and as yet unknown long-term risks of mitomycin C use against those of other alternative procedures (discussed later).

Trabeculectomy surgeons have recently advocated use of a fornix-based conjunctival incision in adults (Chapter 38) and children, noting the decreased avascularity of the resultant blebs and their tendency to be more broad-based than with limbus incisions (**Fig. 40.8**) (115). The long-term differences in mitomycin C–augmented trabeculectomy success using the fornix-based rather than limbus-based incision for refractory pediatric cases await the test of time.

Posttrabeculectomy care of the pediatric patient includes careful long-term follow-up and the gradual tapering of topical steroid, with the prolonged use of nonsteroidal anti-inflammatory agents in selected cases, and the use of topical aqueous suppressants in others (e.g., when the bleb is relatively thin and seems to be enlarging gradually over time). Diligent parental awareness of the lifelong risk for bleb infection and leaks is imperative; for this reason, contact lens use in eyes with functioning trabeculectomy blebs is usually discouraged.

Glaucoma Drainage-Device Surgery

Trabeculectomy, despite recent modifications and use of antiproliferative agents, still fails to control IOP (or is not applicable) in some cases of refractory pediatric glaucoma. Remaining surgical options include cyclodestructive and glaucoma (aqueous) drainage-device procedures. Given the low success with trabeculectomy in infants and in aphakic eyes (92,98,101), and the lifelong risk for bleb leak and infection in eyes with successfully filtering after trabeculectomy, glaucoma drainage-device surgery may be a reasonable option before trabeculectomy in selected patients (103,109,116) (**Fig. 40.9**). Glaucoma drainage devices have also proven useful in the treatment of uveitis-related glaucoma after failed angle surgery (117–120). Although the Molteno implant has been used in children for nearly 2 decades, experience has grown with other devices, including the Baerveldt and the Ahmed drainage implants. Reported success and complication rates vary widely (121–146).

Numerous studies have reported on the success of Molteno drainage-device surgery for childhood glaucoma (131–133,135–138,147–153). Using a two-stage single-plate Molteno implantation procedure, Molteno and colleagues reported a 95% rate of success (defined as IOP < 20 mm Hg) with a low complication rate (10%) in patients with advanced childhood glaucomas (133). In their series of 83 eyes, the average age at surgery was 11 years, and the mean follow-up was 5 years; all patients received systemic corticosteroids, flufenamic acid, and colchicine. Billson and colleagues subsequently reported 78% success (IOP < 21 mm Hg) with the double-plate Molteno device in a two-stage procedure in 23 eyes of 18 patients (age range, 6 months to 46 years) with various childhood glaucomas; no added benefit of systemic antifibrosis was noted (132). Several studies of exclusively younger children have had lower rates of success at pressure control. Lloyd and colleagues achieved a 56% success rate after placement of one or two single-plate Molteno devices in 16 children younger than

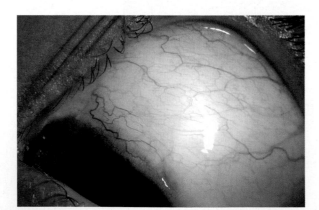

Figure 40.8 Partly avascular filtering bleb after mitomycin C trabeculectomy in an 8-year-old girl with late-recognized end-stage congenital glaucoma. Angle surgery and medications controlled the IOP for 6 years. Pressure is now below 10 mm Hg on no glaucoma medications.

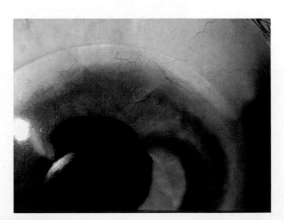

Figure 40.9 Aphakic eye with well-positioned glaucoma drainage device, showing tube in the anterior chamber, and ability to continue contact-lens wear. Ahmed drainage device was implanted into the aphakic eye of this 15-year-old with juvenile idiopathic arthritis–related uveitis and secondary cataract and glaucoma.

13 years; most patients required concurrent use of antiglaucoma medications (134). Hill and coworkers reported a 62% rate of success (IOP > 5 and < 22 mm Hg) after a two-stage, one- or two-plate Molteno implantation procedure in 70 eyes (in patients younger than 21 years) followed up for at least 6 months; nonetheless, 83% of patients needed further glaucoma or other surgery, and complications were common (135). In another relatively large study, of 49 children younger than 12 years, Munoz and colleagues reported a similar, 68% success rate of pressure control with use of a single-plate Molteno device in a one-stage procedure (131). In all these series, Molteno drainage devices were used with ligation or other reversible partial blockade of the connecting tube if single-stage implantation was used.

Complications seen with Molteno drainage-device implantation in children included not only those encountered after trabeculectomy in children (discussed earlier), but also those specific to glaucoma drainage-device surgery. Most common among the latter in many series were contact between the tube and corneal endothelium (tube–cornea touch), erosion of the tube externally through the conjunctiva, migration of the tube, and cataract formation or progression; less commonly, motility disturbance has been reported (136), as has endophthalmitis, although fortunately only rarely (131).

The Baerveldt glaucoma drainage device has also been used in refractory pediatric glaucoma, with fairly high reported success rates (122,127,129,130,140–143). Success rates for implantation of Baerveldt drainage devices range from 80% to 95% at 12 months, decreasing to approximately 50% by 48 months and lower than 50% at 60 months. One retrospective series involving Ahmed and Baerveldt drainage-device implantation reported a 10-year success rate of 55% in patients with aphakic glaucoma and 42% in patients with congenital glaucoma (**Fig. 40.10**)

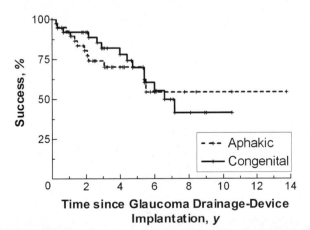

Figure 40.10 Results of Kaplan–Meier analysis showing success of Ahmed or Baerveldt glaucoma drainage devices in eyes of children with aphakic or congenital glaucoma. Success—defined as IOP controlled without serious complication or additional glaucoma surgery—was greater than 75% at 2 years and greater than 60% at 5 years, but fell to less than 50% at 10 years after implantation for both groups. (Modified from O'Malley Schotthoefer E, et al. Aqueous drainage device surgery in refractory pediatric glaucomas: I. Long-term outcomes. *J AAPOS*. 2007;12(1):33–39.)

(127). Rates of success in published series have varied by the type of pediatric glaucoma diagnosis (most series have included refractory primary and secondary cases), the implant size (most using the 250- or 350-mm^2 size), and the location of the tube (anterior chamber vs. pars plana). Complications of Baerveldt glaucoma drainage-device implantation have been similar to those reported with the Molteno device, with all surgeons using tube ligation with an absorbable suture or two-stage implantation to avoid extreme hypotony in the early postoperative period (152). Choroidal hemorrhage, retinal detachment, and phthisis have all been reported, with high incidence among patients with aphakic eyes (126,127). As with other glaucoma drainage devices in children, additional complications have included tube-related problems, corneal damage, uveitis, pupil ectopia, cataract, and motility disturbances (126,127). The Baerveldt implant may be sized to the child's eye, by using the 250- or 350-mm^2 size; the posterior edge of the silicone plate can be trimmed in very short eyes receiving the Baerveldt implant.

The Ahmed glaucoma drainage device, with its flow-regulating valve-like design, has shown promise for the control of refractory childhood glaucoma, with rates of success and complications similar to those reported for the Baerveldt drainage device, although no randomized trials have been conducted to date (121,123–128,144,145). Rates of success after Ahmed drainage-device implantation vary fairly widely among studies, probably the result of differences in patient populations (e.g., age and diagnosis). For example, Chen and Walton reported 12- and 48-month success rates of 85% and 42%, respectively, in a retrospective series composed largely of patients with aphakic and congenital glaucomas. Al-Mobarak and colleagues reported 2-year success of 63% in children younger than 2 years, most of whom had congenital glaucoma. Ou reported fairly low success with Ahmed drainage-device implantation in a study comprising only patients with congenital glaucoma, with a 5-year success rate of only 33%, increasing to 69% with implantation of a second Ahmed device. One study, by Khan and coworkers, compared the S2 (polypropylene) and newer FP-7 (silicone) Ahmed plates in children younger than 2 years at surgery and noted improved success in the latter group, which was made up entirely of patients with primary congenital glaucoma. Complications after Ahmed drainage-device surgery include all those problems reported with Baerveldt drainage-device implantation (121,123–128), with the additional possibility of fibrous ingrowth into the valve chamber as a mechanism not possible with the non-valved Baerveldt and Molteno devices (154). The newer FP-7 silicone plate is not exempt from this problem in pediatric patients (Freedman SF, unpublished data). Endophthalmitis has also been reported after Ahmed implantation in a child's eye (155,156). Glaucoma drainage-device surgery can successfully control glaucoma in children, although many patients require the use of glaucoma medications postoperatively. The most common complications encountered include those related to hypotony in the immediate postoperative period (especially in large, aphakic eyes); those related to the length, position, or blockage of the tube and its sequelae in the anterior segment of the eye in the intermediate term (**Fig. 40.11**); and those

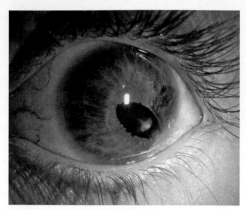

Figure 40.11 A 6-year-old child with drainage-device–related corneal endothelial scar and focal cataract. Patient was born with severe Axenfeld–Rieger–related glaucoma and underwent implantation of an inferior pediatric Ahmed drainage device at 3 months of age. Note inferiorly displaced pupil and focal cataract, and prominent posterior embryotoxon. Pressure is controlled on timolol, with best-corrected vision of 20/60 in this eye. The tube has become shorter in the anterior chamber over time, but the system is still functional.

related to bleb encapsulation and failure of pressure control in the long term. Motility disturbance (**Fig. 40.12**), exposure, infection, retinal detachment, and phthisis also occur and have all been reported with implantation of each type of glaucoma drainage device in children (see the preceding text).

In very young children with refractory glaucoma (younger than 2 years at surgery), IOP appeared to be better controlled with glaucoma drainage-device implantation than with trabeculectomy with mitomycin C (157). A randomized trial comparing mitomycin C–augmented trabeculectomy with mitomycin C–augmented Ahmed drainage-device surgery for pediatric aphakic glaucoma yielded fairly poor, but statistically similar results in one study (40% vs. 67%, respectively, with follow-up of less than 1 year) (158). No randomized trial has compared mitomycin use with nonuse in glaucoma drainage-device surgery for children; one study suggested that use of mitomycin C actually decreased the rate of success of Ahmed device implantation in children younger than 2 years, perhaps because of exuberant capsule fibrosis (159).

The basic surgical technique of glaucoma drainage-device implantation in children is similar to that in adult eyes (see Chapter 39). Glaucoma drainage-device placement is usually preferable in the superotemporal quadrant, although other quadrants may be used in selected cases. Implants may be placed by using a limbus-based or fornix-based conjunctival incision. Placing the plate of the device is usually easier with an incision made in the fornix (limbus-based); this technique seems preferable whenever the conjunctiva is mobile, as it increases patient comfort and decreases the risk for conjunctival retraction postoperatively. There may also be an advantage to avoid limbal incisions in children with tenuous corneal status. Glaucoma drainage-device tubes have been placed under partial-thickness scleral flaps (as with trabeculectomy);

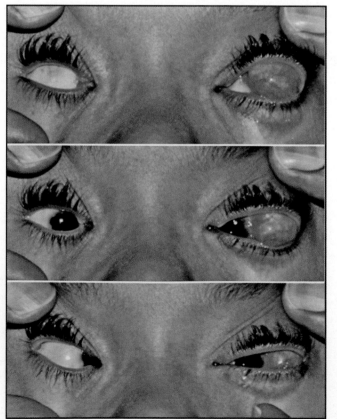

A

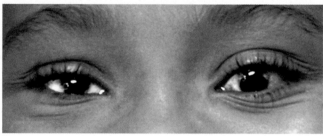

B

Figure 40.12 Restrictive strabismus—before **(A)** versus after **(B)** surgery—secondary to huge bleb formation around anteriorly migrated pediatric Ahmed drainage device in the left eye of a 6-year-old boy with microcornea and aphakic glaucoma. **A:** Note the esotropia in primary gaze (*middle*), and the inability of the left eye to abduct even to the midline (*bottom*), while he can still adduct the eye (*top*). **B:** Removal of the glaucoma drainage device and capsule, with concurrent diode endocyclophotocoagulation, improved the strabismus and maintained IOP control.

alternatively, many surgeons prefer full-thickness donor sclera or similar material, such as fascia lata, to cover the tube (141,145). Although several different glaucoma implant designs and methods of implantation are available, published experience suggests that the Molteno, Baerveldt, and Ahmed glaucoma drainage devices can control IOP in children with refractory glaucomas (especially those with extensive scarring or in whom trabeculectomy has failed). The optimal glaucoma drainage device chosen for a given child's eye depends on several factors, including the urgency of IOP reduction, the size and surgical history of the eye, and the extent of existing optic nerve damage. No known randomized trial has compared the safety and effectiveness of one device style with those of another in pediatric glaucoma cases. The Ahmed glaucoma drainage device may be preferable when immediate IOP reduction is needed, as when corneal edema persists and the infant's eye is rapidly expanding after failure of (or inability to perform) angle surgery. Similarly, some surgeons would prefer the larger Baerveldt device in fairly large eyes of older children, in those who can tolerate delayed IOP reduction (i.e., clear cornea and mild to moderate damage), and in those at risk for choroidal hemorrhage or other severe complications associated with sudden postoperative hypotony (e.g., patients with Sturge–Weber syndrome) (143) (**Fig. 40.13**).

We recommend ligation of the Molteno and Baerveldt drainage-device tubes with a 6-0 Vicryl suture for one-stage implantation (160), with care taken not to cover the suture ligating the tube with the scleral or other patch-graft material. This ligature usually releases at 5 to 6 weeks after surgery, allowing adequate time for formation of a capsule over the plate. Venting slits can be made in the tubing proximal to the Vicryl ligature, by using the needle of the same 9-0 nylon suture (with spatula needle) used to secure the tubing to the patient's sclera (usually three to four slits are made). The Ahmed glaucoma drainage device is usually implanted without ligation in pediatric cases (144,145). The limbus-based incision is currently the authors' preference, except in cases with scarring and inadequate mobility of the Tenon capsule and conjunctiva near the limbus in the

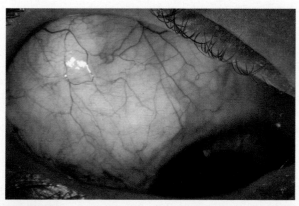

Figure 40.13 Superotemporal quadrant of a 13-year-old patient with Sturge–Weber–associated glaucoma, treated with implantation of a Baerveldt glaucoma drainage device 5 years earlier. Note the visible scleral patch graft, elevation over the plate, and prominent vessel pattern consistent with the episcleral vessels of her condition.

quadrant chosen for device implantation. The tube of the device is secured to the sclera with a 9-0 nylon figure-of-eight suture under a full-thickness donor scleral patch graft (145). The tube should be placed into the anterior chamber in phakic eyes. It can be placed in the posterior chamber (sulcus) or pars plana in aphakic or pseudophakic eyes, although full vitrectomy is recommended for most of the latter cases. It is best to place the tube parallel to the iris, and just above it in phakic cases, because of a tendency for the tube to rotate anteriorly over time in very young children. Use of a 23-gauge needle to make the entry into the eye minimizes leakage of fluid around the tube in the early postoperative period. Two-layer wound closure with 8-0 Vicryl on a vascular needle helps ensure a watertight closure and minimizes the risk for tube exposure.

Combined Filtration–Cataract Surgery

Although surgery for cataract removal in the setting of severe or uncontrolled glaucoma is relatively frequent in adults, the analogous situation in children is rare. Children who present with primary congenital glaucoma usually have clear lenses, whereas those with congenital cataracts usually have normal IOP. Glaucoma most often arises in young children with cataracts some time after cataract surgery has been completed. Children do present with concurrent glaucoma and cataracts in several unusual settings: (a) with primary glaucoma and associated cataracts (i.e., Lowe syndrome), (b) with chronic uveitis and coexisting secondary glaucoma and cataract (as seen in juvenile idiopathic arthritis), and (c) in other unusual cases of secondary glaucoma and cataract (e.g., posttraumatic or steroid-induced).

Great caution is advised regarding combined cataract and glaucoma surgery in children. If trabeculectomy is combined with cataract removal, there is a significant risk of postoperative hypotony and ciliary body shutdown, secondary choroidal detachment, and subsequent bleb scarring and failure (Freedman SF, unpublished data). In nonuveitic cases of cataract and glaucoma, we generally favor gaining control of the glaucoma first, with cataract surgery performed subsequently. In the instance of an older child with cataract, glaucoma, and a quiet eye, one might consider extracapsular cataract removal with preservation of the posterior capsule and concurrent glaucoma drainage-device implantation (161). In patients with uveitic glaucoma and cataract, we generally favor goniotomy (as the initial glaucoma procedure of choice) before cataract surgery. If angle surgery has failed, and additional glaucoma surgery is needed, we recommend either (a) glaucoma drainage-device implantation (if the glaucoma is severe or optic nerve damaged) or (b) removal of the cataract first, followed by the other surgery as a second, staged procedure (118–120).

Cyclodestructive Surgery

The surgical procedures previously described all share the goal of increasing aqueous outflow from the eye, through the angle structures or via a fistula or tube placed into the anterior chamber (or posteriorly). By contrast, cyclodestructive procedures reduce the rate of aqueous production by injuring the ciliary processes; results are often unpredictable, and complications frequent. As with refractory glaucoma in adults, cyclodestruction nonetheless constitutes a valid means of attempting control of otherwise vision-threatening glaucoma in children, once medical and other surgical means have been exhausted or have proven inadequate to the task.

Cyclocryotherapy

Cyclocryotherapy (freezing the ciliary processes from an external approach) has been used as therapy for difficult childhood glaucomas for many years and is applied with a similar technique to that used in adults (see Chapter 41). Reported success using cyclocryotherapy in childhood glaucoma (IOP control without severe visual loss or phthisis) has been fairly poor. al Faran and colleagues reported 30% success after one or more treatments in a large series of children with advanced congenital glaucoma (162). Wagle and associates reported a similar 44% success after an average follow-up of 5 years, although many retreatments were required. Devastating complications in this study were more likely to occur in patients with aniridic glaucoma than in patients with nonaniridic glaucoma (163). In children, cryotherapy should be applied to a maximum of 180 degrees of the circumference of the eye at one session, by using six or seven freezes (45 to 60 seconds each, at −80°C) with the anterior edge of a 2.5-mm diameter cryoprobe placed 1 to 1.5 mm from the limbus (in a nonbuphthalmic eye) (164). Placement of the probe directly over the 3- and 9-o'clock positions should be avoided to minimize damage to the long posterior ciliary vessels. Transillumination can be helpful when the unusual size and anatomy of the eye make it difficult to locate the pars plicata (165,166). In retreatments, at least one quadrant of the ciliary body should be left untouched, because no rescue therapy is available for chronic postoperative hypotony or phthisis (163). In addition to limited success rates, the risks of cyclocryotherapy are similar in both adults and children (Chapter 41) and include not only hypotony or phthisis, but also uveitis, cataract formation, and attendant visual loss.

Transscleral Cyclophotocoagulation

Transscleral cyclophotocoagulation with the Nd:YAG laser has also been used to reduce IOP in adults with refractory glaucoma, with results at least comparable to those of cryotherapy (167). This procedure is performed by using a spherical-tipped probe, placed with its anterior edge 0.5 to 1.5 mm from the limbus and perpendicular to the eye; 32 to 40 applications of 7 to 9 W for 0.5 to 0.7 seconds are applied for 360 degrees, often sparing the 3- and 9-o'clock positions (167). Limited experience with Nd:YAG contact transscleral cyclophotocoagulation in young children with advanced, uncontrolled glaucoma suggests effective pressure reduction in approximately 40% after a single 360-degree treatment (168). Advantages of this laser technique over cyclocryotherapy in adults (and likely also in children) include reduced severity or incidence of a transient postlaser increase in IOP, a less exuberant uveitic response, and reduced pain postoperatively. Risks of serious complication remain, however, with both techniques (169).

Transscleral cyclophotocoagulation has also been performed in children by using the diode laser and the Iris Medical G-probe, with reported success of 30% to 75% after one or more treatments and after fairly short follow-up (170–172). One recommended technique involves placement of 16 to 18 applications (of 2 seconds each) to three quadrants with the Iris G-probe, with variable power settings (mostly 1500 to 2000 MW) (171). Reported success with this technique has been similar to that with a second drainage-device surgery for children with uncontrolled glaucoma after initial drainage-device implantation (173).

Endoscopic Cyclophotocoagulation

Endoscopic cyclophotocoagulation using the diode laser has been applied in children with refractory glaucoma, with modest results (174–177). Investigators used the microendoscopic system incorporating fiber optics for a video monitor, diode laser endophotocoagulation, and illumination all within a 20-gauge probe (Microprobe, Endo Optiks, Little Silver, NJ) (178). In children with aphakic or pseudophakic glaucoma, cumulative success of all procedures at last follow-up was 53% in this series of 34 eyes, after an average of 1.5 treatment sessions, performed via limbal or pars plana approach, with mean follow-up time of 44 months (175). Retinal detachment, hypotony, and visual loss were reported in these series, which included both aphakic and phakic eyes (175,177). A small series of children with refractory glaucoma and corneal opacification reported a low rate of success using endoscopic diode laser cycloablation in these (aphakic) eyes (174).

Cycloablation, despite its limited success and significant complications, does nonetheless play a role in the management of refractory pediatric glaucoma. Its place in the surgical strategy depends on several factors, including the anatomy of the given eye and prior failed surgical interventions, the severity of the glaucoma, and the age of the child (170,171,174,175,177). It may have an appropriate role as an adjunct to prior glaucoma drainage-device surgery after the latter has incompletely controlled the IOP (170,171,173–175,177).

FOLLOW-UP OF CHILDREN WITH GLAUCOMA

Even children whose glaucoma is well controlled after surgical therapy (with or without adjunctive medical therapy) require lifelong follow-up. Loss of IOP control may occur months or even decades after initial successful control with surgery and may be asymptomatic in the older child or young adult. In addition, young children with glaucoma often face vision-threatening difficulties, such as corneal scarring, anisometropia, and resultant amblyopia even after IOP control has been achieved. Children with glaucoma that is controlled without the use of medications should be followed up at least every 6 months, and young children, or those whose IOP has been controlled for less than 2 years, should probably be evaluated at least every 3 or 4 months. During these office examinations, correlates of adequate IOP control include (a) stable visual function, refractive error, and optic nerve appearance; (b) corneas that are free of edema and stable in size; and (c) children who are free of epiphora, excessive photophobia, and blepharospasm. By contrast, even if the IOP is less than 20 mm Hg, deteriorating vision, progressive myopia, progressive optic nerve cupping, or increases in corneal size, edema, or ocular symptoms suggest that glaucoma control may be inadequate for the long term.

KEY POINTS

- Medications can be very useful in the management of pediatric glaucomas but must be administered with awareness of the special susceptibility of children to the systemic side effects of these drugs. Special care is needed when prescribing the β-blockers and brimonidine in young children.

- Many childhood glaucomas require surgical intervention. While angle surgery is usually the first-line surgery for primary congenital and selected other developmental glaucomas, other more resistant cases require filtering surgery, glaucoma drainage-device implantation, or even cyclodestructive procedures. The success of glaucoma surgery in children depends on many factors, and glaucoma control not infrequently requires a combination of surgical and continued medical treatment.

- Medical and surgical therapy for childhood glaucomas has challenged ophthalmologists for many years. Despite tremendous advances in medical, laser, and surgical technology over the past quarter century, we are still humbled by our inability to preserve sight in many children with glaucoma.

REFERENCES

1. deLuise VP, Anderson DR. Primary infantile glaucoma (congenital glaucoma). *Surv Ophthalmol.* 1983;28(1):1–19.
2. Ott EZ, Mills MD, Arango S, et al. A randomized trial assessing dorzolamide in patients with glaucoma who are younger than 6 years. *Arch Ophthalmol.* 2005;123(9):1177–1186.
3. Whitson JT, Roarty JD, Vijaya L, et al. Efficacy of brinzolamide and levobetaxolol in pediatric glaucomas: a randomized clinical trial. *J AAPOS.* 2008;12(3):239–246.
4. Passo MS, Palmer EA, Van Buskirk EM. Plasma timolol in glaucoma patients. *Ophthalmology.* 1984;91(11):1361–1363.
5. Haas J. Principles and problems of therapy in congenital glaucoma. *Invest Ophthalmol.* 1968;7(2):140–146.
6. Dickens CJ, Hoskins HD. Diagnosis and treatment of congenital glaucoma. In: Ritch R, Shields MB, Krupin T, eds. *The Glaucomas.* Vol 2. St. Louis, MO: CV Mosby; 1989:773–785.
7. Walton DS. In: Epstein DL, ed. *Chandler and Grant's Glaucoma.* 3rd ed. Philadelphia, PA: Lea & Febiger; 1986.
8. Portellos M, Buckley EG, Freedman SF. Topical versus oral carbonic anhydrase inhibitor therapy for pediatric glaucoma. *J AAPOS.* 1998;2(1):43–47.
9. Sabri K, Levin AV. The additive effect of topical dorzolamide and systemic acetazolamide in pediatric glaucoma. *J AAPOS.* 2006;10(5):464–468.
10. Walton DS. Primary congenital open angle glaucoma: a study of the anterior segment abnormalities. *Trans Am Ophthalmol Soc.* 1979;77:746–768.
11. Kolker AE, Hetherington J Jr(eds). Congenital glaucoma. In: *Becker-Shaffer's Diagnosis and Therapy of the Glaucomas.* 5th ed. St. Louis, MO: CV Mosby; 1983:317–369.
12. Chandler PA, Grant WM. *Glaucoma.* 2d ed. Philadelphia, PA: Lea & Febiger; 1979.
13. Mann I. *Developmental Abnormalities of the Eye.* 2nd ed. Philadelphia, PA: JB Lippincott; 1957.
14. Boger WP III, Walton DS. Timolol in uncontrolled childhood glaucomas. *Ophthalmology.* 1981;88(3):253–258.
15. Boger WP III. Timolol in childhood glaucoma. *Surv Ophthalmol.* 1983;28(suppl):259–261.
16. Zimmerman TJ, Kooner KS, Morgan KS. Safety and efficacy of timolol in pediatric glaucoma. *Surv Ophthalmol.* 1983;28(suppl):262–264.
17. Hoskins HD Jr, Hetherington J Jr, Magee SD, et al. Clinical experience with timolol in childhood glaucoma. *Arch Ophthalmol.* 1985;103(8):1163–1165.
18. McMahon CD, Hetherington J Jr, Hoskins HD Jr, et al. Timolol and pediatric glaucomas. *Ophthalmology.* 1981;88(3):249–252.
19. Olson RJ, Bromberg BB, Zimmerman TJ. Apneic spells associated with timolol therapy in a neonate. *Am J Ophthalmol.* 1979;88(1):120–122.
20. Raab EL. Congenital glaucoma. *Persp Ophthalmol.* 1978;2:35–41.
21. Becker B, Shaffer RN. *Diagnosis and Therapy of the Glaucomas.* 2nd ed. St. Louis, MO: CV Mosby; 1965.
22. Shields MB. *Textbook of Glaucoma.* 3rd ed. Baltimore, MD: Williams & Wilkins; 1992.
23. Wright TM, Freedman SF. Exposure to topical apraclonidine in children with glaucoma. *J Glaucoma.* 2009;18(5):395–398.
24. Carlsen JO, Zabriskie NA, Kwon YH, et al. Apparent central nervous system depression in infants after the use of topical brimonidine. *Am J Ophthalmol.* 1999;128(2):255–256.
25. Korsch E, Grote A, Seybold M, et al. Systemic adverse effects of topical treatment with brimonidine in an infant with secondary glaucoma. *Eur J Pediatr.* 1999;158(8):685.
26. Enyedi LB, Freedman SF. Safety and efficacy of brimonidine in children with glaucoma. *J AAPOS.* 2001;5(5):281–284.
27. Mungan NK, Wilson TW, Nischal KK, et al. Hypotension and bradycardia in infants after the use of topical brimonidine and beta-blockers. *J AAPOS.* 2003;7(1):69–70.
28. Ong T, Chia A, Nischal KK. Latanoprost in port wine stain related paediatric glaucoma. *Br J Ophthalmol.* 2003;87(9):1091–1093.
29. Enyedi LB, Freedman SF, Buckley EG. The effectiveness of latanoprost for the treatment of pediatric glaucoma. *J AAPOS.* 1999;3(1):33–39.
30. Enyedi LB, Freedman SF. Latanoprost for the treatment of pediatric glaucoma. *Surv Ophthalmol.* 2002;47(suppl 1):S129–S132.
31. Yang CB, Freedman SF, Myers JS, et al. Use of latanoprost in the treatment of glaucoma associated with Sturge–Weber syndrome. *Am J Ophthalmol.* 1998;126(4):600–602.
32. Yanovitch TL, Enyedi LB, Schotthoeffer EO, et al. Travoprost in children: adverse effects and intraocular pressure response. *J AAPOS.* 2009;13(1):91–93.
33. Elgin U, Batman A, Berker N, et al. The comparison of eyelash lengthening effect of latanoprost therapy in adults and children. *Eur J Ophthalmol.* 2006;16(2):247–250.
34. de Vincentiis C. Incisions del angolo irideo nel glaucoma [in Italian]. *Ann Ottalmol.* 1893;22:540–542.
35. Barkan O. Technique of goniotomy. *Arch Ophthalmol.* 1938;19:217–221.
36. Barkan O. Goniotomy for the relief of congenital glaucoma. *Br J Ophthalmol.* 1948;32(9):701–728.
37. Walton DS. Goniotomy. In: Thomas JV, ed. *Glaucoma Surgery.* St. Louis, MO: CV Mosby; 1992:107–121.
38. Yeung HH, Walton DS. Goniotomy for juvenile open-angle glaucoma. *J Glaucoma.* 2010;19(1):1–4.
39. Kanski JJ, McAllister JA. Trabeculodialysis for inflammatory glaucoma in children and young adults. *Ophthalmology.* 1985;92(7):927–930.
40. Freedman SF, Rodriguez-Rosa RE, Rojas MC, et al. Goniotomy for glaucoma secondary to chronic childhood uveitis. *Am J Ophthalmol.* 2002;133(5):617–621.
41. Chen TC, Walton DS. Goniosurgery for prevention of aniridic glaucoma. *Trans Am Ophthalmol Soc.* 1998;96:155–165; discussion 165–169.
42. Walton DS. Aniridic glaucoma: the results of gonio-surgery to prevent and treat this problem. *Trans Am Ophthalmol Soc.* 1986;84:59–70.
43. Freedman SF, Johnston SC. Glaucoma in infancy and early childhood. In: Wilson ME, Saunders RA, Trivedi RH, eds. *Pediatric Ophthalmology: Current Thought and a Practical Guide.* Berlin: Springer-Verlag; 2009.
44. Amoils SP, Simmons RJ. Goniotomy with intraocular illumination. A preliminary report. *Arch Ophthalmol.* 1968;80(4):488–491.
45. Hodapp E, Heuer DK. A simple technique for goniotomy. *Am J Ophthalmol.* 1986;102(4):537.
46. Arnoult JB, Vila-Coro AA, Mazow ML. Goniotomy with sodium hyaluronate. *J Pediatr Ophthalmol Strabismus.* 1988;25(1):18–22.
47. Joos KM, Alward WL, Folberg R. Experimental endoscopic goniotomy. A potential treatment for primary infantile glaucoma. *Ophthalmology.* 1993;100(7):1066–1070.
48. Bayraktar S, Koseoglu T. Endoscopic goniotomy with anterior chamber maintainer: surgical technique and one-year results. *Ophthalmic Surg Lasers.* 2001;32(6):496–502.

49. Medow NB, Sauer HL. Endoscopic goniotomy for congenital glaucoma. *J Pediatr Ophthalmol Strabismus.* 1997;34(4):258–259.

50. Draeger J. New microsurgical techniques to improve chamber angle surgery. *Glaucoma.* 1980;2:403.

51. Buckley EG, Freedman SF, Shields MB. *Atlas of Ophthalmic Surgery.* Vol 3: *Strabismus and Glaucoma Surgery.* St. Louis, MO: Mosby–Year Book; 1995.

52. Litinsky SM, Shaffer RN, Hetherington J, et al. Operative complications of goniotomy. *Trans Sect Ophthalmol Am Acad Ophthalmol Otolaryngol.* 1977;83(1):78–79.

53. Shaffer RN. Prognosis of goniotomy in primary infantile glaucoma (trabeculodysgenesis). *Trans Am Ophthalmol Soc.* 1982;80:321–325.

54. Taylor RH, Ainsworth JR, Evans AR, et al. The epidemiology of pediatric glaucoma: the Toronto experience. *J AAPOS.* 1999;3(5):308–315.

55. Catalano RA, King RA, Calhoun JH, et al. One versus two simultaneous goniotomies as the initial surgical procedure for primary infantile glaucoma. *J Pediatr Ophthalmol Strabismus.* 1989;26(1):9–13.

56. Scheie HG. Goniopuncture—a new filtering operation for glaucoma; preliminary report. *Arch Ophthalmol.* 1950;44(6):761–782.

57. Vannas S, Pohjola S. Modified goniopuncture in the treatment of congenital glaucoma. *Acta Ophthalmol.* 1971;49(1):159–164.

58. Melamed S, Latina MA, Epstein DL. Neodymium:YAG laser trabeculopuncture in juvenile open-angle glaucoma. *Ophthalmology.* 1987;94(2):163–170.

59. Fernandez JL, Galin MA. Technique of direct goniotomy. *Arch Ophthalmol.* 1973;90(4):305–306.

60. Safran MJ, Robin AL, Pollack IP. Argon laser trabeculoplasty in younger patients with primary open-angle glaucoma. *Am J Ophthalmol.* 1984;97(3):292–295.

61. Wilensky JT, Weinreb RN. Early and late failures of argon laser trabeculoplasty. *Arch Ophthalmol.* 1983;101(6):895–897.

62. Burian HM. A case of Marfan's syndrome with bilateral glaucoma. With description of a new type of operation for developmental glaucoma (trabeculotomy ab externo). *Am J Ophthalmol.* 1960;50:1187–1192.

63. Smith R. A new technique for opening the canal of Schlemm. Preliminary report. *Br J Ophthalmol.* 1960;44:370–373.

64. Ikeda H, Ishigooka H, Muto T, et al. Long-term outcome of trabeculotomy for the treatment of developmental glaucoma. *Arch Ophthalmol.* 2004;122(8):1122–1128.

65. McPherson SD Jr. Results of external trabeculotomy. *Am J Ophthalmol.* 1973;76(6):918–920.

66. Shrader CE, Cibis GW. External trabeculotomy. In: Thomas JV, Belcher CD III, Simmons RJ, eds. *Glaucoma Surgery.* St. Louis, MO: CV Mosby; 1992:123–131.

67. Walton DS. Glaucoma in infants and children. In: Nelson L, Calhoun JH, Harley RD, eds. *Pediatric Ophthalmology.* Philadelphia, PA: WB Saunders; 1983.

68. Beck AD, Lynch MG. 360 degrees trabeculotomy for primary congenital glaucoma. *Arch Ophthalmol.* 1995;113(9):1200–1202.

69. Smith R. Nylon filament trabeculotomy in glaucoma. *Trans Ophthalmol Soc U K.* 1962;82:439–454.

70. Mandal AK, Matalia JH, Nutheti R, et al. Combined trabeculotomy and trabeculectomy in advanced primary developmental glaucoma with corneal diameter of 14 mm or more. *Eye (Lond).* 2006;20(2):135–143.

71. Elder MJ. Combined trabeculotomy-trabeculectomy compared with primary trabeculectomy for congenital glaucoma. *Br J Ophthalmol.* 1994;78(10):745–748.

72. Mullaney PB, Selleck C, Al-Awad A, et al. Combined trabeculotomy and trabeculectomy as an initial procedure in uncomplicated congenital glaucoma. *Arch Ophthalmol.* 1999;117(4):457–460.

73. Al-Hazmi A, Awad A, Zwaan J, et al. Correlation between surgical success rate and severity of congenital glaucoma. *Br J Ophthalmol.* 2005;89(4):449–453.

74. Mandal AK. Primary combined trabeculotomy-trabeculectomy for early-onset glaucoma in Sturge–Weber syndrome. *Ophthalmology.* 1999;106(8):1621–1627.

75. Luntz MH. The advantages of trabeculotomy over goniotomy. *J Pediatr Ophthalmol Strabismus.* 1984;21(4):150–153.

76. Hoskins HD Jr, Shaffer RN, Hetherington J. Goniotomy vs trabeculotomy. *J Pediatr Ophthalmol Strabismus.* 1984;21(4):153–158.

77. Anderson DR. Trabeculotomy compared to goniotomy for glaucoma in children. *Ophthalmology.* 1983;90(7):805–806.

78. McPherson SD Jr, Berry DP. Goniotomy vs external trabeculotomy for developmental glaucoma. *Am J Ophthalmol.* 1983;95(4):427–431.

79. Broughton WL, Parks MM. An analysis of treatment of congenital glaucoma by goniotomy. *Am J Ophthalmol.* 1981;91(5):566–572.

80. Draeger J, Wirt H, von Domarus D. Long-term results after goniotomy [in German]. *Klin Monbl Augenheilkd.* 1982;180(4):264–270.

81. Mendicino ME, Lynch MG, Drack A, et al. Long-term surgical and visual outcomes in primary congenital glaucoma: 360 degrees trabeculotomy versus goniotomy. *J AAPOS.* 2000;4(4):205–210.

82. Eustis HS Jr, Walton RC, Ball SF. Pupillary block glaucoma following pediatric cataract extraction. *Ophthalmic Surg.* 1990;21(6):413–415.

83. Peyman GA, Sanders DR, Minatoya H. Pars plana vitrectomy in the management of pupillary block glaucoma following irrigation and aspiration. *Br J Ophthalmol.* 1978;62(5):336–339.

84. Michael AJ, Pesin SR, Katz LJ, et al. Management of late-onset angle-closure glaucoma associated with retinopathy of prematurity. *Ophthalmology.* 1991;98(7):1093–1098.

85. Cadera W, Pachtman MA, Cantor LB, et al. Filtering surgery in childhood glaucoma. *Ophthalmic Surg.* 1984;15(4):319–322.

86. Scheie HG. Results of peripheral iridectomy with scleral cautery in congenital and juvenile glaucoma. *Trans Am Ophthalmol Soc.* 1962;60:116–139.

87. Beauchamp GR, Parks MM. Filtering surgery in children: barriers to success. *Ophthalmology.* 1979;86(1):170–180.

88. Rodrigues AM, Junior AP, Montezano FT, et al. Comparison between results of trabeculectomy in primary congenital glaucoma with and without the use of mitomycin C. *J Glaucoma.* 2004;13(3):228–232.

89. Fulcher T, Chan J, Lanigan B, et al. Long-term follow up of primary trabeculectomy for infantile glaucoma. *Br J Ophthalmol.* 1996;80(6):499–502.

90. Miller MH, Rice NS. Trabeculectomy combined with beta irradiation for congenital glaucoma. *Br J Ophthalmol.* 1991;75(10):584–590.

91. Zalish M, Leiba H, Oliver M. Subconjunctival injection of 5-fluorouracil following trabeculectomy for congenital and infantile glaucoma. *Ophthalmic Surg.* 1992;23(3):203–205.

92. Freedman SF, McCormick K, Cox TA. Mitomycin C-augmented trabeculectomy with postoperative wound modulation in pediatric glaucoma. *J AAPOS.* 1999;3(2):117–124.

93. Kitazawa Y, Kawase K, Matsushita H, et al. Trabeculectomy with mitomycin. A comparative study with fluorouracil. *Arch Ophthalmol.* 1991;109(12):1693–1698.

94. Palmer SS. Mitomycin as adjunct chemotherapy with trabeculectomy. *Ophthalmology.* 1991;98(3):317–321.

95. Mandal AK, Walton DS, John T, et al. Mitomycin C-augmented trabeculectomy in refractory congenital glaucoma. *Ophthalmology.* 1997;104(6):996–1001; discussion 1002–1003.

96. Freedman SF. Discussion of "Mitomycin C-augmented trabeculectomy in refractory congenital glaucoma." *Ophthalmology.* 1997;104:1002–1003.

97. Ehrlich R, Snir M, Lusky M, et al. Augmented trabeculectomy in paediatric glaucoma. *Br J Ophthalmol.* 2005;89(2):165–168.

98. Beck AD, Wilson WR, Lynch MG, et al. Trabeculectomy with adjunctive mitomycin C in pediatric glaucoma. *Am J Ophthalmol.* 1998;126(5):648–657.

99. Sidoti PA, Belmonte SJ, Liebmann JM, et al. Trabeculectomy with mitomycin-C in the treatment of pediatric glaucomas. *Ophthalmology.* 2000;107(3):422–429.

100. al-Hazmi A, Zwaan J, Awad A, et al. Effectiveness and complications of mitomycin C use during pediatric glaucoma surgery. *Ophthalmology.* 1998;105(10):1915–1920.

101. Susanna R Jr, Oltrogge EW, Carani JC, et al. Mitomycin as adjunct chemotherapy with trabeculectomy in congenital and developmental glaucomas. *J Glaucoma.* 1995;4(3):151–157.

102. Agarwal HC, Sood NN, Sihota R, et al. Mitomycin-C in congenital glaucoma. *Ophthalmic Surg Lasers.* 1997;28(12):979–985.

103. Beck AD, Freedman SF. Trabeculectomy with mitomycin-C in pediatric glaucomas. *Ophthalmology.* 2001;108(5):835–837.

104. Paciuc M, Velasco CF. Trabeculectomy with mitomycin-C in pediatric glaucomas. *Ophthalmology.* 2001;108(5):835.

105. Mandal AK, Prasad K, Naduvilath TJ. Surgical results and complications of mitomycin C-augmented trabeculectomy in refractory developmental glaucoma. *Ophthalmic Surg Lasers.* 1999;30(6):473–480.

106. Giampani J Jr, Borges-Giampani AS, Carani JC, et al. Efficacy and safety of trabeculectomy with mitomycin C for childhood glaucoma: a study of results with long-term follow-up. *Clinics (Sao Paulo).* 2008;63(4):421–426.

107. Noe RL, Lynch MG, Beck D. Glaucoma filtering surgery with mitomycin-C in children. *Invest Ophthalmol Vis Sci.* 1994;35(suppl):1431.

108. Sidoti PA, Lopez PF, Michon J, et al. Delayed-onset pneumococcal endophthalmitis after mitomycin-C trabeculectomy: association with cryptic nasolacrimal obstruction. *J Glaucoma.* 1995;4(1):11–15.

109. Waheed S, Ritterband DC, Greenfield DS, et al. Bleb-related ocular infection in children after trabeculectomy with mitomycin C. *Ophthalmology.* 1997;104(12):2117–2120.

110. Mochizuki K, Jikihara S, Ando Y, et al. Incidence of delayed onset infection after trabeculectomy with adjunctive mitomycin C or 5-fluorouracil treatment. *Br J Ophthalmol.* 1997;81(10):877–883.

111. DeBry PW, Perkins TW, Heatley G, et al. Incidence of late-onset bleb-related complications following trabeculectomy with mitomycin. *Arch Ophthalmol.* 2002;120(3):297–300.

112. Greenfield DS, Suner IJ, Miller MP, et al. Endophthalmitis after filtering surgery with mitomycin. *Arch Ophthalmol.* 1996;114(8):943–949.

113. Crooke ST, Bradner WT. Mitomycin C: a review. *Cancer Treat Rev.* 1976;3(3):121–139.

114. Glaubinger D, Ramu A. Antitumor antibiotics. In: Chabner BA, ed. *Pharmacologic Principles of Cancer Treatment.* Philadelphia, PA: WB Saunders; 1982:402–415.

115. Wells AP, Cordeiro MF, Bunce C, et al. Cystic bleb formation and related complications in limbus- versus fornix-based conjunctival flaps in pediatric and young adult trabeculectomy with mitomycin C. *Ophthalmology.* 2003;110(11):2192–2197.

116. Wheeler DT, Stager DR, Weakley DR Jr. Endophthalmitis following pediatric intraocular surgery for congenital cataracts and congenital glaucoma. *J Pediatr Ophthalmol Strabismus.* 1992;29(3):139–141.

117. Kafkala C, Hynes A, Choi J, et al. Ahmed valve implantation for uncontrolled pediatric uveitic glaucoma. *J AAPOS.* 2005;9(4):336–340.

118. Molteno AC, Sayawat N, Herbison P. Otago glaucoma surgery outcome study: long-term results of uveitis with secondary glaucoma drained by Molteno implants. *Ophthalmology.* 2001;108(3):605–613.

119. Hill RA, Nguyen QH, Baerveldt G, et al. Trabeculectomy and Molteno implantation for glaucomas associated with uveitis. *Ophthalmology.* 1993;100(6):903–908.

120. Da Mata A, Burk SE, Netland PA, et al. Management of uveitic glaucoma with Ahmed glaucoma valve implantation. *Ophthalmology.* 1999;106(11):2168–2172.

121. Al-Mobarak F, Khan AO. Complications and 2-year valve survival following Ahmed valve implantation during the first 2 years of life. *Br J Ophthalmol.* 2009;93(6):795–798.

122. Banitt MR, Sidoti PA, Gentile RC, et al. Pars plana Baerveldt implantation for refractory childhood glaucomas. *J Glaucoma.* 2009;18(5):412–417.

123. Chen TC, Bhatia LS, Walton DS. Ahmed valve surgery for refractory pediatric glaucoma: a report of 52 eyes. *J Pediatr Ophthalmol Strabismus.* 2005;42(5):274–283; quiz 304–305.

124. Khan AO, Al-Mobarak F. Comparison of polypropylene and silicone Ahmed valve survival 2 years following implantation in the first 2 years of life. *Br J Ophthalmol.* 2009;93(6):791–794.

125. Morad Y, Donaldson CE, Kim YM, et al. The Ahmed drainage implant in the treatment of pediatric glaucoma. *Am J Ophthalmol.* 2003;135(6):821–829.

126. O'Malley Schotthoefer E, Yanovitch TL, Freedman SF. Aqueous drainage device surgery in refractory pediatric glaucoma: II. Ocular motility consequences. *J AAPOS.* 2008;12(1):40–45.

127. O'Malley Schotthoefer E, Yanovitch TL, Freedman SF. Aqueous drainage device surgery in refractory pediatric glaucomas: I. Long-term outcomes. *J AAPOS.* 2008;12(1):33–39.

128. Ou Y, Yu F, Law SK, et al. Outcomes of Ahmed glaucoma valve implantation in children with primary congenital glaucoma. *Arch Ophthalmol.* 2009;127(11):1436–1441.

129. Rolim de Moura C, Fraser-Bell S, Stout A, et al. Experience with the Baerveldt glaucoma implant in the management of pediatric glaucoma. *Am J Ophthalmol.* 2005;139(5):847–854.

130. van Overdam KA, de Faber JT, Lemij HG, et al. Baerveldt glaucoma implant in paediatric patients. *Br J Ophthalmol.* 2006;90(3):328–332.

131. Munoz M, Tomey KF, Traverso C, et al. Clinical experience with the Molteno implant in advanced infantile glaucoma. *J Pediatr Ophthalmol Strabismus.* 1991;28(2):68–72.

132. Billson F, Thomas R, Aylward W. The use of two-stage Molteno implants in developmental glaucoma. *J Pediatr Ophthalmol Strabismus.* 1989; 26(1):3–8.

133. Molteno AC, Ancker E, Van Biljon G. Surgical technique for advanced juvenile glaucoma. *Arch Ophthalmol.* 1984;102(1):51–57.

134. Lloyd MA, Sedlak T, Heuer DK, et al. Clinical experience with the single-plate Molteno implant in complicated glaucomas. Update of a pilot study. *Ophthalmology.* 1992;99(5):679–687.

135. Hill RA, Heuer DK, Baerveldt G, et al. Molteno implantation for glaucoma in young patients. *Ophthalmology.* 1991;98(7):1042–1046.

136. Christmann LM, Wilson ME. Motility disturbances after Molteno implants. *J Pediatr Ophthalmol Strabismus.* 1992;29(1):44–48.

137. Molteno AC. Children with advanced glaucoma treated by draining implants. *S Afr Arch Ophthalmol.* 1973;1:55–61.

138. Cunliffe IA, Molteno AC. Long-term follow-up of Molteno drains used in the treatment of glaucoma presenting in childhood. *Eye (Lond).* 1998;12(3a):379–385.

139. Heuer DK, Lloyd MA, Abrams DA, et al. Which is better? One or two? A randomized clinical trial of single-plate versus double-plate Molteno implantation for glaucomas in aphakia and pseudophakia. *Ophthalmology.* 1992;99(10):1512–1519.

140. Netland PA, Walton DS. Glaucoma drainage implants in pediatric patients. *Ophthalmic Surg.* 1993;24(11):723–729.

141. Fellenbaum PS, Sidoti PA, Heuer DK, et al. Experience with the Baerveldt implant in young patients with complicated glaucomas. *J Glaucoma.* 1995;4(2):91–97.

142. Donahue SP, Keech RV, Munden P, et al. Baerveldt implant surgery in the treatment of advanced childhood glaucoma. *J AAPOS.* 1997;1(1):41–45.

143. Budenz DL, Sakamoto D, Eliezer R, et al. Two-staged Baerveldt glaucoma implant for childhood glaucoma associated with Sturge–Weber syndrome. *Ophthalmology.* 2000;107(11):2105–2110.

144. Coleman AL, Smyth RJ, Wilson MR, et al. Initial clinical experience with the Ahmed glaucoma valve implant in pediatric patients. *Arch Ophthalmol.* 1997;115(2):186–191.

145. Englert JA, Freedman SF, Cox TA. The Ahmed valve in refractory pediatric glaucoma. *Am J Ophthalmol.* 1999;127(1):34–42.

146. Djodeyre MR, Peralta Calvo J, Abelairas Gomez J. Clinical evaluation and risk factors of time to failure of Ahmed glaucoma valve implant in pediatric patients. *Ophthalmology.* 2001;108(3):614–620.

147. Ah-Chan JJ, Molteno AC, Bevin TH, et al. Otago Glaucoma Surgery Outcome Study: follow-up of young patients who underwent Molteno implant surgery. *Ophthalmology.* 2005;112(12):2137–2142.

148. Adachi M, Dickens CJ, Hetherington J Jr, et al. Clinical experience of trabeculotomy for the surgical treatment of aniridic glaucoma. *Ophthalmology.* 1997;104(12):2121–2125.

149. Airaksinen PJ, Aisala P, Tuulonen A. Molteno implant surgery in uncontrolled glaucoma. *Acta Ophthalmol.* 1990;68(6):690–694.

150. Astle WF, Lin DT, Douglas GR. Bilateral penetrating keratoplasty and placement of a Molteno implant in a newborn with Peters' anomaly. *Can J Ophthalmol.* 1993;28(6):276–282.

151. Billson F, Thomas R, Grigg J. Resiting Molteno implant tubes. *Ophthalmic Surg Lasers.* 1996;27(9):801–803.

152. Molteno AC, Van Biljon G, Ancker E. Two-stage insertion of glaucoma drainage implants. *Trans Ophthalmol Soc N Z.* 1979;31:17–26.

153. Wellemeyer ML, Price FW Jr. Molteno implants in patients with previous cyclocryotherapy. *Ophthalmic Surg.* 1993;24(6):395–398.

154. Trigler L, Proia AD, Freedman SF. Fibrovascular ingrowth as a cause of failure in children. *Am J Ophthalmol.* 2006;141(2):388–389.

155. Al-Torbaq AA, Edward DP. Delayed endophthalmitis in a child following an Ahmed glaucoma valve implant. *J AAPOS.* 2002;6(2):123–125.

156. Gutierrez-Diaz E, Montero-Rodriguez M, Mencia-Gutierrez E, et al. Propionibacterium acnes endophthalmitis in Ahmed glaucoma valve. *Eur J Ophthalmol.* 2001;11(4):383–385.

157. Beck AD, Freedman S, Kammer J, et al. Aqueous shunt devices compared with trabeculectomy with mitomycin-C for children in the first two years of life. *Am J Ophthalmol.* 2003;136(6):994–1000.

158. Pakravan M, Homayoon N, Shahin Y, et al. Trabeculectomy with mitomycin C versus Ahmed glaucoma implant with mitomycin C for treatment of pediatric aphakic glaucoma. *J Glaucoma.* 2007;16(7):631–636.

159. Al-Mobarak F, Khan AO. Two-year survival of Ahmed valve implantation in the first 2 years of life with and without intraoperative mitomycin-C. *Ophthalmology.* 2009;116(10):1862–1865.

160. Molteno AC, Polkinghorne PJ, Bowbyes JA. The Vicryl tie technique for inserting a draining implant in the treatment of secondary glaucoma. *Aust N Z J Ophthalmol.* 1986;14(4):343–354.

161. Tesser R, Hess DB, Freedman SF. Combined intraocular lens implantation and glaucoma implant (tube shunt) surgery in pediatric patients: a case series. *J AAPOS.* 2005;9(4):330–335.

162. al Faran MF, Tomey KF, al Mutlaq FA. Cyclocryotherapy in selected cases of congenital glaucoma. *Ophthalmic Surg.* 1990;21(11):794–798.

163. Wagle NS, Freedman SF, Buckley EG, et al. Long-term outcome of cyclocryotherapy for refractory pediatric glaucoma. *Ophthalmology.* 1998;105(10):1921–1926; discussion 1926–1927.

164. Freedman SF. Medical and surgical treatments for childhood glaucoma. In: Epstein DL, Allingham RR, Schuman JS, eds. *Chandler*

and Grant's Glaucoma. 4th ed. Baltimore, MD: Williams & Wilkins; 1997.

165. Bellows AR, Grant WM. Cyclocryotherapy in advanced inadequately controlled glaucoma. *Am J Ophthalmol.* 1973;75(4):679–684.

166. Bellows AR. Cyclocryotherapy: its role in the treatment of glaucoma. *Perspect Ophthalmol.* 1980;4:139.

167. Schuman JS, Bellows AR, Shingleton BJ, et al. Contact transscleral Nd:YAG laser cyclophotocoagulation. Midterm results. *Ophthalmology.* 1992;99(7):1089–1094; discussion 1095.

168. Phelan MJ, Higginbotham EJ. Contact transscleral Nd:YAG laser cyclophotocoagulation for the treatment of refractory pediatric glaucoma. *Ophthalmic Surg Lasers.* 1995;26(5):401–403.

169. Shields MB, Shields SE. Noncontact transscleral Nd:YAG cyclophotocoagulation: a long-term follow-up of 500 patients. *Trans Am Ophthalmol Soc.* 1994;92:271–283; discussion 283–287.

170. Autrata R, Rehurek J. Long-term results of transscleral cyclophotocoagulation in refractory pediatric glaucoma patients. *Ophthalmologica.* 2003;217(6):393–400.

171. Bock CJ, Freedman SF, Buckley EG, et al. Transscleral diode laser cyclophotocoagulation for refractory pediatric glaucomas. *J Pediatr Ophthalmol Strabismus.* 1997;34(4):235–239.

172. Izgi B, Demirci H, Demirci FY, et al. Diode laser cyclophotocoagulation in refractory glaucoma: comparison between pediatric and adult glaucomas. *Ophthalmic Surg Lasers.* 2001;32(2):100–107.

173. Sood S, Beck AD. Cyclophotocoagulation versus sequential tube shunt as a secondary intervention following primary tube shunt failure in pediatric glaucoma. *J AAPOS.* 2009;13(4):379–383.

174. Al-Haddad CE, Freedman SF. Endoscopic laser cyclophotocoagulation in pediatric glaucoma with corneal opacities. *J AAPOS.* 2007;11(1):23–28.

175. Carter BC, Plager DA, Neely DE, Endoscopic diode laser cyclophotocoagulation in management aphakic and pseudophakic glaucoma in children. *J AAPOS.* 2007;11(1):34–40.

176. Plager DA, Neely DE. Intermediate-term results of endoscopic diode laser cyclophotocoagulation for pediatric glaucoma. *J AAPOS.* 1999;3(3):131–137.

177. Neely DE, Plager DA. Endocyclophotocoagulation for management of difficult pediatric glaucomas. *J AAPOS.* 2001;5(4):221–229.

178. Uram M. Ophthalmic laser microendoscope endophotocoagulation. *Ophthalmology.* 1992;99(12):1829–1832.

Cyclodestructive Surgery

41

The operations discussed in the preceding chapters lower the intraocular pressure (IOP) by improving the rate of aqueous outflow. This is clearly preferred from a physiologic standpoint, in that the aqueous humor can continue to be produced in an unaltered state and fulfill its various functions, including nourishment of intraocular tissues. An alternative approach to reducing IOP, however, is to decrease the rate of aqueous production by partially eliminating the function of the ciliary processes. Historically, these techniques were rarely the first operation of choice, because the results are hard to predict and the complication rate is high because of damage to adjacent ocular structures and the influence of a pronounced inflammatory response. Newer approaches with transscleral and endoscopic diode laser appear to be associated with reasonable efficacy and fewer vision-threatening complications and may be considered earlier in the treatment paradigm.

Cyclodestructive procedures constitute a valuable adjunct in our surgical armamentarium for eyes in which other operations have failed or when the surgeon wishes to avoid incisional surgery, such as in eyes with limited visual potential or with a high risk for intraocular complications with standard outflow procedures. An important exception is endoscopic cyclophotocoagulation (ECP), a procedure that may be a useful adjunct in eyes with reasonable visual potential and whose indications are still evolving.

OVERVIEW OF CYCLODESTRUCTIVE PROCEDURES

Cyclodestructive operations differ according to (a) the destructive energy source and (b) the route by which the energy reaches the ciliary processes. In the 1930s and 1940s, several energy sources were evaluated, including diathermy, β-irradiation, and electrolysis, although only cyclodiathermy achieved clinical acceptance. Cryotherapy was introduced in the 1950s and became the most commonly used cyclodestructive procedure. However, subsequent experience with laser cyclophotocoagulation showed clear advantages over other techniques, and it has become the preferred cyclodestructive operation. Other cyclodestructive techniques include therapeutic ultrasonography and microwave cyclodestruction. Each of these energy sources may be delivered by the transscleral route, in which the destructive element passes through conjunctiva, sclera, and ciliary muscle before reaching the ciliary processes. Transscleral cyclodestructive operations have the advantages of being nonincisional and relatively quick and easy. However, significant disadvantages include the inability to visualize the processes being treated and damage to adjacent tissue, leading to unpredictable results and frequent complications. With the advent of laser energy as the cyclodestructive element, alternative delivery routes, including transpupillary and endoscopic approaches, are now possible.

EARLY CYCLODESTRUCTIVE PROCEDURES

Penetrating Cyclodiathermy

Weve (1) introduced the concept of cyclodestructive surgery in 1933, using nonpenetrating diathermy to produce selective destruction of ciliary processes. Vogt (2,3) modified the technique by using a diathermy probe, which penetrated the sclera, and this became the standard cyclodestructive procedure. One or two rows of diathermy lesions were generally placed 2.5 to 5 mm behind the limbus several millimeters apart for approximately 180 degrees. Early reports of experience with cyclodiathermy were encouraging (4,5). However, subsequent study revealed a low success rate (about 5%) and a significant incidence of hypotony and phthisis (about 5%) (6).

Other Early Cyclodestructive Procedures

β-Irradiation Therapy

In 1948, Haik and coworkers (7) reported the experimental application of radium over the ciliary body in rabbit eyes and in one clinical case. Although this was shown to produce a reduction in the vascular supply of the ciliary body, it also caused damage to the lens, and the technique was never adopted for clinical use.

Cycloelectrolysis

Berens and coworkers (8) in 1949 described a technique that used low-frequency galvanic current to create a chemical reaction within the ciliary body. This led to the formation of sodium hydroxide, which is caustic to the tissue of the ciliary body. Although this was shown in rabbit studies to produce destruction of ciliary processes (9), the procedure did not seem to have significant advantages over penetrating cyclodiathermy and never achieved widespread clinical popularity.

Therapeutic Ultrasonography

In 1964, Purnell and associates (10) introduced the concept of using focused transscleral ultrasonic radiation to produce localized destruction of the ciliary body in rabbit eyes. Coleman and coworkers in 1985 reported the results of rabbit studies and preliminary clinical trials with high-intensity focused ultrasound (11,12). Several clinical trials of therapeutic ultrasonography in patients with refractory glaucomas, similar to those described in studies of other cyclodestructive procedures, have revealed IOP reduction to the low 20s (mm Hg) or less in one half to two thirds of the cases 6 to 12 months after a single treatment (13–15). In a multicenter study involving 880 eyes, success (IOP between 6 and 22 mm Hg) after a single treatment was 48.7% at 6 months (16). With repeated treatments as required, the success rate rose to 79.3% at 1 year. The most common complication was an immediate postoperative IOP increase and mild iritis. Scleral thinning was observed in 2.5%, and phthisis in 1.1%. Decreased visual acuity occurred in approximately 20% of the cases.

Transscleral Microwave Cyclodestruction

The direct application of high-frequency electromagnetic radiation over the conjunctiva in rabbits produced heat-induced damage to the ciliary body with relative sparing of the conjunctiva and sclera (17). In rabbits with experimentally induced glaucoma, the procedure was successful in reducing IOP in all treated eyes for 4 weeks (18).

Excision of the Ciliary Body

In addition to the use of many cyclodestructive elements, as described earlier, other surgeons have sought to reduce aqueous production by removing a portion of the ciliary body. Several studies have revealed reasonable success and complication rates with this basic approach in eyes with unusually refractory glaucomas (19–21).

LASER CYCLODESTRUCTION

Transscleral Cyclophotocoagulation

In 1961, Weekers and associates (22) used light as the cyclodestructive element, using the transscleral application of xenon-arc photocoagulation over the ciliary body. As with other operations that use light energy, however, it was the introduction of the laser that eventually led to the clinical application of cyclophotocoagulation. In 1969, Vucicevic and associates (23) reported the use of a ruby laser to perform transscleral cyclophotocoagulation in rabbits, with an adjunctive cytochemical agent to enhance laser absorption by the ciliary body. Other reports of transscleral laser cyclophotocoagulation

followed (24–26), and in 1984 Beckman and Waeltermann (27) reported results of a 10-year experience with 241 eyes treated by using transscleral ruby laser cyclophotocoagulation. Their overall rate of IOP control was 62%, with 86% in aphakic eyes with glaucoma and 53% in eyes with neovascular glaucoma. Chronic hypotony occurred in 41 eyes, with phthisis in 17 cases, although most eyes retained their preoperative level of vision. However, it was not until the availability of specially designed Nd:YAG (neodymium:yttrium–aluminum–garnet) and, subsequently, semiconductor diode lasers that widespread interest in transscleral cyclophotocoagulation developed.

Instruments
Nd:YAG Lasers

Nd:YAG lasers, with a wavelength of 1064 nm, have been useful for transscleral cyclophotocoagulation because they traverse the sclera with relatively low absorption and scatter. They may be operated in a pulsed, free-running, thermal mode, or a continuous-wave mode, and may be delivered by either a noncontact, slitlamp system, or a contact probe, fiberoptic system. However, these units do not appear to be commercially available for transscleral cyclophotocoagulation. (Readers wishing more information can consult the fifth edition of this book.)

Semiconductor Diode Lasers

Although semiconductor diode lasers, with a range of wavelengths between 750 and 850 nm, do not traverse the sclera as efficiently as Nd:YAG lasers do, they have the advantage of greater absorption by uveal melanin. In addition, they have the advantage of solid-state construction with compact size, low maintenance requirements, and no special requirement for electric outlet or water cooling.

The Oculight SLx (Iris Medical Instruments) is a continuous-wave, contact delivery diode laser with a wavelength of 810 nm, a maximum power output of 2.5 to 3.0 W, and a maximum duration of 9.9 seconds (28–30) (**Fig. 41.1**). The probe (G-Probe) consists of a 600-μm quartz fiberoptic, protruding 0.7 mm from a handpiece, which is fabricated to center the fiberoptic 1.2 mm behind the surgical limbus and parallel to the visual axis (30). The back of the G-Probe pushes the lid away from the surgical site, and the sides can be used to aid in spacing the laser applications (**Fig. 41.2**).

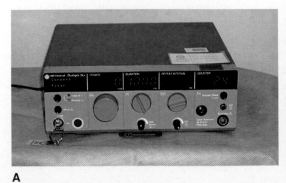
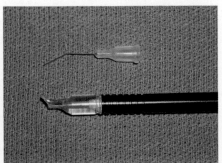

Figure 41.1   **A:** Semiconductor diode laser (IRIS, Oculight, SLx, Iris Medical Inc., Mountain View, CA) for transscleral diode cyclophotocoagulation. **B:** G-Probe handpiece for transscleral diode cyclophotocoagulation. (From Lin SC. Endoscopic and transscleral cyclophotocoagulation for the treatment of refractory glaucoma. *J Glaucoma*. 2008;17: 238–247.)

A   B

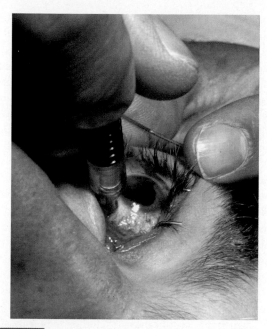

Figure 41.2 Transscleral diode cyclophotocoagulation, showing use of G-Probe to position fiberoptic 1.2 mm from surgical limbus and to space adjacent laser applications.

An ophthalmic laser microendoscope (Endo Optiks Inc., Little Silver, NJ) has also been developed which houses fiberoptics for a video monitor, diode laser endophotocoagulation, and illumination in a 20-gauge probe (31) (**Fig. 41.3**). The diode laser has 1.2 W of power output and is focused visually by means of a 670 nm (2.0 mW) laser aiming beam. Optimal focal distance for the laser is 0.75 mm from the tip of the probe. Depth of focus while viewing is from 0 to 20 mm, and the camera lens has a 70-degree field of view.

Krypton Lasers

Transscleral cyclophotocoagulation has also been performed with a retinal krypton laser, delivered by a contact probe. The shorter wavelength results in poorer scleral transmission but better uveal pigment absorption than with the Nd:YAG laser,

and histologic lesions in rabbits were similar with the two lasers (32). Successful clinical results were reported, using 4 to 5 J of energy, 10-second exposures, and firm compression with the probe (33,34).

Theories of Mechanism

The mechanism by which transscleral cyclophotocoagulation reduces IOP is not fully understood. The prevailing theory is that it reduces aqueous production by damaging the pars plicata, although it is unclear whether this is due to direct destruction of the ciliary epithelium or reduced vascular perfusion. Still other investigators suggest that the primary mechanism may be increased outflow through an effect on the pars plana.

Evidence for Reduced Aqueous Production

Rabbit studies have demonstrated that transscleral application of Nd:YAG laser energy results in coagulative necrosis of the ciliary epithelium, including destruction of ciliary vessels in the overlying area (35).

Studies of human autopsy eyes revealed structural changes of the ciliary body similar to those seen in rabbits. The gross appearance of lesions created by the noncontact, free-running Nd:YAG laser was a white elevation of the ciliary epithelium (36). The histologic correlate was a blister-like elevation of the epithelial layers from the adjacent stroma, with marked disruption primarily of the pigmented epithelium but minimal change in the ciliary muscle and sclera in the path of the laser beam (37,38) (**Fig. 41.4**). In contrast, the histologic appearance of lesions created by the contact, continuous-wave Nd:YAG laser was a smaller, more coagulative effect on the epithelium with less of the blister-like elevation (38,39). One study showed a more full-thickness thermal effect, including sclera (38), while another showed no scleral alteration (39). A videographic study of human autopsy eyes also showed that shorter-duration Nd:YAG laser exposures caused greater tissue disruption, whereas the more prolonged, continuous-wave exposures produced a more coagulative, shrinkage-like lesion (40).

Figure 41.3 **A:** An ECP unit (Uram E2, Endo Optiks, Little Silver, NJ), including laser, monitor, and foot pedal. **B:** An ECP probe (20 gauge). A 27-gauge cannula tip is shown above for size comparison. (From Lin SC. Endoscopic and transscleral cyclophotocoagulation for the treatment of refractory glaucoma. *J Glaucoma.* 2008;17:238–247.)

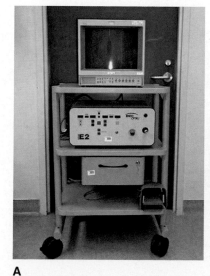

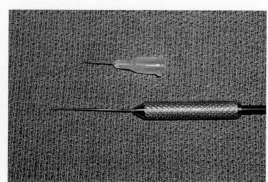

A

B

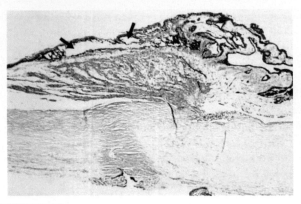

Figure 41.4 Light microscopic view of human autopsy eye treated with transscleral thermal, pulsed Nd:YAG cyclophotocoagulation showing blister-like elevation of disrupted ciliary epithelium (arrows) with minimal ciliary muscle and scleral damage. Defect on scleral surface was created by needle with India ink to mark center of laser track after laser application.

Histologic studies have also been performed on human eyes that were enucleated at some point after transscleral Nd:YAG cyclophotocoagulation. In one series of eyes treated with the noncontact, free-running Nd:YAG laser a few days before scheduled enucleation, the structural changes were the same as those seen in human autopsy eyes with the addition of fibrin and scant inflammatory cells between the disrupted epithelial layers and stroma (41). No changes in ciliary body vasculature were observed. A clinicopathologic study of three eyes enucleated 2 weeks, 8 weeks, and 17 months after noncontact Nd:YAG cyclophotocoagulation revealed destruction of the nonpigmented and pigmented ciliary epithelium, occlusion of capillaries, and stromal necrosis, with subsequent hyperplasia of the epithelial layers, fibrosis, and near–total atrophy of the ciliary processes (42). Histologic evaluation of another eye, which had received the same laser treatment 70 days before enucleation for hypotony and pain, revealed pigment disruption and granulomatous inflammation of the ciliary body (43). Two eyes treated with contact, continuous-wave Nd:YAG transscleral cyclophotocoagulation 1 day before enucleation for melanomas

revealed epithelial necrosis and partial capillary thrombosis of the ciliary body with slight scleral damage (44).

Histologic observations with both light microscopy and scanning electron microscopy reveal that tissue treated with transscleral diode cyclophotocoagulation shows pronounced tissue disruption of the ciliary body muscle and stroma, ciliary processes, and both pigmented and nonpigmented ciliary epithelium. ECP-treated tissue, however, only exhibits pronounced contraction of the ciliary processes with disruption of the ciliary body epithelium, sparing of the ciliary body muscle with less architectural disorganization (**Fig. 41.5**) (45). A study of vascular effects of transscleral compared with ECP in rabbits demonstrated immediate and severely reduced or nonexistent blood flow in the areas of treatment after both types of procedures (46). After 1 week and 1 month, however, transscleral-treated processes remained nonperfused, whereas ECP processes showed some reperfusion that increased over time. The authors concluded that chronic poor perfusion of the ciliary after transscleral diode cyclophotocoagulation may partly account for its efficacy and the significant complications, including hypotony and phthisis. Late reperfusion of this region after ECP may provide some insight into the differences in efficacy and complication rates, compared with transscleral diode cyclophotocoagulation.

Evidence for Increased Aqueous Outflow

Although the aforementioned studies confirm that transscleral cyclophotocoagulation can destroy tissues of the pars plicata, most likely by a direct effect on the ciliary epithelium, this does not prove that direct destruction of the pars plicata is an essential element in the mechanism of IOP reduction. Other studies have shown that more posteriorly placed lesions over the pars plana or even peripheral retina also decrease the IOP (47–50). The explanation for this observation could be reduced aqueous production due to the inflammatory response (47), although it is unlikely that this would be a sustained effect. An alternative explanation is enhanced aqueous outflow, either by transscleral filtration or uveoscleral outflow (48–52). In a monkey study of contact, continuous-wave Nd:YAG cyclophotocoagulation, in which right eyes were treated over the pars plicata, 1 mm behind

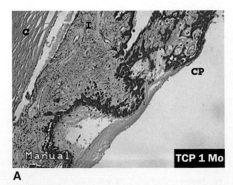

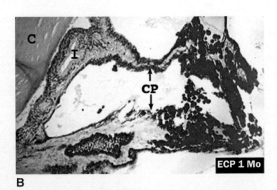

Figure 41.5 **A:** Histopathology of rabbit ciliary processes 1 month after contact transscleral diode cyclophotocoagulation. Note coagulative necrosis of the ciliary tissue with cyclitic membrane formation (×40). **B:** Histopathology of rabbit ciliary processes 1 month after diode laser ECP. Disruption of ciliary architecture is shown but a relatively normal process with patent vessel is seen to the left (×40). C, cornea; CP, ciliary processes; I, iris. (From Lin SC. Endoscopic and transscleral cyclophotocoagulation for the treatment of refractory glaucoma. J Glaucoma. 2008;17:238–247.)

the limbus, and left eyes were treated over the pars plana, 3 mm behind the limbus, IOP reduction occurred in both eyes but returned to baseline by 8 weeks in the former group, whereas the latter group maintained IOP reduction for the 6-month observation period (51). Histology of the latter eyes suggested enhanced uveoscleral outflow by showing tracer elements in enlarged extracellular spaces of the ciliary stroma from the anterior chamber to the suprachoroidal space. In a similar clinical trial in which laser applications were placed either 1.5 mm or 3.0 to 4.0 mm behind the limbus, the latter group had a higher percentage of eyes with sustained IOP reduction, although they also had received more than twice as many laser applications (52). In another clinical trial using noncontact Nd:YAG cyclophotocoagulation in which all treatment parameters were kept constant except for laser placement 1.5 or 3.0 mm posterior to the limbus, the former group had significantly lower IOP and required fewer repeated treatments during 6-month follow-up (53).

In summary, the most likely mechanism of IOP lowering by transscleral cyclophotocoagulation is reduced aqueous production through destruction of ciliary epithelium. However, alternative possibilities, including reduced inflow due to ciliary vascular disruption or chronic inflammation, or increased outflow due to pars plana–transscleral outflow or enhanced uveoscleral outflow, have not been ruled out.

Techniques

Preoperative and Postoperative Management

Unlike most other glaucoma laser procedures, the intraoperative pain associated with transscleral cyclophotocoagulation is such that retrobulbar anesthesia is required, although this has been omitted by some surgeons with the contact, continuous-wave technique (44). Also, unlike most other laser procedures and other transscleral cyclodestructive procedures, postoperative IOP rise is not a frequent problem, and special preoperative and postoperative measures, such as the use of topical apraclonidine, are usually unnecessary. For ECP, peribulbar, topical, or intracameral anesthesia may be selected.

Postoperative inflammation can be a significant problem, requiring special prophylactic measures. One approach is to give a subconjunctival injection of a short-acting steroid at the end of the procedure and to prescribe topical atropine and steroid for approximately 10 days (54). Use of preoperative glaucoma medications is continued, except for miotics, until IOP reduction allows discontinuation. Postoperative pain is typically mild, and a weak analgesic is usually sufficient. IOP is usually checked a few hours after the procedure, the following day, and then thereafter as required.

Laser Settings and Protocols

The histologic studies with human eyes, as previously described, have been used to establish protocols for clinical trials. However, preferred settings differ among surgeons, and the optimum protocols have yet to be established.

Nd:YAG Noncontact, Thermal Mode, and Continuous Wave. These instruments are no longer available but appear to have a similar mechanism of action as contact, thermal mode lasers.

Semiconductor Diode, Continuous Wave. With the Oculight SLx, the G-Probe footplate is placed on conjunctiva with the short side adjacent to the limbus, which positions the fiberoptic tip 1.2 mm behind the limbus. Initial settings are 1750 mW and 2 seconds (30). If a popping sound is heard with the initial application, the power is reduced by increments of 250 mW until no pop is heard. If no pop is heard with the initial application, the power is increased by the same increments until the sound is heard, and then it is reduced by one increment. Videographic studies of human autopsy eyes have shown that this audible indicator represents excessive tissue destruction, whereas a power setting one increment below this level is believed to provide optimum tissue damage (55). Some surgeons prefer lower power and longer duration burns, such as 1250 mW at 4 seconds in heavily pigmented eyes and 1500 mW at 3.5 seconds in lightly pigmented eyes (56). The laser applications are spaced circumferentially by placing the side of the G-Probe footplate adjacent to the indentation mark of the previous fiberoptic placement. The original protocol involved 17 to 19 applications for 270 degrees (30), although 24 applications for 360 degrees may provide more effective IOP reduction. We suggest avoiding the 3- and 9-o'clock positions because this may reduce the chances of occluding the long posterior ciliary vessels and thus reduce the chance of anterior segment ischemia. This procedure can be performed with the patient supine or reclining in an examination chair or positioned at a standard slitlamp.

The G-probe used with transscleral diode cyclophotocoagulation can be reused several times without loss of power, even if cleaned by alcohol each time (57). More research is needed, however, to determine the best sterilization methods for this probe.

For ECP, a limbal or pars plana approach can be used. In the limbal approach, a paracentesis is created (about 2 mm), usually at the temporal side initially, and the anterior chamber is filled with viscoelastic agent (typically a cohesive viscoelastic such as sodium hyaluronate), which is further used to expand the space between the iris and the intraocular lens. This viscoelastic expansion of the posterior chamber allows for easier approach to the pars plicata with the ECP probe. A pars plana approach is preferred if there is an anterior chamber IOL or if the anterior segment structures are disrupted or the view is not good (e.g., with a failed penetrating keratoplasty graft). The pars plan approach can be used if eyes have received a previous complete vitrectomy, or where simultaneous vitrectomy can be done.

After orientation of the probe image outside of the eye (with black lettering on a ruler, suture pack, or label), the ECP probe is inserted through the incision and into the posterior chamber. At this time, the ciliary processes are viewed on the monitor and the surgeon's attention can be turned to the monitor (**Fig. 41.6**). Usually, about five to six processes are viewed and the aiming beam is directed on the apex of the processes. It is important to have the probe oriented as flat as possible (otherwise the aiming beam will focus further posteriorly on the pars plana or ora serrata).

The laser is set at 2000 milliseconds or continuous wave and energy settings with the separate diode laser at 400 to 600 mW (which may need to be adjusted if using the built-in laser). Approximately 120 to 150 degrees of ciliary processes is photoco-

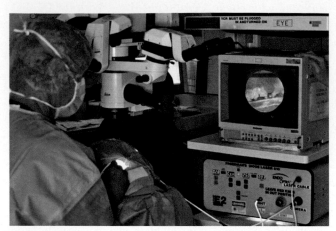

Figure 41.6 Surgeon performing ECP. A video monitor is used to view the ciliary processes during the procedure.

agulated (more can be done with a curved probe). Laser energy is applied to each process until shrinkage and whitening occurs (**Fig. 41.7**). Raised processes and valleys in between are treated (it is important to treat the entire process that is visible, not just the tip). If excessive energy is used, the ciliary process explodes (or "pops") with bubble formation, and this should be avoided. Before closure of the wounds with suture material, viscoelastic is irrigated out with balanced salt solution (ideally by using a manual or automated irrigation and aspiration device), taking care to remove viscoelastic from the anterior and posterior chambers to prevent or minimize postoperative IOP spikes. If further treatment is required, an incision can be made superonasally to access the temporal ciliary processes. Usually, it is best to treat at least 270 to 300 degrees (particularly for high starting pressure) (58).

In the pars plana approach, the entry is made about 3.5 mm behind the limbus, avoiding the 3- and 9-o'clock positions so as not to interfere with the long posterior ciliary arteries. An optional infusion port can be created through the pars plana elsewhere or in the anterior chamber.

With ECP, depending on the degree of postoperative inflammation anticipated, subtenons dexamethasone, methylprednisolone (Depo-Medrol), or triamcinolone (Kenalog) is administered at the end of the procedure. Postoperatively,

antibiotics, cycloplegics, and aqueous suppressants are given. The patient's eye can be patched overnight (e.g., after peribulbar anesthesia) or left unpatched (if topical–intracameral).

Clinical Experience

Indications and General Results

Transscleral cyclophotocoagulation, as with other cyclodestructive procedures, is typically reserved for patients with refractory forms of glaucoma, such as advanced aphakic or pseudophakic glaucoma, neovascular glaucoma, chronic angle-closure glaucoma, inflammatory glaucoma, tumor-associated glaucoma, and in patients with multiple failed filtering procedures or who have had penetrating keratoplasty (59,60). It has also been evaluated—with inconclusive results—as a primary surgical treatment in developing countries where conventional glaucoma therapy is unavailable (61). Maximum pressure reduction is typically achieved in 1 month, and it is usually desirable to wait at least this long before retreating. Results differ somewhat according to the type of glaucoma. In general, patients with aphakic or pseudophakic eyes have more favorable results, and those with neovascular glaucoma tend to do less well. Patients with glaucoma after penetrating keratoplasty have good IOP response to Nd:YAG cyclophotocoagulation, although graft failure is a problem in some cases (62,63). Long-term success with Nd:YAG cyclophotocoagulation appears to be about 50% at 10 years, with most failures (40%) in the first year of treatment (64).

Contact transscleral Nd:YAG and diode laser cyclophotocoagulation have also been shown to be beneficial in children with refractory glaucoma (65,66). Patients with severe uveitis, silicone oil, or severe neovascular glaucoma, and children with glaucoma in an aphakic eye, appear not to do as well in terms of IOP lowering as patients with other indications; in addition, these patients have a higher risk of severe complications, such as inflammation or choroidal detachment (67).

ECP appears to be associated with a lower risk of hypotony, phthisis, and severe vision loss. Hence, it may be considered in eyes with reasonable vision potential where an intraocular procedure would be deemed safe. Some surgeons have advocated using ECP in conjunction with cataract surgery to reduce the burden of medications in patients with glaucoma; further long-term data on efficacy and safety are needed, however.

Figure 41.7 Endoscopic view of ciliary processes. **A:** Untreated processes. **B:** Treated processes, which are white and shrunken. (Courtesy of Martin Uram, MD, MPH. From Weiss HS, Schwartz KS, Schwartz AL. Laser surgery in glaucoma. In: Tasman W, Jaeger EA, eds. *Duane's Clinical Ophthalmology.* Vol 6. Lippincott Williams & Wilkins; 2006:chap 19.)

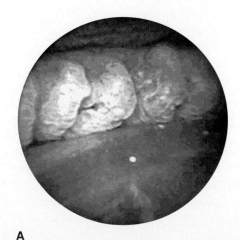
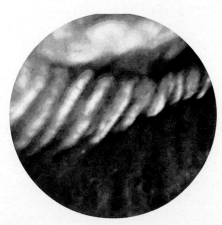

A   B

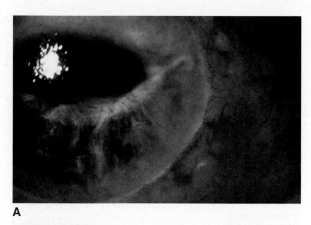
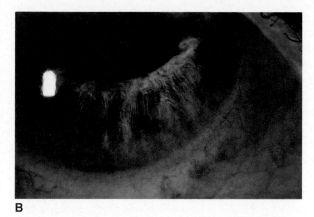

A   **B**

Figure 41.8 An eye of a patient who underwent noncontact transscleral cyclophotocoagulation. **A:** Slitlamp view at postoperative day 1, showing substantial hyperemia. **B:** Slitlamp view at postoperative day 7, by which time the hyperemia has improved considerably.

Complications

Cyclophotocoagulation is frequently associated with mild to moderate conjunctival hyperemia, which typically resolves in a few days (**Fig. 41.8**). Anterior chamber flare and cells are seen in all cases. This is usually mild to moderate, although some patients may develop fibrin clots or hypopyon. Hyphema may also be seen, especially in patients with neovascular glaucoma. The inflammatory response is transient and is routinely managed with postoperative subconjunctival and subsequent topical steroids. Many patients are left with a chronic flare due to a breakdown in the blood–aqueous barrier, but this does not require long-term treatment. A transient IOP rise occurs in a small proportion of patients and usually is clinically insignificant (68). Nevertheless, checking the pressure a few hours after the procedure and the next day is advisable. Postoperative pain also tends to be mild, with many patients requiring no analgesic, and rarely more than a mild pain reliever in the first 24 hours. Inflammation, transient IOP elevation, and pain are all significantly less with laser cyclophotocoagulation, compared with cyclocryotherapy.

Other reported complications have included hypotony with choroidal detachments and a flat anterior chamber (69), vitreous hemorrhages, and cataracts. Several cases of sympathetic ophthalmia have been reported in association with transscleral cyclophotocoagulation (70–74). In most cases, the treated eyes had previously undergone incisional surgery, and the sympathizing eyes typically respond promptly to steroid therapy. Cases of malignant glaucoma after Nd:YAG cyclophotocoagulation have also been reported (75,76). With use of transscleral diode laser, necrotizing scleritis and inadvertent sclerostomy with filtering bleb formation have been reported (77,78).

The most significant complication associated with transscleral cyclophotocoagulation is loss of visual acuity. Some degree of visual loss may occur in as many as 50% of patients. In many cases, this appears to be associated with the underlying disorder, such as a retinopathy or keratopathy. However, at least one half of the cases of visual reduction are thought to occur as a direct result of the laser treatment (79). The precise mechanisms of the latter are not fully understood, but likely causes include macular edema associated with the inflammatory response and possibly a direct phototoxic effect. One histologic study demonstrated that about 3% of 5% of the energy from laser treatment reaches the macula (80). It is advisable to use transscleral cyclophotocoagulation with caution in eyes with good visual potential. When performing the procedure, it is wise to use the lowest power and exposure durations possible and to keep the probe perpendicular to the sclera so that excess energy is transmitted more anteriorly instead of being directed toward the macula.

With ECP, complications include fibrin exudates, postoperative IOP spikes, hyphema, cystoid macular edema, decreased vision, and choroidal detachment; rarely, serious complications, such as retinal detachment and hypotony, may occur, primarily in pediatric cases (81). Although not reported in the literature, endophthalmitis and choroidal hemorrhage are potential severe complications, owing to the intraocular nature of the surgery. On occasion, early postoperative IOP spikes may be related to retained viscoelastic material. Iris hooks may provide a safe alternative for elevation of the iris during ECP treatment and may be particularly advantageous in eyes with aphakia or posterior capsule compromise, in which viscoelastic removal is made more difficult (58).

Influence of Treatment Variables

Exposure Duration. Histologic and in vitro videographic studies of transscleral Nd:YAG cyclophotocoagulation have revealed an influence of exposure duration on tissue responses of the ciliary body. The thermal mode (20 milliseconds) produces an explosive, blister-like lesion, whereas the continuous-wave mode (usually 0.5 to 2.0 seconds) produces a more gradual contraction and coagulation of the tissue (36–40).

Nd:YAG versus Diode Wavelengths. As previously noted, semiconductor diode lasers have the physical advantages of being compact and portable with no special electric outlet or water-cooling requirements and with solid-state construction that is relatively durable and requires minimal maintenance. The different wavelengths of the Nd:YAG (1064 nm) and diode (750 to 850 nm) lasers also impart variable biologic effects, with the latter having less effective scleral transmission and increased light scattering but greater absorption by melanin. In a videographic study of human autopsy eyes that compared contact transscleral continuous-wave Nd:YAG with diode cyclophotocoagulation, the former produced more prominent whitening and contraction of the ciliary epithelium, whereas the latter seemed to produce a deeper tissue contraction. The histologic correlate was predominant coagulation and disruption of the ciliary epithelium with the Nd:YAG laser, whereas the diode treatment was associated with less epithelial effect and more coagulative response in the ciliary muscle. These findings are consistent with results of other studies that revealed coagulative changes in the ciliary epithelium, stroma, and vasculature of human autopsy eyes in response to diode cyclophotocoagulation and deeper, more extensive tissue damage, compared with use of similar energy levels of Nd:YAG treatment in both rabbit eyes and pre-enucleation human eyes (82–84). However, the study involving human eyes revealed similar lesions at lower energy levels (84), and another videographic study of human autopsy eyes revealed similar ciliary body responses to noncontact Nd:YAG and diode laser applications (85). Results of clinical trials suggest that visual loss may be less with transscleral diode cyclophotocoagulation than with the Nd:YAG procedures (86).

Comparisons with Alternative Procedures

Comparisons of transscleral Nd:YAG cyclophotocoagulation with cyclocryotherapy in both rabbit and human eyes have revealed insignificant differences in IOP responses, but less tissue destruction and fewer complications with the laser treatments (87,88). On the basis of these and other reports of the various cyclodestructive operations, transscleral cyclophotocoagulation is now believed to be the cyclodestructive procedure of choice.

A comparison of noncontact transscleral Nd:YAG cyclophotocoagulation with several glaucoma drainage devices revealed better IOP control with the latter techniques (89). Although the laser group had less visual loss in that study, the loss of visual acuity with all transscleral cyclophotocoagulation procedures remains an important concern. In general, filtering surgery with adjunctive antimetabolite therapy or glaucoma drainage-device surgery is preferred in patients with good visual potential, although transscleral cyclophotocoagulation offers a reasonable alternative in the high-risk glaucoma population, especially when the visual potential is poor.

In patients with neovascular glaucoma, ECP has fared well compared with trabeculectomy (90–92). ECP has also fared well when compared with Ahmed valve implantation (93).

Intraocular Cyclophotocoagulation

An alternative to transscleral and transpupillary cyclophotocoagulation in patients with glaucoma in aphakic, or possibly pseudophakic, eyes is intraocular cyclophotocoagulation, by using an endophotocoagulator through a limbal or pars plana incision. Visualization with this technique can usually be accomplished by an endoscope or via the transpupillary route.

Vitreoretinal surgeons have reported the use of argon laser endophotocoagulators via a pars plana incision for the treatment of retinal disorders under transpupillary visualization (94–96). During the course of a vitrectomy in an aphakic eye, it is possible to lower the IOP and use scleral indentation to bring the ciliary processes into transpupillary view for the

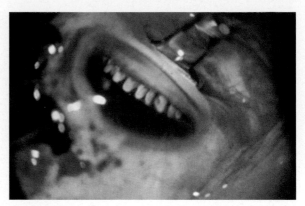

Figure 41.9 Intraocular cyclophotocoagulation with transpupillary visualization. Ciliary processes are brought into view with a scleral depressor and treated with laser endophotocoagulator via a pars plana incision.

purpose of cyclophotocoagulation with the intraocular laser probe (97–99).

After performing the vitrectomy, the vitreous instrument is removed and the endophotocoagulator is inserted through the same opening. Scleral indentation in the opposite quadrants is then used to bring several ciliary processes into view, and the tip of the laser probe is positioned 2 to 3 mm from the processes (**Fig. 41.9**). With an exposure time of 0.1 to 0.2 second, laser therapy is applied to individual ciliary processes by using an energy level sufficient to produce a white reaction and a shallow tissue disruption (usually 1000 mW). Three to five laser exposures are then applied to each process in the two quadrants opposite the entry site.

In one large series with a mean follow-up of 13 months, three fourths of the eyes had an IOP of 21 mm Hg or less with or without use of medications after one or two treatments (99). The primary value of this procedure is as an adjunct to pars plana vitrectomy in eyes with refractory glaucoma.

Transpupillary Cyclophotocoagulation

In 1971, Lee and Pomerantzeff (100) introduced the concept of argon laser cyclophotocoagulation via a transpupillary approach. Histopathologic studies in rabbit and human eyes confirmed the ability of direct laser application to selectively destroy ciliary processes (100,101).

Transpupillary cyclophotocoagulation is limited to eyes in which a sufficient number of ciliary processes can be visualized gonioscopically. This is not possible in most eyes, especially those in which long-term miotic therapy prevents wide dilatation. However, situations such as aniridia, a large iridectomy, or retraction of the iris, as in advanced neovascular glaucoma, may provide adequate visualization of ciliary processes. Special contact lenses with scleral depressors have been developed to rotate the processes into better view. Typical argon laser settings are 0.1 to 0.2 second, 100 to 200 μm, and an energy level that is sufficient to produce white discoloration, as well as a brown concave burn, often with pigment dispersion or gas bubbles (usually 700 to 1000 mW). All visible portions of the ciliary process should be treated, which typically requires three to five applications per process. All visible processes should be treated up to a total of 180 degrees. Additional processes can be treated at subsequent sessions, if required.

The reported results with transpupillary cyclophotocoagulation have been variable (102–107). Those cases in which the procedure fails may be due, in part, to the number of ciliary processes that can be visualized and treated and to the intensity of the laser burns to each process (102,104). However, the number of treated processes and the intensity of treatment do not always correlate with the extent of the IOP reduction (107). Another factor that may contribute to failure of transpupillary cyclophotocoagulation is the angle at which the processes are visualized gonioscopically. Even with scleral indentation, only the anterior tips of the ciliary ridges are usually exposed, preventing destruction of the entire ciliary process (107).

CYCLOCRYOTHERAPY

The use of a freezing source as the cyclodestructive element was suggested by Bietti (108) in 1950. Cyclocryotherapy was generally thought to be somewhat more predictable and less destructive than penetrating cyclodiathermy, and it gradually replaced the latter technique as the most commonly used cyclodestructive operation. It is still used by some surgeons, especially when laser technology is not readily available. Histologic studies of eyes treated with cyclocryotherapy show destruction of vascular, stromal, and epithelial elements of the ciliary processes with replacement by fibrous tissue (109).

Mechanism of Action

Cyclocryotherapy presumably destroys the ability of ciliary processes to produce aqueous humor by the biphasic mechanism of intracellular ice crystal formation and ischemic necrosis (110). Initially, freezing of extracellular fluid concentrates the remaining solutes, which leads to cellular dehydration and is the probable mechanism of cell death associated with a slow freeze. When the rate of cooling is rapid, intracellular ice crystals develop. Although these crystals are not always lethal to the cell, a slow thaw leads to the formation of larger crystals, which are highly destructive to the cell by an uncertain mechanism. Maximum cell death is achieved with a rapid freeze and a slow thaw. A second and later mechanism of cryoinduced cell death is a superimposed hemorrhagic infarction, which results from obliteration of the microcirculation in the frozen tissue. Ischemic necrosis is the histologic hallmark of cryoinjured tissue.

In addition to decreasing the IOP, cyclocryotherapy may provide relief of pain by destroying corneal nerves. Wallerian degeneration of corneal nerve fibers was observed in rabbits following cyclocryotherapy, although regeneration began within 9 to 16 days (111).

Techniques

Cryoinstruments

Nitrous oxide or carbon dioxide gas cryosurgical units may be used. The diameters of the more commonly used cryoprobe tips range from 1.5 to 4 mm, and it has been suggested that 2.5

mm may be optimum for cyclocryotherapy (112). A modified cryoprobe with a curved 3 × 6-mm tip has been developed to reduce the number of applications required (113). An automatic timer to monitor the duration of each application has also been described (114).

Cryoprobe Placement

With the 2.5-mm tip, placement of the anterior edge of the probe 1 mm from the corneolimbal junction temporally, inferiorly, and nasally, and 1.5 mm superiorly is believed to concentrate the maximum freezing effect over the ciliary processes (112) (**Fig. 41.10**). It has also been suggested that transillumination may be helpful by delineating the pars plicata (115,116), although this is not usually necessary unless the anatomic landmarks are distorted, as with an eye that has buphthalmos. The cryoprobe should be applied with firm pressure on the sclera, because this may reduce ciliary blood flow, thereby contributing to faster penetration of the ice ball to the ciliary processes (112).

Number of Cryoapplications

Most surgeons treat two to three quadrants, with three to four cryoapplications per quadrant. A study in cats showed that graded cyclocryotherapy of 90, 180, or 270 degrees produced graded destruction of the ciliary epithelium and proportionally related changes in IOP and aqueous humor dynamics (117). The number of cryolesions may be based to a degree on preoperative parameters, such as the type of glaucoma, the IOP level, and the number of previous cyclocryotherapy procedures. It has also been shown that younger patients generally require a larger number of cryoapplications than older individuals do to achieve satisfactory pressure reduction (118). However, there are no precise guidelines by which an individual patient's response to therapy can be predicted, and it is best to err on the side of undertreatment rather than to run the risk of phthisis. One recommended approach is to limit each treatment session to six applications or fewer over 180 degrees of the globe (115).

Freezing Technique

Studies indicate that temperature levels warmer than –60°C to –80°C or a duration of freeze less than 60 seconds does not provide adequate destruction of the ciliary process, whereas values much greater than these increase the risk of phthisis (112). Most surgeons, therefore, prefer applications of –60°C to –80°C for 60 seconds (119). As previously noted, a rapid freeze and slow, unassisted thaw produce the maximum cell death (110). If the initial procedure does not adequately lower the IOP after approximately 1 month, cyclocryotherapy may be repeated one or more times as required. In one series, 14 of 61 eyes required two or more procedures (119).

Postoperative Management

For approximately the first 24 hours, the patient may experience intense pain, and use of strong analgesics is often required. It has been noted that use of subconjunctival steroids at the end of the procedure also minimizes the postoperative pain (115). In addition, frequent administration of topical corticosteroids and a cycloplegic–mydriatic agent should be used routinely, starting on

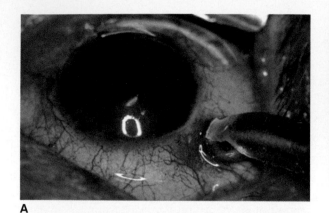

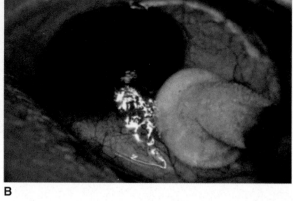

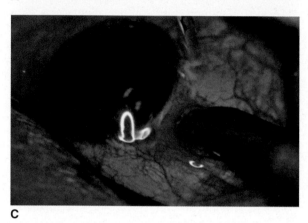

Figure 41.10 Cyclocryotherapy technique. **A:** The probe tip is placed roughly 2.5 mm from the limbus. The temperature at the probe tip is reduced to approximately −80°C and maintained for 60 seconds. **B:** Typical ice ball 30 seconds after initiating freezing. **C:** The probe is irrigated with saline solution before removing the probe from the conjunctiva. Note the hyperemia around the probe tip.

the day of surgery. Because the IOP may remain elevated for 1 or more days after the treatment, it is advisable to keep the patient on the preoperative antiglaucoma medications, with the exception of miotics, until a pressure reduction is observed.

Complications

Transient Intraocular Pressure Elevation

A marked rise in IOP may occur during cyclocryotherapy and in the early postoperative period. In one study, pressures of 60 to 80 mm Hg were recorded in the freezing phase, with return to baseline during the thawing phase (120). The researchers in that study thought this component of IOP elevation was due to volumetric changes, possibly related to scleral contraction, and they described a technique for controlling the complication with manometric regulation of the pressure during surgery. They also noted a second IOP rise that averaged 50 mm Hg and peaked 6 hours after the procedure. The mechanism for this component of the IOP elevation is unclear but is probably associated with the marked inflammatory response. Gonioscopic evaluation after cyclocryotherapy revealed frozen aqueous humor in the anterior chamber angle (121), with the obvious consequences that this may have on the remaining conventional outflow system.

Uveitis

Uveitis occurs in all cases and is usually intense, with the frequent formation of a fibrin clot. Results of one study suggested that the inflammation is prostaglandin induced and might be minimized by pretreatment with aspirin (122). However, a comparison of

topical flurbiprofen, dexamethasone, and placebo suggested that cyclocryotherapy-induced inflammation is difficult to control with any topical medication (123). A chronic aqueous flare usually persists because of permanent disruption of the blood–aqueous barrier (124), but this does not require treatment.

Pain

Pain, as previously noted, may be intense after cyclocryotherapy and may last for days. It is most likely a consequence of the IOP elevation and inflammation, both of which should be treated vigorously, along with the use of strong analgesics.

Hyphema

Hyphema is a common complication, especially in eyes with neovascular glaucoma, and usually clears with conservative management.

Hypotony

A major disadvantage of all cyclodestructive procedures is that nothing can be done to reverse the hypotony or phthisis, if it occurs. Although this complication is less common with cyclocryotherapy than with cyclophotocoagulation, it does occur and is best avoided by treating a limited area each time. It is far better to repeat the treatment several times than to produce phthis as a result of overtreatment.

Other Complications

Other complications associated with cyclocryotherapy include choroidal detachment, which may lead to a flat anterior chamber (125). Intravitreal neovascularization from the ciliary body, with vitreous hemorrhage, may follow cyclocryotherapy and may regress after panretinal photocoagulation (126). Anterior segment ischemia has been reported in eyes with neovascular glaucoma after 360 degrees of cyclocryotherapy (127). Rare complications have included subretinal fibrosis, subluxation, and sympathetic ophthalmia (128–131).

Indications

Although cyclodestruction with laser is preferred to cryotherapy, cyclocryotherapy can be used for situations in which other glaucoma operations have repeatedly failed or in which the surgeon wishes to avoid incisional surgery. Conditions in which this procedure has been reported to have particular value include glaucoma after penetrating keratoplasty, chronic open-angle glaucoma in an aphakic eye, and congenital glaucoma (118,132–136). Cyclocryotherapy is thought by some surgeons to be useful in the management of neovascular glaucoma, although others think that the main benefit of the surgery in this and other disorders is relief of pain.

KEY POINTS

- Cyclodestructive operations decrease IOP by reducing aqueous inflow. The most commonly used methods for cycloablative therapy involve transscleral and endoscopic approaches.
- Transscleral laser methods for cyclodestruction provide more precise tissue destruction with a significant reduction in complications compared with cyclocryotherapy. The opinion of the American Academy of Ophthalmology is that diode laser cyclophotocoagulation "appears to possess the best combination of effectiveness, portability, expense, and ease of use at this time" (56).
- ECP offers distinct advantages over transscleral diode cyclophotocoagulation in the management of refractory pediatric and adult glaucomas. It permits selective treatment of the ciliary epithelium with minimal energy and less damage to underlying tissues. There is less risk of vision loss, hypotony, and phthisis. However, there is the potential for complications related to intraocular surgery.
- Major indications for cyclodestructive surgery include the following:
  - refractory forms of glaucoma associated with neovascularization, trauma, aphakia, congenital glaucoma, uveitis, penetrating keratoplasty, silicone oil, conjunctival scarring, and others;
  - eyes with limited visual potential and uncontrolled IOP (although with ECP, eyes with reasonable visual potential can also be treated);
  - eyes without vision and that have pain, thought to be secondary to elevated IOP.
- Complications associated with cyclodestructive procedures include conjunctival burns, anterior uveitis, vision loss, postoperative pain, hyphema, vitreous hemorrhage, rise in IOP, hypotony, choroidal detachment, phthisis bulbi, malignant glaucoma, cataracts, and, rarely, sympathetic ophthalmia.

REFERENCES

1. Weve H. Die Zyklodiatermie das Corpus ciliare bei Glaukom. *Zentralbl Ophthalmol*. 1933;29:562–569.
2. Vogt A. Versuche zur intraokularen Druckherabsetzung mittels Diatermieschadigung des Corpus ciliare (Zyklodiatermiestichelung). *Klin Monatsbl Augenheilkd*. 1936;97:672–677.
3. Vogt A. Cyclodiathermy puncture in cases of glaucoma. *Br J Ophthalmol*. 1940;24(6):288–297.
4. Albaugh CH, Dunphy EB. Cyclodiathermy. *Arch Ophthalmol*. 1942; 27(3):543–557.
5. Stocker FW. Response of chronic simple glaucoma to treatment with cyclodiathermy puncture. *Arch Ophthalmol*. 1945;34(3):181–186.
6. Walton DS, Grant WM. Penetrating cyclodiathermy for filtration. *Arch Ophthalmol*. 1970;83(1):47–48.
7. Haik GM, Breffeilh LA, Barber A. Beta irradiation as a possible therapeutic agent in glaucoma. *Am J Ophthalmol*. 1948;31(8):945–952.
8. Berens C, Sheppard LB, Duel AB Jr. Cycloelectrolysis for glaucoma. *Trans Am Ophthalmol Soc*. 1949;47:364–382.
9. Sheppard LB. Retrociliary cyclodiathermy versus retrociliary cycloelectrolysis: effects on the normal rabbit eye. *Am J Ophthalmol*. 1958;46 (1 pt 1):27–37.
10. Purnell EW, Sokollu A, Torchia R, et al. Focal chorioretinitis produced by ultrasound. *Invest Ophthalmol*. 1964;3(12):657–664.
11. Coleman DJ, Lizzi FL, Driller J, et al. Therapeutic ultrasound in the treatment of glaucoma. I. Experimental model. *Ophthalmology*. 1985;92(3): 339–346.
12. Coleman DJ, Lizzi FL, Driller J, et al. Therapeutic ultrasound in the treatment of glaucoma. II. Clinical applications. *Ophthalmology*. 1985;92(3): 347–353.
13. Burgess SE, Silverman RH, Coleman DJ, et al. Treatment of glaucoma with high-intensity focused ultrasound. *Ophthalmology*. 1986;93(6):831–838.
14. Maskin SL, Mandell AI, Smith JA, et al. Therapeutic ultrasound for refractory glaucoma: a three-center study. *Ophthalmic Surg*. 1989;20(3):186–192.
15. Valtot F, Kopel J, Haut J. Treatment of glaucoma with high intensity focused ultrasound. *Int Ophthalmol*. 1989;13(1–2):167–170.
16. Silverman RH, Vogelsang B, Rondeau MJ, et al. Therapeutic ultrasound for the treatment of glaucoma. *Am J Ophthalmol*. 1991;11(3)1:327–337.
17. Finger PT, Smith PD, Paglione RW, et al. Transscleral microwave cyclodestruction. *Invest Ophthalmol Vis Sci*. 1990;31(10):2151–2155.
18. Finger PT, Moshfeghi DM, Smith PD, et al. Microwave cyclodestruction for glaucoma in a rabbit model. *Arch Ophthalmol*. 1991;109(7): 1001–1004.
19. Freyler H, Scheimbauer I. Excision of the ciliary body (Sautter procedure) as a last resort in secondary glaucoma [in German]. *Klin Monatsbl Augenheilkd*. 1981;179(6):473–477.
20. Demeler U. Ciliary surgery for glaucoma. *Trans Ophthalmol Soc U K*. 1986;105(pt 2):242–245.
21. Welge-Lussen L, Stadler G. Results with a modified ciliary body excision to reduce intraocular pressure [in German]. *Klin Monatsbl Augenheilkd*. 1986;189(3):199–203.
22. Weekers R, Lavergne G, Watillon M, et al. Effects of photocoagulation of ciliary body upon ocular tension. *Am J Ophthalmol*. 1961;52: 156–163.
23. Vucicevic ZM, Tsou KC, Nazarian IH, et al. A cytochemical approach to the laser coagulation of the ciliary body. *Bibl Ophthalmol*. 1969;8: 467–478.
24. Smith RS, Stein MN. Ocular hazards of transscleral laser radiation: II. Intraocular injury produced by ruby and neodymium lasers. *Am J Ophthalmol*. 1969;67(1):100–110.
25. Beckman H, Kinoshita A, Rota AN, et al. Transscleral ruby laser irradiation of the ciliary body in the treatment of intractable glaucoma. *Trans Am Acad Ophthalmol Otolaryngol*. 1972;76(2):423–436.
26. Beckman H, Sugar HS. Neodymium laser cyclocoagulation. *Arch Ophthalmol*. 1973;90(1):27–28.
27. Beckman H, Waeltermann J. Transscleral ruby laser cyclocoagulation. *Am J Ophthalmol*. 1984;98(6):788–795.
28. Peyman GA, Naguib KS, Gaasterland D. Transscleral application of a semiconductor diode laser. *Laser Surg Med*. 1990;10(6):569–575.
29. Schuman JS, Jacobson JJ, Puliafito CA, et al. Experimental use of semiconductor diode laser in contact transscleral cyclophotocoagulation in rabbits. *Arch Ophthalmol*. 1990;108(8):1152–1157.
30. Gaasterland DE, Pollack IP. Initial experience with a new method of laser transscleral cyclophotocoagulation for ciliary ablation in severe glaucoma. *Trans Am Ophthalmol Soc*. 1992;90:225–243.

31. Uram M. Ophthalmic laser microendoscope endophotocoagulation. *Ophthalmology.* 1992;99(12):1829–1832.

32. Immonen I, Suomalainen VP, Kivel T, et al. Energy levels needed for cyclophotocoagulation: a comparison of transscleral contact cw-YAG and krypton lasers in the rabbit eye. *Ophthalmic Surg.* 1993;24(8): 530–533.

33. Immonen IJ, Puska P, Raitta C. Transscleral contact krypton laser cyclophotocoagulation for treatment of glaucoma. *Ophthalmology.* 1994; 101(5):876–882.

34. Kivelä T, Puska P, Raitta C, et al. Clinically successful contact transscleral krypton laser cyclophotocoagulation: long-term histopathologic and immunohistochemical autopsy findings. *Arch Ophthalmol.* 1995;113(11): 1447–1453.

35. Devenyi RG, Trope GE, Hunter WH. Neodymium-YAG transscleral cyclocoagulation in rabbit eye. *Br J Ophthalmol.* 1987;71(6):441–444.

36. Fankhauser F, van der Zypen E, Kwasniewska S, et al. Transscleral cyclophotocoagulation using a neodymium YAG laser. *Ophthalmic Surg.* 1986;17(2):94–100.

37. Hampton C, Shields MB. Transscleral neodymium-YAG cyclophotocoagulation: a histologic study of human autopsy eyes. *Arch Ophthalmol.* 1988;106(8):1121–1123.

38. Schubert HD. Noncontact and contact pars plana transscleral neodymium:YAG laser cyclophotocoagulation in postmortem eyes. *Ophthalmology.* 1989;96(10):1471–1475.

39. Allingham RR, de Kater AW, Bellows AR, et al. Probe placement and power levels in contact transscleral neodymium:YAG cyclophotocoagulation. *Arch Ophthalmol.* 1990;108(5):738–742.

40. Prum BE Jr, Shields SR, Simmons RB, et al. The influence of exposure duration in transscleral Nd:YAG laser cyclophotocoagulation. *Am J Ophthalmol.* 1992;114(5):560–567.

41. Blasini M, Simmons R, Shields MB. Early tissue response to transscleral neodymium:YAG cyclophotocoagulation. *Invest Ophthalmol Vis Sci.* 1990;31(6):1114–1118.

42. Marsh P, Wilson DJ, Samples JR, et al. A clinicopathologic correlative study of noncontact transscleral Nd:YAG cyclophotocoagulation. *Am J Ophthalmol.* 1993;115(5):597–602.

43. Shields SM, Stevens JL, Kass MA, et al. Histopathologic findings after Nd:YAG transscleral cyclophotocoagulation. *Am J Ophthalmol.* 1988; 106(1):100–101.

44. Brancato R, Leoni G, Trabucchi G, et al. Probe placement and energy levels in continuous wave neodymium-YAG contact transscleral cyclophotocoagulation. *Arch Ophthalmol.* 1990;108(5):679–683.

45. Pantcheva MB, Kahook MY, Schuman JS, et al. Comparison of acute structural and histopathological changes in human autopsy eyes after endoscopic cyclophotocoagulation and trans-scleral cyclophotocoagulation. *Br J Ophthalmol.* 2007;91(2):248–252.

46. Lin SC, Chen MJ, Lin MS, et al. Vascular effects on ciliary tissue from endoscopic versus trans-scleral cyclophotocoagulation. *Br J Ophthalmol.* 2006;90(4):496–500.

47. Schubert HD, Federman JL. The role of inflammation on CW Nd:YAG contact transscleral photocoagulation and cryopexy. *Invest Ophthalmol Vis Sci.* 1989;30(3):543–549.

48. Schubert HD, Federman JL. A comparison of CW Nd:YAG contact transscleral cyclophotocoagulation with cyclocryopexy. *Invest Ophthalmol Vis Sci.* 1989;30(3):536–542.

49. Schubert HD, Agarwala A, Arbizo V. Changes in aqueous outflow after in vitro neodymium:Yttrium aluminum garnet laser cyclophotocoagulation. *Invest Ophthalmol Vis Sci.* 1990;31(9):1834–1838.

50. Schubert HD, Agarwala A. Quantitative CW Nd:YAG pars plana transscleral photocoagulation in postmortem eyes. *Ophthalmic Surg.* 1990; 21(12):835–839.

51. Liu GJ, Mizukawa A, Okisaka S. Mechanism of intraocular pressure decrease after contact transscleral continuous-wave Nd:YAG laser cyclophotocoagulation. *Ophthalmic Res.* 1994;26(2):65–79.

52. Ando F, Kawai T. Transscleral contact cyclophotocoagulation for refractory glaucoma: comparison of the results of pars plicata and pars plana irradiation. *Lasers Light Ophthalmol.* 1993;5:143.

53. Crymes BM, Gross RL. Laser placement in noncontact Nd:YAG cyclophotocoagulation. *Am J Ophthalmol.* 1990;110(6):670–673.

54. Hampton C, Shields MB, Miller KN, et al. Evaluation of a protocol for transscleral neodymium:YAG cyclophotocoagulation in one hundred patients. *Ophthalmology.* 1990;97(7):910–917.

55. Simmons RB, Prum BE Jr, Shields SR, et al. Videographic and histologic comparison of Nd:YAG and diode laser contact transscleral cyclophotocoagulation. *Am J Ophthalmol.* 1994;117(3):337–341.

56. Pastor SA, Singh K, Lee DA, et al. Cyclophotocoagulation: a report by the American Academy of Ophthalmology. *Ophthalmology.* 2001;108(11): 2130–2138.

57. Carrillo MM, Trope GE, Chipman ML, et al. Repeated use of transscleral cyclophotocoagulation laser G-probes. *J Glaucoma.* 2004;13(1): 51–54.

58. Kahook MY, Lathrop KL, Noecker RJ. One-site versus two-site endoscopic cyclophotocoagulation. *J Glaucoma.* 2007;16(6):527–530.

59. Wanner JB, Pasquale LR. Glaucomas secondary to intraocular melanomas [review]. *Semin Ophthalmol.* 2006;21(3):181–189.

60. Ocakoglu O, Arslan OS, Kayiran A. Diode laser transscleral cyclophotocoagulation for the treatment of refractory glaucoma after penetrating keratoplasty. *Curr Eye Res.* 2005;30(7):569–574.

61. Egbert PR, Fiadoyor S, Budenz DL, et al. Diode laser trans-scleral cyclophotocoagulation as a primary surgical treatment for primary open-angle glaucoma. *Arch Ophthalmol.* 2001;119(3):345–350.

62. Hardten DR, Brown JD, Holland EJ. Results of neodymium:YAG laser transscleral cyclophotocoagulation for postkeratoplasty glaucoma. *J Glaucoma.* 1993;2(4):241–245.

63. Threlkeld AB, Shields MB. Noncontact transscleral Nd:YAG cyclophotocoagulation for glaucoma after penetrating keratoplasty. *Am J Ophthalmol.* 1995;120(5):569–576.

64. Lin P, Wollstein G, Glavas IP, et al. Contact transscleral neodymium: yttrium-aluminum-garnet laser cyclophotocoagulation long-term outcome. *Ophthalmology.* 2004;111(11):2137–2143.

65. Phelan MJ, Higginbotham EJ. Contact transscleral Nd:YAG laser cyclophotocoagulation for the treatment of refractory pediatric glaucoma. *Ophthalmic Surg Lasers.* 1995;26(5):401–403.

66. Formińska-Kapuścik M, Pieczara E, Domański R. Diode laser in secondary glaucoma in children—long-term results [in Polish]. *Klin Oczna.* 2005;107(4–6):236–238.

67. Heinz C, Koch JM, Heiligenhaus A. Transscleral diode laser cyclophotocoagulation as primary surgical treatment for secondary glaucoma in juvenile idiopathic arthritis: high failure rate after short term follow up. *Br J Ophthalmol.* 2006;90(6):737–740.

68. Trope GE, Murphy PH. Immediate pressure effects of Nd:YAG cyclocoagulation. *Am J Ophthalmol.* 1991;112(5):603–604.

69. Maus M, Katz LJ. Choroidal detachment, flat anterior chamber, and hypotony as complications of neodymium:YAG laser cyclophotocoagulation. *Ophthalmology.* 1990;97(1):69–72.

70. Edward DP, Brown SV, Higginbotham E, et al. Sympathetic ophthalmia following neodymium:YAG cyclotherapy. *Ophthalmic Surg.* 1989;20(8): 544–546.

71. Brown SV, Higginbotham E, Tessler H. Sympathetic ophthalmia following Nd:YAG cyclotherapy. *Ophthalmic Surg.* 1990;21(10):736–737.

72. Lam S, Tessler HH, Lam BL, et al. High incidence of sympathetic ophthalmia after contact and noncontact neodymium:YAG cyclotherapy. *Ophthalmology.* 1992;99(12):1818–1822.

73. Pastor SA, Iwach A, Nozik RA, et al. Presumed sympathetic ophthalmia following Nd:YAG transscleral cyclophotocoagulation. *J Glaucoma.* 1993;2(1):30–31.

74. Bechrakis NE, Müller-Stolzenburg NW, Helbig H, et al. Sympathetic ophthalmia following laser cyclocoagulation. *Arch Ophthalmol.* 1994;112(1):80–84.

75. Hardten DR, Brown JD. Malignant glaucoma after Nd:YAG cyclophotocoagulation. *Am J Ophthalmol.* 1991;111(2):245–247.

76. Wand M, Schuman JS, Puliafito CA. Malignant glaucoma after contact transscleral Nd:YAG laser cyclophotocoagulation. *J Glaucoma.* 1993;2(2): 110–111.

77. Ganesh SK, Rishi K. Necrotizing scleritis following diode laser transscleral cyclophotocoagulation. *Indian J Ophthalmol.* 2006;54(3): 199–200.

78. Gupta V, Sony P, Sihota R. Inadvertent sclerostomy with encysted bleb following trans-scleral contact diode laser cyclophotocoagulation. *Clin Experiment Ophthalmol.* 2006;34(1):86–87.

79. Shields MB, Shields SE. Noncontact transscleral Nd:YAG cyclophotocoagulation: a long-term follow-up of 500 patients. *Trans Am Ophthalmol Soc.* 1994;92:271–283.

80. Myers JS, Trevisani MG, Imami N, et al. Laser energy reaching the posterior pole during transscleral cyclophotocoagulation. *Arch Ophthalmol.* 1998;116(4):488–491.

81. Neely DE, Plager DA. Endocyclophotocoagulation for management of difficult pediatric glaucomas. *J AAPOS.* 2001;5:221–229.

82. Schuman JS, Noecker RJ, Puliafito CA, et al. Energy levels and probe placement in contact transscleral semiconductor diode laser cyclopho-

tocoagulation in human cadaver eyes. *Arch Ophthalmol.* 1991;109(11): 1534–1538.

83. Brancato R, Leoni G, Trabucchi G, et al. Histopathology of continuous wave neodymium:yttrium aluminum garnet and diode laser contact transscleral lesions in rabbit ciliary body. *Invest Ophthalmol Vis Sci.* 1991;32(5):1586–1592.

84. Brancato R, Trabucchi G, Verdi M, et al. Diode and Nd:YAG laser contact transscleral cyclophotocoagulation in a human eye: a comparative histopathologic study of the lesions produced using a new fiber optic probe. *Ophthalmic Surg.* 1994;25(9):607–611.

85. Assia EI, Hennis HL, Stewart WC, et al. A comparison of neodymium:yttrium aluminum garnet and diode laser transscleral cyclophotocoagulation and cyclocryotherapy. *Invest Ophthalmol Vis Sci.* 1991;32(10): 2774–2778.

86. Lin SC. Endoscopic and transscleral cyclophotocoagulation for the treatment of refractory glaucoma [review]. *J Glaucoma.* 2008;17(3):238–247.

87. Higginbotham EJ, Harrison M, Zou X. Cyclophotocoagulation with the transscleral contact neodymium:YAG laser versus cyclocryotherapy in rabbits. *Ophthalmic Surg.* 1991;22(1):27–30.

88. Suzuki Y, Araie M, Yumita A, et al. Transscleral Nd:YAG laser cyclophotocoagulation versus cyclocryotherapy. *Graefes Arch Clin Exp Ophthalmol.* 1991;229(1):33–36.

89. Noureddin BN, Wilson-Holt N, Lavin M, et al. Advanced uncontrolled glaucoma. Nd:YAG cyclophotocoagulation or tube surgery. *Ophthalmology.* 1992;99(3):430–436.

90. Uram M. Ophthalmic laser microendoscope ciliary process ablation in the management of neovascular glaucoma. *Ophthalmology.* 1992;99(12): 1823–1828.

91. Chen J, Cohn RA, Lin SC, et al. Endoscopic photocoagulation of the ciliary body for treatment of refractory glaucomas. *Am J Ophthalmol.* 1997;124(6):787–796.

92. Kuang TM, Liu CJ, Chou CK, et al. Clinical experience in the management of neovascular glaucoma. *J Chin Med Assoc.* 2004;67(3):131–135.

93. Lima FE, Magacho L, Carvalho DM, et al. A prospective, comparative study between endoscopic cyclophotocoagulation and the Ahmed drainage implant in refractory glaucoma. *J Glaucoma.* 2004;13(3):233–237.

94. Fleishman JA, Schwartz M, Dixon JA. Argon laser endophotocoagulation: an intraoperative trans-pars plana technique. *Arch Ophthalmol.* 1981;99(9):1610–1612.

95. Peyman GA, Salzano TC, Green JL. Argon endolaser. *Arch Ophthalmol.* 1981;99(11):2037–2038.

96. Landers MB III, Trese MT, Stefansson E, et al. Argon laser intraocular photocoagulation. *Ophthalmology.* 1982;89(7):785–788.

97. Shields MB. Cyclodestructive surgery for glaucoma: past, present and future. *Trans Am Ophthalmol Soc.* 1985;83:285–303.

98. Patel A, Thompson JT, Michels RG, et al. Endolaser treatment of the ciliary body for uncontrolled glaucoma. *Ophthalmology.* 1986;93(6):825–830.

99. Zarbin MA, Michels RG, de Bustros S, et al. Endolaser treatment of the ciliary body for severe glaucoma. *Ophthalmology.* 1988;95(12):1639–1648.

100. Lee PF, Pomerantzeff O. Transpupillary cyclophotocoagulation of rabbit eyes: an experimental approach to glaucoma surgery. *Am J Ophthalmol.* 1971;71(4):911–920.

101. Bartl G, Haller BM, Wocheslander E, et al. Light and electron microscopic observations after argon laser photocoagulation of ciliary processes [in German]. *Klin Monatsbl Augenheilkd.* 1982;181(5):414–416.

102. Lee PF. Argon laser photocoagulation of the ciliary processes in cases of aphakic glaucoma. *Arch Ophthalmol.* 1979;97(11):2135–2138.

103. Bernard JA, Haut J, Demailly PH, et al. Coagulation of the ciliary processes with the argon laser: its use in certain types of hypertonia [in French]. *Arch Ophthalmol (Paris).* 1974;34(8–9):577–580.

104. Merritt JC. Transpupillary photocoagulation of the ciliary processes. *Ann Ophthalmol.* 1976;8(3):325–328.

105. Lee PF, Shihab Z, Eberle M. Partial ciliary process laser photocoagulation in the management of glaucoma. *Lasers Surg Med.* 1980;1(1):85–92.

106. Klapper RM, Dodick JM. Transpupillary argon laser cyclophotocoagulation. *Doc Ophthalmol Proc.* 1984;36:197–203.

107. Shields S, Stewart WC, Shields MB. Transpupillary argon laser cyclophotocoagulation in the treatment of glaucoma. *Ophthalmic Surg.* 1988;19(3):171–175.

108. Bietti G. Surgical intervention on the ciliary body: new trends for the relief of glaucoma. *JAMA.* 1950;142(12):889–897.

109. Smith RS, Boyle E, Rudt LA. Cyclocryotherapy: a light and electron microscopic study. *Arch Ophthalmol.* 1977;95(2):285–288.

110. Wilkes TD, Fraunfelder FT. Principles of cryosurgery. *Ophthalmic Surg.* 1979;10(8):21–30.

111. Wener RG, Pinkerton RM, Robertson DM. Cryosurgical induced changes in corneal nerves. *Can J Ophthalmol.* 1973;8(4):548–555.

112. Prost M. Cyclocryotherapy for glaucoma: evaluation of techniques. *Surv Ophthalmol.* 1983;28:93–100.

113. Machemer R. Modified cryoprobe for retinal detachment surgery and cyclocryotherapy. *Am J Ophthalmol.* 1977;83:123.

114. Machemer R, Lashley R. Automatic timer for cryotherapy. *Am J Ophthalmol.* 1977;83:125.

115. Bellows AR. Cyclocryotherapy for glaucoma. *Int Ophthalmol Clin.* 1981;21(1):99–111.

116. Wesley RE, Kielar RA. Cyclocryotherapy in treatment of glaucoma. *Glaucoma.* 1980;3:533–538.

117. Higginbotham EJ, Lee DA, Bartels SP, et al. Effects of cyclocryotherapy on aqueous humor dynamics in cats. *Arch Ophthalmol.* 1988;106(3):396–403.

118. Brindley G, Shields MB. Value and limitations of cyclocryotherapy. *Graefes Arch Clin Exp Ophthalmol.* 1986;224(6):545–548.

119. Bellows AR, Grant WM. Cyclocryotherapy in advanced inadequately controlled glaucoma. *Am J Ophthalmol.* 1973;75(4):679–684.

120. Caprioli J, Sears M. Regulation of intraocular pressure during cyclocryotherapy for advanced glaucoma. *Am J Ophthalmol.* 1986;101(5): 542–545.

121. Strasser G, Haddad R. Gonioscopic changes after cyclocryocoagulation. *Klin Monatsbl Augenheilkd.* 1985;187(5):343–344.

122. Chavis RM, Vygantas CM, Vygantas A. Experimental inhibition of prostaglandin-like inflammatory response after cryotherapy. *Am J Ophthalmol.* 1976;82(2):310–312.

123. Hurvitz LM, Spaeth GL, Zakhour I, et al. A comparison of the effect of flurbiprofen, dexamethasone, and placebo on cyclocryotherapy-induced inflammation. *Ophthalmic Surg.* 1984;15(5):394–399.

124. Haddad R. Cyclocryotherapy: experimental studies of the breakdown of the blood-aqueous barrier and analysis of a long term follow-up study [in German]. *Wien Klin Wochenschr Suppl.* 1981;126:1–18.

125. Kaiden JS, Serniuk RA, Bader BF. Choroidal detachment with flat anterior chamber after cyclocryotherapy. *Ann Ophthalmol.* 1979;11(7): 1111–1113.

126. Gieser RG, Gieser DK. Treatment of intravitreal ciliary body neovascularization. *Ophthalmic Surg.* 1984;15(6):508–510.

127. Krupin T, Johnson MF, Becker B. Anterior segment ischemia after cyclocryotherapy. *Am J Ophthalmol.* 1977;84(3):426–428.

128. Kao SF, Morgan CM, Bergstrom TJ. Subretinal fibrosis following cyclocryotherapy. *Arch Ophthalmol.* 1987;105(9):1175–1176.

129. Pearson PA, Baldwin LB, Smith TJ. Lens subluxation as a complication of cyclocryotherapy. *Ophthalmic Surg.* 1989;20(6):445–446.

130. Sabates R. Choroiditis compatible with the histopathologic diagnosis of sympathetic ophthalmia following cyclocryotherapy of neovascular glaucoma. *Ophthalmic Surg.* 1988;19(3):176–182.

131. Harrison TJ. Sympathetic ophthalmia after cyclocryotherapy of neovascular glaucoma without ocular penetration. *Ophthalmic Surg.* 1993; 24(1):44–46.

132. West CE, Wood TO, Kaufman HE. Cyclocryotherapy for glaucoma pre- or postpenetrating keratoplasty. *Am J Ophthalmol.* 1973;7(4)6:485–489.

133. Binder PS, Abel R Jr, Kaufman HE. Cyclocryotherapy for glaucoma after penetrating keratoplasty. *Am J Ophthalmol.* 1975;79(3):489–492.

134. Bellows AR, Grant WM. Cyclocryotherapy of chronic open-angle glaucoma in aphakic eyes. *Am J Ophthalmol.* 1978;85(5 pt 1):615–621.

135. Frucht-Pery J, Feldman ST, Brown SI. Transplantation of congenitally opaque corneas from eyes with exaggerated buphthalmos. *Am J Ophthalmol.* 1989;107(6):655–658.

136. Al Faran MF, Tomey KF, Al Mutlaq FA. Cyclocryotherapy in selected cases of congenital glaucoma. *Ophthalmic Surg.* 1990;21(11):794–798.

42

Surgical Approaches for Coexisting Glaucoma and Cataract

In the management of a patient with a visually significant cataract and coexisting glaucoma, there are three basic surgical approaches: (a) cataract extraction alone, which may need to be followed by a trabeculectomy later; (b) glaucoma filtering surgery alone, followed by cataract removal later (two-stage approach); and (c) combined cataract and glaucoma surgery. Combined procedures have certain advantages and disadvantages compared with the other two options. Compared with cataract surgery alone—which itself is associated with an increased risk for posterior capsule break in glaucomatous eyes, particularly when exfoliation is present (1–4)—combined procedures are associated with a greater risk for postoperative complications, such as increased inflammation, hyphema, hypotony, shallow anterior chambers, and choroidal detachments; however, they have the advantage of reducing early intraocular pressure (IOP) rise. Compared with filtering surgery alone, with or without subsequent cataract extraction, the combined procedures may have a lower chance of long-term glaucoma control, but have the obvious advantage of a single surgery instead of two. For these reasons, the surgeon should consider each of the basic surgical options, evaluate the severity of the glaucoma, and the visual need and potential for each individual patient, and select the approach that seems most appropriate. With advances in cataract and glaucoma surgery, success rates with combined procedures have improved and relative indications have shifted. We first review the general indications for the three basic surgical approaches and then consider how advances in surgical techniques are influencing the relative indications for these procedures.

INDICATIONS

Predicting Visual Potential

In each case, it is assumed that a cataract is present for which extraction is indicated, independent of the glaucoma. However, the visual significance of the cataract is often difficult to determine in an eye with both a cataract and glaucoma, in which it is hard to know how much the glaucoma is contributing to the reduced vision. Several instruments have been developed to help predict the anticipated postoperative visual acuity. One focuses a miniaturized Snellen visual acuity chart on the retina (potential acuity meter), whereas others project stripe patterns from either a laser or white light source (Visometer). Potential acuity meter measurements do not always show good correlation to postoperative results, particularly for dense cataracts (5,6). In one study, the Visometer gave more

accurate predictions than the potential acuity meter did in patients with cataract and chronic open-angle glaucoma (COAG), even with glaucomatous field loss (7). In other studies, the potential acuity meter was accurate when the glaucomatous damage was mild to moderate and the postoperative visual acuity was 20/40 to 20/50 or better, whereas the results with advanced visual field loss or a worse postoperative vision were unreliable (8,9). Automated perimetry was useful in predicting whether the vision would be better or worse than 20/40. Combining this with the use of the potential acuity meter further increased the predictive value (9).

When it is decided that cataract surgery is needed, the selection of the specific surgical approach is based primarily on the status of the glaucoma.

Cataract Extraction Alone

Most surgeons prefer to perform cataract extraction alone when the IOP is well controlled medically in the presence of mild to moderate glaucomatous optic neuropathy. However, cataract extraction with placement of a posterior chamber intraocular lens (IOL) can be associated with a significant IOP rise during the early postoperative course in patients with preexisting glaucoma, especially when older, extracapsular techniques are used (10–15), or when viscoelastic material is not completely removed from the eye. Although outflow facility seems to improve after phacoemulsification (16), the IOP can still be significantly elevated in the first 24 hours. Peak IOP elevation after cataract extraction often occurs 2 hours postoperatively (17,18). After extracapsular cataract extraction (ECCE) or phacoemulsification with posterior chamber IOL implantation in patients with glaucoma, more than half of patients may have an IOP greater than 25 mm Hg, or even 35 mm Hg, indicating the need for close monitoring and prophylactic medical treatment to prevent postoperative IOP spikes (12,16,19). A significant increase in IOP during the first 5 to 7 hours after surgery has been found after both ECCE and phacoemulsification, with better IOP control seen after phacoemulsification when a sutureless scleral tunnel was used (15). Use of an anterior chamber maintainer instead of viscoelastic substance for lens implantation has been associated with a lower IOP on the first postoperative day (20). Although the pressure can usually be brought under control within the first few postoperative days, patients with advanced glaucomatous damage before surgery may have additional, irreversible loss of vision during this time. Therefore, moderate to advanced glaucomatous optic atrophy and visual field loss may argue against cataract surgery alone, despite the preoperative level of IOP, although the risk may be less with phacoemulsification techniques and thorough removal of viscoelastic material from the eye. Conversely, one study found that an IOP spike greater than 30 mm Hg was almost three times as common in eyes that had a combined procedure as in eyes that had phacoemulsification alone (21).

Several studies have also looked at the IOP course in the intermediate and late postoperative periods after cataract surgery in patients with preexisting glaucoma. In general, the extracapsular techniques with posterior chamber IOLs were better tolerated than intracapsular procedures were (11), although glaucoma control postoperatively can be a problem with either technique. During the first 2 to 4 months after ECCE surgery, many glaucoma patients will have pressures above the preoperative baseline, whereas the IOP in others may be unchanged or even improved (22–24). Patients with preexisting COAG were found to have a small reduction in mean IOP and require use of fewer medications for up to 5 years after ECCE surgery (25–28). A similar trend has been seen in patients with glaucoma after phacoemulsification and IOL implantation, patients with exfoliation, and patients without glaucoma (29–35). The reasons for IOP lowering after phacoemulsification are unclear, but one proposed hypothesis involves an induction of a potential stress response in the trabecular meshwork by the ultrasound (36). Anterior chamber depth increased after cataract extraction with posterior chamber IOL implantation in patients with angle-closure glaucoma and COAG, and IOP was well controlled in most cases (37,38). However, this trend generally reverses with time (28,39). Cataract surgery alone should not be relied on as a means of treating uncontrolled glaucoma. However, as stated, when the IOP is well controlled in the presence of mild glaucomatous damage, cataract surgery alone, especially small-incision phacoemulsification with posterior chamber IOL implantation, is often a reasonable choice.

Filtering Surgery Alone

When the glaucoma is uncontrolled despite maximum tolerable medical therapy and laser trabeculoplasty, the surgical procedure of choice is the one that has the greatest chance of providing immediate and long-term IOP control. In most cases, this is a filtering operation performed alone. In some patients, eliminating the need for IOP-lowering therapy postoperatively may improve quality of life and vision enough to delay the need for cataract surgery. In other patients, the cataract can be removed 4 to 6 months later, after the filtering bleb is well established, as the second part of a two-stage approach. In one study, patients who underwent the two-stage procedure had a greater percentage of long-term IOP reduction than those who had cataract surgery alone or a combined cataract–glaucoma operation (14). Other studies have found no difference in success rates between two-stage procedures and combined phacoemulsification with trabeculectomy (40,41). In a study of 21 patients undergoing ECCE with posterior chamber IOL implantation in eyes with established filtering blebs followed up for a minimum of 2 years, the IOP increased by an average of 3.5 mm Hg, with six eyes

requiring resumption of medical therapy and two requiring repeated filtering surgery (42).

Temporal clear corneal phacoemulsification did not cause a significant difference in IOP control in patients with filtering blebs after 1 year of follow-up in one study (43). In another study, phacoemulsification through a superior clear corneal incision in eyes with previous trabeculectomy increased the IOP within 1 year, but at 2 years, there was no significant difference from baseline in IOP control (44). Retrospective studies have shown that in patients with glaucoma who had trabeculectomy and subsequent cataract surgery, the IOP appeared to be better controlled by phacoemulsification than by ECCE (45,46). However, the bleb is still likely to become smaller and the IOP is likely to increase even after phacoemulsification, especially if the preoperative IOP is greater than 10 mm Hg, the iris is manipulated intraoperatively, or the patient is younger than 50 years (47,48). The IOP usually increases after phacoemulsification in eyes with preexisting hypotony (49), but resolution of the hypotony is unpredictable (48).

Combined Cataract Extraction–Glaucoma Surgery

Between the two extremes already noted—that is, the patients whose glaucoma is well controlled and those whose glaucoma is uncontrolled and poses an immediate threat to vision—there is a third group of patients with borderline glaucoma status and visually significant cataracts. For these patients, a combined procedure may be indicated. A combined approach might be preferred in the following scenarios: (a) glaucoma under borderline control despite maximum tolerable medical therapy and laser trabeculoplasty; (b) adequate IOP control, but significant drug-induced side effects; (c) adequate IOP control on well-tolerated medical therapy, but advanced glaucomatous optic atrophy; or (d) uncontrolled glaucoma, but an urgent need to restore vision or when two operations are infeasible.

The rationale for a combined procedure, as opposed to cataract surgery alone, in eyes with good IOP control but advanced damage, is the risk of a transient pressure rise in the early postoperative period. Even if laser trabeculoplasty has achieved good IOP control, it may still be necessary to combine glaucoma surgery with the cataract extraction, because a good response to laser therapy before cataract surgery does not guarantee postoperative pressure control (50). Studies have shown that the early postoperative pressure rise is significantly less after a combined procedure than after cataract extraction alone (13,14), and this was probably the primary benefit of the combined surgery during the era of ECCE surgery, when long-term glaucoma control after combined procedures was less predictable. However, with the advent of small-incision cataract surgery and the adjunctive use of antimetabolites with the filtering surgery (discussed later in this chapter), the long-term results of combined procedures have improved and the relative indications for this surgical option have expanded (51,52). Nevertheless, there is still a role for each of the three basic surgical options, the selection of which depends not only on the status of the individual patient but also on the results that each surgeon experiences with the various approaches.

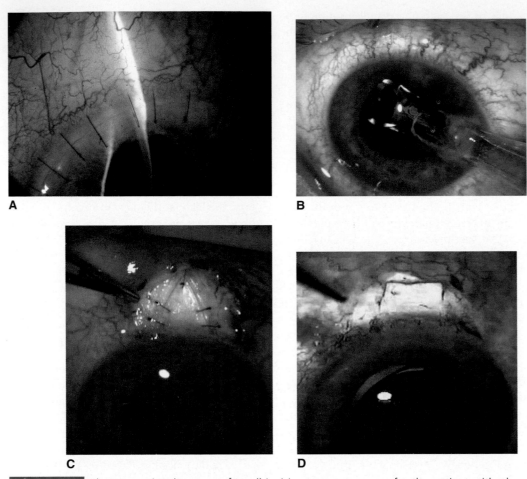

Figure 42.1 The anatomic advantage of small-incision cataract surgery for the patient with glaucoma. **A:** Long-term bleb function with a large cataract incision is difficult to achieve with ECCE–trabeculectomy or trabeculectomy followed later by ECCE. Inflammation, bleeding, and long-term wound healing stimulate fibroblasts, increasing the likelihood of bleb failure. **B,C:** Two-site phacotrabeculectomy has the advantage of modern-day small-incision cataract surgery combined with separate-site trabeculectomy. A smaller incision size results in less inflammation and cataract wound healing that is largely confined to the temporal area. Visual rehabilitation with phacoemulsification and foldable IOL is also faster. The likelihood of long-term filtration is greater with phacotrabeculectomy. **D:** Single-site phacotrabeculectomy is another option. The lens extraction and the trabeculectomy are performed through the same small limbal incision. (From Fellman RL, Starita RJ, Godfrey DG, et al. Cataract extraction in patients with glaucoma. In: Tasman W, Jaeger EA, eds. *Duane's Clinical Ophthalmology.* Vol 6. Philadelphia:Lippincott Williams & Wilkins; 2008:chap 16.)

Cataract extraction by phacoemulsification or ECCE, combined with IOL implantation and trabeculotomy, has been found to be a safe and effective treatment for patients with co-existing glaucoma and cataract (53,54). However, most studies find that the use of the smaller incision with phacotrabeculectomy has a higher success rate and more rapid visual recovery (**Fig. 42.1**). Several retrospective studies have found that the postoperative complication rate and IOP were lower when trabeculectomy was combined with phacoemulsification than with ECCE after 1 to 2 years of follow-up (55,56), and that ECCE may be a risk factor for unsatisfactory late IOP control and filtering bleb appearance. The frequency of fibrin formation and the incidence of an IOP spike of more than 25 mm Hg were lower in one study after the phacoemulsification than after the ECCE (57). More frequent IOL dislocation has been found when trabeculectomy was combined with ECCE than when it was combined with phacoemulsification (58).

Small-incision cataract surgery can be readily combined with trabeculectomy in patients with COAG (59–62). Phacoemulsification and posterior chamber IOL implantation, combined with trabeculectomy, is usually associated with a significant improvement in visual acuity, and with lowering of the IOP and the number of glaucoma medications (63). A retrospective analysis of phacoemulsification with posterior chamber IOL implant, combined with mitomycin C–augmented trabeculectomy with fornix-based conjunctival flaps, has shown that the filtering blebs were large, diffuse, and noncystic, achieving good control of IOP and improvement of visual acuity (64). A meta-analysis of techniques found that two-site surgery had better outcomes compared with single-site surgery.

However, combined cataract and trabeculectomy did not perform as well as trabeculectomy alone did (65).

TECHNIQUES

Cataract Surgery in Eyes with Glaucoma

Miotic Pupil

In some cases, the cataract operation can be performed in the surgeon's usual manner, with no special measures for the coexisting glaucoma. A previously common problem with cataract surgery in the glaucomatous eye, although one that is less common today, is the irreversible miosis from chronic miotic therapy. This became more important with the advent of phacoemulsification, in which adequate pupillary dilatation is needed to perform the surgery safely and effectively. A wide variety of techniques have been described to surgically enlarge the pupil. One approach is to make a sector iridotomy above, often with two inferior sphincterotomies (66), or multiple sphincterotomies and a peripheral iridectomy (67). If a sector iridotomy is made, some surgeons will elect to close it with sutures after implanting the lens (68,69), although it can be left open if the lens haptics are rotated horizontally away from the iridotomy. One study compared patients with sutured and unsutured sector iridotomies and found no difference in glare sensitivity (70). Sector iridectomies and sphincterotomies are less commonly used since the advent of more modern techniques to manage the small pupil (described later).

Several iris retractors have been developed to mechanically enlarge a miotic pupil (71–74). One of these instruments is the three- or four-point Beehler pupil dilator, which has two or three extendable "microfingers" through 2.5- to 3.0-mm incisions and can dilate a 2- to 3-mm pupil to approximately 6 to 7 mm. Flexible nylon hooks and the Malyugin ring are also useful to dilate and control a small pupil during cataract surgery (**Fig. 42.2**) (72,75–77). Other techniques include mechanical stretching of the pupil, various iris suture techniques, a maneuver of tucking the iris pillars of a sector iridectomy, and a pupil-expanding ring (74,78–82). It has also been suggested that phacoemulsification can be performed through a pupil of 4 mm or more if the capsulorrhexis is intact and the nucleus is

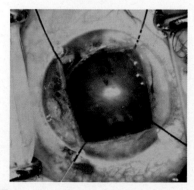

Figure 42.2 Four flexible iris retractors inserted through clear cornea stab incisions are used to dilate a chronically miotic pupil during combined cataract and glaucoma surgery.

fractured into small segments in the capsule (83), although success depends on the skill of the surgeon. In addition to stretching the pupil, the surgeon can insert the iris hooks into the capsular bag under the anterior capsule, after performing capsulorrhexis to stabilize the lens capsule in eyes with weak or damaged zonules (e.g., exfoliation syndrome) (84–87). Pupil stretch during phacoemulsification appears to have no negative effect on best-corrected visual acuity, IOP, inflammation, or other potential complications (88).

Viscoelastic Substances

Viscoelastic substances, such as hyaluronic acid, should be used with caution in eyes with glaucoma. They are especially useful during the anterior capsulotomy, not only for maintaining a deep anterior chamber and protecting corneal endothelium but also for providing additional pupillary dilatation. However, viscoelastic substances increase the risk for early postoperative IOP rise and should be carefully removed at the end of the procedure. There were no significant differences in postoperative IOP spikes in one study when Healon 5, Healon, and Healon GV were used, although viscoelastic substances with lower viscosity appear to cause less elevation in IOP (89).

Capsulorrhexis Size

Making a capsulorrhexis diameter smaller than 5 to 6 mm prevents dislocation of the IOL from the capsular bag into anterior chamber and often eliminates the need for postoperative pupillary constriction. However, if pupillary constriction is needed after lens implantation, intracameral carbachol may be preferable to acetylcholine, because the former has been associated with better early postoperative pressure control (89). In another study, use of a combination of intraoperative acetylcholine and postoperative acetazolamide prevented an acute IOP rise more effectively than use of either agent alone did (90). It has been reported that a flap of anterior lens capsule can be included in the trabeculectomy site to facilitate filtration in combined trabeculectomy with ECCE and posterior chamber IOL implantation (91).

Intraocular Lens Selection

Selection of the proper IOL is also important in eyes with glaucoma. Posterior chamber silicone, polymethylmethacrylate, and acrylic lenses appear to be well tolerated (92), although one study found higher postoperative IOP with the acrylic IOLs than with the silicone lenses (93). Anterior chamber IOLs should, in most cases, be avoided in glaucomatous eyes. However, when loss of capsular support precludes the standard implantation of a posterior chamber IOL, the surgeon usually must decide between a sutured posterior chamber IOL and an anterior chamber IOL. Several techniques have been described for the former option (94–99), most of which use the basic principle of passing two 10-0 Prolene sutures attached to the lens haptics through the ciliary sulcus and sclera, and securing them beneath conjunctival and partial-thickness scleral flaps. These can all be difficult techniques, however, especially if they are not performed frequently, and it has been reported that the much easier procedure of implanting a semiflexible, one-piece, open-loop anterior chamber IOL is associated with reasonable long-term IOP control in most glaucomatous eyes (100); however, the tendency toward increased IOP in eyes with an anterior chamber IOL has also been observed (101,102).

Placing of releasable sutures on the scleral flap has been advocated for the combined procedure (103).

Cataract Extraction after Filtering Surgery

When extraction of the cataract becomes necessary in an eye with a functioning filtering bleb, the cataract incision should be positioned to maximize bleb survival. Phacoemulsification typically has less effect on the postoperative IOP elevation than ECCE does, although both approaches can be associated with an increase in IOP (45,104,105). Intraoperative complications during cataract surgery, especially vitreous loss, have been associated with bleb failure (104). Phacoemulsification with a foldable posterior chamber IOL through a clear corneal incision with or without a corneal suture has become a popular approach for cataract surgery in eyes with an established filtering bleb (**Fig. 42.3**). Most surgeons prefer to use a temporal corneal incision for phacoemulsification (106), although a clear corneal incision elsewhere, depending on the location of the filtering bleb, may be used. These basic methods generally preserve function of the filtering bleb comparably, although most eyes will have a slightly higher IOP postoperatively and many will require more glaucoma medication (44,107,108). As would be expected, eyes with a well-controlled IOP after trabeculectomy appear to have a better prognosis after cataract surgery (109).

Combined Cataract–Glaucoma Surgery

Early combined operations that use full-thickness filtering procedures were associated with an increased risk of a transient shallow or flat anterior chamber, which often led to significant complications in the inflamed eye. For this reason, essentially all combined procedures now use a trabeculectomy, which is less likely to cause loss of the anterior chamber.

Guarded Fistula and Cataract Extraction

The protective scleral flap over a limbal fistula, which reduces the chances of an early postoperative flat anterior chamber, makes the guarded filtering operation particularly desirable for combined procedures. Several techniques were described for combining a trabeculectomy with intracapsular cataract surgery during the 1970s (110–112), but it was not until the popularity of ECCE and posterior chamber IOL implantation (the "triple procedure") in the 1980s and phacoemulsification in the 1990s that combined trabeculectomy and cataract extraction began to provide more consistent long-term glaucoma control (113–116).

Phacoemulsification became the preferred cataract technique for combined procedures in the 1990s, and it appears to be associated with further improvement in the long-term success rates. The procedure can be combined with a trabeculectomy by using the fistula for the cataract incision (117). The incision may be 6 mm to insert a rigid IOL, or less than 3 mm for a foldable lens. The latter has been shown to have a significantly lower incidence of postoperative complications and

Figure 42.3 **A:** Slitlamp view of an eye with functioning glaucoma-filtering bleb in which extracapsular cataract extraction and posterior chamber lens implantation were performed through a clear corneal incision to preserve the preexisting bleb. **B:** Intraoperative view of cataract surgery performed by using a temporal clear corneal incision in a patient with a preexisting bleb. Main wound and paracentesis wounds avoid the area of the bleb.

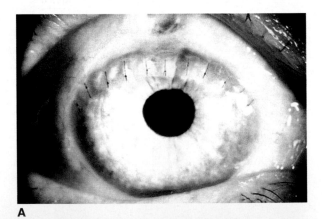

A

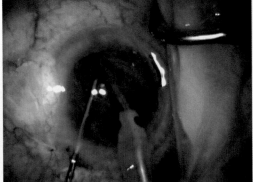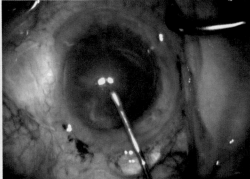

B

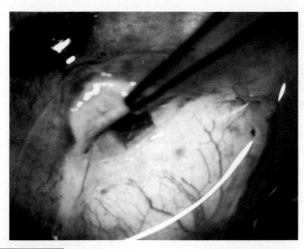

Figure 42.4 Intraoperative view during guarded sclerectomy and phacoemulsification showing excision of fistula from posterior lip of scleral tunnel incision.

better visual acuity in the early postoperative period (118). After creating a superior scleral tunnel and converting the tunnel to a scleral flap, the surgeon creates a limbal fistula under it (single-site technique). If a scleral tunnel incision is used, the fistula can be excised from the posterior lip of the incision, leaving the anterior lip of the tunnel to cover the fistula (119) (**Fig. 42.4**).

One of the commonly used techniques is to perform a phacoemulsification through a separate temporal corneal incision as a first step, followed by a trabeculectomy at the superior limbus (two-site technique) (106,120,121). Prospective studies comparing single-site versus two-site approaches, have shown that patients in the two-site group had 1 to 2 mm Hg greater IOP reduction and required less postoperative medication use, although the differences were statistically insignificant (122–124).

An alternative approach with ECCE involves preparation of the partial-thickness scleral flap and limbal fistula in the usual manner, followed by extension of the corneoscleral incision from either side of the fistula. After a standard ECCE and implantation of the posterior chamber IOL, both scleral flap and corneoscleral or corneal incision are closed with multiple sutures. The conjunctival flap is closed in the manner described for glaucoma filtering procedures (see Chapter 38). A limbal-based versus fornix-based conjunctival flap was found to have no difference on the outcome of trabeculectomy combined with either ECCE or phacoemulsification and posterior chamber IOL (125–131). The use of topical apraclonidine, 1%, before, immediately after, and 12 hours after surgery was shown to provide better IOP control after combined ECCE and trabeculectomy (132), although using apraclonidine, 1%, once after phacoemulsification has not demonstrated significant IOP reduction (133). Use of oral acetazolamide and topical dorzolamide has been shown to control postoperative IOP elevation more effectively than use of apraclonidine does (134,135).

Several studies have compared phacoemulsification with ECCE in combination with a guarded filtering procedure; generally, the former has been associated with fewer complications,

improved long-term IOP control, and better visual outcome (55,119,136).

Adjunctive Use of Antimetabolites

Another factor that may be associated with the improved long-term IOP control with combined procedures is the adjunctive use of antimetabolites to minimize excessive fibrosis. The first of these agents to be evaluated was 5-fluorouracil (5-FU), which is typically administered as several postoperative subconjunctival injections. Although preliminary experience with combined ECCE and trabeculectomy suggested some benefit, subsequent studies showed no significant difference with or without adjunctive 5-FU (137–140). Results of studies with combined phacoemulsification and trabeculectomy have shown little or no benefit of 5-FU use (141–144).

When intraoperative mitomycin C (MMC) was used in conjunction with combined cataract extraction and trabeculectomy, some earlier studies failed to demonstrate a significant benefit of the concomitant use of MMC, although IOP was generally well controlled at 6 to 12 months postoperatively (145–148). Several randomized studies have found greater IOP control with the use of MMC in combined glaucoma and cataract surgery (144,149–152).

Other Combined Techniques

In general, any glaucoma filtering procedure or drainage-device surgery can be combined with cataract removal (**Fig. 42.5**). Techniques have been described in which the surgeon performs a trabeculotomy through a radial incision at 12 o'clock adjacent to a partial-thickness corneoscleral incision before extending the incision full-thickness for the cataract surgery (29,153,154). Combining phacoemulsification with endoscopic laser to perform either goniopuncture or cyclophotocoagulation through a cataract incision has also been proposed as an alternative to combined cataract and trabeculectomy surgery (155–157). Deep sclerectomy and viscocanalostomy combined with phacoemulsification have both been reported to achieve IOP reduction and visual acuity similar to phacoemulsification combined with trabeculectomy, but with fewer complications (158–161). A technique of combining trabecular aspiration with phacoemulsification was proposed as an alternative to the combination of trabeculectomy and phacoemulsification in patients with exfoliative glaucoma, but this technique appeared to provide insufficient postoperative IOP lowering (162).

Cataract surgery has also been combined with implantation of an Ahmed or Baerveldt drainage device and is reported to effectively improve IOP control in certain eyes in which combined trabeculectomy has failed or in which the risk of failure is high—for example, eyes with neovascular or uveitic glaucoma, or with significant conjunctival scarring from previous ocular surgery (163–165). However, complications such as aqueous misdirection, corneal edema, choroidal effusion, and capsular bag distention have been reported (167,168).

Cataract surgery combined with trabeculotomy via an ab interno approach (by using the Trabectome device) and canaloplasty has been used successfully (166–168).

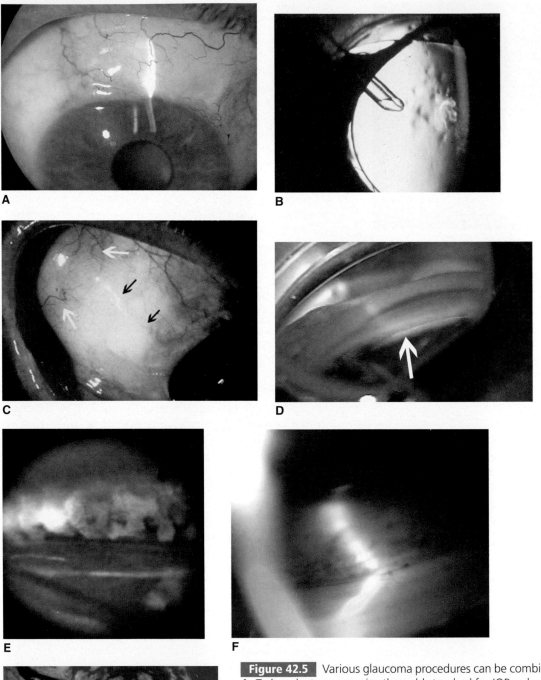

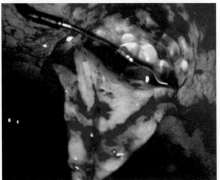

Figure 42.5 Various glaucoma procedures can be combined with cataract extraction. **A:** Trabeculectomy remains the gold standard for IOP reduction in an eye with a pristine blood–aqueous barrier and virgin conjunctiva. **B,C:** Combined cataract extraction and glaucoma drainage-device implantation. Note margins of the equatorial bleb *(yellow arrows)* and the tube covered by a patch graft that prevents erosion *(black arrows)*. **D:** Gonioscopic view of trabeculotomy cleft *(white arrow)* in a patient who has undergone Trabectome surgery combined with cataract extraction. **E:** Endoscopic cyclophotocoagulation performed in conjunction with phacoemulsification. The white area represents coagulation and shrinkage of the ciliary body processes, and the red circle is the aiming beam on the adjacent process. **F:** Gonioscopic view of patient after canaloplasty and phacoemulsification. Note the blue 10-0 Prolene sutures in the Schlemm canal. **G:** Deep sclerectomy and viscocanalostomy are similar forms of nonpenetrating surgery that may also be combined with lens extraction. (From Fellman RL, Starita RJ, Godfrey DG, et al. Cataract extraction in patients with glaucoma. In: Tasman W, Jaeger EA, eds. *Duane's Clinical Ophthalmology*. Vol 6. Philadelphia:Lippincott Williams & Wilkins; 2008:chap 16.)

KEY POINTS

- In an eye with a cataract, for which extraction is believed to be indicated, and coexisting glaucoma, the surgical approach is based primarily on the status of the glaucoma.
- In some eyes, cataract extraction alone may be sufficient, whereas other eyes may require filtering surgery alone with cataract surgery at a later date. In other eyes, a combined glaucoma and cataract operation may be the procedure of choice.
- The preferred technique for the glaucoma portion of a combined procedure is usually some form of guarded filtering surgery. The combination of phacoemulsification with a guarded filtering procedure, possibly in conjunction with antimetabolite therapy, appears to have improved the long-term success rate of the combined procedure.

REFERENCES

1. Abbasoglu OE, Hosal B, Tekeli O, et al. Risk factors for vitreous loss in cataract surgery. *Eur J Ophthalmol.* 2000;10:227–232.
2. Chiselita D, Vancea PP. The effect of the pseudoexfoliative syndrome on the evolution and treatment of pseudoexfoliative glaucoma and senile cataract [in Romanian] *Oftalmologia.* 1996;40:249–260.
3. Fine IH, Hoffman RS. Phacoemulsification in the presence of exfoliation: challenges and options. *J Cataract Refract Surg.* 1997;23:160–165.
4. Drolsum L, Haaskjold E, Sandvig K. Phacoemulsification in eyes with exfoliation. *J Cataract Refract Surg.* 1998;24:787–792.
5. Devereux CJ, Rando A, Wagstaff CM, et al. Potential acuity meter results in cataract patients. *Clin Experiment Ophthalmol.* 2000;28:414–418.
6. Lasa MS, Datiles MB III, Freidlin V. Potential vision tests in patients with cataracts. *Ophthalmology.* 1995;102:1007–1011.
7. Spurny RC, Zaldivar R, Belcher CD III, et al. Instruments for predicting visual acuity: a clinical comparison. *Arch Ophthalmol.* 1986;104:196–200.
8. Asbell PA, Chiang B, Amin A, et al. Retinal acuity evaluation with the potential acuity meter in glaucoma patients. *Ophthalmology.* 1985;92:764–767.
9. Stewart WC, Connor AB, Hunt HH. Prediction of postoperative visual acuity in patients with total glaucomatous cupping using the Potential Acuity Meter and automated perimetry. *Ophthalmic Surg.* 1993;24:730–734.
10. McGuigan LJ, Gottsch J, Stark WJ, et al. Extracapsular cataract extraction and posterior chamber lens implantation in eyes with preexisting glaucoma. *Arch Ophthalmol.* 1986;104:1301–1308.
11. Vu MT, Shields MB. The early postoperative pressure course in glaucoma patients following cataract surgery. *Ophthalmic Surg.* 1988;19:467–470.
12. Gross JG, Meyer DR, Robin AL, et al. Increased intraocular pressure in the immediate postoperative period after extracapsular cataract extraction. *Am J Ophthalmol.* 1988;105:466–469.
13. Krupin T, Feitl ME, Bishop KI. Postoperative intraocular pressure rise in open-angle glaucoma patients after cataract or combined cataract-filtration surgery. *Ophthalmology.* 1989;96:579–584.
14. Murchison JF Jr, Shields MB. An evaluation of three surgical approaches for coexisting cataract and glaucoma. *Ophthalmic Surg.* 1989;20:393–398.
15. Lagreze WD, Bomer TG, Funk J. Effect of surgical technique on the increase in intraocular pressure after cataract extraction. *Ophthalmic Surg Lasers.* 1996;27:169–173.
16. Meyer MA, Savitt ML, Kopitas E. The effect of phacoemulsification on aqueous outflow facility. *Ophthalmology.* 1997;104:1221–1227.
17. Thirumalai B, Baranyovits PR. Intraocular pressure changes and the implications on patient review after phacoemulsification. *J Cataract Refract Surg.* 2003;29:504–507.
18. Shingleton BJ, Rosenberg RB, Teixeira R, et al. Evaluation of intraocular pressure in the immediate postoperative period after phacoemulsification. *J Cataract Refract Surg.* 2007;33:1953–1957.
19. Barak A, Desatnik H, Ma-Naim T, et al. Early postoperative intraocular pressure pattern in glaucomatous and nonglaucomatous patients. *J Cataract Refract Surg.* 1996;22:607–611.
20. Shingleton BJ, Mitrev PV. Anterior chamber maintainer versus viscoelastic material for intraocular lens implantation: case-control study. *J Cataract Refract Surg.* 2001;27:711–714.
21. Tanito M, Ohira A, Chihara E. Factors leading to reduced intraocular pressure after combined trabeculotomy and cataract surgery. *J Glaucoma.* 2002;11:3–9.
22. Hansen TE, Naeser K, Rask KL. A prospective study of intraocular pressure four months after extracapsular cataract extraction with implantation of posterior chamber lenses. *J Cataract Refract Surg.* 1987;13:35–38.
23. Savage JA, Thomas JV, Belcher CD III, et al. Extracapsular cataract extraction and posterior chamber intraocular lens implantation in glaucomatous eyes. *Ophthalmology.* 1985;92:1506–1516.
24. McMahan LB, Monica ML, Zimmerman TJ. Posterior chamber pseudophakes in glaucoma patients. *Ophthalmic Surg.* 1986;17:146–150.
25. Radius RL, Schultz K, Sobocinski K, et al. Pseudophakia and intraocular pressure. *Am J Ophthalmol.* 1984;97:738–742.
26. Handa J, Henry JC, Krupin T, et al. Extracapsular cataract extraction with posterior chamber lens implantation in patients with glaucoma. *Arch Ophthalmol.* 1987;105:765–769.
27. Cinotti DJ, Fiore PM, Maltzman BA, et al. Control of intraocular pressure in glaucomatous eyes after extracapsular cataract extraction with intraocular lens implantation. *J Cataract Refract Surg.* 1988;14:650–653.
28. Shingleton BJ, Pasternack JJ, Hung JW, et al. Three and five year changes in intraocular pressures after clear corneal phacoemulsification in open angle glaucoma patients, glaucoma suspects, and normal patients. *J Glaucoma.* 2006;15:494–498.
29. Gimbel HV, Meyer D, DeBroff BM, et al. Intraocular pressure response to combined phacoemulsification and trabeculotomy ab externo versus phacoemulsification alone in primary open-angle glaucoma. *J Cataract Refract Surg.* 1995;21:653–660.
30. Matsumura M, Mizoguchi T, Kuroda S, et al. Intraocular pressure decrease after phacoemulsification-aspiration intraocular lens implantation in primary open angle glaucoma eyes [in Japanese]. *Nippon Ganka Gakkai Zasshi.* 1996;100:885–889.
31. Hayashi K, Hayashi H, Nakao F, et al. Effect of cataract surgery on intraocular pressure control in glaucoma patients. *J Cataract Refract Surg.* 2001;27:1779–1786.
32. Shingleton BJ, Nguyen BK, Eagan EF, et al. Outcomes of phacoemulsification in fellow eyes of patients with unilateral exfoliation: single-surgeon series. *J Cataract Refract Surg.* 2008;34:274–279.
33. Merkur A, Damji KF, Mintsioulis G, et al. Intraocular pressure decrease after phacoemulsification in patients with exfoliation syndrome. *J Cataract Refract Surg.* 2001;27:528–532.
34. Shingleton BJ, Laul A, Nagao K, et al. Effect of phacoemulsification on intraocular pressure in eyes with exfoliation: single-surgeon series. *J Cataract Refract Surg.* 2008;34:1834–1841.
35. Tennen DG, Masket S. Short- and long-term effect of clear corneal incisions on intraocular pressure. *J Cataract Refract Surg.* 1996;22:568–570.
36. Wang N, Chintala SK, Fini ME, et al. Ultrasound activates the TM ELAM-1/IL-1/NF-κB response: a potential mechanism for intraocular pressure reduction after phacoemulsification. *Invest Ophthalmol Vis Sci.* 2003;44:1977–1981.
37. Hayashi K, Hayashi H, Nakao F, et al. Changes in anterior chamber angle width and depth after intraocular lens implantation in eyes with glaucoma. *Ophthalmology.* 2000;107:698–703.
38. Yang CH, Hung PT. Intraocular lens position and anterior chamber angle changes after cataract extraction in eyes with primary angle-closure glaucoma. *J Cataract Refract Surg.* 1997;23:1109–1113.
39. Sponagel LD, Gloor B. Does implantation of posterior chamber lenses lower intraocular pressure? *Klin Monatsbl Augenheilkd.* 1986;188:495.
40. El-Sayyad FF, Helal MH, Khalil MM, et al. Phacotrabeculectomy versus two-stage operation: a matched study. *Ophthalmic Surg Lasers.* 1999;30:260–265.
41. Donoso R, Rodriguez A. Combined versus sequential phacotrabeculectomy with intraoperative 5-fluorouracil. *J Cataract Refract Surg.* 2000;26:7–41.
42. Dickens MA, Cashwell LF. Long-term effect of cataract extraction on the function of an established filtering bleb. *Ophthalmic Surg Lasers.* 1996;27:9–14.
43. Park HJ, Kwon YH, Weitzman M, et al. Temporal corneal phacoemulsification in patients with filtered glaucoma. *Arch Ophthalmol.* 1997;115:1375–1380.
44. Casson R, Rahman R, Salmon JF. Phacoemulsification with intraocular lens implantation after trabeculectomy. *J Glaucoma.* 2002;11:429–433.

45. Manoj B, Chako D, Khan MY. Effect of extracapsular cataract extraction and phacoemulsification performed after trabeculectomy on intraocular pressure. *J Cataract Refract Surg.* 2000;26:75–78.

46. Casson RJ, Riddell CE, Rahman R, et al. Long-term effect of cataract surgery on intraocular pressure after trabeculectomy: extracapsular extraction versus phacoemulsification. *J Cataract Refract Surg.* 2002;28:2159–2164.

47. Rebolleda G, Munoz-Negrete FJ. Phacoemulsification in eyes with functioning filtering blebs: a prospective study. *Ophthalmology.* 2002;109:2248–2255.

48. Chen PP, Weaver YK, Budenz DL, et al. Trabeculectomy function after cataract extraction. *Ophthalmology.* 1998;105:1928–1935.

49. Doyle JW, Smith MF. Effect of phacoemulsification surgery on hypotony following trabeculectomy surgery. *Arch Ophthalmol.* 2000;118:763–765.

50. Galin MA, Obstbaum SA, Asano Y, et al. Laser trabeculoplasty and cataract surgery. *Trans Ophthalmol Soc U K.* 1985;104(pt 1):72–75.

51. Wand M. Combined phacoemulsification, intraocular lens implant, and trabeculectomy with intraoperative mitomycin-C: comparison between 3.2- and 6.0-mm incisions. *J Glaucoma.* 1996;5:301–307.

52. Rockwood EJ, Larive B, Hahn J. Outcomes of combined cataract extraction, lens implantation, and trabeculectomy surgeries. *Am J Ophthalmol.* 2000;130:704–711.

53. Honjo M, Tanihara H, Negi A, et al. Trabeculotomy ab externo, cataract extraction, and intraocular lens implantation: preliminary report. *J Cataract Refract Surg.* 1996;22:601–606.

54. Kubota T, Touguri I, Onizuka N, et al. Phacoemulsification and intraocular lens implantation combined with trabeculotomy for open-angle glaucoma and coexisting cataract. *Ophthalmologica.* 2003;217:204–207.

55. Chia WL, Goldberg I. Comparison of extracapsular and phacoemulsification cataract extraction techniques when combined with intraocular lens placement and trabeculectomy: short-term results. *Aust N Z J Ophthalmol.* 1998;26:19–27.

56. Tezel G, Kolker AE, Kass MA, et al. Comparative results of combined procedures for glaucoma and cataract: I. Extracapsular cataract extraction versus phacoemulsification and foldable versus rigid intraocular lenses. *Ophthalmic Surg Lasers.* 1997;28:539–550.

57. Yamagami S, Hamada N, Araie M, et al. Risk factors for unsatisfactory intraocular pressure control in combined trabeculectomy and cataract surgery. *Ophthalmic Surg Lasers.* 1997;28:476–482.

58. Shammas HJ. Anterior intraocular lens dislocation after combined cataract extraction trabeculectomy. *J Cataract Refract Surg.* 1996;22:358–361.

59. Nielsen PJ. Combined small-incision cataract surgery and trabeculectomy: a prospective study with 1 year of follow-up. *Ophthalmic Surg Lasers.* 1997;28:21–29.

60. Caprioli J, Park HJ, Weitzman M. Temporal corneal phacoemulsification combined with superior trabeculectomy: a controlled study. *Trans Am Ophthalmol Soc.* 1996;94:451–463.

61. Park HJ, Weitzman M, Caprioli J. Temporal corneal phacoemulsification combined with superior trabeculectomy: a retrospective case-control study. *Arch Ophthalmol.* 1997;115:318–323.

62. Yalvac I, Airaksinen PJ, Tuulonen A. Phacoemulsification with and without trabeculectomy in patients with glaucoma. *Ophthalmic Surg Lasers.* 1997;28:469–475.

63. Mamalis N, Lohner S, Rand AN, et al. Combined phacoemulsification, intraocular lens implantation, and trabeculectomy. *J Cataract Refract Surg.* 1996;22:467–473.

64. Lederer CM Jr. Combined cataract extraction with intraocular lens implant and mitomycin-augmented trabeculectomy. *Ophthalmology.* 1996;103:1025–1034.

65. Friedman DS, Jampel HD, Lubomski LH, et al. Surgical strategies for coexisting glaucoma and cataract: an evidence-based update. *Ophthalmology.* 2002;109:1902–1913.

66. Shields MB. Combined cataract extraction and guarded sclerectomy: reevaluation in the extracapsular era. *Ophthalmology.* 1986;93:366–370.

67. Kolker AE, Stewart RH, LeBlanc RP. Cataract extraction in glaucomatous patients. *Arch Ophthalmol.* 1970;84:63–64.

68. Saito Y, Kiboshi H. A new intra-anterior chamber iris suturing method. *Am J Ophthalmol.* 1988;105:701–703.

69. Whitsett JC, Stewart RH. A new technique for combined cataract/glaucoma procedures in patients on chronic miotics. *Ophthalmic Surg.* 1993;24:481–485.

70. Cahane M, Glovinsky Y, Blumenthal M. Effect of a resutured iridotomy on glare disability in glaucoma patients having cataract surgery. *J Cataract Refract Surg.* 1991;17:58–61.

71. McCuen BW, Hickingbotham D, Tsai M, et al. Temporary iris fixation with a micro-iris retractor. *Arch Ophthalmol.* 1989;107:925–927.

72. de Juan E Jr, Hickingbotham D. Flexible iris retractor. *Am J Ophthalmol.* 1991;111:776–777.

73. Fuller DG, Wilson DL. Translimbal iris hook for pupillary dilation during vitreous surgery. *Am J Ophthalmol.* 1990;110:577.

74. Miller KM, Keener GT Jr. Stretch pupilloplasty for small pupil phacoemulsification. *Am J Ophthalmol.* 1994;117:107–108.

75. Cornetto AD III, de Juan E Jr. Reusable superelastic iris retractor: the Microsurgery Advanced Design Laboratory. *Ophthalmic Surg Lasers.* 1999;30:586–587.

76. Oetting TA, Omphroy LC. Modified technique using flexible iris retractors in clear corneal cataract surgery. *J Cataract Refract Surg.* 2002;28:596–598.

77. Change DF. Use of Malyugin pupil expansion device for intraoperative floppy-iris syndrome: results in 30 consecutive cases. *J Cataract Refract Surg.* 2008;34:835–841.

78. Murray TG, Abrams GW. A new self-sealing needle for iris suture fixation. *Arch Ophthalmol.* 1990;108:746–747.

79. Freeman WR, Feldman ST, Munguia D, et al. The prethreaded pupillary dilating (torpedo) suture for phakic and aphakic eyes. *Arch Ophthalmol.* 1992;110:564–567.

80. Gaudric A. Transpupillary continuous suture for intraoperative mydriasis. *Am J Ophthalmol.* 1993;115:670–671.

81. Johnstone MA. The iris tucking maneuver in cataract surgery for glaucoma patients with miotic pupils. *Am J Ophthalmol.* 1992;113:586–587.

82. Graether JM. Graether pupil expander for managing the small pupil during surgery. *J Cataract Refract Surg.* 1996;22:530–535.

83. Gimbel HV. Nucleofractis phacoemulsification through a small pupil. *Can J Ophthalmol.* 1992;27:115–119.

84. Novak J. Flexible iris hooks for phacoemulsification. *J Cataract Refract Surg.* 1997;23:828–831.

85. Merriam JC, Zheng L. Iris hooks for phacoemulsification of the subluxated lens. *J Cataract Refract Surg.* 1997;23:1295–1297.

86. Lee V, Bloom P. Microhook capsule stabilization for phacoemulsification in eyes with exfoliation-syndrome-induced lens instability. *J Cataract Refract Surg.* 1999;25:1567–1570.

87. Mackool RJ. Capsule stabilization for phacoemulsification. *J Cataract Refract Surg.* 2000;26:629.

88. Shingleton BJ, Campbell CA, O'Donoghue MW. Effects of pupil stretch technique during phacoemulsification on postoperative vision, intraocular pressure, and inflammation. *J Cataract Refract Surg.* 2006;32:1142–1145.

89. Arshinoff SA, Albiani DA, Taylor-Laporte J. Intraocular pressure after bilateral cataract surgery using Healon, Healon 5, and Healon GV. *J Cataract Refract Surg.* 2002;28:617–625.

90. Ruiz RS, Rhem MN, Prager TC. Effects of carbachol and acetylcholine on intraocular pressure after cataract extraction. *Am J Ophthalmol.* 1989;107:7–10.

91. West J, Burke J, Cunliffe I, et al. Prevention of acute postoperative pressure rises in glaucoma patients undergoing cataract extraction with posterior chamber lens implant. *Br J Ophthalmol.* 1992;76:534–537.

92. Anwar M, el-Sayyad F, el-Maghraby A. Lens capsule inclusion in trabeculectomy with cataract extraction. *J Cataract Refract Surg.* 1997;23:1103–1108.

93. Kosmin AS, Wishart PK, Ridges PJ. Silicone versus poly(methyl methacrylate) lenses in combined phacoemulsification and trabeculectomy. *J Cataract Refract Surg.* 1997;23:97–105.

94. Lemon LC, Shin DH, Song MS, et al. Comparative study of silicone versus acrylic foldable lens implantation in primary glaucoma triple procedure. *Ophthalmology.* 1997;104:1708–1713.

95. Hu BV, Shin DH, Gibbs KA, et al. Implantation of posterior chamber lens in the absence of capsular and zonular support. *Arch Ophthalmol.* 1988;106:416–420.

96. Stark WJ, Gottsch JD, Goodman DF, et al. Posterior chamber intraocular lens implantation in the absence of capsular support. *Arch Ophthalmol.* 1989;107:1078–1083.

97. Lindquist TD, Agapitos PJ, Lindstrom RL, et al. Transscleral fixation of posterior chamber intraocular lenses in the absence of capsular support. *Ophthalmic Surg.* 1989;20:769–775.

98. Helal M, el Sayyad F, Elsherif Z, et al. Transscleral fixation of posterior chamber intraocular lenses in the absence of capsular support. *J Cataract Refract Surg.* 1996;22:347–351.

99. Shin DH, Birt CM, O'Grady JM, et al. Transscleral suture fixation of posterior chamber lenses combined with trabeculectomy. *Ophthalmology.* 2001;108:919–929.

100. Wagoner MD, Cox TA, Ariyasu RG, et al. Intraocular lens implantation in the absence of capsular support: a report by the American Academy of Ophthalmology. *Ophthalmology.* 2003;110:840–859.

101. Bergman M, Laatikainen L. Intraocular pressure level in glaucomatous and nonglaucomatous eyes after complicated cataract surgery and implantation of an AC-IOL. *Ophthalmic Surg.* 1992;23:378–382.

102. Bellucci R, Pucci V, Morselli S, et al. Secondary implantation of angle-supported anterior chamber and scleral-fixated posterior chamber intraocular lenses. *J Cataract Refract Surg.* 1996;22:247–252.

103. Drolsum L. Long-term follow-up of secondary flexible, open-loop, anterior chamber intraocular lenses. *J Cataract Refract Surg.* 2003;29:498–503.

104. Morris DA, Peracha MO, Shin DH, et al. Risk factors for early filtration failure requiring suture release after primary glaucoma triple procedure with adjunctive mitomycin. *Arch Ophthalmol.* 1999;117:1149–1154.

105. Seah SK, Jap A, Prata JA Jr, et al. Cataract surgery after trabeculectomy. *Ophthalmic Surg Lasers.* 1996;27:587–594.

106. Wygnanski-Jaffe T, Barak A, Melamed S, et al. Intraocular pressure increments after cataract extraction in glaucomatous eyes with functioning filtering blebs. *Ophthalmic Surg Lasers.* 1997;28:657–660.

107. Mandal AK, Chelerkar V, Jain SS, et al. Outcome of cataract extraction and poster chamber intraocular lens implantation following glaucoma filtration surgery. *Eye.* 2005;19:1000–1008.

108. Swamynathan K, Capistrano AP, Cantor LB, et al. Effect of temporal corneal phacoemulsification on intraocular pressure in eyes with prior trabeculectomy with an antimetabolite. *Ophthalmology.* 2004;111:674–678.

109. Caprioli J, Park HJ, Kwon YH, et al. Temporal corneal phacoemulsification in filtered glaucoma patients. *Trans Am Ophthalmol Soc.* 1997;95:153–167.

110. Mietz H, Andresen A, Welsandt G, et al. Effect of cataract surgery on intraocular pressure in eyes with previous trabeculectomy. *Graefes Arch Clin Exp Ophthalmol.* 2001;239:763–769.

111. Dellaporta A. Combined trepano-trabeculectomy and cataract extraction. *Trans Am Ophthalmol Soc.* 1971;69:113–123.

112. Rich W. Cataract extraction with trabeculectomy. *Trans Ophthalmol Soc U K.* 1974;94:458–467.

113. Johns GE, Layden WE. Combined trabeculectomy and cataract extraction. *Am J Ophthalmol.* 1979;88:973–981.

114. Percival SP. Glaucoma triple procedure of extracapsular cataract extraction, posterior chamber lens implantation, and trabeculectomy. *Br J Ophthalmol.* 1985;69:99–102.

115. Simmons ST, Litoff D, Nichols DA, et al. Extracapsular cataract extraction and posterior chamber intraocular lens implantation combined with trabeculectomy in patients with glaucoma. *Am J Ophthalmol.* 1987;104:465–470.

116. Raitta C, Tarkkanen A. Combined procedure for the management of glaucoma and cataract. *Acta Ophthalmol (Copenh).* 1988;66:667–670.

117. Longstaff S, Wormald RP, Mazover A, et al. Glaucoma triple procedures: efficacy of intraocular pressure control and visual outcome. *Ophthalmic Surg.* 1990;21:786–793.

118. Hansen LL, Hoffmann F. Combination of phacoemulsification and trabeculectomy: results of a retrospective study [in German]. *Klin Monatsbl Augenheilkd.* 1987;190:478–481.

119. Lyle WA, Jin JC. Comparison of a 3- and 6-mm incision in combined phacoemulsification and trabeculectomy. *Am J Ophthalmol.* 1991;111:189–196.

120. Shingleton BJ, Kalina PH. Combined phacoemulsification, intraocular lens implantation, and trabeculectomy with a modified scleral tunnel and single-stitch closure. *J Cataract Refract Surg.* 1995;21:528–532.

121. Weitzman M, Caprioli J. Temporal corneal phacoemulsification combined with separate-incision superior trabeculectomy. *Ophthalmic Surg.* 1995;26:271–273.

122. Park HJ, Kwon YH, Weitzman M, et al. Temporal corneal phacoemulsification in patients with filtered glaucoma. *Arch Ophthalmol.* 1997;115:1375–1380.

123. Borggrefe J, Lieb W, Grehn F. A prospective randomized comparison of two techniques of combined cataract-glaucoma surgery. *Graefes Arch Clin Exp Ophthalmol.* 1999;237:887–892.

124. Rossetti L, Bucci L, Miglior S, et al. Temporal corneal phacoemulsification combined with separate-incision superior trabeculectomy vs. standard phacotrabeculectomy: a comparative study. *Acta Ophthalmol Scand.* 1997;(suppl):39.

125. Wyse T, Meyer M, Ruderman JM, et al. Combined trabeculectomy and phacoemulsification: a one-site vs. a two-site approach. *Am J Ophthalmol.* 1998;125:334–339.

126. Simmons ST, Litoff D, Nichols DA, et al. Extracapsular cataract extraction and posterior chamber intraocular lens implantation combined with trabeculectomy in patients with glaucoma. *Am J Ophthalmol.* 1987;104:465–470.

127. McCartney DL, Memmen JE, Stark WJ, et al. The efficacy and safety of combined trabeculectomy, cataract extraction, and intraocular lens implantation. *Ophthalmology.* 1988;95:754–763.

128. Shingleton BJ, Chaudhry IM, O'Donoghue MW, et al. Phacotrabeculectomy: limbus-based versus fornix-based conjunctival flaps in fellow eyes. *Ophthalmology.* 1999;106:1152–1155.

129. Tezel G, Kolker AE, Kass MA, et al. Comparative results of combined procedures for glaucoma and cataract: II. Limbus-based versus fornix-based conjunctival flaps. *Ophthalmic Surg Lasers.* 1997;28:551–557.

130. Berestka JS, Brown SV. Limbus- versus fornix-based conjunctival flaps in combined phacoemulsification and mitomycin C trabeculectomy surgery. *Ophthalmology.* 1997;104:187–196.

131. Lemon LC, Shin DH, Kim C, et al. Limbus-based vs. fornix-based conjunctival flap in combined glaucoma and cataract surgery with adjunctive mitomycin C. *Am J Ophthalmol.* 1998;125:340–345.

132. Kozobolis VP, Siganos CS, Christodoulakis EV, et al. Two-site phacotrabeculectomy with intraoperative mitomycin-C: fornix- versus limbus-based conjunctival opening in fellow eyes. *J Cataract Refract Surg.* 2002;28:1758–1762.

133. Robin AL. Effect of topical apraclonidine on the frequency of intraocular pressure elevations after combined extracapsular cataract extraction and trabeculectomy. *Ophthalmology.* 1993;100:628–633.

134. Kasetti SR, Desai SP, Sivakumar S, et al. Preventing intraocular pressure increase after phacoemulsification and the role of perioperative apraclonidine. *J Cataract Refract Surg.* 2002;28:2177–2180.

135. Byrd S, Singh K. Medical control of intraocular pressure after cataract surgery. *J Cataract Refract Surg.* 1998;24:1493–1497.

136. Zohdy GA, Rogers ZA, Lukaris A, et al. A comparison of the effectiveness of dorzolamide and acetazolamide in preventing post-operative intraocular pressure rise following phacoemulsification surgery. *J R Coll Surg Edinb.* 1998;43:344–346.

137. Stewart WC, Crinkley CM, Carlson AN. Results of trabeculectomy combined with phacoemulsification versus trabeculectomy combined with extracapsular cataract extraction in patients with advanced glaucoma. *Ophthalmic Surg.* 1994;25:621–627.

138. Cohen JS. Combined cataract implant and filtering surgery with 5-fluorouracil. *Ophthalmic Surg.* 1990;21:181–186.

139. Hennis HL, Stewart WC. The use of 5-fluorouracil in patients following combined trabeculectomy and cataract extraction. *Ophthalmic Surg.* 1991;22:451–454.

140. Wong PC, Ruderman JM, Krupin T, et al. 5-Fluorouracil after primary combined filtration surgery. *Am J Ophthalmol.* 1994;117:149–154.

141. Hurvitz LM. 5-FU-supplemented phacoemulsification, posterior chamber intraocular lens implantation, and trabeculectomy. *Ophthalmic Surg.* 1993;24:674–680.

142. Gandolfi SA, Vecchi M. 5-Fluorouracil in combined trabeculectomy and clear-cornea phacoemulsification with posterior chamber intraocular lens implantation: a one-year randomized, controlled clinical trial. *Ophthalmology.* 1997;104:181–186.

143. O'Grady JM, Juzych MS, Shin DH, et al. Trabeculectomy, phacoemulsification, and posterior chamber lens implantation with and without 5-fluorouracil. *Am J Ophthalmol.* 1993;116:594–599.

144. Jampel HD, Friedman DS, Lubomski LH, et al. Effect of technique on intraocular pressure after combined cataract and glaucoma surgery: an evidence-based review. *Ophthalmology.* 2002;109(12):2215–2224.

145. Shin DH, Simone PA, Song MS, et al. Adjunctive subconjunctival mitomycin C in glaucoma triple procedure. *Ophthalmology.* 1995;102:1550–1558.

146. Ruderman JM, Fundingsland B, Meyer MA. Combined phacoemulsification and trabeculectomy with mitomycin-C. *J Cataract Refract Surg.* 1996;22:1085–1090.

147. Munden PM, Alward WL. Combined phacoemulsification, posterior chamber intraocular lens implantation, and trabeculectomy with mitomycin C. *Am J Ophthalmol.* 1995;119:20–29.

148. Joos KM, Bueche MJ, Palmberg PF, et al. One-year follow-up results of combined mitomycin C trabeculectomy and extracapsular cataract extraction. *Ophthalmology.* 1995;102:76–83.

149. Cohen JS, Greff LJ, Novack GD, et al. A placebo-controlled, double-masked evaluation of mitomycin C in combined glaucoma and cataract procedures. *Ophthalmology.* 1996;103:1934–1942.

150. Carlson DW, Alward WL, Barad JP, et al. A randomized study of mitomycin augmentation in combined phacoemulsification and trabeculectomy. *Ophthalmology.* 1997;104:719–724.

151. Shin DH, Kim YY, Sheth N, et al. The role of adjunctive mitomycin C in secondary glaucoma triple procedure as compared to primary glaucoma triple procedure. *Ophthalmology.* 1998;105:740–745.

152. Shin DH, Ren J, Juzych MS, et al. Primary glaucoma triple procedure in patients with primary open-angle glaucoma: the effect of mitomycin C in patients with and without prognostic factors for filtration failure. *Am J Ophthalmol.* 1998;125:346–352.
153. McPherson SD Jr. Combined trabeculotomy and cataract extraction as a single operation. *Trans Am Ophthalmol Soc.* 1976;74:251–260.
154. Tanito M, Ohira A, Chihara E. Surgical outcome of combined trabeculotomy and cataract surgery. *J Glaucoma.* 2001;10:302–308.
155. Feltgen N, Mueller H, Ott B, et al. Endoscopically controlled erbium:YAG goniopuncture versus trabeculectomy: effect on intraocular pressure in combination with cataract surgery. *Graefes Arch Clin Exp Ophthalmol.* 2003;241:94–100.
156. Uram M. Combined phacoemulsification, endoscopic ciliary process photocoagulation, and intraocular lens implantation in glaucoma management. *Ophthalmic Surg.* 1995;26:346–352.
157. Gayton JL, Van Der KM, Sanders V. Combined cataract and glaucoma surgery: trabeculectomy versus endoscopic laser cycloablation. *J Cataract Refract Surg.* 1999;25:1214–1219.
158. Gianoli F, Mermoud A. Cataract-glaucoma combined surgery: comparison between phacoemulsification combined with deep sclerectomy, or trabeculectomy. *Klin Monatsbl Augenheilkd.* 1997;210:256–260.
159. Gianoli F, Schnyder CC, Bovey E, et al. Combined surgery for cataract and glaucoma: phacoemulsification and deep sclerectomy compared with phacoemulsification and trabeculectomy. *J Cataract Refract Surg.* 1999;25:340–346.
160. Tanito M, Park M, Nishikawa M, et al. Comparison of surgical outcomes of combined viscocanalostomy and cataract surgery with combined trabeculotomy and cataract surgery. *Am J Ophthalmol.* 2002;134:513–520.
161. O'Brart DP, Rowlands E, Islam N, et al. A randomised, prospective study comparing trabeculectomy augmented with antimetabolites with a viscocanalostomy technique for the management of open angle glaucoma uncontrolled by medical therapy. *Br J Ophthalmol.* 2002;86:748–754.
162. Jacobi PC, Dietlein TS, Krieglstein GK. Comparative study of trabecular aspiration vs. trabeculectomy in glaucoma triple procedure to treat exfoliation glaucoma. *Arch Ophthalmol.* 1999;117:1311–1318.
163. Das JC, Chaudhuri Z, Bhomaj S, et al. Combined extracapsular cataract extraction with Ahmed glaucoma valve implantation in phacomorphic glaucoma. *Indian J Ophthalmol.* 2002;50:25–28.
164. Hoffman KB, Feldman RM, Budenz DL, et al. Combined cataract extraction and Baerveldt glaucoma drainage implant: indications and outcomes. *Ophthalmology.* 2002;109:1916–1920.
165. McQueen BR, Margo CE. Capsular bag distention syndrome after combined cataract-lens implant surgery and Ahmed valve implantation. *Am J Ophthalmol.* 2001;132:109–110.
166. Francis BA, Minckler D, Dustin L, et al. Trabectome Study Group. Combined cataract extraction and trabeculotomy by the internal approach for coexisting cataract and open-angle glaucoma: initial results. *J Cataract Refract Surg.* 2008;34:1096–1103.
167. Lewis RA, von Wolff K, Tetz M, et al. Canaloplasty: circumferential viscodilation and tensioning of Schlemm canal using a flexible microcatheter for the treatment of open-angle glaucoma in adults: two-year interim clinical study results. *J Cataract Refract Surg.* 2009;35:814–824.
168. Shingleton B, Tetz M, Korber N. Circumferential viscodilation and tensioning of Schlemm canal (canaloplasty) with temporal clear corneal phacoemulsification cataract surgery for open-angle glaucoma and visually significant cataract: one-year results. *J Cataract Refract Surg.* 2008;34:433–440.

Page numbers followed by f indicate figures; those followed by t indicate tabular material.